Carolyn Smith

metoclopramide HCl	midazolam HCl	morphine sulfate	nalbuphine HCl	pentazocine lactate	pentobarbital Na	perphenazine	phenobarbital Na	prochlorperazine edisylate	promazine HCl	promethazine HCl	ranitidine HCl	scopolamine HBr	secobarbital Na	sodium bicarbonate	thiethylperazine maleate	thiopental Na	
P	Y	P	Y	P	P	Y		P	P	P	Y	P					atropine sulfate
	Y	Y		Y	N		N					Y	N			N	benzquinamide HCl
	Y	Y		Y	N	Y		Y		Y		Y			Y		butorphanol tartrate
P	Y	P		P	N	Y		Y	P	P	Y	P				N	chlorpromazine HCl
	Y	Y	Y	Y	N	Y		Y	Y	Y		Y	N				cimetidine HCl
																	codeine phosphate
P	N	P		P	N	Y		N	N	N	Y	P				N	dimenhydrinate
Y	Y	P		P	N	Y		P	P	P	Y	P				N	diphenhydramine HCl
P	Y	P	Y	P	N	Y		P	P	P		P					droperidol
P	Y	P		P	N	Y		P	P	P	Y	P					fentanyl citrate
	Y	Y		N	N			Y	Y	Y	Y	Y	N	N		N	glycopyrrolate
P(5)		N*		N			P(5)			N							heparin Na
	Y			Y	Y			N*		Y	Y	Y			Y		hydromorphone HCl
P	Y	Y	Y	Y	N			P	P	P	N	Y					hydroxyzine HCl
P	Y	N		P	N	P		P	P	Y	Y	P				N	meperidine HCl
	Y	P		P		P		P	P	P	Y	P		N			metoclopramide HCl
Y		Y	Y		N	N		N	Y	Y	N	Y			Y		midazolam HCl
P	Y			P	N*	Y		P*	P	P*	Y	P				N	m[illegible]ine sulfate
	Y				N			Y		Y	Y	Y			Y	[illegible]	[illegible]ne HCl
P		P			N	Y		P	Y	Y	Y	P		[illegible]	[illegible]	[illegible]	[illegible] lactate
	N	N*	N	N		N		N	N	N		Y		[illegible]	[illegible]	[illegible]	[illegible]Na
P	N	Y		Y	N			Y			Y	[illegible]	[illegible]	[illegible]	[illegible]	[illegible]	[illegible]
											[illegible]	[illegible]	[illegible]	[illegible]	[illegible]	[illegible]	[illegible]
P	N	P*	Y	P	N	Y			P	[illegible]	[illegible]	[illegible]	[illegible]	[illegible]	[illegible]	[illegible]	[illegible]ne edisylate
P	Y	P		Y	N			P		[illegible]	[illegible]	[illegible]	[illegible]	[illegible]	[illegible]	[illegible]	[illegible] HCl
P	Y	P*	Y	Y	N			[illegible]	[illegible]	[illegible]	[illegible]	[illegible]	[illegible]	[illegible]	[illegible]	[illegible]	[illegible]thazine HCl
Y	N	Y	Y	Y		Y	N	[illegible]	[illegible]	[illegible]	[illegible]	[illegible]	[illegible]	[illegible]	[illegible]	[illegible]	[illegible]nitidine HCl
P	Y	P	Y	P	Y			P	[illegible]	[illegible]	[illegible]	[illegible]	[illegible]	[illegible]	[illegible]		scopolamine HBr
									[illegible]	[illegible]	[illegible]	[illegible]	[illegible]	[illegible]			secobarbital Na
N					Y					[illegible]	[illegible]	[illegible]	[illegible]			N	sodium bicarbonate
	Y		Y								[illegible]						thiethylperazine maleate
		N			Y			N		N		Y		N			thiopental Na

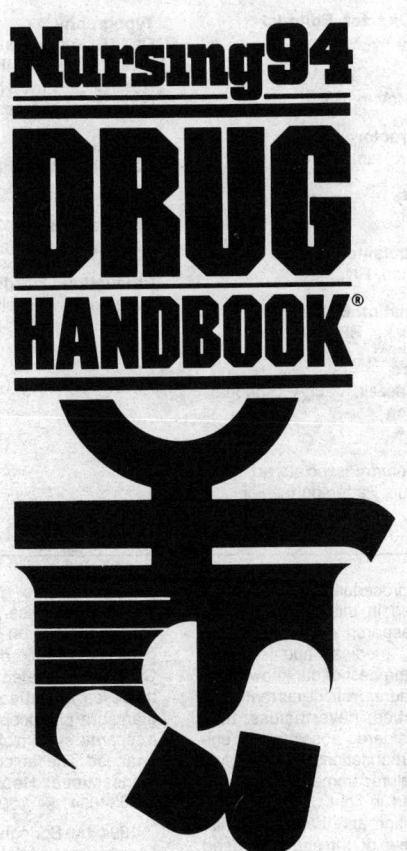

Nursing94 DRUG HANDBOOK®

NURSING94 BOOKS™
SPRINGHOUSE CORPORATION
SPRINGHOUSE, PENNSYLVANIA

STAFF

Executive Director, Editorial
Stanley Loeb

Publisher
Barbara F. McVan, RN

Editorial Director
Helen Klusek Hamilton

Art Director
John Hubbard

Clinical Acquisitions
Joan E. Mason, RN, MEd

Drug Information Editor
George J. Blake, RPh, MS

Copy Editors
Christina Ponczek, Traci A. Ginnona, Mary T. Durkin

Designers
Stephanie Peters (associate art director), Matie Patterson (senior designer)

Typography
David C. Kosten (director), Diane Paluba (manager), Elizabeth Bergman, Joyce Rossi Biletz, Phyllis Marron, Robin Mayer, Valerie Rosenberger

Manufacturing
Deborah C. Meiris (director), Anna Brindisi

Editorial Assistants
Maree DeRosa, Mary Madden

Production Coordination
Margaret A. Rastiello

The clinical procedures described and recommended in this publication are based on research and consultation with nursing, medical, and legal authorities. To the best of our knowledge, these procedures reflect currently accepted practice; nevertheless, they can't be considered absolute and universal recommendations. For individual application, all recommendations must be considered in light of the patient's clinical condition and, before administration of new or infrequently used drugs, in light of the latest package-insert information. The authors and the publisher disclaim responsibility for any adverse effects resulting directly or indirectly from the suggested procedures, from any undetected errors, or from the reader's misunderstanding of the text.

Authorization to photocopy items for internal or personal use, or the internal or personal use of specific clients, is granted by Springhouse Corporation for users registered with the Copyright Clearance Center (CCC) Transactional Reporting Service, provided that the base fee of $00.00 per copy, plus $.75 per page, is paid directly to CCC, 27 Congress St., Salem, Mass. 01970. For those organizations that have been granted a photocopy license by CCC, a separate system of payment has been arranged. The fee code for users of the Transactional Reporting Service is 0874346541/94 $00.00 + $.75.

© 1994 by Springhouse Corporation. All rights reserved. No part of this publication may be used or reproduced in any manner whatsoever without written permission except for brief quotations embodied in critical articles and reviews. Printed in the United States of America. For information, write Springhouse Corporation, 1111 Bethlehem Pike, P.O. Box 908, Springhouse, Pa. 19477-0908.

NGDH-011093
ISSN 0273-320X
ISBN 0-87434-654-1

CONTENTS

Hematologic Agents

Antineoplastic Agents

Immunomodulation Agents

Eye, Ear, Nose, and Throat Drugs

Dermatomucosal Agents

Anesthetic Agents

Nutritional Agents

Miscellaneous Drug Categories

Appendices and Index

CONSULTANTS, REVIEWERS, AND ADVISORS

At the time of publication, the clinical consultants, pharmacy reviewers, and advisors held the following positions.

Clinical Consultants

Mary Ann Cali-Ascani, RNC, MSN, OCN, Oncology Nurse Manager, Easton (Pa.) Hospital
Nancy G. Evans, RN, BSN, CGRN, Nurse Manager, Gastroenterology Department, Daniel Freeman Memorial and Marina Hospitals, Inglewood, Calif.
Walter Carl Faubion, RN, MHSA, Clinical Manager, Home Medicine, University of Michigan Medical Center, Ann Arbor
Terry Matthew Foster, RN, BSN, CCRN, CEN, Emergency Nursing Consultant, Staff Nurse, Emergency Department, Saint Elizabeth Medical Center, Covington, Ky.
Shirley A. Grieshaber, RN, Advanced Clinical Nurse, National Institutes of Health, Bethesda, Md.
Roseann Hendrickson, RN, Nursing Consultant, Emergency Physician Associates, Woodbury, N.J.
Karen Landis, RN, MS, CCRN, Pulmonary Clinical Nurse Specialist, Lehigh Valley Hospital Center, The Allentown (Pa.) Hospital
Rosemarie Marinaro, RN,C, MSN, Perinatal Clinical Nurse Specialist, Frankford Hospital-Perinatal Center, Philadelphia
Chris Platt Moldovanyi, RN, MSN, Nursing Consultant, Cleveland, Ohio
Nancy V. Runta, RN, BSN, CCRN, Infection Control Practitioner, North Penn Hospital, Lansdale, Pa.
Debra L. Ryan, RN, MN, CCRN, Critical Care Clinical Nurse Specialist, Memorial Medical Center, Springfield, Ill.

Pharmacy Reviewers

Douglas R. Allington, RPh, PharmD, Assistant Professor, University of Montana, Missoula
Alan D. Barreuther, RPh, PharmD, Associate Professor, Pharmacy Practice, University of Arizona, Tucson; Manager, Drug Information, Tucson Medical Center
Doyle M. Cummings, RPh, PharmD, FCP, FCCP, Associate Professor of Family Medicine, Clinical Pharmacy Section, East Carolina University School of Medicine, Greenville, N.C.
Mark J. Ellison, RPh, PharmD, FCP, Associate Professor of Family Medicine, Clinical Pharmacy Section, East Carolina University School of Medicine, Greenville, N.C.
Jimmi Hatton, RPh, PharmD, Assistant Professor, University of Kentucky, College of Pharmacy, Lexington
David W. Hawkins, RPh, PharmD, Professor and Assistant Dean, University of Georgia College of Pharmacy, Athens
James R. Hildebrand, RPh, PharmD, Director, Drug Information Center; Associate Professor of Clinical Pharmacy, Philadelphia College of Pharmacy and Science
Arthur I. Jacknowitz, RPh, PharmD, Professor and Chair, Department of Clinical Pharmacy, West Virginia University, Morgantown
Cary E. Johnson, RPh, PharmD, Associate Professor, University of Michigan College of Pharmacy; Clinical Pharmacist, University of Michigan Medical Center, Ann Arbor
Susanne P. Mulligan, RPh, BS, Staff Pharmacist, Presbyterian Medical Center, Philadelphia
Lea Anne O'Brien, RPh, PharmD, Clinical Coordinator of Critical Care, Department of Pharmacy, New York Hospital-Cornell Medical Center, New York
Andrew T. Pennell, RPh, PharmD, Assistant Professor, Auburn (Ala.) University School of Pharmacy
David R. Pipher, RPh, PharmD, Assistant Director, Clinical Services, Forbes Regional Health Center, Monroeville, Pa.
Marc S. Roth, RPh, MS, Clinical Coordinator for Critical Nutrition Support, New York Hospital-Cornell Medical Center, New York
Joanne M. Sica, RPh, MHA, Administrator, Pharmacy Program, Greater Atlantic Health Service, Philadelphia

J. Michael Spivey, RPh, PharmD, Instructor of Family Medicine, East Carolina University School of Medicine, Greenville, N.C.
Joseph F. Steiner, RPh, PharmD, Professor of Clinical Pharmacy, University of Wyoming, Casper

Special thanks to the following, who have made major contributions or have contributed to recent past editions: Michael J. Booth, RN, MA, CRNA; Heather Boyd-Monk, SRN, RN, BSN; Karen E. Burgess, RN, MSN; Nancy Burns, RN, PhD; Carla J. Burton, RN, BS; Bruce D. Clayton RPh, PharmD; Michael Cohen, RPh, MS, FASHP; Charmaine J. Cummings, RN, MSN; Judith Hopfer Deglin, RPh, PharmD; Bruce M. Frey, RPh, PharmD; Larry N. Gever, RPh, PharmD; Joel Glucroft, PhD; Marcia Jo Hill, RN, MSN; Alan Hopefl, RPh, PharmD; Nina E. Jakobowski, RPh, PharmD; Meredith Ann McCord, RN, MS; Helene K. Nawrocki, RN, MSN; Sandra L. Nettina, RNC, MSN, CRNP; Margaret Smellie-Belfield, RN, BSN, CCRN; Marilyn Sawyer Sommers, RN, PhD, CCRN; Julie Tackenberg, RN, MA, CNRN; Kerri J. Vandel, RPh, PharmD; Paul J. Vitale, RPh, PharmD, FASCP.

Advisory Board

Lillian S. Brunner, RN, MSN, ScD, FAAN, Nurse-Author, Berwyn, Pa.
Luther P. Christman, RN, PhD, Nurse Consultant, Chapel Hill, Tenn.
Kathleen A. Dracup, RN, DNSc, Editor, *American Journal of Critical Care;* Professor, University of California School of Nursing, Los Angeles
Stanley J. Dudrick, MD, FACS, Surgeon-in-Chief, Hermann Hospital, Houston; Clinical Professor of Surgery, University of Texas Houston Health Science Center
Halbert E. Fillinger, MD, Forensic Pathologist, Assistant Medical Examiner, Office of the Medical Examiner, Philadelphia
M. Josephine Flaherty, RN, PhD, Principal Nursing Officer, Department of National Health and Welfare, Ottawa
Joyce LeFever Kee, RN, MSN, Associate Professor, College of Nursing, University of Delaware, Newark
Dennis E. Leavelle, MD, Associate Professor, Mayo Medical Laboratories, Mayo Clinic, Rochester, Minn.
Ara G. Paul, PhD, Dean, College of Pharmacy; Professor of Pharmacognosy, University of Michigan, Ann Arbor
Rose Pinneo, RN, MS, Professor Emeritus, University of Rochester (N.Y.) School of Nursing
Thomas E. Rubbert, JD, LLB, BSL, Attorney-at-Law, Pasadena, Calif.
Maryanne Schreiber, RN, BA, Product Manager, Patient Monitoring, Hewlett-Packard Co., Waltham (Mass.) Division
Frances Storlie, RN, PhD, Adult Nurse Practitioner (C); Director, Personal Health Services, Southwest Washington Health District, Vancouver
Claire L. Watson, RN, Clinical Documentation Associate, IVAC Corporation, San Diego

1

How to use *Nursing94 Drug Handbook*

Nursing94 Drug Handbook is meant to fill a very special need. It represents a joint effort by pharmacists and nurses to provide the nursing profession with drug information that focuses on what nurses need to know. With this in mind, it emphasizes clinical aspects and does not attempt to replace detailed pharmacology texts. Also, the information is arranged in a format designed to make it readily accessible.

Introductory information
Following this chapter, Chapter 2 explains, in a general way, how drugs work. It also tells about side effects and adverse reactions and gives general guidelines about drug use in pregnancy and the presence of drugs in breast milk. Chapters 3 and 4 discuss the unique problems of administering drugs to children and elderly patients and offer guidelines to minimize problems in these areas. Chapter 5 discusses drug therapy as it relates to the nursing process.

In the remaining chapters, all drugs are classified according to their approved therapeutic uses. Drugs that have multiple therapeutic uses are classified according to their most common use; they are also listed (with a cross-reference to the major drug entry) in drug groups that share their secondary applications. For example, nadolol, a beta-adrenergic blocker, is described in the chapter that covers antianginals because its major therapeutic application is the management of angina pectoris; because it is less commonly used to treat hypertension, it is listed among the generic drugs grouped as antihypertensives with a cross-reference to Chapter 21, Antianginals.

Such classification by therapeutic use offers several advantages. It helps the reader identify an unknown drug by its clinical application alone. At the same time, it automatically identifies all other drugs that share the same use and provides easy comparison of their dosages and effects. Thereby, it quickly identifies potential pharmacotherapeutic alternatives for patients who cannot tolerate or fail to respond to a particular drug.

Drug information
Each chapter, representing a major therapeutic use, begins with an alphabetically arranged list of the generic names of drugs described in that chapter. This is followed by a list of selected combination products in which these drugs are found. Specific information on each drug is arranged under the following headings: *How Supplied, Mechanism of Action, Indications & Dosage, Adverse Reactions, Interactions,* and *Nursing Considerations.*

In each drug entry, the drug's generic name is immediately followed by an alphabetized list of its brand names. A trade name followed by an open diamond indicates a drug that is available in preparations that do not require a prescription (◇). Brands available *only* in Canada are designated with a dagger (†); those available *only* in Australia, with a double dagger (‡). A brand name with no symbol after it is available in the United States, Canada, and possibly Australia. If a drug is a controlled substance, that is indicated (example: Controlled Substance Schedule II). The mention of a brand name in no way implies endorsement of that product or guarantees its legality.

Each systemically absorbed drug

has been assigned a pregnancy risk category based upon available clinical and preclinical information. The Pregnancy Risk Category parallels the five Pregnancy Categories (A, B, C, D, and X) assigned by the Food and Drug Administration to reflect a drug's potential to cause birth defects. Although it is generally accepted that no drugs should be used during pregnancy, this rating system permits rapid assessment of the risk-benefit ratio should drug administration to a pregnant woman become necessary. Drugs in category A are generally considered safe to use in pregnancy; drugs in category X are generally contraindicated.

- A: Adequate studies in pregnant women have failed to show a risk to the fetus in the first trimester of pregnancy – and there is no evidence of risk in later trimesters.
- B: Animal studies have not shown a risk to the fetus, but there are no adequate clinical studies in pregnant women; or, animal studies have shown an adverse effect on the fetus, but adequate studies in pregnant women have not shown a risk to the fetus during the first trimester of pregnancy and there is no evidence of risk in later trimesters.
- C: Animal studies have shown an adverse effect on the fetus, but there are no adequate studies in humans. The benefits from use in pregnant women may be acceptable despite potential risks; or, there are no animal reproduction studies or adequate human studies. Pregnancy risk is unknown.
- D: There is evidence of risk to the human fetus, but the potential benefits of use in pregnant women may be acceptable despite risks.
- X: Studies in animals or humans show fetal abnormalities, or adverse reaction reports indicate evidence of fetal risk. The risks involved clearly outweigh potential benefits.
- NR: Not rated.

In this volume, the Pregnancy Risk Category has been omitted if the drug is not rated and if such rating is not applicable.

The section titled *How Supplied* lists the preparations available for each drug (for example, tablets, capsules, solutions for injection), specifying available dosage forms and strengths. Preparations that do not require a prescription are marked with an open diamond (◇).

The section titled *Mechanism of Action* succinctly describes *how* each specific drug provides its therapeutic effect. For example, although all antihypertensives lower blood pressure, they don't all do so by the same pharmacologic process.

The section titled *Indications & Dosage* lists general dosage information for adults (including recommended geriatric dosages, when available) and children, as applicable. Children's dosages are usually indicated in terms of mg/kg daily. Dosage instructions reflect current clinical trends in therapeutics and can't be considered as absolute and universal recommendations. For individual application, dosage instructions must be considered in light of the patient's clinical condition.

The section titled *Adverse Reactions* lists each drug's commonly observed adverse reactions (and selected rare ones if life-threatening). For easy reference, the most common adverse reactions are in italics; life-threatening reactions are in bold italics. An exception to this rule is an adverse reaction that, although normally considered hazardous, has been reported to be mild and reversible with the drug in question. For example, thrombocytopenia is considered a life-threatening adverse reaction to plicamycin but a mild and reversible reaction to methyldopa. Hence, thrombocytopenia listed as an adverse reaction to plicamycin is in bold italics, whereas the same reaction under methyldopa is not. Adverse reactions are grouped according to the body system in which they appear.

The next section, *Interactions,* lists each drug's confirmed, *clinically significant* interactions with other drugs (additive effects, potentiated effects, and antagonistic effects) with specific suggestions for avoiding dangerous drug interactions (for example, by reducing doses). Drug interactions are listed under the drug that is adversely affected. For example, magnesium trisilicate, an ingredient in antacids, interacts with tetracycline to cause decreased absorption of tetracycline. Therefore, this interaction is listed under tetracycline. To check on the possible effects of using two or more drugs simultaneously, refer to the interaction entry for *each* of the drugs in question.

The final section, *Nursing Considerations,* lists other useful information, starting with contraindications and precautions, followed by monitoring techniques and suggestions for prevention and treatment of adverse reactions. Also included are suggestions for patient comfort, for patient teaching, and for preparing, administering, and storing each drug. Recommendations for I.V. use are graphically highlighted.

Alcohol and tartrazine content

Many liquid drug preparations for oral use contain alcohol. Although the slight sedative effect that alcohol produces is not harmful in most patients – and can sometimes be beneficial – alcohol ingestion can be undesirable and even dangerous in some circumstances. So, alcohol-containing oral drugs should be given very cautiously, if at all, to patients who are:

- concomitantly taking potent CNS depressants, such as barbiturates
- taking drugs that may produce a disulfiram-type reaction (such as chlorpropamide, metronidazole, and moxalactam)
- taking disulfiram as part of a treatment program for their alcoholism. Such patients, upon ingestion of alcohol, will exhibit severe symptoms that may include blurred vision, confusion, dyspnea, flushing, sweating, and tachycardia.

To help prevent inadvertent exposure to alcohol, this volume signals alcohol content with a single asterisk (*) after each brand of a liquid preparation that may contain it. In many of the preparations so marked, the alcohol content is small. Nevertheless, these drugs should be avoided in patients who are susceptible to adverse effects upon exposure to alcohol.

Tartrazine dye, also known as FD&C Yellow No. 5, is a common coloring agent in some foods and drugs. Usually harmless, it can provoke a severe allergic reaction in susceptible persons. For this reason, most drug manufacturers have begun to eliminate tartrazine from their products, but many drugs still contain it.

The incidence of tartrazine sensitivity is estimated at approximately 1 in 10,000 in the general population but somewhat higher in persons with asthma and/or sensitivity to aspirin. Why this is so is unknown. The most common symptoms of tartrazine sensitivity are urticaria, rhinorrhea, asthma, and angioedema. Acutely sensitive persons may develop allergic vascular purpura, tachycardia, dyspnea, and chest pain. These allergic symptoms generally subside spontaneously upon discontinuation of the tartrazine-containing drug but occasionally require treatment with antihistamines or epinephrine.

Avoiding exposure to tartrazine is not simply a matter of avoiding yellow-colored drugs because this substance may be present in many other color blends, such as turquoise, green, and maroon. To prevent exposure to tartrazine, this volume signals possible tartrazine content with a double asterisk (**) after each brand that may contain it. If you suspect tartrazine sensitivity in a patient receiving such a drug, inform the doctor and contact the manufacturer to determine which dosage forms contain tartrazine.

A guide to abbreviations

AIDS	acquired immunodeficiency syndrome
ALT	alanine aminotransferase
AST	aspartate aminotransferase
AV	atrioventricular
b.i.d.	twice daily
BUN	blood urea nitrogen
CBC	complete blood count
CHF	congestive heart failure
CMV	cytomegalovirus
CNS	central nervous system
COPD	chronic obstructive pulmonary disease
CPK	creatine phosphokinase
CSF	cerebrospinal fluid
CV	cardiovascular
CVA	cerebrovascular accident
DNA	deoxyribonucleic acid
ECG	electrocardiogram
EENT	eyes, ears, nose, throat
FDA	Food and Drug Administration
g	gram
G	gauge
GFR	glomerular filtration rate
GI	gastrointestinal
GU	genitourinary
G6PD	glucose-6-phosphate dehydrogenase
h.s.	at bedtime
ID	intradermal
I.M.	intramuscular
IND	investigational new drug
IPPB	intermittent positive-pressure breathing
IU	international unit
I.V.	intravenous
kg	kilogram
M	molar
m^2	square meter
MAO	monoamine oxidase
mcg	microgram
mEq	milliequivalent
mg	milligram
MI	myocardial infarction
ml	milliliter
Na	sodium
NaCl	sodium chloride
NSAID	nonsteroidal anti-inflammatory drug
OTC	over the counter
PABA	para-aminobenzoic acid
P.O.	by mouth
P.R.	by rectum
p.r.n.	as needed
q	every
q.d.	every day
q.i.d.	four times daily
q.o.d.	every other day
RBC	red blood cell
RDA	recommended daily allowance
REM	rapid eye movement
RNA	ribonucleic acid
RSV	respiratory syncytial virus
SA	sinoatrial
S.C.	subcutaneous
SIADH	syndrome of inappropriate antidiuretic hormone
S.L.	sublingual
t.i.d.	three times daily
UCE	urea cycle enzymopathy
USP	United States Pharmacopeia
WBC	white blood cell

2

Drug actions, reactions, and interactions explained

Administration of any drug provokes a series of physiochemical events within the body. The first event, when a drug combines with cellular drug receptors, is known as the drug action. What follows as a result of this action of the drug is known as the drug effect. Depending on the number of different cellular drug receptors affected by a given drug, a drug effect can be local, systemic, or both. Obviously, a local effect follows application to the skin; however, transdermal absorption can produce systemic effects. Moreover, local effects can follow systemic absorption. For example, the antipeptic ulcer drug cimetidine acts solely by blocking histamine receptor cells in the parietal cells of the stomach. This is known as a local drug effect because the drug action is sharply limited to one area and does not spread to other parts of the body. On the other hand, diphenhydramine produces a systemic effect in that it blocks histamine receptors in widespread areas of the body. In other words, local drug effects are specific to a limited number of organ systems, whereas systemic drug effects are generalized and affect different and diverse organ systems.

Three factors modify drug action

1. Absorption

Before a drug can act within the body, it must be absorbed into the bloodstream – usually after oral administration, the most frequently used route. Before a drug contained in a tablet or capsule can be absorbed, the dosage form must disintegrate, that is, break into smaller particles. Then, these smaller particles can dissolve in gastric juices. Only after so dissolving can a drug be absorbed into the bloodstream. Once absorbed and circulated in the bloodstream, it is said to be bioavailable, or ready to produce a drug effect. Whether such absorption is complete or partial depends on several factors: the drug's physiochemical effects, its dosage form, its route of administration, its interactions with other substances in the GI tract, and various patient characteristics. These same factors also determine the speed of absorption. Thus, oral solutions and elixirs, which bypass the need for disintegration and dissolution, are usually absorbed more rapidly. Some tablets have special (enteric) coatings that prevent disintegration in the acidic environment of the stomach; other may have coatings of varying thickness that delay release of the drug.

Drugs administered intramuscularly must first be absorbed through the muscle into the bloodstream. Rectal suppositories must dissolve to be absorbed through the rectal mucosa. Drugs administered intravenously, which are placed directly into the bloodstream, are completely and immediately bioavailable.

2. Distribution

After absorption, a drug moves from the bloodstream into various fluids and tissues within the body; this is distribution. Individual patient variations can greatly alter the amount of drug that is distributed throughout the body. For example, in an edematous patient, a given dose must be distributed to a larger volume than in a nonedematous patient; the amount of drug must sometimes be increased to account for this. Remember, the dose should be decreased when the edema is corrected. Conversely, in an extremely dehydrated patient, the drug will be distributed to a much smaller volume, so the dose must then be decreased. The total area to which a drug is distributed is known as volume of distribution. Patients who are particularly obese may present another problem when considering drug distribution. Some drugs – such as digoxin, gentamicin, and tobramycin – are not well distributed to fatty tissue. Therefore, dosing based on actual body weight may lead to overdose and serious toxicity. In some cases, dosing must be based on lean body weight, which may be estimated from actuarial tables that give average weight range for height.

3. Metabolism and excretion (drug elimination)
Most drugs are metabolized in the liver and excreted by the kidneys. Hepatic diseases may affect one or more of the metabolic functions of the liver. Therefore, in patients with hepatic disease, the metabolism of a drug may be increased, decreased, or unchanged. Clearly, all patients with hepatic disease must be monitored closely for drug effect and toxicity. Some drugs (digoxin, gentamicin) are eliminated almost unchanged by the kidneys. For safe use of such drugs, renal function must be adequate or the drug will accumulate, producing toxic effects. Some drugs can alter the effect and excretion of other drugs. For example, they can stimulate or inhibit hepatic-metabolizing enzymes to alter the rate of metabolism and change the drug effect. Or they can block or promote renal excretion of other drugs, causing them to accumulate and enhancing their effects, or cause rapid excretion, thereby diminishing their effects. Some slight elimination takes place by way of perspiration, saliva, breast milk, and so on. Certain volatile anesthetics, however – halothane, for instance – are eliminated primarily by exhalation.

The rate at which a drug is metabolized varies with the individual. In some patients, drugs are metabolized so quickly that their blood and tissue levels prove therapeutically inadequate. In others, the rate of metabolism is so slow that ordinary doses can produce toxic results.

Other modifying factors
An important factor that influences a drug's action and effect is its *binding to plasma proteins,* especially albumin, and other tissue components. Because only a free, unbound drug can act in the body, such binding greatly influences effectiveness and duration of effect.

The *patient's age* is another important factor. Elderly patients usually have decreased hepatic function, less muscle mass, and diminished renal function. Consequently, they need lower doses and sometimes longer dosage intervals to avoid toxicity. With similar consequences, neonates have underdeveloped metabolic enzyme systems and inadequate renal function. They need highly individualized dosage and careful monitoring.

Underlying disease can also markedly affect drug action and effect. For example, acidosis may cause insulin resistance. Genetic diseases, such as G6PD deficiency and hepatic porphyria, may turn drugs into toxins with serious consequences. Patients with G6PD deficiency may develop hemolytic anemia when given sulfonamides or a number of other drugs. A genetically susceptible patient can develop an acute porphyria attack if given a barbiturate. Also, patients who have highly active hepatic enzyme systems (for example, rapid acetylators), when treated with isoniazid, can develop hepatitis from the rapid intrahepatic buildup of a toxic metabolite.

Things to consider about administration

• *Dosage forms do matter.* Some tablets and capsules are too large to be easily swallowed by very ill patients. You may then request an oral solution or elixir of the same drug, but bear in mind that because a liquid is more easily and completely absorbed, it produces higher blood levels than a tablet. When a potentially toxic drug (such as digoxin) is given, the increased amount absorbed could cause toxicity. Sometimes a change in dosage form requires a change in dosage.

• *Routes of administration are not therapeutically interchangeable.* For example, phenytoin is readily absorbed orally but is slowly and erratically absorbed intramuscularly. On the other hand, gentamicin must be given parenterally because oral administration yields inadequate blood levels to treat systemic infections.

• *Improper storage can alter a drug's potency.* Most drugs should be stored in tight containers protected from direct sunlight and extremes in temperature and humidity which can cause them to deteriorate. Some may require special storage conditions (such as refrigeration).

• *The timing of drug administration can be important.* Sometimes giving an oral drug during or shortly after mealtime decreases the amount of drug absorbed. This is not clinically significant with most drugs and may in fact be desirable with irritating drugs such as aspirin or phenylbutazone. But penicillins and tetracyclines should not be scheduled for administration at mealtimes because certain foods can inactivate them. If in doubt about the effect of food on a certain drug, check with the pharmacist.

• *Consider the patient's age, height, and weight.* The doctor will need this information when calculating the dosage for many drugs. It should be accurately recorded on the patient's chart. This chart should also include current laboratory data, especially renal and liver function studies, so the doctor can adjust the dosage as needed.

• *Watch for metabolic changes.* Monitor for any physiologic change (depressed respiratory function, acidosis or alkalosis) that might alter drug effect.

• *Know the patient's history.* Whenever possible, obtain a comprehensive family history from the patient or his family. Ask about past reactions to drugs, possible genetic traits that might alter drug response, and the current use of other drugs. Multiple drug therapy can cause drug interactions that can dramatically change the effects of many drugs.

Drug interactions

When one drug administered in combination with or shortly after another drug alters the effect of one or both drugs, this is known as a drug interaction. Usually, the effect of one drug is increased or decreased. For instance, one drug may inhibit or stimulate the metabolism or excretion of the other; or it may release another from plasma protein-binding sites, freeing it for further action.

Combination therapy is based on drug interaction. One drug, for example, may be given to potentiate another. Probenecid, which blocks the excretion of penicillin, is sometimes given with penicillin to maintain adequate blood levels of penicillin for a longer period. Often, two drugs with similar actions are given together precisely because of the additive effect that results. For instance, aspirin and codeine, both analgesics, are often given in combination because together they provide greater pain relief than either alone.

Drug interactions are sometimes used to prevent or antagonize certain adverse reactions. Hydrochlorothiazide and spironolactone, both diuretics, are often administered in combination because the former is potassium-depleting, whereas the latter is potassium-sparing.

But not all drug interactions are beneficial. Multiple drugs can interact to produce effects that are often undesirable and sometimes hazardous. Harmful drug interactions decrease efficacy or increase toxicity. A hypertensive patient well controlled with guanethidine may see his blood pressure rise to its former high level if he takes the antidepressant amitriptyline at the same time. Such a drug effect is known as antagonism. Drug combinations that produce these effects should be avoided if possible. Another kind of inhibiting effect occurs when a tetracycline drug is administered with calcium- or magnesium-containing drugs or foods (such as antacids or milk). These combine with tetracycline in the GI tract and cause inadequate absorption of tetracycline.

Adverse reactions

Any drug effect other than what is therapeutically intended can be called an adverse reaction. It may be expected and benign, or unexpected and potentially harmful. Mild, but *predictable,* adverse reactions are sometimes called side effects. Drowsiness caused by antihistamines is an example of this. During hay fever season, a patient may have to contend with this drowsiness to get relief from hay fever symptoms. In such a case, the dosage may be adjusted up or down to balance therapeutic effects with side effects.

An adverse reaction may be tolerated for a necessary therapeutic effect, or it may be hazardous and unacceptable and require discontinuation of the drug. Some adverse reactions subside with continued use. As an example, the drowsiness associated with methyldopa and the orthostatic hypotension associated with prazosin usually subside after several days, as the patient develops a tolerance to these effects. But many adverse reactions are dosage-related and lessen or disappear only if the dosage is reduced. Although most adverse reactions are not therapeutically desirable, an occasional one can be put to clinical use. An outstanding example of this is the drowsiness associated with diphenhydramine, which makes it clinically useful as a mild hypnotic.

Hypersensitivity, a term sometimes used interchangeably with drug allergy, is the result of an antigen-antibody immune reaction that occurs in the body when a drug is given to a susceptible patient. One of the most dangerous of all drug hypersensitivities is penicillin allergy. In its severest form, penicillin anaphylaxis can rapidly become fatal.

Rarely, idiosyncratic reactions occur. These are highly unpredictable, individual, and unusual. Probably the best known idiosyncratic drug reaction is the aplastic anemia caused by the antibiotic chloramphenicol. This reaction appears in only 1 out of 40,000 patients, but when it does, it is often fatal. A more common idiosyncratic reaction is extreme sensitivity to very low doses of a drug, or insensitivity to higher-than-normal doses.

To deal with adverse reactions correctly, you need to be alert to even minor changes in the patient's clinical status. Such minor changes may be an early warning of pending toxicity. Listen to the patient's complaints about his reactions to a drug, and consider each complaint objectively. You may be able to reduce adverse reactions in several ways. Obviously, dosage reduction often helps. But often so does a simple rescheduling of the same dose. For example, pseudoephedrine may produce stimulation that will be no problem if it's given early in the day; similarly, the drowsiness that occurs with antihistamines or tranquilizers can be totally harmless if the dose is given at bedtime. Most important, your patient needs to be told what adverse reactions to expect so he won't become worried or even stop taking the drug on his own. Of course, the patient should report any unusual or unexpected adverse reactions to the doctor.

Recognizing drug allergies or serious idiosyncratic reactions can sometimes be lifesaving. Ask each patient about drugs he is taking or has taken in the past and what, if any, unusual effects he experienced from taking them. If a patient claims to be allergic to a drug, ask him to tell you exactly what happens when he takes it. He may be calling a harmless side effect such as upset stomach an allergic reaction, or he may have a true tendency toward anaphylaxis. In either case, you and the doctor need to know this. Of course, you must record and report any clinical changes throughout the patient's hospital stay. If you suspect a severe adverse reaction, withhold the drug until you can check with the pharmacist and the doctor.

Toxic reactions

Chronic drug toxicities are generally due to the cumulative effect and resulting buildup of the drug in the body. These effects may be extensions of the desired therapeutic effect. For example, guanethidine-induced norepinephrine depletion produces a desired antihypertensive effect, but in larger doses, this action often produces orthostatic hypotension.

Drug toxicities usually occur when drug blood levels rise due to impaired metabolism or excretion. For example, blood levels of theophylline rise when hepatic dysfunction impairs metabolism of the drug. Similarly, digoxin toxicity can follow impaired renal function because digoxin is eliminated from the body almost exclusively by the kidneys (via glomerular filtration). Of course, toxic blood levels also follow excessive dosage. Aspirin tinnitus (ringing in ears) is usually a sign that the safe dose has been exceeded.

Most drug toxicities are predictable and dosage-related; fortunately, most are also readily reversible upon dosage adjustment. So it's essential to monitor patients carefully for physiologic changes that might alter drug effect. Watch especially for impaired hepatic and renal function. Warn the patient about signs of pending toxicity, and tell him what to do if a toxic reaction occurs. Also, be sure to emphasize the importance of taking a drug exactly as prescribed. Warn the patient about serious problems that could arise if he changes the dose or the schedule for taking it.

Drugs and pregnancy

Ever since the thalidomide tragedy of the late 1950s – when thousands of malformed infants were born after their mothers used this mild sedative-hypnotic during pregnancy – use of drugs during pregnancy has been a source of serious medical concern and controversy. To identify drugs that may cause such teratogenic effects, preclinical drug studies always include tests on pregnant laboratory animals. These tests point out gross teratogenicity but do not clearly establish safety. Because different species react to drugs in different ways, animal studies do not rule out possible teratogenic effects in humans. For example, the preliminary studies on thalidomide gave no warning of teratogenic effects, and it was subsequently released for general use in Europe.

What about the placental barrier? Once thought to protect the fetus from drug effects, the placenta isn't actually much of a barrier at all. Except for drugs with exceptionally large molecular structure, almost every drug administered to a pregnant woman crosses the placenta and enters the fetal circulation. An example of a drug with a large molecular size is heparin, the injectable anticoagulant. Theoretically, then, heparin could be used in a pregnant woman without fear of harming the fetus – but even heparin carries a warning for cautious use in pregnancy. Conversely, just because a drug crosses the placenta doesn't necessarily mean it's harmful to the fetus.

Actually, only one factor – stage of fetal development – seems clearly related to exaggerated risk during pregnancy. During two stages of pregnancy – the first and the third trimesters – the fetus is especially vulnerable to damage from maternal use of drugs. During these times, *all* drugs should be given with extreme caution.

The most sensitive period for drug-induced fetal malformation is the first trimester, when fetal organs are differentiating (organogenesis). During this time, *all* drugs should be withheld unless doing so would jeopardize the mother's health. Theoretically, during this sensitive time, even aspirin could harm the fetus. So, strongly advise your patient to avoid *all* self-prescribed drugs during early pregnancy. The other time of special fetal sensitivity to drugs is the last trimester. The reason? At birth, when separated from his mother, the neonate must rely on his own metabolism to eliminate any remaining drug. Because his detoxifying systems are not fully developed, any residual drug may take a long time to be metabolized – and thus may induce prolonged toxic reactions. Consequently, drugs should be used only when absolutely necessary during the last 3 months of pregnancy.

Of course, in many circumstances, pregnant women must continue to take certain drugs. For example, a woman with a seizure disorder that is well controlled with an anticonvulsant should continue to take the drug even during pregnancy. Similarly, a pregnant woman with a bacterial infection must receive antibiotics. In such cases, the potential risk to the fetus is outweighed by the mother's need. The relative risk to the fetus is expressed by the drug's pregnancy risk category (see Chapter 1).

Following these general guidelines can prevent indiscriminate and potentially harmful use of drugs in pregnancy:

- Before a drug is prescribed for a woman of childbearing age, she should be asked the date of her last menstrual period and whether there is a possibility she is pregnant. If a drug is a known teratogen (for example, isotretinoin), some manufacturers may recommend special precautions to ensure that the drug not be given to a female of childbearing age until pregnancy is ruled out.
- Especially during the first and the third trimesters, a pregnant patient should avoid *all* drugs except those *essential* to maintain the pregnancy or maternal health.
- Topical drugs are not exempt from the warning against indiscriminate use during pregnancy. Many topically applied drugs can be absorbed in large enough amounts to be harmful to the fetus.
- When a pregnant patient needs *any* drug, the doctor should prescribe the *safest* possible drug in the *lowest* possible dose to minimize any harmful effect to the fetus.
- Every pregnant patient should check with her doctor before taking *any* drug.

Drugs and lactation

Most drugs a nursing mother takes appear in breast milk. Drug levels in breast milk tend to be high when blood levels are high – generally, shortly after taking each dose. Therefore, the mother should be advised to breast-feed *before* taking medication, not *after*.

Nevertheless, with very few exceptions, a mother who wishes to breast-feed may continue to do so with her doctor's permission. However, breast-feeding should be temporarily interrupted and replaced with bottle-feeding when the mother must take tetracyclines, chloramphenicol, sulfonamides (during first 2 weeks postpartum), oral anticoagulants, iodine-containing drugs, or antineoplastics.

To protect her infant, a nursing mother should avoid taking drugs indiscriminately. If she needs to take a drug to maintain her own health, she should first check with her doctor to be sure of taking the safest drug at the lowest dose.

What to teach patients about proper use of drugs

Store drugs in their original containers, at room temperature (unless directed otherwise), in places that are not accessible to children or exposed to sunlight. Avoid storage in the bathroom medicine cabinet or the glove compartment or trunk of an automobile, where extremes of temperature and humidity will cause them to deteriorate. Never share prescription drugs with others.

Learn the trade name and generic name of any drug you are taking. Be sure to tell doctors, dentists, or other health care professionals you see regularly that you are taking it. Before taking any drug, be sure you have informed your doctor, nurse, or pharmacist about any unusual reactions you've had to drugs in the past and about your allergies to foods and other substances, any special medical problems, and any drugs you've taken over the last few weeks, including any nonprescription drugs.

Always take any drug exactly as prescribed, at the recommended dosage and for the duration of treatment.

To avoid hazardous mistakes, always read the label before taking any drug. When using a drug prescribed for occasional or prolonged use, check the container for an expiration date (if available).

To avoid potentially harmful changes in effectiveness, do not change brands of a drug without medical approval. Certain generic preparations are not precisely equivalent in effect to brand-name preparations of the same drug.

Never mix different drugs in a single container, and don't remove any drug from its original container or remove the label. Relying on your memory to identify a drug and specific directions for its use is hazardous.

Discard any drugs that are outdated or no longer needed.

Before you have any surgery (including dental surgery), tell the doctor about all of the drugs that you have been taking.

Be sure to tell the doctor, nurse, or pharmacist about any side effects or unpleasant effects you've experienced while taking a drug. Such effects may require medical attention.

If you or someone else has taken an overdose, call your doctor, poison control center, or pharmacist immediately. Keep syrup of ipecac in your home to induce vomiting, but induce vomiting only if one of these professionals has advised you to do so.

Try to have all your prescriptions filled at the same pharmacy. Most pharmacists keep records of all your prescriptions and can quickly identify and warn against potentially harmful drug interactions. Also be sure to check with the pharmacist before taking OTC medications, especially if you're taking any other drugs.

3

Drug therapy in children

A child's absorption, distribution, metabolism, and excretion processes undergo profound changes that affect drug dosage. To ensure optimal drug effect and minimal toxicity, consider these factors when administering drugs to a child.

Absorption

Drug absorption in children depends on the form of the drug; its physical properties; other drugs or substances, such as food, taken simultaneously; physiologic changes; and concurrent disease.

- The pH of neonatal gastric fluid is neutral or slightly acidic and becomes more acidic as the infant matures. This affects drug absorption. For example, nafcillin and penicillin G, erratically absorbed or malabsorbed in an adult due to degradation by gastric acid, are better absorbed in an infant due to low gastric acidity.
- Various infant formulas or milk products may increase gastric pH and impede absorption of acidic drugs. So, if possible, give a child oral medications when his stomach is empty.
- Gastric emptying time and transit time through the small intestine – which is longer in children than in adults – can affect absorption. Also, intestinal hypermotility (as in diarrhea) can diminish the drug's absorption.
- A child's comparatively thin epidermis allows increased absorption of topical drugs.

Distribution

As with absorption, changes in body weight and physiology during childhood can significantly influence a drug's distribution and effects. In a premature infant, body fluid makes up about 85% of total body weight; in a full-term infant, 55% to 70%; and in an adult, 50% to 55%. Extracellular fluid (mostly blood) constitutes 40% of a neonate's body weight, compared with 20% in an adult. Intracellular fluid remains fairly constant throughout life and has little effect on drug dosage.

Since most drugs travel through extracellular fluid to reach their receptors, however, extracellular fluid volume influences a water-soluble drug's concentration and effect. Children have a larger proportion of fluid to solid body weight, so their distribution area is proportionately greater.

Because the proportion of fat to lean body mass increases with age, the distribution of fat-soluble drugs is more limited in children than adults. As a result, a drug's lipid- or water-solubility affects the dosage for a child.

Binding to plasma proteins

As the result of a decrease in albumin concentration or intermolecular attraction between drug and plasma protein, many drugs are less bound to plasma proteins in infants than in adults.

Furthermore, preparations that bind plasma proteins may displace endogenous compounds, such as bilirubin or free fatty acids. Conversely, an endogenous compound may displace a weakly bound drug. For example, displacement of bound bilirubin can cause a rise in unbound bilirubin, which can lead to increased risk of kernicterus at normal bilirubin levels.

Since only an unbound, or free, drug has a pharmacologic effect, any alteration in ratio of a protein-bound to an unbound active drug can greatly influence its effect.

Several diseases and disorders, such as nephrotic syndrome and malnutrition, can also decrease plasma protein and increase the concentration of an unbound drug, intensifying the drug's effect or producing toxicity.

Metabolism

A neonate's ability to metabolize a drug depends on the integrity of his hepatic enzyme system, his intrauterine exposure to the drug, and the nature of the drug itself.

Certain metabolic mechanisms are underdeveloped in neonates. Glucuronidation is a metabolic process that renders most drugs more water soluble, thereby facilitating renal excretion. This process is insufficiently developed to permit full pediatric doses until the infant is 1 month old. Because of this, the use of chloramphenicol in a neonate may cause gray syndrome, illustrating the infant's inability to metabolize the drug. Use of chloramphenicol in neonates, therefore, requires decreased dosage (25 mg/kg/day) and monitoring of blood levels.

Conversely, intrauterine exposure to drugs may induce precocious development of hepatic enzyme mechanisms, increasing the infant's capacity to metabolize potentially harmful substances.

Older children can metabolize some drugs (theophylline, for example) more rapidly than adults. This ability may be due to their increased hepatic metabolic activity. Larger doses than those recommended for adults may be required.

Also, preparations given concurrently to a child may alter hepatic metabolism and induce production of hepatic enzymes. Phenobarbital, for example, can induce hepatic enzyme production and accelerate metabolism of drugs given concurrently.

Excretion

Renal excretion of a drug is the net effect of glomerular filtration, active tubular secretion, and passive tubular reabsorption. Because so many drugs are excreted in the urine, the degree of renal development or presence of renal disease can profoundly affect a child's dosage requirements.

If a child is unable to excrete a drug renally, drug accumulation and possible toxicity may result unless the dosage is reduced.

Physiologically, an infant's kidneys differ from an adult's in that they have:

- high resistance to blood flow and receive a smaller proportion of cardiac output
- incomplete glomerular and tubular development and short, incomplete loops of Henle (A child's glomerular filtration reaches adult values by ages 2½ to 5 months; his tubular secretion may reach adult values by ages 7 to 12 months.)
- low glomerular filtration rate (Penicillins are eliminated by this route.)
- decreased ability to concentrate urine or reabsorb various filtered compounds
- reduced ability of the proximal tubules to secrete organic acids.

Both children and adults have diurnal variations in urine pH that correlate with sleep-wake patterns.

Calculating and monitoring pediatric dosages

When calculating pediatric dosages, don't use formulas that modify adult dosages: a child is not a scaled-down version of an adult. Pediatric dosages should be calculated on the basis of either body weight (mg/kg) or body surface area (mg/m^2).

- Reevaluate dosages at regular intervals to ensure necessary adjustments as the child develops.
- Although useful for adults and older children, don't use dosages based on

body surface area in premature or full-term infants. Use the body weight method instead.

- Don't exceed the maximum adult dosage when calculating amounts per kilogram of body weight (except with certain drugs, such as theophylline, if indicated).
- Obtain an accurate maternal drug history – prescription and nonprescription drugs, vitamins, and herbs or other health foods taken during pregnancy.
- Drugs passed through breast milk can also have adverse effects on the nursing infant. Before a drug is prescribed for a breast-feeding mother, the potential effects on the infant should be investigated. For example, sulfonamides given to a breast-feeding mother for a urinary tract infection appear in breast milk and may cause kernicterus at lower-than-normal levels of unconjugated bilirubin. Also, high concentrations of isoniazid appear in breast milk. Since this drug is metabolized by the liver, an infant's immature hepatic enzyme mechanisms cannot metabolize the drug, and the infant may suffer CNS toxicity.

Oral medications

- *When giving oral medication to an infant,* administer it in liquid form if possible. For accuracy, measure and give the preparation by syringe; never use a vial or cup.
- Lift the patient's head to prevent aspiration of the medication, and press down on his chin to prevent choking.
- You may also place the drug in a nipple and allow the infant to suck the contents.
- *If the patient is a toddler,* explain how you're going to give him the medication. If possible, have the parents enlist the child's cooperation.
- Don't mix medication with food or call it "candy" even if it has a pleasant taste.
- Let the child drink liquid medication from a calibrated medication cup rather than from a spoon: it's easier and more accurate. If the preparation is available only in tablet form, crush it and mix it with a compatible syrup. (Check with the pharmacist to make sure the tablet can be crushed without losing its effectiveness.)
- *If the patient is an older child* who can swallow a tablet or capsule by himself, have him place the medication on the back of his tongue and swallow it with water or fruit juice. Remember, milk or milk products may interfere with drug absorption.

I.V. infusions

When administering I.V. infusions to children, note the following special considerations.

Protecting the insertion site

In infants, use a peripheral vein or a scalp vein in the temporal region for I.V. infusions. The scalp vein is safest in that the needle is not likely to be dislodged; however, the head must be shaved around the site. Temporary disfigurement may also result from the needle and infiltrated fluids. For these reasons, the scalp veins are not used as frequently today as they were in the past.

The extremities are the most accessible insertion sites; however, since patients tend to move about, take these precautions:

- Protect the insertion site to prevent catheter or needle dislodgment.
- Use a padded arm board to minimize dislodgment. Remove the arm board during range-of-motion exercises.
- Place the clamp out of the child's reach; if extension tubing is used to allow the child greater mobility, securely tape the connection.
- Restrain the child only when necessary.
- To allay anxiety, give a simple ex-

planation to the child who must be restrained while asleep.

Maintaining flow rate and fluid balance
While administering a continuous I.V. infusion to a child, monitor flow rate and check the patient's condition and insertion site at least hourly – more frequently when giving drug intermittently.

Adjust the flow rate only while the patient is composed; crying and emotional upset can constrict blood vessels. Flow rate may vary if a pump isn't used. Flow should be adequate because some drugs (calcium, for example) can be very irritating at low flow rates.

Making dilutions
Some drugs are hyperosmolar; in infants, these drugs must be diluted to prevent radical changes in fluid that might induce CNS hemorrhage. Sodium bicarbonate, for example, must be diluted to half-strength to lower osmolality and lessen the risk of CNS bleeding.

In general, however, use the minimum amount of compatible fluid over the shortest recommended period of time. Remember also to check the total daily fluid intake and the amount allotted to medication.

I.M. injections
I.M. injections are preferred when the drug cannot be given by other parenteral routes and rapid absorption is necessary.
• In children under age 2, the vastus lateralis muscle is the preferred injection site; in older children, either the ventrogluteal area or the gluteus medius muscle can be used.
• To determine correct needle size, consider the patient's age, muscle mass, and nutritional status and the drug's viscosity; record and rotate injection sites.
• Explain to the patient that the injection will hurt, but that the medication will help him. Restrain him during the injection, if needed, and comfort him afterward.

Topical medications and inhalants
• Use ear drops warmed to room temperature; cold drops can cause considerable pain and possibly vertigo.
• To administer drops, turn the patient on his side, with the affected ear up. If he is under age 3, pull the pinna down and back; if he is over age 3, pull the pinna up and back.
• Avoid using inhalants in very young children: obtaining their cooperation is difficult.
• Before attempting to administer medication through a metered-dose nebulizer to an older child, explain the inhaler to him. Then have him hold the nebulizer upside down and close his lips around the mouthpiece. Have him exhale; pinch his nostrils shut; and when he starts to inhale, release one dose of medication into his mouth. Tell the patient to continue inhaling until his lungs feel full.
• Most inhaled agents are not useful if taken orally; therefore, if you doubt the patient's ability to use the inhalant correctly, don't use it.
• Use topical corticosteroids with caution because chronic steroid use in children has been associated with delayed growth. When topical corticosteroids are used on the diaper area of infants, avoid covering this area with plastic or rubber pants, which will act as an occlusive dressing and enhance systemic absorption.

Parenteral nutrition
I.V. nutrition is given to patients who can't or won't take adequate food orally and patients with hypermetabolic conditions who need I.V. supplementation. The latter group includes premature infants and children who have burns or other major trauma, in-

tractable diarrhea, malabsorption syndromes, GI abnormalities, emotional disorders (such as anorexia nervosa), and congenital abnormalities.

Before fat emulsions are administered to infants and children, however, potential benefits must be weighed against possible risks.

Fats – supplied as 10% or 20% emulsions – are administered both peripherally and centrally. Their use is limited by the child's ability to metabolize them. An infant or a child with a diseased liver cannot efficiently metabolize fats, for example.

Some fats, however, must be supplied both to prevent essential fatty acid deficiency and to permit normal growth and development. A minimum of calories (2% to 4%) must be supplied as linoleic acid – an essential fatty acid found in lipids. In infants, fats are essential for normal neurologic development.

Nevertheless, fat solutions may decrease oxygen perfusion and may adversely affect children with pulmonary disease. This risk can be minimized by supplying only the minimum fat needed for essential fatty acid requirements and not the usual intake of 40% to 50% of the child's total calories.

Fatty acids can also displace bilirubin bound to serum albumin, causing a rise in free, unconjugated bilirubin and an increased risk of kernicterus. However, fat solutions may interfere with some bilirubin assays and cause falsely elevated levels. To avoid this complication, a blood sample should be drawn 4 hours after infusion of the lipid emulsion; or if the emulsion is introduced over 24 hours, the blood sample should be centrifuged before the assay is performed.

4

Drug therapy in elderly patients

If you're providing drug therapy for elderly patients, you'll want to understand physiologic and pharmacokinetic changes that may alter drug dosage, common adverse reactions, and compliance problems in elderly patients.

Physiologic changes affecting drug action

As a person ages, gradual physiologic changes occur. Some of these age-related changes may alter the therapeutic and toxic effects of medications.

Body composition

Proportions of fat, lean tissue, and water in the body change with age. Total body mass and lean body mass tend to decrease; the proportion of body fat tends to increase.

Varying from person to person, these changes in body composition affect the relationship between a drug's concentration and distribution in the body.

For example, a water-soluble drug, such as gentamicin, is not distributed to fat. Since there's relatively less lean tissue in an elderly person, more drug remains in the blood.

GI function

In elderly patients, decreases in gastric acid secretion and GI motility slow the emptying of stomach contents and the movement of intestinal contents through the entire tract. Furthermore, inconclusive research shows that elderly patients may have more difficulty absorbing medications. This is a particularly significant problem with drugs having a narrow therapeutic range, such as digoxin, in which any change in absorption can be crucial.

Hepatic function

The liver's ability to metabolize certain drugs decreases with age. This is due to diminished blood flow to the liver, which results from the age-related decrease in cardiac output and from the diminished activity of certain liver enzymes. When an elderly patient takes certain sleep medications, such as secobarbital, his liver's reduced ability to metabolize the drug may produce a hangover effect the next morning.

Decreased hepatic function may cause:

- more intense drug effects due to higher blood levels
- longer-lasting drug effects due to prolonged blood concentrations
- greater incidence of drug toxicity.

Renal function

Although an elderly person's renal function is usually sufficient to eliminate excess body fluid and waste, his ability to eliminate some medications may be reduced by 50% or more.

Many medications commonly used by elderly patients, such as digoxin, are excreted primarily through the kidneys. If the kidneys' ability to excrete the drug is decreased, high blood concentrations may result. Digoxin toxicity, therefore, is relatively common in elderly patients who are not receiving a reduced digoxin dosage to account for their decreased renal function.

Drug dosages can be modified to compensate for age-related decreases in renal function. Aided by laboratory tests, such as blood urea nitrogen and serum creatinine, clinical pharmacists may recommend a change and doctors may adjust medication dosages so the patient receives the expected therapeutic benefits without the risk of toxicity. Observe your patient for signs of toxicity. A patient taking digoxin, for example, may experience anorexia, nausea, vomiting, or confusion.

Adverse drug reactions
As compared with younger people, elderly patients experience twice as many adverse drug reactions relating to greater drug consumption, poor compliance, and physiologic changes.

Signs and symptoms of adverse drug reactions – confusion, weakness, and lethargy – are often mistakenly attributed to senility or disease. If the adverse reaction isn't identified, the patient may continue to receive the drug. Furthermore, he may receive unnecessary additional medication to treat complications caused by the original medication. This can sometimes result in the pattern of inappropriate and excessive medication use referred to as "polypharmacy."

Although any medication can cause adverse reactions, most of the serious reactions in the elderly are caused by relatively few medications. Be particularly alert for toxicities resulting from diuretics, antihypertensives, digoxin, corticosteroids, sleeping aids, and nonprescription drugs.

Diuretic toxicity
Because total body water content decreases with age, normal dosages of potassium-wasting diuretics, such as hydrochlorothiazide and furosemide, may result in fluid loss and even dehydration in an elderly patient.

These diuretics may deplete serum potassium, causing weakness in the patient; and they may raise blood uric acid and glucose levels, complicating preexisting gout and diabetes mellitus.

Antihypertensive toxicity
Many elderly people experience lightheadedness or fainting when using antihypertensive medications. This is partially due to the fact that hypertension in elderly patients is partly a response to such changes as atherosclerosis and decreased elasticity of the blood vessels. Antihypertensive drugs lower blood pressure too rapidly, resulting in insufficient blood flow to the brain. This may cause dizziness, fainting, or even stroke.

Consequently, dosages of antihypertensive drugs must be carefully individualized for each patient. In elderly patients, overaggressive treatment of high blood pressure may clearly do more harm than good, so treatment goals should be reasonable. While it may be appropriate to bring blood pressure down to 120/85 mm Hg for a young hypertensive patient, a more reasonable goal for some elderly hypertensive patients might be 150/95 mm Hg.

Digoxin toxicity
As the body's renal function and rate of excretion decline, digoxin concentrations in the blood may build to toxic levels, causing nausea, vomiting, diarrhea, and – most serious – cardiac arrhythmias. Try to prevent severe toxicity by observing your patient for early signs, such as appetite loss, confusion, or depression.

Corticosteroid toxicity
Elderly patients on corticosteroids may experience short-term effects, including fluid retention and psychological manifestations ranging from mild euphoria to acute psychotic reactions. Long-term toxic effects, such as osteoporosis, can be especially severe in elderly patients who have been taking prednisone or related steroidal compounds for months or even years. To prevent serious toxicity, carefully monitor patients on long-term regimens. Observe them for subtle changes in appearance, mood, and

mobility, as well as for signs of impaired healing and fluid and electrolyte disturbances.

Sleeping aid toxicity
Sedatives or sleeping aids, such as flurazepam, may cause excessive sedation or residual drowsiness. Keep in mind that ingestion of alcohol may exaggerate such depressant effects, even if the sleeping aid was taken the previous evening.

Nonprescription drug toxicity
When aspirin and aspirin-containing analgesics are used in moderation, toxicity is minimal, but prolonged ingestion may cause GI irritation and gradual blood loss resulting in severe anemia. Although anemia from chronic aspirin consumption can affect all age-groups, elderly patients may be less able to compensate because of their already reduced iron stores.

Laxatives may cause diarrhea in elderly patients who are extremely sensitive to drugs such as bisacodyl. Chronic oral use of mineral oil as a lubricating laxative may result in lipid pneumonia due to aspiration of small residual oil droplets in the patient's mouth.

Patient noncompliance
Poor compliance is a problem with patients of all ages. However, in elderly patients, specific factors linked to aging – such as diminished visual acuity, hearing loss, forgetfulness, the common need for multiple drug therapy, and various socioeconomic factors – combine to make compliance a special problem. Approximately one-third of elderly patients fail to comply with their prescribed drug therapy. They may fail to take prescribed doses or to follow the correct schedule; they may take medications prescribed for previous disorders, discontinue medications prematurely, or use p.r.n. medications indiscriminately.

Review your patient's medication regimen with him. Be sure he understands the medication amount and the time and frequency of doses. Also, explain how he should take each medication, that is, with food or water or by itself.

Give your patient whatever help you can to avoid drug therapy problems, and refer him to the doctor or pharmacist if he needs further information.

5

Drug therapy and the nursing process

The nursing process guides nursing decisions about drug administration to ensure the patient's safety and meet medical and legal standards. This process, in five steps, provides thorough assessment, appropriate nursing diagnosis, effective planning, correct interventions, and constant evaluation.

First step: Assessment
During assessment, the nurse focuses on direct data collection by:
- obtaining a drug history from the patient, parent, spouse, or significant other
- reviewing the patient's previous medical history
- performing a physical examination
- obtaining relevant laboratory or diagnostic test results.

Drug history
Data collection begins at admission to the hospital or in an outpatient setting with specific questions about the patient's background, including allergies, medical history, habits, socioeconomic status, life-style and beliefs, and sensory deficits. These aspects of the patient's background can significantly influence drug therapy.

Allergies
The patient's allergy profile includes the patient's reactions to both drugs and food. Information about allergic reactions to drugs must specify the drug, when the allergic reaction occurred, the situation and setting at the time of the reaction, a description of the reaction, and any contributing factors. Examples of contributing factors might include the concurrent use of stimulants, tobacco, alcohol, or illicit drugs, or a significant change in nutritional patterns. Asking the patient to describe his allergic reaction is especially important to help determine whether the patient actually reacts adversely to a drug or simply dislikes taking it.

Allergies to foods can also affect a drug therapy. For example, allergies to shellfish can contraindicate use of drugs that contain iodine or are byproducts of shellfish. Allergies to eggs are significant in patients who are to receive vaccines, which are commonly derived from chick embryos.

Prescription drugs
The patient's drug history should explore the following:
- the reason for using the drug
- the patient's knowledge of the appropriate dosage
- the patient's knowedge about determining effectiveness of the drug (if appropriate), potential adverse effects, what to do about adverse effects, and when to contact the doctor
- route of administration
- the pattern of administration at home
- use of OTC drugs
- cognitive status.

Note any special monitoring the patient must perform, such as blood glucose monitoring before insulin administration or checking radial pulse rate before taking digoxin. Make sure the patient is performing such procedures correctly and that the results are within acceptable limits.

Discuss the effects of drug therapy with the patient and determine if new symptoms or unpredicted adverse effects have developed. Noting the patient's pattern of administration may provide insight into why a particular drug regimen succeeds or fails.

Over-the-counter drugs
A comprehensive drug history should also list any OTC drugs the patient is taking. Many OTC drugs can inhibit or potentiate the effects of a prescribed drug. For example, aspirin potentiates the anticoagulant effects of warfarin.

OTC drugs include a wide range of products from common aspirin and nutritional supplements to various sprays and cleansing agents. The patient may not think of all of these products as drugs, so the nurse may have to suggest a general list of products to get an accurate response.

Dosage and frequency of use are just as important as the type of the OTC product the patient is using. One tablet of aspirin taken once a day may have no effect on concomitant drug therapy; however, a higher dosage (such as that used for arthritis) could influence it profoundly.

Medical history
In gathering the medical history, note any chronic diseases or disorders the patient may have and record the following information for each:
- date of diagnosis
- initial prescribed treatment
- current treatment
- the doctor in charge.

Careful attention to this part of the medical history can uncover one of the most important problems with drug therapy – conflicting and incompatible drug regimens. The patient who does not have a family physician to oversee and coordinate all care may seek the care of several specialists who may prescribe drug treatment without knowing what other drugs the patient is taking. A carefully detailed medical history can uncover such problems. The nurse who identifies such conflicting or overlapping drug therapy must call them to the appropriate doctor's attention and then teach the patient about the importance of informing caregivers about all drugs he is taking.

Habits
Carefully consider dietary habits and the nontherapeutic use of drugs.

Certain foods can directly affect the effectiveness of many drugs. For example, a person who is taking the anticoagulant warfarin should not increase his intake of green leafy vegetables because they contain levels of vitamin K that can antagonize the drug's anticoagulant effect.

Nontherapeutic use of drugs can profoundly affect a patient's health and impair the effectiveness of a drug therapy. Consider the possible use of alcohol, tobacco, caffeine, and illicit drugs, such as marijuana, cocaine, and heroin. For example, if the patient uses alcohol, note the frequency of use, the amount, and the type of alcohol consumed. Carefully document the intake of stimulants, such as caffeine, because they significantly affect a patient's cardiovascular status and nervous system. Record the type of stimulant (coffee, tea, soda, or chocolate), the frequency of intake, and the amount consumed.

For the patient who smokes, document the following information:
- the length of time the patient has smoked
- what the patient smokes (cigarettes, cigar, or pipe)
- how many cigarettes or cigars the patient smokes per day
- the brand of cigarettes or cigars the patient smokes or the brand of tobacco and how much he chews per day.

Defining the patient's use of illicit drugs may be difficult. However, the nurse who suspects such use should encourage the patient to discuss it honestly, emphasizing that these drugs have profound effects that may cause serious drug interactions. If the patient admits using illicit drugs, document the drug, the amount and frequency of use, and the route of administration.

Socioeconomic status
Note the patient's age, educational level, occupation, and insurance coverage. These factors may be significant to compliance and to an effective care plan. The patient's age, for example, can determine whom to include in the care plan (parents or other family members) and the level of information that is appropriate for teaching the patient.

Knowing the patient's educational background and occupation helps you select interventions at an appropriate level, plan a drug regimen that fits the patient's daily routine, and encourage compliance. Knowing the patient's insurance status may help you anticipate the need for financial assistance and counseling. Remember that noncompliance frequently results from inability to afford costly medications.

Life-style and beliefs
Support systems, marital status, childbearing status, attitudes toward health and health care, use of the health care system, and daily patterns of activities all affect the plan of care and patient compliance. For example, an 18-year-old single parent, who is a high-school dropout on medical assistance and has no family support, will probably require more teaching and support to gain a commitment and compliance to drug therapy than a 40-year-old affluent professional, with a lot of family support, who can understand why she needs the drug and can readily pay for it.

Sensory deficits
Any sensory deficit can significantly shape an appropriate care plan. For example, impaired vision, paralysis of one or more extremities, loss of a limb, or loss of sensation in an extremity can impair the patient's ability to administer a subcutaneous injection, break a scored tablet, or open a medication container. Color blindness may cause difficulty in distinguishing between two medications. Hearing impairment can prevent effective patient instruction. Any sensory deficit requires careful consideration in any plan of prescribed drug therapy.

Clinical status
Two other factors can profoundly influence drug therapy: the patient's cognitive status and systemic effects of the prescribed drugs. A patient's intact cognitive abilities ensure that he can understand and implement the actions necessary for compliance. During the interview, note if the patient is alert and oriented, if he is able to interact appropriately with people, and if his conversation is appropriate. Consider whether the patient can think clearly and express his thoughts coherently. Finally, check both short-term and long-term memory because the patient needs both to follow a specified drug regimen. If such evaluation identifies a cognitive deficit, determine the probable cause, which can range from a transient drug-related effect to permanent neurologic impairment, and then determine whether or not the patient can carry out the prescribed drug regimen. If not, the nurse must find another way to ensure that the patient receives the prescribed therapy.

After completing the drug history, perform a physical examination to assess those body systems that may be affected by a particular drug the patient is taking or that may be prescribed. Every drug has a desired effect on a body system, but it may have an undesired effect on another. For example, chemotherapeutic agents destroy cancerous cells, but they also affect normal cells and often cause the patient to experience hair loss, diarrhea, or nausea. Therefore, examine the patient for expected drug effects; also closely monitor the patient for potentially harmful adverse effects.

Second step: Formulating a nursing diagnosis
Using information gathered during assessment, define any potential or actual drug-related problems by formulating each in a relevant nursing diagnosis. The most common problem statements related to drug therapy are "Knowledge deficit," "Noncompliance," and "Altered Health Maintenance."

Third step: Planning
Nursing diagnoses provide the framework for planning interventions and outcome criteria (patient goals).

Outcome criteria
Outcome criteria state the desired patient behaviors or responses that should result from nursing care. Outcome criteria should be measurable and objective, concise, realistic for the patient, and attainable by nursing management; they should express patient behavior in terms of expectations and specify a time frame. A typical outcome statement is "The patient verbalizes major adverse effects related to his chemotherapy drugs prior to discharge."

Fourth step: Intervention
After developing the outcome criteria, the nurse determines the interventions needed to help the patient reach the desired behavior or goals. Drug-related interventions may focus on patient teaching for a drug's action, adverse effects, scheduling, steps to avoid or treat a drug reaction, or drug administration techniques.

Appropriate interventions related to drug therapy will also include administration procedures and techniques, legal and ethical concerns, patient teaching, and any concerns related to special groups of patients (geriatric, pediatric, and pregnant or breast-feeding patients). Such interventions may be independent nursing actions, such as turning a bedridden patient every 2 hours, or may be nursing actions that require a doctor's order.

Fifth step: Evaluation
The final component of the nursing process, evaluation, is a formal and systematic process for determining the effectiveness of nursing care. This process enables the nurse to determine whether outcome criteria were met, and thereby make informed decisions about subsequent interventions. For example, if the patient experienced relief of headache within 1 hour after the nurse administered a p.r.n. analgesic, the outcome criterion was met. If the headache was the same or worse, the outcome criterion was not met and requires a new assessment, which may result in a new plan of care or may yield new data that invalidate the nursing diagnosis or suggest new nursing interventions that are more specific or more acceptable to the patient. This assessment could lead to a higher dosage, a different analgesic, or a reevaluation of the cause.

Evaluation enables the nurse to design and implement a revised plan of care, to continuously reevaluate outcome criteria, and to plan again until each nursing diagnosis is resolved.

6

Amebicides and antiprotozoals

chloroquine hydrochloride
(See Chapter 9, ANTIMALARIALS.)
chloroquine phosphate
(See Chapter 9, ANTIMALARIALS.)
eflornithine hydrochloride
emetine hydrochloride
iodoquinol
metronidazole
metronidazole hydrochloride
paromomycin sulfate
pentamidine isethionate

COMBINATION PRODUCTS
None.

eflornithine hydrochloride (DFMO)
Ornidyl
Pregnancy Risk Category: C

HOW SUPPLIED
Injection (concentrate): 200 mg/ml

MECHANISM OF ACTION
Specifically and irreversibly inhibits the enzyme ornithine decarboxylase and limits the availability of substrate for certain amines necessary for cell differentiation and division.

INDICATIONS & DOSAGE
Treatment of the meningoencephalitic stage of Trypanosoma brucei gambiense *(sleeping sickness)* –
Adults: 100 mg/kg by I.V. infusion q 6 hours for 14 days.

ADVERSE REACTIONS
Common reactions are in italics; life-threatening reactions are in bold italics.
Blood: ***anemia, leukopenia, thrombocytopenia, myelosuppression,*** eosinophilia.
CNS: ***seizures,*** *hearing impairment, dizziness, headache, asthenia.*
GI: diarrhea, vomiting, abdominal pain, anorexia.
Other: facial edema, alopecia.

INTERACTIONS
None reported.

NURSING CONSIDERATIONS
- *Use cautiously* in patients with impaired renal function because most (about 80%) of the drug is excreted unchanged in the urine.
- Impose antiseizure precautions because seizures occurred in about 8% of patients receiving the drug during clinical trials.
- Myelosuppression is a common and serious adverse reaction that is reversible when therapy is discontinued. Close patient monitoring is essential. Perform CBC and platelet counts before initiation of therapy, twice weekly during therapy, and weekly after the drug is discontinued until hematologic parameters return to pretreatment levels.
- **I.V. use:** The infusion concentrate is hypertonic and must be diluted before administration. Dilute with sterile water for injection and follow strict aseptic technique. To prepare infusion, dilute one part drug to four parts sterile water for injection by adding 25 ml (5,000 mg or 5 g) of the concentrate to each of four bags containing 100 ml of sterile water. After dilution, the final concentration of each bag will be 5,000 mg/125 ml or 40 mg/ml. Use within 24 hours.
- Administer infusion over 45 minutes. Do not administer other drugs with the infusion.
- To minimize the risk of microbial growth, store diluted drug in refrigerator (39° F [4° C]).
- The undiluted concentrate may be

*Liquid form contains alcohol. **May contain tartrazine.

stored at room temperature (below 86° F [30° C]), but protect from light and freezing.
• Some patients have experienced hearing impairment. Obtain serial audiograms when feasible.
• Patient should be monitored for at least 24 months after treatment.

emetine hydrochloride

Pregnancy Risk Category: X

HOW SUPPLIED
Injection: 65 mg/ml

MECHANISM OF ACTION
Kills *Entamoeba histolytica* by a mechanism related to the inhibition of protein synthesis.

INDICATIONS & DOSAGE
Acute fulminating amebic dysentery –
Adults: 1 mg/kg daily up to 60 mg daily (one or two doses) deep S.C. or I.M. 3 to 5 days (only until symptoms are under control). Give another antiamebic drug simultaneously.
Children: 1 mg/kg daily in two doses I.M. for up to 5 days. Do not exceed 20 mg daily in children over 8 years; do not exceed 10 mg daily in children 8 years and under.
Amebic hepatitis and abscess –
Adults: 60 mg daily (one or two doses) deep S.C. or I.M. for 10 days.

ADVERSE REACTIONS
Common reactions are in italics; life-threatening reactions are in bold italics.
CNS: dizziness, headache, mild sensory disturbances, central or peripheral nerve function changes, neuromuscular symptoms (weakness, aching, stiffness, tenderness, pain, tremors).
CV: ***acute toxicity*** – can occur at any dose (hypotension, tachycardia, precordial pain, dyspnea, *ECG abnormalities,* gallop rhythm, cardiac dilatation, severe acute degenerative myocarditis, pericarditis, congestive failure).
GI: *nausea, vomiting, diarrhea,* abdominal cramps, loss of sense of taste.
Metabolic: decreased serum potassium levels.
Skin: eczematous, urticarial purpuric lesions.
Local: skeletal muscle stiffness, aching, tenderness, *muscle weakness at injection site, cellulitis.*
Other: edema.

INTERACTIONS
None significant.

NURSING CONSIDERATIONS
• *Contraindicated* in cardiac or renal disease, except with amebic abscess or hepatitis not controlled by chloroquine or metronidazole; in patients who have received a course of emetine less than 6 to 8 weeks previously; in children, except for those with severe dysentery unresponsive to other amebicides; and in patients with polyneuropathy or muscle disease.
• *Use cautiously* and in reduced dosage in elderly or debilitated patients, patients with hypotension, or those about to undergo surgery.
• Deep S.C. administration is preferred; I.M. is acceptable, but I.V. route can be cardiotoxic and is contraindicated. Rotate sites and apply warm soaks.
• Record pulse rate and blood pressure 2 to 3 times daily. Discontinue use if drug produces tachycardia, precipitous fall in blood pressure, neuromuscular symptoms, marked GI effects, or considerable weakness. Weakness and muscle symptoms usually precede more serious symptoms and serve as a guide for avoiding toxicity.
• Because of potential for cardiovascular toxicity, don't exceed recommended dose or extend therapy beyond 10 days. Impose bed rest during

treatment and for several days thereafter.

• Drug may alter ECG tracings for 6 weeks. ECG should be taken before therapy, after fifth dose, upon completion, and 1 week after therapy. Patterns can resemble those of myocardial infarction. First and most consistent change is T wave inversion.

• Record intake and output; odor and consistency of stools; and presence of mucus, blood, or other foreign matter. Send warm specimens to lab for analysis. Repeat fecal examinations at 3-month intervals to assure elimination of amebae. Patients with acute amebic dysentery often become asymptomatic carriers. Check family members and suspected contacts.

• Suspect emetine-induced reaction if stools increase in number following initial relief of diarrhea.

• To help prevent reinfestation, teach patient about the need for good personal hygiene, especially handwashing technique. Patient should refrain from preparing food until stools are negative.

• Drug is very irritating. Avoid contact with eyes and mucous membranes. Wear gloves and goggles when preparing injection.

iodoquinol (diiodohydroxyquin)

Diodoquin†, Moebiquin, Yodoxin

Pregnancy Risk Category: C

HOW SUPPLIED

Tablets: 210 mg, 650 mg

MECHANISM OF ACTION

An iodine derivative with amebicidal activity in the intestinal lumen. Its precise mechanism of action is unknown.

INDICATIONS & DOSAGE

Intestinal amebiasis –

Adults: 630 to 650 mg P.O. t.i.d. after meals for 20 days. Total daily dosage should not exceed 2 g.

Children: usual dosage 30 to 40 mg/kg of body weight daily in two to three divided doses for 20 days.

Additional courses of iodoquinol therapy should not be repeated before a resting interval of 2 to 3 weeks.

ADVERSE REACTIONS

Common reactions are in italics; life-threatening reactions are in bold italics.

Blood: ***agranulocytosis.***

CNS: neurotoxicity (dose-related), dysesthesia, weakness, vertigo, malaise, headache, agitation, retrograde amnesia, ataxia, *peripheral neuropathy.*

EENT: *optic neuritis,* optic atrophy, loss of vision.

GI: anorexia, nausea, vomiting, abdominal cramps, diarrhea, increased motility, constipation, epigastric burning and pain, gastritis, anal irritation and itching.

Skin: pruritus, hives, papular and pustular eruptions, urticaria, discoloration of hair and nails.

Other: thyroid enlargement, fever, chills, generalized furunculosis, hair loss.

INTERACTIONS

None significant.

NURSING CONSIDERATIONS

• *Contraindicated* in patients with hypersensitivity to 8-hydroxyquinoline derivatives or iodine-containing preparations. Iodoquinol causes hepatic damage in such patients. Also contraindicated in hepatic or renal disease or preexisting optic neuropathy.

• Patient should have periodic ophthalmologic examinations during treatment.

• Give after meals. Crush tablets and mix with applesauce or chocolate syrup.

• Record intake and output and color

and amount of stool. Send warm specimens to lab for analysis.
- Watch for diarrhea during the first 2 or 3 days of treatment. Notify doctor if it continues past 3 days.
- Advise patient not to discontinue the medication prematurely. Tell him to notify doctor if skin rash occurs.
- May interfere with thyroid function tests for up to 6 months after discontinuation of drug.
- To help prevent reinfestation, teach patient about the need for good personal hygiene, especially handwashing technique. Patient should refrain from preparing food until stools are negative.

metronidazole

Apo-Metronidazole†, Flagyl, Metizol, Metrogyl‡, Metrozine‡, Metryl, Neo-Metric†, Novonidazol†, PMS Metronidazole†, Protostat

metronidazole hydrochloride

Flagyl I.V., Flagyl I.V. RTU, Metro I.V., Novonidazol†

Pregnancy Risk Category: B

HOW SUPPLIED

Tablets: 200 mg‡, 250 mg, 400 mg‡, 500 mg
Oral suspension (benzoyl metronidazole): 200 mg/5 ml‡
Injection: 500 mg/100 ml ready to use
Powder for injection: 500-mg single-dose vials

MECHANISM OF ACTION

A direct-acting trichomonacide and amebicide that works at both intestinal and extraintestinal sites.

INDICATIONS & DOSAGE

Amebic hepatic abscess –
Adults: 500 to 750 mg P.O. t.i.d. for 5 to 10 days.
Children: 35 to 50 mg/kg daily (in three doses) for 10 days.
Intestinal amebiasis –
Adults: 750 mg P.O. t.i.d. for 5 to 10 days.
Children: 35 to 50 mg/kg daily (in three doses) for 10 days. Follow this therapy with oral iodoquinol.
Trichomoniasis –
Adults (both male and female): 250 mg P.O. t.i.d. for 7 days or 2 g P.O. in single dose; 4 to 6 weeks should elapse between courses of therapy.
Refractory trichomoniasis –
Women: 250 mg P.O. b.i.d. for 10 days.
Treatment of bacterial infections caused by anaerobic microorganisms –
Adults: Loading dose is 15 mg/kg I.V. infused over 1 hour (approximately 1 g for a 70-kg adult). Maintenance dose is 7.5 mg/kg I.V. or P.O. q 6 hours (approximately 500 mg for a 70-kg adult). The first maintenance dose should be administered 6 hours following the loading dose. Maximum dosage not to exceed 4 g daily.
Giardiasis –
Adults: 250 mg P.O. t.i.d. for 5 days.
Children: 5 mg/kg P.O. t.i.d. for 5 days.
Prevention of postoperative infection in contaminated or potentially contaminated colorectal surgery –
Adults: 15 mg/kg infused over 30 to 60 minutes and completed approximately 1 hour before surgery. Then, 7.5 mg/kg infused over 30 to 60 minutes at 6 and 12 hours after the initial dose.

ADVERSE REACTIONS

Common reactions are in italics; life-threatening reactions are in bold italics.
Blood: transient leukopenia, neutropenia.
CNS: vertigo, headache, ataxia, incoordination, confusion, irritability, depression, restlessness, weakness, fatigue, drowsiness, insomnia, sen-

sory neuropathy, paresthesia of extremities, psychic stimulation, seizures, neuromyopathy.
CV: ECG change (flattened T wave), edema (with I.V. RTU preparation).
GI: abdominal cramping, stomatitis, *nausea, vomiting, anorexia,* diarrhea, constipation, proctitis, dry mouth.
GU: darkened urine, polyuria, dysuria, pyuria, incontinence, cystitis, decreased libido, dyspareunia, dryness of vagina and vulva, sense of pelvic pressure.
Skin: pruritus, flushing, rash.
Local: *thrombophlebitis after I.V. infusion.*
Other: overgrowth of nonsusceptible organisms, especially *Candida* (glossitis, furry tongue), metallic taste, fever, gynecomastia.

INTERACTIONS
Alcohol: disulfiram-like reaction (nausea, vomiting, headache, cramps, flushing). Don't use together.
Cimetidine: increased risk of metronidazole toxicity by inhibiting hepatic metabolism. Monitor closely.
Disulfiram: acute psychoses and confusional states. Don't use together.
Oral anticoagulants: increased anticoagulant effects. Monitor closely.
Phenytoin, phenobarbital: decreased metronidazole effectiveness because of increased hepatic clearance. Monitor closely.

NURSING CONSIDERATIONS
- *Warning:* This drug has been shown to be carcinogenic in mice and possibly rats. Unnecessary use should be avoided.
- *Use cautiously* in patients with a history of blood dyscrasia or CNS disorder and in patients with retinal or visual field changes. Also use cautiously in hepatic disease or alcoholism and in conjunction with known hepatotoxic drugs.
- If indicated during pregnancy for trichomoniasis, the 7-day regimen is preferred over the 2-g single-dose regimen.
- Tell patient to avoid alcohol or alcohol-containing medications during therapy and for at least 48 hours after therapy is completed.
- Give oral form with meals to minimize GI distress.
- Tell patient metallic taste and dark or red-brown urine may occur.
- Record number and character of stools when used in the treatment of amebiasis. Metronidazole should be used only after *Trichomonas vaginalis* has been confirmed by wet smear or culture or *Entamoeba histolytica* has been identified. Asymptomatic sexual partners of patients being treated for *T. vaginalis* infection should be treated simultaneously to avoid reinfection. Instruct patient in proper hygiene.
- **I.V. use:** The I.V. form should be administered by slow infusion only. Don't give I.V. push.
- Follow package instructions carefully when mixing the I.V. solution.
- Don't refrigerate Flagyl I.V. RTU
- Flagyl I.V. RTU may cause sodium retention. Observe carefully for edema, especially in patients also receiving corticosteroids.

paromomycin sulfate
Humatin

Pregnancy Risk Category: C

HOW SUPPLIED
Capsules: 250 mg

MECHANISM OF ACTION
Acts as an intestinal amebicide. Its specific mechanism of action is unknown.

INDICATIONS & DOSAGE
Intestinal amebiasis, acute and chronic –
Adults and children: 25 to 35 mg/kg

daily P.O. in three doses for 5 to 10 days after meals.
Tapeworms (fish, beef, pork, dog) –
Adults: 1 g P.O. q 15 minutes for four doses.
Children: 11 mg/kg P.O. q 15 minutes for four doses.

ADVERSE REACTIONS
Common reactions are in italics; life-threatening reactions are in bold italics.
Blood: eosinophilia.
CNS: headache, vertigo.
EENT: ototoxicity.
GI: anorexia, *nausea, vomiting, epigastric pain and burning, abdominal cramps,* diarrhea, constipation, increased motility, steatorrhea, pruritus ani, malabsorption syndrome.
GU: hematuria, nephrotoxicity.
Skin: rash, exanthema, pruritus.
Other: overgrowth of nonsusceptible organisms.

INTERACTIONS
None significant.

NURSING CONSIDERATIONS
- *Contraindicated* in patients with impaired renal function or intestinal obstruction.
- *Use cautiously* in patients with ulcerative lesions of the bowel to avoid inadvertent absorption and resulting renal toxicity. Poorly absorbed orally, but will accumulate with renal impairment or ulcerative lesions.
- Ask about history of sensitivity to drug before giving first dose.
- Administer with or after meals.
- To help prevent reinfestation, teach patient about the need for good personal hygiene, especially handwashing technique. Patient should refrain from preparing food until stools are negative.
- Criterion of cure is absence of amebae in stools examined weekly for 6 weeks after treatment and thereafter at monthly intervals for 2 years. Examine feces of family members or suspected contacts.
- Avoid high doses or prolonged therapy.
- Watch for signs of superinfection (continued fever and other signs of new infections, especially monilial infections).

pentamidine isethionate
NebuPent, Pentam 300
Pregnancy Risk Category: C

HOW SUPPLIED
Injection: 300 mg/vial
Aerosol: 300 mg/vial

MECHANISM OF ACTION
Interferes with biosynthesis of DNA, RNA, phospholipids, and proteins in susceptible organisms.

INDICATIONS & DOSAGE
Treatment of pneumonia due to Pneumocystis carinii –
Adults and children: 4 mg/kg I.V. or I.M. once a day for 14 days.
Prevention of Pneumocystis carinii *pneumonia in high-risk individuals* –
Adults: 300 mg by inhalation (using a Respirgard II nebulizer) once every 4 weeks.

ADVERSE REACTIONS
Common reactions are in italics; life-threatening reactions are in bold italics.
Blood: *leukopenia,* thrombocytopenia, anemia.
CNS: confusion, hallucinations.
CV: ***hypotension,*** tachycardia.
Endocrine: ***hypoglycemia,*** hyperglycemia, hypocalcemia.
GI: nausea, anorexia, metallic taste.
GU: *elevated serum creatinine,* renal toxicity.
Hepatic: elevated liver enzymes.
Local: *sterile abscess, pain or induration at injection site.*
Skin: rash, facial flushing, pruritus.
Other: fever.

INTERACTIONS
Aminoglycosides, amphotericin B, cisplatin, vancomycin, zidovudine: increased risk of nephrotoxicity.

NURSING CONSIDERATIONS
- Once the diagnosis of *Pneumocystis carinii* pneumonia has been firmly established, there are no absolute contraindications to pentamidine therapy.
- *Use cautiously* in hypertension, hypotension, hypoglycemia, hypocalcemia, leukopenia, thrombocytopenia, anemia, and hepatic or renal dysfunction.
- Patient should be lying down when receiving the drug because sudden, severe hypotension may develop. Monitor blood pressure during administration and several times thereafter until blood pressure is stable.
- **I.V. use:** When administering I.V., infuse slowly over 60 minutes to minimize risk of hypotension.
- Monitor blood glucose, serum calcium, serum creatinine, and BUN levels daily. After parenteral administration, blood glucose level may decrease initially; hypoglycemia may be severe in 5% to 10% of patients. This may be followed by hyperglycemia and insulin-dependent diabetes mellitus (which may be permanent).
- Pain and induration occur universally with I.M. injection. Administer by deep I.M. injection.
- In patients with AIDS, pentamidine may produce less severe adverse reactions than the alternative treatment co-trimoxazole. Therefore, in some AIDS patients, pentamidine is considered the treatment of choice.
- The aerosol form should be administered only by the Respirgard II nebulizer manufactured by Marquest. Dosage recommendations are based on the particle size and delivery rate of this device. To administer aerosol form, mix the contents of one vial in 6 ml of sterile water for injection. *Do not* use saline because this will cause the drug to precipitate. Do not mix with other drugs.
- Do not use low pressure (< 20 psi) compressors. The flow rate should be 5 to 7 liters/minute from a 40 to 50 psi air or oxygen source.
- Instruct the patient to use the aerosol device until the chamber is empty. (This may take up to 45 minutes).

*Liquid form contains alcohol. **May contain tartrazine.

7

Anthelmintics

mebendazole
niclosamide
oxamniquine
piperazine adipate
piperazine citrate
praziquantel
pyrantel embonate
pyrantel pamoate
quinacrine hydrochloride
thiabendazole

COMBINATION PRODUCTS
None.

mebendazole

Vermox

Pregnancy Risk Category: C

HOW SUPPLIED
Tablets (chewable): 100 mg
Oral suspension: 100 mg/5 ml‡

MECHANISM OF ACTION
Selectively and irreversibly inhibits uptake of glucose and other nutrients in susceptible helminths.

INDICATIONS & DOSAGE
Pinworm –
Adults and children over 2 years: 100 mg P.O. as a single dose. If infection persists 3 weeks later, repeat treatment.
Roundworm, whipworm, hookworm –
Adults and children over 2 years: 100 mg P.O. b.i.d. for 3 days. If infection persists 3 weeks later, repeat treatment.

ADVERSE REACTIONS
Common reactions are in italics; life-threatening reactions are in bold italics.
GI: occasional, transient abdominal pain and diarrhea in massive infection and expulsion of worms.

INTERACTIONS
None significant.

NURSING CONSIDERATIONS
- *Contraindicated* in patients with hypersensitivity to the drug.
- Tablets may be chewed, swallowed whole, or crushed and mixed with food.
- No dietary restrictions, laxatives, or enemas are necessary.
- Treat all family members.
- Teach patient about the need for good personal hygiene, especially good handwashing technique. To avoid reinfection, teach him to wash perianal area daily. Change undergarments and bedclothes daily. Wash hands and clean fingernails before meals and after bowel movements. Advise patient to refrain from preparing food during infestation.

niclosamide

Niclocide, Yomesan‡

Pregnancy Risk Category: B

HOW SUPPLIED
Tablets (chewable): 500 mg

MECHANISM OF ACTION
Inhibits the metabolic process of oxidative phosphorylation in tapeworms.

INDICATIONS & DOSAGE
Tapeworms (fish, beef, and pork) –
Adults: 4 tablets (2 g) chewed thoroughly as a single dose.
Children (more than 34 kg): 3 tablets (1.5 g) chewed thoroughly as a single dose.
Children (11 to 34 kg): 2 tablets (1 g) chewed thoroughly as a single dose.

Dwarf tapeworm –
Adults: 4 tablets chewed thoroughly as a single dose for 7 days.
Children over 2 years (more than 34 kg): 3 tablets chewed thoroughly on the first day, then 2 tablets for the next 6 days.
Children over 2 years (11 to 34 kg): 2 tablets chewed thoroughly on the first day, then 1 tablet daily for the next 6 days.

ADVERSE REACTIONS
Common reactions are in italics; life-threatening reactions are in bold italics.
CNS: drowsiness, dizziness, headache.
EENT: oral irritation, bad taste in mouth.
GI: *nausea, vomiting, anorexia,* diarrhea.
Skin: rash, pruritus ani.

INTERACTIONS
None reported.

NURSING CONSIDERATIONS
- Instruct patient to chew tablets thoroughly and wash down with water; for children, the tablets can be crushed and mixed with water or applesauce.
- Tablets should be taken as a single dose after breakfast.
- A mild laxative should be administered to cleanse the bowel prior to initiation of niclosamide therapy in patients who are constipated.
- When treating dwarf tapeworms, urge patient to drink fruit juices. This helps to eliminate the accumulated intestinal mucus under which they lodge.
- Teach patient about the need for good personal hygiene, especially good handwashing technique. Advise patient to refrain from preparing food during infestation.
- Patient is not considered cured until the stool has been negative for tapeworms for at least 3 months.

oxamniquine
Vansil
Pregnancy Risk Category: C

HOW SUPPLIED
Capsules: 250 mg

MECHANISM OF ACTION
Reduces the egg load of *Schistosoma mansoni,* but its exact mechanism of action is unknown.

INDICATIONS & DOSAGE
Treatment of schistosomiasis caused by Schistosoma mansoni, Western Hemisphere strains –
Adults and children (over 30 kg): 12 to 15 mg/kg given as a single oral dose.
Children (under 30 kg): 10 mg/kg P.O., followed by 10 mg/kg P.O. 2 to 8 hours later.

ADVERSE REACTIONS
Common reactions are in italics; life-threatening reactions are in bold italics.
CNS: seizures, *dizziness, drowsiness, headache.*
GI: nausea, vomiting, abdominal pain, anorexia.
Skin: urticaria.

INTERACTIONS
None significant.

NURSING CONSIDERATIONS
- *Use cautiously* in patients with a history of seizure disorders. Epileptiform seizures have rarely been observed within the first few hours after ingestion.
- Instruct patient to avoid driving and other hazardous activities if he's dizzy or drowsy.
- GI tolerance is improved if the drug is given after meals.
- Although *S. mansoni* infection is rare in the United States and Canada, travelers or immigrants from such areas as Puerto Rico, Latin America,

*Liquid form contains alcohol. **May contain tartrazine.

and Africa may have contracted the infection from contaminated water.

piperazine adipate
Entacyl†

piperazine citrate
Antepar, Bryrel, Pin-Tega Tabs, Pipril, Ta-Verm, Veriga†, Vermirex†, Vermizine

Pregnancy Risk Category: B

HOW SUPPLIED

adipate
Oral suspension: 600 mg/5 ml
Granules: 2 g/packet

citrate
Tablets: 250 mg
Syrup: 500 mg/5 ml

MECHANISM OF ACTION

Blocks neuromuscular action, paralyzing the worm and causing its expulsion by normal peristalsis.

INDICATIONS & DOSAGE

Enterobiasis (pinworm) –
Adults and children: 65 mg/kg P.O. daily 7 to 8 days. Maximum daily dosage is 2.5 g. Alternatively, give adults 2 g P.O. daily for 7 days, and give children 1 g/m² P.O. daily for 7 days. Some clinicians order according to body weight:
Children under 7 kg: 250 mg P.O. daily for 7 days.
Children 7 to 14 kg: 500 mg P.O. daily for 7 days.
Children 14 to 27 kg: 1 g P.O. daily for 7 days.
Children over 27 kg and adults: 2 g P.O. daily for 7 days.
Ascariasis (roundworm) –
Adults: 3.5 g P.O. in single doses for 2 consecutive days.
Children: 75 mg/kg or 2 g/m² P.O. daily in single doses for 2 consecutive days. Maximum daily dosage is 3.5 g. Alternatively, give according to body weight:
Children under 14 kg: 1 g P.O. daily for 2 days.
Children 14 to 23 kg: 2 g P.O. daily for 2 days.
Children 23 to 45 kg: 3 g P.O. daily or 2 days.
Children over 45 kg and adults: 3.5 g P.O. daily or 2 days.
Some clinicians continue treatment for 4 days in patients with massive infestation. May repeat in 1 week if necessary.

ADVERSE REACTIONS

Common reactions are in italics; life-threatening reactions are in bold italics.
CNS: ataxia, tremors, choreiform movements, muscular weakness, myoclonus, hyporeflexia, paresthesias, seizures, sense of detachment, EEG abnormalities, memory defect, *headache, vertigo.*
EENT: nystagmus, blurred vision, paralytic strabismus, cataracts with visual impairment, lacrimation, difficulty in focusing, rhinorrhea.
GI: *nausea, vomiting,* diarrhea, abdominal cramps.
Skin: urticaria, photodermatitis, ***erythema multiforme,*** purpura, eczematous skin reactions.
Other: arthralgia, fever, bronchospasm, ***hemolytic anemia.***

INTERACTIONS

Pyrantel pamoate: possible antagonism. Don't administer together.

NURSING CONSIDERATIONS

- *Contraindicated* in hepatic and/or renal impairment or seizure disorders.
- *Use cautiously* in severe malnutrition or anemia.
- Discontinue if CNS or significant GI reactions occur.
- Because of potential neurotoxicity, avoid prolonged or repeated treatment, especially in children.
- No dietary restrictions, laxatives, or enemas are necessary.
- May be taken with food; but, for

best absorption, tell patient to take on empty stomach.
- Mix powder for oral suspension in 57 ml water, milk, or fruit juice.
- Treat all family members.
- Teach patient about the need for good personal hygiene, especially good handwashing technique. To avoid reinfection, teach him to wash perianal area, to change undergarments and bedclothes daily, and to wash hands and clean fingernails before meals and after bowel movements. Advise patient to refrain from preparing food during infestation.

praziquantel

Biltricide

Pregnancy Risk Category: B

HOW SUPPLIED

Tablets: 600 mg

MECHANISM OF ACTION

Causes a contraction of schistosomes by a specific effect on the permeability of the cell membrane.

INDICATIONS & DOSAGE

Treatment of schistosomiasis caused by Schistosoma mekongi, S. japonicum, S. mansoni, *and* S. haematobium –

Adults and children 4 years and older: 20 mg/kg P.O. t.i.d. as a 1-day treatment. The interval between doses should be between 4 and 6 hours.

ADVERSE REACTIONS

Common reactions are in italics; life-threatening reactions are in bold italics.

CNS: *drowsiness, malaise,* headache, dizziness.

GI: abdominal discomfort, nausea.

Hepatic: minimal increase in liver enzymes.

Skin: urticaria.

Other: fever.

INTERACTIONS

None significant.

NURSING CONSIDERATIONS

- *Contraindicated* with ocular cysticercosis because destruction of the parasite in the eye may cause permanent eye damage.
- May produce drowsiness. Tell patient to avoid hazardous activities that require alertness on the day of treatment and the day after treatment.
- Adverse effects may be more frequent or serious in patients with a heavy worm burden.
- In the event of overdose, give a fast-acting laxative.
- Advise patient to take the tablet during meals and to wash down the unchewed tablet with a liquid.
- Tablets taste very bitter. Keeping them in the mouth may cause gagging or vomiting.
- Praziquantel is effective for several different species of *Schistosoma.*
- May also be effective against liver flukes.

pyrantel embonate

Anthel‡, Combantrin‡, Early Bird‡

pyrantel pamoate

Antiminth, Combantrin†

Pregnancy Risk Category: C

HOW SUPPLIED

embonate

Tablets: 125 mg‡, 250 mg‡

Oral suspension: 50 mg/ml‡

Granules: 100 mg/g‡

Squares (chocolate-flavored): 100 mg‡

pamoate

Tablets: 125 mg†

Oral suspension: 50 mg/ml

MECHANISM OF ACTION

Blocks neuromuscular action, paralyzing the worm and causing its expulsion by normal peristalsis.

*Liquid form contains alcohol. **May contain tartrazine.

INDICATIONS & DOSAGE
Roundworm and pinworm –
Adults and children over 2 years: single dosage of 11 mg/kg P.O. Maximum dosage 1 g. For pinworm, dosage should be repeated in 2 weeks.

ADVERSE REACTIONS
Common reactions are in italics; life-threatening reactions are in bold italics.
CNS: headache, dizziness, drowsiness, insomnia.
GI: anorexia, nausea, vomiting, gastralgia, cramps, diarrhea, tenesmus.
Hepatic: transient elevation of AST (SGOT).
Skin: rashes.
Other: fever, weakness.

INTERACTIONS
Piperazine salts: Possible antagonism; don't give together.

NURSING CONSIDERATIONS
- *Use cautiously* in severe malnutrition or anemia, or in hepatic dysfunction. Treat for anemia, dehydration, or malnutrition before giving drug.
- No dietary restrictions, laxatives, or enemas are necessary.
- May be taken with food, milk, or fruit juices. Shake suspension well.
- Treat all family members.
- Teach patient about the need for good personal hygiene, especially good handwashing technique. To avoid reinfection, teach him to wash perianal area daily, to change undergarments and bedclothes daily, and to wash hands and clean fingernails before meals and after bowel movements. Advise patient to refrain from preparing food during infestation.
- Protect drug from light. Store below 30° C (86° F).

quinacrine hydrochloride (mepacrine hydrochloride)
Atabrine

Pregnancy Risk Category: C

HOW SUPPLIED
Tablets: 100 mg

MECHANISM OF ACTION
Inhibits DNA metabolism in susceptible parasites.

INDICATIONS & DOSAGE
Treatment of giardiasis –
Adults: 300 mg P.O. in 3 divided doses for 5 to 7 days.
Children: 7 mg/kg/day P.O. given in 3 divided doses after meals for 5 days. Maximum 300 mg/day. Dosage may be repeated in 2 weeks.
Tapeworms (beef, pork, and fish) –
Adults and children over 14 years: 4 doses of 200 mg P.O. given 10 minutes apart (800 mg total).
Children 11 to 14 years: 600 mg P.O. total dosage, administered in 3 or 4 divided doses, 10 minutes apart.
Children 5 to 10 years: 400 mg P.O. total dosage, administered in 3 or 4 divided doses, 10 minutes apart.

ADVERSE REACTIONS
Common reactions are in italics; life-threatening reactions are in bold italics.
CNS: *headache, dizziness, nervousness, vertigo, mood shifts, nightmares,* ***seizures.***
GI: *diarrhea, anorexia, nausea, abdominal cramps,* vomiting.
GU: yellow urine.
Skin: pleomorphic skin eruptions, yellow discoloration.

INTERACTIONS
Primaquine: enhanced toxicity of primaquine. Don't use together.

NURSING CONSIDERATIONS
• *Contraindicated* if patient is taking primaquine since primaquine toxicity could be increased.
• *Use with extreme caution* in porphyria or psoriasis; may exacerbate these conditions.
• *Use cautiously* in hepatic, renal, or cardiac disease; alcoholism; psychosis; and G6PD deficiency and in those over 60 years or under 1 year.
• Give after meals with large glass of water, tea, or fruit juice to reduce GI irritation. Bitter taste may be disguised by jam or honey.
• Give a saline cathartic 1 to 2 hours after drug is given, to expel the worm.
• Collect all of stool after treatment. Look for the scolex (attachment organ), which will be stained yellow.
• Warn patient about temporary yellow color of skin and urine.
• Patient should be on a bland, nonfat, semisolid diet for 24 hours, and should fast after the evening meal before treatment.

thiabendazole
Mintezol
Pregnancy Risk Category: C

HOW SUPPLIED
Tablets (chewable): 500 mg
Oral suspension: 500 mg/5 ml

MECHANISM OF ACTION
Unknown.

INDICATIONS & DOSAGE
Systemic infection with pinworm, roundworm, threadworm, whipworm, cutaneous larva migrans, and trichinosis –
Adults or children: 25 mg/kg P.O. in two doses daily for 2 successive days. Maximum dosage is 3 g daily.
Cutaneous infestations with larva migrans (creeping eruption) –
Adults and children: 25 mg/kg P.O. b.i.d. for 2 to 5 days. Maximum 3 g daily. If lesions persist after 2 days, repeat course.
Pinworm – two doses daily for 1 day; repeat in 7 days.
Roundworm, threadworm, whipworm – two doses daily for 2 successive days.
Trichinosis – two doses daily for 2 to 4 successive days.

ADVERSE REACTIONS
Common reactions are in italics; life-threatening reactions are in bold italics.
CNS: impaired mental alertness, impaired physical coordination, *drowsiness, fatigue,* giddiness, *headache,* dizziness.
CV: *hypotension.*
GI: *anorexia, nausea, vomiting,* diarrhea, epigastric distress.
Skin: *rash, pruritus,* ***erythema multiforme.***
Other: lymphadenopathy, fever, flushing, chills.

INTERACTIONS
None significant.

NURSING CONSIDERATIONS
• *Use cautiously* in hepatic or renal dysfunction, severe malnutrition, and anemia and in patients who are vomiting. Supportive therapy indicated for anemic, dehydrated, or malnourished patients. In children under 15 kg, weigh benefits against risks.
• Administer after meals. For oral suspension, shake before measuring dosage. For tablets, advise patient to chew before swallowing.
• No dietary restrictions, laxatives, or enemas are necessary.
• Treat all family members.
• Emphasize the need for good personal hygiene. To avoid reinfection, patient should wash perianal area daily, change undergarments and bedclothes daily, and wash hands and clean fingernails before meals and after bowel movements.

8

Antifungals

amphotericin B
fluconazole
flucytosine
griseofulvin microsize
griseofulvin ultramicrosize
itraconazole
ketoconazole
miconazole
nystatin

COMBINATION PRODUCTS
None.

amphotericin B

Fungilin Oral‡, Fungizone

Pregnancy Risk Category: B

HOW SUPPLIED
Tablets: 100 mg‡
Oral suspension: 100 mg/ml‡
Lozenges: 10 mg‡
Injection: 50-mg lyophilized cake

MECHANISM OF ACTION
Probably acts by binding to sterols in the fungal cell membrane, altering cell permeability and allowing leakage of intracellular components.

INDICATIONS & DOSAGE
Systemic fungal infections (histoplasmosis, coccidioidomycosis, blastomycosis, cryptococcosis, disseminated moniliasis, aspergillosis, phycomycosis), meningitis –
Adults: initially, 1 mg in 250 ml of dextrose 5% in water infused over 2 to 4 hours; or 0.25 mg/kg daily by slow infusion over 6 hours. Increase daily dosage gradually as patient tolerance develops to maximum 1 mg/kg daily. Therapy must not exceed 1.5 mg/kg. If drug is discontinued for 1 week or more, administration must resume with initial dose and again increase gradually.
Intrathecal: 25 mcg/0.1 ml diluted with 10 to 20 ml of cerebrospinal fluid and administered by barbotage 2 or 3 times weekly. Initial dose should not exceed 100 mcg.
Treatment of Candida albicans *infections involving the GI tract –*
Adults: 100 mg P.O. q.i.d. for 2 weeks.
Oral and perioral candidal infections –
Adults: 1 lozenge q.i.d. for 7 to 14 days. The lozenge should be sucked and allowed to dissolve slowly in the mouth.

ADVERSE REACTIONS
Common reactions are in italics; life-threatening reactions are in bold italics.
Blood: normochromic, normocytic anemia.
CNS: headache, peripheral neuropathy; with intrathecal administration – peripheral nerve pain, paresthesias.
CV: hypotension, ***cardiac arrhythmias, asystole.***
GI: *anorexia, weight loss, nausea,* vomiting, dyspepsia, diarrhea, epigastric cramps.
GU: abnormal renal function with hypokalemia, azotemia, hyposthenuria, hypomagnesemia, renal tubular acidosis, nephrocalcinosis; with large doses – permanent renal impairment, anuria, oliguria.
Local: burning, stinging, irritation, tissue damage with extravasation, *thrombophlebitis,* pain at site of injection.
Other: arthralgia, myalgia, muscle weakness secondary to hypokalemia, *fever, chills,* malaise, generalized pain.

INTERACTIONS

Other nephrotoxic antibiotics: may cause additive kidney toxicity. Administer very cautiously.

NURSING CONSIDERATIONS

• *Use cautiously* in patients with impaired renal function.
• Use parenterally only in hospitalized patients, under close supervision, when diagnosis of potentially fatal fungal infection has been confirmed.
• Oral form is not available in the United States.
• Monitor vital signs every 30 minutes; fever, shaking chills, and hypotension may appear 1 to 2 hours after start of I.V. infusion and should subside within 4 hours of discontinuation.
• Monitor intake and output; report change in urine appearance or volume. Monitor BUN and serum creatine (or creatinine clearance) at least weekly during therapy. Renal damage usually reversible if drug is stopped at first sign of dysfunction.
• Obtain liver and renal function studies weekly. If BUN exceeds 40 mg/100 ml, or if serum creatinine exceeds 3 mg/100 ml, doctor may reduce or stop drug until renal function improves. Monitor CBC weekly. Stop drug if alkaline phosphatase or bilirubin levels become elevated.
• Monitor potassium levels closely. Report any signs of hypokalemia. Check calcium and magnesium levels twice weekly. Perform liver and renal function studies and monitor CBCs weekly.
• In the dry state, store at 2° to 8° C (35.6° to 46.4° F). Protect from light. Reconstitute with 10 ml sterile water only. Mixing with solutions containing sodium chloride, other electrolytes, or bacteriostatic agents, such as benzyl alcohol, causes precipitation. Do not use if solution contains precipitate or foreign matter.
• Severity of some adverse reactions can be reduced by premedication with antipyretics, antihistamines, antiemetics, or small doses of corticosteroids; addition of phosphate buffer and heparin to the solution; and alternate-day dose schedule. For severe reactions, drug may have to be discontinued for varying intervals and the doctor notified.
• Appears to be compatible with limited amounts of heparin sodium, hydrocortisone sodium succinate, and methylprednisolone sodium succinate.
• Reconstituted solution is stable for 1 week under refrigeration or 24 hours at room temperature. It has 8-hour stability in room light.
• **I.V. use:** An initial test dose may be prescribed: 1 mg is added to 50 to 250 ml of dextrose 5% in water and infused over 20 to 30 minutes and the patient's pulse, respiratory rate, temperature, and blood pressure are monitored for at least 4 hours. Some clinicians give this test dose more slowly (over a 4-hour period).
• For I.V. infusion, use an infusion pump. An in-line filter with mean pore diameter larger than 1 micron can be used. Infuse very slowly (over 6 hours); rapid infusion may result in cardiovascular collapse. Warn patient of possible discomfort at infusion site and other potential adverse reactions. Advise patient that several months of therapy may be needed to assure adequate response.
• Administer in distal veins. If veins become thrombosed, doctor can change to every-other-day regimen.
• Antibiotics should be given separately; don't mix or piggyback with amphotericin B.

fluconazole

Diflucan

Pregnancy Risk Category: C

*Liquid form contains alcohol. **May contain tartrazine.

HOW SUPPLIED
Tablets: 50 mg, 100 mg, 200 mg
Injection: 200 mg/100 ml, 400 mg/200 ml

MECHANISM OF ACTION
Inhibits fungal cytochrome P-450, an enzyme responsible for fungal sterol synthesis. This results in weakening of fungal cell walls.

INDICATIONS & DOSAGE
Oropharyngeal candidiasis –
Adults: 200 mg P.O. or I.V. on the first day, followed by 100 mg once daily. Therapy should continue for 2 weeks.
Esophageal candidiasis –
Adults: 200 mg P.O. or I.V. on the first day, followed by 100 mg once daily. Higher doses (up to 400 mg daily) have been used, depending upon the patient's condition and tolerance of treatment. Patients should receive the drug for at least 3 weeks and for 2 weeks after symptoms resolve.
Systemic candidiasis –
Adults: 400 mg P.O. or I.V. on the first day, followed by 200 mg once daily. Treatment should continue for at least 4 weeks or for 2 weeks after symptoms resolve.
Cryptococcal meningitis –
Adults: 400 mg P.O. or I.V. on the first day, followed by 200 mg once daily. Higher doses (up to 400 mg daily) may be used. Treatment should continue for 10 to 12 weeks after cultures of the cerebrospinal fluid are negative.
Suppression of relapse of cryptococcal meningitis in patients with AIDS –
Adults: 200 mg P.O. or I.V. daily.

ADVERSE REACTIONS
Common reactions are in italics; life-threatening reactions are in bold italics.
CNS: headache, dizziness.
GI: *nausea,* vomiting, abdominal pain, diarrhea.
Skin: rash, ***Stevens-Johnson syndrome (rare).***
Other: hepatotoxicity (rare), elevated liver enzymes.

INTERACTIONS
Cyclosporine, phenytoin: may cause increased plasma concentrations of these drugs. Monitor serum cyclosporine or phenytoin levels.
Isoniazid, phenytoin, rifampin, valproic acid, oral sulfonylureas: increased incidence of abnormally elevated hepatic transaminases. Monitor closely.
Oral antidiabetic agents (tolbutamide, glyburide, glipizide): may cause increased plasma concentrations of these drugs. Monitor for enhanced hypoglycemic effect.
Rifampin: enhanced metabolism of fluconazole. Monitor for lack of response.
Warfarin: increased risk of bleeding. Monitor prothrombin time.

NURSING CONSIDERATIONS
- *Contraindicated* in patients with hypersensitivity to the drug.
- *Use cautiously* in patients with hypersensitivity to other antifungal azole compounds because there is no information regarding cross-sensitivity.
- The incidence of adverse reactions appears to be greater in human immunodeficiency virus- (HIV-) infected patients.
- Because the drug is excreted unchanged by the kidneys, dosage should be adjusted in patients with renal failure. If creatinine clearance is 21 to 50 ml/minute, dosage should be reduced 50%. If creatinine clearance is 11 to 20 ml/minute, reduce dosage by 75%. Patients receiving regular hemodialysis treatment should receive the usual dose after each dialysis session.
- Oral bioavailability of fluconazole is greater than 90% and is unaffected

by gastric pH. Dosage is the same for oral or I.V. use.

• **I.V. use:** May be administered by continuous infusion at a rate not to exceed 200 mg/hour. Use an infusion pump. Do not connect in series with other infusions to prevent air embolism. Do not add any other drugs to the solution.

• I.V. bags of fluconazole are shipped with a protective overwrap that should not be removed until just before use. This helps ensure product sterility. The plastic container may show some opacity from moisture absorbed during sterilization. This is normal, will not affect the drug, and will diminish over time.

• Safety and effectiveness in children have not been established, but a few children 3 to 13 years have received 3 to 6 mg/kg/day.

flucytosine (5-FC)

Ancobon

Pregnancy Risk Category: C

HOW SUPPLIED

Capsules: 250 mg, 500 mg

MECHANISM OF ACTION

Appears to penetrate fungal cells, where it is converted to fluorouracil, a known metabolic antagonist. Causes defective protein synthesis.

INDICATIONS & DOSAGE

For severe fungal infections caused by susceptible strains of Candida *(including septicemia, endocarditis, urinary tract and pulmonary infections) and* Cryptococcus *(meningitis, pulmonary infection, and possible urinary tract infections)* –

Adults and children over 50 kg: 50 to 150 mg/kg daily P.O. q 6 hours.

Adults and children under 50 kg: 1.5 to 4.5 g/m^2/day P.O. in four divided doses.

Severe infections, such as meningitis, may require doses up to 250 mg/kg.

ADVERSE REACTIONS

Common reactions are in italics; life-threatening reactions are in bold italics.

Blood: anemia, ***leukopenia, bone marrow suppression, thrombocytopenia.***

CNS: dizziness, drowsiness, confusion, headache, vertigo.

GI: *nausea, vomiting, diarrhea,* abdominal bloating.

Hepatic: elevated AST (SGOT), ALT (SGPT).

Metabolic: elevated serum alkaline phosphatase, BUN, serum creatinine.

Skin: occasional rash.

INTERACTIONS

None significant.

NURSING CONSIDERATIONS

• *Use with extreme caution* in patients with impaired hepatic or renal function or bone marrow depression. Patients with renal dysfunction should have dosage based on plasma flucytosine levels.

• Hematologic tests and renal and liver function studies should precede therapy and should be repeated at frequent intervals thereafter. Before treatment, susceptibility tests should establish that organism is flucytosine-sensitive. Tests should be repeated weekly to monitor drug resistance.

• GI adverse reactions are reduced if capsules are given over a 15-minute period.

• Monitor intake and output; report any marked change.

• If possible, blood level assays of drug should be performed regularly to maintain flucytosine at therapeutic level (25 to 120 mcg/ml). Higher blood levels may be toxic.

• Drug is usually combined with amphotericin because they are synergistic.

• Inform patient that adequate therapeutic response may take weeks or months.

griseofulvin microsize

Fulcin‡, Fulvicin-U/F, Grifulvin V, Grisactin, Grisovin‡, Grisovin 500‡, Grisovin-FP

griseofulvin ultramicrosize

Fulvicin P/G, Grisactin Ultra, Griseostatin‡, Gris-PEG

Pregnancy Risk Category: C

HOW SUPPLIED

microsize

Tablets: 250 mg, 500 mg
Capsules: 125 mg, 250 mg
Oral suspension: 125 mg/5ml

ultramicrosize

Tablets: 125 mg, 165 mg, 250 mg, 330 mg

MECHANISM OF ACTION

Arrests fungal cell activity by disrupting its mitotic spindle structure.

INDICATIONS & DOSAGE

Ringworm infections of skin, hair, nails (tinea corporis, tinea pedis, tinea capitis) when caused by Trichophyton, Microsporum, *or* Epidermophyton –

Adults: 500 mg (microsize) P.O. daily in single or divided doses. Severe infections may require up to 1 g daily. Alternatively, may give 330 to 375 mg ultramicrosize in single or divided doses.

Tinea pedis and tinea unguium –

Adults: 0.75 to 1 g (microsize) P.O. daily. Alternatively, may give 660 to 750 mg ultramicrosize P.O. daily.

Children: 11 mg/kg/day (microsize) P.O. Alternatively, may give 7.3 mg/kg/day of the ultramicrosize.

ADVERSE REACTIONS

Common reactions are in italics; life-threatening reactions are in bold italics.

Blood: leukopenia, ***granulocytopenia*** (requires discontinuation of drug).
CNS: headaches (in early stages of treatment), transient decrease in hearing, fatigue with large doses, occasional mental confusion, impaired performance of routine activities, psychotic symptoms, dizziness, insomnia.
GI: nausea, vomiting, excessive thirst, flatulence, diarrhea.
Metabolic: porphyria.
Skin: rash, urticaria, photosensitivity (may aggravate lupus erythematosus).
Other: estrogen-like effects in children, oral thrush.

INTERACTIONS

Alcohol: may cause tachycardia, diaphoresis, and flushing. Avoid alcohol.
Barbiturates: decreased griseofulvin blood levels due to decreased absorption or increased metabolism. Avoid using together or administer griseofulvin t.i.d.
Coumarin anticoagulants: decreased effectiveness. Monitor prothrombin times when used concurrently.
Oral contraceptives: decreased effectiveness. Suggest alternate methods of contraception.

NURSING CONSIDERATIONS

- *Contraindicated* in porphyria or hepatocellular failure. Since griseofulvin is a penicillin derivative, cross-sensitivity is possible. *Use cautiously* in penicillin-sensitive patients. Use only when topical treatment fails to arrest mycotic disease.
- CBC should be repeated regularly.
- Advise patient that prolonged treatment may be needed to control infection and prevent relapse, even if symptoms abate in first few days of therapy. Tell patient to keep skin clean and dry and to maintain good hygiene. Caution him to avoid intense sunlight.
- Most effectively absorbed and causes least GI distress when given after high-fat meal.

• Effective treatment of tinea pedis may require concomitant use of topical agent.
• Diagnosis of infecting organism should be verified in laboratory. Continue drug until clinical and laboratory examinations confirm complete eradication.
• Because griseofulvin ultramicrosize is dispersed in polyethylene glycol (PEG), it is absorbed more rapidly and completely than microsize preparations and is effective at one half to two thirds the usual griseofulvin dose.
• Advise patient to avoid alcoholic beverages.

itraconazole

Sporanox

Pregnancy Risk Category: C

HOW SUPPLIED
Capsules: 100 mg

MECHANISM OF ACTION
Interferes with fungal cell wall synthesis by inhibiting the formation of ergosterol, a vital component. Increased cell wall permeability makes the fungus susceptible to osmotic instability.

INDICATIONS & DOSAGE
Pulmonary and extrapulmonary blastomycosis; histoplasmosis –
Adults: 200 mg P.O. daily. Increase dosage as needed and tolerated in 100-mg increments to a maximum of 400 mg daily. Doses that exceed 200 mg daily should be given in two divided doses. Treatment should continue for a minimum of 3 months. In life-threatening illness, administer a loading dose of 200 mg t.i.d. for 3 days.

ADVERSE REACTIONS
Common reactions are in italics; life-threatening reactions are in bold italics.
GI: nausea, vomiting, diarrhea, abdominal pain, anorexia.
Skin: rash, pruritus.
Other: edema, fatigue, fever, malaise.

INTERACTIONS
Cyclosporine, digoxin: itraconazole may increase plasma levels of these drugs. Monitor plasma levels closely.
H_2-receptor antagonists, antacids, rifampin, phenytoin: coadministration with itraconazole may result in lowered itraconazole plasma levels. Avoid concomitant use.
Isoniazid: may decrease plasma levels of itraconazole. Monitor closely.
Oral anticoagulants: itraconazole may enhance anticoagulant effects. Monitor prothrombin times closely.
Oral antidiabetic agents: similar antifungals have caused hypoglycemia. Monitor blood glucose levels closely.
Terfenadine, astemizole: itraconazole inhibits metabolism of these antihistamines, resulting in elevated blood levels and risk of serious cardiac toxicity. Never administer together.

NURSING CONSIDERATIONS
• *Contraindicated* in patients with hypersensitivity to the drug and in patients receiving terfenadine or astemizole. Because drug is excreted in breast milk, don't use in breast-feeding women.
• *Use cautiously* in patients with hypochlorhydria because these patients may not absorb the drug as readily as patients with normal gastric acidity. Because hypochlorhydria can accompany human immunodeficiency virus (HIV) infection, also use cautiously in HIV-infected patients.
• Itraconazole and its metabolite are highly bound to plasma proteins (greater than 99%). *Use cautiously* in patients receiving other highly bound medications.
• Tell patient to take drug with food to ensure maximal absorption.

• Perform baseline hepatic function tests, and monitor periodically. Patients should know the signs and symptoms of liver disease (anorexia, dark urine, pale stools, unusual fatigue or jaundice) and report them if they occur.

ketoconazole

Nizoral

Pregnancy Risk Category: C

HOW SUPPLIED

Tablets: 200 mg
Oral suspension: 100 mg/5 ml†

MECHANISM OF ACTION

Inhibits purine transport and DNA, RNA, and protein synthesis; increases cell wall permeability, making the fungus more susceptible to osmotic pressure.

INDICATIONS & DOSAGE

Treatment of systemic candidiasis, chronic mucocandidiasis, oral thrush, candiduria, coccidioidomycosis, histoplasmosis, chromomycosis, and paracoccidioidomycosis; severe cutaneous dermatophyte infections resistant to therapy with topical or oral griseofulvin –
Adults and children over 40 kg: initially, 200 mg P.O. daily single dose. Dosage may be increased to 400 mg once daily in patients who don't respond to lower dosage.
Children 2 years and over: 3.3 to 6.6 mg/kg P.O. daily.

ADVERSE REACTIONS

Common reactions are in italics; life-threatening reactions are in bold italics.
CNS: headache, nervousness, dizziness.
GI: *nausea, vomiting,* abdominal pain, diarrhea, constipation.
Hepatic: elevated liver enzymes, ***fatal hepatotoxicity***.
Skin: itching.
Other: gynecomastia with breast tenderness in males.

INTERACTIONS

Antacids, anticholinergics, H_2 blockers: decreased absorption of ketoconazole. Wait at least 2 hours after ketoconazole dose before administering these drugs.
Rifampin, isoniazid: increases ketoconazole metabolism. Monitor for decreased antifungal effect.

NURSING CONSIDERATIONS

• *Contraindicated* in patients with hypersensitivity to the drug.
• *Use cautiously* in patients with hepatic disease and in those who are taking other hepatotoxic drugs.
• Because of the potential of serious liver toxicity, ketoconazole should not be used for less serious conditions, such as fungus infections of the skin or nails.
• Ketoconazole is not effective in patients with achlorhydria because drug requires acidity for dissolution and absorption. Instruct such patients to dissolve each tablet in 4 ml aqueous solution of 0.2 N hydrochloric acid; and, to avoid contact with teeth, to sip the mixture through a straw (glass or plastic). Tell patient to follow with a glass of water.
• Make sure patient understands that treatment should be continued until all clinical and laboratory tests indicate that active fungal infection has subsided. If drug is discontinued too soon, infection will recur. Minimum treatment for candidiasis is 7 to 14 days. Minimum treatment for other systemic fungal infections is 6 months. Minimum treatment for resistant dermatophyte infections is at least 4 weeks.
• Reassure patient that, although nausea is common early in therapy, it will subside. To minimize nausea, you may, with doctor's permission, divide the

daily dosage into 2 doses. Taking with meals also helps to decrease nausea.
• Monitor for elevated liver enzymes and nausea that does not subside, as well as unusual fatigue, jaundice, dark urine, or pale stools. May be signs of hepatotoxicity.
• Much larger doses (up to 800 mg/day) can be used to effectively treat fungal meningitis and intracerebral fungal lesions.

miconazole

Monistat I.V.

Pregnancy Risk Category: C

HOW SUPPLIED
Injection: 10 mg/ml

MECHANISM OF ACTION
Inhibits purine transport and DNA, RNA, and protein synthesis; increases cell wall permeability, making the fungus more susceptible to osmotic pressure.

INDICATIONS & DOSAGE
Treatment of systemic fungal infections (coccidioidomycosis, candidiasis, cryptococcosis, paracoccidioidomycosis), chronic mucocutaneous candidiasis –
Adults: 200 to 3,600 mg/day. Dosages may vary with diagnosis and with infective agent. May divide daily dosage over 3 infusions, 200 to 1,200 mg per infusion. Dilute in at least 200 ml of 0.9% sodium chloride. Repeated courses may be needed because of relapse or reinfection.
Children 1 year and over: 20 to 40 mg/kg/day. Do not exceed 15 mg/kg per infusion.
Fungal meningitis –
Adults: 20 mg intrathecally as an adjunct to intravenous administration, q 3 to 7 days.

ADVERSE REACTIONS
Common reactions are in italics; life-threatening reactions are in bold italics.
Blood: transient decreases in hematocrit, thrombocytopenia.
CNS: dizziness, drowsiness.
GI: *nausea, vomiting,* diarrhea.
Metabolic: *transient decrease in serum sodium.*
Skin: *pruritic rash.*
Local: *phlebitis at injection site.*
Other: fever, chills.

INTERACTIONS
Oral anticoagulants: enhanced anticoagulant effect. Monitor closely.

NURSING CONSIDERATIONS
• *Use cautiously.* Acute cardiorespiratory arrest has occurred with the first dose. The first dose should be given under continuous medical supervision with emergency resuscitative equipment immediately available.
• **I.V. use:** Use of I.V. miconazole has been replaced largely by newer drugs that are better tolerated.
• Rapid injection of undiluted miconazole may produce arrhythmias. Dilute infusion with at least 200 ml of 0.9% sodium chloride solution and infuse over 30 to 60 minutes.
• Premedication with antiemetic may lessen nausea and vomiting.
• Avoid administration at mealtime in order to lessen GI adverse reactions.
• Pruritic rash may persist for weeks after drug is discontinued. Pruritus may be controlled with oral or I.V. diphenhydramine.
• In treatment of fungal meningitis and urinary bladder infections, must be supplemented with intrathecal administration and bladder irrigation, respectively.
• Inform patient that adequate therapeutic response may take weeks or months.
• Monitor levels of hemoglobin, hematocrit, electrolytes, and lipids regularly. Transient elevations in serum

cholesterol and triglycerides may be due to castor oil vehicle.

nystatin

Mycostatin*, Nadostine†, Nilstat, Nystex*

Pregnancy Risk Category: B

HOW SUPPLIED

Tablets: 500,000 units
Oral suspension: 100,000 units/ml
Vaginal suppositories: 100,000 units

MECHANISM OF ACTION

Probably acts by binding to sterols in the fungal cell membrane, altering cell permeability and allowing leakage of intracellular components.

INDICATIONS & DOSAGE

GI infections –
Adults: 500,000 to 1 million units as oral tablets, t.i.d.
Oral, vaginal, and intestinal infections caused by Candida albicans (Monilia) *and other* Candida *species –*
Adults: 400,000 to 600,000 units oral suspension q.i.d. for oral candidiasis.
Children and infants over 3 months: 250,000 to 500,000 units oral suspension q.i.d.
Neonates and premature infants: 100,000 units oral suspension q.i.d.
Vaginal infections –
Adults: 100,000 units, as vaginal tablets, inserted high into vagina, daily or b.i.d. for 14 days.

ADVERSE REACTIONS

Common reactions are in italics; life-threatening reactions are in bold italics.
GI: transient nausea, vomiting, diarrhea (usually with large oral dosage).

INTERACTIONS

None significant.

NURSING CONSIDERATIONS

- Nystatin is virtually nontoxic and nonsensitizing when used orally, vaginally, or topically, but advise patient to report redness, swelling, or irritation.
- Vaginal tablets can be used by pregnant women up to 6 weeks before term to treat maternal infection that may cause thrush in newborns.
- Continue therapy during menstruation.
- Instruct patient to wash applicator thoroughly after each use.
- Explain that use of antibiotics, oral contraceptives, and corticosteroids; diabetes; reinfection by sexual partner; and tight-fitting panty hose are predisposing factors of vaginal infection. Encourage patient to use cotton (not synthetic) underpants.
- For treatment of oral candidiasis (thrush): Be sure the mouth is clean of food debris before administering drug, then tell patient to hold suspension in mouth for several minutes before swallowing. When treating infants, swab medication on oral mucosa. Instruct patient in good oral hygiene techniques. Tell patient overuse of mouthwash or poorly fitting dentures, especially in older patients, may alter flora and promote infection.
- Advise patient to continue medication for at least 2 days after symptoms disappear to ensure against reinfection. Consult doctor for exact length of therapy.
- For treatment of oral candidiasis, immunosuppressed patients sometimes take vaginal tablets (100,000 units) by mouth since this provides prolonged contact with oral mucosa.
- Instruct patient in careful hygiene for affected areas, including cleansing perineal area from front to back after defecation.
- Not effective against systemic infections.

9
Antimalarials

chloroquine hydrochloride
chloroquine phosphate
chloroquine sulphate
hydroxychloroquine sulfate
mefloquine hydrochloride
primaquine phosphate
pyrimethamine
pyrimethamine with sulfadoxine
quinine bisulfate
quinine sulfate

COMBINATION PRODUCTS
ARALEN PHOSPHATE WITH PRIMAQUINE PHOSPHATE: chloroquine phosphate 500 mg (300 mg base) and primaquine phosphate 79 mg (45 mg base).
M-KYA, Q-VEL: quinine sulfate 64.8 mg and vitamin E 400 U (as d,l alpha-tocopheryl acetate) and lecithin

chloroquine hydrochloride
Aralen HCl, Chlorquin‡

chloroquine phosphate
Aralen Phosphate, Chlorquin‡

chloroquine sulphate
Nivaquine‡

Pregnancy Risk Category: C

HOW SUPPLIED
hydrochloride
Injection: 50 mg/ml (40-mg/ml base)
phosphate
Tablets: 250 mg (150-mg base), 500 mg (300-mg base)
sulphate
Tablets: 200 mg (150-mg base)
Syrup: 68 mg (50-mg base)/5 ml

MECHANISM OF ACTION
As an antimalarial, may bind to and alter the properties of DNA in susceptible parasites. As an amebicide, mechanism of action is unknown.

INDICATIONS & DOSAGE
Suppressive prophylaxis and treatment of acute attacks of malaria due to Plasmodium vivax, P. malariae, P. ovale, *and susceptible strains of* P. falciparum –
Adults: initially, 600 mg (base) P.O., then 300 mg P.O. at 6, 24, and 48 hours. Or 160 to 200 mg (base) I.M. initially; repeat in 6 hours if needed. Switch to oral therapy as soon as possible.
Children: initially, 10 mg (base)/kg P.O., then 5 mg (base)/kg dose P.O. at 6, 24, and 48 hours (do not exceed adult dose). Or 5 mg (base)/kg I.M. initially; repeat in 6 hours if needed. Switch to oral therapy as soon as possible.
Malaria suppressive treatment –
Adults and children: 5 mg (base)/kg P.O. (not to exceed 300 mg) weekly on same day of the week (begin 2 weeks before entering endemic area and continue for 8 weeks after leaving). If treatment begins after exposure, double the initial dose (600 mg for adults, 10 mg/kg for children) in two divided doses P.O. 6 hours apart.
Extraintestinal amebiasis –
Adults: 160 to 200 mg chloroquine (hydrochloride) base I.M. daily for no more than 12 days. As soon as possible, substitute 1 g (600 mg base) chloroquine phosphate P.O. daily for 2 days; then 500 mg (300 mg base) daily for at least 2 to 3 weeks. Treatment is usually combined with an effective intestinal amebicide.
Children: 10 mg/kg of chloroquine (hydrochloride) base for 2 to 3 weeks. Maximum 300 mg daily.

*Liquid form contains alcohol. **May contain tartrazine.

Rheumatoid arthritis and lupus erythematosus –
Adults: 250 mg chloroquine phosphate daily with evening meal.

ADVERSE REACTIONS
Common reactions are in italics; life-threatening reactions are in bold italics.
Blood: ***agranulocytosis, aplastic anemia,*** hemolytic anemia, thrombocytopenia.
CNS: mild and transient headache, neuromyopathy, psychic stimulation, fatigue, irritability, nightmares, seizures, dizziness.
CV: hypotension, ECG changes.
EENT: *visual disturbances* (blurred vision; difficulty in focusing; reversible corneal changes; generally irreversible, sometimes progressive or delayed, retinal changes, such as narrowing of arterioles; macular lesions; pallor of optic disk; optic atrophy; patchy retinal pigmentation, often leading to blindness); ototoxicity (nerve deafness, vertigo, tinnitus).
GI: anorexia, abdominal cramps, diarrhea, nausea, vomiting, stomatitis.
Skin: pruritus, lichen planus-like eruptions, skin and mucosal pigmentary changes, pleomorphic skin eruptions.

INTERACTIONS
Cimetidine: decreased hepatic metabolism of chloroquine. Monitor for toxicity.
Magnesium and aluminum salts, kaolin: decreased GI absorption. Separate administration times.

NURSING CONSIDERATIONS
- *Contraindicated* in retinal or visual field changes or porphyria.
- *Use with extreme caution* in presence of severe GI, neurologic, or blood disorders.
- *Use cautiously* in patients with hepatic disease or alcoholism because drug concentrates in liver and in patients with G6PD deficiency or psoriasis because drug may exacerbate these conditions.
- CBCs and liver function studies should be performed periodically during prolonged therapy; if severe blood disorder appears that is not attributable to disease under treatment, drug may need to be discontinued.
- Overdosage can quickly lead to toxic symptoms: headache, drowsiness, visual disturbances, cardiovascular collapse, and seizures, followed by respiratory and cardiac arrest. Children are extremely susceptible to toxicity; avoid long-term treatment.
- Baseline and periodic ophthalmologic examinations needed. Tell patient to report blurred vision, increased sensitivity to light, or muscle weakness. Check periodically for ocular muscle weakness after long-term use. Audiometric examinations recommended before, during, and after therapy, especially if long term.
- For prophylaxis, drug should be taken immediately before or after meals on same day each week to enhance compliance.
- To avoid exacerbated drug-induced dermatoses, warn patient to avoid excessive exposure to sun.

hydroxychloroquine sulfate
Plaquenil

Pregnancy Risk Category: C

HOW SUPPLIED
Tablets: 200 mg (150-mg base)

MECHANISM OF ACTION
May bind to and alter the properties of DNA.

INDICATIONS & DOSAGE
Suppressive prophylaxis of attacks of malaria due to Plasmodium vivax, P. malariae, P. ovale, *and susceptible strains of* P. falciparum –
Adults and children: for suppres-

sion: 5 mg (base)/kg body weight P.O. (not to exceed 310 mg) weekly on same day of the week (begin 2 weeks before entering and continue for 8 weeks after leaving endemic area). If not started before exposure, double initial dose (620 mg for adults, 10 mg/kg for children) in two divided doses P.O. 6 hours apart.

Treatment of acute malarial attacks –

Adults and children over 15 years: initially, 800 mg (sulfate) P.O., then 400 mg after 6 to 8 hours, then 400 mg daily for 2 days (total 2 g sulfate salt).

Children 11 to 15 years: 600 mg (sulfate) P.O. stat, then 200 mg 8 hours later, then 200 mg 24 hours later (total 1 g sulfate salt).

Children 6 to 10 years: 400 mg (sulfate) P.O. stat, then two doses of 200 mg at 8-hour intervals (total 800 mg sulfate salt).

Children 2 to 5 years: 400 mg (sulfate) P.O. stat, then 200 mg 8 hours later (total 600 mg sulfate salt).

Children under 1 year: 100 mg (sulfate) P.O. stat; then three doses of 100 mg 6 to 9 hours apart (total 400 mg sulfate salt).

Lupus erythematosus (chronic discoid and systemic) –

Adults: 400 mg P.O. daily or b.i.d., continued for several weeks or months, depending on response. Prolonged maintenance dosage – 200 to 400 mg P.O. daily.

Rheumatoid arthritis –

Adults: initially, 400 to 600 mg P.O. daily. When good response occurs (usually in 4 to 12 weeks), cut dosage in half.

ADVERSE REACTIONS

Common reactions are in italics; life-threatening reactions are in bold italics.

Blood: ***agranulocytosis, leukopenia,*** thrombocytopenia, ***hemolysis in patients with G6PD deficiency, aplastic anemia.***

CNS: irritability, nightmares, ataxia, seizures, psychic stimulation, toxic psychosis, vertigo, tinnitus, nystagmus, lassitude, fatigue, dizziness, hypoactive deep tendon reflexes, skeletal muscle weakness.

EENT: visual disturbances (blurred vision; difficulty in focusing; reversible corneal changes; generally irreversible, sometimes progressive or delayed, retinal changes, e.g., narrowing of arterioles; macular lesions; pallor of optic disk; optic atrophy; visual field defects; patchy retinal pigmentation, often leading to blindness), ototoxicity (irreversible nerve deafness, tinnitus, labyrinthitis).

GI: anorexia, abdominal cramps, diarrhea, nausea, vomiting.

Skin: pruritus, lichen planus-like eruptions, skin and mucosal pigmentary changes, pleomorphic skin eruptions.

Other: weight loss, alopecia, bleaching of hair.

INTERACTIONS

Cimetidine: decreased hepatic metabolism of hydroxychloroquine. Monitor for toxicity.

Magnesium and aluminum salts, kaolin: Decreased GI absorption. Separate administration times.

NURSING CONSIDERATIONS

- *Contraindicated* in patients with retinal or visual field changes, or porphyria.
- *Use with extreme caution* in presence of severe GI, neurologic, or blood disorders.
- *Use cautiously* in patients with hepatic disease or alcoholism because drug concentrates in liver and in patients with G6PD deficiency or psoriasis because drug may exacerbate these conditions.
- CBCs and liver function studies should be made periodically during prolonged therapy; if severe blood disorder appears that is not attribut-

*Liquid form contains alcohol. **May contain tartrazine.

able to disease under treatment, consider discontinuing.
• Overdosage can quickly lead to toxic symptoms: headache, drowsiness, visual disturbances, cardiovascular collapse, and seizures, followed by respiratory and cardiac arrest. Children are extremely susceptible to toxicity; avoid long-term treatment.
• Baseline and periodic ophthalmologic examinations needed. Tell patient to report blurred vision, increased sensitivity to light, or muscle weakness. Check periodically for ocular muscle weakness after long-term use. Audiometric examinations recommended before, during, and after therapy, especially if long term.
• Drug should be taken immediately before or after meals on same day of each week.

mefloquine hydrochloride

Lariam

Pregnancy Risk Category: C

HOW SUPPLIED

Tablets: 250 mg

MECHANISM OF ACTION

Exact mechanism unknown. Mefloquine is a structural analog of quinine. Antimalarial activity may be related to its ability to form complexes with hemin.

INDICATIONS & DOSAGE

Treatment of acute malaria infections caused by mefloquine-sensitive strains of Plasmodium falciparum *or* Plasmodium vivax –
Adults: 1,250 mg P.O. as a single dose. Patients with *P. vivax* infections should receive subsequent therapy with primaquine or other 8-aminoquinolines to avoid relapse after treatment of the initial infection.
Malaria prophylaxis –
Adults: 250 mg P.O. once weekly. Initiate prophylaxis 1 week before entering endemic area, and continue prophylaxis for 4 weeks after return from such areas. When returning to an area without malaria after a prolonged stay in an endemic area, prophylaxis ends after three doses.

ADVERSE REACTIONS

Common reactions are in italics; life-threatening reactions are in bold italics.
CNS: dizziness, syncope, headache, transient emotional disturbances (rare).
CV: extrasystoles.
EENT: tinnitus.
GI: loss of appetite, vomiting, *nausea,* loose stools, diarrhea, GI discomfort.
Skin: rash.
Other: fatigue, fever, chills.

INTERACTIONS

Quinine, chloroquine: increased risk of seizures.
Quinine, quinidine, beta-adrenergic blocking agents: ECG abnormalities and cardiac arrest may occur.
Valproic acid: decreased valproic acid blood levels and loss of seizure control at start of mefloquine therapy. Monitor anticonvulsant blood levels.

NURSING CONSIDERATIONS

• *Contraindicated* in patients with hypersensitivity to mefloquine or related compounds.
• *Use cautiously* in patients with cardiac disease.
• Advise the patient to take the drug on the same day of the week when using it for prophylaxis.
• Tell the patient not to take the drug on an empty stomach and always to take it with a full glass (at least 8 oz [240 ml]) of water.
• Because the health risks from concomitant administration of quinine and mefloquine are great, mefloquine therapy should not begin sooner than 12 hours after the last dose of quinine or quinidine.

• Advise patients to use caution when performing hazardous activities that require alertness and good coordination because there have been reports of dizziness, a disturbed sense of balance, and neuropsychiatric reactions.
• In cases of suspected overdose, induce vomiting and seek medical advice immediately because there is potential for cardiotoxicity. Animal studies reveal that mefloquine has cardiac actions similar to quinidine and quinine.
• Patients taking mefloquine prophylaxis should discontinue the drug if they notice signs or symptoms of unexplained anxiety, depression, confusion, or restlessness. These symptoms may indicate impending toxicity.
• Periodic ophthalmic examinations are recommended in patients undergoing long-term therapy because ocular lesions have been noted in laboratory animals.
• Periodic liver function tests are recommended.
• Patients with infections caused by *P. vivax* are at high risk of relapse because the drug does not eliminate the hepatic phase (exoerythrocytic parasites). Follow-up therapy is advisable.

primaquine phosphate

Pregnancy Risk Category: D

HOW SUPPLIED
Tablets: 7.5 mg (base)‡, 15 mg (base)

MECHANISM OF ACTION
A gametocidal drug that destroys exoerythrocytic forms and prevents delayed primary attack. Its precise mechanism of action is unknown.

INDICATIONS & DOSAGE
Radical cure of relapsing vivax malaria, eliminating symptoms and infection completely; prevention of relapse –
Adults: 15 mg (base) P.O. daily for 14 days. (26.3 mg tablet = 15 mg of base).

ADVERSE REACTIONS
Common reactions are in italics; life-threatening reactions are in bold italics.
Blood: leukopenia, ***hemolytic anemia in G6PD deficiency,*** methemoglobinemia in NADH methemoglobin reductase deficiency, leukocytosis, mild anemia, ***granulocytopenia, agranulocytosis.***
CNS: headache.
EENT: disturbances of visual accommodation.
GI: nausea, vomiting, epigastric distress, abdominal cramps.
Skin: urticaria.

INTERACTIONS
Magnesium and aluminum salts: Decreased GI absorption. Separate administration times.
Quinacrine: enhanced toxicity of primaquine. Don't use together.

NURSING CONSIDERATIONS
• *Contraindicated* in lupus erythematosus and rheumatoid arthritis and in patients taking bone marrow suppressants and potentially hemolytic drugs.
• Use with a fast-acting antimalarial, such as chloroquine. Use full dose to reduce possibility of drug-resistant strains.
• Light-skinned patients taking more than 30 mg (base) daily, dark-skinned patients taking more than 15 mg (base) daily, and patients with severe anemia or suspected sensitivity should have frequent blood studies and urine examinations. Sudden fall in hemoglobin concentration, erythrocyte or leukocyte count, or marked darkening of the urine suggests impending hemolytic reactions.
• Observe closely for tolerance in patients with previous idiosyncrasy (manifested by hemolytic anemia, methemoglobinemia, or leukopenia); family or personal history of favism;

erythrocytic G6PD deficiency or NADH methemoglobin reductase deficiency.

- Administer drug with meals.

pyrimethamine

Daraprim

pyrimethamine with sulfadoxine

Fansidar

Pregnancy Risk Category: C

HOW SUPPLIED

pyrimethamine

Tablets: 25 mg

pyrimethamine with sulfadoxine

Tablets: pyrimethamine 25 mg, sulfadoxine 500 mg

MECHANISM OF ACTION

Inhibits the enzyme dihydrofolate reductase, thereby impeding reduction of dihydrofolic acid to tetrahydrofolic acid. Sulfadoxine competitively inhibits PABA.

INDICATIONS & DOSAGE

Malaria prophylaxis and transmission control (pyrimethamine) –

Adults and children over 10 years: 25 mg P.O. weekly.

Children 4 to 10 years: 12.5 mg P.O. weekly.

Children under 4 years: 6.25 mg P.O. weekly.

Continue in all age-groups at least 10 weeks after leaving endemic areas.

Acute attacks of malaria (Fansidar) –

Adults: 2 to 3 tablets as a single dose, either alone or in sequence with quinine or primaquine.

Children 9 to 14 years: 2 tablets.

Children 4 to 8 years: 1 tablet.

Children under 4 years: ½ tablet.

Malaria prophylaxis (Fansidar) –

Adults: 1 tablet weekly, or 2 tablets q 2 weeks.

Children 9 to 14 years: ¾ tablet weekly, or 1½ tablets q 2 weeks.

Children 4 to 8 years: ½ tablet weekly, or 1 tablet q 2 weeks.

Children under 4 years: ¼ tablet weekly, or ½ tablet q 2 weeks.

Acute attacks of malaria (pyrimethamine) –

Not recommended alone in nonimmune persons; use with faster-acting antimalarials, such as chloroquine, for 2 days to initiate transmission control and suppressive cure.

Adults and children over 15 years: 25 mg P.O. daily for 2 days.

Children under 15 years: 12.5 mg P.O. daily for 2 days.

Toxoplasmosis (pyrimethamine) –

Adults: initially, 100 mg P.O., then 25 mg P.O. daily for 4 to 5 weeks; during same time give 1 g sulfadiazine P.O. q 6 hours.

Children: initially, 1 mg/kg P.O., then 0.25 mg/kg daily for 4 to 5 weeks, along with 100 mg sulfadiazine/kg P.O. daily, divided q 6 hours.

ADVERSE REACTIONS

Common reactions are in italics; life-threatening reactions are in bold italics.

Blood: ***agranulocytosis, aplastic anemia,*** megaloblastic anemia, bone marrow suppression, leukopenia, thrombocytopenia, pancytopenia.

CNS: stimulation and seizures (acute toxicity).

GI: anorexia, vomiting, diarrhea, atrophic glossitis.

Skin: rashes, ***erythema multiforme (Stevens-Johnson syndrome), toxic epidermal necrolysis.***

INTERACTIONS

Folic acid and para-aminobenzoic acid: decreased antitoxoplasmic effects. May require dosage adjustment.

Sulfonamides, co-trimoxazole, methotrexate: increased adverse effects. Use together cautiously.

NURSING CONSIDERATIONS

- Fansidar is *contraindicated* in porphyria because it contains sulfadoxine, a sulfonamide. *Use cautiously* in impaired hepatic or renal function, severe allergy or bronchial asthma, or G6PD deficiency.
- Pyrimethamine alone is not useful; use the combination drug with sulfadoxine (Fansidar) in chloroquine-resistant malaria. *Use cautiously* in seizure disorders; smaller doses may be needed. Also use cautiously after treatment with chloroquine.
- Warn patient taking Fansidar to stop drug and notify doctor at first sign of skin rash.
- Dosages required to treat toxoplasmosis approach toxic levels. Twice-weekly blood counts, including platelets, are required. If signs of folic or folinic acid deficiency develop, dosage should be reduced or discontinued while patient receives parenteral folinic acid (leucovorin) until blood counts become normal.
- Give with meals to minimize GI distress.
- The first dose of Fansidar, when taken prophylactically, should be taken 1 to 2 days before traveling to an endemic area.
- Because of the possibility of severe skin reactions, Fansidar should be used only in regions where chloroquine-resistant malaria is prevalent and only when the traveler plans to stay in the region longer than 3 weeks.

quinine bisulfate (quinine bisulphate)

Bi-Chinine‡, Biquinate‡, Myoquin‡, Quinbisul‡

quinine sulfate (quinine sulphate)

Chinine‡, Legatrin, Novoquinine†, Quinamm, Quinate‡, Quindan, Quine-200◇, Quine-300, Quinoctal‡, Quiphile, Strema, Sulquin‡

Pregnancy Risk Category: X

HOW SUPPLIED

bisulfate

Tablets: 100 mg, 300 mg

sulfate

Tablets: 260 mg, 325 mg◇

Capsules: 65 mg◇, 130 mg◇, 195 mg◇, 200 mg◇, 260 mg, 300 mg◇, 325 mg◇

MECHANISM OF ACTION

Mechanism of antiprotozoal action is unknown, but the drug is often referred to as a generalized protoplasmic poison. As a muscle relaxant, quinine appears to have a direct effect on muscle fibers that decreases their response to repetitive stimulation.

INDICATIONS & DOSAGE

Malaria due to Plasmodium falciparum *(chloroquine-resistant)* –

Adults: 650 mg P.O. q 8 hours for 10 days, with 25 mg pyrimethamine q 12 hours for 3 days, and with 500 mg sulfadiazine q.i.d. for 5 days.

Nocturnal leg cramps –

Adults: 260 to 300 mg P.O. at bedtime or after the evening meal.

ADVERSE REACTIONS

Common reactions are in italics; life-threatening reactions are in bold italics.

Blood: hemolytic anemia, thrombocytopenia, ***agranulocytosis,*** hypoprothrombinemia.

CNS: severe headache, apprehension, excitement, confusion, delirium, syncope, hypothermia, seizures (with toxic doses).

CV: hypotension, ***CV collapse*** with overdosage or rapid I.V. administration.

EENT: altered color perception, photophobia, blurred vision, night blindness, amblyopia, scotoma, diplopia, mydriasis, optic atrophy, tinnitus, impaired hearing.

GI: epigastric distress, diarrhea, nausea, vomiting.
GU: renal tubular damage, anuria.
Skin: rashes, pruritus.
Local: thrombosis at infusion site.
Other: asthma, flushing.

INTERACTIONS
Antacids containing aluminum: decreased absorption of quinine. Separate administration times by at least 2 hours.
Cimetidine: decreased hepatic metabolism of quinine. Monitor for toxicity.
Digoxin: serum digoxin levels may be increased. Monitor for toxicity.
Mefloquine: risk of seizures, ECG changes, and cardiac arrest. Don't use together.
Neuromuscular blockers: prolonged muscle paralysis. Monitor for respiratory distress or excessive weakness.
Oral anticoagulants: enhanced anticoagulant effect. Monitor for bleeding.
Sodium bicarbonate: elevates quinine levels by decreasing quinine excretion. Use together cautiously.

NURSING CONSIDERATIONS
- *Contraindicated* in G6PD deficiency.
- *Use cautiously* in CV conditions.
- Discontinue if any signs of idiosyncrasy or toxicity occur.
- Quinine is no longer used for acute attacks of malaria due to *Plasmodium vivax* or for suppression of malaria due to organism resistance.
- Administer after meals to minimize GI distress. Do not crush tablets, as the drug is irritating to gastric mucosa.
- When parenteral therapy is necessary or when oral therapy is not feasible, quinine dihydrochloride may be obtained from the Centers for Disease Control. Administer by slow infusion (over at least 1 hour).

10

Antituberculars and antileprotics

capreomycin sulfate
clofazimine
cycloserine
dapsone
ethambutol hydrochloride
ethionamide
isoniazid
pyrazinamide
rifampin
streptomycin sulfate
(See Chapter 11, AMINOGLYCOSIDES.)

COMBINATION PRODUCTS
RIFAMATE: isoniazid 150 mg and rifampin 300 mg.
RIMACTANE/INH DUAL PACK: thirty 300-mg isoniazid tablets and sixty 300-mg rifampin capsules.

capreomycin sulfate
Capastat

Pregnancy Risk Category: C

HOW SUPPLIED
Injection: 1 g/vial

MECHANISM OF ACTION
Unknown (bacteriostatic).

INDICATIONS & DOSAGE
Adjunctive treatment in pulmonary tuberculosis –
Adults: 15 mg/kg/day up to 1 g I.M. daily injected deeply into large muscle mass for 60 to 120 days; then 1 g two to three times weekly for 18 to 24 months. Maximum dosage should not exceed 20 mg/kg daily. Must be given in conjunction with another antitubercular drug.

ADVERSE REACTIONS
Common reactions are in italics; life-threatening reactions are in bold italics.
Blood: eosinophilia, leukocytosis, leukopenia.
CNS: headache, ***neuromuscular blockade.***
EENT: *ototoxicity* (tinnitus, vertigo, hearing loss).
GU: *nephrotoxicity* (elevated BUN and nonprotein nitrogen levels, casts, RBC counts, leukocytes; tubular necrosis; proteinuria; decreased creatinine clearance).
Metabolic: hypokalemia, alkalosis, hepatotoxicity.
Local: pain, induration, excessive bleeding and sterile abscesses at injection site.

INTERACTIONS
None significant.

NURSING CONSIDERATIONS
- *Contraindicated* in patients receiving other ototoxic or nephrotoxic drugs. Drug is never given I.V. because this use may cause neuromuscular blockade.
- *Use cautiously* in patients with impaired renal function, history of allergies, or hearing impairment.
- Considered a "second-line" drug in the treatment of tuberculosis.
- Administer deep into large muscle mass to minimize local reactions. Apply ice to injection site p.r.n. for pain.
- Evaluate patient's hearing before and every 1 to 2 weeks during therapy. Notify doctor if patient complains of tinnitus, vertigo, or hearing impairment.
- Monitor renal function (output, specific gravity, urinalysis, BUN level, and serum creatinine level) before and during therapy; notify doctor of decreasing renal function. Dose must be reduced in renal impairment.
- Straw- or dark-colored solution does

not indicate a loss in potency. Do not administer solutions that contain a precipitate.

clofazimine

Lamprene

Pregnancy Risk Category: C

HOW SUPPLIED

Capsules: 50 mg, 100 mg

MECHANISM OF ACTION

Inhibits mycobacterial growth by binding preferentially to mycobacterial DNA. Also has anti-inflammatory effects that suppress skin reactions of erythema nodosum leprosum.

INDICATIONS & DOSAGE

Treatment of dapsone-resistant leprosy (Hansen's disease) –

Adults: 100 mg P.O. daily in combination with other antileprotics for 3 years. Then, clofazimine *alone,* 100 mg daily.

Erythema nodosum leprosum –

Adults: 100 to 200 mg P.O. daily for up to 3 months. Taper dosage to 100 mg daily as soon as possible. Dosages above 200 mg daily are not recommended.

ADVERSE REACTIONS

Common reactions are in italics; life-threatening reactions are in bold italics.

EENT: conjunctival and corneal pigmentation.

GI: *epigastric pain, diarrhea, nausea, vomiting, GI intolerance, bowel obstruction, GI bleeding.*

Skin: *pink to brownish black pigmentation, ichthyosis and dryness,* rash, itching.

Other: ***splenic infarction,*** discolored body fluids and excrement.

INTERACTIONS

None significant.

NURSING CONSIDERATIONS

- *Use cautiously* in GI dysfunction, such as abdominal pain and diarrhea.
- Advise patient to take the drug with meals.
- Doses that exceed 100 mg daily should be given for as short a period as possible and only under close medical supervision.
- If patient complains of colicky or burning abdominal pain or of any other GI symptom, report this to the doctor, who may reduce the dose or increase the interval between doses.
- Warn patient that clofazimine may discolor skin, body fluids, and excrement. The color ranges from red to brownish black. Reassure patient that the unsightly skin discoloration is reversible but may not disappear until several months or years after drug treatment ends.
- Recommend application of skin oil or cream to help reverse skin dryness or ichthyosis.

cycloserine

Seromycin

Pregnancy Risk Category: C

HOW SUPPLIED

Capsules: 250 mg

MECHANISM OF ACTION

Inhibits cell wall biosynthesis by interfering with the utilization of amino acids (bacteriostatic).

INDICATIONS & DOSAGE

Adjunctive treatment in pulmonary or extrapulmonary tuberculosis –

Adults: initially, 250 mg P.O. q 12 hours for 2 weeks; then, if blood levels are below 25 to 30 mcg/ml and there are no clinical signs of toxicity, dosage is increased to 250 mg P.O. q 8 hours for 2 weeks. If optimum blood levels are still not achieved, and there are no signs of clinical toxicity, then dosage is increased to 250 mg

P.O. q 6 hours. Maximum dosage is 1 g/day. If CNS toxicity occurs, drug is discontinued for 1 week, then resumed at 250 mg daily for 2 weeks. If no serious toxic effects occur, dosage is increased by 250-mg increments q 10 days until blood level of 25 to 30 mcg/ml is obtained.

ADVERSE REACTIONS
Common reactions are in italics; life-threatening reactions are in bold italics.
CNS: ***seizures,*** drowsiness, headache, tremor, dysarthria, vertigo, confusion, loss of memory, ***possible suicidal tendencies*** and other psychotic symptoms, *nervousness, hallucinations, depression,* hyperirritability, paresthesia, paresis, hyperreflexia.
Other: hypersensitivity (allergic dermatitis).

INTERACTIONS
Ethanol or ethionamide: increased risk of CNS toxicity (seizures).
Isoniazid: monitor for CNS toxicity (dizziness or drowsiness).

NURSING CONSIDERATIONS
- *Contraindicated* in seizure disorders, depression or severe anxiety, severe renal insufficiency, or chronic alcoholism.
- *Use cautiously* in impaired renal function; reduced dosage is required.
- Considered a "second-line" drug in the treatment of tuberculosis.
- Obtain specimen for culture and sensitivity tests before therapy begins and periodically thereafter to detect possible resistance.
- Serious neurologic effects can be precipitated by ingestion of alcohol; warn patient to avoid alcohol.
- Toxic reactions may occur with blood levels above 30 mcg/ml.
- Pyridoxine, anticonvulsants, tranquilizers, or sedatives may help to relieve adverse reactions.
- Observe for psychotic symptoms, hallucinations, and possible suicidal tendencies.
- Monitor hematologic tests and renal and liver function studies.
- Instruct patient to take drug exactly as prescribed; warn against discontinuing use without doctor's approval.

dapsone
Avlosulfon†, Dapsone 100‡

Pregnancy Risk Category: C

HOW SUPPLIED
Tablets: 25 mg, 100 mg

MECHANISM OF ACTION
Unknown. May inhibit folic acid biosynthesis in susceptible organisms (bacteriostatic).

INDICATIONS & DOSAGE
All forms of leprosy (Hansen's disease)–
Adults: 100 mg P.O. daily for indefinite period, plus rifampin 600 mg daily for 6 months.
Children: 1.4 mg/kg P.O. daily.
Prophylaxis for leprosy patient's close contacts–
Adults: 50 mg P.O. daily.
Children 6 to 12 years: 25 mg P.O. daily for 3 years.
Children 2 to 5 years: 25 mg P.O. three times weekly for 3 years.
Infants 6 to 23 months: 12 mg P.O. three times weekly for 3 years.
Children under 6 months: 6 mg P.O. three times weekly for 3 years.
Dermatitis herpetiformis–
Adults: 50 mg. P.O. daily; may increase to 400 mg. daily.
Malaria suppression or prophylaxis due to chloroquine-resistant Plasmodium falciparum *when other agents aren't available–*
Adults: 100 mg. P.O. weekly; usually given with pyrimethimine 12.5 mg. P.O. weekly.
Children: 2 mg/kg P.O. weekly, with pyrimethamine 0.25 mg/kg weekly.

*Liquid form contains alcohol. **May contain tartrazine.

Continue prophylaxis during exposure and for 6 weeks after exposure.
Pneumocystis carinii *pneumonia in patients with AIDS* –
Adults: 100 mg P.O. daily in conjunction with trimethoprim 20 mg/kg P.O. daily (usually divided q.i.d.).
Actinomycotic mycetoma –
Adults: 100 mg P.O. b.i.d. Treatment is usually continued for months after clinical symptoms abate.

ADVERSE REACTIONS
Common reactions are in italics; life-threatening reactions are in bold italics.
Blood: ***aplastic anemia, agranulocytosis, hemolytic anemia;*** methemoglobinemia; possible leukopenia.
CNS: insomnia, psychosis, headache, dizziness, lethargy, severe malaise, paresthesia, peripheral neuropathy (with loss of motor function).
EENT: tinnitus, allergic rhinitis.
GI: anorexia, abdominal pain, nausea, vomiting.
Hepatic: hepatitis, cholestatic jaundice.
Skin: allergic dermatitis (generalized or fixed maculopapular rash).

INTERACTIONS
Folic acid antagonists (such as methotrexate): increased risk of adverse hematologic reactions. Avoid concomitant use.
Probenecid: elevates levels of dapsone. Use together with extreme caution.
Rifampin: increased hepatic metabolism of dapsone. Monitor for lack of efficacy.

NURSING CONSIDERATIONS
- *Use cautiously* in chronic renal, hepatic, or CV disease or in refractory types of anemia. Also use cautiously in G6PD deficiency.
- Therapy should be interrupted if generalized, diffuse dermatitis occurs.
- Dapsone dosage should be reduced or temporarily discontinued if hemoglobin falls below 9 g/dl; if leukocyte count falls below 5,000/mm^3; if erythrocyte count falls below 2.5 million/mm^3 or remains low.
- Antihistamines may help to combat dapsone-induced allergic dermatitis.
- Erythema nodosum type of lepra reaction may occur during therapy as a result of *Mycobacterium leprae* bacilli (malaise, fever, painful inflammatory induration in the skin and mucosa, iritis, and neuritis). In severe cases, therapy should be stopped and glucocorticoids given cautiously.
- Obtain CBC before treatment and monitor frequently throughout therapy (weekly for the first month, monthly for 6 months, and semiannually thereafter).
- Also used to treat relapsing polychondritis and as prophylaxis against malaria. Has been used investigationally to treat rheumatoid arthritis, allergic vasculitis, relapsing polychondritis, and postular and inflammatory dermatoses.
- Instruct breast-feeding mothers to report cyanosis in infants, as this indicates high sulfone level.

ethambutol hydrochloride
Etibi†, Myambutol
Pregnancy Risk Category: B

HOW SUPPLIED
Tablets: 100 mg, 400 mg

MECHANISM OF ACTION
Interferes with the synthesis of one or more metabolites of susceptible bacteria, altering cellular metabolism during cell division (bacteriostatic).

INDICATIONS & DOSAGE
Adjunctive treatment in pulmonary tuberculosis –
Adults and children over 13 years: initial treatment for patients who have not received previous antitubercular

therapy is 15 mg/kg P.O. daily single dose.
Re-treatment: 25 mg/kg P.O. daily single dose for 60 days with at least one other antitubercular drug; then decrease to 15 mg/kg P.O. daily single dose.

ADVERSE REACTIONS
Common reactions are in italics; life-threatening reactions are in bold italics.
CNS: headache, dizziness, mental confusion, possible hallucinations, peripheral neuritis (numbness and tingling of extremities).
EENT: optic neuritis (vision loss and loss of color discrimination, especially red and green).
GI: anorexia, nausea, vomiting, abdominal pain.
Metabolic: *elevated uric acid.*
Other: ***anaphylactoid reactions,*** fever, malaise, bloody sputum.

INTERACTIONS
None significant.

NURSING CONSIDERATIONS
- *Contraindicated* in optic neuritis and in children under 13 years.
- *Use cautiously* in impaired renal function, cataracts, recurrent eye inflammations, gout, and diabetic retinopathy.
- Dose must be reduced in renal impairment.
- Perform visual acuity and color discrimination tests before and during therapy.
- Always monitor serum uric acid; observe patient for symptoms of gout.
- Reassure patient that visual disturbances will disappear several weeks to months after drug is stopped.

---

ethionamide
Trecator-SC
Pregnancy Risk Category: D

HOW SUPPLIED
Tablets: 250 mg

MECHANISM OF ACTION
Unknown. Probably inhibits peptide synthesis (bacteriostatic).

INDICATIONS & DOSAGE
Adjunctive treatment in pulmonary or extrapulmonary tuberculosis (when primary therapy with streptomycin or isoniazid cannot be used or has failed) –
Adults: 500 mg to 1 g P.O. daily in divided doses. Concomitant administration of other effective antitubercular drugs and pyridoxine recommended.
Children: 15 to 20 mg/kg P.O. daily in three to four doses. Maximum dosage is 1 g.

ADVERSE REACTIONS
Common reactions are in italics; life-threatening reactions are in bold italics.
Blood: thrombocytopenia.
CNS: asthenia, drowsiness, *peripheral neuritis,* psychic disturbances (especially mental depression).
CV: postural hypotension.
GI: *anorexia,* metallic taste in mouth, nausea, vomiting, sialorrhea, *epigastric distress,* diarrhea, stomatitis, weight loss.
Hepatic: jaundice, hepatitis, elevated AST (SGOT) and ALT (SGPT).
Skin: rash, ***exfoliative dermatitis.***

INTERACTIONS
None significant.

NURSING CONSIDERATIONS
- *Contraindicated* in severe hepatic damage.
- *Use cautiously* in diabetes mellitus.
- Culture and sensitivity tests should be performed before starting therapy. Stop drug if skin rash occurs; may progress to exfoliative dermatitis.
- Monitor hepatic function every 2 to 4 weeks.

• Give with meals or antacids to minimize GI effects. Patient may require antiemetic.
• Pyridoxine may be ordered to prevent neuropathy.
• Instruct patient to take this drug exactly as prescribed; warn against discontinuing drug without doctor's consent.
• Warn patient to avoid excess alcohol ingestion because it may make him more vulnerable to liver damage.

isoniazid (INH)

DOW-Isoniazid, Isotamine†, Laniazid-C.T., Nydrazid**, PMS-Isoniazid†

Pregnancy Risk Category: C

HOW SUPPLIED

Tablets: 50 mg, 100 mg, 300 mg
Oral solution: 50 mg/5 ml
Injection: 100 mg/ml

MECHANISM OF ACTION

Inhibits cell wall biosynthesis by interfering with lipid and DNA synthesis (bactericidal).

INDICATIONS & DOSAGE

Primary treatment against actively growing tubercle bacilli –
Adults: 5 mg/kg P.O. or I.M. daily single dose, up to 300 mg/day, continued for 6 months to 2 years.
Infants and children: 10 to 20 mg/kg P.O. or I.M. daily single dose, up to 300 to 500 mg/day, continued for 18 months to 2 years. Concomitant administration of at least one other effective antitubercular drug is recommended.
Preventive therapy against tubercle bacilli of those closely exposed or those with positive skin test whose chest X-rays and bacteriologic studies are consistent with nonprogressive tuberculous disease –
Adults: 300 mg P.O. daily single dose, continued for 1 year.
Infants and children: 10 mg/kg P.O. daily single dose, up to 300 mg/day, continued for 1 year.

ADVERSE REACTIONS

Common reactions are in italics; life-threatening reactions are in bold italics.
Blood: ***agranulocytosis, hemolytic anemia, aplastic anemia,*** eosinophilia, leukopenia, neutropenia, thrombocytopenia, methemoglobinemia, pyridoxine-responsive hypochromic anemia.
CNS: *peripheral neuropathy* (especially in the malnourished, alcoholics, diabetics, and slow acetylators), usually preceded by paresthesias of hands and feet, psychosis.
GI: nausea, vomiting, epigastric distress, constipation, dryness of the mouth.
Hepatic: ***hepatitis, occasionally severe and sometimes fatal, especially in elderly patients.***
Metabolic: hyperglycemia, metabolic acidosis.
Local: irritation at I.M. injection site.
Other: rheumatic syndrome and systemic lupus erythematosus-like syndrome; hypersensitivity (fever, rash, lymphadenopathy, vasculitis).

INTERACTIONS

Aluminum-containing antacids and laxatives: may decrease the rate and amount of isoniazid absorbed. Give isoniazid at least 1 hour before antacid or laxative.
Carbamazepine: increased risk of isoniazid hepatotoxicity. Use together very cautiously.
Corticosteroids: may decrease therapeutic effectiveness. Monitor need for larger isoniazid dose.
Disulfiram: neurologic symptoms, including changes in behavior and coordination, may develop with concomitant isoniazid use. Avoid concomitant use.

NURSING CONSIDERATIONS

- *Contraindicated* in acute hepatic disease or isoniazid-associated hepatic damage.
- *Use cautiously* in chronic non-isoniazid-associated hepatic disease, seizure disorders (especially those taking phenytoin), severe renal impairment, and chronic alcoholism and in elderly patients.
- Isoniazid pharmacokinetics may vary among patients, since its metabolism occurs in the liver by genetically controlled acetylation. Fast acetylators metabolize the drug up to five times as fast as slow acetylators. About 50% of blacks and whites are slow acetylators; over 80% of Chinese, Japanese, and Eskimos are fast acetylators.
- Monitor hepatic function. Tell patient to notify doctor immediately if symptoms of hepatic impairment occur (loss of appetite, fatigue, malaise, jaundice, dark urine).
- Alcohol may be associated with increased incidence of isoniazid-related hepatitis. Advise against use.
- Pyridoxine should be given to prevent peripheral neuropathy, especially in malnourished patients.
- Instruct patient to take this drug exactly as prescribed; warn against discontinuing drug without doctor's consent.
- Encourage patient to fully comply with treatment, which may take months or years.
- Advise patient to take with food if GI irritation occurs.
- Reportedly effective when used investigationally to treat arthritis and action tremor in multiple sclerosis.

pyrazinamide

PMS Pyrazinamide†, Tebrazid†, Zinamide‡

Pregnancy Risk Category: C

HOW SUPPLIED

Tablets: 500 mg

MECHANISM OF ACTION

Unknown (bacteriostatic).

INDICATIONS & DOSAGE

Adjunctive treatment of tuberculosis (when primary and secondary antitubercular drugs cannot be used or have failed) –

Adults: 20 to 35 mg/kg P.O. daily, divided in three to four doses. Maximum dosage is 3 g daily.

ADVERSE REACTIONS

Common reactions are in italics; life-threatening reactions are in bold italics.

Blood: sideroblastic anemia, possible bleeding tendency due to thrombocytopenia.

GI: anorexia, nausea, vomiting, diarrhea.

GU: dysuria.

Hepatic: hepatitis.

Metabolic: interference with control in diabetes mellitus, *hyperuricemia.*

Other: malaise, fever, arthralgia.

INTERACTIONS

None significant.

NURSING CONSIDERATIONS

- *Contraindicated* in severe hepatic disease.
- *Use cautiously* in diabetes mellitus or gout.
- Nearly 100% excreted in urine; reduced dose needed in patients with renal impairment.
- Perform liver function studies and examination for jaundice, liver tenderness, or enlargement before and frequently during therapy.
- Watch closely for signs of gout and of hepatic impairment (loss of appetite, fatigue, malaise, jaundice, dark urine, and liver tenderness). Notify doctor at once.
- Question doses that exceed 35 mg/kg, as they may cause liver damage.

• Monitor hematopoietic studies and serum uric acid.
• When used with surgical management of tuberculosis, start pyrazinamide 1 to 2 weeks before surgery and continue for 4 to 6 weeks postoperatively.

rifampin (rifampicin)

Rifadin, Rimactane, Rimycin‡, Rofact†

Pregnancy Risk Category: C

HOW SUPPLIED
Capsules: 150 mg, 300 mg
Kit: 60 capsules, 300 mg
Injection: 600 mg

MECHANISM OF ACTION
Inhibits DNA-dependent RNA polymerase, thus impairing RNA synthesis (bactericidal).

INDICATIONS & DOSAGE
Primary treatment in pulmonary tuberculosis –
Adults: 600 mg P.O. or I.V. daily single dose 1 hour before or 2 hours after meals.
Children over 5 years: 10 to 20 mg/kg P.O. or I.V. daily single dose 1 hour before or 2 hours after meals. Maximum dosage is 600 mg daily. Concomitant administration of other effective antitubercular drugs is recommended.
Meningococcal carriers –
Adults: 600 mg P.O. or I.V. b.i.d. for 2 days.
Children 1 month to 12 years: 10 mg/kg P.O. or I.V. b.i.d. for 2 days, not to exceed 600 mg/dose.
Infants under 1 month: 5 mg/kg P.O. or I.V. b.i.d. for 2 days.
Prophylaxis of Haemophilus influenzae *type b –*
Adults and children: 20 mg/kg P.O. daily for 4 days. Do not exceed 600 mg/day.

ADVERSE REACTIONS
Common reactions are in italics; life-threatening reactions are in bold italics.
Blood: eosinophilia, thrombocytopenia, transient leukopenia, ***hemolytic anemia.***
CNS: headache, fatigue, *drowsiness,* ataxia, dizziness, mental confusion, generalized numbness.
GI: epigastric distress, anorexia, nausea, vomiting, abdominal pain, diarrhea, flatulence, sore mouth and tongue.
Metabolic: hyperuricemia.
Hepatic: ***serious hepatotoxicity*** *as well as transient abnormalities in liver function tests.*
Skin: pruritus, urticaria, rash.
Other: flu-like syndrome, discoloration of body fluids.

INTERACTIONS
Alcohol: may increase risk of hepatotoxicity.
Para-aminosalicylate sodium, ketoconazole: may interfere with absorption of rifampin. Give these drugs 8 to 12 hours apart.
Probenecid: may increase rifampin levels. Use cautiously.

NURSING CONSIDERATIONS
• *Contraindicated* in clinically active hepatitis.
• *Use cautiously* in hepatic disease or in those receiving other hepatotoxic drugs.
• Monitor hepatic function, hematopoietic studies, and serum uric acid.
• Watch closely for signs of hepatic impairment (loss of appetite, fatigue, malaise, jaundice, dark urine, liver tenderness). Notify doctor if these occur.
• Warn patient about drowsiness and the possibility of red-orange discoloration of urine, feces, saliva, sweat, sputum, and tears. Soft contact lenses may be permanently stained.
• Rifampin is not considered a teratogen. However, it may cause hemor-

rhaging in neonates of rifampin-treated mothers.

- Advise patient to avoid alcoholic beverages while taking this drug. May increase risk of hepatotoxicity.
- Give 1 hour before or 2 hours after meals for optimal absorption; however, if GI irritation occurs, patient may take rifampin with meals.
- Increases enzyme activity of liver; may require increased doses of warfarin, corticosteroids, oral contraceptives, and oral hypoglycemics. See each drug entry for specific drug interactions.
- Concomitant treatment with at least one other antitubercular drug is recommended.
- **I.V. use:** Reconstitute vial with 10 ml sterile water for injection to make a solution containing 60 mg/ml. Add to 100 ml dextrose 5% in water and infuse over 30 minutes, or add to 500 ml dextrose 5% in water and infuse over 3 hours. When dextrose is contraindicated, drug may be diluted with 0.9% sodium chloride injection. Do not use other I.V. solutions.

*Liquid form contains alcohol. **May contain tartrazine.

11

Aminoglycosides

amikacin sulfate
gentamicin sulfate
kanamycin sulfate
neomycin sulfate
netilmicin sulfate
streptomycin sulfate
tobramycin sulfate

COMBINATION PRODUCTS
NEOSPORIN G.U. IRRIGANT: 40 mg neomycin sulfate and 200,000 units polymixin B sulfate/ml.

amikacin sulfate

Amikin

Pregnancy Risk Category: C

HOW SUPPLIED
Injection: 50 mg/ml, 250 mg/ml

MECHANISM OF ACTION
Inhibits protein synthesis by binding directly to the 30S ribosomal subunit. Generally bactericidal.

INDICATIONS & DOSAGE
Serious infections caused by sensitive Pseudomonas aeruginosa, Escherichia coli, Proteus, Klebsiella, Serratia, Enterobacter, Acinetobacter, Providencia, Citrobacter, Staphylococcus –
Adults and children with normal renal function: 15 mg/kg/day divided q 8 to 12 hours I.M. or I.V. infusion (in 100 to 200 ml dextrose 5% in water run in over 30 to 60 minutes). May be given by direct I.V. push if necessary.
Neonates with normal renal function: initially, 10 mg/kg I.M. or I.V. infusion (in dextrose 5% in water run in over 1 to 2 hours), then 7.5 mg/kg q 12 hours I.M. or I.V. infusion.
Meningitis –
Adults: systemic therapy as above; may also use up to 20 mg intrathecally or intraventricularly daily.
Children: systemic therapy as above; may also use 1 to 2 mg intrathecally daily.
Uncomplicated urinary tract infections –
Adults: 250 mg I.M. or I.V. b.i.d.
Adults with impaired renal function: initially, 7.5 mg/kg. Subsequent doses and frequency determined by blood amikacin levels and renal function studies.

ADVERSE REACTIONS
Common reactions are in italics; life-threatening reactions are in bold italics.
CNS: headache, lethargy, ***neuromuscular blockade.***
EENT: *ototoxicity (tinnitus, vertigo, hearing loss).*
GU: *nephrotoxicity (cells or casts in urine, oliguria, proteinuria, decreased creatinine clearance, increased BUN and serum creatinine levels).*
Other: ***hypersensitivity reactions, hepatic necrosis.***

INTERACTIONS
Cephalothin: increased nephrotoxicity. Use together cautiously.
Dimenhydrinate: may mask symptoms of ototoxicity. Use with caution.
General anesthetics, neuromuscular blocking agents: may potentiate neuromuscular blockade.
I.V. loop diuretics (such as furosemide): increase ototoxicity. Use cautiously.
Other aminoglycosides, amphotericin B, cisplatin, methoxyflurane: increases nephrotoxicity. Use together cautiously.
Parenteral penicillins (such as carben-

icillin and ticarcillin): amikacin inactivation in vitro. Don't mix together in I.V.

NURSING CONSIDERATIONS

- *Use cautiously* in impaired renal function, in neonates and infants, and in elderly patients.
- Obtain specimen for culture and sensitivity tests before first dose. Therapy may begin pending test results.
- Weigh patient and obtain baseline renal function studies before therapy begins.
- Monitor renal function (output, specific gravity, urinalysis, BUN and creatinine levels, and creatinine clearance). Notify doctor of signs of decreasing renal function.
- Patient should be well hydrated while taking drug to minimize chemical irritation of the renal tubules.
- Evaluate patient's hearing before and during therapy. Notify doctor if patient complains of tinnitus, vertigo, or hearing loss.
- Watch for superinfection (continued fever and other signs of new infections, especially of upper respiratory tract).
- Usual duration of therapy is 7 to 10 days. If no response after 3 to 5 days, therapy may be stopped and new specimens obtained for culture and sensitivity.
- Peak blood levels that are above 35 mcg/ml and trough levels that are above 10 mcg/ml may be associated with higher incidence of toxicity.
- **I.V. use:** After I.V. infusion, flush line with normal saline solution or dextrose 5% in water.
- Draw blood for peak amikacin level 1 hour after I.M. injection and 30 minutes to 1 hour after infusion ends; for trough levels, draw blood just before next dose. Don't collect blood in a heparinized tube because heparin is incompatible with aminoglycosides.
- Potency of drug is not affected if solution turns light yellow.

gentamicin sulfate

Cidomycin†‡, Garamycin, Gentafair, Jenamicin

Pregnancy Risk Category: C

HOW SUPPLIED

Injection: 40 mg/ml (adult), 10 mg/ml (pediatric), 2 mg/ml (intrathecal)

MECHANISM OF ACTION

Inhibits protein synthesis by binding directly to the 30S ribosomal subunit. Generally bactericidal.

INDICATIONS & DOSAGE

Serious infections caused by sensitive Pseudomonas aeruginosa, Escherichia coli, Proteus, Klebsiella, Serratia, Enterobacter, Citrobacter, Staphylococcus –

Adults with normal renal function: 3 mg/kg daily in divided doses q 8 hours I.M. or I.V. infusion (in 50 to 200 ml of normal saline solution or dextrose 5% in water infused over 30 minutes to 2 hours). May be given by direct I.V. push if necessary. For life-threatening infections, patient may receive up to 5 mg/kg daily in 3 to 4 divided doses.

Children with normal renal function: 2 to 2.5 mg/kg I.M. or I.V. infusion q 8 hours.

Infants and neonates over 1 week with normal renal function: 2.5 mg/kg q 8 hours I.M. or I.V. infusion.

Neonates under 1 week: 2.5 mg/kg I.V. q 12 hours. For I.V. infusion, dilute in normal saline solution or dextrose 5% in water and infuse over 30 minutes to 2 hours.

Meningitis –

Adults: systemic therapy as above; may also use 4 to 8 mg intrathecally daily.

Children: systemic therapy as above;

*Liquid form contains alcohol. **May contain tartrazine.

may also use 1 to 2 mg intrathecally daily.
Endocarditis prophylaxis for GI or GU procedure or surgery –
Adults: 1.5 mg/kg I.M. or I.V. 30 minutes before procedure or surgery. Maximum dose is 80 mg. Given with ampicillin (vancomycin in penicillin-allergic patients). Repeat in 8 hours.
Children: 2.5 mg/kg I.M. or I.V. 30 minutes before procedure or surgery. Maximum dose should not exceed 80 mg. Given with ampicillin (vancomycin in penicillin-allergic patients). After 8 hours, give half the initial dose.
Patients with impaired renal function: initial dose is same as for those with normal renal function. Subsequent doses and frequency determined by renal function studies and serum concentrations of gentamicin.
Posthemodialysis to maintain therapeutic blood levels –
Adults: 1 to 1.7 mg/kg I.M. or I.V. infusion after each dialysis.
Children: 2 mg/kg I.M. or I.V. infusion after each dialysis.

ADVERSE REACTIONS

Common reactions are in italics; life-threatening reactions are in bold italics.
CNS: headache, lethargy, ***neuromuscular blockade.***
EENT: *ototoxicity (tinnitus, vertigo, hearing loss).*
GU: *nephrotoxicity (cells or casts in the urine; oliguria; proteinuria; decreased creatinine clearance; increased BUN, nonprotein nitrogen, and serum creatinine levels).*
Other: ***hypersensitivity reactions, hepatic necrosis.***

INTERACTIONS

Cephalothin: increases nephrotoxicity. Use together cautiously.
Dimenhydrinate: may mask symptoms of ototoxicity. Use with caution.
General anesthetics, neuromuscular blockers: may potentiate neuromuscular blockade.
I.V. loop diuretics (such as furosemide): increase ototoxicity. Use cautiously.
Other aminoglycosides, methoxyflurane: increase ototoxicity and nephrotoxicity. Use together cautiously.
Parenteral penicillins (such as carbenicillin and ticarcillin): gentamicin inactivation in vitro. Don't combine in I.V.

NURSING CONSIDERATIONS

- *Use cautiously* in impaired renal function and in neonates, infants, and elderly patients.
- Obtain specimen for culture and sensitivity tests before first dose. Therapy may begin pending test results.
- Weigh patient and obtain baseline renal function studies before therapy begins.
- Monitor renal function (output, specific gravity, urinalysis, BUN and creatinine levels, and creatinine clearance). Notify doctor of signs of decreasing renal function.
- Patient should be well hydrated while taking drug to minimize chemical irritation of the renal tubules.
- **I.V. use:** After completing I.V. infusion, flush the line with normal saline solution or dextrose 5% in water.
- Evaluate patient's hearing before and during therapy. Notify doctor if patient complains of tinnitus, vertigo, or hearing loss.
- Watch for superinfection (continued fever and other signs of new infections, especially of upper respiratory tract).
- Usual duration of therapy is 7 to 10 days. If no response in 3 to 5 days, therapy may be stopped and new specimens obtained for culture and sensitivity.
- Peak blood levels above 12 mcg/ml and trough levels (those drawn just before next dose) above 2 mcg/ml

may be associated with higher incidence of toxicity.

- Draw blood for peak gentamicin level 1 hour after I.M. injection and 30 minutes to 1 hour after infusion ends; for trough levels, draw blood just before next dose. Don't collect blood in a heparinized tube because heparin is incompatible with aminoglycosides.
- Hemodialysis (8 hours) removes up to 50% of drug from blood.
- Intrathecal form (without preservatives) should be used when intrathecal administration is indicated.

kanamycin sulfate

Kanasig‡, Kantrex, Klebcil

Pregnancy Risk Category: D

HOW SUPPLIED

Capsules: 500 mg

Injection: 37.5 mg/ml (pediatric), 250 mg/ml, 333 mg/ml

MECHANISM OF ACTION

Inhibits protein synthesis by binding directly to the 30S ribosomal subunit. Generally bactericidal.

INDICATIONS & DOSAGE

Serious infections caused by sensitive Escherichia coli, Proteus, Enterobacter aerogenes, Klebsiella pneumoniae, Serratia marcescens, Acinetobacter –

Adults and children with normal renal function: 15 mg/kg daily divided q 8 to 12 hours deep I.M. into upper outer quadrant of buttocks or I.V. infusion (diluted 500 mg/200 ml of 0.9% sodium chloride solution or dextrose 5% in water infused at 60 to 80 drops/minute). Maximum daily dosage is 1.5 g.

Neonates: 15 mg/kg daily I.M. or I.V. divided q 12 hours.

Adjunctive treatment in hepatic coma –

Adults: 8 to 12 g daily P.O. in divided doses.

Preoperative bowel sterilization –

Adults: 1 g P.O. q 1 hour for four doses, then q 4 hours for four doses; or 1 g P.O. q 1 hour for four doses, then q 6 hours for 36 to 72 hours.

Intraperitoneal irrigation –

500 mg in 20 ml sterile distilled water instilled via catheter into wound after patient is fully recovered from anesthesia and neuromuscular blocker effects.

Wound irrigation –

Up to 2.5 mg/ml in 0.9% sodium chloride solution irrigant.

ADVERSE REACTIONS

Common reactions are in italics; life-threatening reactions are in bold italics.

CNS: headache, lethargy, ***neuromuscular blockade.***

EENT: *ototoxicity (tinnitus, vertigo, hearing loss).*

GU: *nephrotoxicity (cells or casts in the urine, oliguria, proteinuria, decreased creatinine clearance, increased BUN and serum creatinine levels).*

Other: ***hypersensitivity reactions.***

INTERACTIONS

Cephalothin: increases nephrotoxicity. Use together cautiously.

Dimenhydrinate: may mask symptoms of ototoxicity. Use with caution.

General anesthetics, neuromuscular blocking agents: may potentiate neuromuscular blockade.

I.V. loop diuretics (such as furosemide): increase ototoxicity. Use cautiously.

Other aminoglycosides, amphotericin B, cisplatin, methoxyflurane: increases nephrotoxicity. Don't use together.

Parenteral penicillins (such as carbenicillin and ticarcillin): kanamycin inactivation in vitro. Don't combine in I.V.

NURSING CONSIDERATIONS

- *Contraindicated* for oral use in intestinal obstruction and treatment of systemic infection.
- *Use cautiously* in patients with impaired renal function and in elderly patients.
- Obtain specimen for culture and sensitivity tests before first dose. Therapy may begin pending test results.
- Weigh patient and obtain baseline renal function studies before therapy.
- **I.V. use:** Dilute 500 mg of the drug per 200 ml of normal saline solution or dextrose 5% in water and infuse at 60 to 80 drops/minute.
- Monitor renal function (output, specific gravity, urinalysis, BUN and creatinine levels, and creatinine clearance). Notify doctor of signs of decreasing renal function.
- Patient should be well hydrated while taking drug to minimize chemical irritation of the renal tubules.
- Evaluate patient's hearing before and during therapy. Notify doctor if patient complains of tinnitus, vertigo, or hearing loss.
- Watch for superinfection (continued fever and other signs of new infection, especially of upper respiratory tract).
- If no response in 3 to 5 days, therapy may be stopped and new specimens obtained for culture and sensitivity.
- Peak blood levels over 30 mcg/ml and trough levels over 10 mcg/ml may be associated with increased incidence of toxicity.

neomycin sulfate

Mycifradin, Neosulf‡

Pregnancy Risk Category: C

HOW SUPPLIED

Tablets: 500 mg
Oral solution: 125 mg/5 ml

MECHANISM OF ACTION

Inhibits protein synthesis by binding directly to the 30S ribosomal subunit. Generally bactericidal.

INDICATIONS & DOSAGE

Infectious diarrhea caused by enteropathogenic Escherichia coli –
Adults: 50 mg/kg daily P.O. in four divided doses for 2 to 3 days.
Children: 50 to 100 mg/kg daily P.O. divided q 4 to 6 hours for 2 to 3 days.
Suppression of intestinal bacteria preoperatively –
Adults: 1 g P.O. q 1 hour for four doses, then 1 g q 4 hours for the balance of the 24 hours. A saline cathartic should precede therapy.
Children: 40 to 100 mg/kg daily P.O. divided q 4 to 6 hours. First dose should follow saline cathartic.
Adjunctive treatment in hepatic coma –
Adults: 1 to 3 g P.O. q.i.d. for 5 to 6 days; or 200 ml of 1% or 100 ml of 2% solution as enema retained for 20 to 60 minutes q 6 hours.

ADVERSE REACTIONS

Common reactions are in italics; life-threatening reactions are in bold italics.
CNS: headache, lethargy.
EENT: *ototoxicity (tinnitus, vertigo, hearing loss).*
GI: nausea, vomiting.
GU: *nephrotoxicity (cells or casts in the urine, oliguria, proteinuria, decreased creatinine clearance, increased BUN and serum creatinine levels).*
Skin: rash, urticaria.
Other: ***hypersensitivity reactions.***

INTERACTIONS

Cephalothin: Increases nephrotoxicity. Use together cautiously.
Dimenhydrinate: may mask symptoms of ototoxicity. Use with caution.
I.V. loop diuretics (such as furosemide): increase ototoxicity. Use cautiously.

Oral anticoagulants: oral neomycin inhibits vitamin K-producing bacteria and may potentiate anticoagulant effect.
Other aminoglycosides, amphotericin B, cisplatin, methoxyflurane: increases nephrotoxicity. Use together cautiously.

NURSING CONSIDERATIONS

- *Contraindicated* in intestinal obstruction.
- *Use cautiously* in impaired renal function, in ulcerative bowel lesions, and in elderly patients. Never administer parenterally.
- The ototoxic and nephrotoxic properties of neomycin limit its usefulness. Limited absorption prevents substantial systemic effects.
- Nonabsorbable at recommended dosage. However, more than 4 g/day may be systemically absorbed and lead to nephrotoxicity.
- Weigh patient and obtain baseline renal function studies before therapy begins.
- Obtain specimen for culture and sensitivity tests before first dose. Therapy may begin pending test results.
- Watch for superinfection (fever or other signs of new infection).
- Monitor renal function (output, specific gravity, urinalysis, BUN and creatinine levels, and creatinine clearance). Notify doctor of signs of decreasing renal function.
- Patient should be well hydrated while taking drug to minimize chemical irritation of the renal tubules.
- Watch for respiratory depression in patients with renal disease, hypocalcemia, or neuromuscular diseases, such as myasthenia gravis.
- Evaluate hearing of patient with hepatic or renal disease before and during prolonged therapy. Notify doctor if patient complains of tinnitus, vertigo, or hearing loss. Onset of deafness may occur several weeks after drug is stopped.
- An adjunctive treatment of hepatic coma, neomycin is used to decrease ammonia-producing flora in the GI tract. During such treatment, decrease patient's dietary protein and assess neurologic status frequently.
- For preoperative disinfection, provide a low-residue diet and a cathartic immediately before oral administration of neomycin.
- Available in combination with polymyxin B as a urinary bladder irrigant.

netilmicin sulfate

Netromycin

Pregnancy Risk Category: C

HOW SUPPLIED

Injection: 10 mg/ml, 25 mg/ml, 100 mg/ml

MECHANISM OF ACTION

Inhibits protein synthesis by binding directly to the 30S ribosomal subunit. Generally bactericidal.

INDICATIONS & DOSAGE

Serious infections caused by sensitive Pseudomonas aeruginosa, Escherichia coli, Proteus, Klebsiella, Serratia, Enterobacter, Citrobacter, Staphylococcus –
Adults and children over 12 years: 3 to 6.5 mg/kg/day by I.M. injection or I.V. infusion. May be given q 12 hours to treat serious urinary tract infections and q 8 to 12 hours to treat serious systemic infections.
Infants and children 6 weeks to 12 years: 5.5 to 8 mg/kg/day by I.M. injection or I.V. infusion given either as 1.8 to 2.7 mg/kg q 8 hours or as 2.7 to 4 mg/kg q 12 hours.
Neonates under 6 weeks: 4 to 6.5 mg/kg/day by I.M. injection or I.V. infusion given as 2 to 3.25 mg/kg q 12 hours.
Patients with impaired renal func-

*Liquid form contains alcohol. **May contain tartrazine.

tion: Initial dose is the same as for patients with normal renal function. Subsequent doses and frequency are determined by renal function and serum concentration of netilmicin.

ADVERSE REACTIONS
Common reactions are in italics; life-threatening reactions are in bold italics.
CNS: headache, lethargy, ***neuromuscular blockade.***
EENT: *ototoxicity (tinnitus, vertigo, hearing loss).*
GU: *nephrotoxicity (cells or casts in the urine; oliguria; proteinuria; decreased creatinine clearance; increased BUN, nonprotein nitrogen, and serum creatinine levels).*
Other: *hypersensitivity reactions.*

INTERACTIONS
Cephalothin: increases nephrotoxicity. Use together cautiously.
Dimenhydrinate: may mask symptoms of ototoxicity. Use cautiously.
General anesthetics, neuromuscular blocking agents: may potentiate neuromuscular blockade.
I.V. loop diuretics (such as furosemide): increase ototoxicity. Use cautiously.
Other aminoglycosides, amphotericin B, cisplatin, methoxyflurane: increases nephrotoxicity. Use together cautiously.
Parenteral penicillins (such as carbenicillin and ticarcillin): netilmicin inactivation. Don't mix together in I.V.

NURSING CONSIDERATIONS
- *Use cautiously* in impaired renal function and in neonates, infants, and elderly patients.
- Obtain specimen for culture and sensitivity tests before first dose. Therapy may begin pending test results.
- Weigh patient and obtain baseline renal function studies before therapy begins.
- Monitor renal function (output, specific gravity, urinalysis, BUN and creatinine levels, and creatinine clearance). Notify doctor of signs of decreasing renal function.
- Patient should be well hydrated while taking drug to minimize chemical irritation of the renal tubules.
- Watch for superinfection (continued fever and other signs of new infections, especially of upper respiratory tract).
- Usual duration of therapy is 7 to 10 days. If no response in 3 to 5 days, therapy may be stopped and new specimens obtained for culture and sensitivity.
- **I.V. use:** After completing I.V. infusion, flush the line with normal saline solution or dextrose 5% in water.
- Peak blood levels above 16 mcg/ml and trough levels (those drawn just before next dose) above 4 mcg/ml may be associated with higher incidence of toxicity.
- Draw blood for peak netilmicin level 1 hour after I.M. injection and 30 minutes to 1 hour after infusion ends; for trough levels, draw blood just before next dose. Don't draw blood in a heparinized tube because heparin is incompatible with aminoglycosides.
- Evaluate patient's hearing before and during therapy. Notify doctor if patient complains of tinnitus, vertigo, or hearing loss. However, some studies show that this drug is less ototoxic than other aminoglycosides.

streptomycin sulfate

Pregnancy Risk Category: D

HOW SUPPLIED
Injection: 400 mg/ml, 500 mg/ml, 1-g vial, 5-g vial

MECHANISM OF ACTION
Inhibits protein synthesis by binding directly to the 30S ribosomal subunit. Generally bactericidal.

INDICATIONS & DOSAGE

Streptococcal endocarditis–
Adults: 10 mg/kg I.M. (maximum 0.5 g) q 12 hours for 2 weeks with penicillin.
Primary and adjunctive treatment in tuberculosis–
Adults: with normal renal function, 1 g I.M. daily for 2 to 3 months, then 1 g 2 or 3 times a week. Inject deeply into upper outer quadrant of buttocks.
Children: with normal renal function, 20 mg/kg daily in divided doses injected deeply into large muscle mass. Give concurrently with other antitubercular agents, but *not* with capreomycin, and continue until sputum specimen becomes negative.
Patients with impaired renal function: initial dose is same as for those with normal renal function. Subsequent doses and frequency determined by renal function study results.
Enterococcal endocarditis–
Adults: 1 g I.M. q 12 hours for 2 weeks, then 500 mg I.M. q 12 hours for 4 weeks with penicillin.
Tularemia–
Adults: 1 to 2 g I.M. daily in divided doses injected deep into upper outer quadrant of buttocks. Continue until patient is afebrile for 5 to 7 days.

ADVERSE REACTIONS

Common reactions are in italics; life-threatening reactions are in bold italics.
CNS: ***neuromuscular blockade.***
EENT: *ototoxicity (tinnitus, vertigo, hearing loss).*
GU: some nephrotoxicity (not nearly as frequent as with other aminoglycosides).
Local: pain, irritation, and sterile abscesses at injection site.
Skin: ***exfoliative dermatitis.***
Other: ***hypersensitivity*** (rash, fever, urticaria, and angioneurotic edema), headache, ***transient agranulocytosis.***

INTERACTIONS

Cephalothin: increases nephrotoxicity. Use together cautiously.
Dimenhydrinate: may mask symptoms of streptomycin-induced ototoxicity. Use together cautiously.
General anesthetics, neuromuscular blockers: may potentiate neuromuscular blockade.
I.V. loop diuretics (such as furosemide): increase ototoxicity. Use cautiously.

NURSING CONSIDERATIONS

- *Contraindicated* in labyrinthine disease. Never administer I.V.
- *Use cautiously* in impaired renal function and in the elderly.
- Obtain specimen for culture and sensitivity tests before first dose except when treating tuberculosis. Therapy may begin pending test results.
- Patient should be well hydrated while taking drug to minimize chemical irritation of the renal tubules.
- Evaluate patient's hearing before, during, and 6 months after therapy. Notify doctor if patient complains of hearing loss, roaring noises, or fullness in ears.
- Watch for superinfection (continued fever and other signs of new infections).
- Protect hands when preparing. Drug is irritating.
- Endocarditis prophylaxis is recommended for all patients with rheumatic or congenital heart disease or with prosthetic heart valve. Patients should receive prophylactic antibiotics during GI or GU procedures or surgery.
- In primary treatment of tuberculosis, streptomycin is discontinued when sputum becomes negative.
- Draw blood for peak streptomycin level 1 to 2 hours after I.M. injection; for trough levels, draw blood just before next dose. Don't use a heparinized tube because heparin is incompatible with aminoglycosides.

tobramycin sulfate

Nebcin

Pregnancy Risk Category: D

HOW SUPPLIED

Injection: 40 mg/ml, 10 mg/ml (pediatric)

MECHANISM OF ACTION

Inhibits protein synthesis by binding directly to the 30S ribosomal subunit. Generally bactericidal.

INDICATIONS & DOSAGE

Serious infections caused by sensitive strains of Escherichia coli, Proteus, Klebsiella, Enterobacter, Serratia, Staphylococcus aureus, Pseudomonas, Citrobacter, Providencia –

Adults and children with normal renal function: 3 mg/kg I.M. or I.V. daily divided q 8 hours. Up to 5 mg/kg I.M. or I.V. daily divided q 6 to 8 hours for life-threatening infections.

Neonates under 1 week: up to 4 mg/kg I.M. or I.V. daily divided q 12 hours. For I.V. use, dilute in 50 to 100 ml normal saline solution or dextrose 5% in water for adults and in less volume for children. Infuse over 20 to 60 minutes.

Patients with impaired renal function: initial dose is same as for those with normal renal function. Subsequent doses and frequency determined by renal function and serum concentrations of tobramycin.

ADVERSE REACTIONS

Common reactions are in italics; life-threatening reactions are in bold italics.

CNS: headache, lethargy, ***neuromuscular blockade.***

EENT: *ototoxicity (tinnitus, vertigo, hearing loss).*

GU: *nephrotoxicity (cells or casts in the urine, oliguria, proteinuria, decreased creatinine clearance, increased BUN and serum creatinine levels).*

Other: ***hypersensitivity reactions.***

INTERACTIONS

Cephalothin: increase nephrotoxicity. Use together cautiously.

Dimenhydrinate: may mask symptoms of ototoxicity. Use with caution.

General anesthetics, neuromuscular blocking agents: may potentiate neuromuscular blockade.

I.V. loop diuretics (such as furosemide): increase ototoxicity. Use cautiously.

Other aminoglycosides, amphotericin B, cisplatin, methoxyflurane: increases nephrotoxicity. Use together cautiously.

Parenteral penicillins (such as carbenicillin and ticarcillin): tobramycin inactivation in vitro. Don't combine in I.V.

NURSING CONSIDERATIONS

- *Use cautiously* in impaired renal function and in elderly patients.
- Obtain specimen for culture and sensitivity tests before first dose. Therapy may begin pending test results.
- Weigh patient and obtain baseline renal function studies before starting therapy.
- Usual duration of therapy is 7 to 10 days.
- Monitor renal function (output, specific gravity, urinalysis, BUN and creatinine levels, and creatinine clearance). Notify doctor of signs of decreasing renal function.
- Patient should be well hydrated while taking drug to minimize chemical irritation of the renal tubules.
- Evaluate patient's hearing before and during therapy. Notify doctor if patient complains of tinnitus, vertigo, or hearing loss.
- Watch for superinfection (continued fever and other signs of new infections).
- **I.V. use:** Dilute in 50 to 100 ml normal saline solution or dextrose 5% in

water for adults and in less volume for children. Infuse over 20 to 60 minutes. After I.V. infusion, flush line with normal saline solution or dextrose 5% in water.

• Peak blood levels over 12 mcg/ml and trough levels above 2 mcg/ml may be associated with increased incidence of toxicity.

• Draw blood for peak tobramycin level 1 hour after I.M. injection and 30 minutes to 1 hour after infusion ends; draw blood for trough level just before next dose. Don't collect blood in a heparinized tube because heparin is incompatible with aminoglycosides.

12

Penicillins

amoxicillin/clavulanate potassium
amoxicillin trihydrate
ampicillin
ampicillin sodium
ampicillin trihydrate
ampicillin sodium/sulbactam sodium
bacampicillin hydrochloride
carbenicillin indanyl sodium
cloxacillin sodium
dicloxacillin sodium
methicillin sodium
mezlocillin sodium
nafcillin sodium
oxacillin sodium
penicillin G benzathine
penicillin G potassium
penicillin G procaine
penicillin G sodium
penicillin V
penicillin V potassium
piperacillin sodium
ticarcillin disodium
ticarcillin disodium/clavulanate potassium

COMBINATION PRODUCTS

AUGMENTIN, CLAVULIN†: amoxicillin 250 mg and clavulanate potassium 125 mg per tablet; amoxicillin 500 mg and clavulanate potassium 125 mg per tablet; amoxicillin 125 mg and clavulanate potassium 31.5 mg per 5 ml oral suspension; amoxicillin 250 mg and clavulanate potassium 62.5 mg per 5 ml oral suspension; amoxicillin 125 mg and clavulanate potassium 31.5 mg per chewable tablet; amoxicillin 250 mg and clavulanate potassium 62.5 mg per chewable tablet.
POLYCILLIN-PRB: ampicillin trihydrate 3.5 g and probenecid 1g per bottle.
PRINCIPEN WITH PROBENECID: ampicillin trihydrate 3.5 g and probenecid 1 g per 9-capsule regimen.
TIMENTIN INJECTION: ticarcillin disodium 3 g and clavulanate potassium 100 mg per vial.
UNASYN INJECTION: ampicillin sodium 1 g and sulbactam sodium 500 mg per vial; ampicillin sodium 2 g and sulbactam sodium 1 g per vial.

amoxicillin/clavulanate potassium (amoxycillin/clavulanate potassium)

Augmentin, Clavulin†

Pregnancy Risk Category: B

HOW SUPPLIED

Tablets (chewable): 125 mg amoxicillin trihydrate, 31.25 mg clavulanic acid; 250 mg amoxicillin trihydrate, 62.5 mg clavulanic acid
Tablets (film-coated): 250 mg amoxicillin trihydrate, 125 mg clavulanic acid; 500 mg amoxicillin trihydrate, 125 mg clavulanic acid
Oral suspension: 125 mg amoxicillin trihydrate and 31.25 mg clavulanic acid/5 ml (after reconstitution); 250 mg amoxicillin trihydrate and 62.5 mg clavulanic acid/5 ml (after reconstitution)

MECHANISM OF ACTION

An aminopenicillin that acts by preventing bacterial cell wall synthesis during active replication. Clavulanic acid increases amoxicillin effectiveness by inactivating beta lactamases, which destroy amoxicillin.

INDICATIONS & DOSAGE

Lower respiratory infections, otitis media, sinusitis, skin and skin structure infections, and urinary tract infections caused by susceptible strains

of gram-positive and gram-negative organisms –
Adults: 250 mg (based on the amoxicillin component) P.O. q 8 hours. For more severe infections, 500 mg q 8 hours.
Children: 20 to 40 mg/kg (based on the amoxicillin component) P.O. daily given in divided doses q 8 hours.

ADVERSE REACTIONS
Common reactions are in italics; life-threatening reactions are in bold italics.
Blood: anemia, thrombocytopenia, thrombocytopenic purpura, eosinophilia, leukopenia.
GI: *nausea,* vomiting, *diarrhea.*
Other: hypersensitivity (erythematous maculopapular rash, urticaria, ***anaphylaxis***), overgrowth of nonsusceptible organisms.

INTERACTIONS
Allopurinol: increased incidence of skin rash.
Probenecid: increases blood levels of amoxicillin and other penicillins. Probenecid may be used for this purpose.

NURSING CONSIDERATIONS
- *Use cautiously* in patients with other drug allergies, especially to cephalosporins (possible cross-allergenicity), and in mononucleosis (high incidence of maculopapular rash).
- Before giving, ask patient about any allergic reactions to penicillin. However, a negative history doesn't rule out future penicillin allergy.
- Obtain specimen for culture and sensitivity tests before first dose. Therapy may begin pending test results.
- Tell patient to take drug exactly as prescribed, even after he feels better. Patient should take entire quantity prescribed.
- Give with food to prevent GI distress.
- Incidence of diarrhea is greater than with amoxicillin alone.
- With large doses and prolonged therapy, bacterial and fungal superinfection may occur, especially in elderly, debilitated, or immunosuppressed patients. Close observation is essential.
- Both the "250" and "500" tablets contain the same amount of clavulanic acid (125 mg). Therefore, two "250" tablets are not equivalent to one "500" tablet.
- Particularly useful in clinical settings with high prevalence of amoxicillin-resistant organisms.
- Give amoxicillin/clavulanate potassium at least 1 hour before bacteriostatic antibiotics.

amoxicillin trihydrate (amoxycillin trihydrate)

Alphamox‡, Amoxil, Apo-Amoxi†, Axicillin†, Cilamox‡, Ibiamox‡, Moxacin‡, Novamoxin†, Polymox†, Trimox, Utimox, Wymox

Pregnancy Risk Category: B

HOW SUPPLIED
Tablets (chewable): 125 mg, 250 mg
Capsules: 250 mg, 500 mg
Oral suspension: 50 mg/ml (pediatric drops), 125 mg/5 ml, 250 mg/5 ml (after reconstitution)

MECHANISM OF ACTION
An aminopenicillin that is bactericidal against microorganisms by inhibiting cell wall synthesis during active multiplication. Bacteria resist amoxicillin by producing penicillinases – enzymes that hydrolyze amoxicillin.

INDICATIONS & DOSAGE
Systemic infections, acute and chronic urinary tract infections caused by susceptible strains of gram-positive and gram-negative organisms –
Adults: 750 mg to 1.5 g P.O. daily in divided doses given q 8 hours.

*Liquid form contains alcohol. **May contain tartrazine.

Children: 20 to 40 mg/kg P.O. daily in divided doses given q 8 hours.
Uncomplicated gonorrhea –
Adults: 3 g P.O. with 1 g probenecid given as a single dose.
Uncomplicated urinary tract infections caused by susceptible organisms –
Adults: 3 g P.O. given as a single dose.

ADVERSE REACTIONS
Common reactions are in italics; life-threatening reactions are in bold italics.
Blood: anemia, thrombocytopenia, thrombocytopenic purpura, eosinophilia, leukopenia.
GI: *nausea,* vomiting, *diarrhea.*
Other: hypersensitivity (erythematous maculopapular rash, urticaria, ***anaphylaxis***), overgrowth of nonsusceptible organisms.

INTERACTIONS
Allopurinol: increased incidence of skin rash.
Probenecid: increases blood levels of amoxicillin and other penicillins. Probenecid may be used for this purpose.

NURSING CONSIDERATIONS
- *Use cautiously* in patients with other drug allergies, especially to cephalosporins (possible cross-allergenicity), and in mononucleosis – high incidence of maculopapular rash in those receiving amoxicillin.
- Obtain specimen for culture and sensitivity tests before first dose. Therapy may begin pending test results.
- Before giving amoxicillin, ask patient if he's had any allergic reactions to penicillin. However, a negative history of penicillin allergy is no guarantee against a future allergic reaction.
- Tell patient to take medication exactly as prescribed, even after he feels better. Entire quantity prescribed should be taken.
- Give with food to prevent GI distress.
- With large doses and prolonged therapy, bacterial and fungal superinfections may occur, especially in elderly, debilitated, or immunosuppressed patients. Close observation is essential.
- Warn patient never to use leftover amoxicillin for a new illness or to share it with family and friends.
- Trimox oral suspension may be stored at room temperature for up to 2 weeks. Be sure to check individual product labels for storage information.
- Tell patient to call the doctor if rash, fever, or chills develop. A rash is the most common allergic reaction. The rash is most common if the patient is also taking allopurinol.
- Urine glucose determinations may be false-positive with copper sulfate tests (Clinitest); glucose enzymatic tests (Clinistix, Tes-Tape) are not affected.
- Give amoxicillin at least 1 hour before bacteriostatic antibiotics.

ampicillin
Amcill, Ampicin†, Ampilean†, Apo-Ampi†, Novo Ampicillin†, Omnipen, Penbritin†, Principen

ampicillin sodium
Ampicyn Injection‡, Omnipen-N, Polycillin-N, Totacillin-N

ampicillin trihydrate
Amcill, Ampicyn Oral‡, D-Amp, Omnipen, Penamp-250, Penamp-500, Penbritin‡, Polycillin, Principen-250, Principen-500, Totacillin

Pregnancy Risk Category: B

HOW SUPPLIED
Capsules: 250 mg, 500 mg
Oral suspension: 100 mg/ml (pediat-

ric drops), 125 mg/5 ml, 250 mg/5 ml, 500 mg/5 ml (after reconstitution)
Injection: 125 mg, 250 mg, 500 mg, 1 g, 2 g
Infusion: 500 mg, 1 g, 2 g
Pharmacy bulk package: 10-g vial

MECHANISM OF ACTION
An aminopenicillin that is bactericidal against microorganisms by inhibiting cell wall synthesis during active multiplication. Bacteria resist ampicillin by producing penicillinases – enzymes that hydrolyze ampicillin.

INDICATIONS & DOSAGE
Systemic infections, acute and chronic urinary tract infections caused by susceptible strains of gram-positive and gram-negative organisms –
Adults: 1 to 4 g P.O. daily, divided into doses given q 6 hours; 2 to 12 g I.M. or I.V. daily, divided into doses given q 4 to 6 hours.
Children: 50 to 100 mg/kg P.O. daily, divided into doses given q 6 hours; or 100 to 200 mg/kg I.M. or I.V. daily, divided into doses given q 6 hours.
Meningitis –
Adults: 8 to 14 g I.V. daily in divided doses q 3 to 4 hours.
Children: up to 300 mg/kg I.V. daily in divided doses q 3 to 4 hours.
Uncomplicated gonorrhea –
Adults: 3.5 g P.O. with 1 g probenecid given as a single dose.

ADVERSE REACTIONS
Common reactions are in italics; life-threatening reactions are in bold italics.
Blood: anemia, thrombocytopenia, thrombocytopenic purpura, eosinophilia, leukopenia.
GI: *nausea,* vomiting, *diarrhea,* glossitis, stomatitis.
Local: pain at injection site, vein irritation, thrombophlebitis.
Other: hypersensitivity (erythematous maculopapular rash, urticaria, ***anaphylaxis***), overgrowth of nonsusceptible organisms.

INTERACTIONS
Allopurinol: increased incidence of skin rash.
Probenecid: increases blood levels of ampicillin and other penicillins. Probenecid may be used for this purpose.

NURSING CONSIDERATIONS
• *Use cautiously* in patients with other drug allergies, especially to cephalosporins (possible cross-allergenicity), and in mononucleosis – high incidence of maculopapular rash in those receiving ampicillin.
• Obtain specimen for culture and sensitivity tests before first dose. Therapy may begin pending test results.
• Before giving ampicillin, ask patient if he's had any allergic reactions to penicillin. However, a negative history of penicillin allergy is no guarantee against a future allergic reaction.
• Tell patient to take medication exactly as prescribed, even after he feels better. Entire quantity prescribed should be taken.
• Tell the patient to call the doctor if rash, fever, or chills develop. A rash is the most common allergic reaction. Rash is most common if the patient is also taking allopurinol.
• When given orally, drug may cause GI disturbances. Food may interfere with absorption, so give 1 to 2 hours before meals or 2 to 3 hours after.
• Don't give I.M. or I.V. unless infection is severe or patient can't take oral dose.
• Dosage should be altered in patients with impaired renal functions.
• **I.V. use:** When giving I.V., mix with dextrose 5% in water or a saline solution. Don't mix with other drugs or solutions: they might be incompatible.
• Give I.V. intermittently to prevent

*Liquid form contains alcohol. **May contain tartrazine.

vein irritation. Change site every 48 hours.

- With large doses or prolonged therapy, bacterial or fungal superinfections may occur, especially in elderly, debilitated, or immunosuppressed patients. Close observation is essential.
- Intitial dilution in vial is stable for 1 hour. Follow manufacturer's direction for stability data when ampicillin is further diluted for I.V. infusion.
- In pediatric meningitis, may be given concurrently with parenteral chloramphenicol for 24 hours pending cultures.
- Urine glucose determinations may be false-positive with copper sulfate tests (Clinitest); glucose enzymatic tests (Clinistix, Tes-Tape) are not affected.
- Give ampicillin at least 1 hour before bacteriostatic antibiotics.
- Warn patient never to use leftover ampicillin for a new illness or to share it with family and friends.

ampicillin sodium/ sulbactam sodium

Unasyn

Pregnancy Risk Category: C

HOW SUPPLIED

Injection: vials and piggyback vials containing 1.5 g (1 g ampicillin sodium with 500 mg sulbactam sodium) and 3 g (2 g ampicillin sodium with 1 g sulbactam sodium)

MECHANISM OF ACTION

Ampicillin (an aminopenicillin) inhibits cell wall synthesis during active multiplication. Sulbactam inactivates bacterial beta-lactamase, the enzyme that inactivates ampicillin and provides bacterial resistance to it.

INDICATIONS & DOSAGE

Intra-abdominal, gynecologic, and skin and skin structure infections caused by susceptible strains of bacteria –

Adults: dosage expressed as total drug (each 1.5-g vial contains 1 g ampicillin sodium and 0.5 g sulbactam sodium): 1.5 to 3 g I.M. or I.V. q 6 hours. Maximum daily dose is 4 g sulbactam (12 g of the combined drugs).

ADVERSE REACTIONS

Common reactions are in italics; life-threatening reactions are in bold italics.

Blood: anemia, thrombocytopenia, thrombocytopenic purpura, eosinophilia, leukopenia.

GI: *nausea,* vomiting, *diarrhea,* glossitis, stomatitis.

Local: pain at injection site, vein irritation, thrombophlebitis.

Other: *hypersensitivity (erythematous maculopapular rash, urticaria,* ***anaphylaxis****), overgrowth of nonsusceptible organisms.*

INTERACTIONS

Allopurinol: increased incidence of skin rash.

Probenecid: increased levels of ampicillin. Probenecid may be used for this purpose.

NURSING CONSIDERATIONS

- *Use cautiously* in patients with other drug allergies, especially to cephalosporins (possible cross-allergenicity), and in mononucleosis – high incidence of maculopapular rash in those receiving ampicillin.
- Obtain specimen for culture and sensitivity tests before first dose. Therapy may begin pending test results.
- Before giving ampicillin, ask if patient has had any allergic reactions to penicillin. However, a negative history of penicillin allergy is no guarantee against a future allergic reaction.
- **I.V. use:** When preparing I.V. injection, reconstitute powder with any of the following diluents: normal saline solution, dextrose 5% in water, lac-

tated Ringer's injection, 1/6 M sodium lactate, dextrose 5% and 0.45% saline injection, and 10% invert sugar. Stability varies with diluent, temperature, and concentration of solution.

- After reconstitution, allow vials to stand for a few minutes to allow foam to dissipate. This will permit visual inspection of contents for particles.
- Give I.V. dose by slow injection (over 10 to 15 minutes), or dilute in 50 to 100 ml of a compatible diluent and infuse over 15 to 30 minutes. If permitted, give intermittently to prevent vein irritation. Change site every 48 hours.
- When giving I.V., don't add or mix with other drugs: They might be physically or chemically incompatible.
- When administering I.M., give by deep injection. Drug may be reconstituted with sterile water for injection, or 0.5% or 2% lidocaine hydrochloride injection. Add 3.2 ml to a 1.5-g vial (or 6.4 ml to a 3-g vial) to yield a concentration of 375 mg/ml.
- Dosage should be altered in patients with impaired renal function.
- With large doses and prolonged therapy, bacterial and fungal superinfections may occur, especially in elderly, debilitated, or immunosuppressed patients. Close observation is essential.
- Urine glucose determinations may be false-positive with copper sulfate tests (Clinitest); glucose enzymatic tests (Clinistix, Tes-Tape) are not affected.
- Give ampicillin/sulbactam at least 1 hour before bacteriostatic antibiotics.
- Tell the patient to call the doctor if rash, fever, or chills develop. A rash is the most common allergic reaction.

bacampicillin hydrochloride

Penglobe†, Spectrobid

Pregnancy Risk Category: B

HOW SUPPLIED

Tablets: 400 mg
Oral suspension: 125 mg/5 ml (after reconstitution)

MECHANISM OF ACTION

An aminopenicillin that is converted to ampicillin in vivo; each mg of bacampicillin yields 623 to 727 mcg ampicillin. It is bactericidal against microorganisms by inhibiting cell wall synthesis during active multiplication. Bacteria resist bacampicillin by producing penicillinases—enzymes that hydrolyze its active form (ampicillin).

INDICATIONS & DOSAGE

Upper and lower respiratory tract infections due to streptococci, pneumococci, staphylococci, and Haemophilus influenzae; *urinary tract infections due to* Escherichia coli, Proteus mirabilis, *and* Streptococcus faecalis; *skin infections due to streptococci and susceptible staphylococci*–

Adults and children weighing more than 25 kg: 400 to 800 mg P.O. q 12 hours.

Gonorrhea–

Usual dosage is 1.6 g plus 1 g probenecid given as a single dose.

Not recommended for children under 25 kg.

ADVERSE REACTIONS

Common reactions are in italics; life-threatening reactions are in bold italics.

Blood: anemia, thrombocytopenia, thrombocytopenic purpura, eosinophilia, leukopenia.

GI: *nausea,* vomiting, *diarrhea,* glossitis, stomatitis.

Other: hypersensitivity (erythematous maculopapular rash, urticaria, ***anaphylaxis***), overgrowth of nonsusceptible organisms.

INTERACTIONS

Allopurinol: increased incidence of skin rash.

*Liquid form contains alcohol. **May contain tartrazine.

Probenecid: increases blood levels of bacampicillin or other penicillins. Probenecid may be used for this purpose.

NURSING CONSIDERATIONS

- *Use cautiously* in patients with other drug allergies, especially to cephalosporins (possible cross-allergenicity), and in mononucleosis. This drug, like ampicillin, is linked to a high incidence of maculopapular rash.
- Obtain specimen for culture and sensitivity tests before first dose. Therapy may begin pending test results.
- Before giving bacampicillin, ask patient if he's had any previous allergic reactions to penicillin. However, a negative history of penicillin allergy is no guarantee against a future allergic reaction.
- Bacampicillin is especially formulated to produce high blood levels of antibiotic when administered twice daily.
- Diarrhea may occur less frequently with bacampicillin than with ampicillin.
- Tell patient to take medication even after he feels better. Entire quantity prescribed should be taken.
- Tell patient to call the doctor if rash, fever, or chills develop. A rash is the most common allergic reaction.
- With large doses and prolonged therapy, bacterial or fungal superinfections may occur, especially in elderly, debilitated, or immunosuppressed patients. Monitor closely.
- Warn patient never to use leftover bacampicillin for a new illness or to share it with family and friends.
- Unlike ampicillin, bacampicillin tablets may be taken with meals without fear of diminished drug absorption. Give with food to prevent GI distress. However, bacampicillin suspension should be taken on an empty stomach.
- Administer bacampicillin at least 1 hour before bacteriostatic antibiotics.

carbenicillin indanyl sodium

Geocillin, Geopen Oral†

Pregnancy Risk Category: B

HOW SUPPLIED

Tablets: 382 mg

MECHANISM OF ACTION

An extended-spectrum penicillin that is bactericidal against microorganisms by inhibiting cell wall synthesis during active multiplication. Bacteria resist carbenicillin by producing penicillinases – enzymes that hydrolyze its active form.

INDICATIONS & DOSAGE

Urinary tract infection and prostatitis caused by susceptible strains of gram-negative organisms –

Adults: 382 to 764 mg P.O. q.i.d.

Not recommended for children.

ADVERSE REACTIONS

Common reactions are in italics; life-threatening reactions are in bold italics.

Blood: leukopenia, neutropenia, eosinophilia, anemia, ***thrombocytopenia***.

GI: *nausea,* vomiting, *diarrhea, flatulence, abdominal cramps, unpleasant taste.*

Other: hypersensitivity (rash, chills, fever, urticaria, pruritus, ***anaphylaxis***), overgrowth of nonsusceptible organisms.

INTERACTIONS

None significant.

NURSING CONSIDERATIONS

- *Use cautiously* in patients with other drug allergies, especially to cephalosporins (possible cross-allergenicity).
- Obtain specimen for culture and

sensitivity tests before first dose. Therapy may begin pending test results.

- Before giving carbenicillin, ask patient if he's had any allergic reactions to penicillin. However, a negative history of penicillin allergy is no guarantee against a future allergic reaction.
- Tell patient to take medication exactly as prescribed, even after he feels better. Entire quantity prescribed should be taken.
- Give 1 to 2 hours before or 2 to 3 hours after meals because food may interfere with absorption.
- Tell patient to call the doctor if he develops rash, fever, or chills. A rash is the most common allergic reaction.
- With large doses or prolonged therapy, bacterial or fungal superinfections may occur, especially in elderly, debilitated, or immunosuppressed patients. Close observation is essential.
- Warn patient never to use leftover carbenicillin for a new illness or to share it with family and friends.
- Use only in patients whose creatinine clearance is 10 ml/minute or more.
- Excellent treatment for *Pseudomonas* urinary tract infections in ambulatory patients.
- May be useful in treatment of cystitis, but not pyelonephritis.
- Not effective for any systemic infection because blood levels are nil.

cloxacillin sodium

Alclox‡, Apo-Cloxi†, Austrastaph‡, Bactopen†, Cloxapen, Novocloxin†, Orbenin†, Orbenin Injection‡, Tegopen

Pregnancy Risk Category: B

HOW SUPPLIED

Capsules: 250 mg, 500 mg
Oral solution: 125 mg/5 ml (after reconstitution)

MECHANISM OF ACTION

A penicillinase-resistant penicillin that is bactericidal against microorganisms by inhibiting cell wall synthesis during active multiplication. Bacteria resist penicillins by producing penicillinases – enzymes that convert penicillins to inactive penicilloic acid. Cloxacillin resists these enzymes.

INDICATIONS & DOSAGE

Systemic infections caused by penicillinase-producing staphylococci –
Adults: 2 to 4 g P.O. daily, divided into doses given q 6 hours.
Children: 50 to 100 mg/kg P.O. daily, divided into doses given q 6 hours.

ADVERSE REACTIONS

Common reactions are in italics; life-threatening reactions are in bold italics.
Blood: eosinophilia.
GI: *nausea,* vomiting, *epigastric distress, diarrhea.*
Other: *hypersensitivity (rash, urticaria, chills, fever, sneezing, wheezing, **anaphylaxis**),* intrahepatic cholestasis, overgrowth of nonsusceptible organisms.

INTERACTIONS

Probenecid: increases blood levels of cloxacillin and other penicillins. Probenecid may be used for this purpose.

NURSING CONSIDERATIONS

- *Use cautiously* in patients with other drug allergies, especially to cephalosporins (possible cross-allergenicity).
- Obtain specimen for culture and sensitivity tests before first dose. Therapy may begin pending test results.
- Before giving cloxacillin, ask patient if he's had any allergic reactions to penicillin. However, a negative history of penicillin allergy is no guarantee against a future allergic reaction.

• Tell patient to take medication exactly as prescribed, even if he feels better. Entire quantity prescribed should be taken.
• Tell patient to call the doctor if rash, fever, or chills develop. A rash is the most common allergic reaction.
• Drug may cause GI disturbances. Food may interfere with absorption, so give 1 to 2 hours before meals or 2 to 3 hours after.
• Patient should take each dose with a full glass of water, not fruit juice or carbonated beverage, because acid will inactivate the drug.
• With large doses and prolonged therapy, bacterial and fungal superinfections may occur, especially in the elderly, debilitated, or immunosuppressed patients. Close observation is essential.
• Warn patient never to use leftover cloxacillin for a new illness or to share it with family and friends.
• Give cloxacillin at least 1 hour before bacteriostatic antibiotics.

dicloxacillin sodium

Dycill, Dynapen, Pathocil

Pregnancy Risk Category: B

HOW SUPPLIED

Capsules: 125 mg, 250 mg, 500 mg
Oral suspension: 62.5 mg/5 ml (after reconstitution)

MECHANISM OF ACTION

A penicillinase-resistant penicillin that is bactericidal against microorganisms by inhibiting cell wall synthesis during active multiplication. Bacteria resist penicillins by producing penicillinases – enzymes that convert penicillins to inactive penicilloic acid. Dicloxacillin resists these enzymes.

INDICATIONS & DOSAGE

Systemic infections caused by penicillinase-producing staphylococci –
Adults: 1 to 2 g daily P.O., divided into doses given q 6 hours.
Children: 25 to 50 mg/kg P.O. daily, divided into doses given q 6 hours.

ADVERSE REACTIONS

Common reactions are in italics; life-threatening reactions are in bold italics.
Blood: eosinophilia.
CNS: neuromuscular irritability, seizures.
GI: *nausea,* vomiting, *epigastric distress,* flatulence, *diarrhea.*
Other: hypersensitivity (pruritus, urticaria, rash, ***anaphylaxis***), overgrowth of nonsusceptible organisms.

INTERACTIONS

Probenecid: increases blood levels of dicloxacillin and other penicillins. Probenecid may be used for this purpose.

NURSING CONSIDERATIONS

• *Use cautiously* in patients allergic to cephalosporins (possible cross-allergenicity).
• Obtain specimen for culture and sensitivity tests before first dose. Therapy may begin pending test results.
• Before giving dicloxacillin, ask patient if he's had any allergic reactions to penicillin. However, a negative history of penicillin allergy is no guarantee against a future allergic reaction.
• Tell patient to take medication exactly as prescribed, even if he feels better. Entire quantity prescribed should be taken.
• Tell patient to call the doctor if rash, fever, or chills develop. A rash is the most common allergic reaction.
• Drug may cause GI disturbances. Food may interfere with absorption, so give 1 to 2 hours before meals or 2 to 3 hours after.
• With large doses and prolonged therapy, bacterial and fungal superinfections may occur, especially in elderly, debilitated, or immunosup-

pressed patients. Close observation is essential.

- Periodic assessments of renal, hepatic, and hematopoietic function should be made when therapy is prolonged.
- Warn patient never to use leftover dicloxacillin for a new illness or to share it with family and friends.
- Give dicloxacillin at least 1 hour before bacteriostatic antibiotics.

methicillin sodium

Metin‡, Staphcillin

Pregnancy Risk Category: B

HOW SUPPLIED

Injection: 1 g, 4 g, 6 g
I.V. infusion piggyback: 1 g, 4 g
Pharmacy bulk package: 10 g

MECHANISM OF ACTION

A penicillinase-resistant penicillin that is bactericidal against microorganisms by inhibiting cell wall synthesis during active multiplication. Bacteria resist penicillins by producing penicillinases – enzymes that convert penicillins to inactive penicilloic acid. Methicillin resists these enzymes.

INDICATIONS & DOSAGE

Systemic infections caused by penicillinase-producing staphylococci –
Adults: 4 to 12 g I.M. or I.V. daily, divided into doses given q 4 to 6 hours.
Children: 100 to 300 mg/kg I.M. or I.V. daily, divided into doses given q 4 to 6 hours.

ADVERSE REACTIONS

Common reactions are in italics; life-threatening reactions are in bold italics.
Blood: ***agranulocytosis,*** *eosinophilia,* hemolytic anemia, transient neutropenia.
CNS: neuropathy, ***seizures with high doses.***
GI: glossitis, stomatitis.
GU: interstitial nephritis.
Local: *vein irritation, thrombophlebitis.*
Other: *hypersensitivity (chills, fever, edema, rash, urticaria,* ***anaphylaxis****),* overgrowth of nonsusceptible organisms.

INTERACTIONS

Probenecid: increases blood levels of methicillin and other penicillins. Probenecid may be used for this purpose.

NURSING CONSIDERATIONS

- *Use cautiously* in patients with other drug allergies, especially to cephalosporins (possible cross-allergenicity), and in infants.
- Obtain specimen for culture and sensitivity tests before first dose. Therapy may begin pending test results.
- Methicillin-resistant strains of Staphylococci should be treated with vancomycin.
- Before giving methicillin, ask patient if he's had any allergic reactions to penicillin. However, a negative history of penicillin allergy is no guarantee against a future allergic reaction.
- Closely monitor renal function. Urinalysis should be done frequently to detect interstitial nephritis.
- If patient has high blood level of this drug, he may have seizures. Institute seizure precautions.
- **I.V. use:** When giving I.V., mix with a normal saline solution. Don't mix with others because methicillin may be inactivated. Initial dilution must be made with sterile water for injection.
- Give I.V. intermittently to prevent vein irritation. Change site every 48 hours.
- With large doses and prolonged therapy, bacterial and fungal superinfections may occur, especially in elderly, debilitated, or immunosup-

pressed patients. Close observation is essential.
- Periodic assessment of hepatic, renal, and hematopoietic function is required during prolonged therapy.
- Give methicillin at least 1 hour before bacteriostatic antibiotics.

mezlocillin sodium
Mezlin

Pregnancy Risk Category: B

HOW SUPPLIED
Injection: 1 g, 2 g, 3 g, 4 g

MECHANISM OF ACTION
An extended-spectrum penicillin that is bactericidal against microorganisms by inhibiting cell wall synthesis during active multiplication. Bacteria resist mezlocillin by producing penicillinases – enzymes that hydrolyze mezlocillin.

INDICATIONS & DOSAGE
Systemic infections caused by susceptible strains of gram-positive and especially gram-negative organisms (including Proteus, Pseudomonas aeruginosa) –
Adults: 200 to 300 mg/kg daily I.V. or I.M. given in 4 to 6 divided doses. Usual dose is 3 g q 4 hours or 4 g q 6 hours. For very serious infections, up to 24 g daily may be administered.
Children up to 12 years: 50 mg/kg q 4 hours by I.V. infusion or direct I.V. injection.

ADVERSE REACTIONS
Common reactions are in italics; life-threatening reactions are in bold italics.
Blood: ***bleeding with high doses,*** neutropenia, eosinophilia, leukopenia, ***thrombocytopenia.***
CNS: neuromuscular irritability.
GI: nausea, diarrhea.
Metabolic: *hypokalemia.*
Local: pain at injection site, vein irritation, phlebitis.
Other: hypersensitivity (edema, fever, chills, rash, pruritus, urticaria, ***anaphylaxis***), *overgrowth of nonsusceptible organisms.*

INTERACTIONS
Aminoglycoside antibiotics (such as gentamicin and tobramycin): chemically incompatible. Don't mix together in I.V. solution. Give 1 hour apart, especially in patients with renal insufficiency.
Probenecid: increases blood levels of mezlocillin. Probenecid may be used for this purpose.

NURSING CONSIDERATIONS
- *Use cautiously* in patients with hypersensitivity to drugs, especially to cephalosporins (possible cross-hypersensitivity), and in bleeding tendencies, uremia, and hypokalemia.
- Obtain specimen for culture and sensitivity tests before first dose. Therapy may begin pending test results.
- Before giving mezlocillin, ask patient if he's had any allergic reactions to penicillin. A negative history of penicillin allergy, however, is no guarantee against future allergic reaction.
- Dosage should be altered in patients with impaired renal function.
- Check CBC and platelets frequently. Drug may cause thrombocytopenia.
- Monitor serum potassium level.
- Patient with high serum level of this drug may have seizures. Institute seizure precautions.
- **I.V. use:** When giving I.V., mix with dextrose 5% in water or other suitable I.V. fluids.
- Give I.V. intermittently to prevent vein irritation. Change site every 48 hours.
- Almost always used with another antibiotic, such as gentamicin.
- With large doses and prolonged therapy, bacterial and fungal superin-

fections may occur, especially in elderly, debilitated, or immunosuppressed patients. Monitor patient closely.

- Compared with similar antibiotics, such as carbenicillin and ticarcillin, mezlocillin is less likely to cause hypokalemia.
- Drug may be better suited to patients on salt-free diets than carbenicillin and ticarcillin (contains 1.85 mEq Na/g of mezlocillin).
- Give mezlocillin at least 1 hour before bacteriostatic antibiotics.

nafcillin sodium

Nafcil, Nallpen, Unipen

Pregnancy Risk Category: B

HOW SUPPLIED

Tablets: 500 mg
Capsules: 250 mg
Oral solution: 250 mg/5 ml (after reconstitution)
Injection: 500 mg, 1 g, 2 g
I.V. infusion piggyback: 1 g, 1.5 g, 2 g, 4 g
Pharmacy bulk package: 10 g

MECHANISM OF ACTION

A penicillinase-resistant penicillin that is bactericidal against microorganisms by inhibiting cell wall synthesis during active multiplication. Bacteria resist penicillins by producing penicillinases – enzymes that hydrolyze penicillin. Nafcillin resists these enzymes.

INDICATIONS & DOSAGE

Systemic infections caused by penicillinase-producing staphylococci –
Adults: 2 to 4 g P.O. daily, divided into doses given q 6 hours; 2 to 12 g I.M. or I.V. daily, divided into doses given q 4 to 6 hours.
Children: 50 to 100 mg/kg P.O. daily, divided into doses given q 4 to 6 hours; or 100 to 200 mg/kg I.M. or I.V. daily, divided into doses given q 4 to 6 hours.

ADVERSE REACTIONS

Common reactions are in italics; life-threatening reactions are in bold italics.
Blood: transient leukopenia, neutropenia, granulocytopenia, ***thrombocytopenia*** with high doses.
GI: *nausea,* vomiting, diarrhea.
Local: *vein irritation, thrombophlebitis.*
Other: hypersensitivity (chills, fever, rash, pruritus, urticaria, ***anaphylaxis***).

INTERACTIONS

None significant.

NURSING CONSIDERATIONS

- *Use cautiously* in patients with other drug allergies, especially to cephalosporins (possible cross-allergenicity), and in GI distress.
- Obtain specimen for culture and sensitivity tests before first dose. Therapy may begin pending test results.
- Before giving nafcillin, ask patient if he's had any allergic reactions to penicillin. However, a negative history of penicillin allergy is no guarantee against a future allergic reaction.
- Tell patient to take medication exactly as prescribed, even if he feels better. Entire quantity prescribed should be taken.
- Tell patient to call the doctor if rash, fever, or chills develop. A rash is the most common allergic reaction.
- When given orally, drug may cause GI disturbances. Food may interfere with absorption, so give 1 to 2 hours before meals or 2 to 3 hours after.
- **I.V. use:** When giving I.V., mix with dextrose 5% in water or a saline solution.
- Give I.V. intermittently to prevent vein irritation. Change site every 48 hours.
- With large doses and prolonged

therapy, bacterial and fungal superinfections may occur, especially in elderly, debilitated, or immunosuppressed patients. Close observation is essential.
- Give nafcillin at least 1 hour before bacteriostatic antibiotics.

oxacillin sodium
Bactocill, Prostaphlin
Pregnancy Risk Category: B

HOW SUPPLIED
Capsules: 250 mg, 500 mg
Oral solution: 250 mg/5 ml (after reconstitution)
Injection: 250 mg, 500 mg, 1 g, 2 g, 4 g, 10 g
I.V. infusion: 1 g, 2 g, 4 g
Pharmacy bulk package: 4 g, 10 g

MECHANISM OF ACTION
A penicillinase-resistant penicillin that is bactericidal against microorganisms by inhibiting cell wall synthesis during active multiplication. Bacteria resist penicillins by producing penicillinases – enzymes that convert penicillins to inactive penicilloic acid. Oxacillin resists these enzymes.

INDICATIONS & DOSAGE
Systemic infections caused by penicillinase-producing staphylococci –
Adults: 2 to 4 g P.O. daily, divided into doses given q 6 hours; 2 to 12 g I.M. or I.V. daily, divided into doses given q 4 to 6 hours.
Children: 50 to 100 mg/kg P.O. daily, divided into doses given q 6 hours; 100 to 200 mg/kg I.M. or I.V. daily, divided into doses given q 4 to 6 hours.

ADVERSE REACTIONS
Common reactions are in italics; life-threatening reactions are in bold italics.
Blood: granulocytopenia, thrombocytopenia, eosinophilia, ***hemolytic anemia,*** transient neutropenia.
CNS: neuropathy, neuromuscular irritability, seizures.
GI: oral lesions.
GU: interstitial nephritis, transient hematuria, proteinuria.
Hepatic: hepatitis, elevated enzymes.
Local: *thrombophlebitis.*
Other: hypersensitivity (fever, chills, rash, urticaria, ***anaphylaxis***), overgrowth of nonsusceptible organisms.

INTERACTIONS
Probenecid: increases blood levels of oxacillin and other penicillins. Probenecid may be used for this purpose.

NURSING CONSIDERATIONS
- *Use cautiously* in patients with other drug allergies, especially to cephalosporins (possible cross-allergenicity), in premature newborns, and in infants.
- Obtain specimen for culture and sensitivity tests before first dose. Therapy may begin pending test results.
- Before giving oxacillin, ask patient if he's had any allergic reactions to penicillin. However, a negative history of penicillin allergy is no guarantee against a future allergic reaction.
- Tell the patient to take medication exactly as prescribed, even if he feels better. The entire quantity prescribed should be taken.
- Tell patient to call the doctor if rash, fever, or chills develop. A rash is the most common allergic reaction.
- When given orally, drug may cause GI disturbances. Food may interfere with absorption, so give 1 to 2 hours before meals or 2 to 3 hours after.
- Don't give I.M. or I.V. unless infection is severe or patient can't take oral dose.
- Periodic liver function studies are indicated; watch for elevated AST (SGOT) and ALT (SGPT).
- **I.V. use:** When giving I.V., mix with dextrose 5% in water or a saline solution.

- Give I.V. intermittently to prevent vein irritation. Change site every 48 hours.
- With large doses and prolonged therapy, bacterial and fungal superinfections may occur, especially in elderly, debilitated, or immunosuppressed patients. Close observation is essential.
- Give oxacillin at least 1 hour before bacteriostatic antibiotics.

penicillin G benzathine (benzylpenicillin benzathine)

Bicillin L-A, Megacillin

Pregnancy Risk Category: B

HOW SUPPLIED

Tablets: 200,000 units
Injection: 300,000 units/ml, 600,000 units/ml

MECHANISM OF ACTION

A natural penicillin that is bactericidal against microorganisms by inhibiting cell wall synthesis during active multiplication. Bacteria resist penicillin by producing penicillinases – enzymes that convert penicillin to inactive penicilloic acid.

INDICATIONS & DOSAGE

Congenital syphilis –
Children under age 2: 50,000 units/kg I.M. as a single dose.
Group A streptococcal upper respiratory infections –
Adults: 1.2 million units I.M. in a single injection.
Children over 27 kg: 900,000 units I.M. in a single injection.
Children under 27 kg: 300,000 to 600,000 units I.M. in a single injection.
Prophylaxis of poststreptococcal rheumatic fever –
Adults and children: 1.2 million units I.M. once a month or 600,000 units twice a month.
Syphilis of less than 1 year's duration –
Adults: 2.4 million units I.M. in a single dose.
Syphilis of more than 1 year's duration –
Adults: 2.4 million units I.M. weekly for 3 successive weeks.

ADVERSE REACTIONS

Common reactions are in italics; life-threatening reactions are in bold italics.
Blood: eosinophilia, hemolytic anemia, thrombocytopenia, leukopenia.
CNS: neuropathy, seizures with high doses.
Local: pain and sterile abscess at injection site.
Other: hypersensitivity (maculopapular and ***exfoliative dermatitis,*** chills, fever, edema, ***anaphylaxis***).

INTERACTIONS

Probenecid: increases blood levels of penicillin. Probenecid may be used for this purpose.

NURSING CONSIDERATIONS

- *Use cautiously* in patients with other drug allergies, especially to cephalosporins (possible cross-allergenicity).
- Obtain specimen for culture and sensitivity tests before first dose. Therapy may begin pending test results.
- Before giving penicillin, ask patient if he's had any allergic reactions to this drug. However, a negative history of penicillin allergy is no guarantee against a future allergic reaction.
- Tell patient to call the doctor if rash, fever, or chills develop. Fever and eosinophilia are the most common allergic reactions.
- With large doses and prolonged therapy, bacterial and fungal superinfections may occur, especially in elderly, debilitated, or immunosuppressed patients.

• Shake medication well before injection.
• Never give I.V. – inadvertent I.V. administration has caused cardiac arrest and death.
• Very slow absorption time makes allergic reactions difficult to treat.
• Inject deeply into upper outer quadrant of buttocks in adults; in midlateral thigh in infants and small children.
• Give penicillin G benzathine at least 1 hour before bacteriostatic antibiotics.

penicillin G potassium (benzylpenicillin potassium)

Megacillin†, NovoPen-G†, P-50†, Pentids**, Pfizerpen

Pregnancy Risk Category: B

HOW SUPPLIED

Tablets: 200,000 units, 250,000 units, 400,000 units, 500,000 units, 800,000 units
Oral suspension: 200,000 units/5 ml, 250,000 units/5 ml, 400,000 units/5 ml (after reconstitution)
Injection: 200,000 units, 500,000 units, 1 million units, 5 million units, 10 million units, 20 million units

MECHANISM OF ACTION

A natural penicillin that is bactericidal against microorganisms by inhibiting cell wall synthesis during active multiplication. Bacteria resist penicillin by producing penicillinases – enzymes that convert penicillin to inactive penicilloic acid.

INDICATIONS & DOSAGE

Moderate to severe systemic infections –
Adults: 1.6 to 3.2 million units P.O. daily in divided doses given q 6 hours (1 mg = 1,600 units); 1.2 to 24 million units I.M. or I.V. daily in divided doses given q 4 hours.
Children: 25,000 to 100,000 units/kg P.O. daily in divided doses given q 6 hours; or 25,000 to 300,000 units/kg I.M. or I.V. daily in divided doses given q 4 hours.

ADVERSE REACTIONS

Common reactions are in italics; life-threatening reactions are in bold italics.
Blood: hemolytic anemia, leukopenia, thrombocytopenia.
CNS: neuropathy, seizures with high doses.
Metabolic: possible severe potassium poisoning with high doses (hyperreflexia, seizures, coma).
Local: *thrombophlebitis, pain at injection site.*
Other: hypersensitivity (rash, urticaria, maculopapular eruptions, ***exfoliative dermatitis,*** chills, fever, edema, ***anaphylaxis***), overgrowth of nonsusceptible organisms.

INTERACTIONS

Probenecid: increases blood levels of penicillin. Probenecid may be used for this purpose.

NURSING CONSIDERATIONS

• *Use cautiously* in patients with other drug allergies, especially to cephalosporins (possible cross-allergenicity).
• Obtain specimen for culture and sensitivity tests before first dose. Therapy may begin pending test results.
• Before giving penicillin, ask patient if he's had any allergic reactions to this drug. However, a negative history of penicillin allergy is no guarantee against a future allergic reaction.
• Tell patient to take medication exactly as prescribed, even if he feels better, and to take entire amount prescribed.
• Tell patient to call the doctor if rash, fever, or chills develop. A rash is the most common allergic reaction.
• When given orally, drug may cause

GI disturbances. Food may interfere with absorption, so give 1 to 2 hours before meals or 2 to 3 hours after.
- Extremely painful when given I.M. Inject deep into large muscle.
- Patients with poor renal function are predisposed to high blood levels. Monitor renal function closely.
- If patient has high blood level of this drug, he may have seizures. Institute seizure precautions.
- **I.V. use:** When giving I.V., mix with dextrose 5% in water or a saline solution.
- Give I.V. intermittently to prevent vein irritation. Change site every 48 hours.
- With large doses and prolonged therapy, bacterial and fungal superinfections may occur, especially in elderly, debilitated, or immunosuppressed patients. Close observation is essential.
- Warn patient never to use leftover penicillin for a new illness or to share penicillin with family and friends.
- Give penicillin G potassium at least 1 hour before bacteriostatic antibiotics.

penicillin G procaine (benzylpenicillin procaine)

Ayercillin†, Crysticillin A.S., Duracillin A.S., Pfizerpen-AS, Wycillin

Pregnancy Risk Category: B

HOW SUPPLIED
Injection: 300,000 units/ml, 500,000 units/ml, 600,000 units/ml

MECHANISM OF ACTION
Bactericidal against microorganisms by inhibiting cell wall synthesis during active multiplication. Bacteria resist penicillin by producing penicillinases – enzymes that convert penicillin to inactive penicilloic acid.

INDICATIONS & DOSAGE
Moderate to severe systemic infections –
Adults: 600,000 to 1.2 million units I.M. daily given as a single dose.
Children: 300,000 units I.M. daily given as a single dose.
Uncomplicated gonorrhea –
Adults and children over 12 years: give 1 g probenecid; then 30 minutes later give 4.8 million units of penicillin G procaine I.M., divided into two injection sites.
Pneumococcal pneumonia –
Adults and children over 12 years: 300,000 to 600,000 units I.M. daily q 6 to 12 hours.

ADVERSE REACTIONS
Common reactions are in italics; life-threatening reactions are in bold italics.
Blood: thrombocytopenia, hemolytic anemia, leukopenia.
CNS: arthralgia, seizures.
Other: hypersensitivity (rash, urticaria, chills, fever, edema, prostration, ***anaphylaxis***), overgrowth of nonsusceptible organisms.

INTERACTIONS
Probenecid: increases blood levels of penicillin. Probenecid may be used for this purpose.

NURSING CONSIDERATIONS
- *Contraindicated* in patients with hypersensitivity to procaine.
- *Use cautiously* in patients with other drug allergies, especially to cephalosporins (possible cross-allergenicity).
- Obtain specimen for culture and sensitivity tests before first dose. Therapy may begin pending test results.
- Before giving penicillin, ask patient if he's had any allergic reactions to this drug. However, a negative history of penicillin allergy is no guarantee against a future allergic reaction.
- Tell patient to call doctor if rash, fe-

*Liquid form contains alcohol. **May contain tartrazine.

ver, or chills develop. A rash is the most common allergic reaction.
• Give deep I.M. in upper outer quadrant of buttocks in adults; in midlateral thigh in small children. Do not give subcutaneously. Don't massage injection site.
• Never give I.V. – inadvertent I.V. administration has caused death, due to CNS toxicity from procaine.
• Due to slow absorption rate, allergic reactions are hard to treat.
• With large doses and prolonged therapy, bacterial and fungal superinfections may occur, especially in elderly, debilitated, or immunosuppressed patients. Close observation is essential.
• Periodic evaluations of renal and hematopoietic function are recommended.
• Give penicillin G procaine at least 1 hour before bacteriostatic antibiotics.

penicillin G sodium (benzylpenicillin sodium)

Crystapen†

Pregnancy Risk Category: B

HOW SUPPLIED
Injection: 5 million units

MECHANISM OF ACTION
Bactericidal against microorganisms by inhibiting cell wall synthesis during active multiplication. Bacteria resist penicillin by producing penicillinases – enzymes that convert penicillin to inactive penicilloic acid.

INDICATIONS & DOSAGE
Moderate to severe systemic infections –
Adults: 1.2 to 24 million units daily I.M. or I.V., divided into doses given q 4 hours.
Children: 25,000 to 300,000 units/kg daily I.M. or I.V., divided into doses given q 4 hours.
Endocarditis prophylaxis for dental surgery –
Adults: 2 million units I.V. or I.M. 30 to 60 minutes before procedure, then 1 million units 6 hours later.

ADVERSE REACTIONS
Common reactions are in italics; life-threatening reactions are in bold italics.
Blood: hemolytic anemia, leukopenia, thrombocytopenia.
CNS: arthralgia, neuropathy, seizures.
CV: *CHF with high doses.*
Local: *vein irritation, pain at injection site, thrombophlebitis.*
Other: hypersensitivity (chills, fever, edema, maculopapular rash, ***exfoliative dermatitis,*** urticaria, ***anaphylaxis***), overgrowth of nonsusceptible organisms.

INTERACTIONS
Probenecid: increases blood levels of penicillin. Probenecid may be used for this purpose.

NURSING CONSIDERATIONS
• *Contraindicated* in patients on sodium restriction.
• *Use cautiously* in patients with other drug allergies, especially to cephalosporins (possible cross-allergenicity).
• Obtain specimen for culture and sensitivity tests before first dose. Therapy may begin pending test results.
• Before giving penicillin, ask patient if he's had any allergic reactions to this drug. However, a negative history of penicillin allergy is no guarantee against a future allergic reaction.
• If patient has high blood level of this drug, he may have seizures. Institute seizure precautions.
• **I.V. use:** Give I.V. intermittently to prevent vein irritation. Change site every 48 hours.
• With large doses and prolonged therapy, bacterial or fungal superin-

fections may occur, especially in elderly, debilitated, or immunosuppressed patients. Close observation is essential.

• Give penicillin G sodium at least 1 hour before bacteriostatic antibiotics.

penicillin V (phenoxymethyl penicillin)

penicillin V potassium (phenoxymethylpenicillin potassium)

Abbocillin VK‡, Apo-Pen-VK†, Beepen-VK, Betapen-VK, Cilicane VK‡, Ledercillin VK, Nadopen-V†, NovoPen-VK†, PVK‡, Penapar VK, Pen Vee K, PVF K†, Robicillin VK, V-Cillin K, VC-K, Veetids**

Pregnancy Risk Category: B

HOW SUPPLIED

penicillin V

Tablets: 250 mg, 500 mg
Oral suspension: 125 mg/5 ml, 250 mg/5 ml (after reconstitution)

penicillin V potassium

Tablets: 125 mg, 250 mg, 500 mg
Tablets (film-coated): 250 mg, 500 mg
Capsules: 250 mg‡
Oral suspension: 125 mg/5 ml, 250 mg/5 ml (after reconstitution)

MECHANISM OF ACTION

Bactericidal against microorganisms by inhibiting cell wall synthesis during active multiplication. Bacteria resist penicillin by producing penicillinases – enzymes that convert penicillin to inactive penicilloic acid.

INDICATIONS & DOSAGE

Mild to moderate systemic infections –
Adults: 250 to 500 mg (400,000 to 800,000 units) P.O. q 6 hours.
Children: 15 to 50 mg/kg (25,000 to 90,000 units/kg) P.O. daily, divided into doses given q 6 to 8 hours.

Endocarditis prophylaxis for dental surgery –
Adults: 2 g P.O. 30 to 60 minutes before procedure, then 1 g 6 hours after.
Children under 30 kg: half of the adult dose.

ADVERSE REACTIONS

Common reactions are in italics; life-threatening reactions are in bold italics.
Blood: eosinophilia, hemolytic anemia, leukopenia, thrombocytopenia.
CNS: neuropathy.
GI: *epigastric distress,* vomiting, diarrhea, *nausea.*
Other: hypersensitivity (rash, urticaria, chills, fever, edema, ***anaphylaxis***), overgrowth of nonsusceptible organisms.

INTERACTIONS

Neomycin: decreases absorption of penicillin. Give penicillin by injection.
Probenecid: increases blood levels of penicillin. Probenecid may be used for this purpose.

NURSING CONSIDERATIONS

• *Use cautiously* in patients with other drug allergies, especially to cephalosporins (possible cross-allergenicity), and in GI disturbances.
• Obtain specimen for culture and sensitivity tests before first dose. Therapy may begin pending test results.
• Before giving penicillin, ask patient if he's had any allergic reactions to this drug. However, a negative history of penicillin allergy is no guarantee against a future allergic reaction.
• Tell patient to take medication exactly as prescribed, even if he feels better. Entire quantity prescribed should be taken.
• Tell patient to call the doctor if rash, fever, or chills develop. A rash is the most common allergic reaction.
• May cause GI disturbances. Food may interfere with absorption, so give 1 to 2 hours before meals or 2 to 3 hours after.

*Liquid form contains alcohol. **May contain tartrazine.

• Patient should take each dose with a full glass of water, not fruit juice or a carbonated beverage, because acid will inactivate the drug.
• With large doses and prolonged therapy, bacterial and fungal superinfections may occur, especially in elderly, debilitated, or immunosuppressed patients. Close observation is essential.
• Periodic renal and hematopoietic function studies are recommended in patients receiving prolonged therapy.
• Warn patient never to use leftover penicillin for a new illness or to share penicillin with family and friends.
• Give penicillin V at least 1 hour before bacteriostatic antibiotics.

piperacillin sodium
Pipracil, Pipril‡
Pregnancy Risk Category: B

HOW SUPPLIED
Injection: 2 g, 3 g, 4 g
Pharmacy bulk package: 40 g

MECHANISM OF ACTION
Bactericidal against microorganisms by inhibiting cell wall synthesis during active multiplication. Bacteria resist penicillins by producing penicillinases – enzymes that convert penicillin to inactive penicilloic acid.

INDICATIONS & DOSAGE
Systemic infections caused by susceptible strains of gram-positive and especially gram-negative organisms (including Proteus, Pseudomonas aeruginosa*)* –
Adults and children over 12 years: 100 to 300 mg/kg daily divided q 4 to 6 hours I.V. or I.M. Doses for children under 12 years not established.
Prophylaxis of surgical infections –
Adults: 2 g I.V., given 30 to 60 minutes before surgery. Depending on type of surgery, dose may be repeated during surgery, and once or twice more after surgery.

ADVERSE REACTIONS
Common reactions are in italics; life-threatening reactions are in bold italics.
Blood: *bleeding with high doses,* neutropenia, eosinophilia, leukopenia, *thrombocytopenia.*
CNS: neuromuscular irritability, seizures, headache, dizziness.
GI: nausea, diarrhea.
Local: pain at injection site, vein irritation, phlebitis.
Metabolic: *hypokalemia.*
Other: hypersensitivity (edema, fever, chills, rash, pruritus, urticaria, ***anaphylaxis***), overgrowth of nonsusceptible organisms.

INTERACTIONS
Aminoglycoside antibiotics (such as gentamicin and tobramycin): chemically incompatible. Don't mix in the same I.V. container.
Probenecid: increases blood levels of piperacillin. Probenecid may be used for this purpose.

NURSING CONSIDERATIONS
• *Use cautiously* in patients with hypersensitivity to drugs, especially to cephalosporins (possible cross-hypersensitivity), and in bleeding tendencies, uremia, and hypokalemia.
• Cystic fibrosis patients tend to be most susceptible to fever or rash.
• Obtain specimen for culture and sensitivity tests before first dose. Therapy may begin pending test results.
• Before giving piperacillin, ask patient if he's had any allergic reactions to penicillin. A negative history of penicillin allergy, however, is no guarantee against future allergic reaction.
• Dosage should be altered in patients with impaired renal function.
• Check CBC and platelets fre-

quently. Drug may cause thrombocytopenia.
- Monitor serum potassium level.
- Patient with high serum level of this drug may have seizures. Institute seizure precautions.
- **I.V. use:** Give I.V. intermittently to prevent vein irritation. Change site every 48 hours.
- Almost always used with another antibiotic, such as gentamicin.
- With large doses and prolonged therapy, bacterial and fungal superinfections may occur, especially in elderly, debilitated, or immunosuppressed patients. Monitor patient closely.
- Drug may be better suited to patients on sodium-free diets than carbenicillin and ticarcillin (contains 1.85 mEq sodium/g of piperacillin).
- Piperacillin has shown greater activity against *Pseudomonas aeruginosa* than carbenicillin, ticarcillin, or mezlocillin.
- Give piperacillin at least 1 hour before bacteriostatic antibiotics.

ticarcillin disodium

Ticar, Ticillin‡

Pregnancy Risk Category: B

HOW SUPPLIED

Injection: 1 g, 3 g, 6 g
I.V. infusion: 3 g
Pharmacy bulk package: 20 g, 30 g

MECHANISM OF ACTION

Bactericidal against microorganisms by inhibiting cell wall synthesis during active multiplication. Bacteria resist penicillins by producing penicillinases – enzymes that convert penicillin to inactive penicilloic acid.

INDICATIONS & DOSAGE

Severe systemic infections caused by susceptible strains of gram-positive and especially gram-negative organisms (including Pseudomonas, Proteus*)* –
Adults: 18 g I.V. or I.M. daily, divided into doses given q 4 to 6 hours.
Children: 200 to 300 mg/kg I.V. or I.M. daily, divided into doses given q 4 to 6 hours.

ADVERSE REACTIONS

Common reactions are in italics; life-threatening reactions are in bold italics.
Blood: leukopenia, neutropenia, eosinophilia, *thrombocytopenia,* hemolytic anemia.
CNS: seizures, neuromuscular excitability.
GI: nausea, diarrhea.
Metabolic: *hypokalemia*.
Local: pain at injection site, vein irritation, phlebitis.
Other: hypersensitivity (rash, pruritus, urticaria, chills, fever, edema, ***anaphylaxis***), overgrowth of nonsusceptible organisms.

INTERACTIONS

Aminoglycoside antibiotics (such as gentamicin and tobramycin): chemically incompatible. Don't mix together in I.V.
Probenecid: increases blood levels of ticarcillin and other penicillins. Probenecid may be used for this purpose.

NURSING CONSIDERATIONS

- *Use cautiously* in other drug allergies, especially to cephalosporins (possible cross-allergenicity), and in impaired renal function, hemorrhagic conditions, hypokalemia, or sodium restrictions (contains 5.2 mEq sodium/g).
- Obtain specimen for culture and sensitivity tests before first dose. Therapy may begin pending test results.
- Before giving ticarcillin, ask patient if he's had any allergic reactions to penicillin. However, a negative history of penicillin allergy is no guarantee against a future allergic reaction.

• Dosage should be decreased in patients with impaired renal functions.
• Check CBC and platelets frequently. Drug may cause thrombocytopenia.
• If patient has high blood level of this drug, he may develop seizures. Institute seizure precautions.
• **I.V. use:** When giving I.V., mix with dextrose 5% in water or other suitable I.V. fluids.
• Give I.V. intermittently to prevent vein irritation. Change site every 48 hours.
• Administer deep I.M. into large muscle.
• Almost always used with another antibiotic, such as gentamicin.
• With large doses and prolonged therapy, bacterial and fungal superinfections may occur, especially in elderly, debilitated, or immunosuppressed patients. Close observation is essential.
• Monitor serum potassium.
• Give ticarcillin at least 1 hour before bacteriostatic antibiotics.

ticarcillin disodium/ clavulanate potassium

Timentin

Pregnancy Risk Category: B

HOW SUPPLIED

Injection: 3 g ticarcillin and 100 mg clavulanic acid

MECHANISM OF ACTION

Ticarcillin is an extended-spectrum penicillin that inhibits cell wall synthesis during active bacterial replication. Clavulanic acid increases ticarcillin's effectiveness by inactivating beta lactamases, which destroy ticarcillin.

INDICATIONS & DOSAGE

Infections of the lower respiratory tract, urinary tract, bones and joints, skin and skin structure, and septicemia when caused by beta-lactamase-producing strains of bacteria or by ticarcillin-susceptible organisms – **Adults:** 1 vial (ticarcillin 3 g and clavulanate potassium 0.1 g) administered by I.V. infusion q 4 to 6 hours.

ADVERSE REACTIONS

Common reactions are in italics; life-threatening reactions are in bold italics.
Blood: leukopenia, neutropenia, eosinophilia, *thrombocytopenia,* hemolytic anemia.
CNS: seizures, neuromuscular excitability.
GI: nausea, diarrhea.
Metabolic: ***hypokalemia.***
Local: pain at injection site, vein irritation, phlebitis.
Other: hypersensitivity (rash, pruritus, urticaria, chills, fever, edema, ***anaphylaxis***), overgrowth of nonsusceptible organisms.

INTERACTIONS

Aminoglycoside antibiotics (such as gentamicin and tobramycin): chemically incompatible. Don't mix together in I.V.
Probenecid: increases blood levels of ticarcillin. Probenecid may be used for this purpose.

NURSING CONSIDERATIONS

• *Use cautiously* in patients with other drug allergies, especially to cephalosporins (possible cross-allergenicity), and in impaired renal function, hemorrhagic conditions, hypokalemia, or sodium restrictions.
• Obtain specimen for culture and sensitivity tests before first dose. Therapy may begin pending test results.
• Before giving Timentin, ask patient if he's had any allergic reactions to penicillin. However, a negative history of penicillin allergy is no guarantee against a future allergic reaction.
• Dosage should be decreased in patients with impaired renal functions.

- With large doses and prolonged therapy, bacterial and fungal superinfections may occur, especially in elderly, debilitated, or immunosuppressed patients. Close observation is essential.
- Check CBC and platelets frequently. Drug may cause thrombocytopenia.
- Monitor serum potassium.
- **I.V. use:** Administer by I.V. infusion over 30 minutes. Don't give by I.V. push or I.M.
- Particularly useful in clinical settings with a high prevalence of ticarcillin-resistant organisms.
- Give drug at least 1 hour before bacteriostatic antibiotics.

*Liquid form contains alcohol. **May contain tartrazine.

13

Cephalosporins

cefaclor
cefadroxil monohydrate
cefamandole nafate
cefazolin sodium
cefixime
cefmetazole sodium
cefonicid sodium
cefoperazone sodium
cefotaxime sodium
cefotetan disodium
cefoxitin sodium
cefpodoxime proxetil
cefprozil
ceftazidime
ceftizoxime sodium
ceftriaxone sodium
cefuroxime axetil
cefuroxime sodium
cephalexin hydrochloride
cephalexin monohydrate
cephalothin sodium
cephapirin sodium
cephradine
loracarbef
moxalactam disodium

COMBINATION PRODUCTS
None.

---

cefaclor

Ceclor

Pregnancy Risk Category: B

HOW SUPPLIED
Capsules: 250 mg, 500 mg
Oral suspension: 125 mg/5 ml, 250 mg/5 ml, 375 mg/5 ml

MECHANISM OF ACTION
Inhibits cell wall synthesis, promoting osmotic instability. Usually bactericidal.

INDICATIONS & DOSAGE
Infections of respiratory or urinary tracts, skin, and soft tissue; and otitis media due to Haemophilus influenzae, Streptococcus pneumoniae, S. pyogenes, Escherichia coli, Proteus mirabilis, Klebsiella *species, and staphylococci –*
Adults: 250 to 500 mg P.O. q 8 hours. Total daily dose should not exceed 4 g.
Children: 20 mg/kg daily P.O. in divided doses q 8 hours. In more serious infections, 40 mg/kg daily are recommended, not to exceed 1 g daily.

ADVERSE REACTIONS
Common reactions are in italics; life-threatening reactions are in bold italics.
Blood: transient leukopenia, lymphocytosis, anemia, eosinophilia.
CNS: dizziness, headache, somnolence.
GI: *nausea,* vomiting, *diarrhea,* anorexia, pseudomembranous colitis.
GU: red and white cells in urine, vaginal moniliasis, vaginitis.
Skin: *maculopapular rash,* dermatitis.
Other: ***hypersensitivity,*** fever, cholestatic jaundice.

INTERACTIONS
Probenecid: may inhibit excretion and increase blood levels of cefaclor.

NURSING CONSIDERATIONS
• *Contraindicated* in hypersensitivity to other cephalosporins.
• *Use cautiously* in impaired renal function and in those with history of sensitivity to penicillin. Ask patient if he's had any reaction to previous cephalosporin or penicillin therapy before administering first dose.

• Obtain specimen for culture and sensitivity tests before first dose. Therapy may begin pending test results.
• Major clinical use appears to be in treating otitis media caused by *H. influenzae* when resistant to ampicillin or amoxicillin. Drug is a second-generation cephalosporin.
• Tell patient to take medication exactly as prescribed, even after he feels better, and to take entire amount prescribed.
• Call doctor if skin rash develops.
• With large doses or prolonged therapy, monitor for superinfection, especially in high-risk patients.
• Store reconstituted suspension in refrigerator. Stable for 14 days if refrigerated. Shake well before using.
• Drug may be taken with meals.
• Cefaclor is a relatively expensive antibiotic and should be used only when the organism is resistant to other agents.
• If ordered, total daily dose of cefaclor may be administered twice daily (at 12-hour intervals) rather than three times daily with similar therapeutic results.
• Urine glucose determinations may be false-positive with copper sulfate tests (Clinitest); glucose enzymatic tests (Clinistix, Tes-Tape) are not affected.

cefadroxil monohydrate

Duricef, Ultracef

Pregnancy Risk Category: B

HOW SUPPLIED

Tablets: 1 g
Capsules: 500 mg
Oral suspension: 125 mg/5 ml, 250 mg/5 ml, 500 mg/5 ml

MECHANISM OF ACTION

Inhibits cell wall synthesis, promoting osmotic instability. Usually bactericidal.

INDICATIONS & DOSAGE

Urinary tract infections caused by Escherichia coli, Proteus mirabilis, *and* Klebsiella *species; infections of skin and soft tissue; and streptococcal pharyngitis –*
Adults: 500 mg to 2 g P.O. per day, depending on the infection being treated. Usually given in once-daily or b.i.d. dosage.
Children: 30 mg/kg P.O. daily in 2 divided doses.

ADVERSE REACTIONS

Common reactions are in italics; life-threatening reactions are in bold italics.
Blood: transient neutropenia, eosinophilia, leukopenia, anemia.
CNS: dizziness, headache, malaise, paresthesias.
GI: pseudomembranous colitis, *nausea,* anorexia, vomiting, *diarrhea,* glossitis, *dyspepsia,* abdominal cramps, anal pruritus, tenesmus, oral candidiasis (thrush).
GU: genital pruritus, moniliasis.
Skin: *maculopapular and erythematous rashes.*
Other: ***hypersensitivity,*** dyspnea.

INTERACTIONS

Probenecid: may inhibit excretion and increase blood levels of cefadroxil.

NURSING CONSIDERATIONS

• *Contraindicated* in patients with hypersensitivity to other cephalosporins.
• *Use cautiously* in patients with history of sensitivity to penicillin. Ask patient if he's had any reaction to previous cephalosporin or penicillin therapy before administering first dose. Also use cautiously in patients with impaired renal function; dosage adjustments are necessary.
• Obtain specimen for culture and sensitivity tests before first dose. Therapy may begin pending test results.
• If creatinine clearance is below 50 ml/minute, dosage interval should be

lengthened so drug doesn't accumulate.

- Tell patient to take medication exactly as prescribed, even after he feels better, and to take entire amount prescribed.
- Call doctor if skin rash develops.
- Since absorption not delayed by presence of food, tell the patient to take with food or milk to lessen GI discomfort.
- Longer half-life permits once- or twice-daily dosing.
- Urine glucose determinations may be false-positive with copper sulfate tests (Clinitest); glucose enzymatic tests (Clinistix, Tes-Tape) are not affected.
- With large doses or prolonged therapy, monitor for superinfection, especially in high-risk patients.

cefamandole nafate

Mandol

Pregnancy Risk Category: B

HOW SUPPLIED

Injection: 500 mg, 1 g, 2 g, 10 g
Pharmacy bulk package: 10 g

MECHANISM OF ACTION

Inhibits cell wall synthesis, promoting osmotic instability. Usually bactericidal.

INDICATIONS & DOSAGE

Serious infections of respiratory and GU tracts, skin and soft-tissue infections, bone and joint infections, septicemia, and peritonitis due to Escherichia coli *and other coliform bacteria,* S. aureus *(penicillinase- and nonpenicillinase-producing),* S. epidermidis, *group A beta-hemolytic streptococci,* Klebsiella, Haemophilus influenzae, Proteus mirabilis, *and* Enterobacter –

Adults: 500 mg to 1 g q 4 to 8 hours. In life-threatening infections, up to 2 g q 4 hours may be needed.

Infants and children: 50 to 100 mg/kg daily in equally divided doses q 4 to 8 hours. May be increased to total daily dose of 150 mg/kg (not to exceed maximum adult dose) for severe infections.

Total daily dosage is same for I.M. or I.V. administration and depends on susceptibility of organism and severity of infection. In patients with impaired renal function, doses or frequency of administration must be modified according to degree of renal impairment, severity of infection, and susceptibility of organism. Should be injected deep I.M. into a large muscle mass, such as gluteus or lateral aspect of thigh.

ADVERSE REACTIONS

Common reactions are in italics; life-threatening reactions are in bold italics.

Blood: transient neutropenia, eosinophilia, hemolytic anemia, *hypoprothrombinemia,* bleeding.

CNS: headache, malaise, paresthesias, dizziness.

GI: pseudomembranous colitis, nausea, anorexia, vomiting, *diarrhea,* glossitis, dyspepsia, abdominal cramps, tenesmus, anal pruritus, oral candidiasis (thrush).

GU: genital pruritus and moniliasis.

Skin: *maculopapular and erythematous rashes, urticaria.*

Local: *at injection site – pain, induration, sterile abscesses,* temperature elevation, tissue sloughing; *phlebitis and thrombophlebitis with I.V. injection.*

Other: ***hypersensitivity,*** dyspnea, cholestatic jaundice.

INTERACTIONS

Ethyl alcohol: may cause a disulfiram-like reaction. Warn patients not to drink alcohol for several days after discontinuing cefamandole.

Oral anticoagulants, aspirin: increased risk of bleeding.

Probenecid: may inhibit excretion and increase blood levels of cefamandole.

NURSING CONSIDERATIONS

- *Contraindicated* in patients with hypersensitivity to other cephalosporins.
- *Use cautiously* in patients with impaired renal function and in those with history of sensitivity to penicillin. Ask patient if he's had any reaction to previous cephalosporin or penicillin therapy before administering first dose.
- Obtain specimen for culture and sensitivity tests before first dose. Therapy may begin pending test results.
- Not as effective as cefoxitin in treating anaerobic infections.
- For most cephalosporin-sensitive organisms, cefamandole offers little advantage over previously available agents.
- **I.V. use:** Reconstitute 1 g with 10 ml of sterile water for injection, dextrose 5% or 0.9% sodium chloride for injection.
- Don't mix with I.V. infusions containing magnesium or calcium ions; chemically incompatible.
- I.M. cefamandole is not as painful as cefoxitin. Does not require addition of lidocaine.
- After reconstitution, drug remains stable for 24 hours at room temperature or 96 hours under refrigeration.
- The chemical structure of this drug includes the methylthiotetrazole (MTT) side chain that has been associated with bleeding disorders. If bleeding occurs, it can be promptly reversed with administration of vitamin K.
- With large doses or prolonged therapy, monitor for superinfection, especially in high-risk patients.
- Urine glucose determinations may be false-positive with copper sulfate tests (Clinitest); glucose enzymatic tests (Clinistix, Tes-Tape) are not affected.

cefazolin sodium

Ancef, Kefzol

Pregnancy Risk Category: B

HOW SUPPLIED

Injection (parenteral): 250 mg, 500 mg, 1 g, 5 g, 10 g, 20 g
Infusion: 500 mg/100 ml vial, 500-mg or 1-g Redi Vials, Faspaks, or ADD-Vantage vials

MECHANISM OF ACTION

Inhibits cell wall synthesis, promoting osmotic instability. Usually bactericidal.

INDICATIONS & DOSAGE

Serious infections of respiratory, biliary, and GU tracts, skin and soft-tissue infections, bone and joint infections, septicemia, and endocarditis due to Escherichia coli, *Enterobacteriaceae, gonococci,* Haemophilus influenzae, Klebsiella, Proteus mirabilis, Staphylococcus aureus, Streptococcus pneumoniae, *and group A beta-hemolytic streptococci; and perioperative prophylaxis –*
Adults: 250 mg I.M. or I.V. q 8 hours to 1 g q 6 hours. Maximum 12 g/day in life-threatening situations.
Children over 1 month: 25 to 100 mg/kg/day I.M. or I.V. in three or four divided doses.

Total daily dosage is same for I.M. or I.V. administration and depends on susceptibility of organism and severity of infection. In patients with impaired renal function, doses or frequency of administration must be modified according to degree of renal impairment, severity of infection, and susceptibility of organism. Should be injected deep I.M. into a large muscle mass, such as gluteus or lateral aspect of thigh.

ADVERSE REACTIONS

Common reactions are in italics; life-threatening reactions are in bold italics.

*Liquid form contains alcohol. **May contain tartrazine.

Blood: transient neutropenia, leukopenia, eosinophilia, anemia.
CNS: dizziness, headache, malaise, paresthesia.
GI: pseudomembranous colitis, nausea, anorexia, vomiting, *diarrhea,* glossitis, dyspepsia, abdominal cramps, anal pruritus, tenesmus, oral candidiasis (thrush).
GU: genital pruritus and moniliasis, vaginitis.
Skin: *maculopapular and erythematous rashes, urticaria.*
Local: *at injection site–pain, induration, sterile abscesses, tissue sloughing; phlebitis and thrombophlebitis with I.V. injection.*
Other: ***hypersensitivity,*** dyspnea.

INTERACTIONS
Probenecid: may inhibit excretion and increase blood levels of cefazolin.

NURSING CONSIDERATIONS
- *Use cautiously* in impaired renal function and in those with history of sensitivity to penicillin. Ask patient if he's ever had any reaction to cephalosporin or penicillin therapy before administering first dose.
- Avoid doses greater than 4 g daily in patients with severe renal impairment.
- Obtain specimen for culture and sensitivity tests before first dose. Therapy may begin pending test results.
- Because of long duration of effect, most infections can be treated with a dose q 8 hours.
- For I.M. administration, reconstitute with sterile water, bacteriostatic water, or 0.9% sodium chloride solution as follows: 2 ml to 250-mg vial; 2 ml to 500-mg vial; 2.5 ml to 1-g vial. Shake well until dissolved. Resultant concentration: 125 mg/ml, 225 mg/ml, 330 mg/ml, respectively.
- Not as painful as other cephalosporins when given I.M.
- **I.V. use:** Alternate injection sites if I.V. therapy lasts longer than 3 days. Use of small I.V. needles in the larger available veins may be preferable.
- For direct injection, further dilute drug with 10 ml of compatible solution; for intermittent infusion, add reconstituted drug to 50 to 100 ml of compatible solution or use premixed solution.
- Reconstituted cefazolin sodium is stable for 24 hours at room temperature or 96 hours under refrigeration.
- From 40% to 75% of patients receiving cephalosporins show a false-positive direct Coombs' test; only a few of these indicate hemolytic anemia.
- With large doses or prolonged therapy, monitor for superinfection, especially in high-risk patients.
- Considered the first-generation cephalosporin of choice by most authorities.
- Urine glucose determinations may be false-positive with copper sulfate tests (Clinitest); glucose enzymatic tests (Clinistix, Tes-Tape) are not affected.

cefixime
Suprax

Pregnancy Risk Category: B

HOW SUPPLIED
Tablets: 200 mg, 400 mg
Oral suspension: 100 mg/5 ml (after reconstitution)

MECHANISM OF ACTION
Inhibits cell wall synthesis, promoting osmotic instability. Usually bactericidal.

INDICATIONS & DOSAGE
Uncomplicated urinary tract infections caused by Escherichia coli *and* Proteus mirabilis; *otitis media caused by* Haemophilus influenzae *(beta-lactam positive and negative strains,* Moraxella (Branhamella) catarrhalis,

and Streptococcus pyogenes; *pharyngitis and tonsillitis caused by* S. pyogenes; *acute bronchitis and acute exacerbations of chronic bronchitis caused by* S. pneumoniae *and* H. influenzae *(beta-lactamase positive and negative strains)* –
Adults: 400 mg/day P.O. as a single 400-mg tablet or 200 mg q 12 hours.
Children: 8 mg/kg/day suspension P.O. as a single daily dose or 4 mg/kg q 12 hours.

Treat children over age 12 and those who weigh more than 50 kg with the recommended adult dose.
Gonorrhea –
Adults: 400 mg P.O. as a single dose.

ADVERSE REACTIONS
Common reactions are in italics; life-threatening reactions are in bold italics.
Blood: thrombocytopenia, leukopenia, eosinophilia.
CNS: headaches, dizziness.
GI: *diarrhea,* loose stools, abdominal pain, nausea, vomiting, dyspepsia, flatulence, pseudomembranous colitis.
GU: genital pruritus, vaginitis, genital candidiasis.
Skin: pruritus, rash, urticaria.
Other: drug fever, ***hypersensitivity reactions.***

INTERACTIONS
None significant.

NURSING CONSIDERATIONS
- *Contraindicated* in patients with hypersensitivity to other cephalosporins.
- *Use cautiously* and with reduced dosage in patients with renal dysfunction; reduced dosage is necessary in patients with creatinine clearance below 60 ml/minute. Also use cautiously in patients with a history of sensitivity to penicillin. Ask patients if they have had any reactions to previous cephalosporin or penicillin therapy before administering the first dose.
- Obtain specimen for culture and sensitivity tests before first dose. Therapy may begin pending test results.
- Call doctor is skin rash develops.
- Preparation of oral suspension: add required amount of water to powder in two portions. Shake well after each addition. After mixing, suspension is stable for 14 days. It does not require refrigeration, but keep tightly closed. Shake well before using.
- With large doses or prolonged therapy, monitor for superinfection, especially in high-risk patients.
- From 40% to 75% of patients receiving cephalosporins show a false-positive direct Coombs' test, but only a few of these tests indicate hemolytic anemia.
- Urine glucose determinations may be false-positive with copper sulfate tests (Clinitest); glucose enzymatic tests (Clinistix, Tes-Tape) are not affected.

cefmetazole sodium
Zefazone

Pregnancy Risk Category: B

HOW SUPPLIED
Injection: 1 g, 2 g

MECHANISM OF ACTION
Inhibits cell wall synthesis, promoting osmotic instability. Usually bactericidal.

INDICATIONS & DOSAGE
Lower respiratory tract infections caused by Streptococcus pneumoniae, Staphylococcus aureus *(penicillinase- and non-penicillinase-producing strains),* Escherichia coli, *and* Haemophilus influenzae *(non-penicillinase-producing strains; intra-abdominal infections caused by* E. coli *or* Bacteroides fragilis; *skin and skin-structure infections caused by* S. aureus *(penicillinase- and non-penicillinase-producing strains),* S. epider-

*Liquid form contains alcohol. **May contain tartrazine.

midis, Streptococcus pyogenes, S. agalactiae, E. coli, Proteus mirabilis, Klebsiella pneumoniae, *and* B. fragilis –
Adults: 2 g I.V. q 6 to 12 hours for 5 to 14 days.
Urinary tract infections caused by E. coli –
Adults: 2 g I.V. q 12 hours.
Prophylaxis in patients undergoing vaginal hysterectomy –
Adults: 2 g I.V. 30 to 90 minutes before surgery as a single dose; or 1 g I.V. 30 to 90 minutes before surgery, repeated in 8 and 16 hours.
Prophylaxis in patients undergoing abdominal hysterectomy –
Adults: 1 g I.V. 30 to 90 minutes before surgery, repeated in 8 and 16 hours.
Prophylaxis in patients undergoing cesarean section –
Adults: 2 g I.V. as a single dose after clamping cord; or 1 g I.V. after clamping cord, repeated in 8 and 16 hours.
Prophylaxis in patients undergoing colorectal surgery –
Adults: 2 g I.V. as a single dose 30 to 90 minutes before surgery. Some clinicians follow with additional 2-g doses in 8 and 16 hours.
Prophylaxis in patients undergoing cholecystectomy (high risk) –
Adults: 1 g I.V. 30 to 90 minutes before surgery, repeated in 8 and 16 hours.

ADVERSE REACTIONS

Common reactions are in italics; life-threatening reactions are in bold italics.
CNS: headache.
CV: ***shock,*** hypotension.
EENT: epistaxis.
GI: nausea, vomiting, *diarrhea,* epigastric pain, pseudomembranous colitis.
GU: vaginitis.
Respiratory: pleural effusion, dyspnea, respiratory distress.
Skin: rash, pruritus, generalized erythema.
Local: pain at injection site, phlebitis.
Other: fever, bacterial or fungal superinfection, ***hypersensitivity,*** altered color perception.

INTERACTIONS

Alcohol: disulfiram-like reaction. Alcohol should be avoided within 24 hours of administration.
Aminoglycosides: increased risk of nephrotoxicity.

NURSING CONSIDERATIONS

- *Contraindicated* in patients with a history of hypersensitivity to cephalosporins. Ask patient if he's had any reaction to previous cephalosporin or penicillin therapy before administering first dose.
- Obtain specimen for culture and sensitivity before first dose. Therapy may begin pending test results.
- Prolonged use may result in overgrowth of nonsusceptible organisms. Monitor patient for bacterial and fungal superinfections.
- The chemical structure of this drug includes the methylthiotetrazole (MTT) side chain that has been associated with bleeding disorders. However, such bleeding has not been reported with this drug. Monitor prothrombin time and administer vitamin K as ordered.
- Cephalosporins may cause false-positive results for urine glucose with copper sulfate tests (Clinitest). Glucose enzymatic tests (Clinistix, Tes-Tape) are not affected.
- **I.V. use:** Reconstitute with bacteriostatic water for injection, sterile water for injection, or 0.9% sodium chloride for injection. After reconstitution, the drug may be further diluted to concentrations ranging from 1 to 20 mg/ml by adding it to 0.9% sodium chloride injection, dextrose 5% in water, or lactated Ringer's injection. Reconstituted or dilute solutions

are stable for 24 hours at room temperature (77° F [25° C]) or 1 week if refrigerated (46° F [8° C]).

cefonicid sodium

Monocid

Pregnancy Risk Category: B

HOW SUPPLIED

Injection: 500 mg, 1 g
Infusion: 1 g/100 ml
Pharmacy bulk package: 10 g

MECHANISM OF ACTION

Inhibits cell wall synthesis, promoting osmotic instability. Usually bactericidal.

INDICATIONS & DOSAGE

Serious infections of the lower respiratory and urinary tract; skin and skin structure infections; septicemia; bone and joint infections; and perioperative prophylaxis. Susceptible microorganisms include Streptococcus pneumoniae, Klebsiella pneumoniae, Escherichia coli, Haemophilus influenzae, Proteus mirabilis, Staphylococcus aureus and epidermidis, and Streptococcus pyogenes –

Adults: usual dosage is 1 g I.V. or I.M. q 24 hours. In life-threatening infections, 2 g q 24 hours.

Total daily dosage is same for I.M. or I.V. administration and depends on susceptibility of organism and severity of infection. In patients with impaired renal function, doses or frequency of administration must be modified according to degree of renal impairment, severity of infection, and susceptibility of organism. Should be injected deep I.M. into a large muscle mass, such as gluteus or lateral aspect of thigh.

ADVERSE REACTIONS

Common reactions are in italics; life-threatening reactions are in bold italics.

Blood: transient neutropenia, leukopenia, eosinophilia, anemia.
CNS: dizziness, headache, malaise, paresthesia.
GI: pseudomembranous colitis, nausea, anorexia, vomiting, diarrhea, glossitis, dyspepsia, abdominal cramps, anal pruritus, tenesmus, oral candidiasis (thrush).
GU: genital pruritus and moniliasis, vaginitis.
Skin: *maculopapular and erythematous rashes, urticaria.*
Local: *at injection site – pain, induration, sterile abscesses, tissue sloughing; phlebitis and thrombophlebitis with I.V. injection.*
Other: ***hypersensitivity,*** dyspnea.

INTERACTIONS

Probenecid: may inhibit excretion and increase blood levels of cefonicid.

NURSING CONSIDERATIONS

- *Contraindicated* in patients with hypersensitivity to other cephalosporins.
- *Use cautiously* in impaired renal function and in those with history of sensitivity to penicillin. Ask if patient has had any reaction to previous cephalosporin or penicillin therapy before administering first dose.
- Obtain specimen for culture and sensitivity tests before first dose. Therapy may begin pending test results.
- When administering 2-g I.M. doses once daily, divide the dose equally and inject deeply in two large muscle sites.
- **I.V. use:** : Reconstitute 500-mg vial with 2 ml of sterile water for injection (yields a concentration of 220 mg/ml) and 1-g vial with 2.5 ml of sterile water for injection (yields a concentration of 325 mg/ml). Shake well. Reconstitute piggyback vials with 50 to 100 ml of sterile water for injection, bacteriostatic water for injection, or 0.9% sodium chloride.
- With large doses or prolonged ther-

apy, monitor for superinfection, especially in high-risk patients.
• Has been promoted as a cost-effective agent for surgical prophylaxis.

cefoperazone sodium
Cefobid

Pregnancy Risk Category: B

HOW SUPPLIED
Infusion: 1 g, 2 g piggyback
Parenteral: 1 g, 2 g

MECHANISM OF ACTION
Inhibits cell wall synthesis, promoting osmotic instability. Usually bactericidal.

INDICATIONS & DOSAGE
Serious infections of the respiratory tract; intra-abdominal, gynecologic, and skin infections; bacteremia, septicemia. Susceptible microorganisms include Streptococcus pneumoniae *and* S. pyogenes; Staphylococcus aureus *(penicillinase and non-penicillinase-producing) and* S. epidermidis; *enterococcus;* Escherichia coli; Klebsiella; Haemophilus influenzae; Enterobacter; Citrobacter; Proteus; *some* Pseudomonas, *including* Pseudomonas aeruginosa; *and* Bacteroides fragilis –

Adults: usual dosage is 1 to 2 g q 12 hours I.M. or I.V. In severe infections, or infections caused by less sensitive organisms, the total daily dosage or frequency may be increased up to 16 g/day in certain situations.

No dosage adjustment is usually necessary in patients with renal impairment. However, doses of 4 g/day should be given very cautiously in patients with hepatic disease. Should be injected deep I.M. into a large muscle mass, such as gluteus or lateral aspect of the thigh.

ADVERSE REACTIONS
Common reactions are in italics; life-threatening reactions are in bold italics.
Blood: transient neutropenia, eosinophilia, hemolytic anemia, hypoprothrombinemia, bleeding.
CNS: headache, malaise, paresthesias, dizziness.
GI: pseudomembranous colitis, nausea, anorexia, vomiting, *diarrhea,* glossitis, dyspepsia, abdominal cramps, tenesmus, anal pruritus, oral candidiasis (thrush).
Hepatic: mildly elevated liver enzymes.
GU: genital pruritus and moniliasis.
Skin: *maculopapular and erythematous rashes, urticaria.*
Local: *at injection site – pain, induration, sterile abscesses, temperature elevation, tissue sloughing; phlebitis and thrombophlebitis with I.V. injection.*
Other: ***hypersensitivity,*** dyspnea.

INTERACTIONS
Ethyl alcohol: may cause a disulfiram-like reaction. Warn patients not to drink alcohol for several days after discontinuing cefoperazone.
Oral anticoagulants, aspirin: increased risk of bleeding.
Probenecid: may inhibit excretion and increase blood levels of cefoperazone.

NURSING CONSIDERATIONS
• *Contraindicated* in patients with hypersensitivity to other cephalosporins.
• *Use cautiously* in impaired renal function and in those with history of sensitivity to penicillin. Ask if patient has had any reaction to previous cephalosporin or penicillin therapy before administering first dose.
• Obtain specimen for culture and sensitivity tests before first dose. Therapy may begin pending test results.
• Cefoperazone is one of the third-generation cephalosporins. It has greater activity than first-generation

cephalosporins against gram-negative organisms, but less activity against gram-positive organisms.
• Because of high degree of biliary excretion, may cause more diarrhea than other cephalosporins.
• The chemical structure of this drug includes the methylthiotetrazole (MTT) side chain that has been associated with bleeding disorders. If bleeding occurs, it can be promptly reversed with administration of vitamin K. Monitor prothrombin time regularly.
• With large doses or prolonged therapy, monitor for superinfection, especially in high-risk patients.
• Urine glucose determinations may be false-positive with copper sulfate tests (Clinitest); glucose enzymatic tests (Clinistix, Tes-Tape) are not affected.
• **I.V. use:** Infuse by intermittent infusion over 15 to 30 minutes into tubing containing a compatible solution.

cefotaxime sodium

Claforan

Pregnancy Risk Category: B

HOW SUPPLIED

Injection: 500 mg, 1 g, 2 g
Infusion: 1 g, 2 g
Pharmacy bulk package: 10-g vial

MECHANISM OF ACTION

Inhibits cell wall synthesis, promoting osmotic instability. Usually bactericidal.

INDICATIONS & DOSAGE

Serious infections of the lower respiratory and urinary tracts, CNS infections, gynecologic infections, bacteremia, septicemia, skin infections, and perioperative prophylaxis. Among susceptible microorganisms are streptococci, including Streptococcus pneumoniae *and* S. pyogenes; Staphylococcus aureus *(penicillinase- and non-penicillinase-producing) and* S. epidermidis; Escherichia coli; Klebsiella; Haemophilus influenzae; Enterobacter; Proteus; *and* Peptostreptococcus –

Adults: usual dose is 1 g I.V. or I.M. q 6 to 8 hours. Up to 12 g daily can be administered in life-threatening infections.

Total daily dosage is same for I.M. or I.V. administration and depends on susceptibility of organism and severity of infection. In patients with impaired renal function, doses or frequency of administration must be modified according to degree of renal impairment, severity of infection, and susceptibility of organism. Should be injected deep I.M. into a large muscle mass, such as gluteus or lateral aspect of thigh.

Children 1 month to 12 years: 50 to 180 mg/kg/day I.M. or I.V. in 4 to 6 divided doses.

Neonates to 1 week: 50 mg/kg I.V. q 12 hours.

Neonates 1 to 4 weeks: 50 mg/kg I.V. q 8 hours.

ADVERSE REACTIONS

Common reactions are in italics; life-threatening reactions are in bold italics.

Blood: transient neutropenia, eosinophilia, hemolytic anemia.

CNS: headache, malaise, paresthesias, dizziness.

GI: pseudomembranous colitis, nausea, anorexia, vomiting, *diarrhea,* glossitis, dyspepsia, abdominal cramps, tenesmus, anal pruritus, oral candidiasis (thrush).

GU: genital pruritus and moniliasis.

Skin: *maculopapular and erythematous rashes, urticaria.*

Local: *at injection site – pain, induration, sterile abscesses, temperature elevation, tissue sloughing; phlebitis and thrombophlebitis with I.V. injection.*

Other: ***hypersensitivity,*** dyspnea, elevated temperature.

*Liquid form contains alcohol. **May contain tartrazine.

INTERACTIONS

Probenecid: may inhibit excretion and increase blood levels of cefotaxime. Use together cautiously.

NURSING CONSIDERATIONS

- *Contraindicated* in patients with hypersensitivity to other cephalosporins.
- *Use cautiously* in impaired renal function and in those with history of sensitivity to penicillin. Ask if patient has had any reaction to previous cephalosporin or penicillin therapy before administering first dose.
- Obtain specimen for culture and sensitivity tests before first dose. Therapy may begin pending test results.
- With large doses or prolonged therapy, monitor for superinfection, especially in high-risk patients.
- Cefotaxime was the first of the so-called third-generation cephalosporins. It has increased antibacterial activity against gram-negative microorganisms and has an active metabolite.
- Some doctors may prescribe cefotaxime in clinical situations in which they formerly prescribed aminoglycosides. However, this drug is usually not effective against infections caused by *Pseudomonas* organisms.
- Urine glucose determinations may be false-positive with copper sulfate tests (Clinitest); glucose enzymatic tests (Clinistix, Tes-Tape) are not affected.
- **I.V. use:** Reconstitute infusion vials with 50 to 100 ml of dextrose 5% in water or 0.9% sodium chloride. Interrupt flow of primary I.V. solution during infusion.

cefotetan disodium

Cefotan

Pregnancy Risk Category: B

HOW SUPPLIED

Injection: 1 g, 2 g
Infusion: 1 g, 2 g piggyback

MECHANISM OF ACTION

Inhibits cell wall synthesis, promoting osmotic instability. Usually bactericidal.

INDICATIONS & DOSAGE

Serious infections of the urinary and lower respiratory tracts, and gynecologic, skin and skin structure, intra-abdominal, and bone and joint infections, and perioperative prophylaxis. Among susceptible microorganisms are streptococci, Staphylococcus aureus *(penicillinase- and non-penicillinase-producing) and* S. epidermidis, Escherichia coli, Klebsiella, Enterobacter, Proteus, Haemophilus influenzae, Neisseria gonorrhoeae, *and* Bacteroides, *including* B. fragilis –
Adults: 1 to 2 g I.V. or I.M. q 12 hours for 5 to 10 days. Up to 6 g daily in life-threatening infections.

Total daily dosage is same for I.M. or I.V. administration and depends on susceptibility of organism and severity of infection. In patients with impaired renal function, doses or frequency of administration must be modified according to degree of renal impairment, severity of infection, and susceptibility of organism. Should be injected deep I.M. into a large muscle mass, such as gluteus or lateral aspect of thigh.

ADVERSE REACTIONS

Common reactions are in italics; life-threatening reactions are in bold italics.
Blood: transient neutropenia, eosinophilia, hemolytic anemia, hypoprothrombinemia, bleeding.
CNS: headache, malaise, paresthesias, dizziness.
GI: pseudomembranous colitis, nausea, anorexia, vomiting, *diarrhea,* glossitis, dyspepsia, abdominal cramps, tenesmus, anal pruritus.
GU: genital pruritus and moniliasis.
Skin: *maculopapular and erythematous rashes, urticaria.*
Local: *at injection site – pain, indura-*

tion, sterile abscesses, tissue sloughing; phlebitis and thrombophlebitis with I.V. injection.
Other: ***hypersensitivity,*** dyspnea, elevated temperature.

INTERACTIONS
Ethyl alcohol: may cause a disulfiram-like reaction. Warn patients not to drink alcohol for several days after discontinuing cefotetan.
Oral anticoagulants, aspirin: increased risk of bleeding.
Probenecid: may inhibit excretion and increase blood levels of cefotetan.

NURSING CONSIDERATIONS
- *Contraindicated* in patients with hypersensitivity to other cephalosporins.
- *Use cautiously* in impaired renal status and in those with history of sensitivity to penicillin. Ask if patient has had any reaction to previous cephalosporin or penicillin therapy before administering first dose.
- Obtain specimen for culture and sensitivity tests before first dose. Therapy may begin pending test results.
- **I.V. use:** Reconstitute with sterile water for injection. Then, may be mixed with 50 to 100 ml of dextrose 5% in water or 0.9% sodium chloride solution. Interrupt flow of primary I.V. solution during cefotetan infusion.
- I.M. injection may be reconstituted with sterile water or bacteriostatic water for injection, normal saline, 0.5% or 1% lidocaine hydrochloride. Shake to dissolve and let stand until clear.
- Reconstituted solution remains stable for 24 hours at room temperature or 96 hours when refrigerated.
- The chemical structure of this drug includes the methylthiotetrazole (MTT) side chain that has been associated with bleeding disorders. However, such bleeding has not been reported with this drug.
- With large doses or prolonged therapy, monitor for superinfection, especially in high-risk patients.
- Cefotetan is similar to cefoxitin in that it's particularly useful in intra-abdominal and gynecologic infections (highly active against *B. fragilis*).

cefoxitin sodium
Mefoxin
Pregnancy Risk Category: B

HOW SUPPLIED
Injection: 1 g, 2 g
Infusion: 1 g, 2 g in 50-ml or 100-ml container
Pharmacy bulk package: 10 g

MECHANISM OF ACTION
Inhibits cell wall synthesis, promoting osmotic instability. Usually bactericidal.

INDICATIONS & DOSAGE
Serious infections of respiratory and GU tracts, skin and soft-tissue infections, bone and joint infections, bloodstream and intra-abdominal infections, and perioperative prophylaxis. Among susceptible organisms are Escherichia coli *and other coliform bacteria,* Staphylococcus aureus *(penicillinase- and non-penicillinase-producing) and* S. epidermidis, *streptococci,* Klebsiella, Haemophilus influenzae, *and* Bacteroides, *including* B. fragilis—
Adults: 1 to 2 g q 6 to 8 hours for uncomplicated forms of infection. Up to 12 g daily in life-threatening infections.
Children: 80 to 160 mg/kg daily given in 4 to 6 equally divided doses.

Total daily dosage is same for I.M. or I.V. administration and depends on susceptibility of organism and severity of infection. In patients with impaired renal function, doses or frequency of administration must be modified according to degree of renal impairment, severity of infection, and susceptibility of organism. Should be injected deep I.M. into a large muscle mass, such as gluteus or lateral aspect of thigh.

ADVERSE REACTIONS

Common reactions are in italics; life-threatening reactions are in bold italics.

Blood: transient neutropenia, eosinophilia, ***hemolytic anemia.***

CNS: headache, malaise, paresthesias, dizziness.

GI: pseudomembranous colitis, nausea, anorexia, vomiting, *diarrhea,* glossitis, dyspepsia, abdominal cramps, tenesmus, anal pruritus, oral candidiasis (thrush).

GU: genital pruritus and moniliasis.

Skin: *maculopapular and erythematous rashes, urticaria.*

Local: *at injection site – pain, induration, sterile abscesses, tissue sloughing; phlebitis and thrombophlebitis with I.V. injection.*

Other: ***hypersensitivity,*** dyspnea, elevated temperature.

INTERACTIONS

Probenecid: may inhibit excretion and increase blood levels of cefoxitin.

NURSING CONSIDERATIONS

• *Contraindicated* in patients with hypersensitivity to other cephalosporins.

• *Use cautiously* in impaired renal status and in those with history of sensitivity to penicillin. Ask if patient has had any reaction to previous cephalosporin or penicillin therapy before administering first dose.

• Obtain specimen for culture and sensitivity tests before first dose. Therapy may begin pending test results.

• A very useful cephalosporin when anaerobic or mixed aerobic-anaerobic infection is suspected, especially *B. fragilis.*

• Associated with development of thrombophlebitis. Assess I.V. site frequently.

• **I.V. use:** Reconstitute 1 g with at least 10 ml of sterile water for injection, and 2 g with 10 to 20 ml. Solutions of dextrose 5% and 0.9% sodium chloride for injection can also be used. Interrupt flow of primary I.V. solution during infusion.

• I.M. injection can be reconstituted with 0.5% or 1% lidocaine hydrochloride (without epinephrine) to minimize pain.

• After reconstitution, remains stable for 24 hours at room temperature or 1 week under refrigeration.

• With large doses or prolonged therapy, monitor for superinfection, especially in high-risk patients.

• Urine glucose determinations may be false-positive with copper sulfate tests (Clinitest); glucose enzymatic tests (Clinistix, Tes-Tape) are not affected.

cefpodoxime proxetil

Vantin

Pregnancy Risk Category: B

HOW SUPPLIED

Tablets (film-coated): 100 mg, 200 mg
Oral suspension: 50 mg/5 ml, 100 mg/5 ml in 100-ml bottles

MECHANISM OF ACTION

A second-generation cephalosporin that inhibits cell wall synthesis, promoting osmotic instability. Usually bactericidal.

INDICATIONS & DOSAGE

Acute, community-acquired pneumonia caused by non-beta-lactamase-producing strains of Haemophilus influenzae *or* Streptococcus pneumoniae –

Adults: 200 mg P.O. q 12 hours for 14 days.

Uncomplicated gonorrhea in men and

women; rectal gonococcal infections in women –
Adults: 200 mg P.O. as a single dose. Follow with doxycycline 100 mg P.O. b.i.d. for 7 days.
Uncomplicated skin and skin-structure infections caused by Staphylococcus aureus *or* Streptococcus pyogenes –
Adults: 400 mg P.O. q 12 hours for 7 to 14 days.
Acute otitis media caused by S. pneumoniae, H. influenzae, *or* Moraxella (Branhamella) catarrhalis –
Children 6 months and over: 5 mg/kg (not to exceed 200 mg) P.O. q 12 hours for 10 days.
Pharyngitis or tonsillitis caused by S. pyogenes –
Adults: 100 mg P.O. q 12 hours for 10 days.
Children 6 months and over: 5 mg/kg (not to exceed 100 mg) P.O. q 12 hours for 10 days.
Uncomplicated urinary tract infections caused by Escherichia coli, Klebsiella pneumoniae, Proteus mirabilis, *or* Staphylococcus saprophyticus –
Adults: 100 mg P.O. q 12 hours for 7 days.
Dosage adjustment for patients with severe renal impairment –
Adults: when creatinine clearance is below 30 ml/minute/1.73 m^2, dosage interval should be increased to q 24 hours. Patients receiving dialysis should get the drug three times weekly, after dialysis.

ADVERSE REACTIONS

Common reactions are in italics; life-threatening reactions are in bold italics.
CNS: headache.
GI: *diarrhea,* nausea, vomiting, abdominal pain.
GU: vaginal fungal infections.
Skin: rash.
Other: ***anaphylaxis.***

INTERACTIONS

Antacids, H_2 antagonists: decreased absorption of cefpodoxime. Avoid concomitant use.
Probenecid: decreased excretion of cefpodoxime. Monitor for toxicity.

NURSING CONSIDERATIONS

- *Contraindicated* in patients with hypersensitivity to the drug or other cephalosporins. Safety and efficacy in children under age 6 months have not been established.
- *Use cautiously* in patients with a history of penicillin hypersensitivity because of the risk of cross-sensitivity and in patients receiving nephrotoxic drugs because other cephalosporins have been shown to have nephrotoxic potential. Because drug is excreted in human breast milk, also use cautiously in breast-feeding women.
- Dosage frequency should be altered in patients with severe renal impairment. When creatinine clearance is below 30 ml/minute, dosage interval should be increased to q 24 hours. Patients receiving dialysis should get the drug three times weekly, after dialysis.
- Studies have shown that drug's pharmacokinetics aren't altered in patients with hepatic impairment, including those with ascites.
- Absorption of drug is enhanced when it's taken with food.
- Store suspension in the refrigerator (36° to 46° F [2° to 8° C]). Shake well before using. Discard unused portion after 14 days.

cefprozil

Cefzil

Pregnancy Risk Category: B

HOW SUPPLIED

Tablets: 250 mg, 500 mg
Oral suspension: 125 mg/5 ml, 250 mg/5 ml

MECHANISM OF ACTION
A second-generation cephalosporin that interferes with bacterial cell wall synthesis during cell replication, leading to osmotic instability and cell lysis (bactericidal).

INDICATIONS & DOSAGE
Pharyngitis or tonsillitis caused by Streptococcus pyogenes –
Adults: 500 mg P.O. daily for at least 10 days.
Otitis media caused by S. pneumoniae, Haemophilus influenzae, *and* Moraxella (Branhamella) catarrhalis –
Infants and children 6 months to 12 years: 15 mg/kg P.O. q 12 hours for 10 days.
Secondary bacterial infections of acute bronchitis and acute bacterial exacerbation of chronic bronchitis caused by S. pneumoniae, H. influenzae, *and* M. catarrhalis –
Adults: 500 mg P.O. q 12 hours for 10 days.
Uncomplicated skin and skin structure infections caused by Staphylococcus aureus *and* Streptococcus pyogenes –
Adults: 250 mg P.O. b.i.d., or 500 mg P.O. daily to b.i.d.

ADVERSE REACTIONS
Common reactions are in italics; life-threatening reactions are in bold italics.
Blood: decreased leukocyte count, eosinophilia.
CNS: dizziness, hyperactivity, headache, nervousness, insomnia.
GI: *diarrhea, nausea,* vomiting, abdominal pain.
GU: elevated BUN level, elevated serum creatinine level, genital pruritus, vaginitis.
Hepatic: elevated liver enzymes, cholestatic jaundice (rare).
Skin: rash, urticaria, diaper rash.
Other: superinfection, hypersensitivity, ***anaphylaxis***.

INTERACTIONS
None reported.

NURSING CONSIDERATIONS
- *Contraindicated* in patients with hypersensitivity to the drug or any other cephalosporin.
- *Use cautiously* in patients with a history of hypersensitivity to penicillin because up to 10% of these patients will exhibit cross-sensitivity to a cephalosporin or a hypersensitivity reaction to cephalosporins or penicillins. Also use cautiously in patients with impaired hepatic or renal function.
- Oral suspensions contain the drug in a bubble-gum flavored vehicle to improve palatability and compliance in children. Reconstituted suspension should be stored in the refrigerator, and unused drug should be discarded after 14 days.
- Drug is removed by hemodialysis; administer after treatment is completed.
- Obtain specimen for culture and sensitivity tests before first dose. Therapy may begin pending test results.
- May cause overgrowth of nonsusceptible bacteria or fungi. Monitor for signs and symptoms of superinfection.
- Tell patient to shake suspension well before measuring dose.
- Tell patient to take all of the medication prescribed, even after he feels better.

---

ceftazidime
Fortaz, Magnacef†, Tazicef, Tazidime

Pregnancy Risk Category: B

HOW SUPPLIED
Injection: 500 mg, 1 g, 2 g
Infusion: 1 g, 2 g in 100-ml vials and bags
Pharmacy bulk package: 6 g

MECHANISM OF ACTION
Inhibits cell wall synthesis, promoting osmotic instability. Usually bactericidal.

INDICATIONS & DOSAGE
Serious infections of the lower respiratory and urinary tracts, gynecologic infections, bacteremia, septicemia, intra-abdominal infections, CNS infections, and skin infections. Among susceptible microorganisms are streptococci, including Streptococcus pneumoniae *and* S. pyogenes; Staphylococcus aureus *(penicillinase- and nonpenicillinase-producing);* Escherichia coli; Klebsiella; Proteus; Enterobacter; Haemophilus influenzae; Pseudomonas; *and some strains of* Bacteroides –
Adults: 1 g I.V. or I.M. q 8 to 12 hours; up to 6 g daily in life-threatening infections.
Children 1 month to 12 years: 30 to 50 mg/kg I.V. q 8 hours.
Neonates 0 to 4 weeks: 30 mg/kg I.V. q 12 hours.

Total daily dosage is same for I.M. or I.V. administration and depends on susceptibility of organism and severity of infection. In patients with impaired renal function, doses or frequency of administration must be modified according to degree of renal impairment, severity of infection, and susceptibility of organism. Should be injected deep I.M. into a large muscle mass, such as gluteus or lateral aspect of thigh.

ADVERSE REACTIONS
Common reactions are in italics; life-threatening reactions are in bold italics.
Blood: eosinophilia; thrombocytosis, leukopenia.
CNS: headache, dizziness.
GI: pseudomembranous colitis, nausea, vomiting, diarrhea, dysgeusia, abdominal cramps.
GU: genital pruritus and moniliasis.
Hepatic: transient elevation in liver enzymes.
Skin: *maculopapular and erythematous rashes, urticaria.*
Local: *at injection site – pain, induration, sterile abscesses, tissue sloughing; phlebitis and thrombophlebitis with I.V. injection.*
Other: ***hypersensitivity,*** dyspnea, elevated temperature.

INTERACTIONS
Sodium bicarbonate-containing solutions: make ceftazidime unstable. Don't mix together.

NURSING CONSIDERATIONS
- *Contraindicated* in patients with hypersensitivity to other cephalosporins.
- *Use cautiously* in patients with history of sensitivity to penicillin. Ask if patient has had any previous reaction to cephalosporin or penicillin therapy before administering first dose.
- Obtain specimen for culture and sensitivity tests before first dose. Therapy may begin pending test results.
- **I.V. use:** The vials of ceftazidime are supplied under reduced pressure. When the antibiotic is dissolved, carbon dioxide is released and a positive pressure develops. Each brand of ceftazidime includes specific instructions for reconstitution. Read and follow these instructions carefully.
- This third-generation cephalosporin has excellent activity against infections caused by *Pseudomonas aeruginosa.* May be prescribed for these infections, especially when aminoglycosides are potentially too dangerous.
- With large doses or prolonged therapy, monitor for superinfection, especially in high-risk patients.

ceftizoxime sodium
Cefizox

Pregnancy Risk Category: B

HOW SUPPLIED
Injection: 1 g, 2 g, 10g
Infusion: 1 g, 2 g in 100-mg vials or in 50 ml dextrose 5% in water

MECHANISM OF ACTION
Inhibits cell wall synthesis, promoting osmotic instability. Usually bactericidal.

INDICATIONS & DOSAGE
Serious infections of the lower respiratory and urinary tracts, gynecologic infections, bacteremia, septicemia, meningitis, intra-abdominal infections, bone and joint infections, and skin infections. Among susceptible microorganisms are streptococci, including Streptococcus pneumoniae *and* S. pyogenes; Staphylococcus aureus *(penicillinase- and non-penicillinase-producing)* and S. epidermidis; Escherichia coli; Klebsiella; Haemophilus influenzae; Enterobacter; Proteus; *some* Pseudomonas; *and* Peptostreptococcus – **Adults:** usual dosage is 1 to 2 g I.V. or I.M. q 8 to 12 hours. In life-threatening infections, up to 2 g q 4 hours.

Total daily dosage is same for I.M. or I.V. administration and depends on susceptibility of organism and severity of infection. In patients with impaired renal function, doses or frequency of administration must be modified according to degree of renal impairment, severity of infection, and susceptibility of organism. Should be injected deep I.M. into a large muscle mass, such as gluteus or lateral aspect of thigh.

ADVERSE REACTIONS
Common reactions are in italics; life-threatening reactions are in bold italics.
Blood: transient neutropenia, eosinophilia, hemolytic anemia.
CNS: headache, malaise, paresthesias, dizziness.
GI: pseudomembranous colitis, nausea, anorexia, vomiting, *diarrhea,* glossitis, dyspepsia, abdominal cramps, tenesmus, anal pruritus.
GU: genital pruritus and moniliasis.
Skin: *maculopapular and erythematous rashes, urticaria.*
Local: *at injection site – pain, induration, sterile abscesses, tissue sloughing; phlebitis and thrombophlebitis with I.V. injection.*
Other: ***hypersensitivity,*** dyspnea, elevated temperature.

INTERACTIONS
Probenecid: may inhibit excretion and increase blood levels of ceftizoxime.

NURSING CONSIDERATIONS
- *Contraindicated* in patients with hypersensitivity to other cephalosporins.
- *Use cautiously* in impaired renal function and in those with history of sensitivity to penicillin. Ask patient if he's had any reaction to previous cephalosporin or penicillin therapy before administering first dose.
- Obtain specimen for culture and sensitivity tests before first dose. Therapy may begin pending test results.
- With large doses or prolonged therapy, monitor for superinfection, especially in high-risk patients.
- Larger doses (2 g) administered I.M. should be divided into two doses and administered at separate sites in a large muscle.
- Ceftizoxime is a third-generation cephalosporin, which is comparable in activity to cefotaxime, moxalactam, ceftriaxone and cefoperazone. No significant degree of bleeding or disulfiram-type reaction has been reported with its use.
- **I.V. use:** To reconstitute powder, add 10 ml of sterile water to 1-g vial and 20 ml to 2-g vial. Reconstitute piggyback vials with 50 to 100 ml 0.9% sodium chloride or dextrose 5% solution. Shake vial well.

ceftriaxone sodium

Rocephin

Pregnancy Risk Category: B

HOW SUPPLIED

Injection: 250 mg, 500 mg, 1 g, 2 g
Infusion: 1 g, 2 g
Pharmacy bulk package: 10 g

MECHANISM OF ACTION

Inhibits cell wall synthesis, promoting osmotic instability. Usually bactericidal.

INDICATIONS & DOSAGE

Serious infections of the CNS (meningitis), lower respiratory and urinary tracts, gynecologic infections, bone and joint infections, bacteremia, septicemia, intra-abdominal infections, preoperative prophylaxis, and skin infections and Lyme disease. Susceptible microorganisms are streptococci, including Streptococcus pneumoniae *and* S. pyogenes; Staphylococcus aureus *(penicillinase- and non-penicillinase-producing) and* S. epidermidis; Escherichia coli; Klebsiella; Haemophilus influenzae; Neisseria meningitidis; N. gonorrhoeae; Enterobacter; Proteus; Pseudomonas; Peptostreptococcus, *and* Serratia marcescens –
Adults: 1 to 2 g I.M. or I.V. daily or in equally divided doses b.i.d. Total daily dose should not exceed 4 g.
Children: 50 to 75 mg/kg, given in divided doses q 12 hours.
Meningitis –
Adults and children: 100 mg/kg given in divided doses q 12 hours. May give loading dose of 75 mg/kg.

Total daily dose is same for I.M. or I.V. administration and depends on susceptibility of organism and severity of infection. Should be injected deep I.M. into a large muscle mass, such as gluteus or lateral aspect of thigh.

ADVERSE REACTIONS

Common reactions are in italics; life-threatening reactions are in bold italics.
Blood: eosinophilia; thrombocytosis, leukopenia.
CNS: headache, dizziness.
GI: pseudomembranous enterocolitis, nausea, vomiting, diarrhea, dysgeusia, abdominal cramps.
GU: genital pruritus and moniliasis.
Hepatic: transient elevation in liver enzymes.
Skin: *maculopapular and erythematous rashes, urticaria.*
Local: *at injection site – pain, induration, sterile abscesses, tissue sloughing; phlebitis and thrombophlebitis with I.V. injection.*
Other: ***hypersensitivity,*** dyspnea, elevated temperature.

INTERACTIONS

Probenecid: high doses (1 or 2 g/day) may enhance hepatic clearance of ceftriaxone and shorten half-life. Avoid concomitant use.

NURSING CONSIDERATIONS

- *Contraindicated* in patients with hypersensitivity to other cephalosporins.
- *Use cautiously* in history of sensitivity to penicillin. Ask patient if he's had any previous reaction to cephalosporin or penicillin therapy before administering first dose.
- Obtain specimen for culture and sensitivity tests before first dose. Therapy may begin pending test results.
- **I.V. use:** Reconstitute with sterile water for injection, 0.9% sodium chloride injection, dextrose 5% or 10% injection, or a combination of sodium chloride and dextrose injection and other compatible solutions. Reconstitute by adding 2.4 ml diluent to the 250-mg vial, 4.8 ml to the 500-mg vial, 9.6 ml to the 1-g vial, and 19.2 ml to the 2-g vial. All reconstituted solutions yield a concentration that averages 100 mg/ml. After

reconstitution, dilute further for intermittent infusion to desired concentration. I.V. dilutions are stable for 24 hours at room temperature.

• A third-generation cephalosporin with the longest half-life of any available cephalosporin. Allows once-daily dose regimen.

• Dosage adjustment generally not needed in patients with renal insufficiency.

• Commonly used in home antibiotic programs for outpatient treatment of serious infections, such as osteomyelitis.

• With large doses or prolonged therapy, monitor for superinfection, especially in high-risk patients.

cefuroxime axetil
Ceftin

cefuroxime sodium
Kefurox, Zinacef

Pregnancy Risk Category: B

HOW SUPPLIED
axetil
Tablets: 125 mg, 250 mg, 500 mg
sodium
Injection: 750 mg, 1.5 g
Infusion: 750 mg, 1.5 g premixed, frozen solution

MECHANISM OF ACTION
Inhibits cell wall synthesis, promoting osmotic instability. Usually bactericidal.

INDICATIONS & DOSAGE
Injectable form is used for treatment of serious infections of the lower respiratory and urinary tracts; skin and skin structure infections; bone and joint infections, septicemia, meningitis, gonorrhea, and perioperative prophylaxis; oral form is used for otitis media, pharyngitis, tonsillitis, infections of the urinary and lower respiratory tracts, and skin and skin structure infections. Among susceptible organisms are Streptococcus pneumoniae *and* S. pyogenes, Haemophilus influenzae, Klebsiella, Staphylococcus aureus, Escherichia coli, Enterobacter, *and* Neisseria gonorrhoeae – **Adults:** usual dosage of cefuroxime sodium is 750 mg to 1.5 g I.M. or I.V. q 8 hours, usually for 5 to 10 days. For life-threatening infections and infections caused by less susceptible organisms, 1.5 g I.M. or I.V. q 6 hours; for bacterial meningitis, up to 3 g I.V. q 6 hours.

Alternatively, administer cefuroxime axetil 250 mg P.O. q 12 hours. For severe infections or less susceptible organisms, dosage may be increased to 500 mg P.O. q 12 hours.

Children and infants over 3 months: 50 to 100 mg/kg/day cefuroxime sodium I.M. or I.V. Higher doses are administered when treating meningitis. Alternatively, give cefuroxime axetil 125 mg P.O. q 12 hours.

Uncomplicated urinary tract infections –
Adults: 125 to 250 mg P.O. q 12 hours.

Otitis media –
Children under 2 years: 125 mg P.O. q 12 hours.
Children 2 years and over: 250 mg P.O. q 12 hours.

ADVERSE REACTIONS
Common reactions are in italics; life-threatening reactions are in bold italics.

Blood: transient neutropenia, eosinophilia, ***hemolytic anemia,*** decrease in hemoglobin and hematocrit.

CNS: headache, malaise, paresthesia, dizziness.

GI: pseudomembranous colitis, nausea, anorexia, vomiting, *diarrhea,* glossitis, dyspepsia, abdominal cramps, tenesmus, anal pruritus.

GU: genital pruritus and moniliasis.

Skin: *maculopapular and erythematous rashes, urticaria.*

Local: *at injection site – pain, indura-*

tion, sterile abscesses, temperature elevation, tissue sloughing; phlebitis and thrombophlebitis with I.V. injection.
Other: ***hypersensitivity,*** dyspnea.

INTERACTIONS
Probenecid: may inhibit excretion and increase blood levels of cefuroxime.

NURSING CONSIDERATIONS
• *Contraindicated* in hypersensitivity to other cephalosporins.
• *Use cautiously* in patients with impaired renal function; dosage should be reduced. Also use cautiously in those with history of sensitivity to penicillin. Ask patient if he's had any reaction to previous cephalosporin or penicillin therapy before administering first dose.
• **I.V. use:** Give reconstituted drug over 15 to 30 minutes. Administer over 10 to 30 minutes in neonates or children.
• Total daily dosage is same for I.M. or I.V. administration and depends on susceptibility of organism and severity of infection. In patients with impaired renal function, doses or frequency of administration must be modified according to degree of renal impairment, severity of infection, and susceptibility of organism. Should be injected deep I.M. into a large muscle mass, such as gluteus or lateral aspect of thigh.
• Absorption of cefuroxime axetil is enhanced by food.
• Cefuroxime axetil is available only in tablet form, which may be crushed for patients who cannot swallow tablets. However, it has a bitter taste that is difficult to mask, even with food. Until a suitable liquid suspension is developed, alternative therapy may be necessary.
• Obtain specimen for culture and sensitivity tests before first dose. Therapy may begin pending test results.
• With large doses or prolonged therapy, monitor for superinfection, especially in high-risk patients.
• Cefuroxime is a second-generation cephalosporin similar to cefamandole. However, cefuroxime has not been associated with prothrombin deficiency and bleeding as are some of the other cephalosporins. Advantage over some other cephalosporins is that cefuroxime is useful in treating meningitis.

cephalexin hydrochloride
Keftab

cephalexin monohydrate
Ceporex†‡, Keflet, Keflex, Novolexin†

Pregnancy Risk Category: B

HOW SUPPLIED
Tablets: 250 mg, 500 mg, 1 g
Capsules: 500 mg, 1,250 mg
Oral suspension: 100 mg/5 ml, 125 mg/5 ml, 250 mg/5 ml

MECHANISM OF ACTION
Inhibits cell wall synthesis, promoting osmotic instability. Usually bactericidal.

INDICATIONS & DOSAGE
Infections of respiratory and GU tracts, skin and soft-tissue infections, bone and joint infections, and otitis media due to Escherichia coli *and other coliform bacteria, group A beta-hemolytic streptococci,* Haemophilus influenzae, Klebsiella, Proteus mirabilis, Streptococcus pneumoniae, *and staphylococci –*
Adults: 250 mg to 1 g P.O. q 6 hours.
Children: 6 to 12 mg/kg P.O. q 6 hours. Maximum 25 mg/kg q 6 hours.

ADVERSE REACTIONS
Common reactions are in italics; life-threatening reactions are in bold italics.
Blood: transient neutropenia, eosinophilia, anemia.

CNS: dizziness, headache, malaise, paresthesia.
GI: pseudomembranous colitis, *nausea, anorexia,* vomiting, *diarrhea,* glossitis, dyspepsia, abdominal cramps, anal pruritus, tenesmus, oral candidiasis (thrush).
GU: genital pruritus and moniliasis, vaginitis.
Skin: *maculopapular and erythematous rashes, urticaria.*
Other: ***hypersensitivity,*** dyspnea.

INTERACTIONS
Probenecid: may increase blood levels of cephalosporins.

NURSING CONSIDERATIONS
• *Use cautiously* in impaired renal function and in those with history of sensitivity to penicillin. Ask patient if he's had any reaction to previous cephalosporin or penicillin therapy before administering first dose.
• Obtain specimen for culture and sensitivity tests before first dose. Therapy may begin pending test results.
• Tell patient to take medication exactly as prescribed, even after he feels better. Group A beta-hemolytic streptococcal infections should be treated for a minimum of 10 days.
• Tell patient to take with food or milk to lessen GI discomfort.
• Call doctor if skin rash develops.
• Preparation of oral suspension: add required amount of water to powder in two portions. Shake well after each addition. After mixing, store in refrigerator. Stable for 14 days without significant loss of potency. Keep tightly closed and shake well before using.
• With large doses or prolonged therapy, monitor for superinfection, especially in high-risk patients.
• From 40% to 75% of patients receiving cephalosporins show a false-positive direct Coombs' test, but only a few of these indicate hemolytic anemia.
• Urine glucose determinations may be false-positive with copper sulfate tests (Clinitest); glucose enzymatic tests (Clinistix, Tes-Tape) are not affected.

cephalothin sodium
Ceporacin†‡, Keflin
Pregnancy Risk Category: B

HOW SUPPLIED
Injection: 1 g, 2 g, 4 g
Infusion: 1 g/50 ml, 2 g/50 ml, 1 g/dl, 2 g/dl
Pharmacy bulk package: 10 g, 20 g

MECHANISM OF ACTION
Inhibits cell wall synthesis, promoting osmotic instability. Usually bactericidal.

INDICATIONS & DOSAGE
Serious infections of respiratory, GU, or GI tract; skin and soft-tissue infections (including peritonitis); bone and joint infections; septicemia; endocarditis; and perioperative prophylaxis. Susceptible organisms include Escherichia coli *and other coliform bacteria, Enterobacteriaceae, enterococci, gonococci, group A beta-hemolytic streptococci,* Haemophilus influenzae, Klebsiella, Proteus mirabilis, Salmonella, Staphylococcus aureus, Shigella, Streptococcus pneumoniae *and* S. viridans, *and staphylococci*–
Adults: 500 mg to 1 g I.M. or I.V. (or intraperitoneally) q 4 to 6 hours; in life-threatening infections, up to 2 g q 4 hours.
Children: 100 mg/kg/day I.V. in divided doses q 4 or 6 hours. Dose should be proportionately less in accordance with age, weight, and severity of infection.

Dosage schedule is determined by degree of renal impairment, severity of infection, and susceptibility of causative organism. Should be injected deep I.M. into a large muscle mass, such as gluteus or lateral aspect of thigh. I.V. route is preferable in severe or life-threatening infections.

ADVERSE REACTIONS
Common reactions are in italics; life-threatening reactions are in bold italics.
Blood: transient neutropenia, eosinophilia, ***hemolytic anemia.***
CNS: headache, malaise, paresthesias, dizziness.
GI: pseudomembranous colitis, nausea, anorexia, vomiting, *diarrhea,* glossitis, dyspepsia, abdominal cramps, tenesmus, anal pruritus, oral candidiasis (thrush).
GU: nephrotoxicity, genital pruritus and moniliasis.
Skin: *maculopapular and erythematous rashes, urticaria.*
Local: *at injection site – pain, induration, sterile abscesses, tissue sloughing; phlebitis and thrombophlebitis with I.V. injection.*
Other: ***hypersensitivity,*** dyspnea, fever.

INTERACTIONS
Aminoglycosides: increased nephrotoxicity. Monitor kidney function tests carefully.
Probenecid: may increase blood levels of cephalosporins. Use together cautiously.

NURSING CONSIDERATIONS
• *Use cautiously* in impaired renal function and in those with history of sensitivity to penicillin. Ask patient if he's had any reaction to previous cephalosporin or penicillin therapy before administering first dose.
• Obtain specimen for culture and sensitivity tests before first dose. Therapy may begin pending test results.
• Drug causes severe pain when administered I.M.; avoid this route if possible.
• For I.M. administration, reconstitute each gram of cephalothin sodium with 4 ml of sterile water for injection, providing 500 mg in each 2.2 ml. If vial contents do not dissolve completely, add an additional 0.2 to 0.4 ml diluent, and warm contents slightly.
• **I.V. use:** When giving this drug I.V., check frequently for vein irritation and phlebitis. Alternate injection sites if I.V. therapy lasts longer than 3 days. Use of small I.V. needle in the larger available veins may be preferable. Addition of a small concentration of heparin (100 units) or hydrocortisone (10 to 25 mg) may reduce incidence of phlebitis.
• For I.V. administration, dilute contents of 4-g vial with at least 20 ml of sterile water for injection, dextrose 5% injection, or 0.9% sodium chloride injection and add to one of following I.V. solutions: acetated Ringer's injection, dextrose 5% injection, dextrose 5% in lactated Ringer's injection, Ionosol B in dextrose 5% in water, lactated Ringer's injection, Normosol-N in dextrose 5% in water, Plasma-Lyte injection, Plasma-Lyte-N injection in dextrose 5%, Ringer's injection, or 0.9% sodium chloride injection. Choose solution and fluid volume according to patient's fluid and electrolyte status.
• With large doses or prolonged therpay, monitor for superinfection, especially in high-risk patients.
• From 40% to 75% of patients receiving cephalosporins show a false-positive direct Coombs' test; only a few of these indicate hemolytic anemia.
• Urine glucose determinations may be false-positive with copper sulfate tests (Clinitest); glucose enzymatic tests (Clinistix, Tes-Tape) are not affected.

cephapirin sodium
Cefadyl

Pregnancy Risk Category: B

HOW SUPPLIED
Injection: 500-mg, 1-g, 2-g vials; 1-g, 2-g, 4-g piggyback vials; 20-g pharmacy bulk package

MECHANISM OF ACTION
Inhibits cell wall synthesis, promoting osmotic instability. Usually bactericidal.

INDICATIONS & DOSAGE
Serious infections of respiratory, GU, or GI tract; skin and soft-tissue infections; bone and joint infections (including osteomyelitis); septicemia; and endocarditis due to Streptococcus pneumoniae, Escherichia coli, *group A beta-hemolytic streptococci,* Haemophilus influenzae, Klebsiella, Proteus mirabilis, Staphylococcus aureus, *and* Streptococcus viridans – **Adults:** 40 to 80 mg/kg/day I.V. or I.M. in divided doses q 4 to 6 hours. **Children over 3 months:** 10 to 20 mg/kg I.V. or I.M. q 6 hours; dose depends on age, weight, and severity of infection.

Should be injected deep I.M. into a large muscle mass, such as gluteus or lateral aspect of thigh. Depending on causative organism and severity of infection, patients with reduced renal function may be treated adequately with a lower dose (7.5 to 15 mg/kg q 12 hours). Patients with severely reduced renal function and who are to be dialyzed should receive same dose just before dialysis and q 12 hours thereafter.

ADVERSE REACTIONS
Common reactions are in italics; life-threatening reactions are in bold italics.
Blood: transient neutropenia, eosinophilia, anemia.
CNS: dizziness, headache, malaise, paresthesias.
GI: pseudomembranous colitis, nausea, anorexia, vomiting, *diarrhea,* glossitis, dyspepsia, abdominal cramps, tenesmus, anal pruritus, oral candidiasis (thrush).
GU: genital pruritus and moniliasis, vaginitis.
Skin: *maculopapular and erythematous rashes, urticaria.*
Local: *at injection site – pain, induration, sterile abscesses, tissue sloughing; phlebitis and thrombophlebitis with I.V. injection.*
Other: ***hypersensitivity,*** dyspnea.

INTERACTIONS
Probenecid: may increase blood levels of cephalosporins.

NURSING CONSIDERATIONS
- *Use cautiously* in patients with impaired renal function and in those with a history of sensitivity to penicillin. Ask patient if he's had any reaction to previous cephalosporin or penicillin therapy before administering first dose.
- Obtain specimen for culture and sensitivity tests before first dose. Therapy may begin pending test results.
- For I.M. administration, reconstitute 1-g vial with 2 ml sterile water for injection or bacteriostatic water for injection so that 1.2 ml contains 500 mg of cephapirin. I.M. injection is painful; prepare patient for this.
- **I.V. use:** When giving this drug I.V., check frequently for vein irritation and phlebitis. Alternate injection sites if I.V. therapy lasts longer than 3 days. Use of small I.V. needles in the larger available veins may be preferable.
- Prepare I.V. infusion using dextrose injection, sodium chloride injection, or bacteriostatic water for injection as diluent: 20 ml yields 1 g per 10 ml; 50

ml yields 1 g per 25 ml; 100 ml yields 1 g per 50 ml.

- I.V. infusion with Y-tubing: during infusion of cephapirin solution, it is desirable to stop other solution. Check volume of cephapirin solution carefully so that calculated dose is infused. When Y-tubing is used, dilute 4-g vial with 40 ml of diluent.
- Reconstituted cephapirin is stable and compatible for 10 days under refrigeration and for 24 hours at room temperature.
- With large doses or prolonged therapy, monitor for superinfection, especially in high-risk patients.
- From 40% to 75% of patients receiving cephalosporins show a false-positive direct Coombs' test, but only a few indicate hemolytic anemia.
- Urine glucose determinations may be false-positive with copper sulfate tests (Clinitest); glucose enzymatic tests (Clinistix, Tes-Tape) are not affected.

cephradine

Anspor, Velosef**

Pregnancy Risk Category: B

HOW SUPPLIED

Capsules: 250 mg, 500 mg
Oral suspension: 125 mg/5 ml, 250 mg/5 ml
Injection: 250 mg, 500 mg, 1 g, 2 g, 4 g
Infusion: 2 g

MECHANISM OF ACTION

Inhibits cell wall synthesis, promoting osmotic instability. Usually bactericidal.

INDICATIONS & DOSAGE

Serious infections of respiratory, GU, or GI tract; skin and soft-tissue infections; bone and joint infections; septicemia; endocarditis; otitis media; and perioperative prophylaxis. Among susceptible organisms are Escherichia coli *and other coliform bacteria, group A beta-hemolytic streptococci,* Haemophilus influenzae, Klebsiella, Proteus mirabilis, Staphylococcus aureus, Streptococcus pneumoniae *and* S. viridans, *and staphylococci* – **Adults:** 500 mg to 1 g I.M. or I.V. 2 to 4 times daily; do not exceed 8 g daily. Or 250 to 500 mg P.O. q 6 hours. Severe or chronic infections may require larger and/or more frequent doses (up to 1 g P.O. q 6 hours).
Children over 1 year: 6 to 12 mg/kg P.O. q 6 hours. 12 to 25 mg/kg I.M. or I.V. q 6 hours.
Otitis media – 19 to 25 mg/kg P.O. q 6 hours. Do not exceed 4 g daily.

All patients, regardless of age and weight: larger doses (up to 1 g q.i.d.) may be given for severe or chronic infections. Parenteral therapy may be followed by oral. Injections should be given deep I.M. into a large muscle mass, such as gluteus or lateral aspect of thigh.

ADVERSE REACTIONS

Common reactions are in italics; life-threatening reactions are in bold italics.
Blood: transient neutropenia, eosinophilia.
CNS: dizziness, headache, malaise, paresthesias.
GI: pseudomembranous colitis, *nausea, anorexia,* vomiting, heartburn, glossitis, dyspepsia, abdominal cramping, *diarrhea,* tenesmus, anal pruritus, oral candidiasis (thrush).
GU: genital pruritus and moniliasis, vaginitis.
Skin: *maculopapular and erythematous rashes, urticaria.*
Local: *at injection site – pain, induration, sterile abscesses, tissue sloughing; phlebitis and thrombophlebitis with I.V. injection.*
Other: ***hypersensitivity,*** dyspnea.

INTERACTIONS

Probenecid: may increase blood levels of cephalosporins.

*Liquid form contains alcohol. **May contain tartrazine.

NURSING CONSIDERATIONS

- *Contraindicated* in patients with hypersensitivity to other cephalosporins.
- *Use cautiously* in impaired renal function and in those with a history of sensitivity to penicillin. Ask patient if he's had any reaction to previous cephalosporin or penicillin therapy before administering first dose.
- Obtain specimen for culture and sensitivity tests. Therapy may begin pending test results.
- Tell patient to take medication exactly as prescribed, even after he feels better. Group A beta-hemolytic streptococcal infections should be treated for a minimum of 10 days.
- Tell patient to take the oral dosage form with food or milk to lessen GI discomfort.
- I.M. injection is painful.
- For I.M. administration, reconstitute with sterile water or with bacteriostatic water for injection as follows: 1.2 ml to 250-mg vial; 2 ml to 500-mg vial; 4 ml to 1-g vial. I.M. solutions must be used within 2 hours if kept at room temperature and within 24 hours if refrigerated. Solutions may vary in color from light straw to yellow without affecting potency.
- **I.V. use:** When giving this drug I.V., check frequently for vein irritation and phlebitis. Alternate injection sites if I.V. therapy lasts longer than 3 days. Use of small I.V. needle in the larger available veins may be preferable.
- When preparing cephradine for I.V. administration, when available, use preparation specifically supplied for infusion. Follow specific product directions carefully when reconstituting.
- With large doses or prolonged therapy, monitor for superinfection, especially in high-risk patients.
- From 40% to 75% of patients receiving cephalosporins show a false-positive direct Coombs' test, but only a few indicate hemolytic anemia.
- Urine glucose determinations may be false-positive with copper sulfate tests (Clinitest); glucose enzymatic tests (Clinistix, Tes-Tape) are not affected.

loracarbef

Lorabid

Pregnancy Risk Category: B

HOW SUPPLIED

Pulvules: 200 mg
Powder for oral suspension: 100 mg/5 ml, 200 mg/5 ml in 50-ml and 100-ml bottles

MECHANISM OF ACTION

A synthetic beta-lactam antibiotic of the carbacephem class. Actions are similar to the second-generation cephalosporins. Inhibits cell wall synthesis, promoting osmotic instability. Usually bactericidal.

INDICATIONS & DOSAGE

Secondary bacterial infections of acute bronchitis –
Adults: 200 to 400 mg P.O. q 12 hours for 7 days.
Acute bacterial exacerbations of chronic bronchitis –
Adults: 400 mg P.O. q 12 hours for 7 days.
Pneumonia –
Adults: 400 mg P.O. q 12 hours for 14 days.
Pharyngitis or tonsillitis –
Adults: 400 mg P.O. q 12 hours for 10 days.
Children: 15 mg/kg P.O. daily in divided doses q 12 hours for 10 days.
Acute otitis media –
Children: 30 mg/kg (oral suspension) P.O. daily in divided doses q 12 hours for 10 days.
Uncomplicated skin and skin-structure infections –
Adults: 200 mg P.O. q 12 hours for 7 days.
Impetigo –

Children: 15 mg/kg P.O. daily in divided doses q 12 hours for 7 days.
Uncomplicated cystitis –
Adults: 200 mg P.O. daily for 7 days.
Uncomplicated pyelonephritis –
Adults: 400 mg P.O. q 12 hours for 7 days.
Dosage adjustment in patients with renal failure –
Patients with a creatinine clearance greater than or equal to 50 ml/minute/1.73 m^2 don't require dose and interval changes. Patients with a creatinine clearance of 10 to 49 ml/minute/1.73 m^2 should receive half of the usual dose at the same interval; with a creatinine clearance below 10 ml/minute/1.73 m^2, the usual dose q 3 to 5 days. Hemodialysis patients should be given another dose after dialysis.

ADVERSE REACTIONS
Common reactions are in italics; life-threatening reactions are in bold italics.
Blood: transient thrombocytopenia, leukopenia, eosinophilia.
CNS: headache, somnolence, nervousness, insomnia, dizziness.
CV: vasodilation.
GI: diarrhea, nausea, vomiting, abdominal pain, anorexia, pseudomembranous colitis.
GU: vaginal candidiasis or moniliasis, transient increases in BUN and creatinine levels.
Hepatic: transient elevations in AST (SGOT), ALT (SGPT), and alkaline phosphatase levels.
Skin: rash, urticaria, pruritus, ***erythema multiforme.***
Other: hypersensitivity reactions, including ***anaphylaxis.***

INTERACTIONS
Probenecid: decreases excretion of loracarbef, causing increased plasma levels. Monitor for toxicity.

NURSING CONSIDERATIONS
- *Contraindicated* in patients with hypersensitivity to the drug or other cephalosporins and in patients with diarrhea caused by pseudomembranous colitis.
- *Use cautiously* in pregnant or breast-feeding women. Also use cautiously and with dosage adjustments in patients with renal failure. Safety and efficacy have not been established in infants under age 6 months.
- Tell patient to take drug on an empty stomach, at least 1 hour before or 2 hours after eating.
- Beta-lactam antibiotics may trigger seizures in susceptible patients, especially when given without dosage modification to those with renal impairment. If seizures occur, discontinue drug and notify doctor. Administer anticonvulsants as ordered.
- For otitis media, use the more rapidly absorbed oral suspension, which produces higher peak plasma levels than the capsules.
- To reconstitute powder for oral suspension, add 30 ml of water to the 50-ml bottle or 60 ml of water to the 100-ml bottle in two portions; shake after each addition.
- After reconstitution, oral suspension is stable for 14 days at room temperature (59° to 86° F [15° to 30° C]). Instruct patient to discard unused portion after 14 days.

moxalactam disodium (latamoxef disodium)
Moxalactam‡, Moxam

Pregnancy Risk Category: C

HOW SUPPLIED
Parenteral: 1 g, 2 g, 10 g

MECHANISM OF ACTION
Inhibits cell wall synthesis, promoting osmotic instability. Usually bactericidal.

INDICATIONS & DOSAGE
Serious infections of lower respiratory and urinary tracts, CNS infections,

*Liquid form contains alcohol. **May contain tartrazine.

intra-abdominal infections, gynecologic infections, bacteremia, septicemia, bone and joint infections, and skin infections. Susceptible microorganisms include Streptococcus pneumoniae *and* S. pyogenes; Staphylococcus aureus *(penicillinase- and nonpenicillinase-producing) and* S. epidermidis; Escherichia coli; Klebsiella; Haemophilus influenzae; Enterobacter; Proteus; *some* Pseudomonas; *and* Peptostreptococcus –

Adults: usual daily dose is 2 to 6 g I.M. or I.V. administered in divided doses q 8 hours for 5 to 10 days, or up to 14 days. Up to 12 g daily may be needed in life-threatening infections or in infections due to less susceptible organisms.

Children: 50 mg/kg I.M. or I.V. q 6 to 8 hours.

Neonates: 50 mg/kg I.M. or I.V. q 8 to 12 hours.

Total daily dosage is same for I.M. or I.V. administration and depends on susceptibility of organism and severity of infection. In patients with impaired renal function, doses or frequency of administration must be modified according to degree of impairment, severity of infection, and susceptibility of organism. Should be injected deep I.M. into the gluteus or lateral aspect of thigh.

ADVERSE REACTIONS

Common reactions are in italics; life-threatening reactions are in bold italics.

Blood: transient neutropenia, eosinophilia, ***hemolytic anemia,*** hypoprothrombinemia, bleeding.

CNS: headache, malaise, paresthesia, dizziness.

GI: pseudomembranous colitis, nausea, anorexia, vomiting, *diarrhea,* glossitis, dyspepsia, abdominal cramps, tenesmus, pruritus ani, oral candidiasis (thrush).

GU: genital moniliasis.

Skin: *maculopapular and erythematous rashes, urticaria.*

Local: *pain at injection site, induration, sterile abscesses, tissue sloughing; phlebitis and thrombophlebitis with I.V. injection.*

Other: ***hypersensitivity,*** dyspnea, elevated temperature.

INTERACTIONS

Ethyl alcohol: may cause a disulfiram-like reaction. Warn patients not to drink alcohol for several days after discontinuing moxalactam.

Oral anticoagulants, aspirin: increased risk of bleeding.

NURSING CONSIDERATIONS

- *Contraindicated* in patients with hypersensitivity to other cephalosporins.
- *Use cautiously* in patients with impaired renal function and in those with history of sensitivity to penicillin. Before giving first dose, ask patient if he's had any reaction to penicillin.
- Obtain specimen for culture and sensitivity tests before first dose. Therapy may begin pending test results.
- **I.V. use:** For direct intermittent I.V. administration, add 10 ml of sterile water for injection, dextrose 5% injection, or 0.9% NaCl injection/g of moxalactam.
- With large doses or prolonged therapy, monitor for superinfection, especially in high-risk patients.
- Bleeding associated with hypoprothrombinemia can be prevented or treated with vitamin K. Doctor may order 10 mg vitamin K per week to be given prophylactically.
- If a bleeding disorder occurs, monitor prothrombin times regularly.
- Moxalactam does not interfere with urine glucose determinations.

14

Tetracyclines

demeclocycline hydrochloride
doxycycline
doxycycline hyclate
doxycycline hydrochloride
minocycline hydrochloride
oxytetracycline hydrochloride
tetracycline hydrochloride

COMBINATION PRODUCTS

UROBIOTIC-250: oxytetracycline hydrochloride 250 mg, sulfamethizole 250 mg, and phenazopyridine hydrochloride 50 mg.

demeclocycline hydrochloride

Declomycin, Ledermycin‡

Pregnancy Risk Category: D

HOW SUPPLIED

Tablets: 150 mg, 300 mg
Capsules: 150 mg

MECHANISM OF ACTION

Exerts bacteriostatic effect by binding to the 30S ribosomal subunit of microorganisms, thus inhibiting protein synthesis.

INDICATIONS & DOSAGE

Infections caused by susceptible gram-negative and gram-positive organisms, psittacosis, lymphogranuloma venereum, granuloma inguinale, relapsing fever, Mycoplasma pneumoniae, *trachoma, rickettsiae* –
Adults: 150 mg P.O. q 6 hours or 300 mg P.O. q 12 hours.
Children over 8 years: 6 to 12 mg/kg P.O. daily, divided q 6 to 12 hours.
Gonorrhea –
Adults: initially, 600 mg P.O., then 300 mg P.O. q 12 hours for 4 days (total 3 g).
Uncomplicated urethral, endocervical, or rectal infection caused by Chlamydia trachomatis –
Adults: 300 mg P.O. q.i.d. for at least 7 days.
SIADH (a hyposmolar state) –
Adults: 600 to 1,200 mg P.O. daily in divided doses q 6 to 8 hours.

ADVERSE REACTIONS

Common reactions are in italics; life-threatening reactions are in bold italics.
Blood: neutropenia, eosinophilia, thrombocytopenia, ***hemolytic anemia.***
CNS: pseudotumor cerebri.
CV: pericarditis.
EENT: dysphagia, glossitis.
GI: anorexia, *nausea, vomiting, diarrhea,* enterocolitis, anogenital inflammation.
Metabolic: *increased BUN level,* diabetes insipidus syndrome (polyuria, polydipsia, weakness).
Skin: *maculopapular and erythematous rashes, photosensitivity, increased pigmentation, urticaria.*
Other: ***hypersensitivity.***

INTERACTIONS

Antacids (including sodium bicarbonate) and laxatives containing aluminum, magnesium, or calcium; food, milk, or other dairy products: decrease antibiotic absorption. Give antibiotic 1 hour before or 2 hours after any of the above.
Ferrous sulfate and other iron products, zinc: decrease antibiotic absorption. Give demeclocycline 3 hours after or 2 hours before iron administration.
Methoxyflurane: may cause nephrotoxicity with tetracyclines. Monitor carefully.
Oral anticoagulants: increased anticoagulant effect. Monitor prothrom-

bin times and adjust dosage as ordered.
Oral contraceptives: decreased contraceptive effectiveness and increased risk of breakthrough bleeding.

NURSING CONSIDERATIONS

- *Use with extreme caution* in impaired renal or hepatic function. Use of these drugs during last half of pregnancy and in children under 8 years may cause permanent discoloration of teeth, enamel defects, and retardation of bone growth.
- Obtain specimen for culture and sensitivity tests. Therapy may begin pending test results.
- Check expiration date. Outdated or deteriorated demeclocycline has been associated with reversible nephrotoxicity (Fanconi's syndrome).
- Do not expose these drugs to light or heat; store in tight container.
- With large doses or prolonged therapy, monitor for superinfection, especially in high-risk patients.
- Check patient's tongue for signs of monilia infection. Stress good oral hygiene.
- Warn patient to avoid direct sunlight and ultraviolet light. A sunscreen may help prevent photosensitivity reactions. Photosensitivity persists for some time after discontinuation of drug.
- Effectiveness is reduced when taken with milk or other dairy products, food, antacids, or iron products. Explain this to patient. Tell patient to take each dose with a full glass of water on an empty stomach, at least 1 hour before meals or 2 hours afterward and remain standing for 90 seconds after ingestion. Give at least 1 hour before bedtime to prevent esophagitis.
- Instruct patient to take medication for as long as prescribed, exactly as prescribed, even after he feels better, and to take entire amount prescribed.
- May cause false-negative reading of Clinistix or Tes-Tape.

doxycycline
Doxylin‡, Vibramycin

doxycycline hyclate
Doryx, Doxy-100, Doxy-200, Doxy-Caps, Doxychel, Doxy-Lemmon, Doxy-Tabs, Vibramycin, Vibra-Tabs

doxycycline hydrochloride
Cyclidox‡, Doryx‡, Vibramycin‡, Vibramycin IV, Vibra-Tabs 50‡
Pregnancy Risk Category: D

HOW SUPPLIED
doxycycline
Tablets: 50 mg‡, 100 mg‡
Oral suspension: 25 mg/5 ml
Syrup: 50 mg/5 ml
doxycycline hyclate
Tablets: 50 mg, 100 mg
Capsules: 50 mg, 100 mg
Capsules (coated pellets): 100 mg
Injection: 100 mg, 200 mg
doxycycline hydrochloride
Tablets: 50 mg‡, 100 mg‡
Capsules: 50 mg‡, 100 mg‡, 250 mg‡
Injection: 100 mg‡
Powder for injection: 200 mg

MECHANISM OF ACTION
Exerts bacteriostatic effect by binding to the 30S ribosomal subunit of microorganisms, thus inhibiting protein synthesis.

INDICATIONS & DOSAGE
Infections caused by sensitive gram-negative and gram-positive organisms, trachoma, rickettsiae, Mycoplasma, Chlamydia, *and Lyme disease –*
Adults: 100 mg P.O. q 12 hours on first day, then 100 mg P.O. daily; or 200 mg I.V. on first day in one or two infusions, then 100 to 200 mg I.V. daily.
Children over 8 years (under 45

kg): 4.4 mg/kg P.O. or I.V. daily, divided q 12 hours first day, then 2.2 to 4.4 mg/kg daily. For children over 45 kg, dosage is same as adults.

Give I.V. infusion slowly (minimum 1 hour). Infusion must be completed within 12 hours (within 6 hours in lactated Ringer's solution or dextrose 5% in lactated Ringer's solution).

Gonorrhea in patients allergic to penicillin –
Adults: 200 mg P.O. initially, followed by 100 mg P.O. at bedtime, and 100 mg P.O. b.i.d. for 3 days; or 300 mg P.O. initially and repeat dose in 1 hour.

Primary or secondary syphilis in patients allergic to penicillin –
Adults: 300 mg P.O. daily in divided doses for at least 10 days.

Uncomplicated urethral, endocervical or rectal infections caused by Chlamydia trachomatis *or* Ureaplasma urealyticum –
Adults: 100 mg P.O. b.i.d. for at least 7 days.

To prevent "traveler's diarrhea" commonly caused by enterotoxigenic Escherichia coli –
Adults: 100 mg P.O. daily.

ADVERSE REACTIONS

Common reactions are in italics; life-threatening reactions are in bold italics.
Blood: neutropenia, eosinophilia.
CNS: ***intracranial hypertension.***
CV: pericarditis.
EENT: sore throat, glossitis, dysphagia.
GI: anorexia, *epigastric distress, nausea,* vomiting, *diarrhea,* enterocolitis, anogenital inflammation.
Skin: *maculopapular and erythematous rashes, photosensitivity, increased pigmentation, urticaria.*
Local: thrombophlebitis.
Other: ***hypersensitivity.***

INTERACTIONS

Antacids (including sodium bicarbonate) and laxatives containing aluminum, magnesium, or calcium: decrease antibiotic absorption. Give antibiotic 1 hour before or 2 hours after any of the above.
Ferrous sulfate and other iron products, zinc: decrease antibiotic absorption. Give doxycycline 3 hours after or 2 hours before iron administration.
Oral contraceptives: decreased contraceptive effectiveness and increased risk of breakthrough bleeding.
Phenobarbital, carbamazepine, alcohol: decrease antibiotic effect. Avoid if possible.

NURSING CONSIDERATIONS

- Use of these drugs during last half of pregnancy and in children under 8 years may cause permanent discoloration of teeth, enamel defects, and retardation of bone growth.
- Patient may develop thrombophlebitis with I.V. administration.
- Obtain specimen for culture and sensitivity tests before first dose. Therapy may begin pending test results.
- Don't expose drug to light or heat. Protect from sunlight during infusion.
- With large doses or prolonged therapy, monitor for superinfection, especially in high-risk patients.
- Check patient's tongue for signs of monilia infection. Stress good oral hygiene.
- May be taken with milk or food if GI adverse effects develop.
- Do not give with antacids.
- Tell patient to take medication exactly as prescribed, even after he feels better, and to take entire amount prescribed.
- **I.V. use:** Reconstitute powder for injection with sterile water for injection. Use 10 ml in 100-mg vial and 20 ml in 200-mg vial. Dilute solution to 100 to 1,000 ml for I.V. infusion. Do not infuse solutions more concen-

*Liquid form contains alcohol. **May contain tartrazine.

trated than 1 mg/ml. Reconstituted solution is stable for 72 hours refrigerated.

- Doxycycline may be used in patients with renal impairment; does not accumulate or cause a significant rise in BUN.
- Parenteral form may cause false-positive reading of Clinitest. All forms may cause false-negative reading of Clinistix or Tes-Tape.
- Should not be taken within 1 hour of bedtime because of increased incidence of dysphagia.
- Check expiration date. Outdated or deteriorated tetracyclines have been associated with reversible nephrotoxicity (Fanconi's syndrome).

minocycline hydrochloride

Minocin*, Minomycin‡, Minomycin IV‡

Pregnancy Risk Category: D

HOW SUPPLIED

Tablets: 50 mg, 100 mg
Capsules: 50 mg, 100 mg
Oral suspension: 50 mg/5 ml
Injection: 100 mg

MECHANISM OF ACTION

Exerts bacteriostatic effect by binding to the 30S ribosomal subunit of microorganisms, thus inhibiting protein synthesis.

INDICATIONS & DOSAGE

Infections caused by sensitive gram-negative and gram-positive organisms, trachoma, amebiasis –
Adults: 200 mg I.V., then 100 mg I.V. q 12 hours. Do not exceed 400 mg/day. Or, give 200 mg P.O. initially, then 100 mg P.O. q 12 hours. Some clinicians use 100 or 200 mg P.O. initially, followed by 50 mg q.i.d.
Children over 8 years: initially, 4 mg/kg P.O. or I.V., followed by 2 mg/kg q 12 hours.

Give I.V. in 500- to 1,000-ml solution without calcium, and administer over 6 hours.

Gonorrhea in patients sensitive to penicillin –
Adults: initially, 200 mg P.O., then 100 mg q 12 hours for at least 4 days.

Syphilis in patients sensitive to penicillin –
Adults: initially, 200 mg P.O., then 100 mg q 12 hours for 10 to 15 days.

Meningococcal carrier state –
100 mg P.O. q 12 hours for 5 days.

Uncomplicated urethral, endocervical, or rectal infection caused by Chlamydia trachomatis *or* Ureaplasma urealyticam –
Adults: 100 mg P.O. b.i.d. for at least 7 days.

Uncomplicated gonoccocal urethritis in men –
Adults: 100 mg P.O. b.i.d. for 5 days.

ADVERSE REACTIONS

Common reactions are in italics; life-threatening reactions are in bold italics.
Blood: neutropenia, eosinophilia.
CNS: *light-headedness, dizziness from vestibular toxicity.*
CV: pericarditis.
EENT: dysphagia, glossitis.
GI: *anorexia,* epigastric distress, *nausea,* vomiting, *diarrhea,* enterocolitis, inflammatory lesions in anogenital region.
Metabolic: increased BUN.
Skin: *maculopapular and erythematous rashes, photosensitivity, increased pigmentation, urticaria.*
Local: *thrombophlebitis.*
Other: ***hypersensitivity.***

INTERACTIONS

Antacids (including sodium bicarbonate) and laxatives containing aluminum, magnesium, or calcium: decrease antibiotic absorption. Give antibiotic 1 hour before or 2 hours after any of the above.
Ferrous sulfate and other iron products, zinc: decrease antibiotic absorption. Tetracyclines should be given 3

hours after or 2 hours before iron administration.
Methoxyflurane: may cause severe nephrotoxicity with tetracyclines. Monitor carefully.
Oral contraceptives: decreased contraceptive effectiveness and increased risk of breakthrough bleeding.

NURSING CONSIDERATIONS

- *Use with extreme caution* in patients with impaired renal or hepatic function. Use during last half of pregnancy and in children under 8 years may cause permanent discoloration of teeth, enamel defects, and retardation of bone growth.
- Obtain specimen for culture and sensitivity tests before first dose. Therapy may begin pending test results.
- Do not expose these drugs to light or heat. Keep cap tightly closed.
- With large doses or prolonged therapy, monitor for superinfection, especially in high-risk patients.
- Check patient's tongue for signs of monilia infection. Stress good oral hygiene.
- May be taken with food. Tell patient to take medication exactly as prescribed, even after he feels better, and to take entire amount prescribed.
- May cause tooth discoloration in young adults. Observe for brown pigmentation and inform doctor if it occurs.
- **I.V. use:** Reconstitute 100 mg powder with 5 ml sterile water for injection with further dilution of 500 to 1,000 ml for I.V. infusion. Stable for 24 hours at room temperature.
- Patient may develop thrombophlebitis with I.V. administration of this drug. Avoid extravasation.
- Parenteral form may cause false-positive reading of Clinitest. All forms may cause false-negative reading of Clinistix or Tes-Tape.
- Check expiration date. Outdated or deteriorated tetracyclines have been associated with reversible nephrotoxicity (Fanconi's syndrome).

oxytetracycline hydrochloride

E.P. Mycin, Terramycin, Uri-Tet
Pregnancy Risk Category: D

HOW SUPPLIED
Capsules: 250 mg
Injection: 50 mg/ml, 125 mg/ml (with lidocaine 2%)

MECHANISM OF ACTION
Exerts bacteriostatic effect by binding to the 30S ribosomal subunit of microorganisms, thus inhibiting protein synthesis.

INDICATIONS & DOSAGE
Infections caused by sensitive gram-negative and gram-positive organisms, trachoma, rickettsiae –
Adults: 250 mg P.O. q 6 hours; 100 mg I.M. q 8 to 12 hours; 250 mg I.M. as a single dose.
Children over 8 years: 25 to 50 mg/kg P.O. daily, divided q 6 hours; 15 to 25 mg/kg I.M. daily, divided q 8 to 12 hours
Brucellosis –
Adults: 500 mg P.O. q.i.d. for 3 weeks with streptomycin 1 g I.M. q 12 hours first week, once daily second week.
Syphilis in patients sensitive to penicillin –
Adults: 30 to 40 g total dosage P.O., divided equally over 10 to 15 days.
Gonorrhea in patients sensitive to penicillin –
Adults: initially, 1.5 g P.O. followed by 0.5 g q.i.d. for a total of 9 g.

ADVERSE REACTIONS
Common reactions are in italics; life-threatening reactions are in bold italics.
Blood: neutropenia, eosinophilia.
CNS: ***intracranial hypertension.***
CV: pericarditis.

*Liquid form contains alcohol. **May contain tartrazine.

EENT: dysphagia, glossitis.
GI: *anorexia, nausea,* vomiting, *diarrhea,* enterocolitis, anogenital inflammation.
Metabolic: *increased BUN levels.*
Skin: *maculopapular and erythematous rashes, urticaria, photosensitivity, increased pigmentation.*
Local: *irritation after I.M. injection, thrombophlebitis.*
Other: ***hypersensitivity.***

INTERACTIONS

Antacids (including sodium bicarbonate) and laxatives containing aluminum, magnesium, or calcium; food, milk, or other dairy products: decrease antibiotic absorption. Give antibiotic 1 hour before or 2 after.
Ferrous sulfate and other iron products, zinc: decrease antibiotic absorption. Give tetracyclines 3 hours after or 2 hours before iron administration.
Methoxyflurane: may cause severe nephrotoxicity with tetracyclines.
Oral contraceptives: decreased contraceptive effectiveness and increased risk of breakthrough bleeding.

NURSING CONSIDERATIONS

- *Use with extreme caution* in patients with impaired renal or hepatic function. Use during last half of pregnancy and in children under 8 years may cause permanent discoloration of teeth, enamel defects, and retardation of bone growth.
- Obtain specimen for culture and sensitivity tests before first dose. Therapy may begin pending test results.
- Check expiration date. Outdated or deteriorated oxytetracyclines have been associated with reversible nephrotoxicity (Fanconi's syndrome).
- Do not expose these drugs to light or heat.
- Inject I.M. dose deeply. Warn that it may be painful. Rotate sites. I.M. preparations contain a local anesthetic; ask patient about hypersensitivity to local anesthetics.
- With large doses or prolonged therapy, monitor for superinfections, especially in high-risk patients.
- Check patient's tongue for signs of monilia infection. Stress good oral hygiene.
- Warn patient to avoid direct sunlight and ultraviolet light. A sunscreen may help prevent photosensitivity reactions. Photosensitivity persists for considerable time after discontinuation of drug.
- Effectiveness is reduced when taken with milk or other dairy products, food, antacids, or iron products. Explain this to patient. Tell patient to take each dose with a full glass of water on an empty stomach, at least 1 hour before meals or 2 hours afterward. Give at least 1 hour before bedtime to prevent esophagitis.
- Tell patient to take medication exactly as prescribed, even after he feels better, and to take entire amount prescribed.
- Parenteral form may cause false-positive reading of Clinitest. All forms may cause false-negative reading of Clinistix or Tes-Tape.

tetracycline hydrochloride

Achromycin V, Apo-Tetra†, Austramycin V‡, Hostacycline P‡, Nor-Tet, Novotetra†, Panmycin**, Panmycin P‡, Robitet, Sumycin, Tetracap, Tetralan, Tetralean†

Pregnancy Risk Category: D

HOW SUPPLIED

Tablets: 250 mg, 500 mg
Capsules: 100 mg, 250 mg, 500 mg
Oral suspension: 125 mg/5 ml
Injection: 100 mg, 250 mg, 500 mg

MECHANISM OF ACTION

Exerts bacteriostatic effect by binding to the 30S ribosomal subunit of microorganisms, thus inhibiting protein synthesis.

INDICATIONS & DOSAGE

Infections caused by sensitive gram-negative and gram-positive organisms, trachoma, rickettsiae, Mycoplasma, *and* Chlamydia –

Adults: 250 to 500 mg P.O. q 6 hours; 250 mg I.M. daily or 150 mg I.M. q 12 hours; or 250 to 500 mg I.V. q 8 to 12 hours (I.M. and I.V. hydrochloride salt only).

Children over 8 years: 25 to 50 mg/kg P.O. daily, divided q 6 hours; 15 to 25 mg/kg daily (maximum 250 mg) I.M. single dose or divided q 8 to 12 hours; or 10 to 20 mg/kg I.V. daily, divided q 12 hours.

Uncomplicated urethral, endocervical, or rectal infection caused by Chlamydia trachomatis –

Adults: 500 mg P.O. q.i.d. for at least 7 days.

Brucellosis –

Adults: 500 mg P.O. q 6 hours for 3 weeks with streptomycin 1 g I.M. q 12 hours week 1 and daily week 2.

Gonorrhea in patients sensitive to penicillin –

Adults: initially, 1.5 g P.O., then 500 mg q 6 hours for a total dose of 9 g.

Syphilis in patients sensitive to penicillin –

Adults: 30 to 40 g P.O. total in equally divided doses over 10 to 15 days.

Acne –

Adults and adolescents: initially, 250 mg P.O. q 6 hours, then 125 to 500 mg P.O. daily or every other day.

Shigellosis –

Adults: 2.5 g P.O. in 1 dose.

ADVERSE REACTIONS

Common reactions are in italics; life-threatening reactions are in bold italics.

Blood: neutropenia, eosinophilia.

CNS: dizziness, headache, ***intracranial hypertension.***

CV: pericarditis.

EENT: sore throat, glossitis, dysphagia.

GI: anorexia, *epigastric distress, nausea,* vomiting, *diarrhea,* stomatitis, enterocolitis, inflammatory lesions in anogenital region.

Hepatic: *hepatotoxicity* with large doses given I.V.

Metabolic: *increased BUN.*

Skin: *maculopapular and erythematous rashes, urticaria, photosensitivity, increased pigmentation.*

Local: *irritation after I.M. injection, thrombophlebitis.*

INTERACTIONS

Antacids (including sodium bicarbonate) and laxatives containing aluminum, magnesium, or calcium; food, milk, or other dairy products: decrease antibiotic absorption. Give antibiotic 1 hour before or 2 hours after any of the above.

Ferrous sulfate and other iron products, zinc: decrease antibiotic absorption. Give tetracyclines 3 hours after or 2 hours before iron administration.

Lithium carbonate: may alter serum lithium levels.

Methoxyflurane: may cause severe nephrotoxicity with tetracyclines.

Oral contraceptives: decreased contraceptive effectiveness and increased risk of breakthrough bleeding.

NURSING CONSIDERATIONS

- *Use with extreme caution* in patients with impaired renal or hepatic function. Use during last half of pregnancy and in children under 8 years may cause permanent discoloration of teeth, enamel defects, and retardation of bone growth.
- Obtain specimen for culture and sensitivity tests before first dose. Therapy may begin pending test results.
- Effectiveness reduced when taken with milk or other dairy products, food, antacids, or iron products. Explain this to patient. Tell patient to

*Liquid form contains alcohol. **May contain tartrazine.

take each dose with a full glass of water on an empty stomach, at least 1 hour before meals or 2 hours afterward. Give at least 1 hour before bedtime to prevent esophagitis.

- Patient may develop thrombophlebitis with I.V. administration. Avoid extravasation.
- Check expiration date. Outdated or deteriorated tetracyclines have been associated with reversible nephrotoxicity (Fanconi's syndrome).
- For I.M. use, reconstitute 100 mg powder for injection with 2 ml sterile water for injection. Concentration will be 50 mg/ml. Amount of diluent for 250-mg injection varies according to brand. Check with pharmacy or follow manufacturer's instructions.
- Discard I.M. solutions after 24 hours because they deteriorate. Exception: discard Achromycin solution in 12 hours.
- Inject I.M. dose deeply. Warn patient that it may be painful. Rotate sites. I.M. preparations often contain a local anesthetic; ask patient about hypersensitivity to local anesthetics.
- With large doses or prolonged therapy, monitor for superinfection, especially in high-risk patients.
- Check patient's tongue for signs of monilia infection. Stress good oral hygiene.
- Warn patient to avoid direct sunlight and ultraviolet light. A sunscreen may help prevent photosensitivity reactions. Photosensitivity persists after discontinuation of drug.
- Tell patient to take drug exactly as prescribed, even after he feels better, and to take entire amount prescribed.
- **I.V. use:** Reconstitute 100 mg and 250 mg powder for injection with 5 ml sterile water; with 10 ml for 500 mg. Further dilute in 100 to 1,000 ml volume of dextrose 5% in 0.9% saline solution. Refrigerate diluted solution for I.V. use and use within 24 hours. Exception: use Achromycin solution immediately.
- Do not mix tetracycline solution with any other I.V. additive.
- Parenteral form may cause false-positive reading of Clinitest. All forms may cause false-negative reading of Clinistix or Tes-Tape.
- Tetracycline may be used as a pleural sclerosing agent in malignant pleural effusions. Instilled through chest tube.
- Do not expose to light or heat.

15

Sulfonamides

co-trimoxazole
sulfadiazine
sulfamethoxazole
sulfasalazine
sulfisoxazole

COMBINATION PRODUCTS
AZO GANTANOL, AZO SULFAMETHOXAZOLE†, URO GANTANOL†: sulfamethoxazole 500 mg and phenazopyridine hydrochloride 100 mg.
AZO GANTRISIN, AZO SULFISOXAZOLE, SULDIAZO: sulfisoxazole 500 mg and phenazopyridine hydrochloride 50 mg.
PEDIAZOLE: sulfisoxazole 600 mg and erythromycin ethylsuccinate 200 mg per 5 ml.
TRIPLE SULFA: sulfadiazine 167 mg, sulfamerazine 167 mg, and sulfamethazine 167 mg.

co-trimoxazole (sulfamethoxazole-trimethoprim)

Apo-Sulfatrim†, Apo-Sulfatrim DS†, Bactrim*, Bactrim DS, Bactrim I.V. Infusion, Cotrim, Cotrim D.S., Novotrimel†, Novotrimel DS†, Protrin†, Protrin DF†, Resprim‡, Roubac†, Roubac DS†, Septra*, Septra DS, Septra I.V. Infusion, Septrin‡, SMZ-TMP, Sulfamethoprim, Sulfamethoprim DS, Sulmeprim, Trib‡, Uroplus DS, Uroplus SS

Pregnancy Risk Category: C (D if near term)

HOW SUPPLIED
Tablets: trimethoprim 80 mg and sulfamethoxazole 400 mg; trimethoprim 160 mg and sulfamethoxazole 800 mg
Oral suspension: trimethoprim 40 mg and sulfamethoxazole 200 mg/5 ml
Injection: trimethoprim 16 mg and sulfamethoxazole 80 mg/ml (5 ml/ampule)

MECHANISM OF ACTION
The sulfamethoxazole component inhibits the formation of dihydrofolic acid from PABA. The trimethoprim component inhibits dihydrofolate reductase. Both decrease bacterial folic acid synthesis.

INDICATIONS & DOSAGE
Urinary tract infections and shigellosis –
Adults: 160 mg trimethoprim/800 mg sulfamethoxazole (double strength tablet) P.O. q 12 hours for 10 to 14 days in urinary tract infections and for 5 days in shigellosis. For simple cystitis or acute urethral syndrome, may give one to three double strength tablets as a single dose. If indicated, give by I.V. infusion 8 to 10 mg/kg/day (based on trimethoprim component) in two to four divided doses q 6, 8, or 12 hours for up to 14 days. Maximum daily dose is 960 mg trimethoprim.
Children 2 months and over: 8 mg/kg trimethoprim/40 mg/kg sulfamethoxazole P.O. per 24 hours, in two divided doses q 12 hours (10 days for urinary tract infections; 5 days, for shigellosis). If indicated, give by I.V. infusion 8 to 10 mg/kg/day (based on trimethoprim component) in two to four divided doses q 6, 8, or 12 hours. Don't exceed the adult dose.
Treatment of otitis media in patients with penicillin allergy or penicillin-resistant infections –
Children 2 months and over: 8 mg/kg trimethoprim/40 mg/kg sulfamethoxazole P.O. per 24 hours, in two divided doses q 12 hours for 10 days.
Pneumocystis carinii *pneumonitis –*

*Liquid form contains alcohol. **May contain tartrazine.

Adults and children 2 months and over: 20 mg/kg trimethoprim/100 mg/kg sulfamethoxazole P.O. per 24 hours, in equally divided doses q 6 hours for 14 days. If indicated, give by I.V. infusion 15 to 20 mg/kg/day (based on trimethoprim component) in three or four divided doses q 6 to 8 hours for up to 14 days.
Chronic bronchitis –
Adults: 160 mg trimethoprim/800 mg sulfamethoxazole P.O. q 12 hours for 10 to 14 days. Not recommended for infants under 2 months old.
Prophylaxis of traveler's diarrhea –
Adults: 160 mg trimethoprim/800 mg sulfamethoxazole P.O. once daily, beginning on the first day of travel and continuing until 2 days after returning home. Maximum duration of therapy is 2 weeks.
Treatment of traveler's diarrhea –
Adults: 160 mg trimethoprim/800 mg sulfamethoxazole P.O. b.i.d. for 3 to 5 days. Some patients may require 2 days of therapy or less.
Treatment of urinary tract infections in males with prostatitis –
Adults: 160 mg trimethoprim/800 mg sulfamethoxazole P.O. b.i.d. for 3 to 6 months.
Prophylaxis of chronic urinary tract infections –
Adults: 40 mg trimethoprim/200 mg sulfamethoxazole (½ tablet) or 80 mg trimethoprim/400 mg sulfamethoxazole P.O. daily or three times a week for 3 to 6 months.

ADVERSE REACTIONS

Common reactions are in italics; life-threatening reactions are in bold italics.
Blood: ***agranulocytosis, aplastic anemia,*** megaloblastic anemia, thrombocytopenia, leukopenia, ***hemolytic anemia.***
CNS: headache, mental depression, seizures, hallucinations.
GI: *nausea, vomiting, diarrhea,* abdominal pain, anorexia, stomatitis.
GU: ***toxic nephrosis with oliguria and anuria,*** crystalluria, hematuria.
Hepatic: jaundice.
Skin: ***erythema multiforme (Stevens-Johnson syndrome),*** *generalized skin eruption,* ***epidermal necrolysis, exfoliative dermatitis,*** photosensitivity, urticaria, pruritus.
Other: ***hypersensitivity,*** *serum sickness, drug fever,* ***anaphylaxis.***

INTERACTIONS

Ammonium chloride, ascorbic acid: doses sufficient to acidify urine may cause precipitation of sulfonamide and crystalluria. Don't use together.
Oral anticoagulants: increased anticoagulant effect.
Oral contraceptives: decreased contraceptive effectiveness and increased risk of breakthrough bleeding.
Oral hypoglycemic agents: increased hypoglycemic effect.

NURSING CONSIDERATIONS

- *Contraindicated* in porphyria, in megaloblastic anemia caused by folate deficiency, and in pregnancy at term.
- *Use cautiously* and in reduced dosages in impaired hepatic or renal function and in those with severe allergy or bronchial asthma, G6PD deficiency, and blood dyscrasia.
- Adverse reactions, especially hypersensitivity reactions, rash, and fever, occur much more frequently in AIDS patients.
- **I.V. use:** I.V. infusion must be diluted in dextrose 5% in water before administration. Don't mix with other drugs or solutions.
- I.V. infusion also must be infused slowly over 60 to 90 minutes. Don't give by rapid infusion or bolus injection. Must be used within 2 hours of mixing. Do not refrigerate.
- Never administer I.M.
- This combination is often used in extremely ill immunosuppressed patients when prescribed for treatment of *Pneumocystis carinii* pneumonia.

• Note that the "DS" or "DF" product means "double strength."
• Promptly report skin rash, sore throat, fever, or mouth sores – early signs of blood dyscrasia.
• Watch for superinfection (fever or other signs of new infection).
• Obtain specimen for culture and sensitivity tests before first dose. Therapy may begin pending test results.
• Tell patient to take medication exactly as prescribed, even if he feels better, and to take entire amount prescribed.
• Used prophylactically for recurrent urinary tract infections in women and for "traveler's diarrhea."

sulfadiazine

Microsulfon

Pregnancy Risk Category: B (D if near term)

HOW SUPPLIED

Tablets: 500 mg

MECHANISM OF ACTION

Inhibits formation of dihydrofolic acid from PABA, decreasing bacterial folic acid synthesis.

INDICATIONS & DOSAGE

Urinary tract infection –
Adults: initially, 2 to 4 g P.O., then 500 mg to 1 g P.O. q 6 hours.
Children 2 months and over: initially, 75 mg/kg or 2 g/m² P.O., then 150 mg/kg or 4 g/m² P.O. in four to six divided doses daily. Maximum daily dosage is 6 g.
Rheumatic fever prophylaxis, as an alternative to penicillin –
Children over 30 kg: 1 g P.O. daily.
Children under 30 kg: 500 mg P.O. daily.
Adjunctive treatment in toxoplasmosis –
Adults: 4 g P.O. in divided doses q 6 hours for 3 to 4 weeks, discontinued for 1 week; given with pyrimethamine 25 mg P.O. daily for 3 to 4 weeks.
Children: 100 mg/kg P.O. in divided doses q 6 hours for 3 to 4 weeks; given with pyrimethamine 2 mg/kg daily for 3 days, then 1 mg/kg daily for 3 to 4 weeks.

ADVERSE REACTIONS

Common reactions are in italics; life-threatening reactions are in bold italics.
Blood: ***agranulocytosis, aplastic anemia,*** megaloblastic anemia, thrombocytopenia, leukopenia, ***hemolytic anemia.***
CNS: headache, mental depression, convulsions, hallucinations.
GI: *nausea, vomiting, diarrhea,* abdominal pain, anorexia, stomatitis.
GU: ***toxic nephrosis*** with oliguria and anuria, crystalluria, hematuria.
Hepatic: jaundice.
Skin: ***erythema multiforme (Stevens-Johnson syndrome),*** *generalized skin eruption,* ***epidermal necrolysis, exfoliative dermatitis,*** photosensitivity, urticaria, pruritus.
Local: irritation, extravasation.
Other: ***hypersensitivity,*** *serum sickness, drug fever,* ***anaphylaxis.***

INTERACTIONS

Ammonium chloride, ascorbic acid: doses sufficient to acidify urine may cause precipitation of sulfonamide and crystalluria. Don't use together.
Oral anticoagulants: increased anticoagulant effect.
Oral contraceptives: decreased contraceptive effectiveness and increased risk of breakthrough bleeding.
Oral hypoglycemic agents: increased hypoglycemic effect.
PABA-containing drugs: inhibit antibacterial action. Don't use together.

NURSING CONSIDERATIONS

• *Contraindicated* in porphyria or in infants under 2 months (except in congenital toxoplasmosis).
• *Use cautiously* and in reduced doses

*Liquid form contains alcohol. **May contain tartrazine.

in impaired hepatic or renal function, bronchial asthma, history of multiple allergies, G6PD deficiency, and blood dyscrasia.

• Tell patient to drink a full glass of water with each dose and to drink plenty of water throughout the day to prevent crystalluria. Monitor input/output. Intake should be sufficient to produce output of 1,500 ml daily (between 3,000 and 4,000 ml daily for adults). To aid in prevention of crystalluria, sodium bicarbonate may be administered to alkalinize urine. Monitor urine pH daily.
• Watch for superinfection (fever or other signs of new infection).
• Obtain specimen for culture and sensitivity tests before first dose. Therapy may begin pending test results.
• Tell patient to take medication exactly as prescribed, even if he feels better, and to take entire amount prescribed.
• Warn patient to avoid direct sunlight and ultraviolet light to prevent photosensitivity reaction.
• Give drug on schedule to maintain constant blood level.
• Monitor for signs of blood dyscrasia (purpura, ecchymosis, sore throat, fever, and pallor). Report them immediately.
• Monitor urine cultures, CBCs, and urinalyses before and during therapy.
• Folic or folinic acid may be used during rest periods in toxoplasmosis therapy to reverse hematopoietic depression and/or anemia associated with pyrimethamine and sulfadiazine.
• Protect drug from light.

sulfamethoxazole (sulphamethoxazole)

Apo-Sulfamethoxazole†, Gantanol, Gantanol DS

Pregnancy Risk Category: B (D if near term)

HOW SUPPLIED

Tablets: 500 mg, 1,000 mg
Oral suspension: 500 mg/5 ml

MECHANISM OF ACTION

Inhibits formation of dihydrofolic acid from PABA, decreasing bacterial folic acid synthesis.

INDICATIONS & DOSAGE

Urinary tract and systemic infections –
Adults: initially, 2 g P.O., then 1 g P.O. b.i.d. up to t.i.d. for severe infections.
Children and infants over 2 months: initially, 50 to 60 mg/kg P.O., then 25 to 30 mg/kg b.i.d. Maximum dosage should not exceed 75 mg/kg daily.
Lymphogranuloma venereum (genital, inguinal, or anorectal infection) –
Adults: 1 g P.O. daily for at least 3 weeks.

ADVERSE REACTIONS

Common reactions are in italics; life-threatening reactions are in bold italics.
Blood: ***agranulocytosis, aplastic anemia,*** megaloblastic anemia, thrombocytopenia, leukopenia, ***hemolytic anemia.***
CNS: headache, mental depression, seizures, hallucinations.
GI: *nausea, vomiting, diarrhea,* abdominal pain, anorexia, stomatitis.
GU: ***toxic nephrosis with oliguria and anuria,*** crystalluria, hematuria.
Hepatic: jaundice.
Skin: ***erythema multiforme (Stevens-Johnson syndrome),*** *generalized skin eruption,* ***epidermal necrolysis, exfoliative dermatitis,*** photosensitivity, urticaria, pruritus.
Other: ***hypersensitivity,*** *serum sickness, drug fever,* ***anaphylaxis.***

INTERACTIONS

Ammonium chloride, ascorbic acid: doses sufficient to acidify urine may

cause precipitation of sulfonamide and crystalluria. Don't use together.
Oral anticoagulants: increased anticoagulant effect.
Oral contraceptives: decreased contraceptive effectiveness and increased risk of breakthrough bleeding.
Oral hypoglycemic agents: increased hypoglycemic effect.
PABA-containing drugs: inhibit antibacterial action. Don't use together.

NURSING CONSIDERATIONS

- *Contraindicated* in porphyria or in infants under 2 months (except in congenital toxoplasmosis).
- *Use cautiously* and in reduced dosages in impaired hepatic or renal function and in those with severe allergy or bronchial asthma, G6PD deficiency, and blood dyscrasia.
- Tell patient to drink a full glass of water with each dose and to drink plenty of water during the day to prevent crystalluria. Monitor fluid intake/output. Intake should be sufficient to produce output of 1,500 ml daily (between 3,000 and 4,000 ml daily for adults). To aid in prevention of crystalluria, sodium bicarbonate may be administered to alkalinize urine. Monitor urine pH daily.
- Watch for superinfection (fever or other signs of new infection).
- Obtain specimen for culture and sensitivity tests before first dose. Therapy may begin pending test results.
- Tell patient to take medication exactly as prescribed, even if he feels better, and to take entire amount prescribed.
- Warn patient to avoid direct sunlight and ultraviolet light to prevent photosensitivity reaction.
- Monitor urine cultures, CBCs, and urinalyses before and during therapy.
- Sulfamethoxazole is also used in adjunctive therapy for treatment of toxoplasmosis.
- Instruct patient to report early signs of blood dyscrasia (sore throat, fever, and pallor) to doctor immediately.

sulfasalazine (salazosulfapyridine, sulphasalazine)

Azulfidine, Azulfidine EN-Tabs, PMS Sulfasalazine E.C.†, Salazopyrin†‡, Salazopyrin EN-Tabs†‡, S.A.S., S.A.S.-Enteric

Pregnancy Risk Category: B (D if near term)

HOW SUPPLIED

Tablets: 500 mg with or without enteric coating
Oral suspension: 250 mg/5 ml

MECHANISM OF ACTION

Inhibits formation of dihydrofolic acid from PABA, decreasing bacterial folic acid synthesis.

INDICATIONS & DOSAGE

Mild to moderate ulcerative colitis, adjunctive therapy in severe ulcerative colitis –
Adults: initially, 3 to 4 g P.O. daily in evenly divided doses; usual maintenance dosage is 1.5 to 2 g P.O. daily in divided doses q 6 hours. May need to start with 1 to 2 g initially, with a gradual increase in dosage to minimize adverse effects.
Children over 2 years: initially, 40 to 60 mg/kg P.O. daily, divided into 3 to 6 doses; then 30 mg/kg daily in 4 doses. May need to start at lower dose if GI intolerance occurs.

ADVERSE REACTIONS

Common reactions are in italics; life-threatening reactions are in bold italics.
Blood: ***agranulocytosis, aplastic anemia,*** megaloblastic anemia, thrombocytopenia, leukopenia, ***hemolytic anemia.***
CNS: headache, mental depression, ***seizures,*** hallucinations.

*Liquid form contains alcohol. **May contain tartrazine.

GI: *nausea, vomiting, diarrhea,* abdominal pain, anorexia, stomatitis.
GU: ***toxic nephrosis with oliguria and anuria,*** crystalluria, hematuria.
Hepatic: jaundice, hepatotoxicity.
Skin: ***erythema multiforme (Stevens-Johnson syndrome),*** *generalized skin eruption,* ***epidermal necrolysis, exfoliative dermatitis,*** photosensitivity, urticaria, pruritus.
Other: ***hypersensitivity,*** *serum sickness, drug fever,* ***anaphylaxis,*** oligospermia, infertility.

INTERACTIONS
Folic acid: absorption may be decreased.
Oral anticoagulants: increased anticoagulant effect.
Oral contraceptives: decreased contraceptive effectiveness and increased risk of breakthrough bleeding.
Oral hypoglycemic agents: increased hypoglycemic effect.

NURSING CONSIDERATIONS
- *Contraindicated* in patients with porphyria, in intestinal and urinary obstruction, and in patients allergic to salicylates.
- *Use cautiously* and in reduced dosages in impaired hepatic or renal function and in those with severe allergy, bronchial asthma, and G6PD deficiency.
- Watch for superinfection (fever or other signs of new infection).
- Obtain specimen for culture and sensitivity tests before first dose. Therapy may begin pending test results.
- Tell patient to take medication exactly as prescribed, even if he feels better, and to take entire amount prescribed.
- Warn patient to avoid direct sunlight and ultraviolet light to prevent photosensitivity reaction.
- Colors alkaline urine orange-yellow.
- Adverse reactions are usually those affecting GI tract. Minimize symptoms by spacing doses evenly and administering after food intake.

sulfisoxazole (sulfafurazole, sulphafurazole)

Azo-Sulfisoxazole†‡, Gantrisin, Novosoxazole†

Pregnancy Risk Category: B (D if near term)

HOW SUPPLIED
Tablets: 500 mg
Liquid: 500 mg/5 ml

MECHANISM OF ACTION
Inhibits formation of dihydrofolic acid from PABA, decreasing bacterial folic acid synthesis.

INDICATIONS & DOSAGE
Urinary tract and systemic infections–
Adults: initially, 2 to 4 g P.O., then 1 to 2 g P.O. q.i.d.
Children over 2 months: initially, 75 mg/kg P.O. daily or 2 g/m^2 P.O. daily in divided doses q 6 hours, then 150 mg/kg or 4 g/m^2 P.O. daily in divided doses q 6 hours.

ADVERSE REACTIONS
Common reactions are in italics; life-threatening reactions are in bold italics.
Blood: ***agranulocytosis, aplastic anemia,*** megaloblastic anemia, thrombocytopenia, leukopenia, ***hemolytic anemia.***
CNS: headache, mental depression, seizures, hallucinations.
GI: *nausea, vomiting, diarrhea,* abdominal pain, anorexia, stomatitis.
GU: ***toxic nephrosis with oliguria and anuria,*** crystalluria, hematuria.
Hepatic: jaundice.
Skin: ***erythema multiforme (Stevens-Johnson syndrome),*** *generalized skin eruption,* ***epidermal necrolysis, exfo-***

liative dermatitis, photosensitivity, urticaria, pruritus.

Other: ***hypersensitivity,*** *serum sickness, drug fever,* ***anaphylaxis.***

INTERACTIONS

Ammonium chloride, ascorbic acid: doses sufficient to acidify urine may cause crystalluria and precipitation of sulfonamide. Don't use together.

Oral anticoagulants: increased anticoagulant effect.

Oral contraceptives: decreased contraceptive effectiveness and increased risk of breakthrough bleeding.

Oral hypoglycemic agents: increased hypoglycemic effect.

PABA-containing drugs: inhibit antibacterial action. Don't use together.

NURSING CONSIDERATIONS

- *Contraindicated* in porphyria and in infants under 2 months (except in congenital toxoplasmosis).
- *Use cautiously* in impaired hepatic or renal function, severe allergy or bronchial asthma, and G6PD deficiency.
- Tell patient to drink a full glass of water with each dose and to drink plenty of water throughout the day to prevent crystalluria. Monitor intake/output. Intake should be sufficient to produce output of 1,500 ml daily (between 3,000 and 4,000 ml daily for adults). To aid in prevention of crystalluria, sodium bicarbonate may be administered to alkalinize urine. Monitor urine pH daily.
- Watch for superinfection (fever or other signs of new infection).
- Obtain specimen for culture and sensitivity tests before first dose. Therapy may begin pending test results.
- Tell patient to take medication exactly as prescribed, even if he feels better, and to take entire amount prescribed.
- Warn patient to avoid direct sunlight and ultraviolet light to prevent photosensitivity reaction.
- Monitor urine cultures, CBCs, prothrombin time, and urinalyses before and during therapy.
- Sulfisoxazole-pyrimethamine combination is used to treat toxoplasmosis.
- Tell patient to report early signs of blood dyscrasia (sore throat, fever, and pallor) immediately to doctor.
- When given preoperatively, the patient should receive a low-residue diet and a minimal number of enemas and cathartics.
- Although often given, initial loading dose is not necessary.

*Liquid form contains alcohol. **May contain tartrazine.

16

Quinolones

cinoxacin
ciprofloxacin
enoxacin
lomefloxacin hydrochloride
nalidixic acid
norfloxacin
ofloxacin

COMBINATION PRODUCTS
None.

cinoxacin

Cinobac

Pregnancy Risk Category: B

HOW SUPPLIED
Capsules: 250 mg, 500 mg

MECHANISM OF ACTION
Inhibits microbial DNA synthesis.

INDICATIONS & DOSAGE
Treatment of initial and recurrent urinary tract infections caused by susceptible strains of Escherichia coli, Klebsiella, Enterobacter, Proteus mirabilis, Proteus vulgaris, *and* Proteus morgani, Serratia, *and* Citrobacter –
Adults and children over 12 years: 1 g P.O. daily, in two to four divided doses for 7 to 14 days.

Not recommended for children under 12 years.

ADVERSE REACTIONS
Common reactions are in italics; life-threatening reactions are in bold italics.
CNS: *dizziness, headache,* drowsiness, insomnia, seizures.
EENT: photosensitivity, tinnitus.
GI: *nausea, vomiting, abdominal pain,* diarrhea.
Skin: rash, urticaria, pruritus, photosensitivity.

INTERACTIONS
Probenecid: may decrease urine levels of cinoxacin by inhibiting renal tubular secretion. Monitor for increased toxicity and reduced antibacterial effectiveness.

NURSING CONSIDERATIONS
- *Contraindicated* in patients with hypersensitivity to nalidixic acid.
- *Use cautiously* in patients with impaired renal and hepatic function.
- Not effective against *Pseudomonas,* enterococci, or staphylococci.
- Obtain clean-catch urine specimen for culture and sensitivity before starting therapy and repeat p.r.n. Therapy may begin pending test results.
- Remind patient to continue taking this drug, even when he feels better, and to take entire amount prescribed.
- High urine levels permit twice-daily dosing.
- Report CNS adverse reactions to doctor immediately. They indicate serious toxicity and usually mean that administration of drug should be stopped.
- Cinoxacin should be taken with meals to help decrease GI adverse reactions.
- Warn patient about photosensitizing effects of the drug, and advise him to avoid very bright sunlight and use sunblock.

ciprofloxacin

Cipro, Cipro I.V., Ciproxin‡

Pregnancy Risk Category: C

HOW SUPPLIED
Tablets: 250 mg, 500 mg, 750 mg
Infusion (premixed): 200 mg in 100

ml 5% dextrose, 400 mg in 200 ml 5% dextrose
Vials: 200 mg (20 ml); 400 mg (40 ml)

MECHANISM OF ACTION
A broad-spectrum quinolone antibiotic. Exact mechanism is unknown, but bactericidal effects may result from drug's ability to inhibit bacterial DNA gyrase and to prevent DNA replication in susceptible bacteria.

INDICATIONS & DOSAGE
Mild to moderate urinary tract infections –
Adults: 250 mg P.O. or 200 mg I.V. q 12 hours.
Severe or complicated urinary tract infections; mild to moderate bone and joint infections; mild to moderate respiratory tract infections; mild to moderate skin and skin structure infections; infectious diarrhea –
Adults: 500 mg P.O. or 400 mg I.V. q 12 hours.
Severe or complicated bone or joint infections; severe respiratory tract infections; severe skin and skin structure infections –
Adults: 750 mg P.O. q 12 hours.

ADVERSE REACTIONS
Common reactions are in italics; life-threatening reactions are in bold italics.
CNS: headache, restlessness, tremor, light-headedness, confusion, hallucinations, *seizures.*
GI: *nausea, diarrhea,* vomiting, abdominal pain or discomfort, oral candidiasis.
GU: crystalluria.
Local: (with I.V. administration) thrombophlebitis, burning, pruritus, paresthesia, erythema, swelling.
Other: *rash,* eosinophilia, photosensitivity.

INTERACTIONS
Antacids containing magnesium hydroxide or aluminum hydroxide, sucralfate, iron supplements: decreased ciprofloxacin absorption. Separate administration by at least 2 hours.
Probenecid: may elevate serum level of ciprofloxacin.
Theophylline: increased plasma theophylline concentrations and prolonged theophylline half-life. Monitor blood levels of theophylline and observe for adverse effects.

NURSING CONSIDERATIONS
- *Contraindicated* in patients sensitive to quinolone antibiotics, in pregnant or breast-feeding women, and in children under 18 years. Quinolone antibiotics have been shown to produce arthropathy in young laboratory animals.
- *Use with extreme caution* with theophylline. Serious (even fatal) reactions have occurred in patients receiving I.V. theophylline and ciprofloxacin. If a patient must receive theophylline or aminophylline therapy with ciprofloxacin, closely monitor serum theophylline levels and adjust dosage accordingly.
- *Use cautiously* in CNS disorders, such as severe cerebral arteriosclerosis or seizure disorders, and in other patients who are at an increased risk of seizures. May cause CNS stimulation.
- Obtain specimen for culture and sensitivity tests before first dose. Therapy may begin pending test results.
- The preferred time for oral dosing is 2 hours after a meal or 2 hours before or after antacids, sucralfate, or products that contain iron (such as vitamins with mineral supplements). Food does not affect absorption but may delay peak serum levels.
- **I.V. use:** I.V. vials must be diluted before use. Infuse slowly (over 60 minutes) into a large vein.
- Dosage adjustments are necessary in patients with renal dysfunction.
- Prolonged use may result in over-

growth of organisms that are resistant to ciprofloxacin.

- Advise patient that hypersensitivity may occur even after first dose. Patient who notices a skin rash or any allergic-type reaction should stop taking drug immediately and notify his doctor.
- Advise patient to avoid caffeine while taking the drug because of potential for cumulative caffeine effects.
- Drug is excreted in breast milk. Patient should discontinue breast-feeding during treatment or should be treated with another drug.
- May cause dizziness or light-headedness. Warn patient to avoid hazardous tasks that require alertness, such as driving, until CNS effects of the drug are known.
- Advise patient to drink plenty of fluids to reduce the risk of crystalluria.

enoxacin

Penetrex

Pregnancy Risk Category: C

HOW SUPPLIED

Tablets: 200 mg, 400 mg

MECHANISM OF ACTION

A fluoroquinolone that interferes with the action of bacterial DNA gyrase, an enzyme necessary for the synthesis of bacterial DNA. Bactericidal.

INDICATIONS & DOSAGE

Uncomplicated urinary tract infections –

Adults: 200 mg P.O. q 12 hours for 7 days.

Severe or complicated urinary tract infections –

Adults: 400 mg P.O. q 12 hours for 14 days.

Uncomplicated urethral or endocervical gonorrhea –

Adults: 400 mg P.O. as a single dose. Follow with doxycycline therapy to treat possible coexisting chlamydial infection.

ADVERSE REACTIONS

Common reactions are in italics; life-threatening reactions are in bold italics.

CNS: headache, restlessness, tremor, light-headedness, confusion, hallucinations, *seizures.*

GI: *nausea, diarrhea,* vomiting, abdominal pain or discomfort, oral candidiasis.

GU: crystalluria.

Other: *rash,* photosensitivity.

INTERACTIONS

Aminophylline, cyclosporine, caffeine, theophylline: increased levels of these drugs because of decreased metabolism. Use together cautiously.

Antacids containing magnesium hydroxide or aluminum hydroxide, oral iron supplements, sucralfate: decreased enoxacin absorption. Separate administration times by at least 2 hours.

Cimetidine: decreased metabolism of enoxacin. Use together cautiously; dosage adjustment may be necessary.

Oral anticoagulants: increased anticoagulant effect. Use together cautiously.

Probenecid: may elevate serum level of fluoroquinolones. Monitor for adverse reactions.

NURSING CONSIDERATIONS

- *Contraindicated* in patients with hypersensitivity to the drug or other quinolone antibiotics, in pregnant or breast-feeding women, and in children under 18 years because similar drugs have produced arthropathy in young laboratory animals.
- *Use with extreme caution* with theophylline. Serious reactions have occurred in patients receiving I.V. theophylline and enoxacin. If patient must receive theophylline or aminophylline therapy with a quinolone antibiotic, closely monitor serum the-

ophylline levels and adjust dosage accordingly.
- *Use cautiously* in CNS disorders, such as severe cerebral arteriosclerosis or seizure disorders, and in other patients who are at an increased risk for seizures. May cause CNS stimulation.
- *Use cautiously* and with dosage adjustments in patients with impaired renal or hepatic function. If creatinine clearance is 30 ml/minute/1.73 m^2 or less, start therapy with the usual initial dose. Subsequent doses should be decreased by 50%.
- Warn patient not to drink caffeine-containing beverages while taking enoxacin. Drug inhibits the metabolism of caffeine and can result in toxicity.
- Patients being treated for gonorrhea should have an initial serologic test for syphilis at the time of diagnosis. Drug has not been shown to be effective in treating syphilis and may mask signs and symptoms of infection. Repeat the serologic test in 1 to 3 months.
- Obtain specimen for culture and sensitivity tests before first dose. Therapy may begin pending test results.
- Prolonged use may result in superinfection.
- Preferred time for dosing is 2 hours after a meal or 2 hours before or after antacids containing magnesium hydroxide or aluminum hydroxide, sucralfate, or products that contain iron (such as vitamins with mineral supplements).
- Similar drugs have been known to cause severe phototoxicity reactions. Advise patient to avoid overexposure to direct sunlight while taking drug and to use a sunscreen and wear protective clothing while outdoors.
- Advise patient to liberally increase fluid intake while taking drug because similar drugs have caused urine microcrystal formation.
- Warn patient that because drug can cause light-headedness or dizziness, he should avoid driving and other hazardous activities until adverse CNS effects of the drug are known.

lomefloxacin hydrochloride

Maxaquin

Pregnancy Risk Category: C

HOW SUPPLIED

Tablets: 400 mg

MECHANISM OF ACTION

A fluoroquinolone that inhibits bacterial DNA gyrase, an enzyme necessary for bacterial replication (bactericidal).

INDICATIONS & DOSAGE

Acute bacterial exacerbations of chronic bronchitis caused by Haemophilus influenzae *or* Moraxella (Branhamella) catarrhalis –

Adults: 400 mg P.O. daily for 10 days.

Uncomplicated urinary tract infections (cystitis) caused by Escherichia coli, Klebsiella pneumoniae, Proteus mirabilis, *or* Staphylococcus saprophyticus –

Adults: 400 mg P.O. daily for 10 days.

Complicated urinary tract infections caused by Escherichia coli, Klebsiella pneumoniae, P. mirabilis, *or* Pseudomonas aeruginosa; *possibly effective against infections caused by* Citrobacter diversus *or* Enterobacter cloacae –

Adults: 400 mg P.O. daily for 14 days.

Prophylaxis of infections after transurethral surgical procedures –

Adults: 400 mg P.O. as a single dose 2 to 6 hours before surgery.

Dosage adjustment for patients with renal failure –

Adults: Patients with a creatinine clearance of 10 to 40 ml/minute/1.73 m^2 should receive a loading dose of 400 mg P.O. on the first day, followed

*Liquid form contains alcohol. **May contain tartrazine.

by 200 mg daily for the duration of therapy. Periodic determination of blood levels of lomefloxacin are recommended. Hemodialysis removes negligible amounts of the drug.

ADVERSE REACTIONS

Common reactions are in italics; life-threatening reactions are in bold italics.

Blood: thrombocythemia, thrombocytopenia, lymphadenopathy, increased fibrinolysis.

CNS: *dizziness, headache,* abnormal dreams, fatigue, malaise, asthenia, agitation, anorexia, anxiety, confusion, depersonalization, depression, increased appetite, insomnia, nervousness, somnolence, ***seizures, coma,*** hyperkinesia, tremor, vertigo, paresthesia, arthralgia, myalgia, asthenia.

CV: flushing, hypotension, hypertension, edema, syncope, arrhythmia, tachycardia, bradycardia, extrasystoles, cyanosis, angina pectoris, ***MI, cardiac failure, pulmonary embolism,*** cerebrovascular disorder, cardiomyopathy, phlebitis.

EENT: epistaxis, abnormal vision, conjunctivitis, eye pain, earache, tinnitus, tongue discoloration.

GI: *diarrhea, nausea,* dry mouth, intermenstrual bleeding, leukorrhea, vaginitis, abdominal pain, dyspepsia, vomiting, flatulence, constipation, inflammation, dysphagia, bleeding.

GU: dysuria, hematuria, anuria, epididymitis, orchitis, vaginal moniliasis, perineal pain.

Metabolic: hypoglycemia, gout.

Respiratory: cough, dyspnea, ***bronchospasm,*** respiratory disorder, respiratory infection, increased sputum, stridor.

Skin: pruritus, skin disorder, skin exfoliation, eczema, rash, urticaria, *photosensitivity.*

Other: ***anaphylaxis,*** increased sweating, taste perversion, leg cramps, thirst, fatigue, back pain, malaise, chills, allergic reaction, facial edema, influenza-like symptoms, decreased heat tolerance.

INTERACTIONS

Antacids, sucralfate: bind with lomefloxacin in the GI tract and impair its absorption. Administer no less than 4 hours before or 2 hours after a dose.

Cimetidine: other quinolones display a substantial increase in half-life when administered to patients taking cimetidine; lomefloxacin has not been tested. Monitor for toxicity.

Probenecid: decreased excretion of lomefloxacin. Monitor for toxicity.

Warfarin, cyclosporine: other quinolones can increase the effects or serum levels of these agents; lomefloxacin has not been tested. Monitor for toxicity.

NURSING CONSIDERATIONS

- *Contraindicated* in patients with hypersensitivity to lomefloxacin or other quinolones. Also contraindicated in children and adolescents under 18 years and in pregnant and breast-feeding women. Lomefloxacin has caused arthropathy and lameness secondary to permanently damaged cartilage when administered to juvenile animals.
- *Use cautiously* in patients with known or suspected CNS disorders, such as seizure disorder or cerebral arteriosclerosis, that may predispose the patient to seizures.
- While most fluoroquinolones exhibit photosensitizing effects, early studies suggest that photosensitization and phototoxicity are more common with lomefloxacin. Some animal studies suggest that prolonged use of drug may predispose subjects to skin cancers. Advise patient to wear protective clothing, use a sunscreen, and avoid prolonged exposure to sunlight during treatment and for a few days after therapy ends. If sunburn occurs, patient should call the doctor as soon as possible.

• Several bacterial strains have demonstrated resistance to lomefloxacin, including *Streptococcus pneumoniae,* most group A, B, D, and G streptococci, *Pseudomonas cepacia, Ureaplasma urealyticum, Mycoplasma hominis,* and anaerobes.
• Lomefloxacin should not be used for the empiric treatment of acute exacerbations of chronic bronchitis when it is likely that the causative organism is *S. pneumoniae* because this organism demonstrates resistance to the drug. It also should not be used to treat bacteremia caused by *P. aeruginosa* because blood levels of the drug do not readily exceed the minimum inhibitory concentration against the organism. However, lomefloxacin has been used successfully to treat complicated urinary tract infections caused by *P. aeruginosa.*
• Lomefloxacin should be taken on an empty stomach.
• Obtain culture and sensitivity tests before first dose. Therapy may begin pending results.
• Prolonged use may result in overgrowth of organisms resistant to lomefloxacin.
• Advise patient that hypersensitivity may occur even after first dose. Patient who notices skin rash or any allergic-type reaction should stop taking the drug and notify his doctor.
• Drug may cause dizziness or lightheadedness. Warn patient to avoid driving and other hazardous tasks that require alertness until CNS effects of drug are known.

nalidixic acid

NegGram

Pregnancy Risk Category: B

HOW SUPPLIED
Tablets: 250 mg, 500 mg, 1 g
Oral suspension: 250 mg/5 ml

MECHANISM OF ACTION
Inhibits microbial DNA synthesis.

INDICATIONS & DOSAGE
Acute and chronic urinary tract infections caused by susceptible gram-negative organisms (Proteus, Klebsiella, Enterobacter, *and* Escherichia coli) – **Adults:** 1 g P.O. q.i.d. for 7 to 14 days; 2 g daily for long-term use.
Children over 3 months: 55 mg/kg P.O. daily divided q.i.d. for 7 to 14 days; 33 mg/kg daily for long-term use.

ADVERSE REACTIONS
Common reactions are in italics; life-threatening reactions are in bold italics.
Blood: eosinophilia.
CNS: drowsiness, weakness, headache, dizziness, vertigo, ***seizures,*** confusion, hallucinations.
EENT: sensitivity to light, change in color perception, diplopia, blurred vision.
GI: *abdominal pain, nausea, vomiting,* diarrhea.
Skin: pruritus, photosensitivity, urticaria, rash.
Other: angioedema, fever, chills, ***increased intracranial pressure and bulging fontanelles in infants and children.***

INTERACTIONS
Oral anticoagulants: Increased anticoagulant effect.

NURSING CONSIDERATIONS
• *Contraindicated* in seizure disorders.
• *Use with extreme caution* in prepubertal children; erosion of cartilage of immature animals has been reported.
• *Use cautiously* in patients with impaired hepatic or renal function or with severe cerebral arteriosclerosis.
• Not effective against *Pseudomonas* or infections outside of the urinary tract.
• Tell the patient to report visual dis-

*Liquid form contains alcohol. **May contain tartrazine.

turbances; these usually disappear with reduced dose.

- Obtain specimen for culture and sensitivity tests before starting therapy and repeat p.r.n. Therapy may begin pending test results.
- Obtain CBC, renal and liver function studies during long-term therapy.
- Resistant bacteria may emerge within the first 48 hours of therapy.
- May cause a false-positive Clinitest reaction. Use Clinistix or Tes-Tape to monitor urine glucose. Also gives false elevations in urine vanillylmandelic acid (VMA) and 17-ketosteroids. Repeat tests after therapy is completed.
- Avoid undue exposure to sunlight due to photosensitivity. Patient may continue to be photosensitive for as long as 3 months after drug is discontinued.

norfloxacin

Noroxin

Pregnancy Risk Category: C

HOW SUPPLIED

Tablets: 400 mg

MECHANISM OF ACTION

Inhibits bacterial DNA synthesis, mainly by inhibiting DNA gyrase. Bactericidal.

INDICATIONS & DOSAGE

Treatment of complicated or uncomplicated urinary tract infections caused by susceptible strains of Escherichia coli, Klebsiella, Enterobacter, Proteus, Pseudomonas aeruginosa, Citrobacter, Staphylococcus aureus *(and* epidermidis*), and group D streptococci–*

Adults: for uncomplicated infections, 400 mg P.O. b.i.d. for 7 to 10 days. For complicated infections, 400 mg b.i.d. for 10 to 21 days.

ADVERSE REACTIONS

Common reactions are in italics; life-threatening reactions are in bold italics.

Blood: eosinophilia.

CNS: fatigue, somnolence, headache, dizziness.

GI: nausea, constipation, flatulence, heartburn, dry mouth.

Hepatic: transient elevations of AST (SGOT) and ALT (SGPT).

Skin: rash.

Other: ***hypersensitivity reactions*** (rash, anaphylactoid reactions).

INTERACTIONS

Antacids, iron products, sucralfate: may hinder absorption. Separate administration times by 2 hours.

Nitrofurantoin: decreases norfloxacin's effectiveness. Don't use together.

Probenecid: may increase serum levels of norfloxacin by decreasing its excretion.

Theophylline: norfloxacin may impair theophylline metabolism, resulting in increased plasma levels and risk of toxicity. Monitor closely.

NURSING CONSIDERATIONS

- *Contraindicated* in patients with hypersensitivity to nalidixic acid and cinoxacin.
- Warn patients not to exceed the recommended dosages. Advise them to drink several glasses of water throughout the day to maintain hydration and adequate urine output.
- Advise patients to take the drug 1 hour before or 2 hours after meals because food, antacids, iron products, and sucralfate may hinder absorption.
- Because norfloxacin may cause dizziness, patients should avoid hazardous activities that require alertness and good coordination until the CNS effects of the drug are known.

ofloxacin

Floxin

Pregnancy Risk Category: C

HOW SUPPLIED

Tablets: 200 mg, 300 mg, 400 mg

MECHANISM OF ACTION

A broad-spectrum quinolone antibiotic. Bactericidal effects may result from the drug's ability to inhibit bacterial DNA gyrase and to prevent DNA replication in susceptible bacteria.

INDICATIONS & DOSAGE

Lower respiratory tract infections caused by susceptible strains of Haemophilus influenzae *or* Streptococcus pneumoniae –
Adults: 400 mg P.O. q 12 hours for 10 days.
Cervicitis or urethritis caused by Chlamydia trachomatis *or* Neisseria gonorrhoeae –
Adults: 300 mg P.O. q 12 hours for 7 days.
Acute, uncomplicated gonorrhea –
Adults: 400 mg P.O. as a single dose.
Mild-to-moderate skin and skin structure infections caused by susceptible strains of Staphylococcus aureus, S. epidermidis, Streptococcus pyogenes, *or* Proteus mirabilis –
Adults: 400 mg P.O. q 12 hours for 10 days.
Cystitis caused by Escherichia coli *or* Klebsiella pneumoniae –
Adults: 200 mg P.O. q 12 hours for 3 days.
Urinary tract infections caused by susceptible strains of Citrobacter diversus, Enterobacter aerogenes, Escherichia coli, Proteus mirabilis, *or* Pseudomonas aeruginosa –
Adults: 200 mg P.O. q 12 hours for 7 days. Complicated infections may require therapy for 10 days.
Prostatitis caused by E. coli –
Adults: 200 mg P.O. q 12 hours for 6 weeks.
Dosage adjustment for patients with renal failure –
If creatinine clearance is 10 to 50 ml/minute, decrease dosage interval to once q 24 hours. If creatinine clearance is <10 ml/minute, give half the recommended dose q 24 hours.

ADVERSE REACTIONS

Common reactions are in italics; life-threatening reactions are in bold italics.
CNS: headache, dizziness, fatigue, lethargy, malaise, drowsiness, sleep disorders, nervousness, light-headedness, insomnia, seizures.
CV: chest pain.
GI: nausea, anorexia, abdominal pain or discomfort, diarrhea, vomiting, dry mouth, flatulence, dysgeusia.
GU: vaginitis, vaginal discharge, genital pruritus.
Skin: rash, pruritus, photosensitivity.
Other: ***hypersensitivity*** (*anaphylactoid*) reaction, visual disturbances, fever.

INTERACTIONS

Antacids containing aluminum or magnesium hydroxide, iron salts, sucralfate, products containing zinc: may interfere with the GI absorption of ofloxacin. Separate administration times by at least 2 hours.
Anticoagulants: increased effect. Monitor for bleeding and altered prothrombin time.
Antineoplastic agents: may lower serum levels of quinolones.
Theophylline: some quinolones may decrease clearance of theophylline. Monitor theophylline levels.

NURSING CONSIDERATIONS

- *Contraindicated* in children and in breast-feeding women because drug has caused arthropathy or osteochondrosis in young animals. Breast milk concentrations are similar to those in plasma. Use during pregnancy only when benefits outweigh fetal risks. Also contraindicated in hypersensitivity to the drug or other quinolones.

- *Use cautiously* in patients with a history of seizure disorders or other CNS diseases, such as cerebral arteriosclerosis. If patient experiences excessive CNS stimulation (restlessness, tremor, confusion, hallucinations), discontinue medication and notify doctor. Institute seizure precautions.
- Because the drug is mainly eliminated by renal excretion, adjust dosage in patients with renal failure.
- Patients treated for gonorrhea should have a serologic test for syphilis. Drug is not effective against syphilis, and treatment of gonorrhea may mask or delay symptoms of syphilis.
- Patients should use sunscreens and protective clothing to avoid photosensitivity reactions.
- Regular blood studies and hepatic and renal function tests are recommended during prolonged therapy.
- Advise patients to take the drug with plenty of fluids, but not with meals, and to avoid antacids, sucralfate, and products containing iron or zinc for at least 2 hours before or after each dose.
- Because the drug may cause lightheadedness, patient should avoid hazardous tasks such as driving until the adverse CNS effects are known.
- Tell the patient to stop drug and notify the doctor if a rash or other signs of hypersensitivity develop.

17

Antivirals

acyclovir sodium
amantadine hydrochloride
didanosine
foscarnet sodium
ganciclovir
ribavirin
vidarabine monohydrate
zalcitabine
zidovudine

COMBINATION PRODUCTS
None.

acyclovir sodium

Zovirax

Pregnancy Risk Category: C

HOW SUPPLIED
Capsules: 200 mg
Injection: 500 mg/vial, 1 g/vial

MECHANISM OF ACTION
Becomes incorporated into viral DNA and inhibits viral multiplication.

INDICATIONS & DOSAGE
Treatment of initial and recurrent episodes of mucocutaneous herpes simplex virus (HSV-1 and HSV-2) infections in immunocompromised patients; severe initial episodes of herpes genitalis in patients who are not immunocompromised –
Adults and children over 11 years: 5 mg/kg, given at a constant rate over a period of 1 hour by I.V. infusion q 8 hours for 7 days (5 days for herpes genitalis).
Children under 12 years: 250 mg/m^2, given at a constant rate over a period of 1 hour by I.V. infusion q 8 hours for 7 days (5 days for herpes genitalis).
Treatment of initial genital herpes –
Adults: 200 mg P.O. q 4 hours while awake (a total of 5 capsules daily). Treatment should continue for 10 days.
Intermittent therapy for recurrent genital herpes –
Adults: 200 mg P.O. q 4 hours while awake (a total of 5 capsules daily). Treatment should continue for 5 days. Initiate therapy at the first sign of recurrence.
Chronic suppressive therapy for recurrent genital herpes –
Adults: 200 mg P.O. t.i.d. or 400 mg b.i.d. for 6 to 12 months.
Chicken pox –
Adults and children: 20 mg/kg P.O. q.i.d. for 5 days. Start therapy as soon as symptoms appear.

ADVERSE REACTIONS
Common reactions are in italics; life-threatening reactions are in bold italics.
CNS: (associated with I.V. dosage): *headache, encephalopathic changes (lethargy, obtundation, tremor, confusion, hallucinations, agitation,* ***seizures, coma****).*
CV: hypotension.
GI: *nausea, vomiting,* diarrhea.
GU: *transient elevations of serum creatinine levels,* hematuria.
Skin: rash, itching.
Local: *inflammation, vesicular eruptions and phlebitis at injection site.*

INTERACTIONS
Probenecid: increased acyclovir blood levels. Monitor for possible toxicity.
Zidovudine: may cause drowsiness or lethargy. Use together cautiously.

NURSING CONSIDERATIONS
• Some clinicians consider acyclovir therapy of marginal benefit for chicken pox because the disease is usually self-limiting. However, acy-

clovir may be more beneficial in adolescents than in young children.
• Teach patient that drug is effective in managing the disease but does not eliminate or cure it.
• Instruct patient that acyclovir will not prevent spread of infection to others.
• Urge patient to recognize the early symptoms of herpes infection (such as tingling, itching, or pain) so he can take acyclovir before the infection fully develops.
• Don't administer topically, intramuscularly, orally, subcutaneously, or ophthalmically.
• **I.V. use:** Infusion must be administered over at least 1 hour to prevent renal tubular damage. Bolus injection, dehydration (decreased urine output), preexisting renal disease, and the concomitant use of other nephrotoxic drugs increase the risk of renal toxicity.
• Don't give by bolus injection.
• Concentrated solutions (10 mg/ml or more) may be associated with a higher incidence of phlebitis.
• Notify doctor if serum creatinine level does not return to normal within a few days. He may increase hydration, adjust dose, or discontinue acyclovir.
• Encephalopathic changes are more likely in patients with neurologic disorders or in those who have had neurologic reactions to cytotoxic drugs.
• Patient must be adequately hydrated during acyclovir infusion.

amantadine hydrochloride

Antadine‡, Symadine, Symmetrel

Pregnancy Risk Category: C

HOW SUPPLIED

Capsules: 100 mg
Syrup: 50 mg/5 ml

MECHANISM OF ACTION

Interferes with influenza A virus penetration into susceptible cells. Its action in the treatment of parkinsonism is unknown.

INDICATIONS & DOSAGE

Prophylaxis or symptomatic treatment of influenza type A virus, respiratory tract illnesses –
Adults to 64 years and children 10 years and over: 200 mg P.O. daily in a single dose or divided b.i.d.
Children 1 to 9 years: 4.4 to 8.8 mg/kg P.O. daily, as a single dose or divided b.i.d. or t.i.d. Don't exceed 150 mg daily.
Adults over 64 years: 100 mg P.O. once daily.

Treatment should continue for 24 to 48 hours after symptoms disappear. Prophylaxis should start as soon as possible after initial exposure and continue for at least 10 days after exposure. May continue prophylactic treatment up to 90 days for repeated or suspected exposures if influenza vaccine unavailable. If used with influenza vaccine, continue dose for 2 to 3 weeks until protection from vaccine develops.

To treat drug-induced extrapyramidal reactions –
Adults: 100 mg P.O. b.i.d., up to 300 mg daily in divided doses. Patient may benefit from as much as 400 mg daily, but dosages over 200 mg must be closely supervised.

To treat idiopathic parkinsonism, parkinsonian syndrome –
Adults: 100 mg P.O. b.i.d.; in patients who are seriously ill or receiving other antiparkinsonian drugs, 100 mg daily for at least 1 week, then 100 mg b.i.d., p.r.n.

ADVERSE REACTIONS

Common reactions are in italics; life-threatening reactions are in bold italics.
CNS: depression, fatigue, confusion, dizziness, psychosis, hallucinations,

anxiety, *irritability,* ataxia, *insomnia,* weakness, headache, light-headedness, difficulty concentrating.
CV: peripheral edema, orthostatic hypotension, *CHF.*
GI: anorexia, nausea, constipation, vomiting, dry mouth.
GU: urine retention.
Skin: *livedo reticularis* (with prolonged use).

INTERACTIONS
Anticholinergics: increased adverse anticholinergic effects. Use together cautiously.
Triamterene, hydrochlorothiazide: increased levels of amantadine. Use together cautiously.

NURSING CONSIDERATIONS
- *Use cautiously* in seizure disorders, CHF, peripheral edema, hepatic disease, mental illness, eczematoid rash, renal impairment, orthostatic hypotension, and CV disease and in elderly patients. Dosage may need to be adjusted in patients with renal failure.
- For best absorption, drug should be taken after meals.
- Instruct patient to report adverse reactions to the doctor, especially dizziness, depression, anxiety, nausea, and urine retention.
- Elderly patients are more susceptible to neurological adverse effects. Taking the drug in two daily doses rather than single dose may reduce their incidence.
- If orthostatic hypotension occurs, instruct patient not to stand or change positions too quickly.
- If insomnia occurs, dose should be taken several hours before bedtime.
- When prescribed for parkinsonism, warn patient against discontinuing drug abruptly since this might precipitate a parkinsonian crisis.

didanosine (ddI)
Videx
Pregnancy Risk Category: B

HOW SUPPLIED
Tablets (chewable): 25 mg, 50 mg, 100 mg, 150 mg
Powder for oral solution (buffered): 100 mg/packet, 167 mg/packet, 250 mg/packet, 375 mg/packet
Powder for oral solution (pediatric): 10 mg/ml in 2- and 4-g bottles

MECHANISM OF ACTION
A synthetic purine analog of deoxyadenosine. After didanosine enters the cell, it is converted to its active form dideoxyadenosine triphosphate (ddATP), which inhibits replication of human immunodeficiency virus (HIV) by preventing DNA replication. In addition, ddATP inhibits the enzyme HIV-RNA dependent DNA polymerase (reverse transcriptase).

INDICATIONS & DOSAGE
Advanced HIV infection in patients who cannot tolerate or who no longer respond to zidovudine therapy –
Adults 75 kg and over: 300 mg (two 150-mg tablets) P.O. q 12 hours; or 375 mg buffered powder q 12 hours.
Adults 50 to 74 kg: 200 mg (two 100-mg tablets) P.O. q 12 hours; or 250 mg buffered powder q 12 hours.
Adults 35 to 49 kg: 125 mg (one 100-mg and one 25-mg tablet) P.O. q 12 hours; or 167 mg buffered powder q 12 hours.
Children: 200 mg/m^2 P.O. daily in divided doses q 12 hours.

ADVERSE REACTIONS
Common reactions are in italics; life-threatening reactions are in bold italics.
CNS: *headache,* insomnia, dizziness, ***seizures,*** confusion, anxiety, nervousness, hypertonia, abnormal thinking.
CV: hypertension.
GI: *diarrhea, nausea, vomiting, ab-*

*Liquid form contains alcohol. **May contain tartrazine.

dominal pain, ***pancreatitis,*** dry mouth, dyspepsia, flatulence.
Hepatic: liver abnormalities.
Other: *peripheral neuropathy,* rash, pruritus, asthenia, pain, myalgia, arthritis, pneumonia, infection, cough, myopathy.

INTERACTIONS
Antacids containing magnesium or aluminum hydroxides: enhanced adverse effects of the antacid component (including diarrhea or constipation) when administered with didanosine tablets or pediatric suspension. Avoid concomitant use.
Ketoconazole, dapsone, drugs that require gastric acid for adequate absorption: buffering action of didanosine can decrease absorption. Administer these drugs 2 hours before didanosine.
Tetracyclines, fluoroquinolones: decreased absorption because of buffering agents in didanosine tablets or antacids in pediatric suspension.

NURSING CONSIDERATIONS
- *Contraindicated* in patients with a history of hypersensitivity to any component of the formulation. Tablets are buffered with dihydroxyaluminum sodium carbonate, magnesium hydroxide, and sodium citrate and are flavored with aspartame and sugar. Powder for oral solution is buffered with sodium phosphate, sodium citrate, and citric acid and is flavored with sucrose.
- *Use cautiously* in patients with a history of pancreatitis. In early studies, the drug caused pancreatitis in about 9% of all patients; fatalities have occurred. Also use cautiously in patients with peripheral neuropathy, renal or hepatic impairment, or hyperuricemia.
- In early clinical trials, the powder for oral solution was associated with a high incidence of diarrhea. Although there is no evidence to suggest that other formulations may be associated with a lower incidence of diarrhea, the manufacturer suggests switching to the tablet formulation if diarrhea is a problem.
- Patients receiving a sodium-restricted diet should know that each two-tablet dose of didanosine contains 529 mg of sodium; each single packet of buffered powder for oral solution contains 1.38 g of sodium.
- Administer didanosine on an empty stomach, regardless of the dosage form used. Studies have shown that administering the drug with meals can result in a 50% decrease in absorption.
- Most patients should receive two tablets per dose.
- Because they contain buffers that raise stomach pH to levels that prevent degradation of the active drug, the tablets should be thoroughly chewed before swallowing, and the patient should drink at least 1 oz of water with each dose. If the tablets are manually crushed, stir them thoroughly in 1 oz of water to disperse the particles uniformly, then have the patient drink the mixture immediately.
- Children over 1 year should receive a two-tablet dose, and children under 1 year may receive a one-tablet dose.
- Single-dose packets containing buffered powder for oral solution are available. To administer, carefully open the packet and pour contents into 4 oz of water. Do not use fruit juice or other beverages that may be acidic. Stir for 2 or 3 minutes until the powder dissolves completely. Administer immediately.
- Use care when preparing the powder or crushing tablets to avoid excessive dispersal of the powder into the air.
- The pediatric powder for oral solution must be prepared by a pharmacist before dispensing. It must be constituted with Purified Water, USP, then diluted with an antacid (either My-

lanta Double Strength Liquid or Maalox TC Suspension) to a final concentration of 10 mg/ml. The admixture is stable for 30 days if refrigerated (at 36° to 46° F [2° to 8° C]). Be sure to shake the solution well before measuring the dose.

foscarnet sodium (phosphonoformic acid)

Foscavir

Pregnancy Risk Category: C

HOW SUPPLIED

Injection: 24 mg/ml in 250- and 500-ml bottles

MECHANISM OF ACTION

An organic analog of pyrophosphate, an inorganic compound used in many enzymatic reactions. Foscarnet inhibits all known herpesviruses in vitro by blocking the pyrophosphate binding site on DNA polymerases and reverse transcriptases.

INDICATIONS & DOSAGE

CMV retinitis in patients with AIDS –
Adults: initially, 60 mg/kg I.V. as an induction treatment in patients with normal renal function. Administer as an I.V. infusion over 1 hour q 8 hours for 2 to 3 weeks, depending on clinical response. Follow with a maintenance infusion of 90 mg/kg daily administered over 2 hours; this dose may be increased as needed and tolerated to 120 mg/kg daily if the disease shows signs of progression.

Dosage adjustment in patients with renal failure –
Adults: first, calculate the patient's creatinine clearance from this equation:

For male patients: creatinine clearance = (140 – age)/(serum creatinine × 72)

For female patients: multiply the above value by 0.85

Then administer as shown below.

Induction dose –

Creatinine clearance (ml/min/kg)	Dose to be administered q 8 hours (mg/kg)
1.6	60
1.5	57
1.4	53
1.3	49
1.2	46
1.1	42
1	39
0.9	35
0.8	32
0.7	28
0.6	25
0.5	21
0.4	18

Maintenance dose –

Creatinine clearance (ml/min/kg)	Equivalent to 90 mg/kg/day	Equivalent to 120 mg/kg/day
1.4	90	120
1.2 to 1.4	78	104
1 to 1.2	75	100
0.8 to 1	71	94
0.6 to 0.8	63	84
0.4 to 0.6	57	76

ADVERSE REACTIONS

Common reactions are in italics; life-threatening reactions are in bold italics.

Blood: *anemia, granulocytopenia, leukopenia,* ***bone marrow suppression,*** thrombocytopenia, platelet abnormalities, thrombocytosis, WBC count abnormalities, lymphadenopathy.

CNS: *headache,* ***seizures,*** *fatigue, rigors, malaise, asthenia, paresthesia, dizziness, hypoesthesia, neuropathy,* tremor, ataxia, generalized spasms, dementia, stupor, sensory disturbances, meningitis, aphasia, abnormal coordination, EEG abnormalities, vertigo, ***coma***, encephalopathy, abnormal gait, hypertonia, visual field defects, dyskinesia, extrapyramidal reactions, speech disorders, paralysis, peripheral neuropathy, nystagmus, ***cerebral edema.***

*Liquid form contains alcohol. **May contain tartrazine.

CV: *hypertension, palpitations, ECG abnormalities, sinus tachycardia, first-degree AV block, hypotension, flushing.*
EENT: visual disturbances.
GI: *nausea, diarrhea, vomiting, abdominal pain, anorexia,* constipation, dysphagia, rectal hemorrhage, dry mouth, melena, flatulence, ulcerative stomatitis, ***pancreatitis.***
GU: ***abnormal renal function,*** *decreased creatinine clearance and increased serum creatinine levels, albuminuria, dysuria, polyuria, urethral disorder, urine retention, urinary tract infections,* ***acute renal failure.***
Respiratory: *cough, dyspnea,* pneumonitis, sinusitis, pharyngitis, rhinitis, respiratory insufficiency, pulmonary infiltration, stridor, pneumothorax, ***bronchospasm,*** hemoptysis.
Skin: *rash, increased sweating,* pruritus, skin ulceration, erythematous rash, seborrhea, skin discoloration.
Other: fever, pain, infection, sepsis, hypokalemia, hypomagnesemia, hypophosphatemia or hyperphosphatemia, hypocalcemia, leg cramps.

INTERACTIONS

Nephrotoxic drugs such as amphotericin B, aminoglycosides: increased risk of nephrotoxicity. Avoid concomitant use.
Pentamidine: increased risk of nephrotoxicity; severe hypocalcemia has also been reported. Don't use together.
Zidovudine: possible increased incidence or severity of anemia. Monitor blood counts.

NURSING CONSIDERATIONS

- *Contraindicated* in patients with hypersensitivity to the drug.
- *Use cautiously* in patients with abnormal renal function because it will result in accumulation of the drug and enhanced toxicity. Because foscarnet is nephrotoxic, it has the potential to worsen renal impairment. Some degree of nephrotoxicity occurs in most patients treated with the drug.
- Administration of the drug is associated with a transient decrease in ionized serum calcium. This decrease may not always be reflected in the patient's laboratory values, and it is caused by a direct, dose-related chemical effect of the drug on serum calcium. Advise patients to report perioral tingling, numbness in the extremities, and paresthesia.
- Creatinine clearance should be determined before therapy and frequently thereafter because of the drug's adverse effects on renal function. A baseline 24-hour creatinine clearance is recommended, followed by regular determinations two to three times weekly during induction and at least once every 1 to 2 weeks during maintenance. If creatinine clearance falls below 0.4 ml/minute/kg, discontinue the drug.
- Because the drug can adversely affect important serum electrolytes such as potassium, calcium, magnesium, and phosphorus, regular determinations of these electrolytes are recommended using a schedule similar to that established for creatinine clearance. Monitor patient for tetany and seizures associated with abnormal electrolyte levels.
- Anemia is common (in up to 33% of patients treated with the drug). It may be severe enough to require transfusions. Monitor the patient's hemoglobin and hematocrit levels.
- Do not exceed the recommended dosage, infusion rate, or frequency of administration. Know that all doses must be individualized according to the patient's renal function.
- **I.V. use:** An infusion pump must be used to administer foscarnet. To minimize renal toxicity, the patient must be adequately hydrated before and during the infusion.
- Because the drug is highly toxic and toxicity is probably dose-related, the

lowest effective maintenance dose should be used throughout therapy.

- Unlike ganciclovir, foscarnet does not require cellular activation by thymidine kinase or other kinases. Foscarnet may be active against certain CMV strains resistant to ganciclovir.

ganciclovir
Cytovene

Pregnancy Risk Category: C

HOW SUPPLIED
Injection: 500 mg/vial

MECHANISM OF ACTION
Inhibits viral DNA synthesis of CMV.

INDICATIONS & DOSAGE
CMV retinitis treatment of immunocompromised individuals, including patients with AIDS –
Adults: induction treatment – initially, 5 mg/kg I.V. q 12 hours for 14 to 21 days (normal renal function); maintenance treatment – 5 mg/kg I.V. daily for 7 days each week, or 6 mg/kg daily for 5 days each week.

ADVERSE REACTIONS
Common reactions are in italics; life-threatening reactions are in bold italics.
Blood: *granulocytopenia,* ***thrombocytopenia.***
CNS: altered dreams, confusion, ataxia, dizziness, headache.
CV: arrhythmias, hypotension, hypertension.
GI: nausea, vomiting, diarrhea, anorexia.
GU: hematuria.
Local: injection site inflammation, pain, phlebitis.
Other: retinal detachment in CMV retinitis patients.

INTERACTIONS
Cytotoxic agents: additive toxic effects, especially hematologic effects and stomatitis.
Imipenem/cilastatin: reports of seizure activity with concomitant use.
Probenecid: increased ganciclovir blood levels.
Zidovudine: increased incidence of granulocytopenia with concurrent use.

NURSING CONSIDERATIONS
- *Contraindicated* in patients with an absolute neutrophil count below 500/mm³ or a platelet count below 25,000/mm³.
- Dosage of ganciclovir should be reduced in patients with renal dysfunction.
- **I.V. use:** Do not administer S.C. or I.M.
- Infusion must take place over at least 1 hour. Use an infusion pump. Infusions faster than 60 minutes will result in increased toxicity. Do not administer as an I.V. bolus.
- Ganciclovir infusion therapy should be accompanied by adequate hydration.
- Because of the frequency of granulocytopenia and thrombocytopenia, neutrophil and platelet counts should be obtained every 2 days during twice-daily ganciclovir dosing and at least weekly thereafter.
- Use caution when preparing ganciclovir solution, which is alkaline.

ribavirin
Virazole

Pregnancy Risk Category: X

HOW SUPPLIED
Powder to be reconstituted for inhalation: 6 g in 100-ml glass vial

MECHANISM OF ACTION
Inhibits viral activity by an unknown mechanism. Thought to inhibit RNA and DNA synthesis by depleting intracellular nucleotide pools.

INDICATIONS & DOSAGE
Hospitalized infants and young children infected by RSV –
Infants and young children: solution in concentration of 20 mg/ml delivered via the Viratek Small Particle Aerosol Generator (SPAG-2). Treatment is carried out for 12 to 18 hours/day for at least 3, and no more than 7, days.

ADVERSE REACTIONS
Common reactions are in italics; life-threatening reactions are in bold italics.
Blood: anemia, reticulocytosis.
EENT: conjunctivitis.
Respiratory: worsening of respiratory state.
Other: rash or erythema of eyelids.

INTERACTIONS
None significant.

NURSING CONSIDERATIONS
- *Contraindicated* in females who are or may become pregnant during treatment with drug.
- Ribavirin aerosol is indicated only for severe lower respiratory tract infection due to RSV. Although treatment may be started while awaiting diagnostic test results, existence of RSV infection must be eventually documented.
- Most infants and children with RSV infection don't require treatment because the disease is often mild and self-limiting. Infants with underlying conditions, such as prematurity or cardiopulmonary disease, get RSV in its severest form and benefit most from treatment with ribavirin aerosol.
- This treatment must be accompanied by, and does not replace, supportive respiratory and fluid management.
- Ribavirin aerosol *must* be administered by the Viratek Small Particle Aerosol Generator (SPAG-2). Don't use any other aerosol generating device.
- Ribavarin may precipitate in ventilator apparatus which may result in equipment malfunction with serious consequences. The use of ribavirin in ventilator dependent patients is not recommended.
- The water used to reconstitute this drug must not contain any antimicrobial agent. Use sterile USP water for injection, *not* bacteriostatic water.
- Discard solutions placed in the SPAG-2 unit at least every 24 hours before adding newly reconstituted solution.
- Store reconstituted solutions at room temperature for 24 hours.

vidarabine monohydrate (adenine arabinoside, ara-A)
Vira-A

Pregnancy Risk Category: C

HOW SUPPLIED
Concentrate for I.V. infusion: 200 mg/ml in 5-ml vial (equivalent to 187.4 mg vidarabine)

MECHANISM OF ACTION
Becomes incorporated into viral DNA and inhibits viral multiplication.

INDICATIONS & DOSAGE
Herpes simplex virus encephalitis –
Adults and children (including neonates): 15 mg/kg I.V. daily for 10 days. Slowly infuse the total daily dose by I.V. infusion at a constant rate over 12-to 24-hour period. Avoid rapid or bolus injection.
Herpes zoster in immunosuppressed patients –
Adults: 10 mg/kg I.V. daily for 5 days.

ADVERSE REACTIONS
Common reactions are in italics; life-threatening reactions are in bold italics.
Blood: anemia, neutropenia, thrombocytopenia.

CNS: tremor, dizziness, hallucinations, confusion, psychosis, ataxia.
GI: *anorexia, nausea,* vomiting, diarrhea.
Hepatic: elevated AST (SGOT), bilirubin.
Skin: pruritus, rash.
Local: pain at injection site.
Other: weight loss.

INTERACTIONS

Allopurinol: concurrent therapy reduces metabolism of vidarabine and increases risk of adverse CNS effects.

NURSING CONSIDERATIONS

- Can reduce mortality caused by herpes simplex virus encephalitis from about 70% to 28%. Vidarabine is not effective against other viruses.
- Monitor hematologic tests, such as hemoglobin, hematocrit, WBC count, and platelet count during therapy. Also monitor renal and liver function studies.
- Patient with impaired renal function may need dosage adjustment.
- Any I.V. solution is suitable as a diluent.
- **I.V. use:** Use with a 0.45-micron (or smaller) I.V. filter.
- Must be diluted to a concentration of less than 0.5 mg/ml. Because vidarabine is not highly soluble, each milligram of drug requires 2.2 ml of I.V. solution to solubilize; the maximum concentration is 450 mg/liter. Dilute just before using, and use within 48 hours.
- Don't give I.M. or subcutaneously because of low solubility and poor absorption. Because large volumes of solution must be administered, monitor patient for fluid overload.

zalcitabine (dideoxycytidine, ddC)

Hivid

Pregnancy Risk Category: C

HOW SUPPLIED

Tablets: 0.375 mg, 0.75 mg

MECHANISM OF ACTION

A synthetic pyrimidine nucleoside analogue. After zalcitabine enters the cell, it's converted by enzymes to its active metabolite, dideoxycytidine 5′-triphosphate (ddCTP), which inhibits replication of human immunodeficiency virus (HIV) by blocking viral DNA synthesis. It performs this action by acting as an alternate for the enzyme's substrate, deoxycytidine triphosphate (dCTP).

INDICATIONS & DOSAGE

Advanced HIV infection (CD4 + T cell count below 300 cells/mm³) in patients who have demonstrated significant clinical or immunologic deterioration –
Adults 30 kg and over: 0.75 mg P.O. q 8 hours. Must be taken with zidovudine 200 mg P.O. q 8 hours.
Dosage adjustment in patients with renal failure –
Adults: Patients with a creatinine clearance above 40 ml/minute/1.73 m² should receive the usual dose; 10 to 40 ml/minute/1.73 m², the usual dose q 12 hours; below 10 ml/minute/1.73 m², the usual dose q 24 hours.

ADVERSE REACTIONS

Common reactions are in italics; life-threatening reactions are in bold italics.
Note: Limited data regarding drug toxicity are available. Consult current literature for more details.
CNS: *peripheral neuropathy,* headache.
EENT: pharyngitis.
GI: nausea, vomiting, diarrhea, abdominal pain, anorexia, constipation, stomatitis.
Skin: pruritus; night sweats; erythematous, maculopapular, or follicular rash.
Other: myalgia, arthralgia, fatigue,

*Liquid form contains alcohol. **May contain tartrazine.

fever, rigors, chest pain, weight increase, **pancreatitis.**

INTERACTIONS

Aminoglycosides, amphotericin B, foscarnet, and other drugs that may impair renal function: increased risk of nephrotoxicity. Avoid concomitant use.

Chloramphenicol, cisplatin, dapsone, disulfiram, ethionamide, glutethimide, gold salts, hydralazine, iodoquinol, isoniazid, metronidazole, nitrofurantoin, phenytoin, ribavirin, and vincristine as well as other drugs that can cause peripheral neuropathy: increased risk of peripheral neuropathy. Avoid concomitant use.

Pentamidine: increased risk of pancreatitis. Avoid concomitant use.

NURSING CONSIDERATIONS

- *Contraindicated* in patients with hypersensitivity to the drug or any component of the formulation.
- *Use with extreme caution* in patients with preexisting peripheral neuropathy. No data exist regarding toxicity of zalcitabine in these patients because those with preexisting neuropathy were excluded from clinical trials.
- *Use cautiously* in patients with renal impairment (creatinine clearance below 55 ml/minute/1.73 m^2) because they may be at increased risk for toxicity to the drug. Dosage adjustments are necessary in patients with moderate to severe renal failure.
- Also use cautiously in patients with hepatic failure. In clinical trials, the drug regimen (zalcitabine plus zidovudine) exacerbated hepatic dysfunction in patients with preexisting liver impairment.
- Additionally, use cautiously in patients with a history of pancreatitis. Rarely, pancreatitis has been fatal in patients receiving zalcitabine. In patients receiving zalcitabine as the only treatment (monotherapy), the incidence of pancreatitis was less than 1%.
- Peripheral neuropathy, characterized by numbness and burning in the extremities, is the major toxicity to the drug. In clinical trials using zalcitabine monotherapy, peripheral neuropathy occurred in 17% to 31% of patients. If drug isn't withdrawn, peripheral neuropathy can progress to sharp shooting pain or severe continuous burning pain requiring narcotic analgesics. It may or may not be reversible.
- If patient experiences symptoms that resemble peripheral neuropathy, drug should be discontinued if symptoms are bilateral and persist beyond 72 hours. If symptoms persist or worsen beyond 1 week, drug should be permanently discontinued. However, if all findings relevant to peripheral neuropathy have resolved to minor symptoms, the drug may be reintroduced at 0.375 mg P.O. q 8 hours.
- If zalcitabine is discontinued because of toxicity, the patient should resume the recommended dose for zidovudine monotherapy (100 mg q 4 hours).
- Administering the drug with food decreases the rate and extent of absorption.
- Women of childbearing age should use an effective contraceptive while taking this drug.
- Make sure patient understands that drug doesn't cure HIV infection and that opportunistic infections may still occur despite continued use. Review safe sex practices with patient.
- Inform patient that peripheral neuropathy is the major toxicity associated with use of this drug and that pancreatitis is the major life-threatening toxicity. Review the signs and symptoms of these adverse reactions and instruct patient to call promptly if any appear.

zidovudine (azidothymidine, AZT)

Retrovir

Pregnancy Risk Category: C

HOW SUPPLIED

Capsules: 100 mg
Syrup: 50 mg/5 ml
Injection: 20 mg/ml

MECHANISM OF ACTION

Prevents replication of the human immunodeficiency virus (HIV) by inhibiting the enzyme reverse transcriptase.

INDICATIONS & DOSAGE

Patients with AIDS or advanced AIDS-related complex (ARC) who have a history of Pneumocystis carinii *pneumonia or a CD4 lymphocyte count below 200 cells/mm³* –
Adults: initially, 200 mg P.O. q 4 hours around the clock for 1 month, then 100 mg P.O. q 4 hours around the clock.
Children: dosage is individualized and will vary according to treatment IND protocol. Early studies have employed doses between 0.9 and 1.4 mg/kg/hour by continuous I.V. infusion; others have used 100 mg/m² I.V. or P.O. q 6 hours.
Postexposure prophylaxis –
Adults: dosage will vary according to study protocol, but most studies use 200 mg P.O. q 4 hours around the clock for 6 to 8 weeks. Some investigators attempt to initiate therapy within 1 hour of exposure.
Asymptomatic HIV infection –
Adults: 100 mg P.O. q 4 hours while awake (500 mg daily).
Children 3 months to 12 years: 180 mg/m² P.O. q 6 hours (720 mg/m²/day) not to exceed 200 mg q 6 hours.

ADVERSE REACTIONS

Common reactions are in italics; life-threatening reactions are in bold italics.
Blood: ***severe bone marrow depression (resulting in anemia), granulocytopenia, thrombocytopenia.***
CNS: *headache,* ***malaise,*** agitation, restlessness, insomnia, confusion, anxiety.
GI: ***nausea,*** anorexia.
Skin: ***rash,*** itching.
Other: myalgia.

INTERACTIONS

Acyclovir: possible seizures, lethargy, and fatigue. Use together cautiously.
Co-trimoxazole, acetaminophen, aspirin, indomethacin: may impair hepatic metabolism of zidovudine, increasing the drug's toxicity.
Other cytotoxic drugs: additive adverse effects on the bone marrow. Avoid concomitant use.
Pentamidine, dapsone, flucytosine, amphotericin B: increased risk of nephrotoxicity and bone marrow suppression. Monitor closely.
Probenecid: may decrease the renal clearance of zidovudine. Avoid concomitant use.

NURSING CONSIDERATIONS

- Zidovudine frequently causes a low red blood cell count by suppressing the bone marrow. Advise patients that they may need blood transfusions during treatment with zidovudine.
- Frequent monitoring of blood studies (every 2 weeks) is recommended to detect anemia or granulocytopenia. Patients may require dosage reduction or temporary discontinuation of the drug.
- Remind patients that they *must* comply with the every-4-hour dosage schedule. Suggest ways to avoid missing doses, such as the use of alarm clocks.
- Warn patients not to take any other drugs for AIDS (especially from the "street") unless their doctors have approved them. Some purported AIDS "cures" may interfere with zidovudine's effectiveness.

*Liquid form contains alcohol. **May contain tartrazine.

• The drug has been shown to temporarily decrease morbidity and mortality in certain patients with AIDS or AIDS-related complex.
• The optimum duration of treatment, as well as the dosage for optimum effectiveness and minimum toxicity, is not yet known.
• Health-care workers who consider zidovudine prophylaxis following occupational exposure (after needlestick injury, for example) should understand that animal and human studies are insufficient to judge the drug's safety or efficacy. These persons should consider the potential toxicity of the drug, as well as the risk of acquiring HIV following occupational exposure. Some clinicians do not advocate such use of zidovudine.
• **I.V. use:** Dilute before administration. Remove the calculated dose from the vial; add to 5% dextrose injection to achieve a concentration that does not exceed 4 mg/ml. Infuse 1 to 2 mg/kg over 1 hour at a constant rate; give every 4 hours around-the-clock. Avoid rapid infusion or bolus injection. Adding mixture to biological or colloidal fluids (for example, blood products, protein solutions) is not recommended. After drug is diluted, the solution is physically and chemically stable for 24 hours at room temperature and for 48 hours if refrigerated at 35.6° to 46.4° F (2° to 8° C) to minimize the risk of microbial contamination. Store undiluted vials at 59° to 77° F (15° to 25° C) and protect them from light.

18

Miscellaneous anti-infectives

atovaquone
azithromycin
aztreonam
bacitracin
chloramphenicol
chloramphenicol palmitate
chloramphenicol sodium succinate
clarithryomycin
clindamycin hydrochloride
clindamycin palmitate hydrochloride
clindamycin phosphate
erythromycin base
erythromycin estolate
erythromycin ethylsuccinate
erythromycin gluceptate
erythromycin lactobionate
erythromycin stearate
imipenem/cilastatin sodium
lincomycin hydrochloride
methenamine hippurate
methenamine mandelate
methylene blue
nitrofurantoin macrocrystals
nitrofurantoin microcrystals
polymyxin B sulfate
rifabutin
spectinomycin dihydrochloride
trimethoprim
vancomycin hydrochloride

COMBINATION PRODUCTS
CYSTEX: methenamine 165 mg, salicylamide 65 mg, sodium salicylate 97 mg, and benzoic acid 32 mg.
HEXALOL: methenamine 40.8 mg, phenyl salicylate 18.1 mg, atropine sulfate 0.03 mg, hyoscyamine 0.03 mg, benzoic acid 4.5 mg, and methylene blue 5.4 mg.
MACROBID: nitrofurantoin macrocrystals 25 mg and nitrofurantoin monohydrate 75 mg.
THIACIDE: methenamine mandelate 500 mg and potassium acid phosphate 250 mg.
TRAC TABS 2X: methenamine 120 mg, methylene blue 6 mg, phenyl salicylate 30 mg, atropine sulfate 0.06 mg, hyoscyamine sulfate 0.03 mg, and benzoic acid 7.5 mg.
URISEDAMINE: methenamine mandelate 500 mg and hyoscyamine 0.15 mg.
URO-PHOSPHATE: methenamine 300 mg and sodium acid phosphate 500 mg. Sugar coated.
UROQUID-ACID: methenamine mandelate 350 mg and sodium acid phosphate 200 mg.
UROQUID-ACID NO. 2: methenamine mandelate 500 mg and sodium acid phosphate 500 mg.

atovaquone
Mepron
Pregnancy Risk Category: C

HOW SUPPLIED
Tablets: 250 mg

MECHANISM OF ACTION
Interferes with electron transport in protozoal mitochondria, resulting in inhibition of enzymes needed for the synthesis of nucleic acids and adenosine triphosphate.

INDICATIONS & DOSAGE
Mild to moderate Pneumocystis carinii *pneumonia in patients who can't tolerate co-trimoxazole –*
Adults: 750 mg P.O. t.i.d. for 21 days.

ADVERSE REACTIONS
Common reactions are in italics; life-threatening reactions are in bold italics.

*Liquid form contains alcohol. **May contain tartrazine.

CNS: *headache, insomnia,* asthenia, dizziness.
EENT: *cough.*
GI: *nausea, diarrhea, vomiting,* constipation, abdominal pain.
Skin: *rash,* pruritus.
Other: *fever,* oral monilia.

INTERACTIONS
None reported.

NURSING CONSIDERATIONS
• *Contraindicated* in patients with hypersensitivity to the drug.
• *Use cautiously* in breast-feeding women. Animal studies have shown that substantial amounts of drug are excreted in breast milk.
• Because drug is highly bound (greater than 99.9%) to plasma protein, also use cautiously with other highly protein bound drugs.
• Absorption is limited but enhanced significantly when taken with food. Instruct patient to take drug with meals.
• Drug is ineffective in treatment of bacterial, fungal, or viral pneumonia or mycobacterial disease. Because of the risk of other concurrent pulmonary infections, patients should be closely evaluated during therapy.

azithromycin
Zithromax

Pregnancy Risk Category: B

HOW SUPPLIED
Capsules: 250 mg

MECHANISM OF ACTION
A macrolide antibiotic that is a derivative of erythromycin. Binds to the 50S subunit of bacterial ribosomes, blocking protein synthesis. Bacteriostatic or bactericidal, depending on concentration.

INDICATIONS & DOSAGE
Acute bacterial exacerbations of COPD caused by Haemophilus influenzae, Moraxella (Branhamella) catarrhalis, *or* Streptococcus pneumoniae; *mild community-acquired pneumonia caused by* H. influenzae *or* S. pneumoniae; *uncomplicated skin and skin structure infections caused by* Staphylococcus aureus, Streptococcus pyogenes, *or* S. agalactiae; *second-line therapy of pharyngitis or tonsillitis caused by* S. pyogenes –
Adults and adolescents 16 years and over: initially, 500 mg P.O. as a single dose on day 1, followed by 250 mg daily on days 2 through 5. Total dose is 1.5 g.
Nongonococcal urethritis or cervicitis caused by Chlamydia trachomatis –
Adults and adolescents 16 years and over: 1 g P.O. as a single dose.

ADVERSE REACTIONS
Common reactions are in italics; life-threatening reactions are in bold italics.
CNS: dizziness, vertigo, headache, fatigue, somnolence.
CV: palpitations, chest pain.
GI: *nausea, vomiting, diarrhea, abdominal pain,* dyspepsia, flatulence, melena, cholestatic jaundice.
GU: monilia, vaginitis, nephritis.
Skin: rash, photosensitivity.
Other: angioedema, pseudomembranous colitis.

INTERACTIONS
Aluminum- and magnesium-containing antacids: lower peak plasma levels of azithromycin. Separate administration times by at least 2 hours.
Theophylline: other macrolides may increase plasma theophylline levels; effect of azithromycin is unknown. Monitor theophylline levels carefully.
Warfarin: other macrolides may increase prothrombin time (PT); effect of azithromycin is unknown. Monitor PT carefully.

NURSING CONSIDERATIONS

• *Contraindicated* in patients with hypersensitivity to erythromycin or other macrolides. Do not use azithromycin to treat gonorrhea or syphilis; moderate-to-severe pneumonia in patients for whom outpatient oral therapy is inappropriate; nosocomial infections; known or suspected bacteremia; conditions requiring hospitalization; elderly or debilitated patients; or immunocompromised patients (for example, those with cancer or AIDS).
• *Use cautiously* in patients with impaired hepatic function.
• Obtain culture and sensitivity tests before first dose. Therapy can begin before results are obtained.
• Administer 1 hour before or 2 hours after a meal, and do not administer with antacids. Remind patient that the drug should always be taken on an empty stomach because food or antacids will decrease absorption.
• May cause overgrowth of nonsusceptible bacteria or fungi. Monitor for signs and symptoms of superinfection.
• Tell patient to take all of the medication prescribed, even after he feels better.

aztreonam

Azactam

Pregnancy Risk Category: B

HOW SUPPLIED

Injection: 500-mg, 1-g, 2-g vials

MECHANISM OF ACTION

Inhibits bacterial cell wall synthesis, ultimately causing cell wall destruction. Bactericidal.

INDICATIONS & DOSAGE

Treatment of urinary tract infections, lower respiratory tract infections, septicemia, skin and skin structure infections, intra-abdominal infections, surgical infections, and gynecologic infections caused by various aerobic organisms –

Adults: 500 mg to 2 g I.V. or I.M. q 8 to 12 hours. For severe systemic or life-threatening infections, 2 g q 6 to 8 hours may be given. Maximum dosage is 8 g daily.

ADVERSE REACTIONS

Common reactions are in italics; life-threatening reactions are in bold italics.

Blood: neutropenia, anemia.
CNS: seizures, headache, insomnia.
CV: hypotension.
GI: diarrhea, nausea, vomiting.
Hepatic: transient elevations of AST (SGOT) and ALT (SGPT).
Local: thrombophlebitis at I.V. site, discomfort and swelling at I.M. injection site.
Other: hypersensitivity, ***anaphylaxis,*** altered taste, halitosis, rash.

INTERACTIONS

Furosemide, probenecid: increased serum aztreonam levels. Avoid concomitant use.

NURSING CONSIDERATIONS

• *Use cautiously* in elderly patients and in impaired renal function.
• Aztreonam is a narrow-spectrum antibiotic, effective solely against gram-negative organisms. Because it is ineffective against gram-positive and anaerobic organisms, aztreonam must be used with other antibiotics for immediate treatment of life-threatening illnesses.
• Patients who are allergic to penicillins or cephalosporins may not be allergic to aztreonam since there is no cross-allergenicity. However, close monitoring of patients who have had an immediate hypersensitivity reaction to these antibiotics is recommended.
• **I.V. use:** To administer a bolus of aztreonam, inject drug slowly (over 3 to 5 minutes) directly into a vein or

I.V. tubing. Give infusions over 20 minutes to 1 hour.
- I.M. injections should be given deep into a large muscle mass, such as the upper outer quadrant of the gluteus maximus or the lateral part of the thigh. Doses greater than 1 g should be given I.V.
- Obtain specimen for culture and sensitivity tests before first dose. Therapy may begin pending test results.
- Watch for superinfection (fever or other signs of new infection).
- Aztreonam is the first commercially available member of a new antibiotic family, the monobactams. Its effectiveness against gram-negative organisms is comparable to that of the aminoglycoside antibiotics, without the ototoxicity or nephrotoxicity usually associated with the aminoglycosides.

bacitracin

Pregnancy Risk Category: C

HOW SUPPLIED
Injection: 10,000-unit, 50,000-unit vials

MECHANISM OF ACTION
Hinders bacterial cell wall synthesis, damaging the bacterial plasma membrane and making the cell more vulnerable to osmotic pressure.

INDICATIONS & DOSAGE
Pneumonia or empyema caused by susceptible staphylococci –
Infants over 2.5 kg: 1,000 units/kg I.M. daily, divided q 8 to 12 hours.
Infants under 2.5 kg: 900 units/kg I.M. daily, divided q 8 to 12 hours.

Although the FDA approves the use of bacitracin in infants only, adults with susceptible staphylococcal infections may receive 10,000 to 25,000 units I.M. q 6 hours (maximum 25,000 units/dose, 100,000 units daily).

ADVERSE REACTIONS
Common reactions are in italics; life-threatening reactions are in bold italics.
Blood: blood dyscrasia, eosinophilia.
EENT: ototoxicity.
GI: nausea, vomiting, anorexia, diarrhea, rectal itching or burning.
GU: ***nephrotoxicity*** *(albuminuria,* cylindruria, oliguria, anuria, increased BUN, ***tubular and glomerular necrosis****)*.
Skin: urticaria, rash.
Local: *pain at injection site.*
Other: superinfection, fever, ***anaphylaxis, neuromuscular blockade.***

INTERACTIONS
Nephrotoxic drugs (such as aminoglycosides): increased nephrotoxicity. Use together cautiously.
Neuromuscular blockers, inhalational anesthetics: prolonged muscle weakness. Monitor patient for excessive muscle weakness or respiratory distress.

NURSING CONSIDERATIONS
- *Contraindicated* in impaired renal function. *Use cautiously* in myasthenia gravis and neuromuscular disease.
- Obtain specimen for culture and sensitivity tests before first dose. Therapy may begin pending test results.
- For I.M. administration only. Give deep I.M.; injection may be painful.
- Maintain adequate fluid intake, and monitor urine output closely. If intake or output decreases, notify the doctor.
- Obtain baseline renal function studies before starting therapy. Monitor daily during therapy. Notify doctor of any change.
- Concentration of bacitracin should be between 5,000 and 10,000 units/ml. Store in refrigerator. Drug is inactivated if stored at room temperature.
- Report adverse effects to the doctor immediately.
- May be used with neomycin as a

bowel preparation, or in solution as a wound irrigating agent.
• Urine pH should be kept above 6.0 to reduce the risk of nephrotoxicity.
• Prolonged therapy may result in overgrowth of nonsusceptible organisms, especially *Candida albicans.*
• Don't administer by I.V. route; drug is irritating to vein and predisposes patient to severe thrombophlebitis.

chloramphenicol
Chloromycetin, Novochlorocap†

chloramphenicol palmitate
Chloromycetin Palmitate

chloramphenicol sodium succinate
Chloromycetin Sodium Succinate, Pentamycetin†

Pregnancy Risk Category: C

HOW SUPPLIED
chloramphenicol
Capsules: 250 mg, 500 mg
chloramphenicol palmitate
Oral suspension: 150 mg/5 ml
chloramphenicol sodium succinate
Injection: 1-g, 10-g vials

MECHANISM OF ACTION
Inhibits bacterial protein synthesis by binding to the 50S subunit of the ribosome (bacteriostatic).

INDICATIONS & DOSAGE
Haemophilus influenzae *meningitis, acute* Salmonella typhi *infection, and meningitis, bacteremia, or other severe infections caused by sensitive* Salmonella *species,* Rickettsia, *lymphogranuloma, psittacosis, or various sensitive gram-negative organisms –* **Adults and children:** 50 to 100 mg/kg P.O. or I.V. daily, divided q 6 hours. Maximum dosage is 100 mg/kg daily.
Premature infants and neonates 2 weeks or younger: 25 mg/kg P.O. or I.V. once daily. I.V. route must be used to treat meningitis.

ADVERSE REACTIONS
Common reactions are in italics; life-threatening reactions are in bold italics.
Blood: ***aplastic anemia,*** hypoplastic anemia, *granulocytopenia,* thrombocytopenia.
CNS: headache, mild depression, confusion, delirium, peripheral neuropathy with prolonged therapy.
EENT: optic neuritis (in patients with cystic fibrosis), glossitis, decreased visual acuity.
GI: nausea, vomiting, stomatitis, diarrhea, enterocolitis.
Other: infections from nonsusceptible organisms, hypersensitivity reaction (fever, rash, urticaria, ***anaphylaxis***), jaundice, ***gray syndrome in neonates, (abdominal distention, gray cyanosis, vasomotor collapse, respiratory distress, death within a few hours of onset of symptoms).***

INTERACTIONS
Acetaminophen: elevates chloramphenicol levels. Monitor for chloramphenicol toxicity.
Chlorpropamide, dicumarol, phenobarbital, phenytoin, tolbutamide: blood levels of these agents may be increased by chloramphenicol. Monitor for toxicity.
Iron supplements, vitamin B_{12}, folic acid: chloramphenicol may delay the response to these drugs in patients with anemia. Monitor closely.

NURSING CONSIDERATIONS
• *Contraindicated* in patients with hypersensitivity to the drug.
• *Use cautiously* in patients with impaired hepatic or renal function, acute intermittent porphyria, and G6PD deficiency and with other drugs causing bone marrow depression or blood disorders. *Don't use for infections caused by organisms susceptible to other agents or for trivial infections; use*

*Liquid form contains alcohol. **May contain tartrazine.

only when clearly indicated for severe infection.
- Obtain specimen for culture and sensitivity tests before first dose. Therapy may begin pending test results.
- Monitor CBC, platelets, serum iron, and reticulocytes before and every 2 days during therapy. Stop drug immediately if anemia, reticulocytopenia, leukopenia, or thrombocytopenia develops.
- Instruct patient to report adverse reactions to the doctor, especially nausea, vomiting, diarrhea, fever, confusion, sore throat, or mouth sores.
- Tell patient to take medication for as long as prescribed, exactly as directed, even after he feels better.
- **I.V. use:** Give I.V. slowly over at least 1 minute. Check injection site daily for phlebitis and irritation.
- Reconstitute 1-g vial of powder for injection with 10 ml sterile water for injection. Concentration will be 100 mg/ml. Stable for 30 days at room temperature, but refrigeration recommended. Do not use cloudy solutions.
- Monitor for evidence of superinfection by nonsusceptible organisms.
- Therapeutic plasma concentrations are 5 to 25 mcg/ml.

clarithromycin

Biaxin Filmtabs

Pregnancy Risk Category: C

HOW SUPPLIED
Tablets: 250 mg, 500 mg

MECHANISM OF ACTION
A macrolide antibiotic that is a derivative of erythromycin. Binds to the 50S subunit of bacterial ribosomes, blocking protein synthesis. Bacteriostatic or bactericidal, depending on concentration.

INDICATIONS & DOSAGE
Pharyngitis or tonsillitis caused by Streptococcus pyogenes –
Adults: 250 mg P.O. q 12 hours for 10 days.
Acute maxillary sinusitis caused by S. pneumoniae –
Adults: 500 mg P.O. q 12 hours for 14 days.
Acute exacerbations of chronic bronchitis caused by Moraxella (Branhamella) catarrhalis *or* S. pneumoniae; *pneumonia caused by* S. pneumoniae *or* Mycoplasma pneumoniae –
Adults: 250 mg P.O. q 12 hours for 7 to 14 days.
Acute exacerbations of chronic bronchitis caused by Haemophilus influenzae –
Adults: 500 mg P.O. q 12 hours for 7 to 14 days.
Uncomplicated skin and skin structure infections caused by Staphylococcus aureus *or* Streptococcus pyogenes –
Adults: 250 mg P.O. q 12 hours for 7 to 14 days.

ADVERSE REACTIONS
Common reactions are in italics; life-threatening reactions are in bold italics.
CNS: headache.
GI: *diarrhea, nausea, abnormal taste,* dyspepsia, abdominal pain or discomfort.

INTERACTIONS
Carbamazepine: preliminary studies indicate that clarithromycin may increase serum levels of carbamazepine. Monitor blood levels.
Theophylline: other macrolides may increase plasma theophylline levels; effect of clarithromycin is unknown. Monitor theophylline levels carefully.
Warfarin: other macrolides may increase prothrombin time (PT); effect of clarithromycin is unknown. Monitor PT carefully.

NURSING CONSIDERATIONS

- *Contraindicated* in patients with hypersensitivity to erythromycin or other macrolides.
- *Use cautiously* in patients with hepatic or renal impairment.
- Obtain specimen for culture and sensitivity tests before first dose. Therapy may begin pending test results.
- Drug may be taken without regard to meals.
- May cause overgrowth of nonsusceptible bacteria or fungi. Monitor for signs and symptoms of superinfection.
- Tell patient to take all of the medication prescribed, even after he feels better.

---

clindamycin hydrochloride
Cleocin HCl, Dalacin C†‡

clindamycin palmitate hydrochloride
Cleocin Pediatric, Dalacin C Palmitate†‡

clindamycin phosphate
Cleocin Phosphate, Dalacin C†‡, Dalacin C Phosphate

Pregnancy Risk Category: B

HOW SUPPLIED

hydrochloride
Capsules: 75 mg, 150 mg, 300 mg
palmitate hydrochloride
Oral solution: 75 mg/5 ml
phosphate
Injection: 150 mg/ml

MECHANISM OF ACTION

Inhibits bacterial protein synthesis by binding to the 50S subunit of the ribosome.

INDICATIONS & DOSAGE

Infections caused by sensitive staphylococci, streptococci, pneumococci, Bacteroides, Fusobacterium, Clostridium perfringens, *and other sensitive aerobic and anaerobic organisms –*
Adults: 150 to 450 mg P.O. q 6 hours; or 300 mg I.M. or I.V. q 6, 8, or 12 hours. Up to 2,700 mg I.M. or I.V. daily, divided q 6, 8, or 12 hours.
May be used for severe infections.
Children over 1 month: 8 to 20 mg/kg P.O. daily, divided q 6 to 8 hours; or 15 to 40 mg/kg I.M. or I.V. daily, divided q 6 hours.

ADVERSE REACTIONS

Common reactions are in italics; life-threatening reactions are in bold italics.
Blood: transient leukopenia, eosinophilia, thrombocytopenia.
GI: *nausea,* vomiting, abdominal pain, *diarrhea,* pseudomembranous colitis, esophagitis, flatulence, anorexia, *bloody or tarry stools, dysphagia.*
Hepatic: elevated AST (SGOT), alkaline phosphatase, bilirubin.
Skin: maculopapular rash, urticaria.
Local: *pain,* induration, *sterile abscess with I.M. injection;* thrombophlebitis, erythema, and pain after I.V. administration.
Other: unpleasant or bitter taste, ***anaphylaxis.***

INTERACTIONS

Erythromycin: antagonist that may block access of clindamycin to its site of action. Don't use together.
Kaolin: decreased absorption of oral clindamycin. Separate administration times.
Neuromuscular blockers: clindamycin may potentiate neuromuscular blockade. Monitor closely.

NURSING CONSIDERATIONS

- *Contraindicated* in patients with hypersensitivity to the antibiotic congener lincomycin and in patients with history of GI disease, especially colitis.
- *Use cautiously* in neonates and pa-

*Liquid form contains alcohol. **May contain tartrazine.

tients with renal or hepatic disease, asthma, or significant allergies.
• Monitor renal, hepatic, and hematopoietic functions during prolonged therapy.
• Obtain specimen for culture and sensitivity tests before first dose. Therapy may begin pending test results.
• Don't use in meningitis. Drug does not penetrate blood/brain barrier.
• Don't refrigerate reconstituted oral solution, as it will thicken. Drug is stable for 2 weeks at room temperature.
• Instruct patient to report adverse reactions to the doctor, especially diarrhea. Warn patient not to treat such diarrhea himself.
• Advise patients taking the capsule form to take with a full glass of water to prevent dysphagia.
• Don't give diphenoxylate compound (Lomotil) to treat drug-induced diarrhea. May prolong and worsen diarrhea.
• Give deep I.M. Rotate sites. Warn that I.M. injection may be painful. Doses greater than 600 mg per injection are not recommended.
• **I.V. use:** When giving I.V., check site daily for phlebitis and irritation. For I.V. infusion, dilute each 300 mg in 50 ml solution, and give no faster than 30 mg/minute (over 10 to 60 minutes). Never give undiluted as a bolus.
• Watch for superinfection (fever or other signs of new infection).
• I.M. injection may cause creatinine phospokinase level to rise due to muscle irritation.

erythromycin base
Apo-Erythro base†, EMU-V‡, E-Mycin, Eryc, Eryc Sprinkle, Ery-Tab, Erythromid†, Novorythro†, PCE Disperstabs, Robimycin

erythromycin estolate
Ilosone, Novorythro†

erythromycin ethylsuccinate
Apo-Erythro-ES†, E.E.S., EryPed, Erythrocin, Pediamycin

erythromycin gluceptate
Ilotycin

erythromycin lactobionate
Erythrocin

erythromycin stearate
Apo-Erythro-S†, Erythrocin, Novorythro†, Wyamycin S

Pregnancy Risk Category: B

HOW SUPPLIED
base
Tablets (enteric-coated): 250 mg, 333 mg, 500 mg
Capsules (enteric-coated pellets): 250 mg
estolate
Tablets: 500 mg
Capsules: 250 mg
Oral suspension: 125 mg/5 ml, 250 mg/5 ml
ethylsuccinate
Tablets (chewable): 200 mg
Oral suspension: 200 mg/5 ml, 400 mg/5 ml, 100 mg/2.5 ml
gluceptate
Injection: 1-g vials
lactobionate
Injection: 500-mg, 1-g vials
stearate
Tablets (film-coated): 250 mg, 500 mg

MECHANISM OF ACTION
Inhibits bacterial protein synthesis by binding to the 50S subunit of the ribosome.

INDICATIONS & DOSAGE
Acute pelvic inflammatory disease caused by Neisseria gonorrhoeae – **Women:** 500 mg I.V. (erythromycin gluceptate, lactobionate) q 6 hours for

3 days, then 250 mg (erythromycin base, estolate, stearate) or 400 mg (erythromycin ethylsuccinate) P.O. q 6 hours for 7 days.
Endocarditis prophylaxis for dental procedures in patients allergic to penicillin –
Adults: 1 g (base, estolate, stearate) or 800 to 1,600 mg (ethylsuccinate) P.O. 1 hour before procedure, then 500 mg (base, estolate, stearate) or 400 to 800 mg (ethylsuccinate) P.O. 6 hours later.
Intestinal amebiasis –
Adults: 250 mg (base, estolate, stearate) or 400 mg (ethylsuccinate) P.O. q 6 hours for 10 to 14 days.
Children: 30 to 50 mg/kg (base, estolate, ethylsuccinate, stearate) P.O. daily, divided q 6 hours for 10 to 14 days.
Mild-to-moderately severe respiratory tract, skin, and soft-tissue infections caused by sensitive group A beta-hemolytic streptococci, Diplococcus pneumoniae, Mycoplasma pneumoniae, Corynebacterium diphtheriae, Bordetella pertussis, Listeria monocytogenes –
Adults: 250 to 500 mg (erythromycin base, estolate, stearate) P.O. q 6 hours; or 400 to 800 mg (erythromycin ethylsuccinate) P.O. q 6 hours; or 15 to 20 mg/kg I.V. daily, as continuous infusion or divided q 6 hours.
Children: 30 mg/kg to 50 mg/kg (oral erythromycin salts) P.O. daily, divided q 6 hours; or 15 to 20 mg/kg I.V. daily, divided q 4 to 6 hours.
Syphilis –
Adults: 500 mg (erythromycin base, estolate, stearate) P.O. q.i.d. for 15 days.
Legionnaire's disease –
Adults: 500 mg to 1 g I.V. or P.O. (base, estolate, stearate) or 800 to 1,600 mg (ethylsuccinate) q 6 hours for 21 days.
Uncomplicated urethral, endocervical, or rectal infections where tetracyclines are contraindicated –
Adults: 500 mg (base, estolate, stearate) or 800 mg (ethylsuccinate) P.O. q.i.d. for at least 7 days.
Urogenital Chlamydia trachomatis *infections during pregnancy –*
Adults: 500 mg (base, estolate, stearate) P.O. q.i.d. for at least 7 days or 250 mg (base, estolate, stearate) or 400 mg (ethylsuccinate) P.O. q.i.d. for at least 14 days.
Conjunctivitis caused by Chlamydia trachomatis *in newborns –*
Newborns: 50 mg/kg P.O. daily in four divided doses for at least 2 weeks.
Pneumonia of infancy due to Chlamydia trachomatis –
Infants: 50 mg/kg/day in four divided doses for at least 3 weeks.

ADVERSE REACTIONS

Common reactions are in italics; life-threatening reactions are in bold italics.
EENT: hearing loss with high I.V. doses.
GI: *abdominal pain and cramping, nausea, vomiting, diarrhea.*
Hepatic: cholestatic jaundice (with erythromycin estolate).
Skin: urticaria, rashes.
Local: *venous irritation, thrombophlebitis following I.V. injection.*
Other: overgrowth of nonsusceptible bacteria or fungi; ***anaphylaxis;*** fever.

INTERACTIONS

Carbamazepine: increased carbamazepine blood levels and increased risk of toxicity. Monitor closely.
Clindamycin, lincomycin: may be antagonistic. Don't use together.
Oral anticoagulants: increased anticoagulant effects. Monitor prothrombin times closely.
Theophylline: decreased erythromycin blood level and increased theophylline toxicity. Use together cautiously.

NURSING CONSIDERATIONS

- Erythromycin estolate is *contraindicated* in hepatic disease. *Use* other

*Liquid form contains alcohol. **May contain tartrazine.

erythromycin salts *cautiously* in impaired hepatic function.

- Obtain specimen for culture and sensitivity tests before first dose. Therapy may begin pending test results.
- For best absorption, instruct patient to take oral form of drug with a full glass of water 1 hour before or 2 hours after meals. If tablets are coated, they may be taken with meals. Tell patient not to drink fruit juice with medication. Chewable erythromycin tablets should not be swallowed whole.
- Coated forms of erythromycin are associated with lower incidence of GI problems. May be more tolerable in patients who cannot easily tolerate erythromycin.
- When administering suspension, be sure to note the concentration.
- May cause overgrowth of nonsusceptible bacteria or fungi. Monitor for signs and symptoms of superinfection.
- Tell patient to take medication for as long as prescribed, exactly as directed, even after he feels better, and to take entire amount prescribed. Treat streptococcal infections for 10 days.
- Report adverse reactions, especially nausea, abdominal pain, and fever.
- Erythromycin estolate may cause serious hepatotoxicity in adults (reversible cholestatic jaundice). Monitor hepatic function (increased levels of bilirubin, AST [SGOT], ALT [SGPT], and alkaline phosphatase may occur). Other erythromycin salts cause hepatotoxicity to a lesser degree. Patients who develop hepatotoxicity from estolate may react similarly to treatment with any erythromycin preparation.
- **I.V. use:** I.V. dose should be administered over 60 minutes. Reconstitute according to manufacturer's directions and dilute each 250 mg in at least 100 ml 0.9% normal saline solution.
- Erythromycin lactobionate should not be administered with other drugs.

imipenem/cilastatin sodium

Primaxin

Pregnancy Risk Category: C

HOW SUPPLIED

Injection: 250-mg, 500-mg, 750-mg vials

MECHANISM OF ACTION

Imipenem is bactericidal and inhibits bacterial cell wall synthesis. Cilastatin inhibits the enzymatic breakdown of imipenem in the kidney, making it effective in the urinary tract.

INDICATIONS & DOSAGE

Serious infections of the lower respiratory and urinary tracts, intra-abdominal and gynecologic infections, bacterial septicemia, bone and joint infections, skin and soft-tissue infections, and endocarditis. Most known microorganisms are susceptible: Staphylococcus, Streptococcus, Escherichia coli, Klebsiella, Proteus, Enterobacter, Pseudomonas aeruginosa, *and* Bacteroides, *including* B. fragilis – **Adults:** 250 mg to 1 g by I.V. infusion q 6 to 8 hours. Maximum daily dosage is 50 mg/kg/day or 4 g/day, whichever is less.

ADVERSE REACTIONS

Common reactions are in italics; life-threatening reactions are in bold italics.

CNS: *seizures,* dizziness.

CV: hypotension.

GI: nausea, vomiting, diarrhea, *pseudomembranous colitis.*

Skin: rash, urticaria, pruritus.

Local: *thrombophlebitis, pain at injection site.*

Other: ***hypersensitivity.***

INTERACTIONS
Ganciclovir: risk of seizures. Avoid concomitant use.

NURSING CONSIDERATIONS
- *Use cautiously* in patients allergic to penicillins or cephalosporins because this drug is chemically similar. Ask patient if he's had a hypersensitivity reaction to either of these drugs before administering first dose of imipenem.
- *Also use cautiously* in patients who have a history of seizure disorders, especially if they also have compromised renal function. If patient develops seizures that persist despite anticonvulsant therapy, notify doctor. The drug should then be discontinued.
- **I.V. use:** Don't administer by direct I.V. bolus injection. Each 250- or 500-mg dose should be given by I.V. infusion over 20 to 30 minutes. Each 1-g dose should be infused over 40 to 60 minutes. If nausea occurs, the infusion may be slowed.
- When reconstituting powder, shake until the solution is clear. Solutions may range from colorless to yellow and variations of color within this range don't affect the drug's potency. After reconstitution, solution is stable for 10 hours at room temperature and for 48 hours when refrigerated.
- Imipenem/cilastatin has the broadest antibacterial spectrum of any available antibiotic. The drug is most valuable for empiric treatment of infections and for mixed infections that would otherwise require a combination of antibiotics, often including an aminoglycoside.
- Patients with impaired renal function may need lower dosage or longer intervals between doses.
- Obtain specimen for culture and sensitivity tests before first dose. Therapy may begin pending test results.
- Monitor patient for bacterial or fungal superinfections and resistant infections during and after therapy.

lincomycin hydrochloride
Lincocin
Pregnancy Risk Category: B

HOW SUPPLIED
Capsules: 500 mg
Pediatric capsules: 250 mg
Injection: 300 mg/ml in 2-ml and 10-ml vials and 2-ml U-Ject

MECHANISM OF ACTION
Inhibits bacterial protein synthesis by binding to the 50S subunit of the ribosome.

INDICATIONS & DOSAGE
Respiratory tract, skin and soft-tissue, and urinary tract infections; osteomyelitis, septicemia caused by sensitive group A beta-hemolytic streptococci, pneumococci, and staphylococci –
Adults: 500 mg P.O. q 6 to 8 hours (not to exceed 8 g daily); or 600 mg I.M. daily or q 12 hours; or 600 mg to 1 g I.V. q 8 to 12 hours (not to exceed 8 g daily).
Children over 1 month: 30 to 60 mg/kg P.O. daily, divided q 6 to 8 hours; or 10 mg/kg I.M. daily or divided q 12 hours; or 10 to 20 mg/kg I.V. daily, divided q 6 to 8 hours. For I.V. infusion, dilute to 100 ml; infuse over 1 hour to avoid hypotension.

ADVERSE REACTIONS
Common reactions are in italics; life-threatening reactions are in bold italics.
Blood: *neutropenia, leukopenia,* thrombocytopenia, purpura.
CNS: dizziness, headache.
CV: hypotension with rapid I.V. infusion.
EENT: glossitis, tinnitus.
GI: nausea, vomiting, ***pseudomembranous colitis,*** *persistent diarrhea,* abdominal cramps, stomatitis, pruritus ani.

*Liquid form contains alcohol. **May contain tartrazine.

GU: vaginitis.
Hepatic: cholestatic jaundice.
Skin: rashes, urticaria.
Local: pain at injection site.
Other: ***hypersensitivity,*** angioedema.

INTERACTIONS
Antidiarrheals (such as kaolin, pectin, and attapulgite): reduce oral absorption of lincomycin by as much as 90%. Antidiarrheals should be avoided or given at least 2 hours before lincomycin.
Neuromuscular blockers: lincomycin may potentiate neuromuscular blockade.

NURSING CONSIDERATIONS
• *Contraindicated* in patients with hypersensitivity to clindamycin.
• *Use cautiously* in GI disorders (especially colitis), asthma or significant allergies, hepatic or renal disease, and endocrine or metabolic disorders.
• Obtain specimen for culture and sensitivity tests before first dose. Therapy may begin pending test results.
• For best absorption, instruct patient to take drug with a full glass of water 1 hour before or 2 hours after meals.
• Tell patient to take medication exactly as directed, even after he feels better, and to take entire amount prescribed.
• Tell patient to report adverse reactions to doctor, especially diarrhea. Warn him not to treat diarrhea himself because it may reflect the onset of antibiotic associated pseudomembraneous colitis.
• Monitor for signs of bacterial and fungal superinfection, especially when therapy exceeds 10 days.
• Give deep I.M. Rotate sites. Warn that I.M. injection may be painful.
• **I.V. use:** When giving I.V., check site daily for phlebitis and irritation. Rotate infusion sites regularly.
• Rapid I.V. infusion may cause hypotension and syncope. Monitor blood pressure in patients receiving the drug parenterally.
• Monitor hepatic function (increased levels of alkaline phosphatase, AST [SGOT], ALT [SGPT], bilirubin may occur).
• Monitor CBC and platelets. Stop drug immediately if neutropenia, leukopenia, or other blood disorders develop.

methenamine hippurate
Hiprex**, Hip-Rex†, Urex

methenamine mandelate
Mandameth, Mandelamine, Sterine†

Pregnancy Risk Category: C

HOW SUPPLIED
hippurate
Tablets: 1 g
mandelate
Tablets: 500 mg, 1 g
Tablets (enteric-coated): 250 mg, 500 mg, 1 g
Tablets (film-coated): 500 mg, 1 g
Oral suspension: 250 mg/5 ml, 500 mg/5 ml
Granules: 500 mg, 1 g

MECHANISM OF ACTION
In acid urine, methenamines are hydrolyzed to ammonia and to formaldehyde, which is responsible for antibacterial action against gram-positive and gram-negative organisms. Mandelic and hippuric acids, with which methenamines are combined, are also antibacterial by unknown mechanisms.

INDICATIONS & DOSAGE
Long-term prophylaxis or suppression of chronic urinary tract infections –
Adults and children over 12 years: 1 g (hippurate) P.O. q 12 hours.
Children 6 to 12 years: 500 mg to 1 g (hippurate) P.O. q 12 hours.
Urinary tract infections, infected re-

sidual urine in patients with neurogenic bladder –
Adults: 1 g (mandelate) P.O. q.i.d. after meals.
Children 6 to 12 years: 500 mg (mandelate) P.O. q.i.d. after meals.
Children under 6 years: 50 mg/kg (mandelate) P.O. divided in four doses after meals.

ADVERSE REACTIONS
Common reactions are in italics; life-threatening reactions are in bold italics.
GI: nausea, vomiting, diarrhea.
GU: with high doses, urinary tract irritation, dysuria, frequency, albuminuria, hematuria.
Hepatic: elevated liver enzymes.
Skin: rashes.

INTERACTIONS
Acetazolamide: antagonizes methenamine effect. Use together cautiously.
Urine alkalinizing agents: inhibit methenamine action. Don't use together.

NURSING CONSIDERATIONS
• *Contraindicated* in renal insufficiency, severe hepatic disease, or severe dehydration.
• Ineffective against *Candida* infection.
• Oral suspension contains vegetable oil. Administer cautiously to elderly or debilitated patients, because aspiration could cause lipid pneumonia.
• Monitor intake and output. Intake should be at least 1,500 to 2,000 ml daily.
• Obtain a clean-catch urine specimen for culture and sensitivity tests before starting therapy, and repeat p.r.n. Therapy may begin pending test results.
• Limit intake of alkaline foods, such as vegetables, milk, and peanuts. May drink cranberry, plum, and prune juices. These juices or ascorbic acid may be used to acidify urine.
• Warn patient not to take antacids, including Alka-Seltzer and sodium bicarbonate.
• For best results, maintain urine pH at 5.5 or below. Use Nitrazine paper to check pH. Large doses of ascorbic acid (12 g/day) may be necessary to effectively acidify urine.
• *Proteus* and *Pseudomonas* tend to raise urine pH; urine acidifiers are usually necessary when treating these infections.
• Obtain liver function studies periodically during long-term therapy.
• Administer after meals to minimize GI upset.
• If rash appears, withhold dose and contact doctor.

methylene blue
Urolene Blue
Pregnancy Risk Category: C (D if injected intra-amniotically)

HOW SUPPLIED
Tablets: 55 mg, 65 mg
Injection: 10 mg/ml

MECHANISM OF ACTION
Methylene blue is a mildly antiseptic dye. High concentrations convert the ferrous iron of reduced hemoglobin to ferric iron to form methemoglobin. This mechanism is the basis for its use as an antidote in cyanide poisoning. Low concentrations of methylene blue can hasten conversion of methemoglobin to hemoglobin.

INDICATIONS & DOSAGE
Cystitis, urethritis –
Adults: 55 to 130 mg P.O. b.i.d. or t.i.d. after meals with glass of water.
Methemoglobinemia and cyanide poisoning –
Adults and children: 1 to 2 mg/kg of 1% sterile solution slow I.V.

ADVERSE REACTIONS
Common reactions are in italics; life-threatening reactions are in bold italics.

Blood: anemia (long-term use).
GI: nausea, vomiting, diarrhea, blue-green stool.
GU: dysuria, bladder irritation, blue-green urine.
Other: fever (large doses).

INTERACTIONS
None significant.

NURSING CONSIDERATIONS
- *Contraindicated* in renal insufficiency.
- Monitor intake and output carefully. Intake should be at least 2,000 ml daily.
- Monitor hemoglobin; possibility of anemia from accelerated destruction of erythrocytes.
- Turns urine and stool blue-green.
- Seldom used as urinary tract antiseptic.
- **I.V. use:** Use caution when handling injectable form, since the liquid can stain the skin. Avoid extravasation.
- I.V. form has been used to treat nitrite intoxication.
- S.C. injection can cause necrotic abscess formation.

nitrofurantoin macrocrystals
Macrodantin

nitrofurantoin microcrystals
Apo-Nitrofurantoin†, Furadantin, Furalan, Furan, Furanite, Macrodantin, Nephronex†, Nitrofan, Novofuran†

Pregnancy Risk Category: B

HOW SUPPLIED
macrocrystals
Capsules: 25 mg, 50 mg, 100 mg
microcrystals
Tablets: 50 mg, 100 mg
Capsules: 50 mg, 100 mg
Oral suspension: 25 mg/5 ml

MECHANISM OF ACTION
Bacteriostatic in low concentration and possibly bactericidal in high concentration. Interferes with bacterial enzyme systems and possibly with bacterial cell wall formation.

INDICATIONS & DOSAGE
Pyelonephritis, pyelitis, and cystitis due to susceptible Escherichia coli, Staphylococcus aureus, *enterococci; certain strains of* Klebsiella, Proteus, *and* Enterobacter –
Adults and children over 12 years: 50 to 100 mg P.O. q.i.d. with milk or meals.
Children 1 month to 12 years: 5 to 7 mg/kg P.O. daily, divided q.i.d.
Long-term suppression therapy –
Adults: 50 to 100 mg P.O. daily at bedtime.
Children: 1 to 2 mg/kg P.O. daily at bedtime.

ADVERSE REACTIONS
Common reactions are in italics; life-threatening reactions are in bold italics.
Blood: ***hemolysis in patients with G6PD deficiency*** (reversed after stopping drug), ***agranulocytosis,*** thrombocytopenia.
CNS: peripheral neuropathy, headache, dizziness, drowsiness, *ascending polyneuropathy with high doses or renal impairment.*
GI: *anorexia, nausea, vomiting,* abdominal pain, *diarrhea.*
Hepatic: hepatitis.
Skin: maculopapular, erythematous, or eczematous eruption; pruritus; urticaria; ***exfoliative dermatitis; Stevens-Johnson syndrome.***
Other: ***asthmatic attacks in patients with history of asthma; anaphylaxis;*** hypersensitivity; transient alopecia; drug fever; overgrowth of nonsusceptible organisms in the urinary tract; ***pulmonary sensitivity reactions*** *(cough, chest pains, fever, chills, dyspnea).*

INTERACTIONS
Magnesium-containing antacids: decreased nitrofurantoin absorption. Separate administration times by 1 hour.
Nalidixic acid, norfloxacin: possible decreased effectiveness. Avoid using together.
Probenecid, sulfinpyrazone: increased blood levels and decreased urine levels. May result in increased toxicity and lack of therapeutic effect. Don't use together.

NURSING CONSIDERATIONS
• *Contraindicated* in children 1 month and under and in moderate to severe renal impairment, anuria, oliguria, or creatinine clearance under 40 ml/minute.
• *Use cautiously* in G6PD deficiency.
• Hypersensitivity may develop when used for long-term therapy.
• Obtain specimen for culture and sensitivity tests before starting therapy and repeat p.r.n. Therapy may begin pending test results.
• Monitor CBC regularly.
• Give with food or milk to minimize GI distress.
• Some patients may experience fewer GI adverse effects with nitrofurantoin macrocrystals.
• Monitor intake and output carefully. May turn urine brown or darker.
• Store in amber container. Keep away from metals other than stainless steel or aluminum to avoid precipitate formation. Warn patients not to use pillboxes made of these materials.
• Continue treatment for 3 days after sterile urine specimens have been obtained.
• Monitor pulmonary status.
• Has no effect in blood or tissue outside the urinary tract.
• Monitor for superinfection. Use of nitrofurantoin may result in growth of nonsusceptible organisms, especially *Pseudomonas.*
• May cause false-positive results with urine sugar test using copper sulfate reduction method (Clinitest) but not with glucose oxidase tests (Tes-Tape, Diastix, Clinistix).

polymyxin B sulfate
Aerosporin

Pregnancy Risk Category: B

HOW SUPPLIED
Powder for injection: 500,000-unit vials

MECHANISM OF ACTION
Hinders bacterial cell wall synthesis, damaging the bacterial plasma membrane and making the cell more vulnerable to osmotic pressure (bactericidal).

INDICATIONS & DOSAGE
Acute urinary tract infections or septicemia caused by sensitive Pseudomonas aeruginosa, *or when other antibiotics are ineffective or contraindicated; bacteremia caused by sensitive* Enterobacter aerogenes *and* Klebsiella pneumoniae, *or acute urinary tract infections caused by* Escherichia coli –
Adults and children: 15,000 to 25,000 units/kg daily I.V. infusion, divided q 12 hours; or 25,000 to 30,000 units/kg daily, divided q 4 to 8 hours. I.M. not advised due to severe pain at injection site.
Meningitis caused by sensitive P. aeruginosa *or* Haemophilus influenzae *when other antibiotics ineffective or contraindicated* –
Adults and children over 2 years: 50,000 units intrathecally once daily for 3 to 4 days, then 50,000 units every other day for at least 2 weeks after cerebrospinal fluid tests are negative and cerebrospinal fluid sugar is normal.
Children under 2 years: 20,000 units intrathecally once daily for 3 to 4 days, then 25,000 units every other

*Liquid form contains alcohol. **May contain tartrazine.

day for at least 2 weeks after cerebrospinal fluid tests are negative and cerebrospinal fluid sugar is normal.

ADVERSE REACTIONS

Common reactions are in italics; life-threatening reactions are in bold italics.

CNS: irritability, drowsiness, facial flushing, weakness, ataxia, respiratory paralysis, headache and meningeal irritation with intrathecal administration, peripheral and perioral paresthesias, ***seizures, coma.***

EENT: blurred vision.

GU: *nephrotoxicity* (albuminuria, cylindruria, hematuria, proteinuria, decreased urine output, increased BUN level).

Skin: urticaria.

Local: *pain at I.M. injection site.*

Other: hypersensitivity reactions with fever, ***anaphylaxis.***

INTERACTIONS

• *Aminoglycosides, amphotericin B, cisplatin, vancomycin, zidovudine:* increased risk of nephrotoxicity. Avoid concomitant use.

• *Neuromuscular blockers:* polymyxin B may potentiate neuromuscular blockade. Monitor closely.

NURSING CONSIDERATIONS

• *Use cautiously* in impaired renal function or myasthenia gravis.

• Give only to hospitalized patients under constant medical supervision.

• For meningitis, must give intrathecally to achieve adequate cerebrospinal fluid levels.

• Give deep I.M. Warn that injection may be painful.

• Don't give solution containing local anesthetics I.V. or intrathecally.

• **I.V. use:** When giving I.V., check site daily for phlebitis and irritation. Dilute each 500,000 units in 300 to 500 ml dextrose 5% in water; infuse over 60 to 90 minutes. Rotate I.V. sites regularly.

• Parenteral solutions should be refrigerated and used within 72 hours.

• Monitor renal function (BUN, serum creatinine, creatinine clearance, urine output) before and during therapy. Intake should be sufficient to maintain output at 1,500 ml/day (between 3,000 and 4,000 ml/day for adults).

• Obtain specimen for culture and sensitivity tests before first dose. Therapy may begin pending test results.

• Notify doctor immediately if patient develops fever, CNS adverse effects, rash, or symptoms of nephrotoxicity.

• If patient is scheduled for surgery, notify anesthesiologist of preoperative treatment with this drug since it may prolong neuromuscular blockade.

rifabutin

Mycobutin

Pregnancy Risk Category: B

HOW SUPPLIED

Capsules: 150 mg

MECHANISM OF ACTION

Inhibits DNA-dependent RNA polymerase in susceptible bacteria, blocking bacterial protein synthesis.

INDICATIONS & DOSAGE

Prevention of disseminated Mycobacterium avium *complex (MAC) in patients with advanced HIV infection –*
Adults: 300 mg P.O. daily as a single dose or divided b.i.d.

ADVERSE REACTIONS

Common reactions are in italics; life-threatening reactions are in bold italics.

Blood: neutropenia, leukopenia, thrombocytopenia, eosinophilia.

EENT: uveitis.

GI: dyspepsia, eructation, flatulence, nausea, vomiting, abdominal pain.

GU: *discolored urine.*

Skin: *rash.*

Other: fever, myalgia, myositis, taste perversion.

INTERACTIONS

Oral contraceptives: decreased effectiveness. Instruct patient to use nonhormonal forms of birth control.

Zidovudine, drugs metabolized by the liver: rifabutin decreases serum levels of zidovudine. Because rifabutin, like rifampin, induces liver enzymes, it may lower serum levels of many other drugs as well. Although dosage adjustments may be necessary, further study is needed.

NURSING CONSIDERATIONS

- *Contraindicated* in patients with hypersensitivity to the drug or other rifamycin derivatives (such as rifampin). Also contraindicated in patients with active tuberculosis because single-agent therapy with rifabutin increases the risk of inducing bacterial resistance to both rifabutin and rifampin.
- *Use cautiously* in patients with preexisting neutropenia and thrombocytopenia. Perform baseline hematologic studies and repeat periodically.
- Although safety and effectiveness in children have not been fully established, several studies have indicated the maximum daily dose to be 5 mg/kg.
- High-fat meals slow the rate of absorption but don't change the extent. Drug may be mixed with soft foods, such as applesauce, for patients who have difficulty swallowing.
- No evidence exists that drug will provide effective prophylaxis against *M. tuberculosis.* Patients requiring prophylaxis against both *M. tuberculosis* and MAC may require rifampin and rifabutin.
- Drug may rarely cause uveitis; tell patient to report photophobia, excessive lacrimation, or eye pain immediately.
- Be sure patient understands that drug or its metabolites may discolor urine, feces, sputum, saliva, tears, and skin brownish orange. Tell him to avoid wearing soft contact lenses because they may be permanently stained.

spectinomycin dihydrochloride

Trobicin

Pregnancy Risk Category: B

HOW SUPPLIED

Injection: 2-g vial with 3.2-ml diluent; 4-g vial with 6.2-ml diluent
Powder for injection: 2 g, 4 g

MECHANISM OF ACTION

Inhibits protein synthesis by binding to the 30S subunit of the ribosome.

INDICATIONS & DOSAGE

Gonorrhea –

Adults: 2 to 4 g I.M. single dose injected deeply into the upper outer quadrant of the buttock.

ADVERSE REACTIONS

Common reactions are in italics; life-threatening reactions are in bold italics.

CNS: insomnia, dizziness.
GI: nausea.
GU: decreased urine output.
Skin: urticaria.
Local: pain at injection site.
Other: fever, chills (may mask or delay symptoms of incubating syphilis).

INTERACTIONS

None significant.

NURSING CONSIDERATIONS

- *Contraindicated* in patients with hypersensitivity to the drug.
- Not effective in the treatment of syphilis. Serologic test for syphilis should be done before treatment dose and 3 months after.
- Should be reserved for penicillin-resistant strains of gonorrhea.
- Use 20G needle to administer drug.

*Liquid form contains alcohol. **May contain tartrazine.

The 4-g dose (10 ml) should be divided into two 5-ml injections – one in each buttock.
- Shake vial vigorously after reconstitution and before withdrawing dose. Store at room temperature after reconstitution and use within 24 hours.

trimethoprim
Alprin‡, Proloprim, Trimpex, Triprim‡
Pregnancy Risk Category: C

HOW SUPPLIED
Tablets: 100 mg, 200 mg

MECHANISM OF ACTION
Interferes with the action of dihydrofolate reductase, inhibiting bacterial synthesis of folic acid.

INDICATIONS & DOSAGE
Treatment of uncomplicated urinary tract infections caused by susceptible strains of Escherichia coli, Proteus mirabilis, Klebsiella, *and* Enterobacter –
Adults: 100 mg P.O. every 12 hours for 10 days.

Not recommended for children under 12 years.

ADVERSE REACTIONS
Common reactions are in italics; life-threatening reactions are in bold italics.
Blood: thrombocytopenia, leukopenia, megaloblastic anemia, methemoglobinemia.
GI: *epigastric distress, nausea, vomiting,* glossitis.
Skin: *rash, pruritus,* ***exfoliative dermatitis.***
Other: fever.

INTERACTIONS
Phenytoin: trimethoprim may decrease phenytoin metabolism and increase serum levels of phenytoin.

NURSING CONSIDERATIONS
- *Contraindicated* in documented megaloblastic anemia due to folate deficiency.
- Clinical signs such as sore throat, fever, pallor, or purpura may be early indications of serious blood disorders. CBCs should be done routinely. Prolonged use of trimethoprim at high doses may cause bone marrow suppression.
- *Use cautiously* in patients with impaired hepatic function. Dosage should be decreased in patients with severely impaired renal function.
- Obtain specimen for culture and sensitivity tests before first dose. Therapy may begin pending test results.
- Instruct patient to continue taking the drug, even if he feels better, and to take entire amount prescribed.
- Because resistance to trimethoprim develops rapidly when it is used alone, it is usually given in combination with other drugs.

vancomycin hydrochloride
Vancocin, Vancoled
Pregnancy Risk Category: C

HOW SUPPLIED
Powder for oral solution: 1-g, 10-g bottles
Powder for injection: 500-mg, 1-g vials

MECHANISM OF ACTION
Hinders bacterial cell wall synthesis, damaging the bacterial plasma membrane and making the cell more vulnerable to osmotic pressure.

INDICATIONS & DOSAGE
Severe staphylococcal infections when other antibiotics ineffective or contraindicated –
Adults: 500 mg I.V. q 6 hours, or 1 g q 12 hours.

Children: 40 mg/kg I.V. daily, divided q 6 hours.
Neonates: 10 mg/kg I.V. daily, divided q 6 to 12 hours.
Antibiotic-associated pseudomembranous and staphylococcal enterocolitis –
Adults: 125 to 500 mg P.O. q 6 hours for 7 to 10 days.
Children: 40 mg/kg P.O. daily, divided q 6 hours. Maximum daily dosage is 2 g.
Endocarditis prophylaxis for dental procedures –
Adults: 1 g I.V. slowly over 1 hour, starting 1 hour before procedure.

ADVERSE REACTIONS

Common reactions are in italics; life-threatening reactions are in bold italics.
Blood: transient eosinophilia, leukopenia.
EENT: tinnitus, ototoxicity.
GI: nausea.
GU: nephrotoxicity.
Skin: "red-neck" syndrome with rapid I.V. infusion (maculopapular rash on face, neck, trunk, and extremities).
Local: pain or thrombophlebitis with I.V. administration, necrosis.
Other: chills, fever, ***anaphylaxis***, superinfection.

INTERACTIONS

Aminoglycosides, amphotericin B, cisplatin, pentamidine: increased risk of nephrotoxicity. Monitor closely.

NURSING CONSIDERATIONS

- *Use cautiously* in patients receiving other neurotoxic, nephrotoxic, or ototoxic drugs; in patients over 60 years, and in those with impaired hepatic or renal function, preexisting hearing loss, or allergies to other antibiotics. Patients with renal dysfunction require adjustment of dosage or dosing interval.
- Obtain specimen for culture and sensitivity tests before first dose. Therapy may begin pending results.
- Tell patient to take medication exactly as directed, even after he feels better, and to take entire amount prescribed. Treat staphylococcal endocarditis for at least 4 weeks.
- Do not give drug I.M.
- **I.V. use:** For I.V. infusion, dilute in 200 ml sodium chloride injection or 5% glucose solution and infuse over 60 minutes. Check site daily for phlebitis and irritation. Report pain at infusion site. Avoid extravasation. Severe irritation and necrosis can result.
- Refrigerate I.V. solution after reconstitution and use within 96 hours.
- Monitor patient carefully for "red-neck" syndrome. Stop infusion and report this reaction promptly.
- Patients should have hearing tests before and during prolonged therapy.
- Tell patient to stop drug immediately and report adverse reactions, especially fullness or ringing in ears.
- Monitor renal function (BUN, serum creatinine, urinalysis, creatinine clearance, and urine output) before and during therapy. Also monitor for signs of superinfection.
- Oral preparation stable for 2 weeks if refrigerated.

19

Inotropics

amrinone lactate
digitoxin
digoxin
flosequinan
milrinone lactate

COMBINATION PRODUCTS
None.

amrinone lactate
Inocor
Pregnancy Risk Category: C

HOW SUPPLIED
Injection: 5 mg/ml

MECHANISM OF ACTION
Produces inotropic action by increasing cellular levels of cyclic adenosine monophosphate. Produces vasodilation through a direct relaxant effect on vascular smooth muscle.

INDICATIONS & DOSAGE
Short-term management of CHF –
Adults: initially, 0.75 mg/kg I.V. bolus over 2 to 3 minutes. Then begin maintenance infusion of 5 to 10 mcg/kg/minute. Additional bolus of 0.75 mg/kg may be given 30 minutes after start of therapy. Total daily dosage should not exceed 10 mg/kg.

ADVERSE REACTIONS
Common reactions are in italics; life-threatening reactions are in bold italics.
Blood: *thrombocytopenia* (dose dependent).
CV: *arrhythmias,* hypotension.
GI: nausea, vomiting, cramps, dyspepsia, diarrhea.
Hepatic: elevated enzymes, rarely hepatotoxicity.
Local: burning at site of injection.
Other: hypersensitivity reactions (pericarditis, ascites, myositis vasculitis, pleuritis).

INTERACTIONS
Digitalis glycosides: Enhanced inotropic effect. Beneficial drug interaction.
Disopyramide: excessive hypotension. Don't administer concurrently.

NURSING CONSIDERATIONS
- *Contraindicated* in severe aortic or pulmonic valvular disease. Not recommended during acute phase of myocardial infarction.
- *Use cautiously* in idiopathic hypertrophic subaortic stenosis.
- Dosage should be based on clinical response, including assessment of pulmonary artery pressures and cardiac output. Cardiovascular effects begin within 2 to 5 minutes after starting infusion, and may last for 30 minutes to 2 hours after infusion is discontinued.
- Amrinone may be added to digitalis glycoside therapy in atrial fibrillation and flutter since it enhances AV conduction and increases ventricular response rate.
- Monitor blood pressure and heart rate throughout the infusion. Slow or stop infusion and notify doctor if patient's blood pressure falls.
- Monitor platelet count. Platelet count below 150,000/mm³ usually requires a decreased dosage.
- **I.V. use:** Amrinone must be administered with an infusion pump. Administer amrinone as supplied, or dilute in 0.4% or 0.9% saline solution to a concentration of 1 to 3 mg/ml. Use diluted solution within 24 hours. Don't mix other drugs into this solution.
- Don't dilute with solutions containing dextrose because a slow chemical reaction occurs over 24 hours. How-

ever, amrinone can be injected into running dextrose infusions through a Y connector or directly into the tubing.

- Furosemide will form a precipitate with amrinone solutions. Don't mix together.
- Amrinone is primarily prescribed for patients who have not responded to therapy with digitalis, diuretics, and vasodilators.
- Patients with end-stage cardiac disease may receive home treatment with an amrinone drip while awaiting a heart transplant.

digitoxin

Crystodigin

Pregnancy Risk Category: C

HOW SUPPLIED

Tablets: 0.05 mg, 0.1 mg, 0.15 mg, 0.2 mg

MECHANISM OF ACTION

Promotes movement of calcium from extracellular to intracellular cytoplasm and inhibits sodium-potassium activated adenosine triphosphatase. These actions strengthen myocardial contraction.

INDICATIONS & DOSAGE

CHF, paroxysmal supraventricular tachycardia, atrial fibrillation and flutter –

Adults: loading dose is 1.2 to 1.6 mg P.O. in divided doses over 24 hours; average maintenance dosage is 0.15 mg daily (range: 0.05 to 0.3 mg daily).

Children 2 to 12 years: loading dose is 0.03 mg/kg or 0.75 mg/m² P.O. in divided doses over 24 hours; maintenance dosage is one-tenth of loading dose or 0.003 mg/kg or 0.075 mg/m² daily. Monitor closely for toxicity.

Children 1 to 2 years: loading dose is 0.04 mg/kg P.O. over 24 hours in divided doses; maintenance dosage is 0.004 mg/kg daily. Monitor closely for toxicity.

Children 2 weeks to 1 year: loading dose is 0.045 mg/kg P.O. in divided doses over 24 hours; maintenance dosage is 0.0045 mg/kg daily. Monitor closely for toxicity.

Premature infants, neonates, severely ill older infants: loading dose is 0.022 mg/kg or 0.3 to 0.35 mg/m² P.O. in divided doses over 24 hours; maintenance dosage is 0.0022 mg/kg daily. Monitor closely for toxicity.

ADVERSE REACTIONS

Common reactions are in italics; life-threatening reactions are in bold italics.

The following are signs of toxicity that may occur with all cardiac glycosides:

CNS: *fatigue, generalized muscle weakness, agitation, hallucinations,* headache, malaise, dizziness, vertigo, stupor, paresthesia.

CV: ***increased severity of CHF, arrhythmias (most commonly conduction disturbances with or without AV block, premature ventricular contractions, and supraventricular arrhythmias),*** hypotension.

Toxic effects on heart may be life-threatening and require immediate attention.

EENT: *yellow-green halos around visual images, blurred vision,* light flashes, photophobia, diplopia.

GI: *anorexia, nausea,* vomiting, diarrhea.

INTERACTIONS

Amphotericin B, carbenicillin, ticarcillin, corticosteroids, and diuretics (including loop diuretics, chlorthalidone, metolazone, and thiazides): hypokalemia, predisposing patient to digitalis toxicity. Monitor serum potassium.

Antacids, kaolin-pectin: decreased absorption of oral digitoxin. Schedule doses as far as possible from oral digitoxin administration.

Cholestyramine, colestipol, metoclo-

pramide: decreased absorption of oral digitoxin. Monitor for decreased effect and low blood levels. Dosage may have to be increased.
Cimetidine: decreased digitoxin metabolism. Monitor for digitoxin toxicity.
Parenteral calcium, thiazides: hypercalcemia and hypomagnesemia, predisposing patient to digitalis toxicity. Monitor serum calcium and serum magnesium.
Phenylbutazone, phenobarbital, phenytoin, rifampin: faster metabolism and shorter duration of digitoxin. Observe for underdigitalization.
Quinidine, verapamil: Possible increased serum digitoxin levels. Monitor patient closely.

NURSING CONSIDERATIONS

- *Contraindicated* in presence of any digitalis-induced toxicity; ventricular fibrillation; and ventricular tachycardia unless caused by CHF. Administering calcium salts to digitalized patient is also contraindicated. Calcium affects cardiac contractility and excitability in much the same way as glycosides and may lead to serious arrhythmias in digitalized patient.
- *Use with extreme caution* in elderly patients and in acute MI, incomplete AV block, sinus bradycardia, premature ventricular contractions, chronic constrictive pericarditis, idiopathic hypertrophic subaortic stenosis, severe pulmonary disease, and hypothyroidism.
- Hypothyroid patients are very sensitive to glycosides; hyperthyroid patients may need larger doses.
- Obtain baseline data (heart rate and rhythm, blood pressure, and electrolytes) and question patient about recent use of cardiac glycosides (within the previous 2 to 3 weeks) before administering a loading dose. Always divide loading dose over first 24 hours unless clinical situation indicates otherwise.
- Dosage is adjusted to patient's clinical condition and is monitored by serum levels of cardiac glycoside, calcium, potassium, magnesium, and by ECG.
- Before giving, take apical-radial pulse for a full minute. Record and report to doctor any significant changes (sudden increase or decrease in rate, pulse deficit, irregular beats, and particularly regularization of a previously irregular rhythm). Check blood pressure and obtain 12-lead ECG with these changes.
- Excessive slowing of the pulse rate (60 beats/minute or less) may be a sign of digitalis toxicity. Withhold drug and notify doctor.
- Monitor serum potassium carefully. Take corrective action *before* hypokalemia occurs.
- Encourage the patient to eat potassium-rich foods.
- Digitoxin is a long-acting drug; watch for cumulative effects and signs of toxicity, especially in children and elderly patients. Ask patient about nausea, vomiting, anorexia, visual disturbances, and other symptoms of toxicity.
- Instruct patient and responsible family member about drug action, dosage regimen, how to take pulse, reportable signs, and follow-up plans.
- Don't substitute one brand for another.
- Therapeutic blood levels of digitoxin range from 25 to 35 ng/ml.
- Digitoxin toxicity may be treated by administering agents that bind the drug in the intestine (for example, colestipol and cholestyramine). Arrhythmias may be treated with phenytoin I.V. Potentially life-threatening toxicity may be treated by specific antigen-binding fragments (such as digoxin immune FAB).

digoxin

Lanoxicaps, Lanoxin*, Novodigoxin†

Pregnancy Risk Category: C

HOW SUPPLIED

Tablets: 0.125 mg, 0.25 mg, 0.5 mg
Capsules: 0.05 mg, 0.1 mg, 0.2 mg
Elixir: 0.05 mg/ml
Injection: 0.05 mg/ml†, 0.1 mg/ml (pediatric), 0.25 mg/ml

MECHANISM OF ACTION

Promotes movement of calcium from extracellular to intracellular cytoplasm and inhibits sodium-potassium activated adenosine triphosphatase. These actions strengthen myocardial contraction.

INDICATIONS & DOSAGE

CHF, paroxysmal supraventricular tachycardia, atrial fibrillation and flutter –

Adults: loading dose is 0.5 to 1 mg I.V. or P.O. in divided doses over 24 hours; maintenance dosage is 0.125 to 0.5 mg I.V. or P.O. daily (average 0.25 mg). Larger doses are often needed for treatment of arrhythmias, depending on patient response. Smaller loading and maintenance doses should be given in patients with impaired renal function.

Adults over 65 years: 0.125 mg P.O. daily as maintenance dose. Frail or underweight elderly patients may require only 0.0625 mg daily or 0.125 mg every other day.

Children over 2 years: loading dose is 0.02 to 0.04 mg/kg P.O. divided q 8 hours over 24 hours; I.V. loading dose is 0.015 to 0.035 mg/kg; maintenance dosage is 0.012 mg/kg P.O. daily divided q 12 hours.

Children 1 month to 2 years: loading dose is 0.035 to 0.06 mg/kg P.O. in three divided doses over 24 hours; I.V. loading dose is 0.03 to 0.05 mg/kg; maintenance dosage is 0.01 to 0.02 mg/kg P.O. daily divided q 12 hours.

Neonates under 1 month: loading dose is 0.035 mg/kg P.O. divided q 8 hours over 24 hours; I.V. loading dose is 0.02 to 0.03 mg/kg; maintenance dosage is 0.01 mg/kg P.O. daily divided q 12 hours.

Premature infants: loading dose is 0.025 mg/kg I.V. in three divided doses over 24 hours; maintenance dosage is 0.01 mg/kg I.V. daily divided q 12 hours.

ADVERSE REACTIONS

Common reactions are in italics; life-threatening reactions are in bold italics.

The following are signs of toxicity that may occur with all cardiac glycosides:

CNS: *fatigue, generalized muscle weakness, agitation, hallucinations,* headache, malaise, dizziness, vertigo, stupor, paresthesias.

CV: ***increased severity of CHF, arrhythmias (most commonly conduction disturbances with or without AV block, premature ventricular contractions, and supraventricular arrhythmias),*** hypotension.

Toxic effects on heart may be life-threatening and require immediate attention.

EENT: *yellow-green halos around visual images, blurred vision,* light flashes, photophobia, diplopia.

GI: *anorexia, nausea,* vomiting, diarrhea.

INTERACTIONS

Amiloride: inhibits and increases digoxin excretion. Monitor for altered digoxin effect.

Amphotericin B, carbenicillin, ticarcillin, corticosteroids, and diuretics (including loop diuretics, chlorthalidone, metolazone, and thiazides): hypokalemia, predisposing patient to digitalis toxicity. Monitor serum potassium.

Antacids, kaolin-pectin: decreased absorption of oral digoxin. Schedule

*Liquid form contains alcohol. **May contain tartrazine.

doses as far as possible from oral digoxin administration.
Anticholinergics: may increase digoxin absorption of oral tablets. Monitor blood levels and observe for toxicity.
Cholestyramine, colestipol, metoclopramide: decreased absorption of oral digoxin. Monitor for decreased effect and low blood levels. Dosage may have to be increased.
Parenteral calcium, thiazides: hypercalcemia and hypomagnesemia, predisposing patient to digitalis toxicity. Monitor serum calcium and serum magnesium.
Quinidine, diltiazem, amiodarone, nifedipine, verapamil: increased digoxin blood levels. Monitor for toxicity.

NURSING CONSIDERATIONS

- *Contraindicated* in presence of any digitalis-induced toxicity; ventricular fibrillation; and ventricular tachycardia unless caused by CHF. Administering calcium salts to digitalized patient is also contraindicated. Calcium affects cardiac contractility and excitability in much the same way as glycosides and may lead to serious arrhythmias in digitalized patient.
- *Use with extreme caution* in elderly patients and in those with acute myocardial infarction, incomplete AV block, sinus bradycardia, premature ventricular contractions, chronic constrictive pericarditis, idiopathic hypertrophic subaortic stenosis, renal insufficiency, severe pulmonary disease, or hypothyroidism. Dosage must be reduced in renal impairment.
- Hypothyroid patients are very sensitive to glycosides; hyperthyroid patients may need larger doses.
- Obtain baseline data (heart rate and rhythm, blood pressure, and electrolytes) before giving first dose.
- Question patient about recent use of cardiac glycosides (within the previous 2 to 3 weeks) before administering a loading dose. Always divide loading dose over first 24 hours unless clinical situation indicates otherwise.
- Dose is adjusted to patient's clinical condition and is monitored by serum levels of cardiac glycoside, calcium, potassium, magnesium, and by ECG. Obtain blood for digoxin levels 8 hours after last P.O. dose.
- Before giving, take apical-radial pulse for a full minute. Record and report to doctor any significant changes (sudden increase or decrease in rate, pulse deficit, irregular beats, and particularly regularization of a previously irregular rhythm). Check blood pressure and obtain 12-lead ECG with these changes.
- **I.V. use:** Infuse drug slowly over at least 5 minutes.
- Excessive slowing of the pulse rate (60 beats/minute or less) may be a sign of digitalis toxicity. Withhold drug and notify doctor.
- Ask patient about nausea, vomiting, anorexia, visual disturbances, and other symptoms of toxicity.
- Monitor serum potassium carefully. Take corrective action *before* hypokalemia occurs. Encourage patient to eat potassium-rich foods.
- Withhold drug for 1 to 2 days before elective electrocardioversion. Adjust dose after cardioversion.
- Instruct patient and responsible family member about drug action, dosage regimen, how to take pulse, reportable signs, and follow-up plans.
- Don't substitute one brand for another.
- When changing from oral tablets or elixir to parenteral therapy, dosage should be reduced by 20% to 25%. When changing from liquid-filled capsules to parenteral therapy, dosage is about equivalent because absorption is best using liquid-filled capsules. Therefore, when changing from oral tablets or elixir to liquid-filled capsules, reduce dose by 20% to 25%.
- Therapeutic blood levels of digoxin range from 0.5 to 2.0 ng/ml.

flosequinan

Manoplax

Pregnancy Risk Category: C

HOW SUPPLIED

Tablets: 50 mg, 75 mg

MECHANISM OF ACTION

Increases cardiac output by causing vasodilation, which reduces both preload and afterload; flosequinan may also have positive inotropic and chronotropic effects. This action on peripheral arteries and veins is not fully understood, but drug may interfere with the intracellular release of calcium by decreasing levels of inositol triphosphate, inhibiting protein kinase C, or inhibiting phosphodiesterase.

INDICATIONS & DOSAGE

Management of CHF in patients not responding adequately to diuretics (with or without a digitalis glycoside) who can't tolerate or don't respond to therapy with an angiotensin-converting enzyme (ACE) inhibitor–

Adults: 50 mg P.O. daily in the morning. Increase dosage as needed and tolerated to 75 mg daily.

ADVERSE REACTIONS

Common reactions are in italics; life-threatening reactions are in bold italics.

CNS: *headache, dizziness,* depression, insomnia, nervousness, vertigo.

CV: *palpitations,* hypotension, postural hypotension, syncope, tachycardia, ventricular tachycardia, edema.

EENT: rhinitis.

GI: *diarrhea,* nausea, anorexia, vomiting.

GU: urinary tract infection.

Metabolic: gout, hyperglycemia, *hypokalemia.*

Respiratory: cough.

Other: back pain, chills, fever, neck pain, myalgia, tooth disorders, taste perversion.

INTERACTIONS

Anticoagulants: increased risk of bleeding. Monitor patient.

Cimetidine: decreased clearance of flosequinan and decreased rate of conversion to its active metabolite. Clinical significance is unknown; monitor for decreased flosequinan effect.

Diuretics: enhanced potassium-wasting effect. Monitor serum potassium levels.

Vasodilators, ACE inhibitors: increased risk of hypotension. Monitor blood pressure.

NURSING CONSIDERATIONS

- *Contraindicated* in patients with hypersensitivity to the drug.
- *Use cautiously* in patients with a history of hypersensitivity to q uinolone antibiotics (cross-sensitivity reactions have occurred, but their incidence is unknown) and in patients with impaired hepatic or renal function.
- Early results from the Prospective Randomized Flosequinan Longevity Evaluation (PROFILE) trial reveal a higher death rate in patients receiving 100 mg of flosequinan daily. Consequently, the manufacturer recommends that patients do not receive more than 75 mg daily.
- Expect a small, asymptomatic decrease in blood pressure of 1 to 2 mm Hg in patients treated with flosequinan.
- Patients receiving an ACE inhibitor are more likely to experience symptoms such as dizziness, postural hypotension, or syncope.
- Be aware that patients receiving ACE inhibitors should initiate therapy at lower dosage. Notify doctor for dosage adjustment as needed.
- Treat persistent hypotension by placing patient in the supine position and administering an I.V. infusion of 0.9% sodium chloride injection. Occasionally, pressor agents may be nec-

essary. A patient who experiences a hypotensive episode isn't excluded from future treatment; however, after his blood pressure stabilizes, drug should be restarted at a lower dosage.

• Flosequinan has anticoagulant activity similar to oral anticoagulants, such as warfarin. Monitor coagulation studies in patients receiving anticoagulant therapy.

• Monitor serum potassium levels closely in patients receiving diuretics and a digitalis glycoside. Patients with heart failure may experience significant decreases of serum potassium during treatment with flosequinan, and hypokalemia increases the risk and severity of digitalis toxicity.

• Tell patient to immediately report adverse reactions.

milrinone lactate

Primacor

Pregnancy Risk Category: C

HOW SUPPLIED

Injection: 1 mg/ml

MECHANISM OF ACTION

Produces inotropic action by increasing cellular levels of cyclic adenosine monophosphate. Produces vasodilation by directly relaxing vascular smooth muscle.

INDICATIONS & DOSAGE

Short-term treatment of CHF–

Adults: initial loading dose of 50 mcg/kg I.V., slowly administered over 10 minutes, followed by continuous I.V. infusion of 0.375 to 0.75 mcg/kg/minute. Adjust infusion dose according to clinical and hemodynamic responses. Typically given with digoxin and diuretics.

ADVERSE REACTIONS

Common reactions are in italics; life-threatening reactions are in bold italics.

CNS: headache.

CV: ***ventricular arrhythmias,*** *ventricular ectopic activity,* nonsustained ventricular tachycardia, ***sustained ventricular tachycardia.***

INTERACTIONS

Furosemide: immediate precipitation when mixed with I.V. milrinone. Don't administer through same I.V. line.

NURSING CONSIDERATIONS

• *Contraindicated* in patients with hypersensitivity to the drug and in patients with severe obstructive pulmonic or aortic valvular disease in lieu of surgical correction of the obstruction; also avoid use during acute phase of MI because safety and efficacy of such use have not been established.

• *Use cautiously* in patients with atrial flutter or fibrillation because drug slightly shortens AV node conduction time and may increase ventricular response rate. If patient is to receive a digitalis glycoside, such therapy should begin before milrinone.

• Monitor patient concurrently receiving diuretics, especially if such therapy has decreased cardiac filling pressure.

• Be aware that inotropic agents may aggravate outflow tract obstruction in patients with hypertrophic subaortic stenosis.

• Patients treated with milrinone have exhibited supraventricular and ventricular arrhythmias. Studies have shown that milrinone isn't arrhythmogenic; however, patients receiving drug may be taking several other medications concurrently, which may increase potential for arrhythmias. Monitor patients who are at increased risk for arrhythmias.

• Monitor fluid and electrolyte status, blood pressure, heart rate, and renal function during therapy. Excessive decrease in blood pressure requires discontinuation or slower rate of infusion.

- Improvement of cardiac output may result in enhanced urine output. Expect dosage reduction in patient's diuretic therapy as CHF improves. Remember that potassium loss produced by excessive diuresis may predispose patient to digitalis toxicity.
- **I.V. use:** Prepare I.V. infusion solution using 0.45% or 0.9% sodium chloride injection or dextrose 5% in water. Prepare 100 mcg/ml solution by adding 180 ml diluent per 20-mg (20-ml) vial. Prepare 150 mcg/ml solution by adding 113 ml diluent per 20-mg (20-ml) vial. Prepare 200 mcg/ml solution by adding 80 ml diluent per 20-mg (20-ml) vial.
- Dosage adjustments are necessary in patients with renal failure. If creatinine clearance is 50 ml/minute/1.73 m^2 or less, dosage should be carefully titrated to maximum clinical effect and shouldn't exceed 1.13 mg/kg/day. Consult manufacturer's literature for specific infusion rate information.

*Liquid form contains alcohol. **May contain tartrazine.

20

Antiarrhythmics

adenosine
amiodarone hydrochloride
atropine sulfate
bretylium tosylate
disopyramide
disopyramide phosphate
esmolol hydrochloride
flecainide acetate
lidocaine hydrochloride
mexiletine hydrochloride
moricizine hydrochloride
phenytoin
(See Chapter 29, ANTICONVULSANTS.)
phenytoin sodium
(See Chapter 29, ANTICONVULSANTS.)
procainamide hydrochloride
propafenone hydrochloride
propranolol hydrochloride
(See Chapter 21, ANTIANGINALS.)
quinidine bisulfate
quinidine gluconate
quinidine polygalacturonate
quinidine sulfate
sotalol
tocainide hydrochloride

COMBINATION PRODUCTS
None.

adenosine
Adenocard
Pregnancy Risk Category: C

HOW SUPPLIED
Injection: 3 mg/ml in 2-ml vials

MECHANISM OF ACTION
Adenosine is a naturally occurring nucleoside. In the heart, it acts on the AV node to slow conduction and inhibit reentry pathways. Adenosine is also useful for the treatment of paroxysmal supraventricular tachycardia (PSVT) associated with accessory bypass tracts (Wolff-Parkinson-White syndrome).

INDICATIONS & DOSAGE
Conversion of PSVT to sinus rhythm –
Adults: 6 mg I.V. by rapid bolus injection (over 1 to 2 seconds). If PSVT is not eliminated in 1 to 2 minutes, give 12 mg by rapid I.V. push. Repeat 12-mg dose if necessary. Single doses over 12 mg are not recommended.

ADVERSE REACTIONS
Common reactions are in italics; life-threatening reactions are in bold italics.
CNS: apprehension, back pain, blurred vision, burning sensation, dizziness, heaviness in arms, lightheadedness, neck pain, numbness, tingling in arms.
CV: chest pain, *facial flushing,* headache, hypotension, palpitations, sweating.
GI: metallic taste, nausea.
Respiratory: *chest pressure, dyspnea, shortness of breath,* hyperventilation.
Other: *tightness in throat, groin pressure.*

INTERACTIONS
Carbamazepine: higher degrees of heart block may occur.
Dipyridamole: may potentiate the drug's effects. Smaller doses may be necessary.
Methylxanthines: antagonism of the drug's effects. Patients receiving theophylline or caffeine may require higher doses or may not respond to adenosine therapy.

NURSING CONSIDERATIONS
• *Contraindicated* in patients with atrial flutter, atrial fibrillation, and ventricular tachycardia because the

drug is ineffective in the treatment of these arrhythmias. It is also contraindicated in patients allergic to the drug. Because it decreases conduction through the AV node, adenosine may produce a transient first-, second-, or third-degree heart block. For this reason, it is contraindicated in patients with second- or third-degree heart block or sick sinus syndrome, unless the patient has an artificial pacemaker. Because the drug has a very short half-life, these effects are usually transient; however, patients who develop significant block after a dose of adenosine should not receive additional doses.

• In clinical trials, more than half of the patients exhibited new arrhythmias when adenosine was used to convert to normal sinus rhythm. They are usually transient, but may include sinus bradycardia or tachycardia, atrial premature contractions, various degrees of AV block, premature ventricular contractions, and skipped beats.

• Inhaled adenosine will cause bronchoconstriction in asthmatic patients. Asthma attacks have not been reported, but the potential for bronchoconstriction exists.

• There is experimental evidence that high concentrations of adenosine may induce chromosomal damage. The clinical significance of this property is not known.

• **I.V. use:** Rapid I.V. injection is necessary for drug action. Administer directly into a vein if possible; if an I.V. line is used, employ the most proximal port and follow with a rapid saline flush to ensure that the drug reaches the systemic circulation quickly.

• Check solution for crystals, which may occur if solution is cold. If crystals are visible, gently warm solution to room temperature. Do not use solutions that aren't clear.

• Because it contains no preservatives, unused drug should be discarded.

amiodarone hydrochloride

Cordarone, Cordarone X‡

Pregnancy Risk Category: C

HOW SUPPLIED

Tablets: 100 mg†‡, 200 mg

MECHANISM OF ACTION

A class III antiarrhythmic that prolongs the refractory period and action potential duration and decreases repolarization.

INDICATIONS & DOSAGE

Ventricular and supraventricular arrhythmias, including recurrent supraventricular tachycardia (Wolff-Parkinson-White syndrome), atrial fibrillation and flutter, and ventricular tachycardia refractory to other antiarrhythmics –

Adults: give loading dose of 800 to 1,600 mg P.O. daily for 1 to 3 weeks until initial therapeutic response occurs. Maintenance dosage is 200 to 600 mg P.O. daily.

ADVERSE REACTIONS

Common reactions are in italics; life-threatening reactions are in bold italics.

CNS: peripheral neuropathy, extrapyramidal symptoms, headache, *malaise, fatigue.*

CV: bradycardia, hypotension, ***arrhythmias, CHF.***

EENT: *corneal microdeposits,* visual disturbances.

Endocrine: hypothyroidism, hyperthyroidism, gynecomastia.

GI: *nausea, vomiting,* constipation.

Hepatic: *altered liver enzymes,* hepatic dysfunction.

Respiratory: ***severe pulmonary toxicity (pneumonitis, alveolitis).***

Skin: *photosensitivity,* blue-gray skin pigmentation.

Other: muscle weakness.

INTERACTIONS

Antiarrhythmic agents: use with amiodarone may induce torsades de pointes; amiodarone may reduce the hepatic or renal clearance of flecainide, procainamide, and quinidine.

Antihypertensives: increased hypotensive effect. Use together cautiously.

Beta blockers, calcium channel blockers: increased cardiac depressant effects; may potentiate slowing of sinus node and AV conduction. Use together cautiously.

Digitalis glycosides: increased serum digoxin levels.

Phenytoin: phenytoin metabolism may be decreased.

Warfarin: increased anticoagulant effect. Monitor patient closely.

NURSING CONSIDERATIONS

- *Use with extreme caution* in patients receiving class I antiarrhythmics.
- *Use cautiously* in preexisting bradycardia or sinus node disease; conduction disturbances; severely depressed ventricular function; marked cardiomegaly.
- Amiodarone is often effective for treatment of arrhythmias resistant to other drug therapy. However, the high incidence of adverse reactions limits its use.
- Amiodarone has been given I.V., but an injectable preparation is not available in the U.S. The loading dose is 5 to 10 mg/kg by I.V. infusion via a central line, followed by an I.V. infusion of 10 mg/kg/day for 3 to 5 days.
- Most patients treated show corneal microdeposits upon slit-lamp ophthalmologic examination. Onset of this effect from 1 to 4 months after beginning amiodarone therapy. However, only 2% to 3% have actual visual disturbances. To minimize this complication, recommend instillation of methylcellulose ophthalmic solution during amiodarone therapy.
- Monitor carefully for pulmonary toxicity, which can be fatal. Incidence increases in patients receiving more than 400 mg/day.
- Monitor for symptoms of pneumonitis – exertional dyspnea, nonproductive cough, and pleuritic chest pain. Monitor pulmonary function tests and chest X-ray.
- Monitor blood pressure and heart rate and rhythm frequently. Continuous ECG monitoring should be performed during initiation and alteration of dosage. Notify doctor of any significant change.
- Monitor hepatic and thyroid function tests. Monitor serum electrolytes, particularly potassium and magnesium levels.
- Divide oral loading dose into three equal doses and give with meals to decrease GI intolerance. Maintenance dosage may be given once daily, but may be divided into two doses taken with meals if GI intolerance occurs.
- Advise patient to use a sunscreen to prevent photosensitivity. Monitor for burning or tingling skin followed by erythema and possible skin blistering.
- Amiodarone's adverse reactions are more prevalent at high doses but are generally reversible when drug therapy is stopped. Resolution of adverse reactions may take up to 4 months.

atropine sulfate

Pregnancy Risk Category: C

HOW SUPPLIED

Tablets: 0.4 mg, 0.6 mg

Injection: 0.05 mg/ml, 0.1 mg/ml, 0.3 mg/ml, 0.4 mg/ml, 0.5 mg/ml, 0.6 mg/ml, 0.8 mg/ml, 1 mg/ml, 1.2 mg/ml

MECHANISM OF ACTION

An anticholinergic, it inhibits acetylcholine at the parasympathetic neuroeffector junction, blocking vagal effects on the sinoatrial node; this enhances conduction through the AV node and speeds heart rate.

INDICATIONS & DOSAGE
Symptomatic bradycardia, bradyarrhythmia (junctional or escape rhythm) –
Adults: usually 0.5 to 1 mg I.V. push; repeat q 5 minutes, to maximum of 2 mg. Lower doses (less than 0.5 mg) can cause bradycardia.
Children: 0.01 mg/kg I.V. dose up to maximum of 0.4 mg; or 0.3 mg/m^2 dose; may repeat q 4 to 6 hours.
Antidote for anticholinesterase insecticide poisoning –
Adults: 2 to 4 mg I.V. repeated q 5 to 10 minutes until muscarinic symptoms disappear or signs of atropine toxicity appear. Severe poisoning may require up to 6 mg q 1 hour.
Children: 1 mg I.V. or I.M. then 0.5 to 1 mg I.V. or I.M. q 5 to 10 minutes until muscarinic signs disappear or signs of atropine toxicity appear.
Preoperatively for diminishing secretions and blocking cardiac vagal reflexes –
Adults: 0.4 to 0.6 mg I.M. 45 to 60 minutes before anesthesia.
Children: 0.01 mg/kg I.M. up to a maximum dose of 0.4 mg 45 to 60 minutes before anesthesia.
Adjunctive treatment of peptic ulcer disease; treatment of functional GI disorders such as irritable bowel syndrome –
Adults: 0.4 to 0.6 mg P.O. q 4 to 6 hours.
Children: 0.01 mg/kg or 0.3 mg/m^2 (not to exceed 0.4 mg) q 4 to 6 hours.

ADVERSE REACTIONS
Common reactions are in italics; life-threatening reactions are in bold italics.
Blood: leukocytosis.
CNS: *headache, restlessness,* ataxia, disorientation, hallucinations, delirium, coma, *insomnia, dizziness;* excitement, agitation, and confusion (especially in elderly patients).
CV: 1 to 2 mg – *tachycardia, palpitations;* greater than 2 mg – ***extreme tachycardia, angina.***
EENT: 1 mg – *slight mydriasis,* photophobia; 2 mg – *blurred vision, mydriasis.*
GI: *dry mouth (common even at low doses),* thirst, *constipation,* nausea, vomiting.
GU: urine retention.
Skin: hot, flushed skin.

INTERACTIONS
Amantadine, glutethimide, meperidine, antiarrhythmics, antiparkinsonian agents, phenothiazines, tricyclic antidepressants: additive anticholinergic effects. Use together cautiously.
Antacids: decreased absorption of anticholinergics. Separate administration times by at least 1 hour.
Digoxin: increased digoxin levels if slow dissolving tablets are used. Use oral solution or tablets that dissolve rapidly.
Ketoconazole, levodopa: decreased absorption. Avoid concomitant use.
Methotrimeprazine: may produce extrapyramidal symptoms. Monitor patient carefully.
Potassium chloride wax-matrix tablets: increased risk of mucosal lesions. Use cautiously.

NURSING CONSIDERATIONS
- *Contraindicated* in narrow-angle glaucoma, obstructive uropathy, obstructive disease of GI tract, myasthenia gravis, paralytic ileus, intestinal atony, unstable cardiovascular status in acute hemorrhage, and toxic megacolon.
- *Use cautiously* in patients with Down's syndrome because these patients may be more sensitive to the drug.
- Adverse reactions vary considerably with dose. Dry mouth is most common.
- Many of the adverse reactions (such as dry mouth and constipation) are an extension of the drug's pharmacologic activity and may be expected.
- Watch for tachycardia in cardiac pa-

tients. It may precipitate ventricular fibrillation.

- Antidote for atropine overdose is physostigmine salicylate.
- Other anticholinergic drugs may increase vagal blockage.
- **I.V. use:** Administer by direct I.V. into a large vein or I.V. tubing over at least 1 to 2 minutes.
- When given I.V., atropine may cause paradoxical initial bradycardia, especially when small doses (0.4 to 0.6 mg) are given. This is caused by a drug effect in the CNS and usually disappears within 2 minutes.
- Monitor intake and output. Drug causes urine retention and urinary hesitancy; have patient void before receiving the drug.
- Monitor closely for urine retention in elderly men with benign prostatic hypertrophy.

bretylium tosylate

Bretylate†‡, Bretylol

Pregnancy Risk Category: C

HOW SUPPLIED

Injection: 50 mg/ml

MECHANISM OF ACTION

A class III antiarrhythmic that initially exerts transient adrenergic stimulation through release of norepinephrine. Subsequent depletion of norepinephrine causes adrenergic blocking actions to predominate. Repolarization is prolonged; duration of action potential and effective refractory period are increased.

INDICATIONS & DOSAGE

Ventricular fibrillation –
Adults: 5 mg/kg by I.V. push over 1 minute. If necessary, increase dose to 10 mg/kg and repeat q 15 to 30 minutes until 30 mg/kg have been given.
Children: safety and efficacy have not been established, but some clinicians use 2 to 5 mg/kg I.M. as a single dose, or 5 mg/kg I.V. followed by 10 mg/kg I.V. if fibrillation persists.

Other ventricular arrhythmias –
Adults: initially, 500 mg diluted to 50 ml with dextrose 5% in water or 0.9% sodium chloride solution and infused I.V. over more than 8 minutes at 5 to 10 mg/kg. Dose may be repeated in 1 to 2 hours. Thereafter, repeat q 6 to 8 hours.

I.V. maintenance –
Adults: infused in diluted solution of 500 ml dextrose 5% in water or normal saline solution at 1 to 2 mg/minute.

I.M. injection –
Adults: 5 to 10 mg/kg undiluted. Repeat in 1 to 2 hours if needed. Thereafter, repeat q 6 to 8 hours.

ADVERSE REACTIONS

Common reactions are in italics; life-threatening reactions are in bold italics.
CNS: *vertigo, dizziness, light-headedness, syncope* (usually secondary to hypotension).
CV: *severe hypotension (especially orthostatic), bradycardia,* anginal pain, transient arrhythmias, transient hypertension.
GI: severe nausea, vomiting (with rapid infusion).

INTERACTIONS

All antihypertensives: may potentiate hypotension. Monitor blood pressure.
Other antiarrhythmics: additive or antagonistic antiarrhythmic effects. Monitor for additive toxicity.

NURSING CONSIDERATIONS

- *Contraindicated* with use of the commercially available preparation mixed in dextrose 5% in water in patients who are hypersensitive to corn or corn products. There are no contraindications to the use of bretylium in the treatment of ventricular fibrillation or life-threatening arrhythmias.
- *Use cautiously* in patients with fixed cardiac output, aortic stenosis, and

pulmonary hypertension to avoid severe and sudden drop in blood pressure.
• Avoid initiating bretylium therapy concomitantly with digitalis glycoside therapy. Do not use in digitalized patients unless the arrhythmia is life-threatening, not caused by digitalis, and is unresponsive to other drugs.
• **I.V. use:** Infuse in diluted solution of 500 ml dextrose 5% in water or normal saline solution at 1 to 2 mg/minute; however, patients who are hypersensitive to corn or corn products should not receive the commercially available preparation mixed with dextrose 5% in water. Administer continuous infusion at a rate of 1 to 2 mg/minute. When infusing drug intermittently, infuse ordered dose over 10 to 30 minutes. When administering as a direct I.V. injection, use a 20G to 22G needle and inject over about 1 minute into vein or into I.V. line containing a free-flowing, compatible solution.
• Monitor blood pressure and heart rate and rhythm continuously. Notify doctor immediately of any significant change. If supine systolic blood pressure falls below 75 mm Hg, notify doctor; may order norepinephrine, dopamine, or volume expanders to raise blood pressure.
• The initial release of norepinephrine caused by bretylium may induce transient hypertension and arrhythmias. Monitor patient closely.
• Keep patient in the supine position until tolerance to hypotension develops. Tell patient to avoid sudden postural changes.
• Follow dosage directions carefully to avoid nausea and vomiting.
• Rotate I.M. injection sites to prevent tissue damage, and don't exceed 3-ml volume in any one site.
• To be used with other cardiopulmonary resuscitation measures, such as CPR, countershock, epinephrine, sodium bicarbonate, and lidocaine.
• Avoid subtherapeutic doses (less than 5 mg/kg), because such doses may cause hypotension.
• Ventricular tachycardia and other ventricular arrhythmias respond less rapidly to treatment than ventricular fibrillation.
• Dosage should be decreased in renal impairment.
• Monitor carefully if pressor amines (sympathomimetics) are given to correct hypotension, because bretylium potentiates pressor amines.
• Ineffective for atrial arrhythmias.
• Has been used investigationally to treat hypertension.
• Observe for increased anginal pain in susceptible patients.
• Observe patient for adverse reactions and notify doctor if any occur.

disopyramide
Rythmodan†

disopyramide phosphate
Napamide, Norpace, Norpace CR, Rythmodan LA†

Pregnancy Risk Category: C

HOW SUPPLIED
disopyramide
Capsules: 100 mg†, 150 mg†
disopyramide phosphate
Tablets (sustained-release): 250 mg†
Capsules: 100 mg, 150 mg
Capsules (controlled-release): 100 mg, 150 mg

MECHANISM OF ACTION
A class Ia antiarrhythmic that depresses phase O. It prolongs the action potential. All class I drugs have membrane stabilizing effects.

INDICATIONS & DOSAGE
Premature ventricular contractions (unifocal, multifocal, or coupled); ventricular tachycardia not severe enough to require electrocardioversion; to convert atrial fibrillation or flutter to normal sinus rhythm –

*Liquid form contains alcohol. **May contain tartrazine.

Adults: usual maintenance dosage 150 to 200 mg P.O. q 6 hours; for patients who weigh less than 50 kg or those with renal, hepatic, or cardiac impairment – 100 mg P.O. q 6 hours. May give sustained-release capsule q 12 hours.
Children 12 to 18 years: 6 to 15 mg/kg P.O. daily.
Children 4 to 12 years: 10 to 15 mg/kg P.O. daily.
Children 1 to 4 years: 10 to 20 mg/kg P.O. daily.
Children under 1 year: 10 to 30 mg/kg P.O. daily.

All children's dosages should be divided into equal amounts and given q 6 hours.

Recommended dosages in advanced renal insufficiency: if creatinine clearance is 30 to 40 ml/minute, dosing interval is q 8 hours; if creatinine clearance is 15 to 30 ml/minute, dosing interval is q 12 hours; if creatinine clearance is < 15 ml/minute, dosing interval is q 24 hours.

ADVERSE REACTIONS

Common reactions are in italics; life-threatening reactions are in bold italics.
CNS: dizziness, agitation, depression, fatigue, muscle weakness, syncope.
CV: *hypotension, **CHF, heart block,*** edema, weight gain, ***arrhythmias.***
EENT: *blurred vision, dry eyes, dry nose.*
GI: nausea, vomiting, anorexia, bloating, abdominal pain, *constipation, dry mouth.*
GU: urine retention and urinary hesitancy.
Hepatic: cholestatic jaundice.
Metabolic: hypoglycemia.
Skin: rash in 1% to 3% of patients.

INTERACTIONS

Antiarrhythmics: possible additive or antagonized antiarrhythmic effects.
Phenytoin: increases disopyramide's metabolism. Monitor for decreased antiarrhythmic effect.

NURSING CONSIDERATIONS

- *Contraindicated* in cardiogenic shock or second- or third-degree heart block with no pacemaker. Use very cautiously, and avoid, if possible, in CHF.
- *Use cautiously* in underlying conduction abnormalities, urinary tract diseases (especially prostatic hypertrophy), hepatic or renal impairment, myasthenia gravis, or narrow-angle glaucoma. Adjust dosage in renal insufficiency.
- Don't give sustained-release capsule for rapid control of ventricular arrhythmias; when therapeutic blood levels must be rapidly attained; in cardiomyopathy or possible cardiac decompensation; or in severe renal impairment.
- When transferring patient from immediate-release to sustained-release capsules, advise him to begin a sustained-release capsule 6 hours after the last immediate-release capsule was taken.
- Discontinue if heart block develops, if QRS complex widens by more than 25%, or if Q-T interval lengthens by more than 25% above baseline.
- Correct any underlying electrolyte abnormalities before use.
- Watch for recurrence of arrhythmias and check for adverse reactions; notify doctor if any occur.
- Check apical pulse before administering drug. Notify doctor if pulse rate is slower than 60 beats/minute or faster than 120 beats/minute.
- Teach patient the importance of taking drug on time, exactly as prescribed. To do this, he may have to use an alarm clock for night doses.
- Relieve discomfort of dry mouth by chewing gum or hard candy.
- Manage constipation with proper diet or bulk laxatives.
- Use of disopyramide with other an-

tiarrhythmics may cause further myocardial depression.

• Most doctors prefer to prescribe disopyramide for patients not in heart failure who can't tolerate quinidine or procainamide.

• Pharmacist may prepare disopyramide suspension from 100-mg capsules using cherry syrup. Protect suspension from light. It should be dispensed in amber glass bottles. May be best for young children.

esmolol hydrochloride

Brevibloc

Pregnancy Risk Category: C

HOW SUPPLIED

Injection: 10 mg/ml in 10-ml vials; 250 mg/ml in 10-ml ampules

MECHANISM OF ACTION

A class II antiarrhythmic, esmolol is an ultrashort-acting $beta_1$-selective adrenergic blocker. Decreases heart rate, myocardial contractility, and blood pressure.

INDICATIONS & DOSAGE

Supraventricular tachycardia –

Adults: loading dose is 500 mcg/kg/minute by I.V. infusion over 1 minute, followed by a 4-minute maintenance infusion of 50 mcg/kg/minute. If adequate response does not occur within 5 minutes, repeat the loading dose followed by a maintenance infusion of 100 mcg/kg/minute for 4 minutes. Maximum maintenance infusion is 200 mcg/kg/minute.

ADVERSE REACTIONS

Common reactions are in italics; life-threatening reactions are in bold italics.

CNS: dizziness, somnolence, headache, agitation, fatigue.

CV: *hypotension* (sometimes with diaphoresis).

GI: *nausea,* vomiting.

Local: inflammation and induration at infusion site.

Other: bronchospasm.

INTERACTIONS

Digoxin: esmolol may increase serum digoxin levels by 10% to 20%.

Morphine: may increase esmolol blood levels. Titrate esmolol carefully.

Reserpine (and other catecholamine-depleting drugs): may cause additive bradycardia and hypotension. Titrate esmolol carefully.

Succinylcholine: esmolol may prolong neuromuscular blockade.

NURSING CONSIDERATIONS

• *Contraindicated* in sinus bradycardia, heart block greater than first degree, cardiogenic shock, or overt heart failure.

• *Use cautiously* in impaired renal function, diabetes, or bronchospasm.

• **I.V. use:** Don't give esmolol by I.V. push; use a controlled infusion device. Drug must be diluted before infusion.

• Esmolol solutions are incompatible with diazepam, furosemide, sodium bicarbonate, and thiopental sodium.

• Monitor continuous ECG and blood pressure during infusion. Up to 50% of all patients treated with esmolol develop hypotension. Monitor closely, especially if patient's pretreatment blood pressure was low.

• Hypotension can usually be reversed within 30 minutes by decreasing the dose or, if necessary, by stopping the infusion.

• Esmolol is recommended only for short-term use, no longer than 48 hours.

• If a local reaction develops at the infusion site, change to another site. Avoid butterfly needles.

• When patient's heart rate becomes stable, esmolol will be replaced by alternative (longer-acting) antiarrhythmics, such as propranolol, digoxin, or verapamil. As the replacement drug is started, the esmolol infusion should be gradually reduced over 1 hour.

• Esmolol has an extremely short duration of action and can be accurately titrated. Therefore, it has advantages over other beta blockers in treating cardiac arrhythmias.

flecainide acetate

Tambocor

Pregnancy Risk Category: C

HOW SUPPLIED

Tablets: 50 mg, 100 mg, 150 mg

Injection: 10 mg/ml‡

MECHANISM OF ACTION

A class Ic antiarrhythmic that depresses phase O. Unlike class Ia and Ib agents, however, it does not prolong or shorten the action potential. All class I drugs have membrane stabilizing effects.

INDICATIONS & DOSAGE

Treatment of life-threatening ventricular arrhythmias, such as sustained ventricular tachycardia –

Adults: 100 mg P.O. q 12 hours. May be increased in increments of 50 mg b.i.d. q 4 days until efficacy is achieved. Maximum dosage is 400 mg daily for most patients.

Initial dosage for patients with CHF is 50 mg q 12 hours.

Where available, flecainide may be given by I.V. injection –

Adults: 2 mg/kg I.V. push over not less than 10 minutes; or the dose may be diluted with dextrose 5% in water and administered as an infusion. Do not use any other solutions for infusion.

ADVERSE REACTIONS

Common reactions are in italics; life-threatening reactions are in bold italics.

CNS: *dizziness, headache,* fatigue, tremor.

CV: ***new or worsened arrhythmias,*** chest pain, ***CHF, cardiac arrest.***

EENT: *blurred vision and other visual disturbances.*

GI: nausea, constipation, abdominal pain.

Other: *dyspnea,* edema, skin rash.

INTERACTIONS

Amiodarone, cimetidine, digoxin, propranolol: altered pharmacokinetics. Monitor for toxicity.

Digitalis glycosides: flecainide may increase plasma digoxin levels by 15% to 25%.

Propranolol, beta-adrenergic blocking agents: both flecainide and propranolol plasma levels increase by 20% to 30%.

Urine acidifying and alkalinizing agents: extremes of urine pH may substantially alter excretion of flecainide.

NURSING CONSIDERATIONS

• *Contraindicated* in preexisting second- or third-degree AV block or right bundle branch block when associated with a left hemiblock, unless a pacemaker is present, and in cardiogenic shock.

• *Use cautiously* in preexisting CHF, cardiomyopathy, severe renal or hepatic disease, prolonged Q-T interval, sick sinus syndrome, or blood dyscrasia.

• Findings from the Cardiac Arrhythmia Suppression Trial (CAST) include a greater-than-twofold increase in the number of deaths and nonfatal cardiac arrest in patients treated with flecainide. Therefore, it should be used only in immediately life-threatening arrhythmias, such as sustained ventricular tachycardia.

• Flecainide can alter endocardial pacing thresholds. Determine pacing threshold 1 week before and after initiating therapy in patients with pacemakers.

• Hypokalemia or hyperkalemia may alter the effect of flecainide and should be corrected before this drug is given.

- Incidence of adverse effects increases when trough blood levels exceed 1 mcg/ml. Periodically monitor blood levels, especially in patients with renal failure or CHF.
- Most patients can be adequately maintained on an every-12-hour dosage schedule, but some need to receive flecainide every 8 hours.
- Full therapeutic effect of flecainide may take 3 to 5 days. The doctor may order I.V. lidocaine while awaiting full effect.
- **I.V. use:** When administering flecainide by I.V. push, give over at least 10 minutes. For I.V. infusion, mix only with dextrose 5% in water.
- Loading doses may aggravate arrhythmias and are therefore not recommended.
- Twice-daily dosing for flecainide aids patient compliance.
- Therapeutic serum levels of flecainide range from 0.2 to 1 mcg/ml.

lidocaine hydrochloride (lignocaine hydrochloride)

Lido Pen Auto-Injector, Xylocaine, Xylocard†‡

Pregnancy Risk Category: B

HOW SUPPLIED

Injection (for direct I.V. use): 1% (10 mg/ml) in 5-ml (50-mg), 10-ml (100-mg) syringes; 2% (20 mg/ml) in 5-ml (100-mg) vials, syringes, and ampules
Injection (for I.M. use): 10% (100 mg/ml) in 3-ml automatic injection device or 5-ml ampules
Injection (for I.V. admixtures): 4% (40 mg/ml) in 25-ml (1-g) vials and syringes and 50-ml (2-g) vials and syringes; 10% (100 mg/ml) in 10-ml (1-g) vials; 20% (200 mg/ml) in 5-ml (1-g) vials and syringes and 10-ml (2-g) vials and syringes
Infusion (premixed): 0.2% (2 mg/ml) in 500-ml vials; 0.4% (4 mg/ml) in 250-ml, 500-ml, 1,000-ml vials; 0.8% (8 mg/ml) in 250-ml, 500-ml vials

MECHANISM OF ACTION

A class Ib antiarrhythmic that depresses phase O. It shortens the action potential. All class I drugs have membrane stabilizing effects.

INDICATIONS & DOSAGE

Ventricular arrhythmias from myocardial infarction, cardiac manipulation, or cardiac glycosides; ventricular tachycardia –
Adults: 50 to 100 mg (1 to 1.5 mg/kg) I.V. bolus at 25 to 50 mg/minute. Give half this amount to elderly patients or patients under 50 kg, and to those with CHF or hepatic disease. Repeat bolus q 3 to 5 minutes until arrhythmias subside or adverse reactions develop. Don't exceed 300-mg total bolus during a 1-hour period. Simultaneously, begin constant infusion of 20 to 50 mg/kg/minute (1 to 4 mg/minute). If single bolus has been given, repeat smaller bolus 15 to 20 minutes after start of infusion to maintain therapeutic serum level. After 24 hours of continuous infusion, decrease rate by half.
I.M. administration: 200 to 300 mg in deltoid muscle only.
Children: 1mg/kg by I.V. bolus, followed by infusion of 30 mcg/kg/minute.

ADVERSE REACTIONS

Common reactions are in italics; life-threatening reactions are in bold italics.
CNS: *confusion, tremors,* lethargy, somnolence, *stupor, restlessness,* slurred speech, euphoria, depression, *light-headedness,* paresthesias, muscle twitching, ***seizures.***
CV: *hypotension,* bradycardia, ***new or worsened arrhythmias.***
EENT: *tinnitus, blurred or double vision.*
Other: ***anaphylaxis,*** soreness at in-

*Liquid form contains alcohol. **May contain tartrazine.

jection site, sensations of cold, diaphoresis.

INTERACTIONS

Cimetidine, beta blockers: decreased metabolism of lidocaine. Monitor for toxicity.

Phenytoin, procainamide, propranolol or quinidine: additive cardiac depressant effects. Monitor carefully.

NURSING CONSIDERATIONS

- *Contraindicated* in patients who are allergic to related local anesthetics of the amide type, such as Nupercaine, and with epinephrine (for local anesthesia) to treat arrhythmias. Do not use for ventricular escape beats. Atropine should be used instead.
- *Use cautiously* in complete or second-degree heart block or sinus bradycardia and in elderly patients, those with CHF, renal or hepatic disease, or those who weigh less than 50 kg. Such patients will need a reduced dose.
- In many severely ill patients, seizures may be the first clinically apparent sign of toxicity. However, severe reactions usually are preceded by somnolence, confusion, and paresthesias.
- If toxic signs (such as dizziness) occur, stop drug at once and notify doctor. Continued infusion could lead to seizures and coma. Give oxygen via nasal cannula, if not contraindicated. Keep oxygen and CPR equipment readily available.
- **I.V. use:** Patients receiving infusions must be attended *at all times* and be on a cardiac monitor. Use an infusion pump for administering infusion precisely. Do not exceed an infusion rate of 4 mg/minute. A faster rate greatly increases risk of toxicity.
- Monitor patient's response, especially blood pressure and serum electrolytes, BUN, and creatinine. Notify doctor promptly if abnormalities develop.
- Discontinue infusion and notify doctor if arrhythmias worsen or ECG changes, such as widening QRS complex or substantially prolonged PR interval, are evident.
- A bolus dose not followed by infusion will have a short-lived effect.
- A patient who has received lidocaine I.M. will show a sevenfold increase in serum creatinine phosphokinase (CPK) level. Such CPK originates in the skeletal muscle, not the heart. Test isoenzymes if using I.M. route.
- Used investigationally to treat refractory status epilepticus.
- Therapeutic serum levels are 2 to 5 mcg/ml.

mexiletine hydrochloride

Mexitil

Pregnancy Risk Category: C

HOW SUPPLIED

Capsules: 50 mg‡, 100 mg†, 150 mg, 200 mg, 250 mg

Injection: 250 mg/10 ml‡

MECHANISM OF ACTION

A class Ib antiarrhythmic that depresses phase O. It shortens the action potential. All class I drugs have membrane stabilizing effects.

INDICATIONS & DOSAGE

Treatment of refractory ventricular arrhythmias, including ventricular tachycardia and premature ventricular contractions –

Adults: 200 to 400 mg P.O. followed by 200 mg q 8 hours. May increase dose to 400 mg q 8 hours if satisfactory control is not obtained. Some patients may respond well to an every-12-hour schedule. May give up to 450 mg q 12 hours.

Where available, mexiletine may be given I.V. –

Adults: following a loading dose of 200 to 250 mg I.V. at a rate of 25 mg/minute, prepare an infusion solution of 250 mg mexiletine/500 ml dextrose 5% in water. Administer the first 120 ml (60 mg) over 1 hour. If clinical response is inadequate, give another bolus of 200 mg over 10 to 20 minutes. Maintenance dose is 0.5 mg/minute (1 ml/minute of prepared solution).

ADVERSE REACTIONS
Common reactions are in italics; life-threatening reactions are in bold italics.
CNS: *tremor, dizziness,* blurred vision, ataxia, diplopia, confusion, nystagmus, nervousness, headache.
CV: hypotension, bradycardia, widened QRS complex, ***new or worsened arrhythmias.***
GI: nausea, vomiting.
Skin: rash.

INTERACTIONS
Cimetidine: increased mexiletine blood levels. Monitor carefully.
Phenytoin, rifampin, phenobarbital: decreased mexiletine blood levels. Monitor carefully.

NURSING CONSIDERATIONS
• *Contraindicated* in cardiogenic shock or preexisting second- or third-degree AV block (if pacemaker is not present).
• Early sign of mexiletine toxicity is tremor, usually a fine tremor of the hands. This progresses to dizziness and later to ataxia and nystagmus as the drug's blood level increases. Question your patient about these symptoms.
• When changing from lidocaine to mexiletine, stop the infusion when the first mexiletine dose is given. Keep the infusion line open, however, until the arrhythmia appears to be satisfactorily controlled.
• May administer oral dose with meals to lessen GI distress.
• Therapeutic levels range from 0.75 to 2 mcg/ml.
• Monitor blood pressure and heart rate and rhythm frequently. Notify doctor of any significant change.
• Patients who respond well to mexiletine can often be maintained on a q 12 hour schedule. Notify doctor if you feel the patient is a good candidate for q 12 hour therapy. Twice-daily dosage eases compliance.
• **I.V. use:** Mexiletine injection is compatible with 0.9% sodium chloride, dextrose 5% in water, 5% sodium bicarbonate, 1/6 M sodium lactate, and 10% fructose (levulose).

moricizine hydrochloride
Ethmozine
Pregnancy Risk Category: B

HOW SUPPLIED
Tablets: 200 mg, 250 mg, 300 mg

MECHANISM OF ACTION
A class I antiarrhythmic that reduces the fast inward current carried by sodium ions.

INDICATIONS & DOSAGE
Life-threatening ventricular arrhythmias –
Adults: individualized dosage is based on clinical response and patient tolerance. Therapy should begin in the hospital. Most patients respond to 600 to 900 mg P.O. daily, given in divided doses q 8 hours. Increase daily dosage q 3 days by 150 mg until the desired clinical effect is seen.
Hepatic or renal function impairment –
Adults: start therapy at 600 mg P.O. daily or less. Monitor closely and adjust dosage carefully.

ADVERSE REACTIONS
Common reactions are in italics; life-threatening reactions are in bold italics.
CNS: *dizziness, headache, fatigue,* anxiety, hypoesthesia, asthenia, nervousness, paresthesia, sleep disorders.

*Liquid form contains alcohol. **May contain tartrazine.

CV: ***proarrhythmic events,*** *ECG abnormalities (including conduction defects, sinus pause, junctional rhythm, or AV block),* ***CHF,*** *palpitations,* ***sustained ventricular tachycardia,*** *chest pain, sinus bradycardia,* ***sinus arrest.***
EENT: blurred vision.
GI: *nausea, vomiting, abdominal pain, dyspepsia, diarrhea, dry mouth.*
GU: urine retention.
Skin: rash.
Other: dyspnea, drug fever, sweating, musculoskeletal pain.

INTERACTIONS

Cimetidine: increased plasma levels of and decreased clearance of moricizine. Begin moricizine therapy at low dosage (not more than 600 mg daily) and monitor plasma levels and therapeutic effect closely.
Propranolol, digoxin: additive prolongation of the PR interval. Monitor closely.
Theophylline: increased theophylline clearance and reduced plasma levels. Monitor plasma levels and therapeutic response; adjust theophylline dosage as needed.

NURSING CONSIDERATIONS

• *Contraindicated* in patients with preexisting second- or third-degree AV block, right bundle branch block when associated with left hemiblock (bifascicular block) unless a pacemaker is present, in patients with severe hepatic insufficiency, and in patients in cardiogenic shock and those with hypersensitivity to the drug.
• *Use with extreme caution* in patients with sick sinus syndrome. The drug may cause sinus bradycardia or sinus arrest.
• The drug should be used only for patients with life-threatening ventricular arrhythmias.
• When substituting another antiarrhythmic, withdraw previous antiarrhythmic therapy for one to two half-lives of the drug before starting moricizine at recommended dosage. Patients who have shown a tendency to develop life-threatening arrhythmias after withdrawal of drug therapy should be hospitalized during withdrawal and adjustment to morizicine. Start moricizine therapy after:
– disopyramide, 6 to 12 hours after the last dose.
– mexilitine, 8 to 12 hours after the last dose.
– procainamide, 3 to 6 hours after the last dose.
– propafenone, 8 to 12 hours after the last dose.
– quinidine, 6 to 12 hours after the last dose.
– tocainide, 8 to 12 hours after the last dose.
• Hypokalemia, hyperkalemia, and hypomagnesemia may alter the effects of the drug. Determine electrolyte status and correct imbalances before therapy.
• Patients with hepatic or renal dysfunction will exhibit decreased moricizine clearance. Administer cautiously and monitor effects closely. Note ECG intervals before adjusting dosage.
• Note that the drug has been detected in breast milk. A decision should be made to discontinue breast-feeding or discontinue the drug, depending on the drug's potential benefit to the mother.

procainamide hydrochloride

Procan SR, Promine, Pronestyl**, Pronestyl-SR, Rhythmin

Pregnancy Risk Category: C

HOW SUPPLIED

Tablets: 250 mg, 375 mg, 500 mg
Tablets (sustained-release): 250 mg, 500 mg, 750 mg, 1,000 mg
Capsules: 250 mg, 375 mg, 500 mg
Injection: 100 mg/ml, 500 mg/ml

MECHANISM OF ACTION

A class Ia antiarrhythmic that depresses phase O. It prolongs the action potential. All class I drugs have membrane stabilizing effects.

INDICATIONS & DOSAGE

Premature ventricular contractions, ventricular tachycardia, atrial arrhythmias unresponsive to quinidine, paroxysmal atrial tachycardia –
Adults: 100 mg q 5 minutes slow I.V. push, no faster than 25 to 50 mg/minute until arrhythmias disappear, adverse reactions develop, or 1 g has been given. (Usual effective dose is 500 to 600 mg.) When arrhythmias disappear, give continuous infusion of 2 to 6 mg/minute. If arrhythmias recur, repeat bolus as above and increase infusion rate; 0.5 to 1 g I.M. q 4 to 8 hours until oral therapy begins.

Loading dose for atrial fibrillation or paroxysmal atrial tachycardia –
Adults: 1 to 1.25 g P.O. If arrhythmias persist after 1 hour, give additional 750 mg. If no change occurs, give 500 mg to 1 g q 2 hours until arrhythmias disappear or adverse reactions occur.

Loading dose for ventricular tachycardia –
Adults: 1 g P.O. Maintenance dosage is 50 mg/kg daily q 3 hours; average is 250 to 500 mg q 3 hours.

Note: Sustained-release tablet may be used for maintenance dosing when treating ventricular tachycardia, atrial fibrillation, and paroxysmal atrial tachycardia. Dose is 500 mg to 1 g q 6 hours.

ADVERSE REACTIONS

Common reactions are in italics; life-threatening reactions are in bold italics.
Blood: thrombocytopenia, ***neutropenia*** (especially with sustained-release forms), ***agranulocytosis,*** hemolytic anemia, *increased antinuclear antibodies titer.*
CNS: hallucinations, confusion, ***seizures,*** depression.
CV: ***severe hypotension,*** *bradycardia,* AV block, ***ventricular fibrillation (after parenteral use).***
GI: *nausea, vomiting, anorexia, diarrhea, bitter taste.*
Skin: *maculopapular rash.*
Other: *fever,* lupus erythematosus syndrome (especially after prolonged administration), myalgia.

INTERACTIONS

Amiodarone: increased procainamide levels and possible drug toxicity.
Anticholinergics: additive anticholinergic effects.
Anticholinesterase agents: anticholinesterase dosage may need to be increased.
Cimetidine: may increase procainamide blood levels. Monitor for toxicity.
Neuromuscular blocking agents: increased skeletal muscle relaxant effects. Monitor patient closely.

NURSING CONSIDERATIONS

- *Contraindicated* in patients with hypersensitivity to procaine and related drugs; with complete, second-, or third-degree heart block unassisted by electrical pacemaker; or with myasthenia gravis.
- *Use cautiously* in CHF or other conduction disturbances, such as bundle branch block, sinus bradycardia, or cardiac glycoside intoxication, or with hepatic or renal insufficiency.
- **I.V. use:** Patients receiving infusions must be *attended at all times.* Use an infusion pump to administer the infusion precisely.
- Monitor serum electrolytes, especially potassium level. Hypokalemia predisposes patients to arrhythmias.
- Monitor blood pressure and ECG continuously during I.V. administration. Watch for prolonged Q-T and QRS intervals, heart block, or increased arrhythmias. If these occur,

*Liquid form contains alcohol. **May contain tartrazine.

withhold drug, obtain rhythm strip, and notify doctor immediately.
- Keep patient supine for I.V. administration if hypotension occurs.
- If procainamide is administered too rapidly, I.V. hypotension can occur. Watch closely for adverse reactions and notify doctor if they occur. Instruct patient to report fever, rash, muscle pain, diarrhea, bleeding, bruises, or pleuritic chest pain.
- Procainamide solution for injection may become discolored. If so, check with pharmacy and prepare to discard.
- Note that the vials for I.V. injection contain 1 g of drug: 100 mg/ml (10 ml) or 500 mg/ml (2 ml).
- Monitor CBC frequently during first 3 months of therapy, particularly in patients taking sustained-release dosage forms.
- Decrease dose in hepatic and renal dysfunction, and give over 6 hours. Half-life of procainamide is increased as much as threefold in these states.
- N-acetylprocainamide (NAPA), an active metabolite, may accumulate when renal function is decreased. This may add to toxicity.
- Patient with CHF has a lower volume of distribution and can be treated with lower doses.
- Positive antinuclear antibody titer is common in about 60% of patients who don't have symptoms of lupus erythematosus syndrome. This response seems related to prolonged use, not dosage.
- After prolonged atrial fibrillation, restoration of normal rhythm may result in thromboembolism, due to dislodgment of thrombi from atrial wall. Anticoagulation usually advised before restoration of normal sinus rhythm.
- Stress importance of taking drug exactly as prescribed. Patient may have to set an alarm clock for night doses.
- Reassure patients who are taking the extended-release form of procainamide that a wax matrix "ghost" from the tablet may be passed in the stool. The drug is completely absorbed before this occurs.
- Elderly patients may be more likely to develop hypotension. Monitor blood pressure carefully.

propafenone hydrochloride

Rythmol

Pregnancy Risk Category: C

HOW SUPPLIED

Tablets: 150 mg, 300 mg

MECHANISM OF ACTION

A class Ic antiarrhythmic agent that stabilizes cardiac cell membranes, probably by decreasing sodium influx. It also has weak beta-adrenergic blocking properties.

INDICATIONS & DOSAGE

Suppression of life-threatening ventricular arrhythmias, such as sustained ventricular tachycardia – **Adults:** initially, 150 mg P.O. q 8 hours. Dosage may be increased to 225 mg q 8 hours after 3 or 4 days; if necessary, increase dosage to 300 mg q 8 hours. Maximum daily dosage is 900 mg.

ADVERSE REACTIONS

Common reactions are in italics; life-threatening reactions are in bold italics.

CNS: anorexia, anxiety, ataxia, dizziness, drowsiness, fatigue, headache, insomnia, syncope, tremor, weakness.

CV: angina, atrial fibrillation, bradycardia, bundle branch block, ***CHF,*** chest pain, edema, first-degree AV block, hypotension, increased QRS duration, intraventricular conduction delay, palpitations, ***proarrhythmic events (ventricular tachycardia, premature ventricular contractions).***

EENT: blurred vision.

GI: abdominal pain or cramps, constipation, diarrhea, dyspepsia, flatu-

lence, nausea, vomiting, dry mouth, unusual taste.
Respiratory: dyspnea.
Skin: rash.
Other: diaphoresis, joint pain.

INTERACTIONS
Antiarrhythmics: increased potential for CHF.
Cimetidine: decreased metabolism of propafenone.
Digitalis glycosides, oral anticoagulants: propafenone may increase serum levels of these agents, resulting in toxicity.
Local anesthetics: increased risk of CNS toxicity.
Propranolol, metoprolol: propafenone slows the metabolism of these agents. Dosage adjustments may be necessary.
Quinidine: slows the metabolism of propafenone. Avoid concomitant use.

NURSING CONSIDERATIONS
• *Contraindicated* in severe or uncontrolled CHF; cardiogenic shock; SA, AV, or intraventricular disorders of impulse conduction; sinus node dysfunction in the absence of a pacemaker; severe bradycardia (50 beats/minute or less); marked hypotension; bronchospastic disorders; severe obstructive pulmonary disease; severe electrolyte imbalance; severe hepatic failure; and hypersensitivity to the drug.
• *Use cautiously* in patients with CHF because propafenone can exert a negative inotropic effect on the heart, in use with other cardiac depressant drugs, and in hepatic or renal failure.
• Because plasma levels do not increase linearly with dose, dosage should be increased stepwise at 3- to 4-day intervals.
• Some patients metabolize propafenone rapidly, and early studies indicate that the drug may have a plasma half-life of 5 to 6 hours in fast metabolizers and 17 hours or more in slow metabolizers.
• Continuous cardiac monitoring is recommended during initiation of therapy and during dosage adjustments. If PR interval or QRS duration increase by more than 25%, a reduction in dosage may be necessary.
• Administer drug with food to minimize adverse GI reactions.
• During concomitant use with digoxin, frequently monitor ECG and serum digoxin levels because propafenone increases serum digoxin levels by about 35% to 85%.

quinidine bisulfate
(66.4% quinidine base)
Biquin Durules†, Kinidin Durules‡

quinidine gluconate
(62% quinidine base)
Duraquin, Quinaglute Dura-Tabs, Quinalan, Quinate†

quinidine polygalacturonate
(60.5% quinidine base)
Cardioquin

quinidine sulfate
(83% quinidine base)
Apo-Quinidine†, Novoquindin†, Quine, Quinidex Extentabs, Quinora
Pregnancy Risk Category: C

HOW SUPPLIED
bisulfate
Tablets: 250 mg†‡
gluconate
Tablets (sustained-release): 324 mg, 325 mg†, 330 mg
Injection: 80 mg/ml
polygalacturonate
Tablets: 275 mg
sulfate
Tablets: 100 mg, 200 mg, 300 mg
Tablets (sustained-release): 300 mg
Capsules: 200 mg, 300 mg

Injection: 200 mg/ml

MECHANISM OF ACTION
A class Ia antiarrhythmic that depresses phase O. It prolongs the action potential. All class I drugs have membrane stabilizing effects.

INDICATIONS & DOSAGE
Atrial flutter or fibrillation –
Adults: 200 mg quinidine sulfate or equivalent base P.O. q 2 to 3 hours for 5 to 8 doses with subsequent daily increases until sinus rhythm is restored or toxic effects develop. Administer quinidine only after digitalization to avoid increasing AV conduction. Maximum dosage is 3 to 4 g daily.
Paroxysmal supraventricular tachycardia –
Adults: 400 to 600 mg I.M. gluconate q 2 to 3 hours until toxic adverse reactions develop or arrhythmia subsides.
Premature atrial and ventricular contractions; paroxysmal atrioventricular junctional rhythm; paroxysmal atrial tachycardia; paroxysmal ventricular tachycardia; maintenance after cardioversion of atrial fibrillation or flutter –
Adults: test dose is 50 to 200 mg P.O., then monitor vital signs before beginning therapy. Quinidine sulfate or equivalent base 200 to 400 mg P.O. q 4 to 6 hours; or initially, quinidine gluconate 600 mg I.M., then up to 400 mg q 2 hours, p.r.n.; or quinidine gluconate 800 mg (10 ml of the commercially available solution) added to 40 ml dextrose 5% in water, infused I.V. at 16 mg (1 ml)/minute.
Children: test dose is 2 mg/kg; 3 to 6 mg/kg q 2 to 3 hours for 5 doses P.O. daily.
Severe Plasmodium falciparum *malaria –*
Adults: 10 mg/kg I.V. (gluconate) diluted in 250 ml 0.9% sodium chloride injection and infused over 1 to 2 hours followed by a continuous maintenance infusion of 0.02 mg/kg/minute for 72 hours or until parasitemia is reduced to less than 1%.

ADVERSE REACTIONS
Common reactions are in italics; life-threatening reactions are in bold italics.
Blood: ***hemolytic anemia, thrombocytopenia, agranulocytosis.***
CNS: *vertigo, headache, light-headedness,* confusion, restlessness, cold sweat, pallor, fainting, dementia.
CV: ***premature ventricular contractions; severe hypotension;*** *SA and AV block;* ***ventricular fibrillation,*** *tachycardia;* ***aggravated CHF;*** *ECG changes (particularly widening of QRS complex, notched P waves, widened Q-T interval, ST segment depression).*
EENT: *tinnitus,* excessive salivation, blurred vision.
GI: *diarrhea, nausea, vomiting,* anorexia, abdominal pains.
Hepatic: hepatotoxicity including granulomatous hepatitis.
Skin: rash, petechial hemorrhage of buccal mucosa, pruritus.
Other: angioedema, acute asthmatic attack, respiratory arrest, *fever, cinchonism.*

INTERACTIONS
Acetazolamide, antacids, sodium bicarbonate: may increase quinidine blood levels due to alkaline urine. Monitor for increased effect.
Amiodarone, cimetidine: increased serum quinidine levels. Monitor for increased effect.
Barbiturates, phenytoin, rifampin: may antagonize quinidine activity. Monitor for decreased quinidine effect.
Digoxin: increased serum digoxin levels after initiating quinidine therapy. Monitor closely.
Nifedipine: may decrease quinidine blood levels. Monitor carefully.
Other antiarrhythmics, such as lidocaine, phenytoin, procainamide, and

propranolol: increased risk of toxicity. Use together cautiously.
Verapamil: may result in hypotension. Monitor blood pressure.
Warfarin: increased anticoagulant effect. Monitor closely.

NURSING CONSIDERATIONS

- *Contraindicated* in digitalis glycoside toxicity when AV conduction is grossly impaired and in complete AV block with AV nodal or idioventricular pacemaker.
- *Use cautiously* in myasthenia gravis. Anticholinesterase drug doses may have to be increased.
- May increase toxicity of digitalis derivatives. *Use cautiously* in patients previously digitalized. Monitor digoxin levels.
- Monitor liver function tests during the first 4 to 8 weeks of therapy.
- When used to treat severe malaria, patients should be hospitalized in an intensive care setting. Continuous monitoring is necessary. Decrease infusion rate if plasma quinidine level exceeds 6 mcg/ml, uncorrected Q-T interval exceeds 0.6 second, or QRS widening exceeds 25% of baseline.
- Dosage varies – some patients may require drug q 4 hours; others, q 6 hours. Titrate dose by both clinical response and blood levels.
- When changing route of administration, alter dosage to compensate for variations in quinidine base content.
- Dosage should be decreased in CHF and hepatic disease.
- Check apical pulse rate and blood pressure before starting therapy. If you detect extremes in pulse rate, withhold drug and notify doctor at once.
- Lidocaine may be effective in treating quinidine-induced arrhythmias, because it increases AV conduction.
- GI adverse reactions, especially diarrhea, are signs of toxicity. Notify doctor. Check quinidine blood levels, which are toxic when greater than 8 mcg/ml. GI symptoms may be decreased by giving with meals. Monitor patient response carefully.
- Instruct patient to notify doctor if skin rash, fever, unusual bleeding, bruising, ringing in ears, or visual disturbance occurs.
- After long-standing atrial fibrillation, restoration of normal sinus rhythm may result in thromboembolism due to dislodgment of thrombi from atrial wall. Anticoagulation often advised before restoration of normal atrial rhythm.
- Never use discolored (brownish) quinidine solution.
- Store away from heat and direct light.

sotalol

Betapace, Sotacor†
Pregnancy Risk Category: B

HOW SUPPLIED
Tablets: 80 mg, 160 mg, 240 mg

MECHANISM OF ACTION
A nonselective beta-adrenergic blocker that depresses sinus heart rate, slows AV conduction, decreases cardiac output, and lowers systolic and diastolic blood pressure.

INDICATIONS & DOSAGE
Documented, life-threatening ventricular arrhythmias –
Adults: initially, 80 mg P.O. b.i.d. Increase dosage q 2 to 3 days as needed and tolerated; most patients respond to daily dosage of 160 to 320 mg. A few patients with refractory arrhythmias have received as much as 640 mg daily.
Dosage adjustment for patients with renal failure –
Adults: If creatinine clearance is greater than 60 ml/minute/1.73 m^2, no adjustment in dosage interval is necessary. If creatinine clearance is 30 to 60 ml/minute/1.73 m^2, give q 24

*Liquid form contains alcohol. **May contain tartrazine.

hours; 10 to 30 ml/minute/1.73 m^2, q 36 to 48 hours; less than 10 ml/minute/1.73 m^2, individualize dosage.
Hypertension† –
Adults: 80 mg P.O. b.i.d. Increase dosage at weekly intervals in increments of 80 mg b.i.d. as needed and tolerated. Most patients respond to daily dosage of 160 to 320 mg; patients taking 320 mg or less daily may take drug as a single daily dose in the morning.
Angina† –
Adults: 80 mg P.O. b.i.d. Increase dosage at weekly intervals in increments of 80 mg b.i.d. as needed and tolerated. Most patients respond to doses of 160 mg b.i.d.; maximum daily dose is 480 mg.

ADVERSE REACTIONS

Common reactions are in italics; life-threatening reactions are in bold italics.
CNS: *asthenia, headache, dizziness, weakness, fatigue.*
CV: *bradycardia,* ***arrhythmias, CHF, AV block.***
GI: *nausea.*
Respiratory: *dyspnea,* ***bronchospasm.***

INTERACTIONS

Antiarrhythmics: additive effects. Avoid concomitant use.
Antihypertensives; catecholamine-depleting drugs, such as reserpine and guanethidine: enhanced hypotensive effects. Monitor closely.
Calcium channel antagonists: enhanced myocardial depression. Avoid concomitant use.
Clonidine: beta blockers may enhance the rebound effect seen after withdrawal of clonidine. Discontinue sotalol several days before withdrawing clonidine.
General anesthetics: may cause additional myocardial depression. Monitor closely.

NURSING CONSIDERATIONS

- *Contraindicated* in patients with severe sinus node dysfunction, sinus bradycardia, second- and third-degree AV block (unless a functioning pacemaker is present), congenital or acquired long QT syndrome, cardiogenic shock, CHF, hypokalemia, hypomagnesemia, bronchial asthma, and allergic rhinitis.
- *Use cautiously* in patients with renal impairment. Because drug is excreted primarily in the urine, dosage adjustments are necessary; for the same reason, such patients take longer to achieve steady-state levels of drug. Dosage increments should be scheduled to follow administration of five or six doses.
- *Also use cautiously* in patients with diabetes mellitus. Beta-adrenergic blockers may mask signs and symptoms of hypoglycemia.
- Adjust dosage slowly, allowing 2 to 3 days between dosage increments to allow adequate monitoring of QT intervals and for plasma levels of drug to reach steady state.
- Because proarrhythmic events may occur at start of therapy and during dosage adjustments, patient should be hospitalized. Facilities and personnel should be readily available for cardiac rhythm monitoring and interpretation of ECG waveforms.
- Although patients receiving I.V. lidocaine have started sotalol therapy without ill effect, other antiarrhythmic drugs should be withdrawn before therapy with sotalol. Usually, sotalol therapy should be delayed until two or three half-lives of the withdrawn drug have elapsed. After withdrawal of amiodarone, sotalol shouldn't be administered until the QT interval normalizes.
- Monitor serum electrolytes regularly, especially if patient is receiving diuretics. Electrolyte imbalances, such as hypokalemia or hypomagnesemia, may enhance QT prolongation

and increase risk of serious arrhythmias, such as torsades de pointes.

- Teach patient about his disease and therapy. Explain the importance of taking this drug as prescribed, even when he's feeling well. Tell patient not to discontinue drug suddenly. If unpleasant adverse reactions occur, he should call doctor.
- Tell patient to take drug on an empty stomach, 1 hour before or 2 hours after meals, because food can interfere with absorption.

tocainide hydrochloride

Tonocard

Pregnancy Risk Category: C

HOW SUPPLIED

Tablets: 400 mg, 600 mg

MECHANISM OF ACTION

A class Ib antiarrhythmic that depresses phase O. It shortens the action potential. All class I drugs have membrane stabilizing effects.

INDICATIONS & DOSAGE

Suppression of symptomatic ventricular arrhythmias, including frequent premature ventricular contractions and ventricular tachycardia –

Adults: initially, 400 mg P.O. q 8 hours. Usual dosage is between 1,200 and 1,800 mg daily in three divided doses.

ADVERSE REACTIONS

Common reactions are in italics; life-threatening reactions are in bold italics.

Blood: ***blood dyscrasia, including aplastic anemia.***

CNS: *light-headedness, tremors,* restlessness, paresthesias, confusion, dizziness.

CV: hypotension, ***new or worsened arrhythmias, CHF.***

EENT: blurred vision.

GI: *nausea, vomiting, epigastric pain,* constipation, diarrhea, anorexia.

Hepatic: hepatitis.

Respiratory: ***respiratory arrest,*** pulmonary fibrosis, pneumonitis, ***pulmonary edema.***

Skin: rash.

INTERACTIONS

Beta blockers: decreased myocardial contractility; increased CNS toxicity.

NURSING CONSIDERATIONS

- *Contraindicated* in patients with hypersensitivity to lidocaine or other amide-type local anesthetics and in patients with second- or third-degree AV block in the absence of a ventricular pacemaker.
- *Use cautiously* in CHF or diminished cardiac reserve and in hepatic or renal impairment. These patients may often be treated effectively with a lower dose.
- Therapeutic blood levels range from 4 to 10 mcg/ml.
- Adverse reactions are generally mild, transient, and reversible by reducing dosage. GI reactions can be minimized by taking the drug with food.
- Dizziness and falling are more likely to occur in elderly patients.
- Monitor patient for tremor, which may indicate approaching maximum dose.
- Considered by cardiologists as an "oral lidocaine." May ease transition from I.V. lidocaine to oral antiarrhythmic therapy. Monitor patient carefully during this transition period.

21

Antianginals

amlodipine besylate
bepridil hydrochloride
diltiazem hydrochloride
erythrityl tetranitrate
isosorbide dinitrate
isosorbide mononitrate
nadolol
nicardipine
nifedipine
nitroglycerin
pentaerythritol tetranitrate
propranolol hydrochloride
verapamil hydrochloride

COMBINATION PRODUCTS

ANGIJEN NO. 1: pentaerythritol tetranitrate 20 mg and phenobarbital sodium 15 mg.
ARCOTRATE NO. 3: pentaerythritol tetranitrate 20 mg and phenobarbital sodium 8 mg.
BITRATE: pentaerythritol tetranitrate 15 mg and phenobarbital sodium 20 mg.
DIMYCOR: pentaerythritol tetranitrate 10 mg and phenobarbital sodium 15 mg.
NITROTYM-PLUS: nitroglycerin 2.5 mg and butabarbital sodium 48 mg.
PERBUZEM: pentaerythritol tetranitrate 10 mg and butabarbital sodium 15 mg.

---

amlodipine besylate

Norvasc

Pregnancy Risk Category: C

HOW SUPPLIED

Tablets: 2.5 mg, 5 mg, 10 mg

MECHANISM OF ACTION

Inhibits calcium ion influx across cardiac and smooth muscle cells, thus decreasing myocardial contractility and oxygen demand, and dilates coronary arteries and arterioles.

INDICATIONS & DOSAGE

Chronic stable angina; vasospastic angina (Prinzmetal's or variant angina) –
Adults: initially, 10 mg P.O. daily. Small, frail, or elderly patients or patients with hepatic insufficiency should begin therapy at 5 mg daily. Most patients require 10 mg daily for adequate therapy.
Hypertension –
Adults: initially, 5 mg P.O. daily. Small, frail, or elderly patients; patients currently receiving other antihypertensive medications; or patients with hepatic insufficiency should begin therapy at 2.5 mg daily. Adjust dosage according to patient response and tolerance. Maximum dosage is 10 mg daily.

ADVERSE REACTIONS

Common reactions are in italics; life-threatening reactions are in bold italics.
CNS: *headache,* fatigue, somnolence.
CV: *edema,* dizziness, flushing, palpitation.
GI: nausea, abdominal pain.

INTERACTIONS

None reported.

NURSING CONSIDERATIONS

- *Contraindicated* in patients with hypersensitivity to the drug.
- *Use cautiously* in patients receiving other peripheral vasodilators, especially patients with severe aortic stenosis, and in those with CHF. Because drug is metabolized by the liver, also use cautiously and in reduced dosage in patients with severe hepatic disease.

• Some patients, especially those with severe obstructive coronary artery disease, have developed increased frequency, duration, or severity of angina or even acute MI after initiation of calcium channel blocker therapy or at time of dosage increase. Monitor patient carefully.
• Notify doctor if signs of CHF, such as swelling of hands and feet or shortness of breath, occur.
• Sublingual nitroglycerin may be taken as needed when anginal symptoms are acute. If patient continues nitrate therapy during titration of amlodipine dosage, urge continued compliance.
• Monitor blood pressure frequently during initiation of therapy. Because drug-induced vasodilation has a gradual onset, acute hypotension is rare.
• Be sure that patient understands his disease. He should continue taking the drug, even when he's feeling better; watch his diet; and check with the doctor or pharmacist before taking other medications, including OTC drugs.
• Dosage adjustments are necessary in patients with hepatic failure but not renal failure because drug is eliminated primarily by the liver.
• Amlodipine may be taken without regard to meals.

bepridil hydrochloride

Vascor

Pregnancy Risk Category C

HOW SUPPLIED

Tablets: 200 mg, 300 mg, 400 mg

MECHANISM OF ACTION

A calcium channel blocking agent that inhibits calcium ion influx across cardiac and smooth muscle cells.

INDICATIONS & DOSAGE

Treatment of chronic stable angina in patients intolerant of or who fail to respond to other agents –

Adults: initially, 200 mg P.O. daily. After 10 days, increase dosage based on response. Maintenance dosage in most patients is 300 mg/day. Maximum daily dosage is 400 mg.

ADVERSE REACTIONS

Common reactions are in italics; life-threatening reactions are in bold italics.

Blood: ***agranulocytosis.***
CNS: dizziness.
CV: edema, flushing, palpitations, tachycardia, ***ventricular arrhythmias.***
GI: nausea, diarrhea.
Skin: rash.
Other: dyspnea.

INTERACTIONS

Fentanyl anesthesia: severe hypotension has been reported with concomitant use of a beta blocker and a calcium channel blocker. Be sure to inform anesthesiologist that the patient is taking a calcium channel blocker.

NURSING CONSIDERATIONS

• *Contraindicated* in patients with hypersensitivity to the drug.
• *Use cautiously* in patients with CHF, especially if combined with a beta-adrenergic blocking agent.
• Not considered a primary agent because the drug has been associated with severe ventricular arrhythmias, including torsades de pointes; also associated with agranulocytosis.
• Elderly patients may require more frequent monitoring to prevent adverse reactions.
• Tell patients to promptly report any unusual bruising or bleeding or any persistent infections (including sore throat, fever, or malaise).

*Liquid form contains alcohol. **May contain tartrazine.

diltiazem hydrochloride

Cardizem, Cardizem CD, Cardizem SR, Dilacor XR

Pregnancy Risk Category: C

HOW SUPPLIED

Tablets: 30 mg, 60 mg, 90 mg, 120 mg
Capsules (dual-release; Cardizem CD): 120 mg, 180 mg, 240 mg, 300 mg
Capsules (extended-release; Cardizem SR, Dilacor XR): 60 mg, 90 mg, 120 mg
Injection: 5 mg/ml

MECHANISM OF ACTION

Inhibits calcium ion influx across cardiac and smooth muscle cells, decreasing myocardial contractility and oxygen demand, and dilates coronary arteries and peripheral arterioles.

INDICATIONS & DOSAGE

Management of vasospastic (Prinzmetal's or variant) angina and classic chronic stable angina pectoris –
Adults: 30 mg P.O. t.i.d. or q.i.d. before meals and at bedtime. Dosage may be gradually increased to maximum 360 mg/day, in divided doses. Alternatively, use 120 or 180 mg (dual-release capsule). Titrate as needed and tolerated to maximum 480 mg daily.
Hypertension –
Adults: 60 mg P.O. b.i.d. (extended-release capsule). Titrate dosage to effect. Maximum recommended dosage is 360 mg/day; experience with higher doses is limited. Alternatively, initially use 180 to 240 mg daily (dual-release capsule). Maximum effect is seen within 14 days. Adjust dosage as necessary.
Atrial fibrillation or flutter; paroxysmal supraventricular tachycardia –
Adults: 0.25 mg/kg as a bolus injection over 2 minutes. If response is inadequate, a dose of 0.35 mg/kg may be given after 15 minutes and followed with a continuous infusion of 10 mg/hour. Some patients may respond to infusion rates of 5 mg/hour; do not exceed the maximum dose of 15 mg/hour. Infusions lasting longer than 24 hours are not recommended.

ADVERSE REACTIONS

Common reactions are in italics; life-threatening reactions are in bold italics.
CNS: *headache, fatigue, drowsiness,* dizziness, nervousness, depression, insomnia, confusion.
CV: *edema, **arrhythmias,*** flushing, bradycardia, hypotension, conduction abnormalities, ***CHF***.
GI: *nausea,* vomiting, diarrhea.
GU: nocturia, polyuria.
Hepatic: transient elevation of liver enzymes.
Skin: *rash,* pruritus.
Other: photosensitivity.

INTERACTIONS

Cimetidine: may inhibit diltiazem metabolism. Monitor for toxicity.
Cyclosporine: diltiazem may increase serum cyclosporine levels, possibly by decreasing its metabolism, leading to increased risk of cyclosporine toxicity. Avoid concomitant use.
Digoxin: diltiazem may increase serum levels of digoxin. Monitor for toxicity.
Furosemide: forms a precipitate when mixed with diltiazem injection. Administer through separate I.V. lines.
Propranolol (and other beta blockers): may prolong cardiac conduction time. Use together cautiously.

NURSING CONSIDERATIONS

- *Contraindicated* in sick sinus syndrome, unless a functioning ventricular pacemaker is present; hypotension when systolic blood pressure is less than 90 mm Hg; and second- or third-degree AV block.
- *Use cautiously* in elderly patients because duration of action may be

prolonged; in impaired ventricular function or conduction abnormalities; and in impaired hepatic or renal function.

- Monitor blood pressure during initiation of therapy and dosage adjustments. Assist patients with ambulation during initiation of diltiazem therapy because dizziness may occur.
- If systolic pressure is less than 90 mm Hg, or heart rate is less than 60 beats/minute, withhold dose and notify doctor.
- If nitrate therapy is prescribed during titration of diltiazem dosage, urge patient to continue compliance. Sublingual nitroglycerin, especially, may be taken concomitantly as needed when anginal symptoms are acute.
- Of the available calcium antagonists, diltiazem may offer the lowest risk of adverse reactions.
- Dual-release capsules (Cardizem CD) provide therapeutic levels of the drug over 24 hours. These capsules contain two types of drug-impregnated beads that differ by the thickness of their encapsulating copolymer membranes. Drug is released from 40% of the beads within the first 12 hours; from the remaining 60%, over the second 12 hours after ingestion.
- May be useful as migraine prophylaxis in some patients. However, diltiazem itself may cause headaches.

erythrityl tetranitrate

Cardilate

Pregnancy Risk Category: C

HOW SUPPLIED

Tablets (chewable): 10 mg
Tablets (oral, sublingual, buccal): 5 mg, 10 mg

MECHANISM OF ACTION

Reduces cardiac oxygen demand by decreasing left ventricular end-diastolic pressure (preload) and, to a lesser extent, systemic vascular resistance (afterload). Also increases blood flow through the collateral coronary vessels.

INDICATIONS & DOSAGE

Prophylaxis and long-term management of frequent or recurrent anginal pain, reduced exercise tolerance associated with angina pectoris –
Adults: 5 mg orally, sublingually, or buccally t.i.d., increasing in 2 to 3 days if needed.

ADVERSE REACTIONS

Common reactions are in italics; life-threatening reactions are in bold italics.
CNS: *headache, sometimes with throbbing; dizziness;* weakness.
CV: *orthostatic hypotension, tachycardia, flushing, palpitations,* fainting.
GI: nausea, vomiting.
Skin: cutaneous vasodilation.
Local: sublingual burning.
Other: hypersensitivity reactions.

INTERACTIONS

None significant.

NURSING CONSIDERATIONS

- *Contraindicated* in hypersensitivity to nitrites, head trauma, cerebral hemorrhage, or severe anemia.
- *Use cautiously* in hypotension.
- Monitor blood pressure and intensity and duration of response to drug.
- May cause headaches, especially at first. Treat headache with aspirin or acetaminophen. Dosage may need to be reduced temporarily, but tolerance usually develops.
- Tell patient to take medication regularly, even long-term, if ordered, and to keep it easily accessible at all times. Physiologically necessary but not habit-forming.
- Additional dose may be taken before anticipated stress or at bedtime if angina is nocturnal.
- Advise patient to avoid alcoholic

beverages; may produce increased hypotension.

- May cause orthostatic hypotension. To minimize it, patient should change to upright position slowly. He should go up and down stairs carefully, and lie down at the first sign of dizziness.
- Teach patient to take sublingual tablet at first sign of attack. He should wet the tablet with saliva, place it under the tongue until completely absorbed, and sit down and rest. Dose may be repeated every 10 to 15 minutes for a maximum of three doses. If no relief, patient should call doctor or go to hospital emergency room. If patient complains of tingling sensation with drug placed sublingually, he may try holding tablet in buccal pouch.
- Teach patient to take oral tablet on empty stomach, either half an hour before or 1 to 2 hours after meals, and to swallow oral tablets whole.
- Drug should not be discontinued abruptly – coronary vasospasm may occur.
- Store drug in cool place, in a tightly closed container, away from light. To ensure freshness, replace supply every 3 months. Remove cotton from container, since it absorbs drug.

isosorbide dinitrate

Apo-ISDN†, Cedocard-SR†, Coronex†, Dilatrate-SR, Iso-Bid, Isonate, Isorbid, Isordil, Isotrate, Nitro-Spray‡, Novosorbide†, Sorbitrate, Sorbitrate SA

isosorbide mononitrate

Ismo

Pregnancy Risk Category: C

HOW SUPPLIED

isosorbide dinitrate

Tablets: 5 mg, 10 mg, 20 mg, 30 mg, 40 mg
Tablets (chewable): 5 mg, 10 mg
Tablets (sublingual): 2.5 mg, 5 mg, 10 mg
Tablets (sustained-release): 40 mg
Capsules: 40 mg
Capsules (sustained-release): 40 mg
Topical spray: 10%‡, 12.5 mg/metered spray‡

isosorbide mononitrate

Tablets: 20 mg

MECHANISM OF ACTION

Reduces cardiac oxygen demand by decreasing left ventricular end-diastolic pressure (preload) and, to a lesser extent, systemic vascular resistance (afterload). Also increases blood flow through the collateral coronary vessels.

Most of the pharmacologic activity of isosorbide dinitrate is attributed to its active metabolite, isosorbide mononitrate.

INDICATIONS & DOSAGE

Treatment of acute anginal attacks (sublingual and chewable tablets of isosorbide dinitrate only); prophylaxis in situations likely to cause anginal attacks; treatment of chronic ischemic heart disease (by preload reduction) – **Adults:** *Sublingual form* – 2.5 to 10 mg under the tongue for prompt relief of anginal pain, repeated q 5 to 10 minutes (maximum of three doses per 30-minute period). For prophylaxis, 2.5 to 10 mg under the tongue q 2 to 3 hours.

Chewable form – 5 to 10 mg, p.r.n., for acute attack or q 2 to 3 hours for prophylaxis but only after initial test dose of 5 mg to determine risk of severe hypotension.

Oral form (isosorbide dinitrate) – 5 to 30 mg P.O. q.i.d. for prophylaxis only (use smallest effective dose); 40 mg P.O. (sustained-release form) q 6 to 12 hours.

Oral form (isosorbide mononitrate) – 20 mg P.O. b.i.d., usually 7 hours apart (the first dose upon awakening).

Topical form (where available) – initially, 2 sprays to the chest in the morning from a distance of about 20

cm. Rub solution in. Dosage is gradually increased as needed to 2 to 5 sprays, daily or b.i.d. (in the morning and h.s.).
Adjunct with other vasodilators, such as hydralazine and prazosin, in treatment of severe chronic CHF–
Adults: *Oral or chewable form* – 20 to 40 mg q 4 hours.

ADVERSE REACTIONS
Common reactions are in italics; life-threatening reactions are in bold italics.
CNS: *headache, sometimes with throbbing; dizziness;* weakness.
CV: *orthostatic hypotension, tachycardia, palpitations, ankle edema,* fainting.
GI: nausea, vomiting.
Skin: cutaneous vasodilation, *flushing.*
Local: sublingual burning.
Other: hypersensitivity reactions.

INTERACTIONS
Antihypertensives: possibly increased hypotensive effects. Monitor closely during initial therapy.

NURSING CONSIDERATIONS
- *Contraindicated* in hypersensitivity to nitrites, head trauma, cerebral hemorrhage, or severe anemia.
- *Use cautiously* in hypotension.
- Monitor blood pressure and intensity and duration of response to drug.
- May cause headaches, especially at first. Treat headache with aspirin or acetaminophen. Dosage may need to be reduced temporarily, but tolerance usually develops.
- Tell patient to take medication regularly, even long-term, if ordered, and to keep it easily accessible at all times. Physiologically necessary but not habit-forming.
- Tell patient taking isosorbide dinitrate to take additional dose before anticipated stress or at bedtime if angina is nocturnal.
- Advise patient to avoid alcoholic beverages; they may produce increased hypotension.
- May cause orthostatic hypotension. To minimize it, patient should change to upright position slowly. He should go up and down stairs carefully, and lie down at the first sign of dizziness.
- Teach patient to take sublingual tablet at first sign of attack. He should wet the tablet with saliva, place it under the tongue until completely absorbed, and sit down and rest. Dose may be repeated every 10 to 15 minutes for a maximum of three doses. If no relief, patient should call doctor or go to hospital emergency room. If patient complains of tingling sensation with drug placed sublingually, he may try holding tablet in buccal pouch.
- Warn patient not to confuse sublingual with oral form.
- Teach patient taking oral form of isosorbide dinitrate to take oral tablet on empty stomach, either half an hour before or 1 to 2 hours after meals; to swallow oral tablets whole; and to chew chewable tablets thoroughly before swallowing.
- The dosage regimen for isosorbide mononitrate (one tablet upon awakening; the second dose in 7 hours) is intended to minimize nitrate tolerance by providing a substantial nitrate-free interval.
- Drug should not be discontinued abruptly – coronary vasospasm may occur.
- Store in cool place, in tightly closed container, away from light.
- Has been used investigationally in treatment of diffuse esophageal spasms.

nadolol
Corgard
Pregnancy Risk Category: C

HOW SUPPLIED
Tablets: 20 mg, 40 mg, 80 mg, 120 mg, 160 mg

*Liquid form contains alcohol. **May contain tartrazine.

MECHANISM OF ACTION

A beta-adrenergic blocker that reduces cardiac oxygen demand by blocking catecholamine-induced increases in heart rate, blood pressure, and force of myocardial contraction. Depresses renin secretion.

INDICATIONS & DOSAGE

Management of angina pectoris –
Adults: 40 mg P.O. once daily, initially. Dosage may be increased in 40- to 80-mg increments until optimum response occurs. Usual maintenance dosage range is 40 to 240 mg once daily.
Treatment of hypertension –
Adults: 40 mg P.O. once daily, initially. Dosage may be increased in 40- to 80-mg increments until optimum response occurs. Usual maintenance dosage range is 40 to 320 mg once daily. Doses of 640 mg may be necessary in rare cases.

ADVERSE REACTIONS

Common reactions are in italics; life-threatening reactions are in bold italics.
CNS: fatigue, lethargy.
CV: *bradycardia, hypotension,* ***CHF,*** peripheral vascular disease.
GI: nausea, vomiting, diarrhea.
Metabolic: hypoglycemia without tachycardia (in diabetic patients).
Skin: rash.
Other: *increased airway resistance,* fever.

INTERACTIONS

Antihypertensive agents: enhanced antihypertensive effect.
Cardiac glycosides: excessive bradycardia and increased depressant effect on myocardium. Use together cautiously.
Epinephrine: severe vasoconstriction and reflex bradycardia. Monitor blood pressure and observe patient carefully.
Indomethacin: decreased antihypertensive effect. Monitor blood pressure and adjust dosage.
Insulin, hypoglycemic drugs (oral): can alter dosage requirements in previously stabilized diabetics. Observe patient carefully.

NURSING CONSIDERATIONS

- *Contraindicated* in bronchial asthma, sinus bradycardia and greater than first-degree conduction block, and cardiogenic shock.
- *Use cautiously* in patients with heart failure, chronic bronchitis, renal or hepatic insufficiency, or emphysema. Elderly patients may experience enhanced adverse reactions. Dose may need to be adjusted.
- Always check patient's apical pulse before giving this drug. If slower than 60 beats/minute, withhold drug and call doctor.
- Monitor blood pressure frequently. If patient develops severe hypotension, administer a vasopressor, as ordered.
- Don't discontinue abruptly; can exacerbate angina and myocardial infarction. Gradually reduce dosage over 1 to 2 weeks.
- Teach patient about his disease and therapy. Explain the importance of taking this drug as prescribed, even when he's feeling well. Tell outpatient not to discontinue drug suddenly, but to call doctor if unpleasant adverse reactions occur.
- Has been used in a limited number of patients with atrial flutter or fibrillation. Also has been used for a few patients in the treatment of migraine headaches.
- This drug masks common signs of shock, hyperthyroidism, and hypoglycemia.
- May be given without regard to meals.

nicardipine

Cardene, Cardene SR

Pregnancy Risk Category: C

HOW SUPPLIED

Capsules (immediate-release): 20 mg, 30 mg
Capsules (sustained-release): 30 mg, 45 mg, 60 mg

MECHANISM OF ACTION

Inhibits calcium ion influx across cardiac and smooth muscle cells, thus decreasing myocardial contractility and oxygen demand, and dilates coronary arteries and arterioles.

INDICATIONS & DOSAGE

Chronic stable angina (used alone or in combination with beta blockers) –
Adults: initially, 20 mg P.O. t.i.d. (immediate-release only). Titrate dosage according to patient response. Usual dosage range is 20 to 40 mg t.i.d.
Hypertension –
Adults: initially, 20 to 40 mg P.O. t.i.d. (immediate-release) or 30 mg b.i.d. (sustained-release). Increase dosage according to patient response.

ADVERSE REACTIONS

Common reactions are in italics; life-threatening reactions are in bold italics.
CNS: dizziness or light-headedness, headache, paresthesias, drowsiness, asthenia.
CV: peripheral edema, palpitations, angina, tachycardia.
GI: nausea, abdominal discomfort, dry mouth.
Skin: rash, flushing.

INTERACTIONS

Antihypertensive agents: enhanced antihypertensive effect.
Beta-adrenergic blocking agents: may increase cardiac depressant effects. Monitor patient closely.
Cimetidine: may decrease metabolism of calcium channel blocking agents. Monitor for increased pharmacologic effect.
Cyclosporine: nicardipine may increase plasma levels of cyclosporine. Monitor for toxicity.
Theophylline: pharmacologic effects of theophylline may be enhanced. Monitor for toxicity.

NURSING CONSIDERATIONS

- *Contraindicated* in patients with hypersensitivity to nicardipine and in advanced aortic stenosis.
- *Use cautiously* in cardiac conduction disturbances, hypotension, and CHF.
- Some patients may experience increased frequency, severity, or duration of chest pain at beginning of therapy or during dosage adjustments. The mechanism for this adverse reaction is not known. Advise patient to report chest pain immediately.
- Patients with renal impairment should be titrated slowly to optimal response. Begin therapy with 20 mg P.O. t.i.d.
- Patients with hepatic impairment should receive lower initial doses (20 mg P.O. b.i.d.) and be carefully titrated to optimal response.
- Allow at least 3 days between dosage adjustments to achieve steady plasma levels.
- Measure blood pressure frequently during initial therapy. Maximum blood pressure response occurs about 1 hour after dosing with the immediate-release form and 2 to 4 hours after the sustained-release form. Check for potential orthostatic hypotension. Because large swings in blood pressure may occur based on blood level of drug, assess adequacy of antihypertensive effect 8 hours after dosing.
- When switching patients from the immediate-release form to the sustained-release preparation, the total daily dosage of the immediate-release form may be used as a guide; how-

ever, in many patients, it isn't a useful predictor of the total daily dosage of sustained-release drug. Individualize therapy and monitor closely.

nifedipine

Adalat, Adalat P.A.†, Apo-Nifed, Novo-Nifedin, Procardia, Procardia XL

Pregnancy Risk Category: C

HOW SUPPLIED

Tablets (sustained-release): 30 mg, 60 mg, 90 mg
Capsules: 10 mg, 20 mg

MECHANISM OF ACTION

Inhibits calcium ion influx across cardiac and smooth muscle cells, decreasing myocardial contractility and oxygen demand, and dilates coronary arteries and arterioles.

INDICATIONS & DOSAGE

Management of vasospastic (also called Prinzmetal's or variant) angina and classic chronic stable angina pectoris; Raynaud's disease –
Adults: starting dose is 10 mg P.O. t.i.d. Usual effective dose range is 10 to 20 mg t.i.d. Some patients may require up to 30 mg q.i.d. Maximum daily dosage is 180 mg.
Hypertension –
Adults: 30 or 60 mg P.O. (sustained-release form only) once daily. Titrate over a 7- to 14-day period.

ADVERSE REACTIONS

Common reactions are in italics; life-threatening reactions are in bold italics.
CNS: *dizziness, light-headedness, flushing, headache,* weakness, syncope.
CV: peripheral edema, hypotension, palpitations.
EENT: nasal congestion.
GI: *nausea, heartburn,* diarrhea.
Metabolic: hypokalemia.
Other: muscle cramps, dyspnea.

INTERACTIONS

Cimetidine, ranitidine: decreased nifedipine metabolism.
Propranolol (and other beta blockers): may cause hypotension and heart failure. Use together cautiously.

NURSING CONSIDERATIONS

- *Use cautiously* in CHF or hypotension and in elderly patients because duration of action may be prolonged.
- Monitor blood pressure regularly, especially in patients who are also taking beta blockers or antihypertensives.
- Monitor serum potassium level regularly.
- Patient may briefly develop anginal exacerbation when beginning drug therapy or when dosage is increased. Reassure him that this symptom is temporary.
- Although rebound effect hasn't been observed when drug is stopped, dosage should still be reduced slowly under doctor's supervision.
- If patient is kept on nitrate therapy while drug dosage is being titrated, urge him to continue his compliance. Sublingual nitroglycerin, especially, may be taken as needed when anginal symptoms are acute.
- Instruct patient to swallow the capsule whole without breaking, crushing, or chewing it. The sustained-release tablets should never be chewed, crushed, or broken.
- Sublingual form of nifedipine is not available. However, the liquid in the oral capsule can be withdrawn by puncturing the capsule with a needle. Instill the drug into the buccal pouch.
- Sublingual nifedipine may be useful in decreasing blood pressure during hypertensive emergencies. Continuous blood pressure and ECG monitoring is recommended.
- Protect capsules from direct light and moisture and store at room temperature.

nitroglycerin (glyceryl trinitrate)

Deponit, Klavikordal, Niong, Nitradisc‡, Nitro-Bid, Nitro-Bid I.V., Nitrocap, Nitrocap T.D., Nitrocine, Nitrodisc, Nitro-Dur, Nitro-Dur II, Nitrogard, Nitrogard SR, Nitrol, Nitrolate Ointment‡, Nitrolin, Nitrolingual, Nitrol TSAR, Nitronet, Nitrong, Nitrong S.R., Nitrospan, Nitrostat, Nitrostat I.V., NTS, Transderm-Nitro, Tridil

Pregnancy Risk Category: C

HOW SUPPLIED

Tablets (buccal): 1 mg, 2 mg, 3 mg
Tablets (sublingual): 0.15 mg (1/400 gr), 0.3 mg (1/200 gr), 0.4 mg (1/150 gr), 0.6 mg (1/100 gr)
Tablets (sustained-release): 2.6 mg, 6.5 mg, 9 mg
Capsules (sustained-release): 6.5 mg, 9 mg
I.V.: 0.5 mg/ml, 0.8 mg/ml, 5 mg/ml
Aerosol (translingual): 0.4 mg/metered spray
Topical: 2% ointment
Transdermal: 2.5 mg, 5 mg, 7.5 mg, 10 mg, 15 mg/24 hour systems

MECHANISM OF ACTION

Reduces cardiac oxygen demand by decreasing left ventricular end-diastolic pressure (preload) and, to a lesser extent, systemic vascular resistance (afterload). Also increases blood flow through the collateral coronary vessels.

INDICATIONS & DOSAGE

Prophylaxis against chronic anginal attacks –

Adults: 2.5 mg sustained-release (capsule) q 8 to 12 hours; or 2% ointment: Start with ½″ ointment, increasing by ½″ increments until headache occurs, then decreasing to previous dose. Range of dosage with ointment is 2″ to 5″. Usual dose is 1″ to 2″. Alternatively, transdermal disc or pad (Nitrodisc, Nitro-Dur, or Transderm-Nitro) may be applied to hairless site once daily.

Relief of acute angina pectoris, prophylaxis to prevent or minimize anginal attacks when taken immediately before stressful events –

Adults: 1 sublingual tablet (gr 1/400, 1/200, 1/150, 1/100) dissolved under the tongue or in the buccal pouch immediately upon indication of anginal attack. May repeat q 5 minutes for 15 minutes. Or, using Nitrolingual spray, spray one or two doses into mouth, preferably onto or under the tongue. May repeat q 3 to 5 minutes to a maximum of 3 doses within a 15-minute period. Or, transmucosally, 1 to 3 mg q 3 to 5 hours during waking hours.

To control hypertension associated with surgery; to treat CHF associated with myocardial infarction (MI); to relieve angina pectoris in acute situations; to produce controlled hypotension during surgery (by I.V. infusion) –

Adults: initial infusion rate is 5 mcg/minute. May be increased by 5 mcg/minute q 3 to 5 minutes until a response is noted. If a 20 mcg/minute rate doesn't produce a response, dosage may be increased by as much as 20 mcg/minute q 3 to 5 minutes.

ADVERSE REACTIONS

Common reactions are in italics; life-threatening reactions are in bold italics.

CNS: *headache, sometimes with throbbing; dizziness;* weakness.
CV: *orthostatic hypotension, tachycardia, flushing, palpitations,* fainting.
GI: nausea, vomiting.
Skin: cutaneous vasodilation.
Local: sublingual burning.
Other: hypersensitivity reactions.

INTERACTIONS

Antihypertensives: possibly enhanced hypotensive effect. Monitor closely.

*Liquid form contains alcohol. **May contain tartrazine.

NURSING CONSIDERATIONS

- *Contraindicated* in hypersensitivity to nitrites, head trauma, cerebral hemorrhage, hypertrophic cardiomyopathy, or severe anemia.
- *Use cautiously* in hypotension.
- Tolerance can occur with prolonged use and is associated with high or sustained blood levels. Tolerance can be minimized with a 10- to 12-hour nitrate-free interval. This can be achieved by removing transdermal systems in the early evening and applying a new system the next morning or by omitting the last daily dose of a buccal, sustained-release, or ointment form. Check with the doctor for alterations in dosage regimen if tolerance is suspected.
- Monitor blood pressure and intensity and duration of response to drug.
- May cause headaches, especially at first. Treat headache with aspirin or acetaminophen. Dosage may need to be reduced temporarily, but tolerance usually develops.
- Tell patient to take medication regularly, even long-term, if ordered, and to keep it easily accessible at all times. Physiologically necessary but not habit-forming.
- Additional dose may be taken before anticipated stress or at bedtime if angina is nocturnal.
- Advise patient to avoid alcoholic beverages; may produce increased hypotension.
- May cause orthostatic hypotension. To minimize it, patient should change to upright position slowly. He should go up and down stairs carefully, and lie down at the first sign of dizziness.
- Teach patient to take sublingual tablet at first sign of attack. He should wet the tablet with saliva, place it under the tongue until completely absorbed, and sit down and rest. Dose may be repeated every 10 to 15 minutes for a maximum of three doses. If no relief, patient should call doctor or go to hospital emergency room. If patient complains of tingling sensation with drug placed sublingually, he may try holding tablet in buccal pouch.
- Although a burning sensation used to be an indication of tablet potency, today many brands don't produce this sensation.
- Store drug in cool, dark place in a tightly closed container. To ensure freshness, replace supply of sublingual tablets every 3 months. Remove cotton from container, since it absorbs drug.
- Tell patient to store nitroglycerin sublingual tablets in original container or other container specifically approved for this use.
- Advise patient not to carry bottle close to body. Patient should carry it in jacket pocket or purse.
- Teach patient to take oral tablet on empty stomach, either half an hour before or 1 to 2 hours after meals; to swallow oral tablets whole; and to chew chewable tablets thoroughly before swallowing.
- To apply ointment, spread uniform, thin layer on any nonhairy area. Do not rub in. Cover with plastic film to aid absorption and to protect clothing. If using Tape-Surrounded Appli-Ruler (TSAR) system, keep the TSAR on skin to protect patient's clothing and to ensure that ointment remains in place.
- Be sure to remove all excess ointment from previous site before applying the next dose.
- Avoid getting ointment on fingers.
- Transdermal dosage forms can be applied to any hairless part of the skin except distal parts of the arms or legs, because absorption will not be maximal at these sites.
- Be sure to remove transdermal patch before defibrillation. Because of its aluminum backing, the electric current may cause the patch to explode.
- When terminating transdermal treatment of angina, gradually reduce

the dosage and frequency of application over 4 to 6 weeks.
• Instruct patient to use caution when wearing transdermal patch near microwave oven. Leaking radiation may heat patch's metallic backing and cause burns.
• The various brands of transdermal nitroglycerin products can be interchanged to achieve the prescribed dose. Now, standardized labels specify the amount of nitroglycerin released over 24 hours.
• If nitroglycerin lingual aerosol (Nitrolingual) has been prescribed for patient, instruct him how to use this device correctly. Remind him he should *not* inhale the spray, but should release the spray onto or under the tongue. Also tell him not to swallow immediately after administering the spray – wait about 10 seconds or so before swallowing.
• The transmucosal dosage form may be used to provide relief from an acute anginal attack as well as for prophylaxis.
• Tell patient to place the transmucosal tablet between lip and gum above the incisors, or between cheek and gum. Tell him not to swallow or chew tablet; this will make it ineffective.
• **I.V. use:** Always administer with an infusion pump and titrate to desired response. Always mix in glass bottles and avoid use of I.V. filters because the drug binds to plastic. Regular polyvinyl chloride (PVC) tubing can bind up to 80% of the drug, making it necessary to infuse higher dosages. A special nonabsorbing (non-PVC) tubing is available from the manufacturer; patients receive more drug when these infusion sets are used. Always use the same type of infusion set when changing I.V. lines.
• Closely monitor vital signs during infusion. Be particularly aware of blood pressure, especially if the drug is being used in a patient with an MI. Excessive hypotension may worsen the MI.

pentaerythritol tetranitrate

Dilar, Duotrate, Naptrate, Pentritol, Pentylan, Peritrate, Peritrate Forte†, Peritrate SA, PETN

Pregnancy Risk Category: C

HOW SUPPLIED

Tablets: 10 mg, 20 mg, 40 mg, 80 mg
Tablets (sustained-release): 80 mg
Capsules (sustained-release): 30 mg, 45 mg, 80 mg

MECHANISM OF ACTION

Reduces cardiac oxygen demand by decreasing left ventricular end-diastolic pressure (preload) and, to a lesser extent, systemic vascular resistance (afterload). Also increases blood flow through the collateral coronary vessels.

INDICATIONS & DOSAGE

Prophylaxis against angina pectoris –
Adults: 10 to 20 mg P.O. q.i.d.; may be titrated upward to 40 mg P.O. q.i.d. half an hour before or 1 hour after meals and h.s.; or 30 to 80 mg sustained-release preparations P.O. b.i.d.

ADVERSE REACTIONS

Common reactions are in italics; life-threatening reactions are in bold italics.
CNS: *headache, sometimes with throbbing; dizziness;* weakness.
CV: *orthostatic hypotension, tachycardia, flushing, palpitations,* fainting.
GI: nausea, vomiting.
Skin: cutaneous vasodilation.
Other: hypersensitivity reactions.

INTERACTIONS

None significant.

NURSING CONSIDERATIONS

• *Contraindicated* in head trauma, cerebral hemorrhage, or severe anemia.

*Liquid form contains alcohol. **May contain tartrazine.

• *Use cautiously* in hypotension and glaucoma.
• Monitor blood pressure and intensity and duration of response to drug.
• May cause headaches, especially at first. Treat with aspirin or acetaminophen. Dosage may need to be reduced temporarily, but tolerance usually develops.
• Medication should be taken regularly, even long-term, if ordered. Physiologically necessary but not habit-forming.
• Additional doses may be taken before anticipated stress or at bedtime for nocturnal angina.
• Not to be used for relief of acute anginal attacks.
• May cause orthostatic hypotension. To minimize it, patient should change to upright position slowly. He should go up and down stairs carefully, and lie down at the first sign of dizziness.
• Advise patient to avoid alcoholic beverages; may exacerbate hypotension.
• Drug should not be discontinued abruptly – coronary vasospasm may occur.
• Store in cool place, in a tightly covered container away from light.

propranolol hydrochloride

Apo-Propranolol†, Deralin‡, Detensol†, Inderal, Inderal LA, Ipran, Novopranol†, PMS-Propranolol†

Pregnancy Risk Category: C

HOW SUPPLIED

Tablets: 10 mg, 20 mg, 40 mg, 60 mg, 80 mg, 90 mg
Capsules (sustained-release): 60 mg, 80 mg, 120 mg, 160 mg
Oral solution: 4 mg/ml, 8 mg/ml, 80 mg/ml (concentrate)
Injection: 1 mg/ml

MECHANISM OF ACTION

A beta-adrenergic blocker that reduces cardiac oxygen demand by blocking catecholamine-induced increases in heart rate, blood pressure, and force of myocardial contraction. Depresses renin secretion. Also prevents vasodilation of the cerebral arteries.

INDICATIONS & DOSAGE

Management of angina pectoris –
Adults: 10 to 20 mg P.O. t.i.d. or q.i.d. Or, one 80-mg sustained-release capsule daily. Dosage may be increased at 7- to 10-day intervals. The average optimum dosage is 160 mg daily.
To reduce mortality following myocardial infarction –
Adults: 180 to 240 mg P.O. daily in divided doses. Usually administered t.i.d. to q.i.d.
Supraventricular, ventricular, and atrial arrhythmias; tachyarrhythmias caused by excessive catecholamine action during anesthesia, hyperthyroidism, and pheochromocytoma –
Adults: 1 to 3 mg by slow I.V. push, not to exceed 1 mg/minute. After 3 mg have been given, another dose may be given in 2 minutes; subsequent doses, no sooner than q 4 hours. Drug may be given by direct injection or diluted in 50 ml dextrose 5% in water or normal saline solution and infused slowly. Usual maintenance dose is 10 to 80 mg P.O. t.i.d. to q.i.d.
Hypertension –
Adults: initial treatment of hypertension: 80 mg P.O. daily in two to four divided doses or the sustained-release form once daily. Increase at 3- to 7-day intervals to maximum daily dosage of 640 mg. Usual maintenance dosage for hypertension is 160 to 480 mg daily.
Prevention of frequent, severe, uncontrollable, or disabling migraine or vascular headache –

Adults: initially, 80 mg P.O. daily in divided doses or 1 sustained-release capsule daily. Usual maintenance dosage is 160 to 240 mg daily, divided t.i.d. or q.i.d.

ADVERSE REACTIONS

Common reactions are in italics; life-threatening reactions are in bold italics.

CNS: *fatigue, lethargy,* vivid dreams, hallucinations.

CV: *bradycardia, hypotension,* ***CHF,*** peripheral vascular disease.

GI: nausea, vomiting, diarrhea.

Metabolic: hypoglycemia without tachycardia (in diabetic patients).

Skin: rash.

Other: *increased airway resistance,* fever, arthralgia.

INTERACTIONS

Aminophylline: antagonized beta-blocking effects of propranolol. Use together cautiously.

Cardiac glycosides, verapamil: excessive bradycardia and increased depressant effect on myocardium. Use together cautiously.

Cimetidine: inhibits propranolol's metabolism. Monitor for greater beta-blocking effect.

Epinephrine: severe vasoconstriction. Monitor blood pressure and observe patient carefully.

Insulin, hypoglycemic drugs (oral): can alter requirements for these drugs in previously stabilized diabetics. Monitor for hypoglycemia.

Isoproterenol, glucagon: antagonized propranolol effect. May be used therapeutically and in emergencies.

NURSING CONSIDERATIONS

- *Contraindicated* in diabetes mellitus, asthma, or allergic rhinitis; during ethyl ether anesthesia; with sinus bradycardia and in heart block greater than first degree; in cardiogenic shock; and with right ventricular failure secondary to pulmonary hypertension.
- *Use cautiously* in patients with CHF or respiratory disease and in patients taking other antihypertensive drugs.
- Elderly patients may experience enhanced adverse reactions. Dosage may need to be adjusted.
- Always check patient's apical pulse before giving this drug. If you detect extremes in pulse rates, withhold drug and call the doctor immediately.
- Monitor blood pressure, ECG, and heart rate and rhythm frequently, especially during I.V. administration. If patient develops severe hypotension, notify doctor. He may prescribe a vasopressor.
- After prolonged atrial fibrillation, restoration of normal sinus rhythm may result in thromboembolism due to dislodgment of thrombi from atrial wall. Anticoagulation often advised before restoration of normal atrial rhythm.
- Teach patient about his disease and therapy. Explain the importance of taking this drug as prescribed, even when he's feeling well. Tell outpatient not to discontinue his drug suddenly; abrupt discontinuation can exacerbate angina and myocardial infarction. Tell patient to call doctor if unpleasant adverse reactions occur.
- This drug masks common signs of shock and hypoglycemia.
- Food may increase the absorption of propranolol. Give consistently with meals.
- Compliance may be improved by administering this drug twice daily, or by sustained-release capsule. Check with doctor.
- Has also been used to treat aggression and rage, stage fright, recurrent GI bleeding, and menopausal symptoms.
- *Don't discontinue before surgery for pheochromocytoma.* Before any surgical procedure, notify anesthesiologist that patient is receiving propranolol.
- **I.V. use:** Double-check dose and

*Liquid form contains alcohol. **May contain tartrazine.

route. I.V. doses are much smaller than P.O.

- For overdose, I.V. isoproterenol or atropine may be given; refractory cases may require a pacemaker. Glucagon is sometimes used.

verapamil hydrochloride

Calan, Calan SR, Cordilox Oral‡, Isoptin, Isoptin SR, Veradil‡, Verelan

Pregnancy Risk Category: C

HOW SUPPLIED

Tablets: 40 mg, 80 mg, 120 mg
Tablets (sustained-release): 120 mg, 180 mg, 240 mg
Injection: 2.5 mg/ml

MECHANISM OF ACTION

Inhibits calcium ion influx across cardiac and smooth muscle cells, thus decreasing myocardial contractility and oxygen demand, and dilates coronary arteries and arterioles.

INDICATIONS & DOSAGE

Management of vasospastic (also called Prinzmetal's or variant) angina and classic chronic, stable angina pectoris; chronic atrial fibrillation –
Adults: starting dose is 80 mg P.O. t.i.d. or q.i.d. Dosage may be increased at weekly intervals. Some patients may require up to 480 mg daily.
Treatment of supraventricular arrhythmias –
Adults: 0.075 to 0.15 mg/kg (5 to 10 mg) I.V. push over 2 minutes with ECG and blood pressure monitoring. Repeat dose in 30 minutes if no response.
Children 1 to 15 years: 0.1 to 0.3 mg/kg as I.V. bolus over 2 minutes.
Children under 1 year: 0.1 to 0.2 mg/kg as I.V. bolus over 2 minutes under continuous ECG monitoring.

Dose can be repeated in 30 minutes if no response.
Migraine headache prophylaxis –
Adults: 80 mg P.O. q.i.d.
Treatment of hypertension –
Adults: 240-mg sustained-release tablet once daily in the morning. If response is not adequate, may give an additional half tablet in the evening or one tablet q 12 hours. Alternatively, may give 80-mg immediate-release tablet t.i.d. or q.i.d.

ADVERSE REACTIONS

Common reactions are in italics; life-threatening reactions are in bold italics.
CNS: dizziness, headache, fatigue.
CV: *transient hypotension,* ***CHF,*** bradycardia, AV block, ***ventricular asystole,*** peripheral edema.
GI: *constipation,* nausea (primarily from oral form).
Hepatic: elevated liver enzymes.

INTERACTIONS

Carbamazepine, digitalis glycosides: verapamil may increase the serum levels of these drugs. Monitor patient for toxicity.
Lithium: verapamil may decrease serum lithium levels. Monitor closely.
Propranolol (and other beta blockers, including ophthalmic timolol), disopyramide, flecainide: may cause heart failure. Use together cautiously.
Quinidine, antihypertensives: may result in hypotension. Monitor blood pressure.
Rifampin: may decrease oral bioavailability of verapamil. Monitor patient for lack of effect.

NURSING CONSIDERATIONS

- *Contraindicated* in advanced heart failure, AV block, severe left ventricular dysfunction, cardiogenic shock, sinus node disease, and severe hypotension. Also contraindicated in patients hypersensitive to the drug.
- *Use cautiously* in elderly patients because duration of action may be prolonged; in MI followed by coronary occlusion, sick sinus syndrome, impaired AV conduction, heart failure

with atrial tachyarrhythmia; and in hepatic or renal disease. Also use cautiously in patients with a history of CHF, especially if combined with a beta-adrenergic blocking agent.

- **I.V. use:** Administer I.V. doses over at least 3 minutes to minimize the risk of adverse reactions.
- All patients receiving I.V. verapamil should be on a cardiac monitor. Monitor the R-R interval.
- Patients with severely compromised cardiac function or those receiving beta blockers should receive lower doses of verapamil. Monitor these patients closely. Do not administer I.V. beta blockers at the same time as I.V. verapamil.
- If verapamil is being used to terminate supraventricular tachycardia, the doctor may have patient perform vagal maneuvers after receiving the drug.
- Notify doctor if such signs of CHF as swelling of hands and feet or shortness of breath occur.
- If patient continues nitrate therapy during titration of oral verapamil dosage, urge him to continue compliance. Sublingual nitroglycerin, especially, may be taken as needed when anginal symptoms are acute.
- Taking extended-release tablets with food may decrease rate and extent of absorption, but allows smaller fluctuations of peak and trough blood levels.
- Monitor blood pressure at start of therapy and during dosage adjustments. Assist patient with ambulation because dizziness may occur.
- Preliminary studies show verapamil to be highly effective in the prophylaxis of migraine headache.
- Liver function should be monitored during prolonged treatment.
- Encourage patient to increase fluid and fiber intake to combat constipation. Administer a stool softener as ordered.

*Liquid form contains alcohol. **May contain tartrazine.

22

Antihypertensives

acebutolol
amlodipine besylate
(See Chapter 21, ANTIANGINALS.)
atenolol
benazepril hydrochloride
betaxolol hydrochloride
captopril
carteolol
clonidine hydrochloride
deserpidine
diazoxide
diltiazem hydrochloride
(See Chapter 21, ANTIANGINALS.)
doxazosin mesylate
enalaprilat
enalapril maleate
felodipine
fosinopril sodium
guanabenz acetate
guanadrel sulfate
guanethidine sulfate
guanfacine hydrochloride
hydralazine hydrochloride
isradipine
labetalol hydrochloride
lisinopril
mecamylamine hydrochloride
methyldopa
methyldopate hydrochloride
metoprolol tartrate
metyrosine
minoxidil
nadolol
(See Chapter 21, ANTIANGINALS.)
nicardipine
(See Chapter 21, ANTIANGINALS.)
nifedipine
(See Chapter 21, ANTIANGINALS.)
nitroprusside sodium
penbutolol sulfate
phenoxybenzamine hydrochloride
phentolamine mesylate
pindolol
prazosin hydrochloride
propranolol hydrochloride
(See Chapter 21, ANTIANGINALS.)
quinapril hydrochloride
ramipril
rauwolfia serpentina
rescinnamine
reserpine
terazosin hydrochloride
timolol maleate
trimethaphan camsylate
verapamil hydrochloride
(See Chapter 21, ANTIANGINALS.)

COMBINATION PRODUCTS

ALDOCLOR-150: chlorothiazide 150 mg and methyldopa 250 mg.
ALDOCLOR-250: chlorothiazide 250 mg and methyldopa 250 mg.
ALDORIL-15: hydrochlorothiazide 15 mg and methyldopa 250 mg.
ALDORIL-25: hydrochlorothiazide 25 mg and methyldopa 250 mg.
ALDORIL D30: hydrochlorothiazide 30 mg and methyldopa 500 mg.
ALDORIL D50: hydrochlorothiazide 50 mg and methyldopa 500 mg.
APRESAZIDE 25/25: hydrochlorothiazide 25 mg and hydralazine hydrochloride 25 mg.
APRESAZIDE 50/50: hydrochlorothiazide 50 mg and hydralazine hydrochloride 50 mg.
APRESAZIDE 100/50: hydrochlorothiazide 50 mg and hydralazine hydrochloride 100 mg.
APRESODEX: hydrochlorothiazide 15 mg and hydralazine hydrochloride 25 mg.
APRESOLINE-ESIDRIX: hydrochlorothiazide 15 mg and hydralazine hydrochloride 25 mg.
CAM-AP-ES: hydrochlorothiazide 15 mg, hydralazine hydrochloride 25 mg, and reserpine 0.1 mg.
CAPOZIDE 25/15: hydrochlorothiazide 15 mg and captopril 25 mg.

†Available in Canada only. ‡Available in Australia only. ◇Available OTC.

CAPOZIDE 25/25: hydrochlorothiazide 25 mg and captopril 25 mg.
CAPOZIDE 50/15: hydrochlorothiazide 15 mg and captopril 50 mg.
CAPOZIDE 50/25: hydrochlorothiazide 25 mg and captopril 50 mg.
CHERAPAS: hydrochlorothiazide 15 mg, hydralazine hydrochloride 25 mg, and reserpine 0.1 mg.
COMBIPRES 0.1: chlorthalidone 15 mg and clonidine hydrochloride 0.1 mg.
COMBIPRES 0.2: chlorthalidone 15 mg and clonidine hydrochloride 0.2 mg.
CORZIDE: nadolol 40 mg or 80 mg and bendroflumethiazide 5 mg.
DEMI-REGROTON: chlorthalidone 25 mg and reserpine 0.125 mg.
DIUPRES-250: chlorothiazide 250 mg and reserpine 0.125 mg.
DIUPRES-500: chlorothiazide 500 mg and reserpine 0.125 mg.
DIURESE-R: trichlormethiazide 4 mg and reserpine 0.1 mg.
DIURIGEN WITH RESERPINE: chlorothiazide 250 mg and reserpine 0.125 mg.
DIUTENSEN: methyclothiazide 2.5 mg and cryptenamine 2 mg (as tannate).
DIUTENSEN-R: methyclothiazide 2.5 mg and reserpine 0.1 mg.
ENDURONYL: methyclothiazide 5 mg and deserpidine 0.25 mg.
ENDURONYL-FORTE: methyclothiazide 5 mg and deserpidine 0.5 mg.
ESIMIL: hydrochlorothiazide 25 mg and guanethidine sulfate 10 mg.
EUTRON FILMTABS: methyclothiazide 5 mg and pargyline hydrochloride 25 mg.
EXNA-R TABLETS: benzthiazide 50 mg and reserpine 0.125 mg.
H.H.R.: hydrochlorothiazide 15 mg, hydralazine hydrochloride 25 mg, and reserpine 0.1 mg.
HYDROMOX-R: quinethazone 50 mg and reserpine 0.125 mg.
HYDROPINE: hydroflumethiazide 25 mg and reserpine 0.125 mg.
HYDROPINE HP: hydroflumethiazide 50 mg and reserpine 0.125 mg.
HYDROPRES-25: hydrochlorothiazide 25 mg and reserpine 0.125 mg.
HYDRO-RESERP: hydrochlorothiazide 25 or 50 mg and reserpine 0.125 mg.
HYDRO-SERP: hydrochlorothiazide 25 or 50 mg and reserpine 0.125 mg.
HYDROSERPINE: hydrochlorothiazide 25 or 50 mg and reserpine 0.125 mg.
HYDROTENSIN-25 TABLETS: hydrochlorothiazide 25 mg and reserpine 0.125 mg.
INDERIDE 40/25: propranolol hydrochloride 40 mg and hydrochlorothiazide 25 mg.
INDERIDE 80/25: propranolol hydrochloride 80 mg and hydrochlorothiazide 25 mg.
INDERIDE LA 80/50: propranolol hydrochloride 80 mg and hydrochlorothiazide 50 mg.
LOPRESSOR HCT 50/25: metoprolol tartrate 50 mg and hydrochlorothiazide 25 mg.
LOPRESSOR HCT 100/25: metoprolol tartrate 100 mg and hydrochlorothiazide 25 mg.
MAXZIDE: triamterene 75 mg and hydrochlorothiazide 50 mg.
METATENSIN TABLETS #2 or #4: trichlormethiazide 2 or 4 mg and reserpine 0.1 mg.
MINIZIDE 1: polythiazide 0.5 mg and prazosin hydrochloride 1 mg.
MINIZIDE 2: polythiazide 0.5 mg and prazosin hydrochloride 2 mg.
MINIZIDE 5: polythiazide 0.5 mg and prazosin hydrochloride 5 mg.
NAQUIVAL: trichlormethiazide 4 mg and reserpine 0.1 mg.
NATURETIN W/K 2.5 mg: bendroflumethiazide 2.5 mg and potassium chloride 500 mg.
NATURETIN W/K 5 mg: bendroflumethiazide 5 mg and potassium chloride 500 mg.
NORMOZIDE 100/25: labetalol hydrochloride 100 mg and hydrochlorothiazide 25 mg.
NORMOZIDE 200/25: labetalol hydro-

*Liquid form contains alcohol. **May contain tartrazine.

chloride 200 mg and hydrochlorothiazide 25 mg.
NORMOZIDE 300/25: labetalol hydrochloride 300 mg and hydrochlorothiazide 25 mg.
ORETICYL 25: hydrochlorothiazide 25 mg and deserpidine 0.125 mg.
ORETICYL 50: hydrochlorothiazide 50 mg and deserpidine 0.125 mg.
ORETICYL FORTE: hydrochlorothiazide 25 mg and deserpidine 0.25 mg.
RAUZIDE**: bendroflumethiazide 4 mg and powdered rauwolfia serpentina 50 mg.
REGROTON: chlorthalidone 50 mg and reserpine 0.25 mg.
RENESE-R: polythiazide 2 mg and reserpine 0.25 mg.
REZIDE: hydrochlorothiazide 15 mg, hydralazine hydrochloride 25 mg, and reserpine 0.1 mg.
R-HCTZ-H: hydrochlorothiazide 15 mg, hydralazine hydrochloride 25 mg, and reserpine 0.1 mg.
SALUTENSIN: hydroflumethiazide 50 mg and reserpine 0.125 mg.
SALUTENSIN DEMI: hydroflumethiazide 25 mg and reserpine 0.125 mg.
SER-A-GEN: hydrochlorothiazide 15 mg, hydralazine hydrochloride 25 mg, and reserpine 0.1 mg.
SERALAZIDE: hydrochlorothiazide 15 mg, hydralazine hydrochloride 25 mg, and reserpine 0.1 mg.
SER-AP-ES: hydrochlorothiazide 15 mg, reserpine 0.1 mg, and hydralazine hydrochloride 25 mg.
SERPASIL-APRESOLINE #1**: reserpine 0.1 mg and hydralazine hydrochloride 25 mg.
SERPASIL-APRESOLINE #2: reserpine 0.2 mg and hydralazine hydrochloride 50 mg.
SERPASIL-ESIDRIX #1: hydrochlorothiazide 25 mg and reserpine 0.1 mg (called Serpasil-Esidrix 25 in Canada).
SERPASIL ESIDRIX #2: hydrochlorothiazide 50 mg and reserpine 0.1 mg.
SERPAZIDE: hydrochlorothiazide 15 mg, hydralazine hydrochloride 25 mg, and reserpine 0.1 mg.
TENORETIC 50: atenolol 50 mg and chlorthalidone 25 mg.
TENORETIC 100: atenolol 100 mg and chlorthalidone 25 mg.
TIMOLIDE 10/25: timolol maleate 10 mg and hydrochlorothiazide 25 mg.
TRI-HYDROSERPINE: hydrochlorothiazide 15 mg, hydralazine hydrochloride 25 mg, and reserpine 0.1 mg.
UNIPRES: hydrochlorothiazide 15 mg, reserpine 0.1 mg, and hydralazine hydrochloride 25 mg.
VASERETIC: enalapril maleate 10 mg and hydrochlorothiazide 25 mg.

acebutolol

Monitan†, Sectral

Pregnancy Risk Category: B

HOW SUPPLIED

Capsules: 200 mg, 400 mg

MECHANISM OF ACTION

A beta-selective blocking agent, acebutolol decreases myocardial contractility and decreases heart rate. It has mild intrinsic sympathomimetic activity.

INDICATIONS & DOSAGE

Treatment of hypertension –
Adults: 400 mg P.O. either as a single daily dosage or divided b.i.d. Patients may receive as much as 1,200 mg daily.
Ventricular arrhythmias –
Adults: 400 mg P.O. daily divided b.i.d. Dosage is then increased to provide an adequate clinical response. Usual dosage is 600 to 1,200 mg daily.

ADVERSE REACTIONS

Common reactions are in italics; life-threatening reactions are in bold italics.
CNS: *fatigue,* headache, dizziness, insomnia.

CV: chest pain, edema, bradycardia, ***CHF, hypotension.***
GI: nausea, constipation, diarrhea, dyspepsia.
Metabolic: hypoglycemia without tachycardia.
Respiratory: dyspnea, ***broncho-spasm.***
Skin: rash.
Other: fever.

INTERACTIONS

Digitalis glycosides: excessive bradycardia and increased depressant effect on myocardium. Use together cautiously.
Indomethacin: decreased antihypertensive effect. Monitor blood pressure and adjust dosage.
Insulin, hypoglycemic drugs (oral): can alter dosage requirements in previously stabilized diabetics. Observe patient carefully.

NURSING CONSIDERATIONS

- *Contraindicated* in persistently severe bradycardia, second- and third-degree heart block, overt cardiac failure, and cardiogenic shock.
- *Use cautiously* in patients with cardiac failure.
- Similar to metoprolol, acebutolol is a cardioselective beta blocker. This drug should be used with caution in patients with bronchospastic diseases such as asthma and emphysema.
- Dosage should be reduced in patients with decreased renal function.
- Elderly patients may require lower acebutolol doses. For such patients, dosage should not exceed 800 mg daily.
- Always check patient's apical pulse before giving this drug; if slower than 60 beats/minute, hold drug and call doctor.
- Acebutolol may mask the signs of hyperthyroidism and hyperglycemia, and potentiate insulin-induced hypoglycemia.
- Before surgery, notify anesthesiologist if patient is receiving this drug.
- Do not discontinue abruptly; can exacerbate angina and myocardial infarction.
- Teach patient about his disease and therapy. Explain the importance of taking this drug as prescribed, even when he's feeling well. Tell patient not to discontinue drug suddenly, but to call the doctor if unpleasant adverse reactions occur.
- Instruct patient to check with doctor or pharmacist before taking OTC medications.

atenolol

Noten‡, Tenormin
Pregnancy Risk Category: C

HOW SUPPLIED

Tablets: 50 mg, 100 mg
Injection: 5 mg/10 ml

MECHANISM OF ACTION

Blocks response to beta stimulation and depresses renin secretion.

INDICATIONS & DOSAGE

Treatment of hypertension –
Adults: initially, 50 mg P.O. daily as a single dose. Dosage may be increased to 100 mg once daily after 7 to 14 days. Dosages greater than 100 mg are unlikely to produce further benefit. Dosage adjustment is necessary in patients with creatinine clearance below 35 ml/minute.
Angina pectoris –
Adults: 50 mg P.O. once daily. May increase to 100 mg daily after 7 days for optimal effect. May give as much as 200 mg daily.
To reduce cardiovascular mortality and risk of reinfarction in patients with acute myocardial infarction –
Adults: 5 mg I.V. over 5 minutes, followed by another 5 mg I.V. 10 minutes later. After an additional 10 minutes, administer 50 mg P.O., followed

by 50 mg P.O. in 12 hours. Thereafter, give 100 mg P.O. daily (as a single dose or 50 mg b.i.d.) for at least 7 days.
To reduce the incidence of supraventricular tachycardia in patients undergoing coronary artery bypass –
Adults: 50 mg P.O. daily starting 3 days before surgery.

ADVERSE REACTIONS
Common reactions are in italics; life-threatening reactions are in bold italics.
CNS: fatigue, lethargy.
CV: *bradycardia, hypotension,* ***CHF,*** peripheral vascular disease.
GI: nausea, vomiting, diarrhea.
Respiratory: dyspnea, ***bronchospasm.***
Skin: rash.
Other: fever.

INTERACTIONS
Antihypertensives: enhanced hypotensive effect. Use together cautiously.
Digitalis glycosides: excessive bradycardia and increased depressant effect on myocardium. Use together cautiously.
Indomethacin: decrease in antihypertensive effect. Monitor blood pressure and adjust dosage.
Insulin, oral hypoglycemic drugs: can alter dosage requirements in previously stabilized diabetics. Observe patient carefully.

NURSING CONSIDERATIONS
- *Contraindicated* in sinus bradycardia and greater than first-degree conduction block, and cardiogenic shock.
- *Use cautiously* in cardiac failure.
- Similar to metoprolol, atenolol is a cardioselective beta blocker. Although atenolol can be used in patients with bronchospastic diseases such as asthma and emphysema, the drug should still be used cautiously in such patients – especially when 100 mg are given. Twice-daily dosing may help minimize this risk.
- Dosage should be reduced if patient has renal insufficiency. Patients with a creatinine clearance of 15 to 35 ml/min/1.73 m^2 should receive a maximum of 50 mg daily; if creatinine clearance is < 15 ml/min/1.73 m^2, the maximum dosage is 50 mg every other day. Hemodialysis patients should receive 50 mg after each dialysis session, but close supervision is mandatory because of the risk of marked decreases in blood pressure.
- **I.V. use:** I.V. doses may be mixed with 5% dextrose, sodium chloride injection, or dextrose and sodium chloride injection. The solution is stable for 48 hours after mixing.
- Once-a-day dosage encourages patient compliance. Counsel your patient to take the drug at a regular time every day. Drug can be dispensed in a 28-day calendar pack.
- Full antihypertensive effect may not appear for 1 to 2 weeks after initiating therapy.
- Always check patient's apical pulse before giving this drug; if slower than 60 beats/minute, hold drug and call doctor.
- Monitor blood pressure frequently.
- Don't discontinue abruptly; can exacerbate angina and myocardial infarction. Drug should be withdrawn gradually over a 2-week period.
- Teach patient about his disease and therapy. Explain the importance of taking this drug as prescribed, even when he's feeling well. Tell patient not to discontinue drug suddenly, but to call the doctor if unpleasant adverse reactions occur.
- Instruct patient to check with doctor or pharmacist before taking OTC medications.
- This drug masks common signs of shock and hypoglycemia. However, atenolol doesn't potentiate insulin-induced hypoglycemia or delay recovery of blood glucose to normal levels.
- Has been prescribed effectively in the treatment of angina pectoris and

in patients with alcohol withdrawal syndrome.

benazepril hydrochloride

Lotensin

Pregnancy Risk Category: C (X in 2nd and 3rd trimesters)

HOW SUPPLIED

Tablets: 5 mg, 10 mg, 20 mg, 40 mg

MECHANISM OF ACTION

Benazepril and its active metabolite, benazeprilat, inhibit angiotensin-converting enzyme (ACE), preventing conversion of angiotensin I to angiotensin II, a potent vasoconstrictor. Reduced formation of angiotensin II decreases peripheral arterial resistance, which results in decreased aldosterone secretion. This reduces sodium and water retention and lowers blood pressure. Benazepril also has antihypertensive activity in patients with low-renin hypertension.

INDICATIONS & DOSAGE

Hypertension –

Adults: initially, 10 mg daily. Titrate dosage as needed and tolerated; most patients take 20 to 40 mg daily in one or two doses.

ADVERSE REACTIONS

Common reactions are in italics; life-threatening reactions are in bold italics.

CNS: headache, dizziness, lightheadedness, anxiety, amnesia, ***seizures,*** depression, insomnia, malaise, nervousness, neuralgia, neuropathy, paresthesia, somnolence, tremor, vertigo.

CV: symptomatic hypotension, syncope, angina, arrhythmia, chest pain, palpitations, ***MI.***

EENT: epistaxis.

GI: nausea, vomiting, abdominal pain, anorexia, constipation, diarrhea, dry mouth, dyspepsia, dysphagia, gastroenteritis, increased salivation, taste disturbance.

Respiratory: dry, persistent, tickling, nonproductive cough; dyspnea.

Skin: hypersensitivity reactions, rash, dermatitis, pruritus, photosensitivity, purpura.

Other: angioedema, arthralgia, arthritis, edema, impotence, increased sweating, myalgia, weight gain, asthenia.

INTERACTIONS

Diuretics, other antihypertensives: risk of excessive hypotension. Discontinue diuretic or lower dose of benazepril as needed.

Lithium: increased serum lithium levels and lithium toxicity have been reported. Avoid concomitant use.

Potassium-sparing diuretics, potassium supplements, sodium substitutes containing potassium: risk of hyperkalemia. Avoid concomitant use.

NURSING CONSIDERATIONS

- *Contraindicated* in patients with hypersensitivity to ACE inhibitors or with a history of angioneurotic edema.
- *Use cautiously* in patients with impaired renal or hepatic function, in diabetes mellitus, and with use of potassium-sparing diuretics, potassium supplements, and sodium substitutes containing potassium because of risk of hyperkalemia.
- Avoid use during pregnancy because ACE inhibitors can cause fetal or neonatal injury or death. When pregnancy is detected, ACE inhibitors should be discontinued as soon as possible.
- Blood pressure measurements should be made when drug levels are at peak (2 to 6 hours after dosing) and at trough (just before a dose) to verify adequate blood pressure control.
- Excessive hypotension can occur when drug is given with diuretics. If possible, diuretic therapy should be

*Liquid form contains alcohol. **May contain tartrazine.

discontinued 2 to 3 days before starting benazepril to decrease potential for excessive hypotensive response. If benazepril does not adequately control blood pressure, diuretic may be reinstituted with care. If the diuretic cannot be discontinued, initiate benazepril therapy at 5 mg P.O. daily. Monitor for hypotension.

- Like other ACE inhibitors, drug may cause dry, persistent, tickling, nonproductive cough, which is reversible when therapy is discontinued.
- Assess renal and hepatic function before and periodically throughout therapy. Also monitor CBC and serum potassium levels.
- Tell patient to take drug on an empty stomach because meals, particularly high-fat meals, can impair absorption.
- Tell patient to stop taking drug and notify doctor if any signs or symptoms of angioedema occur: swelling of face, eyes, lips, tongue, or difficulty in breathing.
- Light-headedness can occur, especially during the first few days of therapy. Tell patient to rise slowly to minimize this effect and to report symptoms to doctor. If syncope (fainting) occurs, tell patient to stop drug immediately and call doctor.
- Inadequate fluid intake, vomiting, diarrhea, and excessive perspiration can lead to light-headedness and syncope. Tell patient to use caution in hot weather and during periods of exercise.
- Tell patient to avoid sodium substitutes because they contain potassium and can cause hyperkalemia.
- Other ACE inhibitors have been associated with granulocytosis and neutropenia. Tell patient to report immediately any signs of infection (sore throat, fever) or of easy bruising or bleeding.

betaxolol hydrochloride

Kerlone

Pregnancy Risk Category: C

HOW SUPPLIED

Tablets: 10 mg, 20 mg

MECHANISM OF ACTION

A $beta_1$-selective blocking agent that decreases blood pressure, probably by slowing heart rate and decreasing cardiac output.

INDICATIONS & DOSAGE

Management of hypertension (used alone or with other antihypertensives) –

Adults: initially, 10 mg P.O. once daily. After 7 to 14 days, full antihypertensive effect should be seen. If necessary, may double dosage to 20 mg P.O. once daily.

ADVERSE REACTIONS

Common reactions are in italics; life-threatening reactions are in bold italics.

CV: bradycardia, chest pain, hypotension, worsening of angina, peripheral vascular insufficiency, ***CHF,*** edema, syncope, postural hypotension, conduction disturbances.

CNS: dizziness, fatigue, headache, lethargy, anxiety.

GI: flatulence, constipation, nausea, diarrhea, dry mouth, vomiting, anorexia.

Respiratory: dyspnea, wheezing, ***bronchospasm.***

Skin: rash.

INTERACTIONS

Calcium channel blocking agents: increased risk of hypotension, left ventricular failure, and AV conduction disturbances. I.V. calcium antagonists should be used with caution.

General anesthetics: increased hypotensive effects. Observe carefully for excessive hypotension or bradycardia, or orthostatic hypotension.

Lidocaine: beta blockers may increase the effects of lidocaine.
Reserpine, catecholamine-depleting drugs: may have an additive effect when administered with a beta blocker.

NURSING CONSIDERATIONS
• *Contraindicated* in patients with severe bradycardia, greater than first-degree heart block, cardiogenic shock, or uncontrolled CHF.
• *Use cautiously* in patients with CHF controlled by digitalis and diuretics because beta-adrenergic blocking agents do not block the inotropic effects of digitalis.
• Note that asymptomatic patients with a history of CHF may exhibit signs of cardiac decompensation with beta blocker therapy.
• Patients with bronchospastic disease (including asthma, chronic bronchitis, emphysema) should avoid beta blocker therapy because some $beta_2$ receptor antagonism may be associated with cardioselective agents such as betaxolol. However, some clinicians will use cardioselective beta blockers in such patients if the patients cannot tolerate other antihypertensives.
• Patients with unrecognized coronary artery disease may exhibit signs of angina pectoris upon withdrawal of the drug.
• Beta-blockade may inhibit glycogenolysis and the signs and symptoms of hypoglycemia (such as tachycardia and blood pressure changes).
• Beta blocking agents may mask tachycardia associated with hyperthyroidism. In patients with suspected thyrotoxicosis, beta blocker therapy should be withdrawn gradually to avoid thyroid storm.
• The anesthesiologist should be advised that the patient is receiving a beta blocking agent so that isoproterenol or dobutamine is made readily available for reversal of the cardiac effects of the drug.
• Withdrawal of beta blocker therapy before surgery is controversial. Some clinicians advocate withdrawal to prevent any impairment of cardiac responsiveness to reflex stimuli and decreased responsiveness to administration of catecholamines.
• Advise the patient to take the drug exactly as prescribed and not to discontinue the drug suddenly. Emphasize the importance of promptly reporting shortness of breath or difficulty breathing, unusually fast heartbeat, cough, or fatigue with exertion.

captopril
Capoten

Pregnancy Risk Category: C (D in 2nd and 3rd trimesters)

HOW SUPPLIED
Tablets: 12.5 mg, 25 mg, 50 mg, 100 mg

MECHANISM OF ACTION
By inhibiting angiotensin-converting enzyme (ACE), prevents conversion of angiotensin I to angiotensin II.

INDICATIONS & DOSAGE
Hypertension –
Adults: 25 mg P.O. b.i.d. or t.i.d. initially. If blood pressure isn't satisfactorily controlled in 1 to 2 weeks, dosage may be increased to 50 mg t.i.d. If not satisfactorily controlled after another 1 to 2 weeks, a diuretic should be added to regimen. If further blood pressure reduction is necessary, dosage may be raised to as high as 150 mg t.i.d. while continuing the diuretic. Maximum dosage is 450 mg daily. Daily dose may also be administered b.i.d.
Congestive heart failure –
Adults: 6.25 to 12.5 mg P.O. t.i.d. initially. May be gradually increased

to 50 mg t.i.d. Maximum dosage is 450 mg daily.

ADVERSE REACTIONS

Common reactions are in italics; life-threatening reactions are in bold italics.
Blood: ***leukopenia, agranulocytosis, pancytopenia.***
CNS: dizziness, fainting.
CV: *tachycardia, hypotension,* angina pectoris, ***CHF,*** pericarditis.
EENT: *loss of taste (dysgeusia).*
GI: anorexia.
GU: *proteinuria, nephrotic syndrome, membranous glomerulopathy, renal failure* (patients with preexisting renal disease or patients receiving high dosages), urinary frequency.
Metabolic: hyperkalemia.
Skin: *urticarial rash, maculopapular rash,* pruritus.
Other: fever, angioedema of face and extremities, transient increases in liver enzymes, persistent cough.

INTERACTIONS

Antacids: decreased captopril effect. Separate administration times.
Digitalis glycosides: may increase serum digoxin concentration by 15% to 30%.
Insulin, oral hypoglycemic agents: risk of hypoglycemia when captopril therapy is initiated. Monitor closely.
NSAIDs: may reduce antihypertensive effect. Monitor blood pressure.
Potassium supplements, potassium-sparing diuretics: increased risk of hyperkalemia. Avoid these agents unless hypokalemic blood levels are confirmed.

NURSING CONSIDERATIONS

- *Contraindicated* during pregnancy because ACE inhibitors can cause fetal and neonatal injury or death. These problems have not been detected when fetal exposure has been limited to the first trimester. When pregnancy is detected, ACE inhibitors should be discontinued as soon as possible.
- *Use cautiously* in impaired renal function or serious autoimmune disease (particularly systemic lupus erythematosus) or in patients who have been exposed to other drugs known to affect WBC counts or immune response.
- Proteinuria and nephrotic syndrome may occur in patients who are on captopril therapy. Those who develop persistent proteinuria or proteinuria that exceeds 1 g daily should have their captopril therapy reevaluated.
- Monitor patient's blood pressure and pulse rate frequently.
- Perform WBC and differential counts before starting treatment, every 2 weeks for the first 3 months of therapy, and periodically thereafter.
- Advise patients to report any sign of infection (sore throat, fever).
- Although captopril can be used alone, its beneficial effects are increased when a thiazide diuretic is added.
- May cause dizziness or fainting, especially during initiation of therapy. Advise patient to avoid sudden postural changes.
- Teach patient about his disease and therapy. Explain the importance of taking this drug as prescribed, even when he's feeling well. Tell outpatient not to discontinue drug suddenly, but to call the doctor if unpleasant adverse reactions occur.
- Instruct patient to check with doctor or pharmacist before taking OTC medications.
- Elderly patients may be more sensitive to the drug's hypotensive effects.
- Should be taken 1 hour before meals since food in the GI tract may reduce absorption.
- Has been prescribed to treat rheumatoid arthritis.

carteolol

Cartrol

Pregnancy Risk Category: C

HOW SUPPLIED

Tablets: 2.5 mg, 5 mg

MECHANISM OF ACTION

A nonselective beta-adrenergic blocking agent with intrinsic sympathomimetic activity (ISA). Its antihypertensive effects are probably caused by decreased sympathetic outflow from the brain and decreased cardiac output. Carteolol does not have a consistent effect on renin output.

INDICATIONS & DOSAGE

Hypertension –

Adults: initially, 2.5 mg P.O. as a single daily dose. Gradually increase dosage as required to 5 mg or 10 mg daily as a single dose.

ADVERSE REACTIONS

Common reactions are in italics; life-threatening reactions are in bold italics.

CNS: weakness, lassitude, tiredness, fatigue, somnolescence.

CV: conduction disturbances.

Other: *muscle cramps, asthenia.*

INTERACTIONS

Calcium channel blocking agents: increased risk of hypotension, left ventricular failure, and AV conduction disturbances. I.V. calcium antagonists should be used with caution.

General anesthetics: increased hypotensive effects. Observe carefully for excessive hypotension or bradycardia, or orthostatic hypotension.

Insulin, oral hypoglycemic agents: hypoglycemic response may be altered by beta blockers. Dosage adjustments may be necessary.

Reserpine, catecholamine-depleting drugs: may have an additive effect when administered with a beta blocker.

NURSING CONSIDERATIONS

- *Contraindicated in* patients with bronchial asthma, severe bradycardia, greater than first-degree heart block, cardiogenic shock, or uncontrolled CHF.
- *Use cautiously* in patients with CHF controlled by digitalis and diuretics because beta-adrenergic blocking agents do not block the inotropic effects of digitalis.
- Food may slow the rate, but not the extent, of carteolol absorption. Under normal circumstances, the patient may take the drug without regard to meals.
- Patients with substantial renal failure should receive the usual dose of carteolol at increased intervals. If creatinine clearance is > 60 ml/minute, the drug is given at 24-hour intervals; if creatinine clearance is 20 to 60 ml/minute, the drug is given at 48-hour intervals; if creatinine clearance is < 20 ml/minute, the drug is given at 72-hour intervals.
- Note that asymptomatic patients with a history of CHF may exhibit signs of cardiac decompensation with beta blocker therapy.
- Patients with unrecognized coronary artery disease may exhibit signs of angina pectoris upon withdrawal of the drug.
- Beta blockade may inhibit glycogenolysis and the signs and symptoms of hypoglycemia (such as tachycardia and blood pressure changes). It may also attenuate insulin release.
- Beta blocking agents may mask tachycardia associated with hyperthyroidism. In patients with suspected thyrotoxicosis, beta blocker therapy should be withdrawn gradually to avoid thyroid storm.
- Withdrawal of beta blocker therapy before surgery is controversial. Some clinicians advocate withdrawal to prevent any impairment of cardiac responsiveness to reflex stimuli and decreased responsiveness to administra-

tion of catecholamines. However, the beta blocking effects of carteolol may persist for weeks, and discontinuing the drug before surgery may be impractical.

- The anesthesiologist should be advised that the patient is receiving a beta blocking agent so that isoproterenol or dobutamine is made readily available for reversal of the cardiac effects of the drug.
- Dosages that exceed 10 mg daily do not produce a greater response and may actually decrease response.
- Advise the patient to take the drug exactly as prescribed, and not to discontinue the drug suddenly. Emphasize the importance of reporting shortness of breath or difficulty breathing, unusually fast heartbeat, cough, or fatigue with exertion.

clonidine hydrochloride

Catapres, Catapres-TTS, Dixarit†‡

Pregnancy Risk Category: C

HOW SUPPLIED

Tablets: 0.025 mg†‡, 0.1 mg, 0.2 mg, 0.3 mg
Transdermal: TTS-1 (releases 0.1 mg/24 hours), TTS-2 (releases 0.2 mg/24 hours), TTS-3 (releases 0.3 mg/24 hours)

MECHANISM OF ACTION

Inhibits the central vasomotor centers, thereby decreasing sympathetic outflow.

INDICATIONS & DOSAGE

Essential, renal, and malignant hypertension –
Adults: initially, 0.1 mg P.O. b.i.d. Then increase by 0.1 to 0.2 mg daily on a weekly basis. Usual dosage range is 0.2 to 0.8 mg daily in divided doses; infrequently, dosages as high as 2.4 mg daily. No dosing recommendations for children.

Or, apply transdermal patch to a hairless area of intact skin on the upper arm or torso, once every 7 days.

Prophylactic treatment of migraine; treatment of menopausal flushing –
Adults: 0.025 mg P.O. b.i.d. If there has been no remission after 2 weeks, increase dosage to 0.050 mg b.i.d.

To suppress abstinence symptoms during narcotics withdrawal –
Adults: 0.1 mg P.O. t.i.d.

ADVERSE REACTIONS

Common reactions are in italics; life-threatening reactions are in bold italics.
CNS: *drowsiness,* dizziness, fatigue, sedation, nervousness, headache, vivid dreams.
CV: orthostatic hypotension, bradycardia, ***severe rebound hypertension.***
EENT: *dry mouth.*
GI: *constipation.*
GU: urine retention, impotence.
Metabolic: transient glucose intolerance (after large doses).
Skin: *pruritus, dermatitis* (from transdermal patch).

INTERACTIONS

CNS depressants: enhanced CNS depression. Use together cautiously.
Propranolol and other beta blockers: paradoxical hypertensive response. Monitor carefully.
Tricyclic antidepressants and MAO inhibitors: may decrease antihypertensive effect. Use together cautiously.

NURSING CONSIDERATIONS

- *Contraindicated* in patients with hypersensitivity to the drug. The transdermal form is contraindicated in patients with hypersensitivity to any component of the adhesive layer of the transdermal system.
- *Use cautiously* in patients with severe coronary insufficiency, diabetes, myocardial infarction, cerebrovascular disease, chronic renal failure, or history of depression or in those taking other antihypertensives.
- Monitor blood pressure and pulse

†Available in Canada only. ‡Available in Australia only. ◇Available OTC.

rate frequently. Dosage is usually adjusted to patient's blood pressure and tolerance.
• May be given to rapidly lower blood pressure in some hypertensive emergency situations.
• Discontinuing clonidine for surgery is not recommended.
• Reduce dosage gradually over 2 to 4 days. If discontinued abruptly, this drug may cause severe hypertension.
• In patients receiving both clonidine and a beta blocker, the beta blocker should be gradually withdrawn before clonidine to minimize adverse reactions.
• Teach patient about his disease and therapy. Explain the importance of taking this drug exactly as prescribed, even when he's feeling well. Tell outpatient not to discontinue this drug suddenly because this can cause severe rebound hypertension, but to call the doctor if unpleasant adverse reactions occur. Warn that this drug can cause drowsiness, but that tolerance to this side effect will develop.
• Instruct patient to check with doctor or pharmacist before taking OTC medications.
• Observe for tolerance to the drug's therapeutic effects that may require an increased dosage.
• Inform patient that orthostatic hypotension can be minimized by rising slowly and avoiding sudden position changes.
• Periodic eye examinations are recommended.
• Elderly patients may be more sensitive to hypotensive effects.
• Last dose should be taken immediately before retiring.
• Transdermal patch provides antihypertensive activity for up to 7 days. Available in three strengths: TTS-1 contains 2.5 mg of clonidine and releases 0.1 mg/24 hours; TTS-2 contains 5 mg of clonidine and releases 0.2 mg/24 hours; TTS-3 contains 7.5 mg of clonidine and releases 0.3 mg/24 hours.
• Transdermal patch usually adheres despite showering and other routine daily activities. An adhesive "overlay" is available to provide additional skin adherence if necessary. Instruct the patient to place the patch at a different site each week.
• Antihypertensive effects of transdermal clonidine may take 2 to 3 days to become apparent. Oral antihypertensive therapy may have to be continued in the interim.
• Remove patch before defibrillation to prevent arcing.
• Has been used investigationally to treat dysmenorrhea. May also suppress craving for nicotine in nicotine addiction.

deserpidine

Harmonyl

Pregnancy Risk Category: C

HOW SUPPLIED

Tablets: 0.25 mg

MECHANISM OF ACTION

Acts peripherally, inhibiting norepinephrine release and depleting norepinephrine stores in adrenergic nerve endings.

INDICATIONS & DOSAGE

Mild essential hypertension –
Adults: 0.25 mg P.O. once daily. No dosing recommendations for children.

ADVERSE REACTIONS

Common reactions are in italics; life-threatening reactions are in bold italics.
CNS: mental confusion, *depression, drowsiness, nervousness, paradoxical anxiety,* nightmares, *sedation, extrapyramidal symptoms.*
CV: bradycardia.
EENT: *dry mouth, nasal stuffiness,* glaucoma.

*Liquid form contains alcohol. **May contain tartrazine.

GI: *hypersecretion of gastric acid, nausea, vomiting,* GI bleeding.
Skin: pruritus, rash.
Other: *impotence, weight gain.*

INTERACTIONS
MAO inhibitors: may cause excitability and hypertension. Avoid concomitant use if possible.

NURSING CONSIDERATIONS
- *Contraindicated* in mental depression.
- *Use cautiously* in severe cardiac or cerebrovascular disease, peptic ulcer, ulcerative colitis, gallstones, or mental depressive disorders; in patients undergoing surgery; and in patients taking other antihypertensives or anticonvulsants.
- Monitor patient's blood pressure and pulse rate frequently.
- Teach patient about his disease and therapy. Explain the importance of taking this drug as prescribed, even when he's feeling well. Tell outpatient not to discontinue this drug suddenly, but to call the doctor if unpleasant adverse reactions, such as mental depression, insomnia, or loss of appetite, occur. Warn that drug can cause drowsiness.
- Instruct patient to check with doctor or pharmacist before taking OTC medications.
- Advise patients to have periodic eye examinations.
- Watch patient closely for signs of mental depression. Warn him to notify doctor promptly if he experiences nightmares.
- Tell patient to avoid alcohol and to follow prescribed diet.
- Dry mouth can be relieved with chewing gum, sour hard candy, or ice chips. Tell patient to contact doctor if relief is needed for nasal stuffiness.
- Give this drug with meals to increase absorption.
- Patient should weigh himself daily and notify doctor of any significant weight gain.

diazoxide
Hyperstat

Pregnancy Risk Category: C

HOW SUPPLIED
Injection: 300 mg/20 ml

MECHANISM OF ACTION
Directly relaxes arteriolar smooth muscle.

INDICATIONS & DOSAGE
Hypertensive crisis –
Adults and children: 1 to 3 mg/kg I.V. bolus (up to a maximum of 150 mg) q 5 to 15 minutes until adequate response is seen. Repeat at intervals q 4 to 24 hours p.r.n.

ADVERSE REACTIONS
Common reactions are in italics; life-threatening reactions are in bold italics.
CNS: *headaches,* dizziness, lightheadedness, euphoria.
CV: *sodium and water retention, orthostatic hypotension,* sweating, flushing, warmth, angina, myocardial ischemia, arrhythmias, ECG changes.
GI: *nausea, vomiting,* abdominal discomfort.
Metabolic: *hyperglycemia,* hyperuricemia.
Local: inflammation and pain from extravasation.

INTERACTIONS
Hydralazine: may cause severe hypotension. Use together cautiously.
Thiazide diuretics: may increase the effects of diazoxide. Use together cautiously.

NURSING CONSIDERATIONS
- *Use cautiously* in patients with impaired cerebral or cardiac function, diabetes, or uremia, or in those taking other antihypertensives.

• **I.V. use:** Monitor blood pressure and ECG continuously. Patient should be supine or in Trendelenberg's position during and for 1 hour after infusion. Notify doctor immediately if severe hypotension develops. Keep norepinephrine available.
• Monitor patient's intake and output carefully. If fluid or sodium retention develops, doctor may want to order diuretics.
• Check patient's standing blood pressure before discontinuing close monitoring for hypotension.
• Take care to avoid extravasation.
• This drug may alter requirements for insulin, diet, or oral hypoglycemic drugs in previously controlled diabetics. Monitor blood glucose daily.
• Weigh patient daily. Notify doctor of any weight increase.
• Watch diabetics closely for signs of severe hyperglycemia or hyperosmolar nonketotic coma. Insulin may be needed.
• Check patient's uric acid levels frequently. Report abnormalities to doctor.
• Inform patient that orthostatic hypotension can be minimized by rising slowly and avoiding sudden position changes. Instruct patient to remain supine for 30 minutes after injection.
• Infusion of diazoxide has been shown to be as effective as a bolus in some patients.
• Protect I.V. solutions from light. Darkened I.V. solutions of diazoxide are subpotent and should not be used.

doxazosin mesylate
Cardura

Pregnancy Risk Category: B

HOW SUPPLIED
Tablets: 1 mg, 2 mg, 4 mg, 8 mg

MECHANISM OF ACTION
An alpha-adrenergic blocking agent that acts on the peripheral vasculature to produce vasodilation.

INDICATIONS & DOSAGE
Essential hypertension –
Adults: initiate dosage at 1 mg P.O. daily and determine effect on standing and supine blood pressure at 2 to 6 hours and 24 hours after dosing. If necessary, increase dose to 2 mg daily. To minimize adverse reactions, titrate dosage slowly (usually increased dosage only q 2 weeks). Dose may be increased to a daily dose of 4 mg, then 8 mg if necessary. Maximum daily dosage is 16 mg, but dosage that exceeds 4 mg daily is associated with a greater incidence of adverse reactions.

ADVERSE REACTIONS
Common reactions are in italics; life-threatening reactions are in bold italics.
CNS: dizziness, vertigo, headache, somnolence, drowsiness, fatigue, malaise, syncope, paresthesia.
CV: *orthostatic hypotension,* hypotension, edema, palpitations, ***arrhythmias,*** tachycardia, peripheral ischemia.
Skin: rash, pruritus.
Other: arthralgia, myalgia, muscle weakness, rhinitis.

INTERACTIONS
None reported.

NURSING CONSIDERATIONS
• *Contraindicated* in patients with hypersensitivity to the drug and quinazoline derivatives (including prazosin and terazosin).
• *Use cautiously* in patients with impaired hepatic function.
• Dosage increase must be titrated gradually, with adjustments every 2 weeks. The 2-, 4- and 8-mg tablets are not indicated for initial therapy.
• Patients taking doxazosin are sus-

ceptible to a "first-dose" effect similar to that produced by other alpha-adrenergic blocking agents; marked orthostatic hypotension may be accompanied by dizziness or syncope. Orthostatic hypotension is most common after the first dose, but can also occur when therapy is interrupted for a few days and during periods of dosage adjustment. Warn the patient that dizziness or fainting may occur. Advise him to avoid driving and other hazardous activities or situations.

- If syncope occurs, place patient in a recumbent position and treat supportively. A transient hypotensive response is not considered a contraindication to continued therapy.
- Warn patient that the drug may cause drowsiness. Tell patient to avoid driving and other hazardous activities that require alertness until the adverse CNS effects of the drug are known.

enalaprilat
Vasotec I.V.

enalapril maleate
Amprace‡, Renitec‡, Vasotec

Pregnancy Risk Category: C (D in 2nd and 3rd trimesters)

HOW SUPPLIED
Tablets: 2.5 mg, 5 mg, 10 mg, 20 mg
Injection: 1.25 mg/ml in 2-ml vials

MECHANISM OF ACTION
By inhibiting angiotensin-converting enzyme (ACE), prevents conversion of angiotensin I to angiotensin II.

INDICATIONS & DOSAGE
Treatment of hypertension –
Adults: initially, 5 mg P.O. once daily, then adjust according to response. Usual dosage range is 10 to 40 mg daily as a single dose or two divided doses. Alternatively, give by I.V. infusion 1.25 mg q 6 hours over 5 minutes.

To convert from I.V. therapy to oral therapy –
Adults: initially, 5 mg P.O. once a day. Adjust dosage to response.

To convert from oral therapy to I.V. therapy –
Adults: 1.25 mg I.V. over 5 minutes q 6 hours. Higher doses have not demonstrated greater efficacy.

Adjunctive treatment of heart failure (with diuretics and digitalis) –
Adults: initially, 2.5 mg P.O. b.i.d. Adjust dosage based on clinical or hemodynamic response. Usual range is 5 to 20 mg daily in two divided doses; maximum dosage is 40 mg/day.

ADVERSE REACTIONS
Common reactions are in italics; life-threatening reactions are in bold italics.
Blood: ***neutropenia, agranulocytosis.***
CNS: *headache, dizziness, fatigue,* insomnia.
CV: *hypotension.*
GI: diarrhea, nausea.
GU: decreased renal function (patients with bilateral renal artery stenosis or CHF).
Skin: rash.
Other: persistent cough, ***angioedema.***

INTERACTIONS
Insulin, oral hypoglycemic agents: risk of hypoglycemia, especially at initiation of enalapril therapy. Monitor closely.
Lithium: lithium toxicity can occur. Monitor lithium levels.
NSAIDs: may reduce antihypertensive effect. Monitor blood pressure.
Potassium supplements, potassium-sparing diuretics: increased risk of hyperkalemia. Avoid these agents unless hypokalemic blood levels are confirmed.

NURSING CONSIDERATIONS
- *Contraindicated* during pregnancy because ACE inhibitors can cause fe-

tal and neonatal injury or death. These problems have not been detected when fetal exposure has been limited to the first trimester. When pregnancy is detected, ACE inhibitors should be discontinued as soon as possible.

• *Use cautiously* in preexisting renal impairment or collagen vascular disease. Diabetic patients, patients with impaired renal function or CHF, and patients receiving drugs that can increase serum potassium may develop hyperkalemia. Monitor potassium intake and serum potassium level.

• If patient is taking a diuretic, it should be discontinued 2 to 3 days before beginning enalapril therapy. This will reduce the risk of hypotension. Then, if enalapril does not control blood pressure, diuretic therapy may be added.

• When used to treat heart failure, monitor patient closely for hypotension, especially after the initial dose. Observe the patient for at least 2 hours and then for at least 1 hour after blood pressure has stabilized.

• A response to I.V. enalaprilat is usually seen in 15 minutes, but peak effects may not be seen for up to 4 hours.

• Teach patient about his disease and therapy. Explain the importance of taking this drug as prescribed, even when he's feeling well. Tell outpatient not to discontinue drug suddenly, but to call the doctor if unpleasant adverse reactions occur.

• Instruct patient to check with doctor or pharmacist before taking OTC medications.

• Angioedema (including laryngeal edema) may occur, especially after the first enalapril dose. Advise patient to report any signs or symptoms such as swelling of face, eyes, lips, tongue, or breathing difficulty.

• Advise patient to report light-headedness, especially during the first few days of therapy, when it's most likely to occur.

• Advise patient to report any sign of infection.

• Enalapril is similar to captopril, another ACE inhibitor, but has a longer duration of action. Many patients may get satisfactory therapeutic results by taking enalapril once daily.

felodipine

Plendil

Pregnancy Risk Category: C

HOW SUPPLIED

Tablets (extended-release): 5 mg, 10 mg

MECHANISM OF ACTION

A dihydropyridine-derivative calcium channel blocker that blocks the entry of calcium ions into vascular smooth muscle and cardiac cells; shows some selectivity for smooth muscle as compared with cardiac muscle.

INDICATIONS & DOSAGE

Hypertension –

Adults: initially, 5 mg P.O. daily. Adjust dosage according to patient response, generally at intervals not less than 2 weeks. The usual dose is 5 to 10 mg daily; the maximum recommended dose is 20 mg daily.

Elderly patients and patients with impaired hepatic function: 5 mg P.O. daily; adjust dosage as for adults. Maximum recommended dose is 10 mg daily.

ADVERSE REACTIONS

Common reactions are in italics; life-threatening reactions are in bold italics.

CNS: headache, dizziness, paresthesia, asthenia.

CV: *peripheral edema,* chest pain, palpitations, increased heart rate.

EENT: cough, rhinorrhea.

GI: dyspepsia, abdominal pain, nausea, constipation, diarrhea.

Respiratory: upper respiratory infection, pharyngitis.
Skin: rash, *flushing*.
Other: muscle cramps, back pain, gingival hyperplasia.

INTERACTIONS
Cimetidine: decreases the clearance of felodipine. Use lower doses of felodipine.
Digoxin: decreased peak levels of digoxin, but total absorbed drug is unchanged. Clinical significance is unknown.
Metoprolol: felodipine may alter the pharmacokinetics of metoprolol. No dosage adjustment appears necessary; monitor for adverse effects.

NURSING CONSIDERATIONS
- *Contraindicated* in patients with hypersensitivity to the drug.
- *Use cautiously* in patients with heart failure, particularly those receiving beta-adrenergic blockers, and in patients with impaired hepatic function because clearance of drug from the blood is dependent on the liver. Although felodipine metabolites accumulate in the plasma of patients with renal disease, these metabolites are inactive.
- Also *use cautiously* in patients with angina. A reflex increase in heart rate is frequently seen during the first week of therapy. This increased rate, which may precipitate chest pain in certain patients, gradually diminishes over time, but heart rate increases of 5 to 10 beats/minute may persist with chronic dosing. Administration of beta-adrenergic blockers will attenuate this effect.
- Peripheral edema appears to be both dose- and age-dependent: it's more common in patients taking higher doses, especially those over age 60.
- Felodipine may be administered without regard to meals. In a small study, bioavailability of the drug was increased more than twofold when taken with doubly concentrated grape juice as compared with water or orange juice.
- Tell the patient to observe good oral hygiene and to see a dentist regularly because drug has been associated with mild gingival hyperplasia.
- Tell the patient to swallow the tablets whole and not to crush or chew them.
- Be sure the patient understands his disease. He should continue taking the drug, even when he's feeling better; watch his diet; and check with the doctor or pharmacist before taking any other medications, including OTC drugs.

fosinopril sodium
Monopril

Pregnancy Risk Category: D

HOW SUPPLIED
Tablets: 10 mg, 20 mg

MECHANISM OF ACTION
Inhibits angiotensin-converting enzyme (ACE), preventing conversion of angiotensin I to angiotensin II, a potent vasoconstrictor. Reduced formation of angiotensin II decreases peripheral arterial resistance, which results in decreased aldosterone secretion. This reduces sodium and water retention and lowers blood pressure. Fosinopril also has antihypertensive activity in patients with low-renin hypertension.

INDICATIONS & DOSAGE
Hypertension –
Adults: initially, 10 mg P.O. daily; adjust dose based on blood pressure response at peak and trough levels. Usual dose is 20 to 40 mg, up to 80 mg. Dose may be divided.

ADVERSE REACTIONS

Common reactions are in italics; life-threatening reactions are in bold italics.

CNS: headache, dizziness, fatigue, light-headedness, syncope, memory disturbances, mood change, paresthesia, sleep disturbance, drowsiness, weakness, ***CVA***.

CV: chest pain, angina, ***MI, hypertensive crisis,*** rhythm disturbances, palpitations, hypotension, flushing, claudications, orthostatic hypotension.

EENT: tinnitus, vision disturbances, eye irritation, epistaxis.

GI: nausea, vomiting, diarrhea, pancreatitis, hepatitis, dysphagia, abdominal distention, abdominal pain, flatulence, constipation, heartburn, appetite change, weight change, dry mouth.

GU: sexual dysfunction, decreased libido, urinary frequency, renal insufficiency, acute renal failure.

Respiratory: cough, ***bronchospasm,*** pharyngitis, sinusitis, rhinitis, laryngitis, hoarseness.

Skin: urticaria, rash, photosensitivity, pruritus.

Other: ***angioedema,*** fever, arthralgia, musculoskeletal pain, myalgia, jaundice, gout.

INTERACTIONS

Antacids: may impair absorption. Separate administration times by at least 2 hours.

Diuretics, other antihypertensives: risk of excessive hypotension. Discontinue diuretic or lower dose of fosinopril as needed.

Lithium: increased serum lithium levels and lithium toxicity have been reported. Avoid concomitant use.

Potassium-sparing diuretics, potassium supplements, sodium substitutes containing potassium: risk of hyperkalemia. Avoid concomitant use.

NURSING CONSIDERATIONS

- *Contraindicated* in patients with hypersensitivity to ACE inhibitors or with a history of angioedema.
- *Use cautiously* in patients with impaired renal or hepatic function and in renal insufficiency, in diabetes mellitus, and with use of potassium-sparing diuretics, potassium supplements, and sodium substitutes containing potassium because of risk of hyperkalemia.
- Avoid use during pregnancy because ACE inhibitors can cause fetal or neonatal injury or death. When pregnancy is detected, ACE inhibitors should be discontinued as soon as possible.
- Avoid use of fosinopril in breast-feeding women because detectable levels of the drug have been found in breast milk.
- Excessive hypotension can occur when drug is given with diuretics. If possible, diuretic therapy should be discontinued 2 to 3 days before starting fosinopril to reduce potential for excessive hypotensive response. If fosinopril does not adequately control blood pressure, diuretic may be reinstituted with care.
- Absorption may be slowed by presence of food in the GI tract. Tell patient that drug should be taken on an empty stomach, 1 hour before or 2 hours after meals. If taking antacids, wait for 2 hours after a dose.
- Like other ACE inhibitors, drug may cause dry, persistent, tickling, nonproductive cough that is reversible when therapy is discontinued.
- Assess renal and hepatic function before and periodically throughout therapy. Monitor CBC with differential counts before and every 2 weeks for the first 3 months of therapy, and periodically thereafter. Monitor potassium levels.
- Inadequate fluid intake, vomiting, diarrhea, and excessive perspiration can lead to light-headedness and syn-

cope. Tell patient to use cautiously in hot weather and during periods of exercise.

- Tell patient to avoid sodium substitutes because they contain potassium and can cause hyperkalemia.
- Other ACE inhibitors have been associated with agranulocytosis and neutropenia.
- Tell patient to call the doctor if any of the following signs or symptoms occur: any signs of infection (such as fever, sore throat); easy bruising or bleeding; swelling of tongue, lips, face, mucous membranes, eyes, lips, or extremities; difficulty swallowing or breathing; and hoarseness.

guanabenz acetate

Wytensin

Pregnancy Risk Category: C

HOW SUPPLIED

Tablets: 4 mg, 8 mg

MECHANISM OF ACTION

Inhibits the central vasomotor centers, thereby decreasing sympathetic outflow.

INDICATIONS & DOSAGE

Treatment of hypertension –

Adults: initially, 4 mg P.O. b.i.d. Dosage may be increased in increments of 4 to 8 mg/day q 1 to 2 weeks. Maximum dosage is 32 mg b.i.d. To ensure adequate overnight blood pressure control, give last dose h.s.

ADVERSE REACTIONS

Common reactions are in italics; life-threatening reactions are in bold italics.

CNS: *drowsiness, sedation, dizziness, weakness,* headache, ataxia, depression.

CV: ***severe rebound hypertension.***

EENT: *dry mouth.*

GU: sexual dysfunction.

INTERACTIONS

CNS depressants: may cause increased sedation. Use together cautiously.

Tricyclic antidepressants, MAO inhibitors: may decrease antihypertensive effect.

NURSING CONSIDERATIONS

- *Use cautiously* in vascular insufficiency, coronary insufficiency, recent MI, cerebrovascular disease, or severe hepatic or renal failure.
- Don't stop guanabenz therapy abruptly. Rebound hypertension may occur.
- Advise patient to avoid driving and other hazardous tasks that require alertness until the CNS effects of the drug are known.
- Elderly patients may be more sensitive to hypotensive effects.
- Warn patient that his tolerance to alcohol or other CNS depressants may be diminished.
- Guanabenz can be used alone or in combination with a thiazide diuretic.
- Teach patient about his disease and therapy. Explain the importance of taking this drug as prescribed, even when he's feeling well. Tell outpatient not to discontinue drug suddenly, but to call the doctor if unpleasant adverse reactions occur.
- Instruct patient to check with doctor or pharmacist before taking OTC medications.
- To relieve dry mouth, tell patient to chew sugarless gum or dissolve ice chips in the mouth.
- Has been used investigationally as an adjunct in the treatment of opiate withdrawal (4 mg P.O. b.i.d.).

guanadrel sulfate

Hylorel

Pregnancy Risk Category: B

HOW SUPPLIED

Tablets: 10 mg, 25 mg

MECHANISM OF ACTION
Acts peripherally, inhibiting norepinephrine release and depleting norepinephrine stores in adrenergic nerve endings.

INDICATIONS & DOSAGE
Treatment of hypertension –
Adults: initially, 5 mg P.O. b.i.d. Dosage can be adjusted until blood pressure is controlled. Most patients require doses of 20 to 75 mg/day, usually given b.i.d.; however, tolerance to hypotensive effect may necessitate upward titration of dosage to 100 to 400 mg daily, given in three to four divided doses.

ADVERSE REACTIONS
Common reactions are in italics; life-threatening reactions are in bold italics.
CNS: *fatigue, dizziness,* drowsiness, faintness.
CV: *orthostatic hypotension,* edema.
GI: diarrhea.
Other: impotence, ejaculation disturbances.

INTERACTIONS
MAO inhibitors, ephedrine, norepinephrine, methylphenidate, tricyclic antidepressants, amphetamines, phenothiazines: may inhibit the antihypertensive effect of guanadrel. Adjust dose accordingly.

NURSING CONSIDERATIONS
• *Contraindicated* in known or suspected pheochromocytoma or frank CHF.
• *Use cautiously* in known peripheral vascular disease, asthma, and history of peptic ulcer disease.
• Guanadrel should be discontinued 48 to 72 hours before surgery to minimize the risk of vascular collapse during anesthesia.
• Don't give concurrently or within 1 week of therapy with an MAO inhibitor.
• Patient response varies widely with this drug and dosage must be individualized. Monitor both supine and standing blood pressure, especially during the period of dosage adjustment.
• Teach patient about his disease and therapy. Explain the importance of taking this drug as prescribed, even when he's feeling well. Tell patient not to discontinue this drug suddenly, but to call the doctor if unpleasant adverse reactions occur.
• Instruct patient to check with doctor or pharmacist before taking OTC medications.
• Tell outpatient to avoid strenuous exercise, and warn that hot showers may cause hypotensive reaction.
• Inform patient that orthostatic hypotension can be minimized by rising slowly from a supine position and by avoiding sudden position changes.
• Elderly patients may be more sensitive to hypotensive effects.

guanethidine sulfate
Apo-Guanethidine†, Ismelin
Pregnancy Risk Category: C

HOW SUPPLIED
Tablets: 10 mg, 25 mg

MECHANISM OF ACTION
Acts peripherally, inhibiting norepinephrine release and depleting norepinephrine stores in adrenergic nerve endings.

INDICATIONS & DOSAGE
For moderate to severe hypertension; usually used in combination with other antihypertensives –
Adults: initially, 10 mg P.O. daily. Increase by 10 mg at weekly to monthly intervals, p.r.n. Usual dose is 25 to 50 mg daily. Some patients may require up to 300 mg.
Children: initially, 200 mcg/kg P.O. daily. Increase gradually q 1 to 3

weeks to maximum of 8 times initial dose.

ADVERSE REACTIONS
Common reactions are in italics; life-threatening reactions are in bold italics.
CNS: *dizziness, weakness, syncope.*
CV: *orthostatic hypotension, bradycardia,* ***CHF, arrhythmias.***
EENT: *nasal stuffiness.*
GI: *diarrhea.*
Other: *edema, weight gain, inhibition of ejaculation.*

INTERACTIONS
Levodopa, alcohol: may increase hypotensive effect of guanethidine. Use together cautiously.
MAO inhibitors, ephedrine, norepinephrine, methylphenidate, tricyclic antidepressants, amphetamines, phenothiazines: may inhibit the antihypertensive effect of guanethidine. Adjust dose accordingly.

NURSING CONSIDERATIONS
- *Contraindicated* in pheochromocytoma.
- *Use cautiously* in severe cardiac disease, recent myocardial infarction, cerebrovascular disease, peptic ulcer, impaired renal function, or bronchial asthma, or in patients taking other antihypertensives.
- Full antihypertensive effect may not appear for 1 to 3 weeks.
- Discontinue drug 2 to 3 weeks before elective surgery to reduce the possibility of vascular collapse and cardiac arrest during anesthesia.
- Teach patient about his disease and therapy. Explain the importance of taking this drug as prescribed, even when he's feeling well. Tell patient not to discontinue this drug suddenly, but to call the doctor if unpleasant adverse reactions occur.
- Instruct patient to check with doctor or pharmacist before taking OTC medications.
- Tell outpatient to avoid strenuous exercise, and warn that hot showers may cause hypotensive reaction.
- A hot environment may also potentiate the hypotensive effects of guanethidine.
- Patient should receive instruction on low-sodium diet. Monitor for possible weight gain and edema.
- Inform patient that orthostatic hypotension can be minimized by rising slowly and avoiding sudden position changes. Dry mouth can be relieved with sugarless chewing gum, sour hard candy, or ice chips.
- Elderly patients may be more sensitive to hypotensive effects.
- If patient develops diarrhea, doctor may prescribe atropine or paregoric.

guanfacine hydrochloride
Tenex

Pregnancy Risk Category: B

HOW SUPPLIED
Tablets: 1 mg

MECHANISM OF ACTION
Inhibits the central vasomotor center, thereby decreasing sympathetic outflow.

INDICATIONS & DOSAGE
Treatment of mild to moderate hypertension –
Adults: initially, 0.5 to 1 mg P.O. daily, h.s. Average dose is 1 to 3 mg daily.

ADVERSE REACTIONS
Common reactions are in italics; life-threatening reactions are in bold italics.
CNS: *drowsiness, dizziness,* fatigue, headache, insomnia.
CV: bradycardia, orthostatic hypotension, rebound hypertension.
EENT: dry mouth.
GI: *constipation,* diarrhea, nausea.
Skin: dermatitis, pruritus.

INTERACTIONS
None significant.

NURSING CONSIDERATIONS
- *Use cautiously* in severe coronary insufficiency, recent myocardial infarction, cerebrovascular disease, or chronic renal or hepatic insufficiency.
- Warn patients not to discontinue therapy abruptly. Rebound hypertension is less common than with similar drugs, such as clonidine, but may occur.
- Guanfacine reportedly has no adverse effect on blood lipids.
- May be used alone or with a diuretic.
- The incidence and severity of adverse reactions increase with higher dosages.
- Teach patient about his disease and therapy. Explain the importance of taking this drug as prescribed, even when he's feeling well. Tell outpatient not to discontinue drug suddenly, but to call the doctor if unpleasant adverse reactions occur.
- Instruct patient to check with doctor or pharmacist before taking OTC medications.
- Because guanfacine causes drowsiness, advise patient to avoid activities that require alertness until response to the drug is established.
- Guanfacine appears to be as effective as methyldopa and clonidine; long half-life permits once-daily dosing.

hydralazine hydrochloride
Alazine, Apresoline**, Novo-Hylazin†, Supres‡

Pregnancy Risk Category: C

HOW SUPPLIED
Tablets: 10 mg, 25 mg, 50 mg, 100 mg
Injection: 20 mg/ml

MECHANISM OF ACTION
Directly relaxes arteriolar smooth muscle.

INDICATIONS & DOSAGE
Essential hypertension (oral, alone or in combination with other antihypertensives); to reduce afterload in severe CHF (with nitrates); and severe essential hypertension (parenteral to lower blood pressure quickly) –
Adults: initially, 10 mg P.O. q.i.d.; gradually increased to 50 mg q.i.d. Maximum recommended dosage is 200 mg daily, but some patients may require 300 to 400 mg daily. Can be given b.i.d. for CHF.
I.V. – 10 to 20 mg given slowly and repeated as necessary, generally q 4 to 6 hours. Switch to oral antihypertensives as soon as possible.
I.M. – 20 to 40 mg repeated as necessary, generally q 4 to 6 hours. Switch to oral antihypertensives as soon as possible.
Children: initially, 0.75 mg/kg P.O. daily in four divided doses (25 mg/m^2 daily). May increase gradually to 10 times this dosage, if necessary.
I.V. – give slowly 1.7 to 3.5 mg/kg daily or 50 to 100 mg/m^2 daily in four to six divided doses.
I.M. – 1.7 to 3.5 mg/kg daily or 50 to 100 mg/m^2 daily in four to six divided doses.

ADVERSE REACTIONS
Common reactions are in italics; life-threatening reactions are in bold italics.
Blood: neutropenia, leukopenia.
CNS: peripheral neuritis, *headache,* dizziness.
CV: orthostatic hypotension, *tachycardia,* arrhythmias, *angina, palpitations, sodium retention.*
GI: *nausea, vomiting, diarrhea, anorexia.*
Skin: rash.
Other: *lupus erythematosus-like syndrome (especially with high doses), weight gain.*

INTERACTIONS
Diazoxide, MAO inhibitors: may cause severe hypotension. Use together cautiously.

NURSING CONSIDERATIONS
- *Use cautiously* in cardiac disease, CVA, or severe renal impairment and in those taking other antihypertensives.
- Monitor patient's blood pressure, pulse rate, and body weight frequently. Some clinicians combine hydralazine therapy with diuretics and beta-adrenergic blocking agents to decrease sodium retention and tachycardia, and to prevent anginal attacks.
- Watch patient closely for signs of lupus erythematosus-like syndrome (sore throat, fever, muscle and joint aches, skin rash). Call doctor immediately if any of these develop.
- Teach patient about his disease and therapy. Explain the importance of taking this drug as prescribed, even when he's feeling well. Tell outpatient not to discontinue this drug suddenly, but to call the doctor if unpleasant adverse reactions occur.
- Instruct patient to check with doctor or pharmacist before taking OTC medications.
- Inform patient that orthostatic hypotension can be minimized by rising slowly and avoiding sudden position changes.
- Elderly patients may be more sensitive to hypotensive effects.
- Give this drug with meals to increase absorption.
- Compliance may be improved by administering this drug b.i.d. Check with doctor.
- CBC, lupus erythematosus cell preparation, and antinuclear antibody titer determinations should be done before therapy and periodically during long-term therapy.
- Has been prescribed during pregnancy for treatment of eclampsia. Administered I.V.
- **I.V. use:** Give slowly and repeat as necessary, generally q 4 to 6 hours. Switch to oral antihypertensives as soon as possible.

isradipine
DynaCirc
Pregnancy Risk Category: C

HOW SUPPLIED
Capsules: 2.5 mg, 5 mg

MECHANISM OF ACTION
A calcium channel blocking agent that inhibits calcium ion influx across cardiac and smooth muscle cells, thus decreasing arteriolar resistance and reducing blood pressure.

INDICATIONS & DOSAGE
Essential hypertension –
Adults: initially, 2.5 mg P.O. b.i.d given alone or with a thiazide diuretic. Adjust dosage based on tolerance and response to a maximum of 20 mg daily.

ADVERSE REACTIONS
Common reactions are in italics; life-threatening reactions are in bold italics.
CNS: dizziness.
CV: edema, flushing, palpitations, tachycardia.
GI: nausea, diarrhea.
GU: frequent urination.
Skin: rash.
Other: dyspnea.

INTERACTIONS
Fentanyl anesthesia: severe hypotension has been reported with concomitant use of a beta blocker and a calcium channel blocker. Be sure to inform anesthesiologist that the patient is taking a calcium channel blocker.

NURSING CONSIDERATIONS
- *Contraindicated* in patients with hypersensitivity to the drug.
- *Use cautiously* in patients with

CHF, especially if combined with a beta blocker.
- Isradipine has diuretic activity; the mechanism is not fully understood. Patients may note an increased need to void.
- Like other calcium channel blockers, isradipine is known to cause symptomatic hypotension; however, syncope and severe dizziness have not been reported. Most adverse reactions are mild and transient and related to vasodilation (dizziness, edema, flushing, palpitations, and tachycardia).
- Initial therapy produces antihypertensive effect in 2 to 3 hours; however, maximal response usually develops after 2 to 4 weeks of continuous therapy.
- Increase dosage by gradual titration. If response is inadequate after first 2 to 4 weeks, increase dosage to 5 mg b.i.d. Continue increasing at 5-mg/day intervals every 2 to 4 weeks to a maximum of 10 mg b.i.d. Most patients show no additional response at dosages over 10 mg daily (5 mg b.i.d.).
- The bioavailability of isradipine is increased in elderly patients and those with impaired hepatic function. However, the starting dosage should still be 2.5 mg b.i.d.
- Teach patient to take his blood pressure.

labetalol hydrochloride

Normodyne, Presolol‡, Trandate

Pregnancy Risk Category: C

HOW SUPPLIED

Tablets: 100 mg, 200 mg, 300 mg
Injection: 5 mg/ml

MECHANISM OF ACTION

Blocks response to alpha and beta stimulation and depresses renin secretion.

INDICATIONS & DOSAGE

Treatment of hypertension –
Adults: 100 mg P.O. b.i.d. with or without a diuretic. Dose may be increased to 200 mg b.i.d. after 2 days. Further dose increases may be made q 1 to 3 days until optimum response is reached. Usual maintenance dosage is 200 to 400 mg b.i.d.

For severe hypertension and hypertensive emergencies –
Adults: Dilute 200 mg to 200 ml with dextrose 5% in water. Infuse at 2 mg/minute until satisfactory response is obtained. Then stop the infusion. May repeat q 6 to 8 hours.

Alternatively, administer by repeated I.V. injection: Initially, give 20 mg I.V. slowly over 2 minutes. May repeat injections of 40 to 80 mg q 10 minutes until maximum dose of 300 mg is reached.

ADVERSE REACTIONS

Common reactions are in italics; life-threatening reactions are in bold italics.
CNS: vivid dreams, fatigue, headache.
CV: *orthostatic hypotension and dizziness,* peripheral vascular disease, bradycardia.
EENT: nasal stuffiness.
Endocrine: hypoglycemia without tachycardia.
GI: nausea, vomiting, diarrhea.
GU: sexual dysfunction, urine retention.
Skin: rash.
Other: increased airway resistance, transient scalp tingling.

INTERACTIONS

Cimetidine: may enhance labetalol's effect. Give together cautiously.
Halothane: additive hypotensive effect.
Insulin, oral hypoglycemic drugs: can alter dosage requirements in previously stabilized diabetics. Observe patient carefully.

*Liquid form contains alcohol. **May contain tartrazine.

NURSING CONSIDERATIONS

- *Contraindicated* in bronchial asthma.
- *Use cautiously* in CHF, hepatic failure, chronic bronchitis, emphysema, preexisting peripheral vascular disease, and pheochromocytoma.
- Monitor blood pressure frequently.
- Teach patient about his disease and therapy. Explain the importance of taking this drug as prescribed, even when he's feeling well. Tell outpatient not to discontinue this drug suddenly; abrupt discontinuation can exacerbate angina and myocardial infarction. Tell patient to call the doctor if unpleasant adverse reactions occur.
- Instruct patient to check with doctor or pharmacist before taking OTC medications.
- This drug masks common signs of shock and hypoglycemia.
- Labetalol is a beta-adrenergic blocker that also has unique alpha-adrenergic blocking effects.
- Unlike other beta blockers, labetalol does not decrease heart rate or cardiac output.
- Dizziness is the most troublesome adverse reaction and tends to occur in early stages of treatment, in patients also receiving diuretics, and in patients receiving higher dosages. Inform patient that this can be minimized by rising slowly and avoiding sudden position changes. Taking a dose at bedtime or taking smaller doses t.i.d. will also help minimize this adverse reaction. Discuss changes in medication schedule with doctor.
- Transient scalp tingling occurs occasionally at the beginning of labetalol therapy. This usually subsides quickly.
- **I.V. use:** Labetalol injection should be administered with a controlled infusion pump. Monitor blood pressure closely: q 5 minutes for 30 minutes, then q 30 minutes for 2 hours, then hourly for 6 hours. Patient should remain supine for 3 hours after infusion.
- When administered I.V. for hypertensive emergencies, labetalol produces a rapid, predictable fall in blood pressure within 5 to 10 minutes.

lisinopril

Prinivil, Zestril

Pregnancy Risk Category: C (D in 2nd and 3rd trimesters)

HOW SUPPLIED

Tablets: 5 mg, 10 mg, 20 mg

MECHANISM OF ACTION

Inhibits angiotensin-converting enzyme (ACE), preventing conversion of angiotensin I to angiotensin II, a potent vasoconstrictor. This decreases peripheral arterial resistance and aldosterone secretion, thereby reducing sodium and water retention and blood pressure.

INDICATIONS & DOSAGE

Mild to severe hypertension –
Adults: initially, 10 mg P.O. daily. Most patients are well controlled on 20 to 40 mg daily as a single dose.

ADVERSE REACTIONS

Common reactions are in italics; life-threatening reactions are in bold italics.
Blood: neutropenia.
CNS: *dizziness, headache, fatigue,* depression, somnolence, paresthesia.
CV: hypotension, *orthostatic hypotension,* chest pain.
EENT: *nasal congestion.*
GI: *diarrhea,* nausea, dyspepsia, dysgeusia.
GU: impotence.
Metabolic: hyperkalemia.
Skin: rash.
Other: *upper respiratory symptoms, cough, muscle cramps,* ***angioedema,*** decreased libido.

INTERACTIONS
Diuretics: excessive hypotension.
Indomethacin: attenuated hypotensive effect.
Insulin, oral hypoglycemic agents: risk of hypoglycemia, especially at initiation of lisinopril therapy. Monitor closely.
Potassium-sparing diuretics, potassium supplements, potassium-containing sodium substitutes: possible hyperkalemia.

NURSING CONSIDERATIONS
- *Contraindicated* during pregnancy because ACE inhibitors can cause fetal and neonatal injury or death. These problems have not been detected when fetal exposure has been limited to the first trimester. When pregnancy is detected, ACE inhibitors should be discontinued as soon as possible.
- Lower dosage is necessary in patients with impaired renal function.
- Lisinopril absorption is unaffected by food.
- Lisinopril attenuates potassium loss of thiazide diuretics. If patient is taking a diuretic, the diuretic should be discontinued 2 to 3 days before lisinopril therapy, or lisinopril dosage should be reduced to 5 mg once daily.
- If drug does not adequately control blood pressure, diuretics may be added.
- Teach patient about his disease and therapy. Explain the importance of taking this drug as prescribed, even when he's feeling well. Tell outpatient not to discontinue drug suddenly, but to call the doctor if unpleasant adverse reactions occur.
- Instruct patient to check with doctor or pharmacist before taking OTC medications.
- Review WBC and differential counts before treatment every 2 weeks for 3 months, and periodically thereafter.
- Beneficial effects of lisinopril may require several weeks of therapy.
- Tell patient to report light-headedness, especially in first few days of treatment, so dose can be adjusted; signs of infection such as sore throat or fever, because drugs may decrease WBC count; facial swelling or difficulty breathing, because drug may cause angioedema; and loss of taste, which may necessitate discontinuation of drug.
- Advise patient to avoid sudden postural changes to minimize orthostatic hypotension.
- Has been used investigationally in the treatment of CHF.

mecamylamine hydrochloride
Inversine
Pregnancy Risk Category: C

HOW SUPPLIED
Tablets: 2.5 mg

MECHANISM OF ACTION
A ganglionic blocker; competes with acetylcholine for ganglionic cholinergic receptors.

INDICATIONS & DOSAGE
For moderate to severe essential hypertension and uncomplicated malignant hypertension –
Adults: initially, 2.5 mg P.O. b.i.d. Increase by 2.5 mg daily q 2 days. Average daily dose is 25 mg given in three divided doses. No dosing recommendations for children.

ADVERSE REACTIONS
Common reactions are in italics; life-threatening reactions are in bold italics.
CNS: *paresthesias,* sedation, *fatigue, tremor, choreiform movements,* seizures, psychic changes, dizziness, *weakness, headaches.*
CV: *orthostatic hypotension.*

*Liquid form contains alcohol. **May contain tartrazine.

EENT: *dry mouth,* glossitis, dilated pupils, *blurred vision.*
GI: *anorexia, nausea, vomiting, constipation, adynamic ileus, diarrhea.*
GU: urine retention, impotence.
Other: decreased libido.

INTERACTIONS
Alcohol, bethanecol: excessive hypotension. Don't use together.
Sodium bicarbonate, acetazolamide: may increase effect of mecamylamine. Use together cautiously. Watch for increased hypotensive effects and toxicity.

NURSING CONSIDERATIONS
- *Contraindicated* in recent myocardial infarction, uremia, or chronic pyelonephritis.
- *Use cautiously* in lower urinary tract pathology, renal insufficiency, glaucoma, pyloric stenosis, coronary insufficiency, or in patients taking other antihypertensives. Mecamylamine is usually reserved for moderate to severe hypertension that is refractory to other drugs.
- Effects of this drug are increased by high environmental temperature, fever, stress, or severe illness.
- Don't withdraw this drug suddenly; rebound hypertension may occur.
- Frequently monitor patient's standing blood pressure.
- Give with meals for more gradual absorption. Schedule the administration consistently with meals. Don't restrict sodium intake.
- If patient develops constipation from this drug, the doctor may want him to take milk of magnesia. Instruct patient to avoid bulk laxatives.
- Teach the patient about his disease and therapy. Explain the importance of taking this drug as prescribed, even when he's feeling well. Tell outpatient to call the doctor if unpleasant adverse reactions develop. Warn him against discontinuing the drug suddenly because this may cause severe rebound hypertension.
- Instruct patient to check with doctor or pharmacist before taking OTC medications.
- Inform patient that orthostatic hypotension can be minimized by rising slowly and avoiding sudden position changes. Dry mouth can be relieved with sugarless chewing gum, sour hard candy, or ice chips.

methyldopa
Aldomet, Aldomet M‡, Apo-Methyldopa†, Dopamet†, Hydopa‡, Novomedopa†

methyldopate hydrochloride
Aldomet, Aldomet Ester Injection‡
Pregnancy Risk Category: B

HOW SUPPLIED
methyldopa
Tablets: 125 mg, 250 mg, 500 mg
Oral suspension: 250 mg/5 ml
methyldopate hydrochloride
Injection: 250 mg/5 ml in 5-ml vials

MECHANISM OF ACTION
Inhibits the central vasomotor centers, thereby decreasing sympathetic outflow.

INDICATIONS & DOSAGE
For sustained mild to severe hypertension; should not be used for acute treatment of hypertensive emergencies –
Adults: initially, 250 mg P.O. b.i.d. to t.i.d. in first 48 hours. Then increase as needed q 2 days. May give entire daily dosage in the evening or h.s. Dosages may need adjustment if other antihypertensive drugs are added to or deleted from therapy. Maintenance dosage is 500 mg to 2 g daily in two to four divided doses. Maximum recommended daily dosage is 3 g.

I.V. – 250 to 500 mg q 6 hours, diluted in dextrose 5% in water and administered over 30 to 60 minutes. Maximum dosage is 1 g q 6 hours. Switch to oral antihypertensives as soon as possible.
Children: initially, 10 mg/kg P.O. daily in two to three divided doses; or 20 to 40 mg/kg I.V. daily in four divided doses. Increase dose daily until desired response occurs. Maximum daily dose is 65 mg/kg, 2 g/m^2, or 3 g/day, whichever is least.

ADVERSE REACTIONS
Common reactions are in italics; life-threatening reactions are in bold italics.
Blood: ***hemolytic anemia,*** reversible granulocytopenia, thrombocytopenia.
CNS: *sedation,* headache, asthenia, weakness, dizziness, *decreased mental acuity,* involuntary choreoathetotic movements, psychic disturbances, depression, nightmares.
CV: bradycardia, *orthostatic hypotension,* aggravated angina, myocarditis, *edema, and weight gain.*
EENT: *dry mouth, nasal stuffiness.*
GI: diarrhea, pancreatitis.
Hepatic: ***hepatic necrosis.***
Other: gynecomastia, lactation, skin rash, ***drug-induced fever,*** impotence.

INTERACTIONS
Levodopa: additive hypotensive effects; possible increased CNS adverse reactions.
Norepinephrine, phenothiazines, tricyclic antidepressants, amphetamines: possible hypertensive effects. Monitor carefully.

NURSING CONSIDERATIONS
• *Use cautiously* in patients receiving other antihypertensives or MAO inhibitors and in patients with impaired hepatic function. Monitor blood pressure and pulse rate frequently.
• Methyldopa is frequently used to treat hypertension in pregnant women, apparently without ill effects to the fetus if the patient is closely monitored. Some clinicians recommend that therapy not begin between 16 and 20 weeks' gestation, if possible.
• **I.V. use:** Observe for involuntary choreoathetoid movements. Report to doctor; he may discontinue drug.
• Observe patient for adverse reactions, particularly unexplained fever. Report adverse reactions to doctor.
• After dialysis, monitor patient for hypertension. Patient may need an extra dose of methyldopa.
• If patient has received this drug for several months, positive reaction to direct Coombs' test indicates hemolytic anemia.
• If patient requires blood transfusion, make sure he gets direct and indirect Coombs' tests to avoid cross-matching problems.
• Monitor blood studies (CBC) before and during therapy. Monitor hepatic function periodically, especially during the first 6 to 12 weeks of therapy.
• Weigh patient daily. Notify doctor of any weight increase. Sodium and water retention may occur but can be relieved with diuretics.
• Teach patient about his disease and therapy. Explain the importance of taking this drug as prescribed, even when he's feeling well. Tell outpatient not to stop this drug suddenly, but to call the doctor if unpleasant adverse reactions occur. Check dosage schedule with doctor.
• Warn patient that this drug may impair ability to perform tasks that require mental alertness, particularly at start of therapy. Once-daily dosage given at bedtime will minimize daytime drowsiness.
• Instruct patient to check with doctor or pharmacist before taking OTC medications.
• Inform patient that orthostatic hypotension can be minimized by rising slowly and avoiding sudden position changes. Dry mouth can be relieved

with sugarless chewing gum, sour hard candy, or ice chips.

- Tell patient that urine may turn dark in toilet bowls treated with bleach.
- Elderly patients are more likely to experience sedation and hypotension.

metoprolol tartrate

Apo-Metoprolol†, Betaloc†‡, Betaloc Durules†, Lopresor†, Lopresor SR†, Lopressor, Novometoprol†

Pregnancy Risk Category: B

HOW SUPPLIED

Tablets: 50 mg, 100 mg
Tablets (sustained-release): 100 mg†, 200 mg†
Injection: 1 mg/ml in 5-ml ampules or refilled syringes

MECHANISM OF ACTION

Blocks cardiac beta receptors and depresses renin secretion.

INDICATIONS & DOSAGE

For hypertension; may be used alone or in combination with other antihypertensives –
Adults: 50 mg b.i.d. or 100 mg once daily P.O. initially. Up to 200 to 400 mg daily in two to three divided doses. No dosage recommendations for children.
Early intervention in acute myocardial infarction –
Adults: Three injections of 5-mg I.V. boluses q 2 minutes. Then, 15 minutes after last dose, administer 50 mg P.O. q 6 hours for 48 hours. Maintenance dosage is 100 mg P.O. b.i.d.
Angina pectoris –
Adults: initially, 100 mg P.O. daily as a single dose. Increase dosage at weekly intervals until an adequate response or a pronounced decrease in heart rate is seen. Daily dosage beyond 400 mg has not been studied.

ADVERSE REACTIONS

Common reactions are in italics; life-threatening reactions are in bold italics.
CNS: fatigue, lethargy, dizziness.
CV: *bradycardia, hypotension, **CHF,*** peripheral vascular disease.
GI: nausea, vomiting, diarrhea.
Skin: rash.
Respiratory: dyspnea, ***bronchospasm.***
Other: fever, arthralgia.

INTERACTIONS

Barbiturates, rifampin: increased metabolism of metoprolol. Monitor for decreased effect.
Chlorpromazine, cimetidine, verapamil: decreased hepatic clearance. Monitor for greater beta-blocking effect.
Digitalis glycosides: excessive bradycardia and increased depressant effect on myocardium. Use together cautiously.
Indomethacin: decrease in antihypertensive effect. Monitor blood pressure and adjust dosage.
Insulin, oral hypoglycemic drugs: can alter dosage requirements in previously stabilized diabetics. Observe patient carefully.

NURSING CONSIDERATIONS

- *Contraindicated* in patients with hypersensitivity to the drug or other beta blockers and in patients with sinus bradycardia, heart block greater than first degree, cardiogenic shock, or overt cardiac failure.
- *Use cautiously* in heart failure, diabetes, respiratory or hepatic disease, or in patients taking other antihypertensives. Always check patient's apical pulse rate before giving this drug. If it's slower than 60 beats/minute, hold drug and call doctor immediately.
- Although most patients with asthma and bronchitis can take this drug without fear of worsening their condition,

doses over 100 mg daily should be used cautiously.

• Monitor blood pressure frequently.
• Teach patient about his disease and therapy. Explain the importance of taking this drug as prescribed, even when he's feeling well. Tell outpatient not to discontinue this drug suddenly because this can exacerbate angina and myocardial infarction. Drug must be withdrawn gradually over 1 to 2 weeks. Instruct patient to call doctor if unpleasant adverse reactions occur.
• Instruct patient to check with doctor or pharmacist before taking OTC medications.
• This drug masks common signs of shock and hypoglycemia. However, metoprolol doesn't potentiate insulin-induced hypoglycemia or delay recovery of blood glucose to normal levels.
• Food may increase absorption of metoprolol. Give consistently with meals.
• Patient should have periodic eye examinations while taking drug.
• Store drug at room temperature and protect from light. Discard solution if it's discolored or contains particles.

metyrosine

Demser

Pregnancy Risk Category: C

HOW SUPPLIED

Capsules: 250 mg

MECHANISM OF ACTION

Inhibits the enzyme tyrosine hydroxylase, thus inhibiting endogenous catecholamine synthesis.

INDICATIONS & DOSAGE

Preoperative preparation of patients with pheochromocytoma; management of such patients when surgery is contraindicated; to control or prevent hypertension before or during pheochromocytomectomy –

Adults and children over 12 years: 250 mg P.O. q.i.d. May be increased by 250 to 500 mg q day to a maximum of 4 g daily in divided doses. When used for preoperative preparation, optimally effective dosage should be given for at least 5 to 7 days. In normotensive patients, doses are adjusted to produce a 50% reduction in urinary metanephrines and vanillylmandelic acid.

ADVERSE REACTIONS

Common reactions are in italics; life-threatening reactions are in bold italics.

CNS: *sedation,* extrapyramidal symptoms, such as speech difficulty and tremors, disorientation.

GI: *diarrhea,* nausea, vomiting, abdominal pain.

GU: *crystalluria,* hematuria.

Other: impotence, hypersensitivity.

INTERACTIONS

Phenothiazines and haloperidol: increased inhibition of catecholamine synthesis may result in extrapyramidal symptoms. Use cautiously.

NURSING CONSIDERATIONS

• During surgery, monitor blood pressure and ECG continuously. If a serious arrhythmia occurs during anesthesia and surgery, treatment with a beta-blocking drug or lidocaine may be necessary.
• Warn patient that sedation almost always occurs in those treated with metyrosine. Sedation usually subsides after several days' treatment.
• Instruct patient to increase daily fluid intake to prevent crystalluria. Daily urine volume should be 2,000 ml or more.
• Insomnia may occur when metyrosine is stopped.
• If patient's hypertension is not adequately controlled by metyrosine, an alpha-adrenergic blocking agent, such as phenoxybenzamine, should be added to the regimen.

minoxidil

Loniten, Minodyl

Pregnancy Risk Category: C

HOW SUPPLIED

Tablets: 2.5 mg, 10 mg, 25 mg‡

MECHANISM OF ACTION

Produces direct arteriolar vasodilation.

INDICATIONS & DOSAGE

Treatment of severe hypertension –
Adults: 5 mg P.O. initially as a single dose. Effective dosage range is usually 10 to 40 mg daily. Maximum dosage is 100 mg daily.
Children under 12 years: 0.2 mg/kg as a single daily dose. Effective dosage range usually is 0.25 to 1 mg/kg daily. Maximum dosage is 50 mg.

ADVERSE REACTIONS

Common reactions are in italics; life-threatening reactions are in bold italics.
CV: *edema, tachycardia, pericardial effusion and tamponade,* ***CHF,*** ECG changes.
Skin: rash, ***Stevens-Johnson syndrome.***
Other: *hypertrichosis* (elongation, thickening, and enhanced pigmentation of fine body hair), breast tenderness.

INTERACTIONS

Guanethidine: severe orthostatic hypotension. Advise patient to stand up slowly.

NURSING CONSIDERATIONS

- *Contraindicated* in pheochromocytoma. Patients with malignant hypertension should be hospitalized during initial therapy.
- A potent vasodilator: use only when other antihypertensives have failed.
- Instruct patient to take his own pulse. Patient should report an increase greater than 20 beats/minute to the doctor.
- Closely monitor blood pressure and pulse at beginning of therapy.
- Monitor intake and output and check for weight gain and edema. Tell outpatients to weigh themselves at least weekly and report substantial weight gain (more than 5 lb per week).
- Elderly patients may be more sensitive to hypotensive effects.
- About 8 out of 10 patients will experience hypertrichosis within 3 to 6 weeks of beginning treatment. Unwanted hair can be controlled with a depilatory or shaving. Assure patient that extra hair will disappear within 1 to 6 months of stopping minoxidil. Advise patient, however, not to discontinue drug without doctor's approval.
- Drug is usually prescribed with a beta-blocking drug to control tachycardia and a diuretic to counteract fluid retention. Make sure patient complies with total treatment regimen.
- Teach patient about his disease and therapy. Explain the importance of taking this drug as prescribed, even when he's feeling well. Tell outpatient not to discontinue drug suddenly, but to call the doctor if unpleasant adverse reactions occur.
- A patient package insert has been prepared by the manufacturer of minoxidil, describing in layman's terms the drug and its adverse reactions. Be sure your patient receives this insert and reads it thoroughly. Provide an oral explanation also.
- Instruct patient to check with doctor or pharmacist before taking OTC medications.
- Prescribed in various topical forms for treatment of some types of male pattern baldness.
- Minoxidil is removed by hemodialysis. Be sure to administer dose after dialysis.

nitroprusside sodium

Nipride, Nitropress

Pregnancy Risk Category: C

HOW SUPPLIED

Injection: 50 mg/vial in 2-ml, 5-ml vials

MECHANISM OF ACTION

Relaxes both arteriolar and venous smooth muscle.

INDICATIONS & DOSAGE

To lower blood pressure quickly in hypertensive emergencies; to control hypotension during anesthesia; to reduce preload and afterload in cardiac pump failure or cardiogenic shock; may be used with or without dopamine –
Adults: 50-mg vial diluted with 2 to 3 ml of dextrose 5% in water I.V. and then added to 250, 500, or 1,000 ml dextrose 5% in water. Infuse at 0.5 to 10 mcg/kg/minute. Average dose is 3 mcg/kg/minute. Maximum infusion rate is 10 mcg/kg/minute.

Patients taking other antihypertensive drugs along with nitroprusside are very sensitive to this drug. Adjust dosage accordingly.

ADVERSE REACTIONS

Common reactions are in italics; life-threatening reactions are in bold italics.
The following adverse reactions usually indicate overdosage:
CNS: *headache, dizziness,* ataxia, loss of consciousness, coma, weak pulse, absent reflexes, widely dilated pupils, *restlessness, muscle twitching, diaphoresis.*
CV: distant heart sounds, palpitations, dyspnea, shallow breathing.
GI: *vomiting, nausea, abdominal pain.*
Metabolic: acidosis.
Skin: pink color.

INTERACTIONS

None significant.

NURSING CONSIDERATIONS

- *Use cautiously* in hypothyroidism or hepatic or renal disease, or in patients receiving other antihypertensives. Keep patient supine when initiating or titrating nitroprusside therapy.
- Because of light sensitivity, wrap I.V. solution in foil. It's not necessary to wrap the tubing in foil. Fresh solution should have faint brownish tint. Discard after 24 hours.
- Don't use bacteriostatic water for injection or sterile saline solution for reconstitution.
- Obtain baseline vital signs before giving this drug, and find out what parameters the doctor wants to achieve.
- **I.V. use:** Infuse with a continuous infusion pump. This drug is best run piggyback through a peripheral line with no other medication. Don't adjust rate of main I.V. line while drug is running. Even small bolus of nitroprusside can cause severe hypotension.
- Check blood pressure every 5 minutes at start of infusion and every 15 minutes thereafter. If severe hypotension occurs, turn off I.V. nitroprusside – effects of drug quickly reverse. Notify doctor. If possible, an arterial pressure line should be started. Regulate drug flow to specified level.
- Excessive doses or rapid infusion (> 15 mcg/kg/minute) of this drug can cause cyanide toxicity, so check serum thiocyanate levels every 72 hours. Thiocyanate levels of greater than 100 mcg/ml are associated with toxicity. Watch for signs of thiocyanate toxicity: profound hypotension, metabolic acidosis, dyspnea, headache, loss of consciousness, ataxia, vomiting. If these occur, discontinue drug immediately and notify doctor.
- Sometimes used with a direct-acting cardiac stimulant such as dopamine in patients with refractory heart failure.

penbutolol sulfate

Levatol

Pregnancy Risk Category: C

HOW SUPPLIED

Tablets: 20 mg

MECHANISM OF ACTION

Blocks both $beta_1$- and $beta_2$-adrenergic receptors.

INDICATIONS & DOSAGE

Treatment of mild to moderate hypertension –

Adults: 20 mg P.O. once daily. Usually given with other antihypertensive agents, such as thiazide diuretics.

ADVERSE REACTIONS

Common reactions are in italics; life-threatening reactions are in bold italics.

CNS: syncope, *dizziness,* vertigo, headache, fatigue, mental depression, paresthesias, hypoesthesia or hyperesthesia, lethargy, anxiety, nervousness, diminished concentration, sleep disturbances, nightmares, bizarre or frequent dreams, sedation, changes in behavior, reversible mental depression, catatonia, hallucinations, alteration of time perception, memory loss, emotional lability, light-headedness.

CV: *bradycardia,* chest pain, ***CHF,*** asymptomatic hypotension, peripheral ischemia, worsening of angina or arterial insufficiency, peripheral vascular insufficiency, claudication, edema, ***pulmonary edema,*** vasodilation, symptomatic postural hypotension, tachycardia, palpitations, conduction disturbances, first-degree and third-degree heart block, intensification of AV block.

EENT: dry mouth.

GI: gastric pain, flatulence, nausea, constipation, heartburn, vomiting, taste alteration.

GU: impotence, nocturia, urine retention.

Metabolic: hyperglycemia, hypoglycemia.

Respiratory: pharyngitis, laryngospasm, respiratory distress, shortness of breath.

Skin: pallor, flushing, rash.

Other: allergic reactions, eye discomfort, decreased libido.

INTERACTIONS

Clonidine: may cause paradoxical hypertension when combined with beta-adrenergic blocking agents. Also, beta blockers may enhance rebound hypertension when clonidine is withdrawn.

Insulin, oral hypoglycemic agents: beta-adrenergic blocking agents may alter the hypoglycemic response to these drugs. Monitor patient closely.

NSAIDs: possibly decreased antihypertensive effects.

Prazosin, terazosin: beta blockers may enhance the "first dose" orthostatic hypotension seen with these drugs.

Sympathomimetics, including isoproterenol, dopamine, dobutamine, or norepinephrine: decreased hypotensive response.

Theophylline: possibly decreased bronchodilator effect.

NURSING CONSIDERATIONS

- *Contraindicated* in patients allergic to penbutolol or other beta blockers; in sinus bradycardia, cardiogenic shock, CHF, and overt cardiac failure; in patients with greater than first-degree heart block; in patients with pheochromocytoma unless alpha-adrenergic blocking agents are also used; and in those with chronic airway disease, such as chronic bronchitis or emphysema.
- *Use cautiously* in patients with a history of CHF controlled by digitalis glycosides and diuretics and with a history of bronchospastic disease.
- Advise patients not to discontinue the drug abruptly, because sudden withdrawal of other beta blockers has

precipitated angina and myocardial infarction. However, clinical experience has shown that withdrawal of beta blocker therapy in patients who have had a myocardial infarction does not present major problems.
- Teach patient the signs and symptoms of CHF (edema and pulmonary congestion). Advise them to contact the doctor if these symptoms occur.
- Always check patient's apical pulse before giving this drug. If you detect extremes in pulse rates, hold drug and call doctor immediately.
- Monitor blood pressure, ECG, and heart rate and rhythm frequently.
- Teach patient about his disease and therapy. Explain the importance taking this drug, even when he's feeling well. Tell patient to call doctor if unpleasant adverse reactions occur.
- Advise patient to check with his doctor or pharmacist before taking OTC medications.

phenoxybenzamine hydrochloride

Dibenyline‡, Dibenzyline

Pregnancy Risk Category: C

HOW SUPPLIED

Capsules: 10 mg

MECHANISM OF ACTION

An alpha-adrenergic blocker that noncompetitively blocks the effect of catecholamines on alpha-adrenergic receptors.

INDICATIONS & DOSAGE

To control hypertension and sweating secondary to pheochromocytoma; may be used in combination with propranolol to control excessive tachycardia –

Adults: initially, 10 mg P.O. daily. Increase by 10 mg daily q 4 days. Maintenance dosage is 20 to 60 mg daily.

Children: initially, 0.2 mg/kg or 6 mg/m² P.O. daily in a single dose. Maintenance dosage is 12 to 36 mg/m² daily as a single dose or in divided doses.

To control Raynaud's disease, frostbite, acrocyanosis –

Adults: initially, 10 mg P.O., then increase by 10 mg q 4 days to a maximum of 60 mg daily.

ADVERSE REACTIONS

Common reactions are in italics; life-threatening reactions are in bold italics.

CNS: lethargy, drowsiness.

CV: *orthostatic hypotension, tachycardia,* shock.

EENT: *nasal stuffiness, dry mouth, miosis.*

GI: vomiting, abdominal distress.

Other: *impotence, inhibition of ejaculation.*

INTERACTIONS

Antihypertensives: excessive hypotension. Use together cautiously.

NURSING CONSIDERATIONS

- *Use cautiously* in cerebrovascular or coronary insufficiency, advanced renal disease, or respiratory disease.
- Watch patient closely for side effects, and call doctor promptly if they occur. If severe hypotension develops, patient may require norepinephrine to counteract effect.
- Nasal congestion, inhibition of ejaculation, and impotence usually decrease with continued therapy.
- Patient with tachycardia may require concurrent propranolol therapy.
- Monitor patient's heart rate and blood pressure frequently.
- This drug may take several weeks to achieve optimal effect.
- Monitor respiratory status carefully. This drug may aggravate symptoms of pneumonia and asthma.
- Teach patient about his disease and therapy. Explain the importance of taking this drug as prescribed, even when he's feeling well. Tell outpatient not to discontinue this drug suddenly,

*Liquid form contains alcohol. **May contain tartrazine.

but to call the doctor if unpleasant adverse reactions occur.

- Instruct patient to check with doctor or pharmacist before taking OTC medications.
- Inform patient that orthostatic hypotension can be minimized by rising slowly and avoiding sudden position changes.
- Dry mouth can be relieved with sugarless chewing gum, sour hard candy, or ice chips. GI distress can be relieved by taking the drug in divided doses or with milk.
- Used investigationally to treat chronic urine retention.
- Small initial doses are increased gradually until desired effect is obtained. Patient should be observed after each dose for at least 4 days.

phentolamine mesylate

Regitine, Rogitine†

Pregnancy Risk Category: C

HOW SUPPLIED

Injection: 5 mg/ml in 1-ml vials, 10 mg/ml‡

MECHANISM OF ACTION

An alpha-adrenergic blocker that competitively blocks the effects of catecholamines on alpha-adrenergic receptors.

INDICATIONS & DOSAGE

To aid in diagnosis of pheochromocytoma; to control or prevent hypertension before or during pheochromocytomectomy –

Adults: I.V. diagnostic dose is 5 mg, with close monitoring of blood pressure.

Before surgical removal of tumor, give 2 to 5 mg I.M. or I.V. During surgery, patient may need small I.V. doses (1 mg) or small I.M. doses (3 mg).

Children: I.V. diagnostic dose is 0.1 mg/kg or 3 mg/m² as single dose, with close monitoring of blood pressure.

Before surgical removal of tumor, give 1 mg I.V. or 3 mg I.M. During surgery, patient may need small I.V. doses (1 mg).

To treat extravasation –

Adults and children: infiltrate area with 5 to 10 mg phentolamine in 10 ml normal saline solution or give half the dosage through the infiltrated I.V. and the other half around the site. Must be done within 12 hours.

ADVERSE REACTIONS

Common reactions are in italics; life-threatening reactions are in bold italics.

CNS: *dizziness, weakness, flushing.*

CV: *hypotension,* shock, *arrhythmias,* palpitations, *tachycardia,* angina pectoris.

GI: *diarrhea,* abdominal pain, *nausea, vomiting,* hyperperistalsis.

Other: *nasal stuffiness,* hypoglycemia.

INTERACTIONS

Epinephrine: excessive hypotension. Don't use together.

NURSING CONSIDERATIONS

- *Contraindicated* in angina, coronary artery disease, and history of myocardial infarction.
- *Use cautiously* in gastritis or peptic ulcer and in patients receiving other antihypertensives.
- Don't administer epinephrine to treat phentolamine-induced hypotension. May cause additional fall in blood pressure ("epinephrine reversal"). Use norepinephrine instead.
- When this drug is given as a diagnostic test for pheochromocytoma, check patient's blood pressure first; check blood pressure frequently during administration.
- Test is positive for pheochromocytoma if I.V. test dose causes severe hypotension.
- Don't give sedatives or narcotics 24

hours before diagnostic test. Rauwolfia alkaloids should be withdrawn at least 4 weeks before such testing.

• Has been used experimentally, alone or with papaverine, to treat impotence. Patients are taught to self-administer this drug by intercavernosal injection.

pindolol

Barbloc‡, Visken

Pregnancy Risk Category: B

HOW SUPPLIED

Tablets: 5 mg, 10 mg, 15 mg‡

MECHANISM OF ACTION

Blocks response to beta stimulation.

INDICATIONS & DOSAGE

Treatment of hypertension –

Adults: initially, 5 mg P.O. b.i.d. Dosage may be increased by 10 mg/day q 2 to 3 weeks up to a maximum of 60 mg/day.

ADVERSE REACTIONS

Common reactions are in italics; life-threatening reactions are in bold italics.

CNS: *insomnia, fatigue, dizziness, nervousness,* vivid dreams, hallucinations, lethargy.

CV: *edema,* bradycardia, ***CHF,*** peripheral vascular disease, hypotension.

EENT: visual disturbances.

GI: *nausea,* vomiting, diarrhea.

Metabolic: hypoglycemia without tachycardia.

Skin: rash.

Other: *increased airway resistance, muscle pain, joint pain,* chest pain.

INTERACTIONS

Digitalis glycosides: excessive bradycardia and increased depressant effect on myocardium. Use together cautiously.

Epinephrine: severe vasoconstriction. Monitor blood pressure and observe patient carefully.

Indomethacin: decreased antihypertensive effect. Monitor blood pressure and adjust dosage.

Insulin, hypoglycemic drugs (oral): can alter requirements for these drugs in previously stabilized diabetics. Monitor for hypoglycemia.

NURSING CONSIDERATIONS

• *Contraindicated* in diabetes mellitus, asthma, allergic rhinitis; during ethyl ether anesthesia; in sinus bradycardia and heart block greater than first degree; in cardiogenic shock; and in right ventricular failure secondary to pulmonary hypertension.

• *Use cautiously* in CHF or respiratory disease and in patients taking other antihypertensives.

• Always check patient's apical pulse rate before giving this drug. If you detect extremes in pulse rates, hold medication and call doctor immediately.

• Monitor blood pressure frequently. If patient develops severe hypotension, notify doctor. He may prescribe a vasopressor.

• Teach patient about his disease and therapy. Explain the importance of taking this drug as prescribed, even when he's feeling well. Tell outpatient not to discontinue this drug suddenly; abrupt discontinuation can exacerbate angina and myocardial infarction. Tell patient to call doctor if unpleasant adverse reactions occur.

• Instruct patient to check with doctor or pharmacist before taking OTC medications.

• This drug masks common signs of shock and hypoglycemia.

• Pindolol may be taken without any special regard for meals.

• Many patients respond favorably to a dose of 5 mg t.i.d.

• The first commercially available beta blocker with partial beta-*agonist* activity. In other words, pindolol also

stimulates beta-adrenergic receptors as well as blocks them. Therefore, it decreases cardiac output less than other beta-adrenergic blockers.
• May be advantageous for patients who develop bradycardia with other beta blockers.
• Withdraw drug gradually (over 1 to 2 weeks) after long-term administration.

prazosin hydrochloride

Minipress

Pregnancy Risk Category: C

HOW SUPPLIED
Capsules: 1 mg, 2 mg, 5 mg

MECHANISM OF ACTION
Relaxes both arteriolar and venous smooth muscle probably by blocking postsynaptic alpha receptors.

INDICATIONS & DOSAGE
For mild to moderate hypertension; used alone or in combination with a diuretic or other antihypertensive drugs; also used to decrease afterload in severe chronic CHF –
Adults: P.O. test dose is 1 mg given before bedtime to prevent "first-dose syncope." Initial dose is 1 mg t.i.d. Increase dosage slowly. Maximum daily dosage is 20 mg. Maintenance dosage is 3 to 20 mg daily in three divided doses. A few patients have required dosages larger than this (up to 40 mg daily). If other antihypertensive drugs or diuretics are added to this drug, decrease prazosin dosage to 1 to 2 mg t.i.d. and retitrate.

ADVERSE REACTIONS
Common reactions are in italics; life-threatening reactions are in bold italics.
CNS: *dizziness,* headache, drowsiness, weakness, *"first-dose syncope,"* depression.
CV: orthostatic hypotension, *palpitations.*
EENT: blurred vision, dry mouth.
GI: vomiting, diarrhea, abdominal cramps, constipation, *nausea.*
GU: priapism, impotence.

INTERACTIONS
Propranolol and other beta blockers: syncope with loss of consciousness may occur more frequently. Advise patient to sit or lie down if he feels dizzy.

NURSING CONSIDERATIONS
• *Use cautiously* in patients receiving other antihypertensives.
• Monitor patient's blood pressure and pulse rate frequently.
• If initial dose is greater than 1 mg, patient may develop severe syncope with loss of consciousness (first-dose syncope). Increase dosage slowly. Instruct patient to sit or lie down if he experiences dizziness.
• Elderly patients may be more sensitive to hypotensive effects.
• Teach patient about his disease and therapy. Explain the importance of taking this drug as prescribed, even when he's feeling well. Tell outpatient not to discontinue this drug suddenly, but to call the doctor if unpleasant adverse reactions occur.
• Instruct patient to check with doctor or pharmacist before taking OTC medications.
• Inform patient that orthostatic hypotension can be minimized by rising slowly and avoiding sudden position changes. Dry mouth can be relieved with sugarless chewing gum, sour hard candy, or ice chips.
• Compliance *may* be improved by giving this drug once a day. Check with doctor.
• Has been used to treat Raynaud's disease.

quinapril hydrochloride
Accupril
Pregnancy Risk Category: D

HOW SUPPLIED
Tablets: 5 mg, 10 mg, 20 mg, 40 mg

MECHANISM OF ACTION
Quinapril and its active metabolite, quinaprilat, inhibit angiotensin-converting enzyme (ACE), preventing conversion of angiotensin I to angiotensin II, a potent vasoconstrictor. Reduced formation of angiotensin II decreases peripheral arterial resistance, which results in decreased aldosterone secretion. This reduces sodium and water retention and lowers blood pressure. Quinapril also has antihypertensive activity in patients with low-renin hypertension.

INDICATIONS & DOSAGE
Hypertension –
Adults: initially, 10 mg daily. Adjust dosage based on patient response at intervals of about 2 weeks. Most patients are controlled at 20, 40, or 80 mg daily, as a single dose or in two divided doses.

ADVERSE REACTIONS
Common reactions are in italics; life-threatening reactions are in bold italics.
CNS: somnolence, vertigo, lightheadedness, syncope, nervousness, depression.
CV: palpitations, vasodilation, tachycardia, heart failure, ***MI, hypertensive crisis, CVA,*** angina, orthostatic hypotension, cardiac rhythm disturbances.
EENT: cough, dry mouth or throat.
GI: abdominal pain, constipation, GI hemorrhage, pancreatitis.
Skin: sweating, pruritus, ***exfoliative dermatitis,*** *photosensitivity.*
Other: hyperkalemia, back pain, malaise, elevated liver enzymes.

INTERACTIONS
Diuretics, other antihypertensives: risk of excessive hypotension. Discontinue diuretic or lower dose of quinapril as needed.
Lithium: increased serum lithium levels and lithium toxicity have been reported. Avoid concomitant use.
Potassium-sparing diuretics, potassium supplements, sodium substitutes containing potassium: risk of hyperkalemia. Avoid concomitant use.

NURSING CONSIDERATIONS
- *Contraindicated* in patients with hypersensitivity to ACE inhibitors or with a history of angioneurotic edema.
- *Use cautiously* in patients with impaired renal or hepatic function, in diabetes mellitus, and with use of potassium-sparing diuretics, potassium supplements, and sodium substitutes containing potassium because of risk of hyperkalemia.
- Avoid use during pregnancy because ACE inhibitors can cause fetal or neonatal injury or death. When pregnancy is detected, ACE inhibitors should be discontinued as soon as possible.
- Excessive hypotension can occur when drug is given with diuretics. If possible, diuretic therapy should be discontinued 2 to 3 days before starting quinapril to decrease potential for excessive hypotensive response. If quinapril does not adequately control blood pressure, diuretic may be reinstituted with care. If diuretic cannot be discontinued, initiate therapy with quinapril at 5 mg P.O. daily.
- Like other ACE inhibitors, drug may cause dry, persistent, tickling, nonproductive cough, which is reversible when therapy is discontinued.
- Assess renal and hepatic function before and periodically throughout therapy.
- Drug may be taken without regard

to meals. Bioavailability is not affected by presence of food.

- Periodically monitor renal function, CBC, and serum potassium levels.
- Tell patient to stop taking drug and notify doctor immediately if any signs or symptoms of angioedema occur: swelling of face, eyes, lips, tongue, or difficulty in breathing.
- Light-headedness can occur, especially during the first few days of therapy. Tell patient to rise slowly to minimize effect and to report symptoms to doctor. If drug causes fainting, patient should stop taking it and notify doctor promptly.
- Inadequate fluid intake, vomiting, diarrhea, and excessive perspiration can lead to light-headedness and syncope. Tell patient to use caution in hot weather and during periods of exercise.
- Tell patient to avoid sodium substitutes because they contain potassium and can cause hyperkalemia.
- Other ACE inhibitors have been associated with agranulocytosis and neutropenia. Tell patient to report immediately any signs of infection (sore throat, fever) or of easy bruising or bleeding.
- Has been used investigationally in the treatment of CHF.

ramipril

Altace

Pregnancy Risk Category: D

HOW SUPPLIED

Capsules: 1.25 mg, 2.5 mg, 5 mg, 10 mg

MECHANISM OF ACTION

Inhibits angiotensin-converting enzyme (ACE), preventing the conversion of angiotensin I to angiotensin II, a potent vasoconstrictor. Reduced formation of angiotensin II decreases aldosterone secretion, reducing sodium and water retention and lowering blood pressure.

INDICATIONS & DOSAGE

Treatment of essential hypertension (alone or in combination with diuretics) –

Adults: initially, 2.5 mg P.O. once daily. Increase dosage as necessary based on patient response. Maintenance dose is 2.5 to 20 mg daily as a single dose or in divided doses.

ADVERSE REACTIONS

Common reactions are in italics; life-threatening reactions are in bold italics.

CNS: headache, dizziness, fatigue, asthenia, malaise, light-headedness, anxiety, amnesia, ***seizures,*** depression, insomnia, nervousness, neuralgia, neuropathy, paresthesia, somnolence, tremor, vertigo.

CV: orthostatic hypotension, syncope, angina, ***arrhythmia,*** chest pain, palpitations, ***MI.***

EENT: epistaxis.

GI: nausea, vomiting, abdominal pain, anorexia, constipation, diarrhea, dry mouth, dyspepsia, dysphagia, gastroenteritis, increased salivation, taste disturbance.

GU: impotence.

Respiratory: dry, persistent, tickling, nonproductive cough; dyspnea.

Skin: hypersensitivity reactions, rash, dermatitis, pruritus, photosensitivity, purpura.

Other: ***angioedema,*** arthralgia, arthritis, edema, increased sweating, myalgia, weight gain.

INTERACTIONS

Diuretics: excessive hypotension, especially at the start of therapy. Before ramipril therapy begins, discontinue diuretic at least 3 days earlier, increase sodium intake, or reduce the starting dose of ramipril.

Insulin, oral hypoglycemic agents: risk of hypoglycemia, especially at initia-

tion of ramipril therapy. Monitor closely.
Lithium: increased serum lithium levels. Use together cautiously and monitor serum lithium levels.
Potassium-sparing diuretics, potassium supplements, sodium substitutes containing potassium: increased risk of hyperkalemia because ramipril attenuates potassium loss. Avoid concomitant use or monitor plasma potassium closely.

NURSING CONSIDERATIONS

- *Contraindicated* in patients with a history of angioedema and hypersensitivity to ramipril; also during pregnancy because ACE inhibitors can cause fetal morbidity and mortality. Use of ACE inhibitors during the second and third trimesters has been associated with oligohydramnios, neonatal hypotension, renal failure, skull hypoplasia, and death.
- *Use cautiously* in patients with renal insufficiency or diabetes mellitus, in patients receiving potassium supplements or potassium-sparing diuretics, and in patients using potassium-containing sodium substitutes because these patients are at a higher risk for developing hyperkalemia.
- Patients with renal insufficiency (creatinine clearance < 40 ml/min/1.73 m^2) should start therapy at 1.25 mg P.O. daily. Dosage should be titrated gradually according to response. Maximum daily dosage is 5 mg.
- Patients with severe CHF whose renal function depends on the angiotensin-aldosterone system have experienced acute renal failure during ACE inhibitor therapy. Hypertensive patients with renal artery stenosis may also show signs of worsening renal function at start of therapy. Closely assess renal function in such patients during first few weeks of therapy.
- Regular assessment of renal function (serum creatinine and BUN levels) is advisable.
- Monitor WBC counts in patients with impaired renal function or collagen vascular diseases (systemic lupus erythematosus or scleroderma) because such patients have developed agranulocytosis and bone marrow depression after therapy with other ACE inhibitors.
- Ramipril can be taken without regard to meals.
- Tell patient to continue taking the drug even if he feels better. He should always check with the doctor or pharmacist before taking nonprescription medications.
- Advise patient to avoid sudden position changes to prevent orthostatic hypotension, especially at the start of therapy.
- Like other ACE inhibitors, ramipril may cause neutropenia or agranulocytosis. Tell the patient to report lightheadedness, sore throat, fever, or any sign of infection; difficulty breathing, signs of edema or swelling; or any unusual bruising or bleeding.
- Tell the patient to avoid sodium substitutes containing potassium unless recommended by doctor.

rauwolfia serpentina

Raudixin**, Rauverid, Wolfina

Pregnancy Risk Category: D

HOW SUPPLIED

Tablets: 50 mg, 100 mg

MECHANISM OF ACTION

Acts peripherally, inhibiting norepinephrine release and depleting norepinephrine stores in adrenergic nerve endings.

INDICATIONS & DOSAGE

Mild to moderate hypertension –
Adults: initially and for 1 to 3 weeks thereafter, 200 to 400 mg P.O. daily

*Liquid form contains alcohol. **May contain tartrazine.

as a single dose or in two divided doses.

Maintenance dosage is 50 to 300 mg daily. No dosing recommendations for children.

ADVERSE REACTIONS

Common reactions are in italics; life-threatening reactions are in bold italics.

CNS: mental confusion, *depression, drowsiness, nervousness, paradoxical anxiety,* nightmares, sedation, headache, extrapyramidal symptoms.

CV: orthostatic hypotension, bradycardia, syncope.

EENT: *dry mouth, nasal stuffiness,* glaucoma.

GI: *hypersecretion of gastric acid, nausea, vomiting,* GI bleeding.

Skin: pruritus, rash.

Other: impotence, weight gain.

INTERACTIONS

Digitalis glycosides: rauwolfia may predispose patients to digitalis-induced arrhythmias. Use together cautiously.

MAO inhibitors: may cause excitability and hypertension. Use together cautiously.

NURSING CONSIDERATIONS

- *Contraindicated* in depression.
- *Use cautiously* in severe cardiac or cerebrovascular disease, impaired renal function, peptic ulcer, ulcerative colitis, gallstones; in those undergoing surgery; in elderly or debilitated patients; and in those taking other antihypertensives or tricyclic antidepressants.
- Monitor patient's blood pressure and pulse rate frequently.
- Teach patient about his disease and therapy. Explain the importance of taking this drug as prescribed, even when he's feeling well. Tell outpatient not to discontinue this drug suddenly, but to call the doctor if unpleasant adverse reactions occur.
- Instruct patient to check with doctor or pharmacist before taking OTC medications.
- Warn that this drug can cause drowsiness. Patient should not drive or perform other activities that require alertness and good coordination until CNS effects are known.
- Watch patient closely for signs of mental depression. Warn him to notify doctor promptly if he experiences nightmares.
- Inform patient that orthostatic hypotension can be minimized by rising slowly and avoiding sudden position changes. Dry mouth can be relieved with sugarless chewing gum, sour hard candy, or ice chips. Tell patient to contact doctor if relief is needed for nasal stuffiness.
- Give this drug with meals.
- Patient should weigh himself daily and notify doctor of any weight gain.
- Effects of this drug may last for 10 days after it's discontinued.
- Advise patient to have periodic eye examinations.

rescinnamine

Moderil

Pregnancy Risk Category: D

HOW SUPPLIED

Tablets: 0.25 mg, 0.5 mg

MECHANISM OF ACTION

Acts peripherally, inhibiting norepinephrine release and depleting norepinephrine stores in adrenergic nerve endings.

INDICATIONS & DOSAGE

For mild to moderate hypertension; may be used alone or in combination with other antihypertensives –

Adults: initially, 0.5 mg P.O. b.i.d. Maintenance dosage is 0.25 to 0.5 mg daily. No dosing recommendations for children.

ADVERSE REACTIONS
Common reactions are in italics; life-threatening reactions are in bold italics.
CNS: mental confusion, *depression, drowsiness, nervousness, anxiety, nightmares,* sedation, parkinsonism.
CV: *orthostatic hypotension, bradycardia, syncope.*
EENT: *dry mouth, nasal stuffiness,* glaucoma.
GI: *hypersecretion of gastric acid, nausea, vomiting,* GI bleeding.
Skin: pruritus, rash.
Other: *impotence, weight gain.*

INTERACTIONS
MAO inhibitors: may cause excitability and hypertension. Use together cautiously.

NURSING CONSIDERATIONS
- *Contraindicated* in depression.
- *Use cautiously* in severe cardiac or cerebrovascular disease, peptic ulcer, ulcerative colitis, or gallstones; in patients undergoing surgery; and in elderly or debilitated patients. Also use cautiously in patients taking other antihypertensives.
- Monitor patient's blood pressure and pulse rate frequently.
- Teach patient about his disease and therapy. Explain the importance of taking this drug as prescribed, even when he's feeling well. Tell outpatient not to discontinue this drug suddenly, but to call the doctor if unpleasant adverse reactions develop.
- Instruct patient to check with doctor or pharmacist before taking OTC medications.
- Warn that this drug can cause drowsiness. Patients should not drive or perform other tasks that require alertness and coordination until the adverse CNS effects of the drug are known.
- Watch patient closely for signs of mental depression. Warn him to notify doctor promptly if he experiences nightmares.
- Inform patient that orthostatic hypotension can be minimized by rising slowly and avoiding sudden position changes. Dry mouth can be relieved with sugarless chewing gum, sour hard candy, or ice chips. Tell patient to contact doctor if relief is needed for nasal stuffiness.
- Give this drug with meals.
- Patient should weigh himself daily and notify doctor of any weight gain.
- Effects of this drug may last for 10 days after it's discontinued.
- Advise patient to have periodic eye examinations.

reserpine
Novoreserpine†, Serpalan, Serpasil*
Pregnancy Risk Category: C

HOW SUPPLIED
Tablets: 0.1 mg, 0.25 mg, 1 mg

MECHANISM OF ACTION
Acts peripherally, inhibiting norepinephrine release and depleting norepinephrine stores in adrenergic nerve endings.

INDICATIONS & DOSAGE
Mild to moderate essential hypertension –
Adults: 0.1 to 0.25 mg P.O. daily.
Children: 5 to 20 mcg/kg P.O. daily.

ADVERSE REACTIONS
Common reactions are in italics; life-threatening reactions are in bold italics.
CNS: mental confusion, *depression, drowsiness, nervousness, paradoxical anxiety, nightmares,* extrapyramidal symptoms, sedation.
CV: *orthostatic hypotension, bradycardia, syncope.*
EENT: *dry mouth, nasal stuffiness,* glaucoma.
GI: *hyperacidity, nausea, vomiting,* GI bleeding.
Skin: pruritus, rash.

*Liquid form contains alcohol. **May contain tartrazine.

Other: *impotence, weight gain.*

INTERACTIONS
MAO inhibitors: may cause excitability and hypertension. Use together cautiously.

NURSING CONSIDERATIONS
- *Contraindicated* in depression.
- *Use cautiously* in severe cardiac or cerebrovascular disease, history of seizures, peptic ulcer, ulcerative colitis, gallstones, or mental depressive disorders; in patients undergoing surgery; and in those taking other antihypertensive drugs.
- Monitor patient's blood pressure and pulse rate frequently.
- Teach patient about his disease and therapy. Explain the importance of taking this drug as prescribed, even when he's feeling well. Tell outpatient not to discontinue this drug suddenly, but to call doctor if unpleasant adverse reactions occur.
- Instruct patient to check with doctor or pharmacist before taking OTC medications.
- Warn patient that this drug can cause drowsiness. Tell him to avoid hazardous activities that require alertness and coordination until CNS effects of the drug are known.
- Warn female patient to notify doctor if she becomes pregnant.
- Watch patient closely for signs of mental depression. Warn him to notify doctor promptly if he experiences nightmares.
- Inform patient that orthostatic hypotension can be minimized by rising slowly and avoiding sudden position changes. Dry mouth can be relieved with sugarless chewing gum, sour hard candy, or ice chips. Tell patient to contact doctor if relief is needed for nasal stuffiness.
- Give this drug with meals.
- Patient should weigh himself daily and notify doctor of any weight gain.
- Effects of this drug may last for 10 days after it's discontinued.
- Advise patient to have periodic eye examinations.

terazosin hydrochloride
Hytrin

Pregnancy Risk Category: C

HOW SUPPLIED
Tablets: 1 mg, 2 mg, 5 mg

MECHANISM OF ACTION
Decreases blood pressure by vasodilation produced in response to blockade of $alpha_1$ adrenergic receptors.

INDICATIONS & DOSAGE
Hypertension –
Adults: initial dose is 1 mg P.O. h.s., gradually increased according to patient response. Usual dosage range is 1 to 5 mg daily. Maximum recommended dosage is 20 mg/day.

ADVERSE REACTIONS
Common reactions are in italics; life-threatening reactions are in bold italics.
CNS: asthenia, *dizziness,* headache, nervousness, paresthesia, somnolence, decreased libido.
CV: *palpitations,* postural hypotension, tachycardia, *peripheral edema.*
EENT: *nasal congestion,* sinusitis, blurred vision.
GI: *nausea.*
Respiratory: dyspnea.
Other: back pain, muscle pain, weight gain, impotence.

INTERACTIONS
Antihypertensives: excessive hypotension. Use together cautiously.

NURSING CONSIDERATIONS
- Do not exceed initial dose of 1 mg.
- Instruct patient to avoid hazardous activities that require mental alertness (such as driving or operating heavy ma-

chinery) for 12 hours after the first dose.

- If terazosin is discontinued for several days, patient will need to be retitrated using initial dosing regimen (1 mg P.O. at bedtime).
- Teach patient about his disease and therapy. Explain the importance of taking this drug as prescribed, even when he's feeling well. Tell outpatient not to discontinue drug suddenly, but to call the doctor if unpleasant adverse reactions occur.
- Instruct patient to check with doctor or pharmacist before taking OTC medications.

timolol maleate

Apo-Timol†, Blocadren

Pregnancy Risk Category: C

HOW SUPPLIED

Tablets: 5 mg, 10 mg, 20 mg

MECHANISM OF ACTION

Blocks response to beta stimulation and depresses renin secretion.

INDICATIONS & DOSAGE

Hypertension –

Adults: initially, 10 mg P.O. b.i.d. Usual daily maintenance dosage is 20 to 40 mg. Maximum daily dosage is 60 mg. Drug is used either alone or in combination with diuretics.

Myocardial infarction (long-term prophylaxis in patients who have survived acute phase) –

Adults: Recommended dosage for long-term prophylaxis in survivors of acute myocardial infarction (MI) is 10 mg P.O. b.i.d.

Migraine headache prophylaxis –

Adults: initially, 20 mg P.O. daily as a single dose or in divided doses b.i.d. Increase dosage to maximum 30 mg daily as needed and tolerated. Discontinue treatment if no response after 6 to 8 weeks treatment at maximum dosage.

Prophylaxis of angina pectoris –

Adults: dosage is highly individualized; dosages of 15 to 45 mg P.O. daily in three or four divided doses have been used. Dosage is adjusted to maintain clinical response and keep patient's resting heart rate at 55 to 60 beats/minute.

ADVERSE REACTIONS

Common reactions are in italics; life-threatening reactions are in bold italics.

CNS: fatigue, lethargy, vivid dreams.

CV: *bradycardia, hypotension, **CHF,*** peripheral vascular disease.

GI: nausea, vomiting, diarrhea.

Metabolic: hypoglycemia without tachycardia.

Respiratory: dyspnea, ***bronchospasm.***

Skin: rash.

Other: *increased airway resistance,* fever.

INTERACTIONS

Digitalis glycosides: excessive bradycardia and increased depressant effect on myocardium. Use together cautiously.

Indomethacin: decreased antihypertensive effect. Monitor blood pressure and adjust dosage.

Insulin, hypoglycemic drugs (oral): can alter requirements for these drugs in previously stabilized diabetics. Monitor for hypoglycemia.

NURSING CONSIDERATIONS

- *Contraindicated* in diabetes mellitus, asthma, allergic rhinitis; during ethyl ether anesthesia; in sinus bradycardia and heart block greater than first degree; in cardiogenic shock; and in right ventricular failure secondary to pulmonary hypertension.
- *Use cautiously* in CHF; hepatic, renal, or respiratory disease; and in patients taking other antihypertensives.
- Always check patient's apical pulse rate before giving this drug. If you detect extremes in pulse rates, withhold

*Liquid form contains alcohol. **May contain tartrazine.

medication and call the doctor immediately.
• Monitor blood pressure frequently.
• Teach patient about his disease and therapy. Explain the importance of taking drug as prescribed, even when he's feeling well. Tell patient not to discontinue drug suddenly because this can exacerbate angina and MI. Tell patient to call doctor if unpleasant adverse reactions occur.
• Instruct patient to check with doctor or pharmacist before taking OTC medications.
• This drug masks common signs of shock and hypoglycemia.
• Warn patient who is taking drug for hypertension not to increase the dose without first consulting the doctor. At least 7 days should elapse between increases in dosage.
• Do not discontinue drug abruptly. Reduce dosage gradually over 1 to 2 weeks.
• Timolol is the first beta blocker approved for use in post-MI patients. Like other beta blockers, it prolongs survival after MI.

trimethaphan camsylate

Arfonad

Pregnancy Risk Category: C

HOW SUPPLIED

Injection: 50 mg/ml in 10-ml ampules, 250 mg/vial‡

MECHANISM OF ACTION

A ganglionic blocker that stabilizes postsynaptic membranes.

INDICATIONS & DOSAGE

To lower blood pressure quickly in hypertensive emergencies; for controlled hypotension during surgery –
Adults: 500 mg (10 ml) diluted in 500 ml dextrose 5% in water to yield concentration of 1 mg/ml I.V. Start I.V. drip at 1 to 2 mg/minute and titrate to achieve desired hypotensive response. Range is 0.3 mg to 6 mg/minute.

ADVERSE REACTIONS

Common reactions are in italics; life-threatening reactions are in bold italics.
CNS: dilated pupils, *extreme weakness.*
CV: *severe orthostatic hypotension, tachycardia.*
GI: anorexia, *nausea, vomiting, dry mouth.*
GU: urine retention.
Other: respiratory depression.

INTERACTIONS

Anesthetics, diuretics, procainamide: Increased hypotensive effect. Monitor patient closely.

NURSING CONSIDERATIONS

• *Contraindicated* in anemia and respiratory insufficiency.
• *Use cautiously* in arteriosclerosis; cardiac, hepatic, or renal disease; degenerative CNS disorders; Addison's disease; and diabetes and in patients receiving glucocorticoids or other antihypertensives.
• Monitor patient's blood pressure and vital signs continuously.
• Patient should be supine during drug administration. May require elevation of the head of the bed for maximal effect to avoid cerebral anoxia. Do not elevate bed more than 30°.
• Watch closely for respiratory distress, especially if large doses are used. Large doses have caused apnea and respiratory arrest.
• If extreme hypotension occurs, discontinue drug and call doctor. Use phenylephrine or mephentermine to counteract hypotension.
• Patient should receive oxygen therapy during use of this agent.
• Use continuous infusion pump to administer this drug slowly and precisely.
• Discontinue drug before wound closure in surgery to allow blood pressure to return to normal.

23
Vasodilators

amyl nitrite
cyclandelate
dipyridamole
ethaverine hydrochloride
isoxsuprine hydrochloride
nimodipine
nylidrin hydrochloride
papaverine hydrochloride
tolazoline hydrochloride

COMBINATION PRODUCTS
None.

amyl nitrite
Pregnancy Risk Category: C

HOW SUPPLIED
Ampules (crushable): 0.18 ml, 0.3 ml

MECHANISM OF ACTION
Reduces cardiac oxygen demand by decreasing left ventricular end-diastolic pressure (preload) and systemic vascular resistance (afterload). Also increases blood flow through the collateral coronary vessels. Converts hemoglobin to methemoglobin (which binds cyanide) to treat cyanide poisoning.

INDICATIONS & DOSAGE
Relief of angina pectoris; relief of renal or gallbladder colic –
Adults and children: 0.2 to 0.3 ml by inhalation (one glass ampule inhaler), p.r.n.
Antidote for cyanide poisoning –
0.2 or 0.3 ml by inhalation for 30 to 60 seconds q 5 minutes until conscious.

ADVERSE REACTIONS
Common reactions are in italics; life-threatening reactions are in bold italics.
Blood: methemoglobinemia.
CNS: *headache, sometimes with throbbing;* dizziness; weakness.
CV: *orthostatic hypotension, tachycardia,* flushing, palpitations, fainting.
GI: nausea, vomiting.
Skin: cutaneous vasodilation.
Other: hypersensitivity reactions.

INTERACTIONS
None significant.

NURSING CONSIDERATIONS
- *Contraindicated* in hypersensitivity to nitrites and during acute MI.
- *Use cautiously* in cerebral hemorrhage, hypotension, head injury, or glaucoma.
- Watch for orthostatic hypotension. Have patient sit down and avoid rapid position changes while inhaling drug.
- Extinguish all cigarettes before use, or ampule may ignite.
- Wrap ampule in cloth and crush. Hold near patient's nose and mouth so vapor is inhaled.
- Effective within 30 seconds but has a short duration of action (3 to 5 minutes).
- Keeping the head low, deep breathing, and movement of extremities may help relieve dizziness, syncope, or weakness from orthostatic hypotension.
- Drug is often abused. Claimed to have aphrodisiac benefits. Street name is "Amy."
- Seldom, if ever, used for treatment of angina because it is expensive, inconvenient, and frequently causes adverse reactions.
- Sometimes used to induce changes in heart murmurs. Patient inhales the drug until reflex tachycardia is induced, then discontinues.
- Store away from light.

*Liquid form contains alcohol. **May contain tartrazine.

cyclandelate

Cyclan, Cyclospasmol

Pregnancy Risk Category: C

HOW SUPPLIED

Tablets: 200 mg, 400 mg
Capsules: 200 mg, 400 mg

MECHANISM OF ACTION

Directly relaxes smooth muscle due to the inhibition of phosphodiesterase, resulting in increased concentrations of cyclic adenosine monophosphate.

INDICATIONS & DOSAGE

Adjunct in intermittent claudication, arteriosclerosis obliterans, vasospasm and muscular ischemia associated with thrombophlebitis, nocturnal leg cramps, Raynaud's phenomenon, selected cases of ischemic cerebral vascular disease –
Adults: initially, 1.2 to 1.6 g P.O. daily, in divided doses before meals and at bedtime. For maintenance, decrease dosage by 200 mg/day to the lowest effective level. Maintenance dosage is usually 400 to 800 mg daily in two to four divided doses.

ADVERSE REACTIONS

Common reactions are in italics; life-threatening reactions are in bold italics.
CNS: *headache, tingling of the extremities, dizziness.*
CV: *mild flushing,* tachycardia.
GI: pyrosis, eructation, nausea, heartburn.
Other: *sweating.*

INTERACTIONS

None significant.

NURSING CONSIDERATIONS

- *Use with extreme caution* in severe obliterative coronary artery or cerebrovascular disease because circulation to these diseased areas may be compromised by vasodilatory effects of the drug elsewhere (coronary steal syndrome).
- *Use cautiously* in glaucoma or hypotension.
- Give with food or antacids to lessen GI distress.
- Use with, not as a substitute for, appropriate medical or surgical therapy for peripheral or cerebrovascular disease.
- Short-term therapy is of little benefit. Instruct patient to expect long-term treatment and to continue to take medication.
- Adverse reactions usually disappear after several weeks of therapy.

dipyridamole

Apo-Dipyridamole†, Persantin 100‡, Persantine**

Pregnancy Risk Category: C

HOW SUPPLIED

Tablets: 25 mg, 50 mg, 75 mg
Injection: 10 mg/2 ml†

MECHANISM OF ACTION

Inhibits platelet adhesion. Also inhibits the enzymes adenosine deaminase and phosphodiesterase.

INDICATIONS & DOSAGE

Inhibition of platelet adhesion in prosthetic heart valves, in combination with warfarin or aspirin –
Adults: 75 to 100 mg P.O. q.i.d.
Transient ischemic attack –
Adults: 400 to 800 mg P.O. daily in divided doses.
As an alternative to exercise in the evaluation of coronary artery disease during thallium myocardial perfusion imaging –
Adults: 0.57 mg/kg as an I.V. infusion at a constant rate over 4 minutes (0.142 mg/kg/minute). Do not give more than 60 mg.
Acute coronary insufficiency‡ –
Adults: 10 mg I.V. or I.M.

ADVERSE REACTIONS

Common reactions are in italics; life-threatening reactions are in bold italics.

CNS: *headache, dizziness,* weakness.

CV: flushing, fainting, *hypotension; chest pain,* ***ECG abnormalities,*** *blood pressure lability, hypertension* (with I.V. infusion).

GI: *nausea,* vomiting, diarrhea.

Local: irritation (with undiluted injection).

Skin: rash.

INTERACTIONS

None significant.

NURSING CONSIDERATIONS

- *Use cautiously* in hypotension and in patients receiving anticoagulant therapy.
- Observe for adverse reactions, especially with large doses. Monitor blood pressure.
- Administer 1 hour before meals. May administer with meals if patient develops GI distress.
- Watch for signs of bleeding, prolonged bleeding time (large doses, long-term).
- **I.V. use:** When given as a diagnostic agent, dilute in 0.45% or 0.9% sodium chloride injection or dextrose 5% in water in at least a 1:2 ratio for a total volume of 20 to 50 ml. Inject thallium-201 within 5 minutes after completion of the 4-minute dipyridamole infusion.
- Dipyridamole should not be used alone for the prophylaxis of thromboembolism in postoperative prosthetic valve patients; it should be used with oral anticoagulants. Its value as part of an antithrombotic regimen is controversial and may not be significantly better than aspirin alone.

ethaverine hydrochloride

Ethaquin, Ethatab, Ethavex-100, Isovex

Pregnancy Risk Category: C

HOW SUPPLIED

Tablets: 100 mg
Capsules: 100 mg

MECHANISM OF ACTION

Directly relaxes smooth muscle due to the inhibition of phosphodiesterase, resulting in increased concentrations of cyclic adenosine monophosphate.

INDICATIONS & DOSAGE

Long-term treatment of peripheral and cerebrovascular insufficiency associated with arterial spasm; spastic conditions of GI and GU tracts–
Adults: 100 to 200 mg P.O. t.i.d.

ADVERSE REACTIONS

Common reactions are in italics; life-threatening reactions are in bold italics.

CNS: *headache,* drowsiness.

CV: *hypotension, flushing,* sweating, vertigo, cardiac depression, arrhythmias.

GI: *nausea, anorexia, abdominal distress, dry throat,* constipation, diarrhea.

Hepatic: jaundice, altered liver function tests.

Skin: rash.

Other: respiratory depression, malaise, lassitude.

INTERACTIONS

None significant.

NURSING CONSIDERATIONS

- *Contraindicated* in complete AV dissociation and severe hepatic disease.
- *Use cautiously* in women who are pregnant or of childbearing age and in glaucoma or pulmonary embolus; may precipitate arrhythmias.
- Withhold dose and call doctor if

signs of hepatic hypersensitivity develop (GI symptoms, altered liver function tests, jaundice, and eosinophilia).
- The FDA has announced this drug may not be effective for disease states indicated.

isoxsuprine hydrochloride
Duvadilan‡, Vasodilan, Vasoprine

Pregnancy Risk Category: C

HOW SUPPLIED
Tablets: 10 mg, 20 mg

MECHANISM OF ACTION
Stimulates beta receptors and may also be a direct-acting peripheral vasodilator.

INDICATIONS & DOSAGE
Adjunct for relief of symptoms associated with cerebrovascular insufficiency, peripheral vascular diseases (such as arteriosclerosis obliterans, thromboangiitis obliterans, Raynaud's disease) –
Adults: 10 to 20 mg P.O. t.i.d. or q.i.d.

ADVERSE REACTIONS
Common reactions are in italics; life-threatening reactions are in bold italics.
CV: tachycardia, hypotension.
GI: vomiting, abdominal distress, intestinal distention.
Skin: severe rash.

INTERACTIONS
None significant.

NURSING CONSIDERATIONS
- *Contraindicated* in immediate postpartum period and arterial bleeding. Use with caution in cardiovascular or cerebrovascular disease.
- Safe use in pregnancy and lactation not established, although drug has been used to inhibit contractions in premature labor.
- Isoxsuprine has also been used to minimize cramping in patients with severe primary dysmenorrhea.
- Discontinue if rash develops.
- Instruct patient to avoid sudden position changes to minimize the risk of orthostasis.

nimodipine
Nimotop

Pregnancy Risk Category: C

HOW SUPPLIED
Capsules: 30 mg

MECHANISM OF ACTION
Inhibits calcium ion influx across cardiac and smooth muscle cells, thus decreasing myocardial contractility and oxygen demand, and dilates coronary and cerebral arteries and arterioles. Initially thought to relieve vasospasm in patients after subarachnoid hemorrhage, its mechanism of action is not fully known; blockade of calcium influx into cerebral neurons may contribute to the drug's effect.

INDICATIONS & DOSAGE
Improvement of neurologic deficits in patients after subarachnoid hemorrhage from ruptured congenital aneurysms –
Adults: 60 mg P.O. q 4 hours for 21 days. Therapy should begin within 96 hours after subarachnoid hemorrhage.

ADVERSE REACTIONS
Common reactions are in italics; life-threatening reactions are in bold italics.
CNS: headaches.
CV: decreased blood pressure, flushing, edema.

INTERACTIONS
Antihypertensives: possible enhanced hypotensive effect.
Calcium channel blockers: possible enhanced cardiovascular effects.

NURSING CONSIDERATIONS

- There are no known contraindications to nimodipine therapy, and the drug was relatively well tolerated in clinical trials. Nimodipine should be reserved for patients who are in good neurologic condition postictus (for example, Hunt and Hess grades I to III).
- Patients with hepatic failure should receive lower doses. Begin therapy at 30 mg P.O. every 4 hours, with close monitoring of blood pressure and heart rate.
- Monitor blood pressure and heart rate in all patients, especially at the initiation of therapy.

nylidrin hydrochloride

Adrin, Arlidin, Arlidin Forte†, PMS Nylidrin†

Pregnancy Risk Category: C

HOW SUPPLIED

Tablets: 6 mg, 12 mg

MECHANISM OF ACTION

Stimulates beta receptors and may directly relax vascular smooth muscle.

INDICATIONS & DOSAGE

To increase blood supply in vasospastic disorders (arteriosclerosis obliterans, thromboangiitis obliterans, diabetic vascular disease, night leg cramps, Raynaud's phenomenon and disease, ischemic ulcer, frostbite, acrocyanosis, acroparesthesia, sequelae of thrombophlebitis) and in circulatory disturbances of the middle ear (primary cochlear ischemia, cochlear striae, vascular ischemia, macular or ampullar ischemia); other disturbances caused by labyrinth artery spasm or obstruction –

Adults: 3 to 12 mg P.O. t.i.d. or q.i.d.

ADVERSE REACTIONS

Common reactions are in italics; life-threatening reactions are in bold italics.

CNS: trembling, *nervousness,* weakness, *dizziness (not associated with labyrinth artery insufficiency).*

CV: *palpitations, hypotension,* flushing.

GI: nausea, vomiting.

INTERACTIONS

None significant.

NURSING CONSIDERATIONS

- *Contraindicated* in acute myocardial infarction, paroxysmal tachycardia, angina pectoris, or thyrotoxicosis.
- *Use cautiously* in uncompensated heart disease or peptic ulcer.
- Advise patient to avoid tasks that require mental alertness (such as driving or operating heavy machinery) until CNS effects of the drug are known.
- Instruct patient to avoid sudden posture changes to minimize the risks of orthostasis.

papaverine hydrochloride

Cerespan, Genabid, Pavabid, Pavabid HP Capsulets, Pavabid Plateau Caps, Pavarine Spancaps, Pavasule, Pavatine, Pavatym, Paverolan Lanacaps

Pregnancy Risk Category: C

HOW SUPPLIED

Tablets: 30 mg, 60 mg, 100 mg, 150 mg, 200 mg, 300 mg
Tablets (timed-release): 200 mg
Capsules (timed-release): 150 mg
Injection: 30 mg/ml

MECHANISM OF ACTION

Directly relaxes smooth muscle from the inhibition of phosphodiesterase, resulting in increased concentrations of cyclic adenosine monophosphate.

INDICATIONS & DOSAGE

Relief of cerebral and peripheral ischemia associated with arterial spasm and myocardial ischemia; treatment

*Liquid form contains alcohol. **May contain tartrazine.

of smooth muscle spasm (coronary occlusion, angina pectoris, sequelae of peripheral and pulmonary embolism, certain cerebral angiospastic states) and visceral spasms (biliary, ureteral, or GI colic) –
Adults: 60 to 300 mg P.O. 1 to 5 times daily, or 150- to 300-mg sustained-release preparations q 8 to 12 hours; 30 to 120 mg I.M. or I.V. q 3 hours, as indicated.

ADVERSE REACTIONS
Common reactions are in italics; life-threatening reactions are in bold italics.
CNS: *headache.*
CV: *increased heart rate, increased blood pressure* (with parenteral use), depressed AV and intraventricular conduction, hypotension, ***arrhythmias.***
GI: constipation, *nausea.*
Other: *sweating, flushing,* malaise, ***hepatic damage,*** increased depth of respiration.

INTERACTIONS
Levodopa: papaverine may interfere with the therapeutic effects of levodopa in patients with Parkinson's disease.

NURSING CONSIDERATIONS
- *Contraindicated* for I.V. use in patients with Parkinson's disease or complete AV block.
- *Use cautiously* in glaucoma.
- Monitor blood pressure and heart rate and rhythm, especially in cardiac disease. Withhold dose and notify doctor immediately if changes occur.
- Not often used parenterally, except when immediate effect is desired.
- Give I.V. slowly (over 1 to 2 minutes) to avoid serious adverse reactions.
- Most effective when given early in the course of a disorder.
- Tell patient to take medication regularly; long-term therapy is required.
- Monitor for adverse hepatic reactions in patients receiving long-term therapy.
- Do not add lactated Ringer's injection to the injectable form; will precipitate.
- Advise patient to avoid tasks that require mental alertness (such as driving or operating heavy machinery) until CNS effects of the drug are known.
- Instruct patient to avoid sudden posture changes to minimize the risks of orthostatic hypotension.
- The FDA has announced this drug may not be effective for disease states indicated.
- Has been used experimentally, alone or with phenoxybenzamine, to treat impotence in males. Patients are taught to self-administer by intercavernosal injection.

tolazoline hydrochloride
Priscoline

Pregnancy Risk Category: C

HOW SUPPLIED
Injection: 25 mg/ml

MECHANISM OF ACTION
Direct-acting vasodilator. May have some alpha receptor blocking effects.

INDICATIONS & DOSAGE
Persistent pulmonary hypertension of the newborn –
Neonates: initially, 1 to 2 mg/kg I.V. over 10 minutes, followed by infusion of 1 to 2 mg/kg/hour.
Peripheral vasospastic disorders –
Adults: 10 to 50 mg I.M. or I.V. q.i.d.

ADVERSE REACTIONS
Common reactions are in italics; life-threatening reactions are in bold italics.
CV: ***arrhythmias,*** anginal pain, *hypertension, flushing,* transient postural vertigo, palpitations, *orthostatic hypotension.*
GI: *nausea, vomiting, diarrhea, epi-*

gastric discomfort, exacerbation of peptic ulcer.
Local: burning at injection site.
Other: weakness, paradoxical response in seriously damaged limbs, increased pilomotor activity, tingling, chilliness, apprehension, pulmonary hemorrhage.

INTERACTIONS

Ethyl alcohol: possible disulfiram reaction from accumulation of acetaldehyde. Use together cautiously.
Vasopressors (epinephrine, norepinephrine): may cause a paradoxical fall in blood pressure.

NURSING CONSIDERATIONS

- *Contraindicated* in coronary artery disease or active peptic ulcer, or following CVA.
- *Use cautiously* in patients with history of peptic ulcer disease, gastritis, or known or suspected mitral stenosis.
- **I.V. use:** Response to treatment of persistent pulmonary hypertension of the newborn should be evident within 30 minutes. There is little information regarding infusions lasting longer than 48 hours.
- Keep patient warm during parenteral administration to increase response.
- Patient should be supine during infusion.
- Appearance of flushing usually indicates maximum tolerable dose.
- Monitor vital signs. Watch especially for blood pressure changes and arrhythmias.
- Instruct patient to avoid sudden posture changes to minimize risks of orthostatic hypotension.
- Instruct patient to avoid alcohol; chills and flushing may occur.
- Warn patient against exposure to cold, which can aggravate tissue damage.
- Often used to distinguish between functional (vasospastic) and organic (obstructive) forms of peripheral vascular disease.

24

Antilipemics

cholestyramine
clofibrate
colestipol hydrochloride
dextrothyroxine sodium
gemfibrozil
lovastatin
niacin
(See Chapter 92, VITAMINS AND MINERALS.)
pravastatin sodium
probucol
simvastatin

COMBINATION PRODUCTS
None.

cholestyramine

Cholybar, Questran**
Pregnancy Risk Category: C

HOW SUPPLIED
Bar: 4 g
Powder: 378-g cans, 9-g single-dose packets. Each scoop of powder or single-dose packet contains 4 g of cholestyramine resin.

MECHANISM OF ACTION
Combines with bile acid to form an insoluble compound that is excreted. The liver must synthesize new bile acid from cholesterol; this leads to reduced low-density-lipoprotein cholesterol levels.

INDICATIONS & DOSAGE
Primary hyperlipidemia, pruritus, and diarrhea due to excess bile acid; as adjunctive therapy for the reduction of elevated serum cholesterol in patients with primary hypercholesterolemia; and to reduce the risks of atherosclerotic coronary artery disease and myocardial infarction –
Adults: 4 g before meals and h.s., not to exceed 32 g daily. Each scoop or packet of Questran contains 4 g cholestyramine. Also available as Cholybar, a chewable candy bar (raspberry or caramel flavored) containing 4 g cholestyramine.
Children: 240 mg/kg daily P.O. in three divided doses with beverage or food. Safe dosage not established for children under 6 years.

ADVERSE REACTIONS
Common reactions are in italics; life-threatening reactions are in bold italics.
GI: *constipation,* fecal impaction, hemorrhoids, *abdominal discomfort,* flatulence, *nausea,* vomiting, steatorrhea.
Skin: *rashes,* irritation of skin, tongue, and perianal area.
Other: *vitamin A, D, and K deficiency from decreased absorption;* hyperchloremic acidosis with long-term use or very high dosage.

INTERACTIONS
Acetaminophen, coumarin anticoagulants, beta-adrenergic blocking agents, corticosteroids, digitalis glycosides, fat-soluble vitamins (A, D, E, and K), iron preparations, thiazide diuretics, thyroid hormone: absorption may be substantially decreased by cholestyramine. Separate administration times by at least 2 hours.

NURSING CONSIDERATIONS
- *Contraindicated* in patients with hypersensitivity to bile acid sequestering resins and in patients with complete biliary obstruction.
- *Use cautiously* in patients predisposed to constipation and in patients with conditions that may be aggravated by constipation, such as severe, symptomatic coronary artery disease. Long-term use may be associated with

deficiency of vitamins A, D, E, and K and folic acid.

• Patients who are taking this drug to reduce the risks of atherosclerotic heart disease should be encouraged to be aware of other cardiac disease risk factors. Recommend weight control and stop-smoking programs.

• Monitor serum cholesterol and triglyceride levels regularly during cholestyramine therapy. Teach the patient about proper dietary management (restricting total fat and cholesterol intake), weight control, and exercise. Explain their importance in controlling elevated serum lipids.

• To mix powder, sprinkle powder on surface of preferred beverage or wet food. Let stand a few minutes, then stir to obtain uniform suspension.

• Mixing with carbonated beverages may result in excess foaming. Use large glass and mix slowly.

• Administer all other medications at least 1 hour before or 4 to 6 hours after cholestyramine to avoid blocking their absorption.

• Monitor bowel habits; treat constipation as needed. Encourage a diet high in fiber and fluids. If severe constipation develops, decrease dosage, add a stool softener, or discontinue drug.

• Monitor cardiac glycosides in patients receiving both medications concurrently. Should cholestyramine therapy be discontinued, cardiac glycoside toxicity may result unless dosage is adjusted.

• Watch for signs of folic acid and vitamin A, D, E, and K deficiency.

• May bind many drugs and cause decreased absorption. Check drug interactions of individual drugs.

clofibrate

Arterioflexin‡, Atromid-S, Claripex†, Novofibrate†

Pregnancy Risk Category: C

HOW SUPPLIED

Capsules: 500 mg

MECHANISM OF ACTION

Seems to inhibit biosynthesis of cholesterol at an early stage, but the exact mechanism is unknown.

INDICATIONS & DOSAGE

Hyperlipidemia and xanthoma tuberosum; type III hyperlipidemia that does not respond adequately to diet; treatment of patients with very high serum triglyceride levels (type IV or V hyperlipidemia) –

Adults: 2 g P.O. daily in two or four divided doses. Some patients may respond to lower doses as assessed by serum lipid monitoring.

Should not be used in children.

ADVERSE REACTIONS

Common reactions are in italics; life-threatening reactions are in bold italics.

Blood: leukopenia.

CNS: fatigue, weakness.

CV: ***arrhythmias.***

GI: *nausea, diarrhea, vomiting,* stomatitis, *dyspepsia,* flatulence.

GU: impotence and decreased libido, acute renal failure.

Hepatic: gallstones, *transient and reversible elevations of liver function tests.*

Skin: rashes, urticaria, pruritus, dry skin and hair.

Other: myalgias and arthralgias, resembling a flu-like syndrome; *weight gain; polyphagia;* fever, decreased libido.

INTERACTIONS

Furosemide, sulfonylureas: clofibrate may potentiate the clinical effect of these agents. Monitor patient closely.

Lovastatin, simvastatin, pravastatin: risk of myositis, rhabdomyolysis, and renal failure. Avoid concomitant use.

Oral anticoagulants: clofibrate may potentiate the anticoagulant effects of

*Liquid form contains alcohol. **May contain tartrazine.

warfarin or dicumarol. Decreased anticoagulant dosage is necessary.
Oral contraceptives, rifampin: may antagonize clofibrate's lipid-lowering effect. Monitor serum lipids.
Probenecid: increased clofibrate effect. Monitor for toxicity.

NURSING CONSIDERATIONS

• *Contraindicated* in severe renal or hepatic disease.
• Warn patient to report flu-like symptoms to doctor immediately.
• Monitor renal and hepatic function, blood counts, and serum electrolyte and blood glucose levels. If liver function tests show steady rise, clofibrate should be discontinued.
• Should not be used indiscriminately. May pose increased risk of gallstones, heart disease, and cancer.
• Used to treat patients with high serum triglyceride levels (type IV or V hyperlipidemia). These patients typically have serum triglyceride levels over 2,000 mg/dl.
• Monitor serum cholesterol and triglycerides regularly during clofibrate therapy.
• Teach patient about proper dietary management (restricting total fat and cholesterol intake), weight control, and exercise. Explain their importance in controlling elevated serum lipids.
• If significant lipid lowering is not achieved within 3 months, drug should be discontinued.
• Clofibrate has been used investigationally to treat diabetes insipidus at doses of 1.5 to 2 g daily.

colestipol hydrochloride

Colestid

Pregnancy Risk Category: C

HOW SUPPLIED

Granules: 500-g bottles, 5-g packets

MECHANISM OF ACTION

Combines with bile acid to form an insoluble compound that is excreted. The liver must synthesize new bile acid from cholesterol; this leads to reduced low-density-lipoprotein cholesterol levels.

INDICATIONS & DOSAGE

Primary hypercholesterolemia and xanthomas –
Adults: 5 to 30 g P.O. daily in two to four divided doses.

ADVERSE REACTIONS

Common reactions are in italics; life-threatening reactions are in bold italics.
CNS: headache, dizziness.
GI: *constipation (common, may require decreasing the dosage),* fecal impaction, hemorrhoids, abdominal discomfort, flatulence, nausea, vomiting, steatorrhea.
Skin: rashes, irritation of skin, tongue, and perianal area.
Other: vitamin A, D, and K deficiency from decreased absorption; hyperchloremic acidosis with long-term use or very high dosage.

INTERACTIONS

Oral hypoglycemics: may antagonize response to colestipol. Monitor serum lipids.
Orally administered drugs: absorption may be decreased by colestipol. Separate administration times: other drugs should be taken at least 1 hour before or 4 hours after colestipol.

NURSING CONSIDERATIONS

• *Contraindicated* in patients with hypersensitivity to bile acid sequestering resins and in patients with complete biliary obstruction.
• *Use cautiously* in patients predisposed to constipation and in patients with conditions that may be aggravated by constipation, such as severe, symptomatic coronary artery disease. Long-term use may be associated with

deficiency of vitamins A, D, E, and K and folic acid.
• Administer all other medications at least 1 hour before or 4 to 6 hours after colestipol to avoid blocking their absorption.
• Monitor cardiac glycoside levels in patients receiving both medications concurrently. Should colestipol therapy be discontinued, cardiac glycoside toxicity may result unless dosage is adjusted.
• Watch for signs of vitamin A, D, and K deficiency.
• Lowering dosage, increasing dietary fiber, or adding stool softener may relieve constipation.
• May bind many drugs and cause decreased absorption. Check drug interaction list of individual drugs.
• Administer this drug in at least 3 oz (90 ml) of juice, milk, or water. After drinking this preparation, patient should swirl a small additional amount of liquid in the same glass and then drink it to ensure ingestion of the entire dose.
• Palatability may be enhanced if the next daily dose is mixed and refrigerated the previous evening.
• Teach patient about proper dietary management (restricting total fat and cholesterol intake), weight control, and exercise. Explain their importance in controlling elevated serum lipids.

dextrothyroxine sodium (d-thyroxine sodium)

Choloxin**

Pregnancy Risk Category: C

HOW SUPPLIED

Tablets: 1 mg, 2 mg, 4 mg, 6 mg

MECHANISM OF ACTION

Accelerates hepatic catabolism of cholesterol and increases bile secretion to lower cholesterol levels.

INDICATIONS & DOSAGE

Hyperlipidemia in euthyroid patients, especially when cholesterol and triglyceride levels are elevated –
Adults: initial dose 1 to 2 mg P.O. daily, increased by 1 to 2 mg daily at monthly intervals to a total of 4 to 8 mg daily.
Children: initial dose 0.05 mg/kg P.O. daily, increased by 0.05 mg/kg daily at monthly intervals to a maximum of 4 mg daily. Alternatively, give 1.5 mg/m² P.O. daily, increased by 1.5 mg/m² daily at monthly intervals. Maximum daily dose is 4 mg. The usual maintenance dose is 0.1 mg/kg or 3 mg/m² daily in euthyroid children.

ADVERSE REACTIONS

Common reactions are in italics; life-threatening reactions are in bold italics.
CV: palpitations, angina pectoris, ***arrhythmias,*** ischemic myocardial changes on ECG, ***MI.***
EENT: visual disturbances, ptosis.
GI: nausea, vomiting, diarrhea, constipation, decreased appetite.
Metabolic: *insomnia, weight loss, sweating,* flushing, hyperthermia, hair loss, menstrual irregularities.

INTERACTIONS

Digitalis glycosides: dextrothyroxine may enhance clinical effect. Use together cautiously.
Oral anticoagulants: dextrothyroxine may potentiate the anticoagulant effect of warfarin or dicumarol.
Sympathomimetics: dextrothyroxine may precipitate arrhythmias or coronary insufficiency in patients with cardiac disease.

NURSING CONSIDERATIONS

• *Contraindicated* in hepatic or renal disease, or iodism. Patients with history of cardiac disease, including arrhythmias, hypertension, or angina pectoris, should receive very small doses.

*Liquid form contains alcohol. **May contain tartrazine.

• May increase need for insulin, diet therapy, or oral hypoglycemics in patients with diabetes.
• If the use of anticoagulants is being considered, discontinue drug 2 weeks before surgery to avoid possible potentiation of anticoagulant effect.
• Observe patient for signs of hyperthyroidism, such as nervousness, insomnia, and weight loss. If these occur, dosage should be decreased or drug discontinued.
• Teach patient about proper dietary management (restricting total fat and cholesterol intake), weight control, and exercise. Explain their importance in controlling elevated serum lipids.

gemfibrozil
Lopid
Pregnancy Risk Category: B

HOW SUPPLIED
Tablets: 600 mg
Capsules: 300 mg

MECHANISM OF ACTION
Inhibits peripheral lipolysis and also reduces triglyceride synthesis in the liver. Lowers serum triglyceride levels and increases high-density-lipoprotein cholesterol levels.

INDICATIONS & DOSAGE
Treatment of type IV hyperlipidemia (hypertriglyceridemia) and severe hypercholesterolemia unresponsive to diet and other drugs; to reduce the risk of coronary heart disease in patients intolerant of or refractory to treatment with bile acid sequestrants or niacin –
Adults: 1,200 mg P.O. administered in two divided doses. Usual dosage range is 900 to 1,500 mg daily. If no beneficial effect is seen after 3 months of therapy, drug should be discontinued.

ADVERSE REACTIONS
Common reactions are in italics; life-threatening reactions are in bold italics.
Blood: anemia, leukopenia.
CNS: blurred vision, headache, dizziness.
GI: *abdominal and epigastric pain, diarrhea, nausea,* vomiting, flatulence.
Hepatic: bile duct obstruction, elevated enzymes.
Skin: rash, dermatitis, pruritus.
Other: painful extremities.

INTERACTIONS
Oral anticoagulants: gemfibrozil may enhance the clinical effects of oral anticoagulants. Monitor patient closely.

NURSING CONSIDERATIONS
• *Contraindicated* in hepatic or severe renal dysfunction – including primary biliary cirrhosis – and preexisting gallbladder disease.
• CBC and liver function tests should be done periodically during the first 12 months of therapy.
• Gemfibrozil is very closely related to clofibrate both chemically and pharmacologically.
• Instruct patient to take drug half an hour before breakfast and dinner.
• Should not be used indiscriminately. May pose risk of gallstones, heart disease, and cancer.
• Observe bowel movements for evidence of steatorrhea or other signs of bile duct obstruction.
• Because of possible dizziness and blurred vision, patient should avoid driving or other hazardous activities until CNS effects of the drug are known.
• Teach patient about proper dietary management (restricting total fat and cholesterol intake), weight control, and exercise. Explain their importance in controlling elevated serum lipids.

lovastatin

Mevacor

Pregnancy Risk Category: X

HOW SUPPLIED

Tablets: 20 mg

MECHANISM OF ACTION

Lovastatin inhibits 3-hydroxy-3-methylglutaryl-coenzyme A (HMG-CoA) reductase. This enzyme is an early (and rate-limiting) step in the synthetic pathway of cholesterol.

INDICATIONS & DOSAGE

Reduction of low-density lipoprotein and total cholesterol levels in patients with primary hypercholesterolemia (types IIa and IIb) –

Adults: initially, 20 mg P.O. once daily with the evening meal. For patients with severely elevated cholesterol levels (for example, over 300 mg/dl), the initial dose should be 40 mg. The recommended range is 20 to 80 mg in single or divided doses.

ADVERSE REACTIONS

Common reactions are in italics; life-threatening reactions are in bold italics.

CNS: headache, dizziness.

EENT: blurred vision, dysgeusia.

GI: constipation, diarrhea, dyspepsia, flatus, abdominal pain or cramps, heartburn, nausea.

Metabolic: elevated serum transaminase levels, abnormal liver test results.

Skin: rash, pruritus.

Other: peripheral neuropathy, muscle cramps, myalgia, myositis, ***rhabdomyolysis***.

INTERACTIONS

Cholestyramine, clofibrate: enhanced lipid-reducing effects.

Immunosuppressive agents, gemfibrozil: possible increased risk of polymyositis and rhabdomyolysis. Maximum recommended lovastatin dosage is 20 mg daily; monitor patient closely.

NURSING CONSIDERATIONS

• *Contraindicated* in patients with hypersensitivity to the drug, active liver disease, or conditions associated with unexplained persistent elevations of serum transaminase; in pregnant and breast-feeding women; and in women of childbearing age unless there is no risk of pregnancy.

• Initiate lovastatin only after diet and other nonpharmacologic therapies have proven ineffective. Patient should be on a standard low-cholesterol diet during therapy.

• Give lovastatin with the evening meal; absorption is enhanced and cholesterol biosynthesis is greater in the evening.

• Therapeutic response occurs in about 2 weeks, with maximum effects in 4 to 6 weeks. Effects of long-term use are unknown.

• Watch for signs of myositis.

• Liver function tests should be performed frequently at start of therapy and periodically thereafter.

• Store tablets at room temperature in a light-resistant container.

• Tell patient to restrict alcohol intake.

• Tell patient to advise doctor of any adverse reactions, particularly muscle aches and pains.

• Advise patient to have periodic eye examinations.

• Teach patient about proper dietary management, weight control, and exercise. Explain their importance in controlling elevated serum lipids.

pravastatin sodium

Pravachol

Pregnancy Risk Category: X

HOW SUPPLIED

Tablets: 10 mg, 20 mg

MECHANISM OF ACTION
Inhibits the enzyme 3-hydroxy-3-methylglutaryl-coenzyme A (HMG-CoA) reductase. This hepatic enzyme is an early (and rate-limiting) step in the synthetic pathway of cholesterol.

INDICATIONS & DOSAGE
Reduction of low-density lipoprotein and total cholesterol levels in patients with primary hypercholesterolemia (types IIa and IIb) –
Adults: initially, 5 to 10 mg daily h.s. Adjust dosage q 4 weeks based on patient tolerance and response; maximum daily dosage is 40 mg. Most elderly patients respond to a daily dosage of 20 mg or less.

ADVERSE REACTIONS
Common reactions are in italics; life-threatening reactions are in bold italics.
CNS: headache, fatigue, dizziness.
CV: chest pain.
EENT: rhinitis.
GI: vomiting, diarrhea, heartburn, nausea.
Respiratory: cough.
Skin: rash.
Other: influenza, localized muscle pain, myalgia, cold.

INTERACTIONS
Cholestyramine, colestipol: concomitant administration decreases plasma levels of pravastatin. Administer pravastatin 1 hour before or 4 hours after these drugs.
Drugs that decrease levels or activity of endogenous steroids (such as cimetidine, spironolactone, ketoconazole): may increase risk of developing endocrine dysfunction. No intervention appears necessary; take complete drug history in patients who develop endocrine dysfunction.
Gemfibrozil: decreases protein-binding and urinary clearance of pravastatin. Avoid concomitant use.
Hepatotoxic drugs, chronic alcohol abuse: increased risk of hepatotoxicity. Avoid concomitant use.
Immunosuppressive agents (such as cyclosporine), fibric acid derivatives (such as clofibrate or gemfibrozil), high doses of niacin (nicotinic acid; 1 g or more daily), erythromycin: may increase the risk of rhabdomyolysis. Monitor patient closely if concomitant use cannot be avoided.

NURSING CONSIDERATIONS
- *Contraindicated* in patients with hypersensitivity to the drug, in patients with active liver disease or conditions that have unexplained persistent elevations of serum transaminase, in pregnant and breast-feeding women, and in women of childbearing age unless there is no risk of pregnancy.
- Administer the recommended dosage in the evening, preferably at bedtime. Drug may be given without regard to meals.
- Dosage adjustments should be made about every 4 weeks. If cholesterol level falls below the target range, dosage may be reduced.
- Perform liver function tests frequently at start of therapy and periodically thereafter.
- Clinical evidence of liver dysfunction may occur in up to 1.3% of patients. Drug should be discontinued and patient monitored closely. A liver biopsy may be performed if enzyme elevations persist.
- Watch for signs of myositis. Myopathy, marked elevations of CPK, possibly leading to rhabdomyolysis, and renal failure secondary to myoglobinuria have been reported rarely.
- Drug should be temporarily discontinued in any patient with an acute condition that suggests a developing myopathy or in patients with risk factors that may predispose them to the development of renal failure secondary to rhabdomyolysis: severe acute infection; severe endocrine, metabolic, or electrolyte disorders; hypo-

tension; major surgery; or uncontrolled seizures.
- Initiate drug only after diet and other nonpharmacologic therapies have proven ineffective. Patients should continue a cholesterol-lowering diet during therapy.
- Because of drug's possible impact on liver function, advise patient to restrict alcohol intake.
- Tell patient to inform doctor of any adverse reactions, particularly muscle aches and pains.
- Teach patient about proper dietary management, weight control, and exercise. Explain their importance in controlling serum lipids.

probucol

Lorelco, Lurselle‡

Pregnancy Risk Category: B

HOW SUPPLIED

Tablets: 250 mg, 500 mg

MECHANISM OF ACTION

Inhibits cholesterol transport from the intestine, prevents oxidation of low-density lipoprotein, and may also decrease cholesterol synthesis. Appears to be more effective in patients with mild cholesterol elevations than in those with severe hypercholesterolemia.

INDICATIONS & DOSAGE

Primary hypercholesterolemia – **Adults:** 500 mg P.O. b.i.d. with morning and evening meals. Do not exceed 1 g/day.

Not recommended for children.

ADVERSE REACTIONS

Common reactions are in italics; life-threatening reactions are in bold italics.

CV: prolonged QT interval, arrhythmias.

GI: *diarrhea, flatulence, abdominal pain, nausea, vomiting.*

Other: *hyperhidrosis,* fetid sweat, ***angioneurotic edema.***

INTERACTIONS

Clofibrate: additive pharmacologic effects.

Tricyclic antidepressants, class Ia antiarrhythmics, phenothiazines, beta blockers, digitalis glycosides, calcium channel blocking agents: increased risk of arrhythmias.

NURSING CONSIDERATIONS
- *Contraindicated* in patients with arrhythmias. Drug should be stopped in any patient whose ECG shows prolonged Q-T interval. Monitor ECG periodically.
- Drug's effect is enhanced when taken with food.
- Teach patient about proper dietary management, weight control, and exercise. Explain their importance in controlling elevated serum lipids.
- If female patient wishes to become pregnant, withdrawal of drug and effective contraception is recommended for 6 months due to the persistence of the drug in the body.

simvastatin

Zocor

Pregnancy Risk Category: X

HOW SUPPLIED

Tablets: 5 mg, 10 mg, 20 mg, 40 mg

MECHANISM OF ACTION

Inhibits the enzyme 3-hydroxy-3-methylglutaryl-coenzyme A (HMG-CoA) reductase. This hepatic enzyme is an early (and rate-limiting) step in the synthetic pathway of cholesterol.

INDICATIONS & DOSAGE

Reduction of low-density lipoprotein and total cholesterol levels in patients with primary hypercholesterolemia (types IIa and IIb) –
Adults: initially, 5 to 10 mg daily in

the evening. Adjust dosage q 4 weeks based on patient tolerance and response; maximum daily dosage is 40 mg.

ADVERSE REACTIONS

Common reactions are in italics; life-threatening reactions are in bold italics.
CNS: headache, asthenia.
GI: abdominal pain, constipation, diarrhea, dyspepsia, flatulence, nausea.
Other: upper respiratory infection.

INTERACTIONS

Digoxin: simvastatin may slightly elevate digoxin levels. Closely monitor plasma digoxin levels at initiation of simvastatin therapy.
Drugs that decrease levels or activity of endogenous steroids (such as cimetidine, spironolactone, ketoconazole): may increase risk of developing endocrine dysfunction. No intervention appears necessary; take complete drug history in patients who develop endocrine dysfunction.
Hepatotoxic drugs, chronic alcohol abuse: increased risk of hepatotoxicity. Avoid concomitant use.
Immunosuppressive agents (such as cyclosporine), fibric acid derivatives (such as clofibrate or gemfibrozil), high doses of niacin (nicotinic acid; 1 g or more daily), erythromycin: may increase the risk of rhabdomyolysis. Monitor patient closely if concomitant use cannot be avoided. Limit daily dosage of simvastatin to 10 mg if patient must take cyclosporine.
Warfarin: anticoagulant effect may be slightly enhanced. Monitor patient's prothrombin time at start of therapy and during dosage adjustments.

NURSING CONSIDERATIONS

- *Contraindicated* in patients with hypersensitivity to the drug, in patients with active liver disease or conditions that have unexplained persistent elevations of serum transaminase, in pregnant and breast-feeding women, and in women of childbearing age unless there is no risk of pregnancy.
- Recommended dosage should be administered in the evening. Drug may be given without regard to meals.
- Dosage adjustments should be made about every 4 weeks. If the cholesterol level falls below the target range, dosage may be reduced.
- Perform liver function tests frequently at start of therapy and periodically thereafter.
- Clinical evidence of liver dysfunction may occur in up to 1% of patients. The drug should be discontinued and patient monitored closely. A liver biopsy may be performed if enzyme elevations persist.
- Watch for signs of myositis. Myopathy, marked elevations of CPK, possibly leading to rhabdomyolysis, and renal failure secondary to myoglobinuria have been reported rarely.
- Drug should be temporarily discontinued in any patient with an acute condition that suggests a developing myopathy or risk factors that may predispose the patient to renal failure secondary to rhabdomyolysis: severe acute infection; severe endocrine, metabolic, or electrolyte disorders; hypotension; major surgery; or uncontrolled seizures.
- Initiate drug only after diet and other nonpharmacologic therapies have proven ineffective. Patients should continue a cholesterol-lowering diet during therapy.
- Because of drug's possible impact on liver function, advise patient to restrict alcohol intake.
- Tell patient to inform doctor of any adverse reactions, particularly muscle aches and pains.
- Teach patient about proper dietary management, weight control, and exercise. Explain their importance in controlling serum lipids.

25

Nonnarcotic analgesics and antipyretics

acetaminophen
aspirin
choline magnesium trisalicylate
choline salicylate
diflunisal
magnesium salicylate
methotrimeprazine hydrochloride
(See Chapter 28, SEDATIVE-HYPNOTICS.)
phenazopyridine hydrochloride
salsalate
sodium salicylate
sodium thiosalicylate

COMBINATION PRODUCTS

ALLEREST NO DROWSINESS TABLETS◇, COLDRINE◇, ORNEX NO DROWSINESS CAPLETS◇, SINUTAB MAXIMUM STRENGTH WITHOUT DROWSINESS◇: acetaminophen 325 mg and pseudoephedrine hydrochloride 30 mg.
AMAPHEN, ANOQUAN, BUTACE, DOLMAR, ENDOLOR ESGIC, EZOL, FEBRIDYNE, FEMCET, FIORICET, ISOPAP, MEDIGESIC, PACAPS, REPAN, ROGESIC, SEMCET, TENCET, TRIAD, TWO-DYNE: acetaminophen 325 mg, caffeine 40 mg, and butalbital 50 mg.
ARTHRALGEN: acetaminophen 250 mg and salicylamide 250 mg.
ASCRIPTIN: aspirin 325 mg, magnesium hydroxide 50 mg, aluminum hydroxide 50 mg, and calcium carbonate 50 mg.
ASCRIPTIN A/D: aspirin 325 mg, magnesium hydroxide 75 mg, aluminum hydroxide 75 mg, and calcium carbonate 75 mg.
AXOTAL: aspirin 650 mg and butalbital 50 mg.
BC POWDER: aspirin 650 mg, salicylamide 195 mg, and caffeine 32 mg.
BC TABLETS: aspirin 325 mg, salicylamide 95 mg, and caffeine 16 mg.
CAMA, ARTHRITIS STRENGTH: aspirin 500 mg, magnesium oxide 150 mg, and aluminum hydroxide 150 mg.
COPE◇: aspirin 421 mg, caffeine 32 mg, magnesium hydroxide 50 mg, and aluminum hydroxide 25 mg.
DURADYNE◇: acetaminophen 180 mg, aspirin 230 mg, and caffeine 15 mg.
EXCEDRIN P.M.◇: acetaminophen 500 mg and diphenhydramine citrate 38 mg.
EXCEDRIN TABLETS◇: aspirin 250 mg, acetaminophen 250 mg, caffeine 65 mg.
FARBITAL, FIORINAL, ISOBUTAL, ISOLLYL, LANIROIF, LANORINAL, MARNAL: aspirin 325 mg, caffeine 40 mg, and butalbital 50 mg.
FEMCAPS◇: acetaminophen 324 mg, caffeine 32 mg, ephedrine sulfate 8 mg, and atropine sulfate 0.0325 mg.
G-1: acetaminophen 500 mg, caffeine 40 mg, and butalbital 50 mg.
GEMNISYN◇: aspirin 325 mg and acetaminophen 325 mg.
MAXIMUM STRENGTH MIDOL FOR CRAMPS◇: aspirin 500 mg, caffeine 32.4 mg, and cinnamedrine hydrochloride 14.9 mg.
MIDOL◇: aspirin 454 mg, caffeine 32.4 mg, and cinnamedrine hydrochloride 14.9 mg.
MIDOL PMS◇: acetaminophen 500 mg, pamabrom 25 mg, pyrilamine maleate 15 mg.
PAC NEW REVISED FORMULA◇: aspirin 400 mg and caffeine 32 mg.
PHRENILIN: acetaminophen 325 mg and butalbital 50 mg.
PHRENILIN FORTE: acetaminophen 650 mg and butalbital 50 mg.
SINUS EXCEDRIN NO DROWSINESS◇: acetaminophen 500 mg and pseudoephedrine hydrochloride 30 mg.
SINUTAB◇: acetaminophen 325 mg,

*Liquid form contains alcohol. **May contain tartrazine.

chlorpheniramine 2 mg, and pseudoephedrine hydrochloride 30 mg.
SINUTAB MAXIMUM STRENGTH◇: acetaminophen 500 mg, pseudoephedrine hydrochloride 30 mg, and chlorpheniramine maleate, 2 mg.
TECNAL†: aspirin 330 mg, caffeine 40 mg, and butalbital 50 mg.
TRIGESIC◇: acetaminophen 125 mg, aspirin 230 mg, and caffeine 30 mg.
TRILISATE: choline salicylate 293 mg and magnesium salicylate 362 mg.
VANQUISH◇: aspirin 227 mg, acetaminophen 194 mg, caffeine 33 mg, aluminum hydroxide 25 mg, and magnesium hydroxide 50 mg.

acetaminophen (paracetamol)

Acephen◇, Aceta*◇, Ace-Tabs†◇, Acetaminophen Uniserts◇, Actamin◇, Actamin Extra◇, Anuphen◇, Apacet◇, Apacet Extra Strength◇, Apacet Oral Solution◇, APAP◇, Apo-Acetaminophen†◇, Atasol†◇, Atasol Forte†◇, Banesin◇, Campain†◇, Ceetamol‡, Children's Apacet◇, Children's Genapap◇, Children's Panadol◇, Children's Tylenol◇, Children's Ty-Pap◇, Children's Ty-Tab◇, Dapa◇, Datril◇, Datril Extra Strength◇, Dolanex*◇, Dymadon‡, Exdol†◇, Exdol Strong†◇, Genapap◇, Genebs◇, Genebs Extra Strength◇, Gentabs◇, Halenol◇, Infant's Apacet◇, Infant's Tylenol◇, Infants' Ty-Pap◇, Junior Disprol‡, Liquiprin◇, Meda Cap◇, Meda Tab◇, Myapap◇, Neopap◇, Oraphen-PD◇, Panadol◇, Panadol Junior Strength◇, Panamax‡, Panex◇, Paraphen†◇, Parmol‡, Pedric*◇, Phenaphen◇, Robigesic†◇, Rounox†◇, Suppap◇, Tapanol◇, Tapanol Extra Strength◇, Tempra◇, Tenol◇, Ty Caplets◇, Ty Caps◇, Tylenol*, Tylenol Extra Strength◇, Ty-Tab◇, Valadol*◇, Valorin◇

Pregnancy Risk Category: B

HOW SUPPLIED

Tablets: 160 mg◇, 325 mg◇, 500 mg◇, 650 mg◇
Tablets (chewable): 80 mg◇
Capsules: 325 mg◇, 500 mg◇
Oral solution: 100 mg/ml◇
Oral suspension: 120 mg/5 ml‡
Oral liquid: 160 mg/5 ml◇, 500 mg/15 ml◇
Elixir: 120 mg/5 ml*◇, 160 mg/5 ml*◇, 320 mg/5 ml*◇
Wafers: 120 mg◇
Effervescent granules: 325 mg/capful◇
Suppositories: 120 mg◇, 125 mg◇, 135 mg◇, 650 mg◇

MECHANISM OF ACTION

Produces analgesia by blocking generation of pain impulses, probably by inhibition of prostaglandin synthesis or inhibition of the synthesis or action of other substances that sensitize pain receptors to mechanical or chemical stimulation. It relieves fever by central action in the hypothalamic heat-regulating center.

INDICATIONS & DOSAGE

Mild pain or fever –
Adults and children over 11 years: 325 to 650 mg P.O. q 4 hours; or 1 g q.i.d. p.r.n. Maximum dosage should not exceed 4 g daily. Dosage for long-term therapy should not exceed 2.6 g daily.
Children 11 years and under: 10 mg/kg P.O. q 4 hours. Do not exceed five doses q 24 hours. Alternatively, use the following guidelines.
Children 11 years: 480 mg/dose.
Children 9 to 10 years: 400 mg/dose.
Children 6 to 8 years: 320 mg/dose.
Children 4 to 5 years: 240 mg/dose.
Children 2 to 3 years: 160 mg/dose.
Children 12 to 23 months: 120 mg/dose.
Children 4 to 11 months: 80 mg/dose.

†Available in Canada only. ‡Available in Australia only. ◇Available OTC.

Children up to 3 months: 40 mg/dose.
Mild pain or fever in patients who can't tolerate oral medication –
Adults: 650 mg P.R. q 4 to 6 hours. Give no more than 6 suppositories in 24 hours.
Children age 6 to 12: 325 mg P.R. q 4 to 6 hours. Give no more than 2.6 g in 24 hours.
Children age 3 to 6: 120 mg P.R. q 4 to 6 hours.
Children under age 3: consult a doctor.

ADVERSE REACTIONS
Common reactions are in italics; life-threatening reactions are in bold italics.
Hepatic: ***severe liver damage with toxic doses.***
Skin: rash, urticaria.

INTERACTIONS
Barbiturates, carbamazepine, hydantoins, rifampin, sulfinpyrazone: high doses or long-term use of these drugs may enhance the hepatotoxic effects of acetaminophen. Avoid concomitant use.
Caffeine: may enhance analgesic effects of acetaminophen.
Diflunisal: increases acetaminophen blood levels. Don't use together.
Ethanol: increased risk of hepatic damage.
Warfarin: increased hypoprothrombinemic effect with chronic acetaminophen use.
Zidovudine: conflicting evidence suggests possible impaired zidovudine metabolism. Monitor patient closely.

NURSING CONSIDERATIONS
- *Contraindicated* for repeated use in anemia, or renal or hepatic disease.
- *Use cautiously* in patients with a history of chronic alcohol abuse because hepatotoxicity has occurred at therapeutic doses. Limit daily intake to 2 g.
- Consult a doctor before administering this drug to children under age 2.
- This drug is only for short-term use. Tell patients to consult a doctor if administering to children for more than 5 days or adults for more than 10 days.
- Has no significant anti-inflammatory effect.
- Should not be used for self-medication of marked fever (over 103.1° F [39.5° C]), fever persisting longer than 3 days, or recurrent fever unless directed by doctor.
- When used for antipyretic effects, consider additional methods to help cool the patient: tepid baths, loosened clothing, and lowered environmental temperature. However, excessive cooling may cause the patient to shiver.
- Many nonprescription products contain acetaminophen. Be aware of this when calculating total daily dosages.
- Recommend the liquid form for children and for all patients who have difficulty swallowing.
- Acetaminophen crosses the placenta, but is apparently safe for short-term use at therapeutic doses during pregnancy. It is routinely used during all stages of pregnancy for the treatment of pain and fever.
- Acetaminophen is found in breast milk in low concentrations (less than 1% of a dose). It is safe to use during breast-feeding provided it is used only for short-term therapy and recommended doses are not exceeded.
- Warn patient that high doses or unsupervised chronic use can cause hepatic damage. Excessive ingestion of alcoholic beverages may increase the risk of hepatotoxicity.
- Acetaminophen may interfere with certain laboratory tests for urinary 5-hydroxyindoleacetic acid. It may also produce false-positive decreases in blood glucose levels in home monitor-

*Liquid form contains alcohol. **May contain tartrazine.

ing systems using Chemstrip bG, Dextrostix, or Visidex II.

aspirin (acetylsalicylic acid)

Ancasal†◇, Arthrinol†◇, Artria SR◇, ASA◇, ASA Enseals◇, Aspergum◇, Aspro‡, Astrin†◇, Bayer Aspirin◇, Bex‡, Coryphen†◇, Easprin◇, Ecotrin◇, Empirin◇, Entrophen†◇, Measurin◇, Norwich Aspirin◇, Novasen†◇, Riphen-10†◇, Sal-Adult†◇, Sal-Infant†◇, Solprin‡, Supasa†◇, Triaphen-10†◇, Vincent's Powders‡, Winsprin Capsules‡, ZORprin◇

Pregnancy Risk Category: C (D in 3rd trimester)

HOW SUPPLIED

Tablets◇*:* 65 mg, 75 mg, 81 mg, 300 mg, 325 mg, 500 mg, 600 mg, 650 mg
Tablets (chewable): 81 mg◇
Tablets (enteric-coated): 325 mg◇, 500 mg◇, 650 mg◇, 975 mg
Tablets (extended-release): 800 mg
Tablets (timed-release): 650 mg◇
Capsules: 325 mg◇, 500 mg◇
Powder: 500 mg
Chewing gum: 227.5 mg◇
Suppositories: 60 to 120 mg◇

MECHANISM OF ACTION

- Produces analgesia by an ill-defined effect on the hypothalamus (central action) and by blocking generation of pain impulses (peripheral action). The peripheral action may involve inhibition of prostaglandin synthesis.
- Exerts its anti-inflammatory effect by inhibiting prostaglandin synthesis, may also inhibit the synthesis or action of other mediators of the inflammatory response.
- Relieves fever by acting on the hypothalamic heat-regulating center to produce peripheral vasodilation. This increases peripheral blood supply and promotes sweating, which leads to loss of heat and to cooling by evaporation.
- Also appears to impede clotting by blocking prostaglandin synthesis, which prevents formation of the platelet-aggregating substance thromboxane A_2.

INDICATIONS & DOSAGE

Adults:
Arthritis – 2.6 to 5.4 g P.O. daily in divided doses.
Mild pain or fever – 325 to 650 mg P.O. or P.R. q 4 hours, p.r.n.
Thromboembolic disorders – 325 to 650 mg P.O. daily or b.i.d.
Transient ischemic attacks in men – 650 mg P.O. b.i.d. or 325 mg q.i.d.
To reduce the risk of heart attack in patients with previous myocardial infarction (MI) or unstable angina – several protocols have been studied; most employ doses of 80 to 325 mg P.O. daily or 325 mg every other day.
Children: *Arthritis* – 90 to 130 mg/kg P.O. daily divided q 4 to 6 hours.
Fever – 40 to 80 mg/kg P.O. or P.R. daily divided q 6 hours, p.r.n.
Mild pain – 65 to 100 mg/kg P.O. or P.R. daily divided q 4 to 6 hours, p.r.n.

ADVERSE REACTIONS

Common reactions are in italics; life-threatening reactions are in bold italics.
Blood: *prolonged bleeding time.*
EENT: *tinnitus and hearing loss.*
GI: *nausea, vomiting, GI distress, occult bleeding.*
Hepatic: abnormal liver function studies, hepatitis.
Skin: *rash,* bruising.
Other: ***hypersensitivity manifested by anaphylaxis or asthma.***

INTERACTIONS

Alcohol, steroids, other NSAIDs: increased risk of GI bleeding. Avoid concomitant use.
NSAIDs, including diflunisal, fenoprofen, ibuprofen, indomethacin, pi-

†Available in Canada only. ‡Available in Australia only. ◇Available OTC.

roxicam, meclofenamate, naproxen: altered pharmacokinetics of these agents, leading to lowered serum levels and decreased effectiveness. Avoid concomitant use.
Ammonium chloride (and other urine acidifiers): increased blood levels of aspirin products. Monitor for aspirin toxicity.
Antacids in high doses (and other urine alkalinizers): decreased levels of aspirin products. Monitor for decreased aspirin effect.
Antihypertensives: decreased antihypertensive effect. Avoid long-term aspirin ingestion if patient is taking antihypertensives.
Corticosteroids: enhance salicylate elimination. Monitor for decreased salicylate effect.
Methotrexate: increased risk of methotrexate toxicity. Avoid concomitant use.
Oral anticoagulants, heparin: increased risk of bleeding. Avoid using together if possible.
Oral hypoglycemic agents: increased hypoglycemic effect. Monitor closely.
Probenecid, sulfinpyrazone: decreased uricosuric effect. Avoid aspirin during therapy with these agents.

NURSING CONSIDERATIONS

- *Contraindicated* in GI ulcer, GI bleeding, patients with bleeding disorders, or aspirin hypersensitivity.
- *Use cautiously* in patients with hypoprothrombinemia, renal failure, or vitamin K deficiency and in asthmatics with nasal polyps (may cause severe bronchospasm).
- Consult a doctor before administering this drug to children under age 12.
- When used to treat inflammatory conditions, rheumatic fever, and thrombosis, aspirin is administered on a scheduled, rather than p.r.n., basis. During prolonged therapy, hematocrit, prothrombin levels, and renal function should be assessed periodically.
- Tell patients they should consult a doctor if administering to children for more than 5 days or adults for more than 10 days.
- Avoid aspirin during pregnancy. Evidence exists that the drug may increase the risk of hemorrhage in both neonate and mother; limited evidence suggests that it may contribute to congenital heart disease or other malformations.
- Because of epidemiologic association with Reye's syndrome, the Centers for Disease Control and Prevention recommends that children or teenagers with chicken pox or influenza-like illness should not be given salicylates.
- Febrile, dehydrated children can develop toxicity rapidly.
- Elderly patients may be more susceptible to aspirin's toxic effects.
- Give with food, milk, antacid, or large glass of water to reduce GI adverse reactions.
- Because of the many possible drug interactions involving aspirin, warn patients taking prescription drugs to check with doctor or pharmacist before taking OTC combinations containing aspirin.
- Therapeutic blood salicylate level in arthritis is 10 to 30 mg/100 ml. Tinnitus may occur at plasma levels of 30 mg/100 ml and above, but this is not a reliable indicator of toxicity, especially in very young patients and those over age 60. With chronic therapy, mild toxicity may occur at plasma levels of 20 mg/100 ml.
- May cause an increase in serum levels of AST (SGOT), ALT (SGPT), alkaline phosphatase, and bilirubin.
- Keep out of reach of children—aspirin is one of the leading causes of poisoning in children. Encourage use of child-resistant containers in households with children.
- Advise patients receiving prolonged treatment with large doses of aspirin to watch for petechiae, bleeding

*Liquid form contains alcohol. **May contain tartrazine.

gums, and signs of GI bleeding and to maintain adequate fluid intake. Encourage the use of a soft toothbrush. Obtain hemoglobin and prothrombin tests periodically.

- Enteric-coated products are slowly absorbed and are not suitable for acute effects. They do cause less GI bleeding and may be more suited for long-term therapy, such as arthritic therapy.
- Aspirin rectal suppositories are available for patients who can't tolerate oral medications. Watch for rectal mucosal irritation or bleeding.
- Aspirin reduces the risk of recurrent MI and transient ischemic attacks in men; data regarding safety and efficacy in women are not available, but investigations continue.
- There is some evidence that aspirin may prevent sunburn and treat sunburn pain by preventing cells from manufacturing prostaglandins.
- Aspirin irreversibly inhibits platelet aggregation. If possible, aspirin should be discontinued 5 to 7 days before elective surgery to allow time for the production and release of new platelets.
- For patients with swallowing difficulties, aspirin can be crushed and combined with soft food or dissolved in liquid. After mixing it with a liquid, administer it immediately because the drug doesn't stay in solution. Don't crush enteric-coated aspirin.
- Aspirin tablets that have a strong vinegar-like odor should be discarded.

choline magnesium trisalicylate (choline salicylate and magnesium salicylate)

Trilisate

Pregnancy Risk Category: C

HOW SUPPLIED

Tablets: 500 mg, 750 mg, 1,000 mg of salicylate

Solution: 500 mg of salicylate/5 ml

MECHANISM OF ACTION

- Produces analgesia by an ill-defined effect on the hypothalamus (central action) and by blocking generation of pain impulses (peripheral action). The peripheral action may involve inhibition of prostaglandin synthesis.
- Exerts its anti-inflammatory effect by inhibiting prostaglandin synthesis.
- Relieves fever by acting on the hypothalamic heat-regulating center to produce peripheral vasodilation. This increases peripheral blood supply and promotes sweating, which leads to loss of heat and to cooling by evaporation.

INDICATIONS & DOSAGE

Arthritis, mild–

Adults: 1 to 2 teaspoonfuls or tablets P.O. b.i.d. Total daily dosage can also be given at one time (usually h.s.)

Rheumatoid arthritis and osteoarthritis–

Adults: initially, 3 g P.O. daily either as a single dose h.s. or b.i.d. Dosage is adjusted according to patient response. Dosage range is 1 to 4.5 g daily.

Juvenile rheumatoid arthritis–

Children (12 to 37 kg): 50 mg/kg/day P.O. in divided doses.

Children (more than 37 kg): 2,250 mg P.O. in divided doses.

Mild to moderate pain and fever–

Adults: 2 to 3 g P.O. daily divided b.i.d.

Children (12 to 37 kg): 50 mg/kg/day P.O. in divided doses.

ADVERSE REACTIONS

Common reactions are in italics; life-threatening reactions are in bold italics.

EENT: tinnitus and hearing loss.

GI: GI distress.

Skin: rash.

Other: ***hypersensitivity manifested by anaphylaxis (rare).***

INTERACTIONS

Alcohol, steroids, and other NSAIDs: enhanced risk of adverse GI effects.
Ammonium chloride (and other urine acidifiers): increased blood levels of salicylates. Monitor for salicylate toxicity.
Antacids in high doses (and other urine alkalinizers): decreased levels of salicylates. Monitor for decreased salicylate effect.
Corticosteroids: enhance salicylate elimination. Monitor for decreased salicylate effect.
Methotrexate: increased risk of methotrexate toxicity. Avoid concomitant use.
Oral anticoagulants: increased risk of bleeding. Use together cautiously.

NURSING CONSIDERATIONS

- *Use cautiously* in chronic renal failure, peptic ulcer disease, and gastritis and in patients with a known allergy to salicylates.
- Each 500-mg tablet or teaspoonful is equal in salicylate content to 650 mg aspirin; each 750-mg tablet, 975 mg aspirin; each 1,000-mg tablet, 1,300 mg aspirin.
- Because of epidemiologic association with Reye's syndrome, the Centers for Disease Control and Prevention recommends that children or teenagers with chicken pox or influenza-like illness should not be given salicylates.
- Causes less GI distress than aspirin. If antacid is needed, give it 2 hours after meals and give choline magnesium trisalicylate before meals.
- Anti-inflammatory, analgesic, and antipyretic effects of salicylate salts are comparable to those of aspirin; however, they do not affect platelet function. Therefore, do not substitute these agents for aspirin during antithrombotic therapy.
- Tell patient to take tablets with food or a full glass of water. Solution may be mixed with fruit juice, but not antacids.
- Febrile, dehydrated children can develop toxicity rapidly.
- Therapeutic blood salicylate level in arthritis is 10 to 30 mg/100 ml. Tinnitus may occur at plasma levels of 30 mg/100 ml and above, but this is not a reliable indicator of toxicity, especially in very young patients and those over age 60. With chronic therapy, mild toxicity may occur at plasma levels of 20 mg/100 ml.
- Periodically monitor hemoglobin and prothrombin tests in patients receiving long-term treatment with large doses.

choline salicylate

Arthropan, Teejel†*

Pregnancy Risk Category: C

HOW SUPPLIED

Liquid: 870 mg/5 ml◊
Gel: 87 mg/g†*

MECHANISM OF ACTION

- Produces analgesia by an ill-defined effect on the hypothalamus (central action) and by blocking generation of pain impulses (peripheral action). The peripheral action may involve inhibition of prostaglandin synthesis.
- Exerts its anti-inflammatory effect by inhibiting prostaglandin synthesis.
- Relieves fever by acting on the hypothalamic heat-regulating center to produce peripheral vasodilation. This increases peripheral blood supply and promotes sweating, which leads to loss of heat and to cooling by evaporation.

INDICATIONS & DOSAGE

Rheumatoid arthritis, osteoarthritis, minor pain or fever–
Adults and children over 12 years: 1 teaspoonful (870 mg choline salicy-

*Liquid form contains alcohol. **May contain tartrazine.

late) P.O. q 3 to 4 hours p.r.n. If tolerated and needed, dosage may be increased to 2 teaspoonfuls. Do not exceed 6 teaspoonfuls daily.
Relief of pain from inflamed gums –
Adults and children over 2 years: apply 1 cm of gel to affected area q 3 to 4 hours and h.s., p.r.n.

ADVERSE REACTIONS
Common reactions are in italics; life-threatening reactions are in bold italics.
EENT: tinnitus and hearing loss.
GI: nausea, vomiting, GI distress.
Skin: rash.
Other: ***hypersensitivity manifested by anaphylaxis (rare).***

INTERACTIONS
Alcohol, steroids, and other NSAIDs: enhanced risk of adverse GI reactions.
Ammonium chloride (and other urine acidifiers): increased blood levels of salicylates. Monitor for salicylate toxicity.
Antacids in high doses (and other urine alkalinizers): decreased levels of salicylates. Monitor for decreased salicylate effect.
Corticosteroids: enhance salicylate elimination. Monitor for decreased salicylate effect.
Methotrexate: increased risk of methotrexate toxicity. Avoid concomitant use.

NURSING CONSIDERATIONS
- *Use cautiously* in chronic renal failure, peptic ulcer disease, and gastritis and in patients with a known allergy to salicylates.
- Because of epidemiologic association with Reye's syndrome, the Centers for Disease Control and Prevention recommends that children or teenagers with chicken pox or influenza-like illness should not be given salicylates.
- Causes less GI distress than aspirin. If antacid is needed, give it 2 hours after meals and give choline salicylate before meals.
- May mix drug with water, fruit juice, or carbonated drinks, but not antacids.
- Febrile, dehydrated children can develop toxicity rapidly.
- Therapeutic blood salicylate level in arthritis is 10 to 30 mg/100 ml. Tinnitus may occur at plasma levels of 30 mg/100 ml and above, but this is not a reliable indicator of toxicity, especially in very young patients and those over age 60. With chronic therapy, mild toxicity may occur at plasma levels of 20 mg/100 ml.
- Periodically monitor hemoglobin and prothrombin tests in patients receiving long-term treatment with large doses.
- Anti-inflammatory, analgesic, and antipyretic effects of salicylate salts are comparable to those of aspirin; however, they do not affect platelet function. Therefore, do not substitute these agents for aspirin during antithrombotic therapy.

diflunisal
Dolobid

Pregnancy Risk Category: C

HOW SUPPLIED
Tablets: 250 mg, 500 mg

MECHANISM OF ACTION
Mechanism of action is unknown, but it is probably related to inhibition of prostaglandin synthesis.

INDICATIONS & DOSAGE
Mild to moderate pain and osteoarthritis –
Adults: 500 to 1,000 mg P.O. daily in two divided doses, usually q 12 hours. Maximum dosage 1,500 mg daily.
Adults over 65: start with one-half the usual adult dose.

ADVERSE REACTIONS

Common reactions are in italics; life-threatening reactions are in bold italics.

CNS: *dizziness,* somnolence, insomnia, *headache,* fatigue.

EENT: *tinnitus, visual disturbances (rare).*

GI: *nausea, dyspepsia, GI pain, diarrhea,* vomiting, constipation, flatulence.

GU: renal impairment, hematuria, interstitial nephritis.

Skin: *rash,* pruritus, sweating, dry mucous membranes, stomatitis.

INTERACTIONS

Acetaminophen, hydrochlorothiazide: diflunisal may substantially increase blood levels, increasing the risk of toxicity. Avoid concomitant use.

Aspirin, antacids: decreased diflunisal blood levels. Monitor for possible decreased therapeutic effect.

Cyclosporine: diflunisal may enhance the nephrotoxicity of cyclosporine. Avoid concomitant use.

Methotrexate: diflunisal may enhance the toxicity of methotrexate. Avoid concomitant use.

Oral anticoagulants, thrombolytic agents: diflunisal may enhance pharmacologic effects of these agents. Use together cautiously.

Sulindac: diflunisal decreases blood levels of sulindac's active metabolite. Monitor for decreased pharmacologic effect.

NURSING CONSIDERATIONS

- *Contraindicated* in patients for whom acute asthmatic attacks, urticaria, or rhinitis are precipitated by aspirin or other NSAIDs.
- *Use cautiously* in patients with active GI bleeding or history of peptic ulcer disease, renal impairment, liver disease, and compromised cardiac function or in those taking anticoagulants.
- Similar to aspirin, diflunisal is a salicylic acid derivative but is metabolized differently. Anti-inflammatory, analgesic, and antipyretic effects are comparable to those of aspirin; however, platelet function is not affected. Do not substitute for aspirin during antithrombotic therapy.
- May be administered with water, milk, or meals.
- Avoid the use of diflunisal in children and teenagers with viral illnesses and flu because of possible association with Reye's syndrome.

magnesium salicylate

Extra-Strength Doan's◇, Magan◇, Mobidin◇, Original Doan's◇

Pregnancy Risk Category: C

HOW SUPPLIED

Tablets: 545 mg, 600 mg
Caplets: 325 mg◇, 500 mg◇

MECHANISM OF ACTION

- Produces analgesia by an ill-defined effect on the hypothalamus (central action) and by blocking generation of pain impulses (peripheral action). The peripheral action may involve inhibition of prostaglandin synthesis.
- Exerts its anti-inflammatory effect by inhibiting prostaglandin synthesis.
- Relieves fever by acting on the hypothalamic heat-regulating center to produce peripheral vasodilation. This increases peripheral blood supply and promotes sweating, which leads to loss of heat and to cooling by evaporation.

INDICATIONS & DOSAGE

Arthritis –
Adults: 545 mg to 1.2 g P.O. t.i.d. or q.i.d. not to exceed 4.8 g daily.
Mild pain or fever –
Adults: 300 to 600 mg P.O. q 4 hours, not to exceed 3.5 g/24 hours.

ADVERSE REACTIONS

Common reactions are in italics; life-threatening reactions are in bold italics.

EENT: *tinnitus and hearing loss.*
GI: *nausea, vomiting, GI distress.*
Hepatic: abnormal liver function studies, hepatitis.
Skin: *rash,* bruising.
Other: ***hypersensitivity manifested by anaphylaxis or asthma (rare).***

INTERACTIONS
Alcohol, steroids, other NSAIDs: increased risk of GI bleeding. Avoid concomitant use.
Ammonium chloride (and other urine acidifiers): increased blood levels of salicylates. Monitor for salicylate toxicity.
Antacids in high doses (and other urine alkalinizers): decreased levels of salicylates. Monitor for decreased salicylate effect.
Corticosteroids: enhance salicylate elimination. Monitor for decreased salicylate effect.
Methotrexate: increased risk of methotrexate toxicity. Avoid concomitant use.
Oral anticoagulants, heparin: increased risk of bleeding. Avoid using together if possible.

NURSING CONSIDERATIONS
- *Contraindicated* in severe chronic renal insufficiency because of risk of magnesium toxicity; GI ulcer; GI bleeding; or aspirin hypersensitivity.
- *Use cautiously* in hypoprothrombinemia, vitamin K deficiency, and bleeding disorders.
- Because of epidemiologic association with Reye's syndrome, the Centers for Disease Control and Prevention recommends that children or teenagers with chicken pox or influenza-like illness should not be given salicylates.
- Febrile, dehydrated children can develop toxicity rapidly.
- Give with food, milk, antacid, or large glass of water to reduce GI adverse reactions.
- Therapeutic blood salicylate level in arthritis is 10 to 30 mg/100 ml. Tinnitus may occur at plasma levels of 30 mg/100 ml and above, but this is not a reliable indicator of toxicity, especially in very young patients and those over age 60. With chronic therapy, mild toxicity may occur at plasma levels of 20 mg/100 ml.
- May cause an increase in serum levels of AST (SGOT), ALT (SGPT), alkaline phosphatase, and bilirubin.
- Monitor hemoglobin and prothrombin tests in patients receiving long-term treatment with large doses.
- Anti-inflammatory, analgesic, and antipyretic effects of salicylate salts are comparable to those of aspirin; however, they do not affect platelet function. Therefore, do not substitute these agents for aspirin during antithrombotic therapy.

phenazopyridine hydrochloride

Azo-Standard◊, Baridium◊, Di-Azo◊, Eridium◊, Geridium◊, Phenazo†, Phenazodine◊, Pyrazodine◊, Pyridiate◊, Pyridin◊, Pyridium, Pyronium†, Urodine◊, Urogesic◊, Viridium◊

Pregnancy Risk Category: B

HOW SUPPLIED
Tablets: 100 mg◊, 200 mg

MECHANISM OF ACTION
Exerts local anesthetic action on urinary mucosa through unknown mechanism.

INDICATIONS & DOSAGE
Pain with urinary tract irritation or infection –
Adults: 100 to 200 mg P.O. t.i.d.
Children: 100 mg P.O. t.i.d.

ADVERSE REACTIONS
Common reactions are in italics; life-threatening reactions are in bold italics.
CNS: headache, vertigo.

GI: nausea.
Skin: rash.

INTERACTIONS
None significant.

NURSING CONSIDERATIONS
- *Contraindicated* in renal and hepatic insufficiency.
- Colors urine red or orange. May stain fabrics.
- Taking the drug with meals may minimize GI distress.
- Use only as analgesic. Use with antibiotic to treat urinary tract infection.
- Drug may be stopped in 3 days if pain is relieved.
- May alter Clinistix or Tes-Tape results. Use Clinitest for accurate urine glucose test results.
- Stop drug if skin or sclera becomes yellow-tinged. May indicate accumulation caused by impaired renal excretion.

salsalate

Arthra-G, Disalcid, Mono-Gesic, Salflex, Salgesic, Salsitab

Pregnancy Risk Category: C

HOW SUPPLIED
Tablets: 500 mg, 750 mg
Capsules: 500 mg

MECHANISM OF ACTION
- The salicylic ester of salicylic acid, each molecule of salsalate is hydrolyzed to two molecules of salicylate in vivo.
- Produces analgesia by an ill-defined effect on the hypothalamus (central action) and by blocking generation of pain impulses (peripheral action). The peripheral action may involve inhibition of prostaglandin synthesis.
- Exerts its anti-inflammatory effect by inhibiting prostaglandin synthesis; may also inhibit the synthesis or action of other mediators of the inflammatory response.

INDICATIONS & DOSAGE
Arthritis –
Adults: 3 g P.O. daily, divided b.i.d. or t.i.d. Usual maintenance dose is 2 to 4 g daily.

ADVERSE REACTIONS
Common reactions are in italics; life-threatening reactions are in bold italics.
EENT: *tinnitus and hearing loss.*
GI: ***nausea, vomiting, GI distress, occult bleeding (rare).***
Hepatic: abnormal liver function studies, hepatitis.
Skin: *rash,* bruising.
Other: *hypersensitivity manifested by anaphylaxis and asthma.*

INTERACTIONS
Alcohol, steroids, other NSAIDs: increased risk of GI bleeding. Avoid concomitant use.
Ammonium chloride (and other urine acidifiers): increased blood levels of salicylates. Monitor for salicylate toxicity.
Antacids in high doses (and other urine alkalinizers): decreased levels of salicylates. Monitor for decreased salicylate effect.
Corticosteroids: compete for binding sites. Monitor for decreased salicylate effect.
Methotrexate: increased risk of methotrexate toxicity. Avoid concomitant use.
Oral anticoagulants: possible increased risk of bleeding. Avoid using together if possible.

NURSING CONSIDERATIONS
- *Contraindicated* in salsalate hypersensitivity.
- *Use cautiously* in GI bleeding, aspirin hypersensitivity, and renal insufficiency and in hypoprothrombinemia, vitamin K deficiency, and bleeding disorders.
- Because of epidemiologic association with Reye's syndrome, the Centers for Disease Control and Preven-

tion recommends that children or teenagers with chicken pox or influenza-like illness should not be given salicylates.

• Give with food, milk, antacid, or large glass of water to reduce possible GI adverse reactions.

• Therapeutic blood salicylate level in arthritis is 10 to 30 mg/100 ml. Tinnitus may occur at plasma levels of 30 mg/100 ml and above, but this is not a reliable indicator of toxicity, especially in very young patients and those over age 60. With chronic therapy, mild toxicity may occur at plasma levels of 20 mg/100 ml.

• May cause an increase in serum levels of AST (SGOT), ALT (SGPT), alkaline phosphatase, and bilirubin.

• Advise patients receiving long-term treatment with large doses to watch for petechiae, bleeding gums, and signs of GI bleeding, and to maintain adequate fluid intake. Obtain hemoglobin and prothrombin tests periodically.

sodium salicylate

Uracel-5◇

Pregnancy Risk Category: C

HOW SUPPLIED

Tablets: 325 mg◇, 650 mg◇
Tablets (enteric-coated): 324 mg◇, 325 mg◇, 650 mg◇
Injection: 1 g/10 ml

MECHANISM OF ACTION

• Produces analgesia by an ill-defined effect on the hypothalamus (central action) and by blocking generation of pain impulses (peripheral action). The peripheral action may involve inhibition of prostaglandin synthesis.

• Exerts its anti-inflammatory effect by inhibiting prostaglandin synthesis; may also inhibit the synthesis or action of other mediators of the inflammatory response.

• Relieves fever by acting on the hypothalamic heat-regulating center to produce peripheral vasodilation. This increases peripheral blood supply and promotes sweating, which leads to loss of heat and to cooling by evaporation.

INDICATIONS & DOSAGE

Minor pain or fever –
Adults: 325 to 650 mg P.O. q 4 to 6 hours, p.r.n., or 500 mg slow I.V. infusion over 4 to 8 hours. Maximum dosage is 1 g daily.
Arthritis –
Adults: 3.5 to 5.4 g P.O. daily in divided doses.

ADVERSE REACTIONS

Common reactions are in italics; life-threatening reactions are in bold italics.
EENT: *tinnitus, hearing loss.*
GI: *nausea, vomiting, GI distress.*
Hepatic: abnormal liver function studies, hepatitis.
Skin: *rash.*
Local: thrombophlebitis (from I.V.).
Other: ***hypersensitivity manifested by anaphylaxis or asthma (rare).***

INTERACTIONS

Alcohol, steroids, other NSAIDs: increased risk of GI distress. Avoid concomitant use.
Ammonium chloride (and other urine acidifiers): increased blood levels of salicylates. Monitor for salicylate toxicity.
Antacids in large doses (and other urine alkalinizers): decreased levels of salicylates. Monitor for decreased salicylate effect.
Corticosteroids: enhance salicylate elimination. Monitor for decreased salicylate effect.
Methotrexate increased risk of methotrexate toxicity. Avoid concomitant use.
Oral anticoagulants: increased risk of bleeding. Avoid using together if possible.

NURSING CONSIDERATIONS

- *Contraindicated* in GI ulcer, GI bleeding, or aspirin hypersensitivity. Use cautiously in hypoprothrombinemia, vitamin K deficiency, bleeding disorders, and asthma with nasal polyps (may cause severe bronchospasm).
- *Use cautiously* in CHF and hypertension because of increased sodium load.
- Because of epidemiologic association with Reye's syndrome, the Centers for Disease Control and Prevention recommends that children or teenagers with chicken pox or influenza-like illness should not be given salicylates.
- Febrile, dehydrated children can develop toxicity rapidly.
- Give with food, milk, antacid, or large glass of water to reduce adverse GI reactions.
- Therapeutic salicylate level in arthritis is 10 to 30 mg/100 ml. Tinnitus may occur at plasma levels of 30 mg/100 ml and above, but this is not a reliable indicator of toxicity, especially in very young patients and those over age 60. With chronic therapy, mild toxicity may occur at plasma levels of 20 mg/100 ml.
- May cause an increase in serum levels of AST (SGOT), ALT (SGPT), alkaline phosphatase, and bilirubin.
- Advise patients receiving long-term treatment with large doses to watch for petechiae, bleeding gums, and signs of GI bleeding, and to maintain adequate fluid intake. Obtain hemoglobin and prothrombin tests periodically.
- Unlike aspirin, sodium salicylate does not inhibit platelet aggregation.

---

sodium thiosalicylate

Asproject, Rexolate, Tusal

Pregnancy Risk Category: C

HOW SUPPLIED

Injection: 50 mg/ml in 2-ml ampules or 30-ml vials.

MECHANISM OF ACTION

- Produces analgesia by an ill-defined effect on the hypothalamus (central action) and by blocking generation of pain impulses (peripheral action). The peripheral action may involve inhibition of prostaglandin synthesis.
- Relieves fever by acting on the hypothalamic heat-regulating center to produce peripheral vasodilation. This increases peripheral blood supply and promotes sweating, which leads to loss of heat and to cooling by evaporation.

INDICATIONS & DOSAGE

Mild pain –
Adults: 50 to 100 mg daily or every other day, I.M. or slow I.V.
Acute gout –
Adults: 100 mg I.M. or slow I.V. q 3 to 4 hours for 2 days; then 100 mg daily.
Rheumatic fever –
Adults: 100 to 150 mg I.M. or slowly I.V. q 4 to 6 hours for 3 days, followed by 100 mg b.i.d. until asymptomatic.

ADVERSE REACTIONS

Common reactions are in italics; life-threatening reactions are in bold italics.
EENT: *tinnitus and hearing loss.*
GI: *nausea, vomiting, GI distress, occult bleeding.*
Hepatic: abnormal liver function studies, hepatitis.
Skin: *rash,* bruising.
Other: ***hypersensitivity manifested by anaphylaxis or asthma (rare).***

INTERACTIONS

Ammonium chloride (and other urine acidifiers): increased blood levels of salicylates. Monitor for salicylate toxicity.
Antacids in large doses (and other urine alkalinizers): decreased levels

of salicylates. Monitor for decreased salicylate effect.
Corticosteriods: enhance salicylate elimination. Monitor for decreased salicylate effects.
Oral anticoagulants, heparin: increased risk of bleeding. Avoid using together if possible.

NURSING CONSIDERATIONS

- *Contraindicated* in GI ulcer, GI bleeding, or aspirin sensitivity.
- *Use cautiously* in hypoprothrombinemia, vitamin K deficiency, bleeding disorders, and asthma with nasal polyps (may cause severe bronchospasm).
- Because of epidemiologic association with Reye's syndrome, the Centers for Disease Control and Prevention recommends that children or teenagers with chicken pox or influenza-like illness should not be given salicylates.
- Tinnitus, headache, dizziness, confusion, fever, sweating, thirst, drowsiness, dim vision, hyperventilation, and tachycardia are signs of mild toxicity.
- May cause an increase in serum levels of AST (SGOT), ALT (SGPT), alkaline phosphatase, and bilirubin.
- I.M. route is preferred because of increased risk of complications associated with I.V. use.

26

Nonsteroidal anti-inflammatory drugs

diclofenac sodium
etodolac
fenoprofen calcium
flurbiprofen
ibuprofen
indomethacin
indomethacin sodium trihydrate
ketoprofen
ketorolac tromethamine
meclofenamate
mefenamic acid
nabumetone
naproxen
naproxen sodium
oxaprozin
oxyphenbutazone
phenylbutazone
piroxicam
sulindac
tolmetin sodium

COMBINATION PRODUCTS
ADVIL COLD & SINUS◊, DRISTAN SINUS CAPLETS◊: pseudoephedrine hydrochloride 30 mg and ibuprofen 200 mg.

diclofenac sodium
Voltaren, Voltaren SR†

Pregnancy Risk Category: B

HOW SUPPLIED
Tablets (enteric-coated): 25 mg, 50 mg, 75 mg
Tablets (slow-release): 100 mg†
Suppositories: 50 mg†, 100 mg†

MECHANISM OF ACTION
Produces anti-inflammatory, analgesic, and antipyretic effects, possibly through inhibition of prostaglandin synthesis.

INDICATIONS AND DOSAGE
Ankylosing spondylitis –
Adults: 25 mg P.O. q.i.d. and h.s.
Osteoarthritis –
Adults: 50 mg P.O. b.i.d. or t.i.d., or 75 mg P.O. b.i.d.
Rheumatoid arthritis –
Adults: 75 to 100 mg P.O. b.i.d., or 50 to 100 mg P.R. (where available) h.s. as a substitute for the last oral dose of the day. Do not exceed 200 mg daily.

ADVERSE REACTIONS
Common reactions are in italics; life-threatening reactions are in bold italics.
CNS: anxiety, depression, drowsiness, insomnia, irritability, *headache.*
CV: ***CHF,*** hypertension.
EENT: *tinnitus,* laryngeal edema, swelling of the lips and tongue.
GI: *abdominal pain or cramps, constipation, diarrhea, indigestion, nausea,* abdominal distention, flatulence, peptic ulceration, ***GI bleeding,*** melena, bloody diarrhea, appetite change, colitis.
GU: azotemia, proteinuria, acute renal failure, oliguria, interstitial nephritis, papillary necrosis, ***nephrotic syndrome,*** *fluid retention.*
Hepatic: elevated hepatic enzymes, jaundice, hepatitis, ***hepatotoxicity.***
Respiratory: asthma.
Skin: rash, pruritus, urticaria, eczema, dermatitis, alopecia, photosensitivity, bullous eruption, ***Stevens-Johnson syndrome (rare),*** allergic purpura.
Other: ***anaphylaxis,*** anaphylactoid reactions, angioedema.

INTERACTIONS
Anticoagulants (including warfarin): possible increased incidence of bleeding. Monitor patient closely.

Aspirin: concomitant use not recommended by manufacturer.
Cyclosporine, digoxin, lithium, methotrexate: diclofenac may reduce renal clearance of these drugs and increase risk of toxicity. Monitor patient closely.
Diuretics: diclofenac may decrease the effectiveness of diuretics.
Insulin, oral hypoglycemic agents: diclofenac may alter requirements for hypoglycemic agents. Monitor patient closely.
Potassium-sparing diuretics: diclofenac may enhance potassium retention and increase serum potassium levels.

NURSING CONSIDERATIONS

- *Contraindicated* in patients with hypersensitivity to diclofenac, aspirin, or other NSAIDs and in patients with a history of asthma, urticaria, or other allergic reactions after taking these drugs. Not recommended for use during pregnancy or breast-feeding.
- *Use cautiously* in patients with a history of peptic ulcer disease, hepatic dysfunction, cardiac disease, or other conditions associated with fluid retention or impaired renal function.
- Elevations of liver tests may occur during therapy. Measure serum transaminase, especially ALT (SGPT), periodically in patients undergoing long-term therapy. The first serum transaminase measurement should be made no later than 8 weeks after initiation of therapy.
- Tell patient to take diclofenac with milk or meals to minimize GI distress.
- Peptic ulceration and GI bleeding have occurred in patients taking NSAIDs despite the absence of GI symptoms. Teach patient the signs and symptoms of GI bleeding, and tell him to contact the doctor promptly if these symptoms appear.
- Teach patient the signs and symptoms of hepatotoxicity, including nausea, fatigue, lethargy, pruritus, jaundice, right upper quadrant tenderness, and flulike symptoms. Tell him to contact doctor immediately if these symptoms appear.
- Tablets are enteric-coated. Do not crush, break, or chew.
- Because of their antipyretic and anti-inflammatory actions, NSAIDs may mask the signs and symptoms of infection.

etodolac (ultradol)
Lodine

Pregnancy Risk Category: C

HOW SUPPLIED
Capsules: 200 mg, 300 mg

MECHANISM OF ACTION
Unknown, but believed to be associated with inhibition of prostaglandin biosynthesis.

INDICATIONS & DOSAGE
Acute and chronic management of osteoarthritis and pain –
Adults: for acute pain, give 200 to 400 mg P.O. q 6 to 8 hours p.r.n., not to exceed 1,200 mg daily. For patients weighing 132 lb (60 kg) or under, total daily dose should not exceed 20 mg/kg.

ADVERSE REACTIONS
Common reactions are in italics; life-threatening reactions are in bold italics.
CNS: *asthenia, malaise,* dizziness, depression, nervousness.
CV: anemia, hypertension, ***CHF,*** flushing, palpitations, edema.
EENT: blurred vision, tinnitus, photophobia.
GI: *dyspepsia, flatulence, abdominal pain, diarrhea, nausea,* constipation, gastritis, melena, vomiting, anorexia, peptic ulcer with or without bleeding or perforation, ulcerative stomatitis, thirst, dry mouth.

GU: dysuria, urinary frequency.
Respiratory: asthma.
Skin: pruritus, rash.
Other: chills, fever, hepatitis.

INTERACTIONS

Antacids: may decrease peak levels of the drug. Monitor for decreased effect of etodolac.
Aspirin: reduces etodolac's protein-binding without altering its clearance. Clinical significance unknown.
Cyclosporine: impaired elimination and increased risk of nephrotoxicity. Avoid concomitant use.
Digoxin, lithium, methotrexate: etodolac may impair elimination of these drugs, resulting in increased levels and risk of toxicity. Monitor blood levels.
Warfarin: etodolac decreases the protein-binding of warfarin but does not change its clearance. Although no dosage adjustment is necessary, monitor prothrombin times closely and watch for bleeding.

NURSING CONSIDERATIONS

- *Contraindicated* in patients with hypersensitivity to the drug and in patients with a history of NSAID-induced asthma, rhinitis, urticaria, or other allergic reactions.
- *Use cautiously* in patients with a history of GI bleeding, ulceration, and perforation and renal or hepatic impairment. Also use cautiously with concurrent use of diuretics in patients with cardiac, renal, or hepatic failure.
- Drug is not recommended for patients with rheumatoid arthritis. Clinical trials have shown that other currently available NSAIDs are more effective.
- No apparent drug interaction occurs when etodolac is administered with diuretics, phenytoin, or glyburide.
- Etodolac appears to cause few GI problems. Minimal GI blood loss has been reported at doses up to 1,200 mg daily; in clinical trials, endoscopy scores were comparable to placebo at doses up to 1,000 mg daily. Etodolac 1,200 mg daily was shown to cause less GI bleeding than ibuprofen 2,400 mg daily, indomethacin 200 mg daily, naproxen 750 mg daily, or piroxicam 20 mg daily. However, GI ulceration or bleeding can occur with any NSAID, sometimes without warning. Patients receiving chronic therapy should be closely watched for signs and symptoms of GI bleeding.
- When reviewing diagnostic tests, know that metabolites of etodolac may cause a false-positive test for urinary bilirubin. Decreased serum uric acid levels and borderline elevations of one or more liver tests may occur.
- Peptic ulcer and GI bleeding have occurred in patients taking NSAIDs despite the absence of GI symptoms. Teach patient the signs and symptoms of GI bleeding, and tell him to contact the doctor if these symptoms appear.
- Tell patient to take etodolac with milk or meals to minimize GI discomfort.

fenoprofen calcium

Nalfon

Pregnancy Risk Category: B (D in 3rd trimester)

HOW SUPPLIED

Tablets: 600 mg
Capsules: 200 mg, 300 mg, 600 mg

MECHANISM OF ACTION

Produces anti-inflammatory, analgesic, and antipyretic effects, possibly through inhibition of prostaglandin synthesis.

INDICATIONS & DOSAGE

Rheumatoid arthritis and osteoarthritis –
Adults: 300 to 600 mg P.O. q.i.d. Maximum dosage is 3.2 g daily.

Mild to moderate pain –
Adults: 200 mg P.O. q 4 to 6 hours, p.r.n.

ADVERSE REACTIONS
Common reactions are in italics; life-threatening reactions are in bold italics.
Blood: prolonged bleeding time, anemia.
CNS: *headache, drowsiness, dizziness, somnolence* .
CV: peripheral edema.
GI: *epigastric distress, nausea,* ***GI bleeding,*** vomiting, occult blood loss, peptic ulceration, constipation, anorexia.
GU: reversible renal failure.
Hepatic: elevated enzymes.
Skin: *pruritus,* rash, urticaria.

INTERACTIONS
Alcohol, corticosteroids: increased risk of adverse GI reactions. Avoid concomitant use.
Aspirin: decreases fenoprofen half-life; may also increase GI toxicity. Avoid concomitant use.
Oral anticoagulants, sulfonylureas: fenoprofen enhances pharmacologic effects of these drugs. Use together cautiously.
Phenobarbital: enhanced metabolism of fenoprofen. Monitor for lack of effectiveness.

NURSING CONSIDERATIONS
- *Contraindicated* in patients with hypersensitivity to the drug, aspirin, or other NSAIDs.
- *Use cautiously* in elderly patients; in patients with GI disorders, angioedema, or cardiovascular disease; and in those with a history of peptic ulcer disease.
- Serious GI toxicity can occur at any time in patients taking chronic NSAID therapy. Teach patient signs and symptoms of GI bleeding. Tell patient to report any signs or symptoms to doctor immediately.
- Tell patient that full therapeutic effect for arthritis may be delayed for 2 to 4 weeks.
- Check renal, hepatic, and auditory function periodically in long-term therapy. Stop drug if abnormalities occur.
- Give dose 30 minutes before or 2 hours after meals. If adverse GI reactions occur, give with milk or meals.
- Prothrombin time may be prolonged in patients receiving coumarin-type anticoagulants. Fenoprofen decreases platelet aggregation and may prolong bleeding time.
- Because fenoprofen may cause somnolence, warn the patient to avoid driving and other hazardous activities that require alertness until adverse CNS effects of the drug are known.
- Because of their antipyretic and anti-inflammatory actions, NSAIDs may mask the signs and symptoms of infection.
- Fenoprofen may cause false elevations in free and total serum triiodothyronine (T_3) levels as measured by the Amerlex-T assay. Fenoprofen or its metabolite may cross-react with the antibody used in the Amerlex-M assay. Limited data suggest that drug may alter free and total T_3 concentrations determined by the Corning method.

flurbiprofen
Ansaid
Pregnancy Risk Category: B

HOW SUPPLIED
Tablets: 50 mg, 100 mg

MECHANISM OF ACTION
Interferes with prostaglandin synthesis.

INDICATIONS AND DOSAGE
Rheumatoid arthritis and osteoarthritis –
Adults: 200 to 300 mg P.O. daily, divided b.i.d. to q.i.d.

ADVERSE REACTIONS
Common reactions are in italics; life-threatening reactions are in bold italics.
CNS: *headache,* anxiety, insomnia, increased reflexes, tremors, amnesia, asthenia, drowsiness, malaise, depression, dizziness.
CV: *edema.*
EENT: rhinitis, tinnitus, visual changes.
GI: *dyspepsia, diarrhea, abdominal pain, nausea,* constipation, ***GI bleeding,*** flatulence, vomiting.
GU: *symptoms suggesting urinary tract infection.*
Hepatic: elevated liver enzymes.
Skin: rash.
Other: weight changes.

INTERACTIONS
Aspirin: decreased flurbiprofen levels. Concomitant use is not recommended.
Diuretics: possible decreased diuretic effect. Monitor patient closely.
Oral anticoagulants: increased bleeding tendencies. Monitor patient closely.

NURSING CONSIDERATIONS
- *Contraindicated* in patients with hypersensitivity, including asthma or urticaria, to aspirin or NSAIDs.
- Serious GI toxicity can occur at any time with patients taking chronic NSAID therapy. Teach patient the signs and symptoms of GI bleeding, and tell him to discontinue the drug and call the doctor if these symptoms appear.
- Elderly or debilitated patients and patients with impaired hepatic or renal function should be closely monitored and probably should receive lower doses. These patients may be at risk for renal toxicity. Periodically monitor renal function.
- Patients receiving long-term therapy should have periodic liver function studies, eye examinations, and hematocrit determinations.
- Tell patient to take drug with food, milk, or antacid if GI upset occurs.
- Advise patient to avoid hazardous activities that require mental alertness until the CNS effects of the drug are known.
- Tell patient to call doctor immediately if edema, substantial weight gain, black stools, skin rash, itching, or visual disturbances occur.

ibuprofen

Aches-N-Pain◇, Advil◇, Amersol†, Apo-Ibuprofen†, Brufen‡, Cap-Profen◇, Children's Advil, Genpril◇, Haltran◇, Ibuprin◇, Inflam‡, Medipren Caplets◇, Medipren Tablets◇, Midol-200◇, Motrin, Motrin IB◇, Novoprofen†, Nuprin◇, Pamprin-IB◇, PediaProfen, Rafen‡, Rufen, Trendar◇

Pregnancy Risk Category: B (D in 3rd trimester)

HOW SUPPLIED
Tablets: 200 mg◇, 300 mg, 400 mg, 600 mg, 800 mg
Caplets: 200 mg◇
Oral suspension: 100 mg/5 ml

MECHANISM OF ACTION
Produces anti-inflammatory, analgesic, and antipyretic effects, possibly through inhibition of prostaglandin synthesis.

INDICATIONS & DOSAGE
Mild to moderate pain, arthritis, primary dysmenorrhea, gout, postextraction dental pain –
Adults: 200 to 800 mg P.O. t.i.d. or q.i.d. not to exceed 3.2 g/day.
Juvenile arthritis –
Children: 20 to 40 mg/kg P.O. daily in three or four divided doses.
Fever –
Adults: 200 to 400 mg P.O. q 4 to 6 hours. Do not exceed 1.2 g daily or take longer than 3 days.

*Liquid form contains alcohol. **May contain tartrazine.

Children 1 to 12 years: if fever is below 102.5° F (39.2° C), the recommended dose is 5 mg/kg P.O. q 6 to 8 hours. Treat higher fevers with 10 mg/kg q 6 to 8 hours. Do not exceed 40 mg/kg daily.

ADVERSE REACTIONS
Common reactions are in italics; life-threatening reactions are in bold italics.
Blood: prolonged bleeding time.
CNS: *headache, drowsiness, dizziness,* aseptic meningitis.
CV: *peripheral edema.*
EENT: visual disturbances, *tinnitus.*
GI: *epigastric distress, nausea, occult blood loss, peptic ulceration.*
GU: reversible renal failure.
Hepatic: elevated enzymes.
Skin: pruritus, rash, urticaria.
Other: ***bronchospasm,*** edema.

INTERACTIONS
Aspirin: may decrease serum levels of ibuprofen. Avoid concomitant use.
Furosemide, thiazide diuretics: ibuprofen may decrease the effectiveness of diuretics.
Oral anticoagulants, lithium: ibuprofen may increase plasma levels or pharmacologic effects of these agents. Monitor for toxicity.

NURSING CONSIDERATIONS
- *Contraindicated* in patients with hypersensitivity to the drug, other NSAIDs, or aspirin.
- *Use cautiously* in GI disorders, history of peptic ulcer disease, angioedema, asthmatics with nasal polyps, hepatic or renal disease, cardiac decompensation, or known intrinsic coagulation defects.
- Tell patient that full therapeutic effect for arthritis may be delayed for 2 to 4 weeks. Analgesic effect occurs at low dosage levels. However, anti-inflammatory effect does not occur at dosages below 400 mg q.i.d.
- Check renal and hepatic function periodically in long-term therapy. Stop drug if abnormalities occur.
- Serious GI toxicity can occur at any time in patients taking chronic NSAID therapy. Teach patient signs and symptoms of GI bleeding, and tell patient to report these to the doctor immediately.
- Give with meals or milk to reduce adverse GI reactions.
- Concomitant use with aspirin, alcohol, or steroids may increase the risk of GI adverse reactions.
- Drug is available OTC in several brands (200-mg strength). Instruct patient not to exceed 1.2 g daily, give to children under age 12, or self-medicate for extended periods without consulting doctor.
- Because of their antipyretic and anti-inflammatory actions, NSAIDs may mask the signs and symptoms of infection.

indomethacin
Apo-Indomethacin†, Arthrexin‡, Indameth, Indocid†‡, Indocid SR†, Indocin, Indocin SR, Indomed, Novomethacin†, Rheumacin‡, Zendole

indomethacin sodium trihydrate
Apo-Indomethacin†, Indocid†, Indocin I.V., Indometh, Novomethacin†

Pregnancy Risk Category: B (D in 3rd trimester)

HOW SUPPLIED
Capsules: 10 mg, 25 mg, 50 mg, 75 mg
Capsules (sustained-release): 75 mg
Oral suspension: 25 mg/5 ml
Injection: 1-mg vials
Suppositories: 50 mg

MECHANISM OF ACTION
Produces anti-inflammatory, analgesic, and antipyretic effects, possibly

through inhibition of prostaglandin synthesis.

INDICATIONS & DOSAGE
Moderate to severe arthritis, ankylosing spondylitis –
Adults: 25 mg P.O. or P.R. b.i.d. or t.i.d. with food or antacids; may increase dosage by 25 mg daily q 7 days up to 200 mg daily. Alternatively, sustained-release capsules (75 mg) may be given: 75 mg P.O. to start, in the morning or h.s., followed, if necessary, by 75 mg b.i.d.
Acute gouty arthritis –
Adults: 50 mg P.O. t.i.d. Reduce dose as soon as possible, then discontinue. Sustained-release capsules shouldn't be used for this condition.
To close a hemodynamically significant patent ductus arteriosus in premature infants (I.V. form only) –
Neonates under 48 hours: 0.2 mg/kg I.V. followed by two doses of 0.1 mg/kg at 12- to 24-hour intervals.
Neonates 2 to 7 days: 0.2 mg/kg I.V. followed by two doses of 0.2 mg/kg at 12- to 24-hour intervals.
Neonates over 7 days: 0.2 mg/kg I.V. followed by two doses of 0.25 mg/kg at 12- to 24-hour intervals.

ADVERSE REACTIONS
Common reactions are in italics; life-threatening reactions are in bold italics.
Oral form:
Blood: ***hemolytic anemia, aplastic anemia, agranulocytosis,*** leukopenia, thrombocytopenic purpura, iron deficiency anemia.
CNS: *headache, dizziness,* depression, drowsiness, confusion, peripheral neuropathy, seizures, psychic disturbances, syncope, *vertigo.*
CV: hypertension, *edema.*
EENT: *blurred vision, corneal and retinal damage,* hearing loss, tinnitus.
GI: *nausea, vomiting,* anorexia, *diarrhea, peptic ulceration,* ***GI bleeding.***
GU: hematuria, hyperkalemia, ***acute renal failure.***
Hepatic: elevated enzymes.
Skin: pruritus, urticaria, ***Stevens-Johnson syndrome.***
Other: hypersensitivity (shocklike symptoms, rash, respiratory distress, ***angioedema***).
I.V. form:
Blood: decreased platelet aggregation.
GI: ***bleeding,*** vomiting.
GU: ***renal dysfunction.***
Metabolic: ***hyponatremia, hyperkalemia, hypoglycemia.***

INTERACTIONS
Alcohol, corticosteroids: increased risk of GI toxicity. Don't use together.
Aminoglycosides, cyclosporine, methotrexate: indomethacin may enhance the toxicity of these agents. Avoid concomitant use.
Antihypertensive agents: reduced antihypertensive effect. Monitor closely.
Aspirin: decreased blood levels of indomethacin. Avoid concomitant use.
Diflunisal, probenecid: decreases indomethacin excretion; watch for increased incidence of indomethacin adverse reactions.
Digoxin: indomethacin may prolong the half-life of digoxin. Use together cautiously.
Lithium: increased plasma lithium levels. Monitor for toxicity.
Thiazide diuretics, furosemide: impaired response to both drugs. Avoid using together if possible.
Triamterene: possible nephrotoxicity. Don't use together.

NURSING CONSIDERATIONS
Oral form:
- *Contraindicated* in patients with hypersensitivity to the drug, other NSAIDs, or aspirin and in those with active peptic ulcer disease.
- *Use cautiously* in seizure disorders, coagulation disorders, parkinsonism, hepatic or renal disease, cardiovascular disease, infection, and history of mental illness and in elderly patients.

*Liquid form contains alcohol. **May contain tartrazine.

- Severe headache may occur. Decrease dose if headache persists.
- Has an antipyretic effect.
- Tell patient to notify doctor immediately if any visual or hearing changes occur. Patients taking drug long-term should have regular eye examinations, hearing tests, CBC, and renal function tests to monitor for toxicity.
- Serious GI toxicity can occur at any time in patients taking chronic NSAID therapy. Teach patient signs and symptoms of GI bleeding, and tell patient to report these to the doctor immediately.
- Concomitant use with aspirin, alcohol, or steroids may increase the risk of adverse GI reactions.
- Adverse CNS reactions are more common and serious in elderly patients.
- Monitor for bleeding in patients receiving anticoagulants, patients with coagulation defects, and neonates.
- Causes sodium retention; monitor for weight gain (especially in elderly patients) and increased blood pressure in patients with hypertension.
- Used as prophylaxis for gout when colchicine is not well tolerated.
- Because of high incidence of adverse effects during chronic use, indomethacin should not be used routinely as an analgesic or antipyretic.
- Tell the patient to take the drug with food, milk, or antacid if GI upset occurs.
- Because of their antipyretic and anti-inflammatory actions, NSAIDs may mask the signs and symptoms of infection.

I.V. form:

- *Contraindicated* in infants with untreated infection, active bleeding, coagulation defects or thrombocytopenia, necrotizing enterocolitis, or impaired renal function.
- **I.V. use:** Don't administer second or third scheduled dose if anuria or marked oliguria is evident.
- If ductus arteriosus reopens, a second course of one to three doses may be given. If ineffective, surgery may be necessary.
- Indomethacin may enhance the hypothalamic-pituitary-adrenal axis response to the dexamethasone suppression test. Inform clinical laboratory personnel that patient is taking indomethacin.
- Monitor carefully for bleeding and for reduced urine output. Discontinue drug and notify doctor if either occurs.

ketoprofen

Orudis, Orudis E†, Orudis SR†‡

Pregnancy Risk Category: B (D in 3rd trimester)

HOW SUPPLIED

Tablets (sustained-release): 200 mg†
Capsules: 25 mg, 50 mg, 75 mg
Suppositories: 100 mg†

MECHANISM OF ACTION

Produces anti-inflammatory, analgesic, and antipyretic effects, possibly through inhibition of prostaglandin synthesis.

INDICATIONS & DOSAGE

Rheumatoid arthritis and osteoarthritis –

Adults: 150 to 300 mg P.O. in three or four divided doses. Usual dosage is 75 mg t.i.d. Maximum dosage is 300 mg/day.

Alternatively, may use suppository where available.

Adults: 100 mg P.R. b.i.d.; or 1 suppository h.s. (in conjunction with oral ketoprofen during the day).

Mild to moderate pain; dysmenorrhea –

Adults: 25 to 50 mg P.O. q 6 to 8 hours p.r.n.

ADVERSE REACTIONS
Common reactions are in italics; life-threatening reactions are in bold italics.
Blood: prolonged bleeding time.
CNS: *headache,* dizziness, *CNS inhibition or excitation.*
EENT: tinnitus, visual disturbances.
GI: *nausea, abdominal pain, diarrhea, constipation, flatulence,* ***peptic ulceration,*** anorexia, vomiting, stomatitis.
GU: ***nephrotoxicity,*** *elevated BUN.*
Hepatic: elevated enzymes.
Skin: rash.

INTERACTIONS
Hydrochlorothiazide, other diuretics: decreased diuretic effectiveness. Monitor for lack of effect.
Methotrexate, lithium: increased levels of these drugs, leading to toxicity. Monitor closely.
Oral anticoagulants: increased risk of bleeding. Monitor closely.
Probenecid, aspirin: decreased plasma levels of ketoprofen. Avoid concomitant use.

NURSING CONSIDERATIONS
• *Contraindicated* in patients with hypersensitivity to the drug, aspirin, or other NSAIDs.
• *Use cautiously* in patients with history of peptic ulcer disease or renal dysfunction.
• Serious GI toxicity can occur at any time in patients taking chronic NSAID therapy. Teach patient signs and symptoms of GI bleeding, and tell patient to report these to the doctor immediately.
• Tell patient to report visual or auditory adverse reactions immediately.
• Concomitant use with aspirin, alcohol, or steroids may increase the risk of adverse GI reactions.
• Tell patient that full therapeutic effect may be delayed for 2 to 4 weeks.
• Check renal and hepatic function every 6 months or as indicated during long-term therapy.
• Give dose 30 minutes before or 2 hours after meals. If adverse GI reactions occur, give with milk or meals.
• Ketoprofen may interfere with some laboratory determinations of blood glucose and serum iron levels, depending on the testing method used.
• Because of their antipyretic and anti-inflammatory actions, NSAIDs may mask the signs and symptoms of infection.

ketorolac tromethamine
Toradol

Pregnancy Risk Category: B

HOW SUPPLIED
Tablets: 10 mg
Injection: 15 mg, 30 mg, 60 mg

MECHANISM OF ACTION
Acts by inhibiting the synthesis of prostaglandins.

INDICATIONS & DOSAGE
Short-term management of pain –
Adults: initially, give 30 or 60 mg I.M as a loading dose, followed by half of the loading dose (15 or 30 mg) I.M. q 6 hours on a regular schedule or p.r.n. Subsequent dosage should be based on patient response. If pain returns before 6 hours, dosage may be increased by as much as 50% (up to 60 mg); if pain relief continues for 8 to 12 hours, increase interval between doses to q 8 to 12 hours, or reduce dose. The recommended maximum dosage is 150 mg I.M. on the first day and 120 mg daily thereafter.

Alternatively, the drug may be used orally on a short-term basis. Give 10 mg P.O. q 4 to 6 hours p.r.n. Do not give more than 40 mg daily, and use the drug *only* for a short time.

ADVERSE REACTIONS
Common reactions are in italics; life-threatening reactions are in bold italics.

*Liquid form contains alcohol. **May contain tartrazine.

CNS: *drowsiness,* dizziness, headache, sweating.
CV: edema.
GI: *nausea, dyspepsia, GI pain,* diarrhea.
Local: pain at the injection site.

INTERACTIONS
Lithium: NSAIDs increase lithium levels. Monitor closely.
Methotrexate: NSAIDs decrease methotrexate clearance and increase its toxicity. Don't use together.
Salicylates, warfarin: ketorolac may increase the levels of free (unbound) salicylates or warfarin in the blood. Clinical significance is unknown.

NURSING CONSIDERATIONS
- *Contraindicated* in patients with hypersensitivity to the drug and in patients with the complete or partial triad syndrome: nasal polyps, angioedema, and bronchospasm after use of other NSAIDs or aspirin.
- *Use cautiously* in patients with hepatic or renal impairment.
- This drug is intended solely for short-term management of pain. The rate and severity of adverse reactions should be less than that observed in patients taking NSAIDs on a chronic basis.
- When switching patients from injectable to oral ketorolac, do not exceed a total dose of 120 mg of drug on the day of transition, including the maximum of 40 mg P.O.
- Because NSAIDs can cause fluid retention and edema, use ketorolac cautiously in patients with cardiac disease or hypertension.
- Carefully observe patients with coagulopathies and those who are taking anticoagulants. Ketorolac inhibits platelet aggregation and can prolong bleeding time. This effect will disappear within 48 hours of discontinuing the drug. It will not alter platelet count, partial thromboplastin time, or prothrombin time.
- I.M. administration may cause pain at the injection site. Holding pressure over the site for 15 to 30 seconds after the injection may minimize local effects.
- GI ulceration, bleeding, and perforation can occur at any time, with or without warning, in any patient taking NSAIDs on a chronic basis. Teach patients the signs and symptoms of GI bleeding.
- Use lower initial doses in patients who are over age 65 or who weigh less than 110 lb (50 kg).
- Because of their antipyretic and anti-inflammatory actions, NSAIDs may mask the signs and symptoms of infection.
- Trace amounts of the drug have been detected in breast milk. Use with caution in breast-feeding women.

meclofenamate
Meclomen

Pregnancy Risk Category: B (D in 3rd trimester)

HOW SUPPLIED
Tablets: 50 mg, 100 mg
Capsules: 50 mg, 100 mg

MECHANISM OF ACTION
Produces anti-inflammatory, analgesic, and antipyretic effects, possibly through inhibition of prostaglandin synthesis.

INDICATIONS & DOSAGE
Rheumatoid arthritis and osteoarthritis –
Adults: 200 to 400 mg/day P.O. in three or four equally divided doses.
Mild to moderate pain –
Adults: 50 to 100 mg P.O. q 4 to 6 hours. Maximum dose is 400 mg/day.

ADVERSE REACTIONS
Common reactions are in italics; life-threatening reactions are in bold italics.
Blood: leukopenia, thrombocyto-

penia, ***agranulocytosis, aplastic anemia.***
CNS: fatigue, malaise, insomnia, *dizziness,* nervousness, *headache.*
CV: edema.
EENT: blurred vision, eye irritation.
GI: *abdominal pain, flatulence,* ***peptic ulceration,*** nausea, vomiting, *diarrhea,* hemorrhage.
GU: dysuria, hematuria, nephrotoxicity.
Hepatic: ***hepatotoxicity.***
Skin: rash, urticaria.

INTERACTIONS
Aspirin: decreased plasma levels of meclofenamate.
Oral anticoagulants: enhanced anticoagulant effect. Monitor for toxicity.

NURSING CONSIDERATIONS
- *Contraindicated* in GI ulceration or inflammation.
- *Use cautiously* in hepatic or renal disease, cardiovascular disease, blood dyscrasia, diabetes mellitus, and a history of peptic ulcer disease; in asthmatics with nasal polyps; and in elderly patients, who are more likely to experience adverse reactions.
- Serious GI toxicity can occur at any time in patients taking chronic NSAID therapy. Teach patient signs and symptoms of GI bleeding, and tell patient to report these to the doctor immediately.
- Concomitant use with other NSAIDs, alcohol, or steroids may increase the risk of GI adverse reactions.
- Warn patient against activities that require alertness until CNS effects of drug are known.
- Stop drug if rash,visual disturbances, or diarrhea develops.
- Administer with food to minimize GI adverse reactions.
- False-positive reactions for urine bilirubin using the diazo tablet test have been reported.
- Patients taking drug long-term should test CBC and renal and hepatic function every 6 months or as indicated.
- Because of their anti-inflammatory and antipyretic actions, NSAIDs may mask the signs and symptoms of infection.

mefenamic acid
Ponstan†, Ponstel
Pregnancy Risk Category: C

HOW SUPPLIED
Capsules: 250 mg

MECHANISM OF ACTION
Produces anti-inflammatory, analgesic, and antipyretic effects, possibly through inhibition of prostaglandin synthesis.

INDICATIONS & DOSAGE
Mild to moderate pain, dysmenorrhea –
Adults and children over 14 years: Initially 500 mg P.O., then 250 mg q 6 hours, p.r.n. Maximum therapy 1 week.

ADVERSE REACTIONS
Common reactions are in italics; life-threatening reactions are in bold italics.
Blood: leukopenia, thrombocytopenia, *agranulocytosis, aplastic anemia.*
CNS: *drowsiness, dizziness,* nervousness, headache.
CV: edema.
EENT: blurred vision, eye irritation.
GI: nausea, vomiting, *diarrhea,* ***peptic ulceration,*** hemorrhage.
GU: dysuria, hematuria, ***nephrotoxicity.***
Hepatic: ***hepatotoxicity.***
Skin: rash, urticaria.

INTERACTIONS
Oral anticoagulants, sulfonylureas, and other drugs that are highly protein bound: increased risk of toxicity.

NURSING CONSIDERATIONS
- *Contraindicated* in GI ulceration or inflammation.
- *Use cautiously* in hepatic or renal disease, cardiovascular disease, blood dyscrasia, diabetes mellitus, and a history of peptic ulcer disease, and in asthmatics with nasal polyps.
- Serious GI toxicity can occur at any time in patients taking chronic NSAID therapy. Teach patient signs and symptoms of GI bleeding, and tell patient to report these to the doctor immediately.
- Concomitant use with aspirin, alcohol, or steroids may increase the risk of GI adverse reactions.
- Warn patient against hazardous activities that require alertness until CNS effects of the drug are known.
- Severe hemolytic anemia may occur with prolonged use. Monitor CBC every 4 to 6 months or as indicated.
- Stop drug if rash, visual disturbances, or diarrhea develops.
- Should not be administered for more than 1 week at a time, because risk of toxicity increases.
- Administer with food to minimize GI adverse reactions.
- Because of their anti-inflammatory and antipyretic actions, NSAIDs may mask the signs and symptoms of infection.
- False-positive reactions for urine bilirubin using the diazo tablet test have been reported.

nabumetone

Relafen

Pregnancy Risk Category: C

HOW SUPPLIED
Tablets: 500 mg, 750 mg

MECHANISM OF ACTION
Probably acts by inhibiting the synthesis of prostaglandins.

INDICATIONS & DOSAGE
Acute and chronic treatment of rheumatoid arthritis or osteoarthritis –
Adults: initially, 1,000 mg P.O. daily as a single dose or in divided doses b.i.d. Maximum daily dose is 2,000 mg.

ADVERSE REACTIONS
Common reactions are in italics; life-threatening reactions are in bold italics.
CNS: *dizziness, headache,* fatigue, increased sweating, insomnia, nervousness, somnolence.
CV: vasculitis.
GI: *diarrhea, dyspepsia, abdominal pain, constipation, flatulence, nausea,* dry mouth, gastritis, stomatitis, vomiting.
Skin: *pruritus, rash.*
Other: *tinnitus, edema.*

INTERACTIONS
Drugs that are highly bound to plasma proteins (such as warfarin): increased risk of adverse effects from displacement of drug by nabumetone. Use cautiously.

NURSING CONSIDERATIONS
- *Contraindicated* in patients with hypersensitivity to the drug and in patients with asthma, urticaria, or other allergic reactions to nabumetone, other NSAIDs, or aspirin.
- *Use cautiously* in patients with renal or hepatic impairment; CHF, hypertension, or other conditions that may predispose the patient to fluid retention; and a history of peptic ulcer disease.
- Administer with food, milk, or antacids. Drug is absorbed more rapidly when administered with food or milk.
- Because NSAIDs impair the synthesis of renal prostaglandins, they can decrease renal blood flow and lead to reversible renal impairment, especially in patients with preexisting renal failure, liver dysfunction, or heart failure; in elderly patients; and

in those taking diuretics. Monitor these patients closely during therapy.
• Serious GI toxicity, such as bleeding and ulceration, can occur in patients receiving chronic NSAID therapy. Such toxicity can occur at any time, sometimes without warning. Stress the importance of follow-up examinations to detect these adverse reactions. Teach patient signs and symptoms of GI bleeding, and tell him to notify the doctor immediately if these symptoms appear.
• During chronic therapy, periodically monitor renal and liver function, CBC, and hematocrit. Assess these patients for signs and symptoms of GI bleeding.
• Advise patient to limit alcohol intake because of the risk of additive GI toxicity.

naproxen
Apo-Naproxen†, Naprosyn, Naxen†‡, Novonaprox†

naproxen sodium
Anaprox, Anaprox DS, Naprogesic‡

Pregnancy Risk Category: B (D in 3rd trimester)

HOW SUPPLIED
naproxen
Tablets: 250 mg, 375 mg, 500 mg
Oral suspension: 125 mg/5 ml
Suppositories: 500 mg‡
naproxen sodium
Tablets (film-coated): 275 mg, 550 mg
Note: 275 mg naproxen sodium = 250 mg naproxen

MECHANISM OF ACTION
Produces anti-inflammatory, analgesic, and antipyretic effects, possibly through inhibition of prostaglandin synthesis.

INDICATIONS & DOSAGE
Arthritis, primary dysmenorrhea (free base) –
Adults: 250 to 500 mg P.O. b.i.d.
Alternatively, may use suppository where available –
Adults: 500 mg P.R. h.s. with oral naproxen during the day.
Maximum dosage is 1,250 mg daily.
Mild to moderate pain, primary dysmenorrhea (naproxen sodium) –
Adults: 2 tablets (275 mg each tablet) P.O. to start, followed by 275 mg q 6 to 8 hours p.r.n. Maximum daily dosage should not exceed 1,375 mg.

ADVERSE REACTIONS
Common reactions are in italics; life-threatening reactions are in bold italics.
Blood: prolonged bleeding time, ***agranulocytosis,*** neutropenia.
CNS: *headache,* drowsiness, *dizziness,* tinnitus.
CV: peripheral edema, dyspnea.
EENT: visual disturbances.
GI: *epigastric distress, occult blood loss, nausea,* ***peptic ulceration.***
GU: nephrotoxicity.
Hepatic: elevated enzymes.
Skin: *pruritus, rash,* urticaria.

INTERACTIONS
Oral anticoagulants, sulfonylureas, and drugs that are highly protein-bound: increased risk of toxicity. Monitor closely.
Probenecid: decreased elimination of naproxen. Monitor for toxicity.
Methotrexate: increased risk of toxicity. Monitor closely.

NURSING CONSIDERATIONS
• *Contraindicated* in patients with hypersensitivity to the drug, aspirin, or other NSAIDs.
• *Use cautiously* in elderly patients and in patients with renal disease, cardiovascular disease, GI disorders, hepatic disease, a history of peptic ulcer disease, or angioedema.

- Serious GI toxicity can occur at any time in patients taking chronic NSAID therapy. Teach patient signs and symptoms of GI bleeding, and tell patient to report these to the doctor immediately.
- Concomitant use with aspirin, alcohol, or steroids may increase the risk of adverse GI reactions.
- Monitor CBC and renal and hepatic function every 4 to 6 months or as indicated during long-term therapy. Advise patient to have periodic eye examinations.
- Tell patient taking naproxen that full therapeutic effect may be delayed 2 to 4 weeks.
- Advise patient to take drug with food or milk to minimize GI upset.
- Warn patient against taking both naproxen and naproxen sodium at the same time because both circulate in the blood as the naproxen anion.
- Naproxen sodium is more rapidly absorbed.
- Naproxen and naproxen sodium have also been used to manage pain of vascular headache, osteitis deformans (Paget's disease) of the bone, and Bartter's syndrome.
- Naproxen may interfere with certain urinary assays of 5-hydroxyindoleacetic acid and may cause false elevations of urinary 17-ketosteroid concentrations. Inform clinical laboratory personnel that patient is taking naproxen.
- Because of their antipyretic and anti-inflammatory actions, NSAIDs may mask the signs and symptoms of infection.

oxaprozin

Daypro

Pregnancy Risk Category: C

HOW SUPPLIED

Caplets: 600 mg

MECHANISM OF ACTION

Produces anti-inflammatory, analgesic, and antipyretic effects, possibly through inhibition of prostaglandin synthesis.

INDICATIONS & DOSAGE

Acute and long-term use in the management of signs and symptoms of osteoarthritis or rheumatoid arthritis –
Adults: initially, 1,200 mg P.O. daily. Individualize dosage to the smallest effective dose to minimize adverse reactions. Smaller patients or those with mild symptoms may require only 600 mg daily. Maximum is 1,800 mg or 26 mg/kg, whichever is lower, in divided doses.

ADVERSE REACTIONS

Common reactions are in italics; life-threatening reactions are in bold italics.
CNS: depression, sedation, somnolence, confusion, sleep disturbances.
GI: *nausea, dyspepsia, diarrhea, constipation,* abdominal pain or distress, anorexia, flatulence, vomiting.
GU: dysuria, urinary frequency.
Skin: *rash.*
Other: tinnitus.

INTERACTIONS

Alcohol, aspirin, corticosteroids: increased risk of adverse GI reactions. Avoid concomitant use.
Antihypertensives: decreased antihypertensive effect. Periodically monitor blood pressure and adjust dosage of antihypertensive as ordered.
Aspirin: oxaprozin displaces salicylates from plasma protein-binding sites, increasing risk of salicylate toxicity. Avoid concomitant use.
Oral anticoagulants: although problems haven't been reported, there is an increased risk of bleeding. Use together cautiously.

NURSING CONSIDERATIONS

- *Contraindicated* in patients with hypersensitivity to the drug, aspirin, or other NSAIDs.
- *Use cautiously* in patients with a history of peptic ulcer disease or hepatic or renal dysfunction.
- Serious GI toxicity can occur at any time in patients taking chronic NSAID therapy. Teach patient signs and symptoms of GI bleeding, and tell him to report these to doctor immediately.
- Because renal prostaglandins play a role in the maintenance of renal perfusion, patients with preexisting conditions that lead to a reduction in renal blood flow may experience renal toxicity with NSAID therapy. Those at greatest risk are elderly patients, patients taking diuretics, and those with impaired renal, hepatic, or cardiac function. Closely monitor renal function in these patients, and discontinue NSAID therapy if problems develop.
- Like other NSAIDs, elevations of liver function tests can occur after chronic use in up to 15% of patients. These abnormal findings may persist, worsen, or resolve with continued therapy. Rarely, patients may progress to severe hepatic dysfunction. Periodically monitor liver function tests in patients receiving long-term therapy, and closely monitor patients with abnormal test results.
- Tell patient to report visual or auditory adverse reactions immediately.
- Tell patient that full therapeutic effect may be delayed for 2 to 4 weeks.
- Give dose 30 minutes before or 2 hours after meals. If adverse GI reactions occur, give with milk or meals.
- Because of their antipyretic and anti-inflammatory actions, NSAIDs may mask the signs and symptoms of infection.
- Oxaprozin has been associated with photosensitivity reactions. Advise patient to use a sunscreen, wear protective clothing, and avoid prolonged exposure to sunlight.

oxyphenbutazone

Pregnancy Risk Category: D

HOW SUPPLIED

Tablets: 100 mg

MECHANISM OF ACTION

Produces anti-inflammatory, analgesic, and antipyretic effects, possibly through inhibition of prostaglandin synthesis.

INDICATIONS & DOSAGE

Pain, inflammation in arthritis, bursitis, superficial venous thrombosis –
Adults: 100 to 200 mg P.O. with food or milk t.i.d. or q.i.d.

Acute gouty arthritis –
Adults: 400 mg initially as single dose, then 100 mg q 4 hours for 4 days or until relief is obtained.

Note: Do not continue therapy for longer than 1 week.

ADVERSE REACTIONS

Common reactions are in italics; life-threatening reactions are in bold italics.

Blood: ***bone marrow suppression (fatal aplastic anemia, agranulocytosis, thrombocytopenia), hemolytic anemia,*** leukopenia.
CNS: restlessness, confusion, lethargy.
CV: hypertension, pericarditis, myocarditis, ***cardiac decompensation.***
EENT: optic neuritis, blurred vision, retinal hemorrhage or detachment, hearing loss.
GI: *nausea, vomiting, diarrhea,* ***peptic ulceration,*** *occult blood loss.*
GU: proteinuria, hematuria, glomerulonephritis, nephrotic syndrome, ***renal failure.***
Hepatic: ***hepatitis.***
Metabolic: toxic and nontoxic goiter, respiratory alkalosis, metabolic acidosis.

Skin: petechiae, pruritus, purpura, various dermatoses from rash to ***toxic necrotizing epidermolysis.***

INTERACTIONS

Insulin, oral hypoglycemic agents: enhanced hypoglycemic effect. Monitor patient closely.
Oral anticoagulants: enhanced risk of bleeding. Monitor patient closely.
Phenytoin, lithium: increased plasma levels after oxyphenbutazone administration.

NURSING CONSIDERATIONS

- *Contraindicated* in children under 14 years and in patients with senility, GI ulcer, blood dyscrasia, and renal, hepatic, cardiac, and thyroid disease. Should not be used in patients receiving long-term anticoagulant therapy.
- This drug should be used only if less toxic alternatives are ineffective or contraindicated.
- Tell patient to stop drug and notify doctor immediately if fever, sore throat, mouth ulcers, GI discomfort, black or tarry stools, bleeding, bruising, rash, or weight gain occurs.
- Give with food, milk, or antacids.
- Complete physical examination and laboratory evaluation are recommended before therapy. Warn patient to remain under close medical supervision and to keep all doctor and laboratory appointments.
- Monitor CBC before therapy and after 3 days.
- Record patient's weight and intake/output daily. May cause sodium retention and edema.
- Response should be seen in 2 or 3 days. Stop drug if no response seen within 1 week.
- Patients over 60 years should not receive drug for longer than 1 week.
- Has antipyretic effect.
- Because of their anti-inflammatory and antipyretic actions, NSAIDs may mask the signs and symptoms of infection.

phenylbutazone

Apo-Phenylbutazone†, Azolid, Butazolidin, Butazone, Intrabutazone†, Novobutazone†

Pregnancy Risk Category: D

HOW SUPPLIED

Tablets: 100 mg
Capsules: 100 mg

MECHANISM OF ACTION

Produces anti-inflammatory, analgesic, and antipyretic effects, possibly through inhibition of prostaglandin synthesis.

INDICATIONS & DOSAGE

Pain, inflammation in arthritis, bursitis, acute superficial thrombophlebitis –
Adults: initially, 100 to 200 mg P.O. t.i.d. or q.i.d. Maximum dosage is 600 mg daily. When improvement is obtained, decrease dosage to 100 mg t.i.d. or q.i.d.
Acute, gouty arthritis –
Adults: 400 mg P.O. initially as single dose, then 100 mg q 4 hours for 4 days or until relief is obtained.

Note: Do not continue therapy for longer than 1 week.

ADVERSE REACTIONS

Common reactions are in italics; life-threatening reactions are in bold italics.
Blood: ***bone marrow suppression (fatal aplastic anemia, agranulocytosis, thrombocytopenia), hemolytic anemia,*** leukopenia.
CNS: agitation, confusion, lethargy.
CV: hypertension, edema, pericarditis, myocarditis, ***cardiac decompensation.***
EENT: optic neuritis, blurred vision, retinal hemorrhage or detachment, hearing loss.
GI: *nausea, vomiting, diarrhea,* ***peptic ulceration,*** *occult blood loss.*
GU: proteinuria, hematuria, glomer-

ulonephritis, nephrotic syndrome, ***renal failure.***
Hepatic: ***hepatitis.***
Metabolic: hyperglycemia, toxic and nontoxic goiter, respiratory alkalosis, metabolic acidosis.
Skin: petechiae, pruritus, purpura, various dermatoses from rash to ***toxic necrotizing epidermolysis.***

INTERACTIONS
Alcohol: increased risk of toxicity. Avoid concomitant use.
Antihypertensives: decreased effectiveness. Monitor blood pressure closely.
Cholestyramine: may alter phenylbutazone absorption. Give 1 hour before cholestyramine.
Insulin, oral hypoglycemics: enhanced hypoglycemic effect. Monitor patient closely.
Oral anticoagulants: enhanced risk of bleeding. Monitor patient closely.
Phenytoin, lithium: increased plasma levels after phenylbutazone administration. Monitor for toxicity.

NURSING CONSIDERATIONS
- *Contraindicated* in patients with hypersensitivity to the drug, other NSAIDs, or aspirin; in children under age 14; and in patients with senility, GI ulcer, blood dyscrasias, or moderate to severe renal, hepatic, cardiac, or thyroid disease.
- *Use cautiously* in patients with mild cardiac, renal, hepatic, or thyroid disease; in GI disorders or a history of peptic ulcer disease; and in patients who may be predisposed to fluid retention.
- Should not be used in patients receiving long-term anticoagulant therapy, hepatotoxic or nephrotoxic drugs, or thrombolytic therapy.
- This drug should be used only if less toxic alternatives are ineffective or contraindicated.
- Warn patient to stop taking drug and notify doctor immediately if fever, sore throat, mouth ulcers, GI discomfort, black or tarry stools, bleeding, bruising, rash, or weight gain occur.
- Give with food, milk, or antacids.
- Complete physical examination and laboratory evaluation are recommended before therapy. Patient should remain under close medical supervision and keep all doctor and laboratory appointments.
- Monitor hepatic, renal, and thyroid function and CBC before therapy. Check CBC again after 3 days and assess for bleeding.
- Record patient's weight and intake and output daily. May cause sodium retention and edema.
- Response should be seen in 3 to 4 days. Discontinue drug if no response within 1 week.
- Patients over age 60 should not receive this drug for longer than 1 week.
- This drug has limited use because it produces severe adverse reactions in up to 45% of patients.
- Phenylbutazone may interfere with thyroid function studies by competing for thyroxine binding sites and blocking uptake of iodine into the thyroid.
- Because of their antipyretic and anti-inflammatory actions, NSAIDs may mask the signs and symptoms of infection.

piroxicam
Apo-Piroxicam†, Feldene, Novopirocam†

Pregnancy Risk Category: C

HOW SUPPLIED
Capsules: 10 mg, 20 mg

MECHANISM OF ACTION
Produces anti-inflammatory, analgesic, and antipyretic effects, possibly through inhibition of prostaglandin synthesis.

*Liquid form contains alcohol. **May contain tartrazine.

INDICATIONS & DOSAGE

Osteoarthritis and rheumatoid arthritis –

Adults: 20 mg P.O. daily. If desired, the dose may be divided.

ADVERSE REACTIONS

Common reactions are in italics; life-threatening reactions are in bold italics.

Blood: prolonged bleeding time, anemia.

CNS: headache, drowsiness, dizziness.

CV: peripheral edema.

GI: *epigastric distress, nausea, occult blood loss,* ***peptic ulceration, severe GI bleeding.***

GU: ***nephrotoxicity.***

Hepatic: elevated enzymes.

Skin: pruritus, rash, urticaria, *photosensitivity.*

INTERACTIONS

Alcohol, corticosteroids: increased risk of GI toxicity. Avoid concomitant use.

Aspirin: decreased plasma levels of piroxicam. Avoid concomitant use.

Lithium: increased plasma lithium levels. Monitor for toxicity.

Oral anticoagulants: enhanced risk of bleeding. Monitor patient closely.

Oral hypoglycemic agents: enhanced hypoglycemic effects. Monitor patient closely.

NURSING CONSIDERATIONS

- *Contraindicated* in patients with hypersensitivity to the drug, other NSAIDs, or aspirin.
- *Use cautiously* in elderly patients and in patients with angioedema, GI disorders, history of renal or peptic ulcer disease, or cardiac disease.
- Serious GI toxicity can occur at any time in patients taking chronic NSAID therapy. Teach patient signs and symptoms of GI bleeding, and tell him to report these immediately.
- Tell patient full therapeutic effect may be delayed for 2 to 4 weeks.
- Causes adverse skin reactions more often than other drugs in its class. Photosensitivity reactions are the most common.
- Check renal, hepatic, and auditory function and CBC periodically during prolonged therapy. Drug should be discontinued if abnormalities occur.
- If adverse GI reactions occur, give with milk, antacids, or meals.
- Because of their antipyretic and anti-inflammatory actions, NSAIDs may mask the signs and symptoms of infection.

sulindac

Clinoril

Pregnancy Risk Category: B (D in 3rd trimester)

HOW SUPPLIED

Tablets: 100 mg◊, 150 mg, 200 mg

MECHANISM OF ACTION

Produces anti-inflammatory, analgesic, and antipyretic effects, possibly through inhibition of prostaglandin synthesis.

INDICATIONS & DOSAGE

Osteoarthritis, rheumatoid arthritis, ankylosing spondylitis –

Adults: initially, 150 mg P.O. b.i.d.; may increase to 200 mg b.i.d.

Acute subacromial bursitis or supraspinatus tendinitis, acute gouty arthritis –

Adults: 200 mg P.O. b.i.d. for 7 to 14 days. Dose may be reduced as symptoms subside.

ADVERSE REACTIONS

Common reactions are in italics; life-threatening reactions are in bold italics.

Blood: prolonged bleeding time, ***aplastic anemia.***

CNS: dizziness, headache, nervousness.

EENT: tinnitus, transient visual disturbances.

GI: *epigastric distress,* ***peptic ulceration,*** *occult blood loss, nausea.*
Hepatic: elevated enzymes.
Skin: rash, pruritus.
Other: edema.

INTERACTIONS

Anticoagulants: increased risk of bleeding. Monitor prothrombin time closely.
Aspirin, other salicylates, diflunisal, dimethyl sulfoxide: decreased metabolism of sulindac to its active metabolite, reducing its effectiveness. Don't use together.
Cyclosporine: increased nephrotoxicity of cyclosporine. Avoid concomitant use.
Methotrexate: increased methotrexate toxicity. Avoid concomitant use.
Probenecid: increased plasma levels of sulindac and its active metabolite. Monitor for toxicity.
Sulfonamides, sulfonylureas, other highly protein-bound drugs: possible displacement of these drugs from plasma protein-binding sites, leading to increased toxicity. Monitor closely.

NURSING CONSIDERATIONS

- *Contraindicated* in acute asthmatics whose conditions are precipitated by other NSAIDs or by aspirin and in patients who have active ulcers and GI bleeding.
- *Use cautiously* in patients with a history of ulcers and GI bleeding, renal dysfunction, compromised cardiac function, or hypertension and in those receiving oral anticoagulants or oral hypoglycemic agents.
- To reduce adverse GI reactions, give with food, milk, or antacids.
- Serious GI toxicity can occur at any time in patients taking chronic NSAID therapy. Teach patient signs and symptoms of GI bleeding, and tell him to report these immediately.
- Patient should notify doctor and have complete eye examination if any visual disturbances occur.
- Periodically monitor hepatic and renal function and CBC in patients receiving long-term therapy.
- Tell patient to notify doctor immediately if easy bruising or prolonged bleeding occurs.
- Drug causes sodium retention but is thought to have the least effect on the kidneys as compared to all other NSAIDs. Patient should report edema and have blood pressure checked monthly.
- Because of their antipyretic and anti-inflammatory actions, NSAIDs may mask the signs and symptoms of infection.

tolmetin sodium

Tolectin, Tolectin DS

Pregnancy Risk Category: B (D in 3rd trimester)

HOW SUPPLIED

Tablets: 200 mg
Capsules: 400 mg

MECHANISM OF ACTION

Produces anti-inflammatory, analgesic, and antipyretic effects, possibly through inhibition of prostaglandin synthesis.

INDICATIONS & DOSAGE

Rheumatoid arthritis, osteoarthritis, gout, dysmenorrhea, juvenile rheumatoid arthritis –
Adults: 400 mg P.O. t.i.d. or q.i.d. Maximum dosage is 2 g daily.
Children 2 years or over: 15 to 30 mg/kg P.O. daily in divided doses.

ADVERSE REACTIONS

Common reactions are in italics; life-threatening reactions are in bold italics.
Blood: prolonged bleeding time.
CNS: headache, dizziness, drowsiness.
GI: *epigastric distress,* ***peptic ulceration,*** *occult blood loss, nausea.*

*Liquid form contains alcohol. **May contain tartrazine.

GU: ***nephrotoxicity,*** pseudoproteinuria.
Skin: rash, urticaria, pruritus.
Other: sodium retention, edema.

INTERACTIONS
Oral anticoagulants: increased risk of bleeding. Monitor patient closely.

NURSING CONSIDERATIONS
- *Contraindicated* in patients with hypersensitivity to the drug, other NSAIDs, or aspirin.
- *Use cautiously* in cardiac and renal disease, GI bleeding, and history of peptic ulcer disease.
- Serious GI toxicity can occur at any time in patients taking chronic NSAID therapy. Teach patient signs and symptoms of GI bleeding and tell him to report these immediately.
- Tell patient to notify doctor immediately if any visual or hearing changes occur. During prolonged therapy, patients should have regular eye examinations, hearing tests, CBCs, and renal function tests to monitor for toxicity.
- Give with food, milk, or antacids to reduce adverse GI reactions.
- Tell patient therapeutic effect should begin within 1 week, but full effect may be delayed 2 to 4 weeks.
- Prolonged therapy requires periodic eye examinations and liver and renal function studies.
- Tolmetin may interfere with certain tests for urinary proteins; it does not interfere with dye-impregnated reagent strips.
- Because of their antipyretic and anti-inflammatory actions, NSAIDs may mask the signs and symptoms of infection.

27

Narcotic and opioid analgesics

alfentanil hydrochloride
buprenorphine hydrochloride
butorphanol tartrate
codeine phosphate
codeine sulfate
dezocine
fentanyl citrate
fentanyl transdermal system
hydromorphone hydrochloride
levorphanol tartrate
meperidine hydrochloride
methadone hydrochloride
morphine hydrochloride
morphine sulfate
nalbuphine hydrochloride
oxycodone hydrochloride
oxycodone pectinate
oxymorphone hydrochloride
pentazocine hydrochloride
pentazocine hydrochloride and naloxone hydrochloride
pentazocine lactate
propoxyphene hydrochloride
propoxyphene napsylate
sufentanil citrate

COMBINATION PRODUCTS

222†: aspirin 375 mg, codeine phosphate 8 mg, and caffeine citrate 30 mg.
222 FORTE†: aspirin 500 mg, codeine phosphate 8 mg, and caffeine citrate 30 mg.
282†: aspirin 375 mg, codeine phosphate 15 mg, and caffeine citrate 30 mg.
292†: aspirin 375 mg, codeine phosphate 30 mg, and caffeine citrate 30 mg.
293†: aspirin 375 mg, codeine phosphate 30 mg, codeine phosphate (slow-release) 30 mg, and caffeine citrate 30 mg.
692†: aspirin 375 mg, propoxyphene hydrochloride 65 mg, and caffeine 30 mg.
A.C.&C.†: aspirin 375 mg, codeine phosphate 8 mg, and caffeine 30 mg.
ACETACO, ACETA WITH CODEINE, EMPRACET-30†, EMTEC-30†, M-GESIC, PYREGESIC-C, TYLAPRIN WITH CODEINE: acetaminophen 300 mg and codeine phosphate 30 mg.
ALLAY, ANOLOR DH5, BANCAP-HC, DOLACET, HYCOMED, HYCO-PAP, HYDROCET, HYDROGESIC, LORCET-HD, MEGAGESIC, POLYGESIC, PRO-PAIN-HC, ROGESIC NO. 3, SENEFEN III, ULTRAGESIC, ZYDONE: acetaminophen 500 mg and hydrocodone bitartrate 5 mg.
AMACODONE, ANEXSIA, ANODYNOS DHC, CO-GESIC, DUOCET, DURADYNE DHC, HY-5, HYCOPAP, HY-PHEN, LORTAB 5, NORCET, VAPOCET, VICODIN: acetaminophen 500 mg and hydrocodone bitartrate 5 mg.
ANACIN WITH CODEINE†: aspirin 325 mg, codeine phosphate 8 mg, and caffeine 32 mg.
ANCASAL 8†, C2 WITH CODEINE†: aspirin 375 mg, codeine phosphate 8 mg, and caffeine 15 mg.
ANCASAL 15†: aspirin 375 mg, codeine phosphate 15 mg, and caffeine 15 mg.
ANCASAL 30†: aspirin 375 mg, codeine phosphate 30 mg, and caffeine 15 mg.
ANEXSIA 7.5, LORCET PLUS, NORCET 7.5: acetaminophen 650 mg and hydrocodone bitartrate 7.5 mg.
BEXOPHENE, COTANAL-65, DARVON COMPOUND-65, DORAPHEN COMPOUND-65, DOXAPHENE COMPOUND, MARGESIC A-C, PRO POX PLUS: aspirin 389 mg, propoxyphene hydrochloride 65 mg, and caffeine 32.4 mg.
BUFF-A-COMP NO. 3: aspirin 325 mg, codeine phosphate 30 mg, caffeine 40 mg, and butalbital 50 mg.

*Liquid form contains alcohol. **May contain tartrazine.

CAPITAL WITH CODEINE, MYAPAP WITH CODEINE*, TYLENOL WITH CODEINE ELIXIR*, TY-PAP WITH CODEINE ELIXIR*: acetaminophen 120 mg and codeine phosphate 12 mg/5 ml.
CODALAN NO. 1: acetaminophen 500 mg, codeine phosphate 8 mg, and caffeine 30 mg.
CODALAN NO. 2: acetaminophen 500 mg, codeine phosphate 15 mg, and caffeine 30 mg.
CODALAN NO. 3: acetaminophen 500 mg, codeine phosphate 30 mg, and caffeine 30 mg.
CODAMINOPHEN†: acetaminophen 300 mg, codeine phosphate 8 mg, and caffeine 30 mg.
DARVOCET-N 50: acetaminophen 325 mg and propoxyphene napsylate 50 mg.
DARVOCET-N 100, DOXAPAP-N, PROPACET 100: acetaminophen 650 mg and propoxyphene napsylate 100 mg.
DARVON COMPOUND: aspirin 325 mg, propoxyphene hydrochloride 32 mg, and caffeine 32. 4 mg.
DARVON-N COMPOUND: aspirin 375 mg, propoxyphene napsylate 100 mg, and caffeine 30 mg.
DARVON-N WITH ASA: aspirin 325 mg and propoxyphene napsylate 100 mg.
DARVON WITH ASA: aspirin 325 mg and propxyphene hydrochloride 65 mg.
DEMEROL-APAP: acetaminophen 300 mg and meperidine hydrochloride 50 mg.
DOLENE-AP-65, D-REX-65, E-LOR, GENAGESIC, PRO POX WITH APAP, WYGESIC: acetaminophen 650 mg and propoxyphene hydrochloride 65 mg.
EMCODEINE NO. 2, EMPIRIN WITH CODEINE NO. 2: aspirin 325 mg and codeine phosphate 15 mg.
EMCODEINE NO. 3, EMPIRIN WITH CODEINE NO. 3: aspirin 325 mg and codeine phosphate 30 mg.
EMCODEINE NO. 4, EMPIRIN WITH CODEINE NO. 4: aspirin 325 mg and codeine phosphate 60 mg.
EMPRACET-60†: acetaminophen 300 mg and codeine phosphate 60 mg.
ENDOCAN†, OXYCODAN†, PERCODAN†: aspirin 325 mg and oxycodone hydrochloride 5 mg.
ENDOCET†, OXYCOCET†, PERCOCET, ROXICET: acetaminophen 325 mg and oxycodone hydrochloride 5 mg.
HYCODAN: hydrocodone bitartrate 5 mg and homatropine methylbromide 1.5 mg/5 ml.
HYCOTUSS*: hydrocodone bitartrate 5 mg and guaifenesin 100 mg/5 ml.
INNOVAR INJECTION: droperidol 2.5 mg and fentanyl citrate 0.05 mg/ml.
LENOLTEC WITH CODEINE NO. 1†, NOVAGESIC C8†: acetaminophen 300 mg, codeine phosphate 8 mg, and caffeine 15 mg.
LORTAB: acetaminophen 500 mg and hydrocodone bitartrate 2.5 mg.
LORTAB 7: acetaminophen 500 mg and hydrocodone bitartrate 7.5 mg.
LORTAB ORAL SOLUTION: acetaminophen 120 mg and hydrocodone bitartrate 2.5 mg/5 ml.
NOVOPROPOXYN COMPOUND: aspirin 375 mg, propoxyphene hydrochloride 65 mg, and caffeine 30 mg.
PANTOPON INJECTION: hydrochlorides of opium alkaloids; 20 mg is therapeutically equivalent to morphine 15 mg.
PERCODAN-DEMI: aspirin 325 mg, oxycodone hydrochloride 2.25 mg, and oxycodone terephthalate 0.19 mg.
PERCODAN-DEMI†: aspirin 325 mg and oxycodone hydrochloride 2.5 mg.
PERCODAN, ROXIPRIN: aspirin 325 mg, oxycodone hydrochloride 4.5 mg, and oxycodone terephthalate 0.38 mg.
PHENAPHEN-650 WITH CODEINE: acetaminophen 650 mg and codeine phosphate 30 mg.

PHENAPHEN WITH CODEINE NO. 2: acetaminophen 325 mg and codeine phosphate 15 mg.
PHENAPHEN WITH CODEINE NO. 3: acetaminophen 325 mg and codeine phosphate 30 mg.
PHENAPHEN WITH CODEINE NO. 4: acetaminophen 325 mg and codeine phosphate 60 mg.
ROUNOX AND CODEINE 15†: acetaminophen 325 mg and codeine phosphate 15 mg.
ROUNOX AND CODEINE 30†: acetaminophen 325 mg and codeine phosphate 30 mg.
ROUNOX AND CODEINE 60†: acetaminophen 325 mg and codeine phosphate 60 mg.
ROXICET 5/500: acetaminophen 500 mg and oxycodone hydrochloride 5 mg.
ROXICET ORAL SOLUTION*: acetaminophen 325 mg and oxycodone hydrochloride 5 mg/5 ml.
TALACEN: acetaminophen 650 mg and pentazocine 25 mg.
TALWIN COMPOUND: aspirin 325 mg and pentazocine 12.5 mg.
TYLENOL WITH CODEINE NO. 1: acetaminophen 300 mg and codeine phosphate 7.5 mg.
TYLENOL WITH CODEINE NO. 2, TY-TAB WITH CODEINE NO. 2: acetaminophen 300 mg and codeine phosphate 15 mg.
TYLENOL WITH CODEINE NO. 3, TY-TAB WITH CODEINE NO. 3: acetaminophen 300 mg and codeine phosphate 30 mg.
TYLENOL WITH CODEINE NO. 4, TY-TAB WITH CODEINE NO. 4: acetaminophen 300 mg and codeine phosphate 60 mg.
TYLOX: acetaminophen 500 mg and oxycodone hydrochloride 5 mg.
VICODIN ES: acetaminophen 750 mg and hydrocodone bitartrate 7.5 mg.

alfentanil hydrochloride

Alfenta
Controlled Substance Schedule II
Pregnancy Risk Category: B (D for prolonged use or use of high doses at term)

HOW SUPPLIED

Injection: 500 mcg/ml

MECHANISM OF ACTION

Binds with opiate receptors at many sites in the CNS (brain, brain stem, and spinal cord), altering both perception of and emotional response to pain through an unknown mechanism.

INDICATIONS & DOSAGE

Adjunct to general anesthetic –
Adults: initially, 8 to 50 mcg/kg I.V., then give increments of 3 to 15 mcg/kg I.V.
As a primary anesthetic –
Adults: initially, 130 to 245 mcg/kg I.V., then give 0.5 to 1.5 mcg/kg/minute I.V.

ADVERSE REACTIONS

Common reactions are in italics; life-threatening reactions are in bold italics.
CNS: blurred vision, *confusion.*
CV: hypotension, hypertension, bradycardia, tachycardia.
GI: nausea, vomiting.
Skin: itching.
Other: ***chest wall rigidity,*** intraoperative muscle movement, ***respiratory depression,*** hypercapnia.

INTERACTIONS

Alcohol, CNS depressants: additive effects. Use together cautiously.

NURSING CONSIDERATIONS

- *Contraindicated* in patients with hypersensitivity to the drug or other opiate analgesics.
- *Use cautiously* in patients with head injury, pulmonary disease, or decreased respiratory reserve.

*Liquid form contains alcohol. **May contain tartrazine.

- Should be administered only by persons specifically trained in the use of I.V. anesthetics.
- As a primary anesthetic, alfentanil may be prescribed for induction of anesthesia for general surgery requiring endotracheal intubation and medical ventilation.
- **I.V. use:** Discontinue infusion at least 10 to 15 minutes before the end of surgery.
- To administer small volumes of alfentanil accurately, use a tuberculin syringe.
- Keep narcotic antagonist (naloxone) and resuscitative equipment available when giving drug I.V.
- Dose should be reduced in elderly and debilitated patients.
- Periodically monitor postoperative vital signs and bladder function. Because drug decreases both rate and depth of respirations, monitoring of arterial oxygen saturation may aid in assessing respiratory depression.

buprenorphine hydrochloride

Buprenex, Temgesic Injection‡
Controlled Substance Schedule V

Pregnancy Risk Category: C (D for prolonged use or use of high doses at term)

HOW SUPPLIED

Injection: 0.324 mg (equivalent to 0.3 mg base)/ml.

MECHANISM OF ACTION

Binds with opiate receptors at many sites in the CNS (brain, brain stem, and spinal cord), altering both perception of and emotional response to pain through an unknown mechanism.

INDICATIONS & DOSAGE

Moderate to severe pain –
Adults: 0.3 mg I.M. or slow I.V. q 6 hours, p.r.n. or around the clock. May administer up to 0.6 mg/dose if necessary.

ADVERSE REACTIONS

Common reactions are in italics; life-threatening reactions are in bold italics.
CNS: *dizziness, sedation, headache,* confusion, nervousness, euphoria.
CV: hypotension.
EENT: *miosis.*
GI: *nausea,* vomiting, constipation.
Skin: pruritus, *sweating.*
Other: ***respiratory depression,*** hypoventilation.

INTERACTIONS

Alcohol, CNS depressants, MAO inhibitors: additive effects. Use together cautiously.
Narcotic analgesics: avoid concomitant use. Possible decreased analgesic effect.

NURSING CONSIDERATIONS

- *Contraindicated* in patients with hypersensitivity to the drug or other opiate analgesics.
- *Use cautiously* in head injury and increased intracranial pressure; severe respiratory, liver, and kidney impairment; CNS depression; thyroid irregularities; adrenal insufficiency; and prostatic hypertrophy.
- Naloxone will not completely reverse the respiratory depression caused by buprenorphine overdose. Therefore, an overdose may necessitate mechanical ventilation. Larger than customary doses of naloxone (more than 0.4 mg) and doxapram may also be ordered.
- When used postoperatively, encourage turning, coughing, and deep breathing to prevent atelectasis.
- Psychological and physical addiction may occur.
- If dependence occurs, withdrawal symptoms may appear up to 14 days after drug is stopped.
- Drug has narcotic antagonist properties. May precipitate abstinence

syndrome in narcotic-dependent patients.
- S.C. administration not recommended.
- Buprenorphine 0.3 mg is equal to 10 mg morphine and 75 mg meperidine in analgesic potency. Has longer duration of action than morphine or meperidine.
- Warn the patient to avoid driving and other hazardous activities that require mental alertness until adverse CNS effects of the drug are known.

butorphanol tartrate

Stadol, Stadol NS

Pregnancy Risk Category: B (D for prolonged use or use of high doses at term)

HOW SUPPLIED

Injection: 1 mg/ml, 2 mg/ml
Nasal spray: 10 mg/ml

MECHANISM OF ACTION

Binds with opiate receptors at many sites in the CNS (brain, brain stem, and spinal cord), altering both perception of and emotional response to pain through an unknown mechanism.

INDICATIONS & DOSAGE

Moderate to severe pain –
Adults: 1 to 4 mg I.M. q 3 to 4 hours, p.r.n. or around the clock; or 0.5 to 2 mg I.V. q 3 to 4 hours, p.r.n. or around the clock. Alternatively, give 1 mg by nasal spray q 3 to 4 hours (1 spray in one nostril). Repeat in 60 to 90 minutes if pain relief is inadequate.

ADVERSE REACTIONS

Common reactions are in italics; life-threatening reactions are in bold italics.
CNS: *sedation, headache, vertigo, floating sensation,* lethargy, confusion, nervousness, unusual dreams, agitation, euphoria, hallucinations, flushing.
CV: palpitations, fluctuation in blood pressure.
EENT: diplopia, blurred vision.
GI: *nausea,* vomiting, dry mouth, constipation.
Skin: rash, hives, *clamminess, excessive sweating.*
Other: ***respiratory depression.***

INTERACTIONS

Alcohol, CNS depressants: additive effects. Use together cautiously.
Narcotic analgesics: avoid concomitant use. Possible decreased analgesic effect.

NURSING CONSIDERATIONS

- *Contraindicated* in narcotic addiction; may precipitate narcotic abstinence syndrome.
- *Use cautiously* in head injury, increased intracranial pressure, acute MI, ventricular dysfunction, coronary insufficiency, respiratory disease or depression, and renal or hepatic dysfunction.
- Psychological and physical addiction may occur.
- Drug has narcotic antagonist properties. May precipitate abstinence syndrome in narcotic-dependent patients.
- Respiratory depression apparently does not increase with increased dosage.
- S.C. route not recommended.
- Periodically monitor postoperative vital signs and bladder function. Because drug decreases both rate and depth of respirations, monitoring of arterial oxygen saturation may aid in assessing respiratory depression.
- Also used as a preoperative medication, as the analgesic component of balanced anesthesia, and for relief of postpartum pain.
- Warn the patient to avoid driving and other hazardous activities that require mental alertness until adverse CNS effects of the drug are known.

codeine phosphate
Paveral†

codeine sulfate
Controlled Substance Schedule II
Pregnancy Risk Category: C (D for prolonged use or use of high doses at term)

HOW SUPPLIED
phosphate
Oral solution: 15 mg/5 ml, 10 mg/ml†
Injection: 30 mg/ml, 60 mg/ml
sulfate
Tablets: 15 mg, 30 mg, 60 mg
Soluble tablets: 15 mg, 30 mg, 60 mg

MECHANISM OF ACTION
Binds with opiate receptors at many sites in the CNS (brain, brain stem, and spinal cord), altering both perception of and emotional response to pain through an unknown mechanism. Also suppresses the cough reflex by direct action on the cough center in the medulla.

INDICATIONS & DOSAGE
Mild to moderate pain –
Adults: 15 to 60 mg P.O. or 15 to 60 mg (phosphate) S.C. or I.M. q 4 hours, p.r.n. or around the clock.
Children: 3 mg/kg P.O. daily divided q 4 hours, p.r.n. or around the clock.
Nonproductive cough –
Adults: 10 to 20 mg P.O. q 4 to 6 hours. Maximum dosage is 120 mg/24 hours.
Children 6 to 12 years: 5 to 10 mg P.O. q 4 to 6 hours. Maximum dosage is 60 mg/24 hours.
Children 2 to 6 years: 2.5 to 5 mg P.O. q 4 to 6 hours. Do not exceed 30 mg in 24 hours.

ADVERSE REACTIONS
Common reactions are in italics; life-threatening reactions are in bold italics.
CNS: *sedation, clouded sensorium, euphoria,* dizziness, seizures with large doses.
CV: *hypotension,* bradycardia.
GI: *nausea, vomiting, constipation, dry mouth,* ileus.
GU: *urine retention.*
Skin: pruritus, flushing.
Other: ***respiratory depression,*** physical dependence.

INTERACTIONS
Alcohol, CNS depressants: additive effects. Use together cautiously.

NURSING CONSIDERATIONS
- *Contraindicated* in patients with hypersensitivity to the drug or other opiate analgesics.
- *Use with extreme caution* in head injury, increased intracranial pressure, increased CSF pressure, hepatic or renal disease, hypothyroidism, Addison's disease, acute alcoholism, seizures, severe CNS depression, bronchial asthma, COPD, respiratory depression, and shock and in elderly or debilitated patients.
- Warn ambulatory patient to avoid hazardous activities that require alertness.
- Oral administration may cause GI upset. Advise patient to take drug with milk or meals to minimize GI distress.
- Monitor respiratory and circulatory status and bowel function.
- For full analgesic effect, give before patient has intense pain.
- Codeine and aspirin or acetaminophen are often prescribed together to provide enhanced pain relief.
- Do not administer discolored injection solution.
- If used with general anesthetics, other narcotic analgesics, tranquilizers, sedatives, hypnotics, alcohol, tricyclic antidepressants, or MAO inhibitors, CNS depression is increased. Use together with extreme caution. Monitor patient response.
- An antitussive; don't use when

cough is a valuable diagnostic sign or beneficial (as after thoracic surgery).

- Monitor cough type and frequency.
- Opiates may cause constipation. Assess bowel function and need for stool softeners or laxatives. Constipating effect makes codeine useful in the treatment of diarrhea.
- The abuse potential of codeine is much less than that of morphine.

dezocine

Dalgan

Pregnancy Risk Category: C

HOW SUPPLIED

Injection: 5 mg/ml, 10 mg/ml, 15 mg/ml

MECHANISM OF ACTION

A synthetic opioid agonist-antagonist that produces postoperative analgesia qualitatively similar to morphine.

INDICATIONS & DOSAGE

Management of moderate to severe pain–

Adults: 5 to 20 mg I.M. q 3 to 6 hours or 2.5 to 10 mg I.V. q 2 to 4 hours. Maximum recommended single I.M. dose is 20 mg, with a maximum daily dosage of 120 mg. Maximum dosage for I.V. use has not been determined.

Dosage in renal and hepatic failure: Limited studies suggest that the drug should be used with caution and in lower doses. The half-life increases hepatic failure. The primary means of drug elimination is renal excretion of the metabolite.

ADVERSE REACTIONS

Common reactions are in italics; life-threatening reactions are in bold italics.

Blood: low hemoglobin.

CNS: *sedation, dizziness, vertigo,* anxiety, mood disorders, sleep disturbances, headache, slurred speech.

CV: edema, hypotension, irregular heartbeat, hypertension, chest pain.

GI: *nausea, vomiting,* dry mouth, constipation, diarrhea, abdominal distress.

Skin: rash, pruritus, *local irritation at the injection site.*

Other: sweating, chills, flushing, pallor, thrombophlebitis.

INTERACTIONS

Alcohol or other CNS depressants: may increase the risk of CNS depression.

Opiates: patients receiving chronic opioid therapy (opioid-dependent patients) may experience withdrawal symptoms after receiving dezocine. May increase the risk of CNS depression.

NURSING CONSIDERATIONS

- *Contraindicated* in patients with hypersensitivity to the drug.
- *Use with extreme caution* in patients with head injury because drug's CNS depressant effects may obscure clinical signs. Related drugs have caused elevations of CSF pressure in head injury patients.
- *Use cautiously* and in lower doses in patients with chronic respiratory disease and in patients undergoing biliary surgery. Related drugs have caused significant increases in pressure within the common bile duct.
- Like other potent analgesics, dezocine should be administered with caution to elderly patients.
- Dezocine produces a dose-dependent respiratory depression similar to that of morphine, usually peaking within 15 minutes of administration. Use only in clinical settings where adequate respiratory support and an opiate antagonist (naloxone) is available to reverse respiratory depressant effects.
- Use of dezocine is not recommended in patients who are opioid-dependent because it may precipitate

a withdrawal syndrome. Also not recommended for patients with chronic pain because of limited experience and because drug can precipitate an abstinence syndrome in patients with substantial tolerance to opiates.
• **I.V. use:** When giving by direct injection, infuse over at least 5 minutes. Note that the injection contains sulfite preservatives, which may cause allergic reactions in certain sensitive patients.
• Plasma concentrations higher than 45 ng/ml are associated with an increased incidence of adverse reactions.
• Warn patient to avoid driving and other hazardous activities that require alertness until adverse CNS effects of the drug are known. Advise patient to move about cautiously because drug may cause dizziness.
• Although currently not a controlled substance, dezocine will replace morphine in animal drug-dependence studies. However, tolerance or physical dependance has not been reported in humans. Nevertheless, in persons with a history of opiate use or dependence, abuse of this drug is a potential risk.
• Because it is not known if the drug is excreted in breast milk, breastfeeding is not recommended during therapy with dezocine.

fentanyl citrate
Sublimaze

fentanyl transdermal system
Duragesic-25, Duragesic-50, Duragesic-75, Duragesic-100

Controlled Substance Schedule II
Pregnancy Risk Category: B (D for prolonged use or use of high doses at term)

HOW SUPPLIED
Injection: 50 mcg/ml
Transdermal system: patches designed to release 25 mcg, 50 mcg, 75 mcg, or 100 mcg of fentanyl/hour.

MECHANISM OF ACTION
Binds with opiate receptors at many sites in the CNS (brain, brain stem, and spinal cord), altering both perception of and emotional response to pain through an unknown mechanism.

INDICATIONS & DOSAGE
Adjunct to general anesthetic –
Adults: 0.05 to 0.1 mg I.V. repeated q 2 to 3 minutes, p.r.n. Dose should be reduced in elderly and high-risk patients.
Postoperatively –
Adults: 0.05 to 0.1 mg I.M. q 1 to 2 hours p.r.n.
Preoperatively –
Adults: 0.05 to 0.1 mg I.M. 30 to 60 minutes before surgery.
Children 2 to 12 years: 1.7 to 3.3 mcg/kg I.M.
Management of chronic pain –
Adults: apply one transdermal system to a portion of the upper torso on an area of skin that is not irritated and has not been irradiated. Initiate therapy with the 25-mcg/hour system; adjust dosage as needed and tolerated. Each system may be worn for 72 hours.

ADVERSE REACTIONS
Common reactions are in italics; life-threatening reactions are in bold italics.
CNS: *sedation, somnolence, clouded sensorium, euphoria,* dizziness, seizures with large doses.
CV: *hypotension,* bradycardia.
GI: nausea, vomiting, *constipation,* ileus.
GU: *urine retention.*
Local: reaction at application site (erythema, papules, edema).
Other: ***respiratory depression,*** mus-

cle rigidity, physical dependence, *pruritus.*

INTERACTIONS

Alcohol, CNS depressants: additive effects. Use together cautiously.

NURSING CONSIDERATIONS

- *Contraindicated* in patients who have received MAO inhibitors within 14 days and in those with myasthenia gravis.
- *Use cautiously* in head injury, increased CSF pressure, asthma, COPD, respiratory depression, seizures, hepatic or renal disease, hypothyroidism, Addison's disease, alcoholism, increased intracranial pressure, CNS depression, and shock and in elderly or debilitated patients.
- Keep narcotic antagonist (naloxone) and resuscitative equipment available when giving drug I.V.
- **I.V. use:** Only staff trained in administration of I.V. anesthetics and managing their potential adverse reactions should administer I.V. fentanyl.
- Epidural injection or infusion has been used for postoperative analgesia, chronic pain management, or postpartum pain control. May be administered with local anesthetics such as bupivicaine to enhance analgesic effects.
- Monitor respirations of neonates exposed to drug during labor.
- Use as postoperative analgesic only in recovery room. Make sure another analgesic is ordered for later use.
- Often used I.V. with droperidol (Innovar) to produce neuroleptanesthesia.
- Monitor circulatory and respiratory status and urinary function carefully. Drug may cause respiratory depression, hypotension, urine retention, nausea, vomiting, ileus, or altered level of consciousness without regard to route of administration.
- Respiratory depression, hypotension, profound sedation, and coma may result if used with other narcotic analgesics, general anesthetics, tranquilizers, alcohol, sedatives, hypnotics, tricyclic antidepressants, or MAO inhibitors. Fentanyl citrate dose should be reduced by one-fourth to one-third. Also give above drugs in reduced dosages.
- Periodically monitor postoperative vital signs and bladder function. Because drug decreases both rate and depth of respirations, monitoring of arterial oxygen saturation (SaO_2) may aid in assessing respiratory depression. Immediately report respiratory rate below 12 breaths/minute, decreased respiratory volume, or decreased SaO_2.
- For better analgesic effect, give before patient has intense pain.
- When used postoperatively, encourage turning, coughing, and deep breathing to prevent atelectasis.
- Pruritus is common, especially after intraspinal administration. Give diphenhydramine as ordered. Some doctors treat severe pruritus with low doses of naloxone S.C.
- High doses can produce muscle rigidity, which can be reversed with neuromuscular blockers; however, patient must be artificially ventilated.

Transdermal form:

- Transdermal fentanyl is not recommended for postoperative pain.
- Dosage equivalent charts are available to calculate the fentanyl transdermal dose based on the daily morphine intake. An approximation: for every 90 mg of oral morphine or 15 mg of I.M. morphine per 24 hours, 25 mcg/hour of transdermal fentanyl is required.
- Dosage adjustments in patients using the transdermal system should be made gradually. Reaching steady-state levels of a new dose may take up to 6 days; patients should delay adjusting dose until after at least two applications. Use supplemental analge-

sics as a guide to calculating the dosage adjustment: for every 90 mg of supplemental oral morphine ingested per 24 hours, the dosage of the transdermal system should be increased by 25 mcg/hour. Some patients will require alternative means of opiate administration when the dose exceeds 300 mcg/hour.

• Patients who discontinue using the transdermal system because of adverse reactions should be monitored closely for at least 12 hours after removal. Serum levels of fentanyl decline very gradually after transdermal use and may take as long as 17 hours to decline by 50%.

• Most patients experience good control of pain for 3 days while wearing the transdermal system, but a few may need a new application after 48 hours. Because serum fentanyl concentration rises for the first 24 hours after application, analgesic effect cannot be evaluated for the first day. Be sure the patient has adequate supplemental analgesic to prevent breakthrough pain.

• When reducing opiate therapy or switching to a different analgesic, patients using the transdermal system will require gradual withdrawal of the drug. Because the serum level of fentanyl declines very gradually after removal, give half of the equianalgesic dose of the new analgesic 12 to 18 hours after removal.

• Teach patient proper application of the transdermal system. Clip hair at the application site. Do not use a razor because shaving may irritate the skin. Wash area with clear water if necessary, but do not use soaps, oils, lotions, or alcohol or any other substance that may irritate the skin or interfere with the adhesive. Be sure area is completely dry before applying.

• Remove transdermal system from package only immediately before applying. Hold in place for 10 to 20 seconds, and be sure the edges of the system are in contact with the patient's skin.

• Teach patient to dispose of the transdermal system by folding the system so the adhesive side adheres to itself and then flushing the system down the toilet.

• If another transdermal system is needed after 72 hours, it should be applied to a new site.

hydromorphone hydrochloride

Dilaudid, Dilaudid HP

Controlled Substance Schedule II

Pregnancy Risk Category: B (D for prolonged use or use of high doses at term)

HOW SUPPLIED

Tablets: 1 mg, 2 mg, 3 mg, 4 mg
Injection: 1 mg/ml, 2 mg/ml, 3 mg/ml, 4 mg/ml, 10 mg/ml
Suppositories: 3 mg

MECHANISM OF ACTION

Binds with opiate receptors at many sites in the CNS (brain, brain stem, and spinal cord), altering both perception of and emotional response to pain through an unknown mechanism. Also suppresses the cough reflex by direct action on the cough center in the medulla.

INDICATIONS & DOSAGE

Moderate to severe pain –
Adults: 1 to 6 mg P.O. q 4 to 6 hours, p.r.n. or around the clock; or 2 to 4 mg I.M., S.C., or I.V. q 4 to 6 hours, p.r.n., or q 6 to 8 hours around the clock (I.V. dose should be given over 3 to 5 minutes); or 3 mg rectal suppository h.s., p.r.n., or q 6 to 8 hours around the clock.

Cough –
Adults: 1 mg P.O. q 3 to 4 hours p.r.n.
Children 6 to 12 years: 0.5 mg P.O. q 3 to 4 hours p.r.n.

ADVERSE REACTIONS
Common reactions are in italics; life-threatening reactions are in bold italics.
CNS: *sedation, somnolence, clouded sensorium,* dizziness, *euphoria,* seizures with large doses.
CV: *hypotension,* bradycardia.
GI: *nausea, vomiting, constipation,* ileus.
GU: *urine retention.*
Local: induration with repeated S.C. injections.
Other: ***respiratory depression,*** physical dependence.

INTERACTIONS
Alcohol, CNS depressants: additive effects. Use together cautiously.

NURSING CONSIDERATIONS
- *Contraindicated* in patients with hypersensitivity to the drug or other opiate analgesics and in those with status asthmaticus.
- *Use with extreme caution* in patients with increased CSF pressure, respiratory depression, hepatic or renal disease, hypothyroidism, shock, Addison's disease, acute alcoholism, seizures, head injury, severe CNS depression, brain tumor, bronchial asthma, and COPD and in elderly or debilitated patients.
- Monitor respiratory and circulatory status and bowel function.
- Keep narcotic antagonist (naloxone) available.
- **I.V. use:** Respiratory depression and hypotension can occur with I.V. administration. Give very slowly and monitor constantly. Keep resuscitative equipment available.
- Rotate injection sites to avoid induration with S.C. injection.
- Commonly abused narcotic.
- Use with general anesthetics, other narcotic analgesics, tranquilizers, sedatives, hypnotics, alcohol, tricyclic antidepressants, or MAO inhibitors increases CNS depression. Hydromorphone dose should be reduced. Use together with extreme caution. Monitor patient response.
- Warn ambulatory patient to avoid hazardous activities that require mental alertness and physical coordination.
- Oral dosage form is particularly convenient for patients with chronic pain because tablets are available in 1 mg, 2 mg, 3 mg, and 4 mg. This enables these patients to titrate dosage.
- For better analgesic effect, give before patient has intense pain.
- When used postoperatively, encourage turning, coughing, and deep breathing to avoid atelectasis.
- May worsen or mask gallbladder pain.
- Dilaudid HP, a highly concentrated form (10 mg/ml), may be administered in smaller volumes, preventing the discomfort associated with large-volume I.M. or S.C. injections.
- Epidural injection or infusion has been used for management of chronic pain.

levorphanol tartrate
Levo-Dromoran
Controlled Substance Schedule II
Pregnancy Risk Category: B (D for prolonged use or use of high doses at term)

HOW SUPPLIED
Tablets: 2 mg
Injection: 2 mg/ml

MECHANISM OF ACTION
Binds with opiate receptors at many sites in the CNS (brain, brain stem, and spinal cord), altering both perception of and emotional response to pain through an unknown mechanism.

INDICATIONS & DOSAGE
Moderate to severe pain –
Adults: 2 to 3 mg P.O. or S.C. q 6 to 8 hours, p.r.n. or around the clock.

ADVERSE REACTIONS
Common reactions are in italics; life-threatening reactions are in bold italics.
CNS: *sedation, somnolence, clouded sensorium,* dizziness, *euphoria,* seizures with large doses.
CV: *hypotension,* bradycardia.
GI: *nausea, vomiting, constipation,* ileus.
GU: urine retention.
Other: ***respiratory depression,*** physical dependence.

INTERACTIONS
Alcohol, CNS depressants: additive effects. Use together cautiously.

NURSING CONSIDERATIONS
- *Contraindicated* in patients with hypersensitivity to the drug or other opiate analgesics, acute alcoholism, bronchial asthma, increased intracranial pressure, respiratory depression, and anoxia.
- *Use with extreme caution* in hepatic or renal disease, hypothyroidism, Addison's disease, seizures, head injury, severe CNS depression, brain tumor, COPD, and shock and in elderly or debilitated patients.
- Warn ambulatory patient to avoid hazardous activities that require mental alertness and physical coordination.
- Monitor circulatory and respiratory status and bowel function.
- Protect from light.
- Keep narcotic antagonist (naloxone) available.
- Use with general anesthetics, other narcotic analgesics, tranquilizers, sedatives, hypnotics, alcohol, tricyclic antidepressants, or MAO inhibitors increases CNS depression. Reduce levorphanol dose. Use together with extreme caution. Monitor patient response.
- For better analgesic effect, give before patient has intense pain.
- When used postoperatively, encourage turning, coughing, and deep breathing to prevent atelectasis.
- Warn patient drug has bitter taste.

meperidine hydrochloride (pethidine hydrochloride)
Demerol
Controlled Substance Schedule II
Pregnancy Risk Category: B (D for prolonged use or use of high doses at term)

HOW SUPPLIED
Tablets: 50 mg, 100 mg
Syrup: 50 mg/ml
Injection: 10 mg/ml, 25 mg/ml, 50 mg/ml, 75 mg/ml, 100 mg/ml

MECHANISM OF ACTION
Binds with opiate receptors at many sites in the CNS (brain, brain stem, and spinal cord), altering both perception of and emotional response to pain through an unknown mechanism.

INDICATIONS & DOSAGE
Moderate to severe pain –
Adults: 50 to 150 mg P.O., I.M., or S.C. q 3 to 4 hours, p.r.n. or around the clock; or 15 to 35 mg/hour by continuous I.V. infusion.
Children: 1 to 1.8 mg/kg P.O., I.M., or S.C. q 4 to 6 hours. Maximum dosage is 100 mg q 4 hours, p.r.n. or around the clock.
Preoperatively –
Adults: 50 to 100 mg I.M. or S.C. 30 to 90 minutes before surgery.
Children: 1 to 2.2 mg/kg I.M. or S.C. 30 to 90 minutes before surgery.

ADVERSE REACTIONS
Common reactions are in italics; life-threatening reactions are in bold italics.
CNS: *sedation, somnolence, clouded sensorium, euphoria,* paradoxical excitement, tremor, dizziness, seizures with large doses.
CV: *hypotension,* bradycardia, tachycardia.

GI: *nausea, vomiting, constipation,* ileus.
GU: *urine retention.*
Local: pain at injection site, local tissue irritation and induration after S.C. injection; phlebitis after I.V. use.
Other: ***respiratory depression,*** physical dependence, muscle twitching.

INTERACTIONS

Alcohol, CNS depressants: additive effects. Use together cautiously.
MAO inhibitors, barbiturates, isoniazid: increased CNS excitation or depression can be severe or fatal. Don't use together.
Phenytoin: decreased blood levels of meperidine. Monitor for decreased analgesia.

NURSING CONSIDERATIONS

• *Contraindicated* in patients with hypersensitivity to the drug or other opiate analgesics and in patients who have received MAO inhibitors within 14 days.
• *Use with extreme caution* in patients with increased intracranial pressure, increased CSF pressure, shock, CNS depression, head injury, asthma, COPD, respiratory depression, supraventricular tachycardias, seizures, acute abdominal conditions, hepatic or renal disease, hypothyroidism, Addison's disease, urethral stricture, prostatic hypertrophy, and alcoholism; in children under 12 years; and in elderly or debilitated patients.
• May be used in some patients allergic to morphine.
• Meperidine and active metabolite normeperidine accumulate. Monitor for increased toxic effect, especially in patients with impaired renal function.
• Because meperidine toxicity often appears after several days of treatment, this drug is not recommended for treatment of chronic pain.
• **I.V. use:** Meperidine may be given slow I.V., preferably as a diluted solution. Keep narcotic antagonist (naloxone) available when giving this drug I.V.
• S.C. injection is not recommended because it is very painful.
• Warn ambulatory patient to avoid hazardous activities that require mental alertness or physical coordination.
• Monitor respirations of neonates exposed to drug during labor. Have resuscitation equipment and naloxone available.
• P.O. dose less than half as effective as parenteral dose. Give I.M. if possible. When changing from parenteral to P.O. route, dose should be increased.
• Syrup has local anesthetic effect. Give with full glass of water.
• Chemically incompatible with barbiturates. Don't mix together.
• Monitor respiratory and cardiovascular status carefully. Don't give if respirations are below 12 breaths/minute, if respiratory rate or depth is decreased, or if change in pupils is noted.
• Monitor bladder function in postoperative patients.
• Monitor bowel function. Patient may need a laxative or stool softener.
• Watch for withdrawal symptoms if drug is discontinued abruptly after long-term use.
• If used with other narcotic analgesics, general anesthetics, phenothiazines, sedatives, hypnotics, tricyclic antidepressants, or alcohol, respiratory depression, hypotension, profound sedation, or coma may occur. Reduce meperidine dose. Use together with extreme caution.
• For better analgesic effect, give before patient has intense pain. Initially, administration on a fixed schedule may result in better pain control with a smaller daily dose by reducing patient anxiety. Once good pain control has been achieved, adjust scheduling per individual requirements.
• Alternating a centrally active nar-

cotic with a more peripherally active nonnarcotic analgesic (aspirin, acetaminophen, or NSAID) may improve pain control while requiring lower narcotic doses.

• When used postoperatively, encourage turning, coughing, and deep breathing and use of an incentive spirometer to prevent atelectasis.

methadone hydrochloride

Dolophine, Methadose, Physeptone‡

Controlled Substance Schedule II

Pregnancy Risk Category: B (D for prolonged use or use of high doses at term)

HOW SUPPLIED

Tablets: 5 mg, 10 mg
Dispersible tablets (for methadone maintenance therapy): 40 mg
Oral solution: 5 mg/5 ml, 10 mg/5 ml, 10 mg/ml (concentrate)
Injection: 10 mg/ml

MECHANISM OF ACTION

Binds with opiate receptors at many sites in the CNS (brain, brain stem, and spinal cord), altering both perception of and emotional response to pain through an unknown mechanism.

INDICATIONS & DOSAGE

Severe pain –
Adults: 2.5 to 10 mg P.O., I.M., or S.C. q 6 to 8 hours, p.r.n. or around the clock.
Narcotic abstinence syndrome –
Adults: 15 to 40 mg P.O. daily (highly individualized). Maintenance dosage is 20 to 120 mg P.O. daily. Adjust dose as needed. Daily dosages greater than 120 mg require special state and federal approval.

ADVERSE REACTIONS

Common reactions are in italics; life-threatening reactions are in bold italics.
CNS: *sedation, somnolence, clouded sensorium, euphoria,* dizziness, seizures with large doses.
CV: *hypotension,* bradycardia.
GI: *nausea, vomiting, constipation,* ileus.
GU: *urine retention.*
Local: pain at injection site, tissue irritation, induration following S.C. injection.
Other: ***respiratory depression,*** decreased libido, sweating, physical dependence.

INTERACTIONS

Alcohol, CNS depressants: additive effects. Use together cautiously.
Ammonium chloride and other urine acidifiers, phenytoin: may reduce methadone effect. Monitor for decreased pain control.
Rifampin: withdrawal symptoms; reduced blood levels of methadone. Use together cautiously.

NURSING CONSIDERATIONS

• Contraindicated in patients with hypersensitivity to the drug or other opiate analgesics.
• *Use with extreme caution* in elderly or debilitated patients or in patients with acute abdominal conditions, severe hepatic or renal impairment, hypothyroidism, Addison's disease, prostatic hypertrophy, urethral stricture, head injury, increased intracranial pressure, asthma, COPD, respiratory depression, and CNS depression.
• When used as an adjunct in the treatment of narcotic addiction ("maintenance"), withdrawal will usually be delayed and mild.
• Safe use as maintenance drug in adolescent addicts not established.
• Once-daily dosage is adequate for maintenance. No advantage to divided doses.
• Oral liquid form legally required in maintenance programs. Completely dissolve tablets in 120 ml of orange juice or powdered citrus drink.

- Oral dose is half as potent as injected dose.
- Rotate injection sites.
- Has cumulative effect; marked sedation can occur after repeated doses.
- Monitor circulatory and respiratory status and bladder and bowel function. Patient may need a laxative.
- Warn ambulatory patient to avoid activities that require mental alertness or physical coordination.
- Regimented scheduling (around the clock) beneficial in severe, chronic pain. When used for severe, chronic pain, tolerance may develop with long-term use, requiring a higher dose to achieve the same degree of analgesia. This is *not* a sign of addiction.
- Patient treated for narcotic abstinence syndrome will usually require an additional analgesic if pain control is necessary.
- Use with general anesthetics, tranquilizers, sedatives, hypnotics, alcohol, tricyclic antidepressants, or MAO inhibitors may cause respiratory depression, hypotension, profound sedation, or coma. Use together with extreme caution. Monitor patient response.

morphine hydrochloride

Morphitec†, M.O.S.†, M.O.S.-S.R.†

morphine sulfate

Astramorph, Astramorph P.F., Duramorph PF, Epimorph†, Morphine H.P.†, MS Contin, MSIR, RMS Uniserts, Roxanol, Roxanol SR, Statex†

Controlled Substance Schedule II

Pregnancy Risk Category: B (D for prolonged use or use of high doses at term)

HOW SUPPLIED

hydrochloride

Tablets: 10 mg†, 20 mg†, 40 mg†, 60 mg†

Oral solution†: 1 mg/ml, 5 mg/ml, 10 mg/ml, 20 mg/ml, 50 mg/ml

Syrup: 1 mg/ml†, 5 mg/ml†

Suppositories: 20 mg†, 30 mg†

sulfate

Tablets: 15 mg, 30 mg

Tablets (controlled-release): 30 mg, 60 mg

Soluble tablets: 10 mg, 15 mg, 30 mg

Oral solution: 10 mg/5 ml, 20 mg/5 ml, 20 mg/ml (concentrate)

Syrup: 1 mg/ml, 5 mg/ml

Injection (with preservative): 1 mg/ml, 2 mg/ml, 3 mg/ml, 4 mg/ml, 5 mg/ml, 8 mg/ml, 10 mg/ml, 15 mg/ml

Injection (without preservative): 500 mcg/ml, 1 mg/ml

Suppositories: 5 mg, 10 mg, 20 mg, 30 mg

MECHANISM OF ACTION

Binds with opiate receptors at many sites in the CNS (brain, brain stem, and spinal cord), altering both perception of and emotional response to pain through an unknown mechanism.

INDICATIONS & DOSAGE

Severe pain –

Adults: 4 to 15 mg S.C. or I.M.; or 30 to 60 mg P.O. or rectally q 4 hours, p.r.n. or around the clock. May be injected slow I.V. (over 4 to 5 minutes) diluted in 4 to 5 ml water for injection. May also administer controlled-release tablets q 8 to 12 hours. As an epidural injection, 5 mg via an epidural catheter q 24 hours.

Children: 0.1 to 0.2 mg/kg dose S.C. or I.M. q 4 hours. Maximum dosage is 15 mg.

In some situations, morphine may be administered by continuous I.V. infusion or by intraspinal and intrathecal injection.

ADVERSE REACTIONS

Common reactions are in italics; life-threatening reactions are in bold italics.

CNS: *sedation, somnolence, clouded sensorium, euphoria,* seizures with

large doses, dizziness, *nightmares* (with long-acting oral forms).
CV: *hypotension,* bradycardia.
GI: *nausea, vomiting, constipation,* ileus.
GU: *urine retention.*
Other: ***respiratory depression,*** *physical dependence, pruritus and skin flushing (with epidural administration).*

INTERACTIONS
Alcohol, CNS depressants: additional effects. Use together cautiously.

NURSING CONSIDERATIONS
• *Contraindicated* in patients with hypersensitivity to the drug or other opiate analgesics.
• *Use with extreme caution* in head injury, increased intracranial pressure, seizures, asthma, COPD, alcoholism, prostatic hypertrophy, severe hepatic or renal disease, acute abdominal conditions, hypothyroidism, Addison's disease, increased CSF pressure, urethral stricture, cardiac arrhythmias, reduced blood volume, and toxic psychosis and in elderly or debilitated patients.
• Monitor circulatory, respiratory, bladder, and bowel functions carefully. Drug may cause respiratory depression, hypotension, urine retention, nausea, vomiting, ileus, or altered level of consciousness without regard to route of administration. Hold dose and notify doctor if respirations are below 12 breaths/minute.
• Warn ambulatory patient to avoid hazardous activities that require mental alertness or physical coordination.
• Constipation often severe with maintenance. Make sure stool softener or other laxative is ordered.
• Drug of choice in relieving pain of MI. May cause transient decrease in blood pressure.
• Keep narcotic antagonist (naloxone) and resuscitative equipment available.
• Respiratory depression, hypotension, profound sedation, or coma may occur if used with general anesthetics, tranquilizers, sedatives, hypnotics, alcohol, tricyclic antidepressants, or MAO inhibitors. Reduce morphine dose. Use together with extreme caution. Monitor patient response.
• Around-the-clock scheduling helpful in severe, chronic pain.
• When used postoperatively, encourage turning, coughing, and deep breathing and use of the incentive spirometer to prevent atelectasis.
• Oral solutions of various concentrations are available, as well as an intensified oral solution (20 mg/ml). Carefully note the strength you are administering.
• Do not crush or break controlled-release tablets.
• Sublingual administration may be ordered. Measure out oral solution with tuberculin syringe. Administer dose a few drops at a time to allow maximal sublingual absorption and to minimize swallowing.
• Refrigeration of rectal suppository is not necessary. Note that in some patients, rectal and oral absorption may not be equivalent.
• Preservative-free preparations are available for epidural and intrathecal administration. Use of the epidural route is increasing.
• When given epidurally, monitor closely for respiratory depression up to 24 hours after the injection. Check respiratory rate and depth every 30 to 60 minutes for 24 hours.
• May worsen or mask gallbladder pain.

nalbuphine hydrochloride
Nubain

Pregnancy Risk Category: B (D for prolonged use or use of high doses at term)

HOW SUPPLIED
Injection: 10 mg/ml, 20 mg/ml

MECHANISM OF ACTION
Binds with opiate receptors at many sites in the CNS (brain, brain stem, and spinal cord), altering both perception of and emotional response to pain through an unknown mechanism.

INDICATIONS & DOSAGE
Moderate to severe pain –
Adults: 10 to 20 mg S.C., I.M., or I.V. q 3 to 6 hours, p.r.n. or around the clock. Maximum daily dosage is 160 mg.

ADVERSE REACTIONS
Common reactions are in italics; life-threatening reactions are in bold italics.
CNS: *headache, sedation,* dizziness, nervousness, depression, restlessness, crying, euphoria, hostility, unusual dreams, confusion, hallucinations, delusions.
GI: cramps, dyspepsia, bitter taste, *nausea, vomiting,* constipation.
GU: urinary urgency.
Skin: itching; burning; urticaria; *sweaty, clammy feeling.*
Other: ***respiratory depression.***

INTERACTIONS
Alcohol, CNS depressants: additive effects. Use together cautiously.
Narcotic analgesics: avoid concomitant use. Possible decreased analgesic effect.

NURSING CONSIDERATIONS
• *Contraindicated* in patients with hypersensitivity to the drug, emotional instability, history of drug abuse, head injury, or increased intracranial pressure.
• *Use cautiously* in hepatic and renal disease. These patients may overreact to customary doses.
• Causes respiratory depression, which at 10 mg is equal to the respiratory depression produced by 10 mg of morphine.
• Monitor respirations of neonates exposed to the drug during labor.
• Respiratory depression, hypotension, profound sedation, or coma may occur if used with general anesthetics, tranquilizers, sedatives, hypnotics, alcohol, tricyclic antidepressants, or other CNS depressants. Use together with extreme caution. Monitor patient response.
• **I.V. use:** Inject slowly (over at least 2 to 3 minutes) into a vein or into an I.V. line containing a compatible free-flowing I.V. solution, such as dextrose 5% in water, 0.9% sodium chloride, or lactated Ringer's injection.
• Respiratory depression can be reversed with naloxone. Keep resuscitative equipment available, particularly when administering I.V.
• Psychological and physical dependence may occur.
• Monitor circulatory and respiratory status and bladder and bowel function. Hold dose and notify doctor if respirations are shallow or rate is below 12 breaths/minute.
• Constipation often severe with maintenance. Make sure stool softener or other laxative is ordered.
• Also acts as a narcotic antagonist; may precipitate abstinence syndrome. For patients who have chronically received opiates, administer 25% of the usual dose initially. Observe for signs of withdrawal.
• Warn patient to avoid hazardous activities that require alertness until CNS effects of the drug are known.

oxycodone hydrochloride
Endone‡, Roxicodone, Supeudol†
Controlled Substance Schedule II

oxycodone pectinate
Proladone‡

Pregnancy Risk Category: B (D for prolonged use or use of high doses at term)

*Liquid form contains alcohol. **May contain tartrazine.

HOW SUPPLIED
hydrochloride
Tablets: 5 mg
Oral solution: 5 mg/5 ml
Suppositories: 10 mg, 20 mg
pectinate
Suppositories: 30 mg‡

MECHANISM OF ACTION
Binds with opiate receptors at many sites in the CNS (brain, brain stem, and spinal cord), altering both perception of and emotional response to pain through an unknown mechanism.

INDICATIONS & DOSAGE
Moderate to severe pain–
Adults: available in combination with other drugs, such as aspirin (Percodan, Percodan-Demi) or acetaminophen (Percocet, Tylox). One to 2 tablets P.O. q 6 hours, p.r.n. or around the clock. Or 5 mg (5 ml) of oxycodone oral solution P.O. q 6 hours.
Adults: (Supeudol) 1 to 3 suppositories rectally daily, p.r.n. or around the clock.
Children: (Percodan-Demi) ¼ to ½ tablet P.O. q 6 hours, p.r.n. or around the clock.

ADVERSE REACTIONS
Common reactions are in italics; life-threatening reactions are in bold italics.
CNS: *sedation, somnolence, clouded sensorium, euphoria,* dizziness, ***seizures*** with large doses.
CV: *hypotension,* bradycardia.
GI: *nausea, vomiting, constipation,* ileus.
GU: *urine retention.*
Other: ***respiratory depression,*** physical dependence.

INTERACTIONS
Alcohol, CNS depressants: additive effects. Use together cautiously.
Anticoagulants: oxycodone hydrochloride products containing aspirin may increase anticoagulant effect. Monitor clotting times. Use together cautiously.

NURSING CONSIDERATIONS
- *Contraindicated* in patients with hypersensitivity to the drug or other opiate analgesics.
- *Use with extreme caution* in head injury, increased intracranial pressure, increased CSF pressure, seizures, asthma, COPD, alcoholism, prostatic hypertrophy, severe hepatic or renal disease, acute abdominal conditions, urethral stricture, hypothyroidism, Addison's disease, cardiac arrhythmias, reduced blood volume, and toxic psychosis and in elderly or debilitated patients.
- Don't give to children, except for Percodan-Demi and Percocet-Demi.
- Warn ambulatory patient to avoid hazardous activities that require mental alertness or physical coordination.
- Monitor circulatory and respiratory status and bladder and bowel function. Hold dose and notify doctor if respirations are shallow or if respiratory rate falls below 12 breaths/minute.
- Because drug has a constipating effect, patient may require a laxative.
- For full analgesic effect, give before patient has intense pain.
- To minimize GI upset, give after meals or with milk.
- Single-agent oxycodone solution or tablets are especially good for patients who shouldn't take aspirin or acetaminophen.
- Concomitant use with general anesthetics, other narcotic analgesics, tranquilizers, sedatives, hypnotics, alcohol, tricyclic antidepressants, or MAO inhibitors can result in increased CNS depression. Reduce oxycodone dose and use together with extreme caution. Monitor patient's response.

oxymorphone hydrochloride

Numorphan
Controlled Substance Schedule II
Pregnancy Risk Category: B (D for prolonged use or use of high doses at term)

HOW SUPPLIED
Injection: 1 mg/ml, 1.5 mg/ml
Suppositories: 5 mg

MECHANISM OF ACTION
Binds with opiate receptors at many sites in the CNS (brain, brain stem, and spinal cord), altering both perception of and emotional response to pain through an unknown mechanism.

INDICATIONS & DOSAGE
Moderate to severe pain –
Adults: 1 to 1.5 mg I.M. or S.C. q 4 to 6 hours, p.r.n. or around the clock; or 0.5 mg I.V. q 4 to 6 hours, p.r.n. or around the clock; or 2.5 to 5 mg rectally q 4 to 6 hours, p.r.n. or around the clock.

ADVERSE REACTIONS
CNS: *sedation, somnolence, clouded sensorium, euphoria,* dizziness, seizures with large doses.
CV: *hypotension,* bradycardia.
GI: *nausea, vomiting, constipation,* ileus.
GU: *urine retention.*
Other: ***respiratory depression,*** physical dependence.

INTERACTIONS
Alcohol, CNS depressants: additive effects. Use together cautiously.

NURSING CONSIDERATIONS
- *Contraindicated* in patients with hypersensitivity to the drug or other opiate analgesics.
- *Use with extreme caution* in head injury, increased intracranial pressure, seizures, asthma, COPD, alcoholism, increased CSF pressure, acute abdominal conditions, prostatic hypertrophy, severe hepatic or renal disease, urethral stricture, CNS depression, respiratory depression, hypothyroidism, Addison's disease, cardiac arrhythmias, reduced blood volume, and toxic psychosis and in elderly or debilitated patients.
- Warn ambulatory patient to avoid activities that require mental alertness or physical coordination.
- Monitor cardiovascular and respiratory status and bladder and bowel function. Hold dose and notify doctor if respirations decrease or rate is below 12 breaths/minute.
- Patient may need laxative.
- Well absorbed rectally. Alternative to narcotics with limited dosage forms.
- Keep narcotic antagonist (naloxone) and resuscitative equipment available.
- If used with general anesthetics, tranquilizers, sedatives, hypnotics, alcohol, tricyclic antidepressants, or MAO inhibitors, CNS depression is increased. Reduce oxymorphone dose. Use together with extreme caution. Monitor patient's response.
- For better analgesic effect, give before patient has intense pain.
- When used postoperatively, encourage turning, coughing, and deep breathing and use of the incentive spirometer to avoid atelectasis.
- Not intended for mild to moderate pain. May worsen gallbladder pain.

pentazocine hydrochloride

Fortral†‡, Talwin†

pentazocine hydrochloride and naloxone hydrochloride

Talwin Nx
Controlled Substance Schedule IV

*Liquid form contains alcohol. **May contain tartrazine.

pentazocine lactate

Fortral‡, Talwin
Controlled Substance Schedule IV
Pregnancy Risk Category: B (D for prolonged use or use of high doses at term)

HOW SUPPLIED
pentazocine hydrochloride
Tablets: 25 mg‡, 50 mg†‡
pentazocine hydrochloride and naloxone hydrochloride
Tablets: 50 mg pentazocine hydrochloride and 500 mcg naloxone hydrochloride
pentazocine lactate
Injection: 30 mg/ml

MECHANISM OF ACTION
Binds with opiate receptors at many sites in the CNS (brain, brain stem, and spinal cord), altering both perception of and emotional response to pain through an unknown mechanism.

INDICATIONS & DOSAGE
Moderate to severe pain–
Adults: 50 to 100 mg P.O. q 3 to 4 hours, p.r.n. or around the clock. Maximum oral dosage is 600 mg daily. Alternatively, may give 30 mg I.M., I.V., or S.C. q 3 to 4 hours, p.r.n. or around the clock. Maximum parenteral dosage is 360 mg daily. Single doses above 30 mg I.V. or 60 mg I.M. or S.C. not recommended.

ADVERSE REACTIONS
Common reactions are in italics; life-threatening reactions are in bold italics.
CNS: *sedation,* visual disturbances, *hallucinations,* drowsiness, *dizziness, light-headedness,* confusion, euphoria, headache, *psychotomimetic effects.*
GI: *nausea, vomiting,* dry mouth, constipation.
GU: *urine retention.*
Local: induration, nodules, sloughing, and sclerosis of injection site.
Other: ***respiratory depression,*** physical and psychological dependence.

INTERACTIONS
Alcohol, CNS depressants: additive effects. Use together cautiously.
Narcotic analgesics: avoid concomitant use. Possible decreased analgesic effect.

NURSING CONSIDERATIONS
- *Contraindicated* in patients with hypersensitivity to the drug, emotional instability, drug abuse, head injury, and increased intracranial pressure. Injectable form contains sulfites, which may precipitate allergic reactions in some patients with hypersensitivity.
- *Use cautiously* in hepatic or renal disease, and in patients with acute MI.
- Tablets not well absorbed.
- Possesses narcotic antagonist properties. May precipitate abstinence syndrome in narcotic-dependent patients.
- Psychological and physical dependence may occur.
- Respiratory depression can be reversed with naloxone.
- Do not mix in same syringe with soluble barbiturates.
- Warn ambulatory patient to avoid activities that require alertness.
- Pentazocine may interfere with certain laboratory tests for urinary 17-hydroxycorticosteroids.
- Talwin Nx, the oral pentazocine available in the U.S., contains the narcotic antagonist naloxone. This prevents illicit I.V. use.

propoxyphene hydrochloride (dextropropoxyphene hydrochloride)

Darvon, Dolene, Doraphen, Doxaphene, Novopropoxyn†, Pro-Pox, Propoxycon, 642†

propoxyphene napsylate (dextropropoxyphene napsylate)

Darvocet-N, Darvon-N, Doloxene‡, Doloxene Co‡

Controlled Substance Schedule IV
Pregnancy Risk Category: C (D for prolonged use)

HOW SUPPLIED

hydrochloride
Capsules: 32 mg, 65 mg
napsylate
Tablets: 100 mg
Capsules: 50 mg, 100 mg
Oral suspension: 10 mg/ml

MECHANISM OF ACTION

Binds with opiate receptors at many sites in the CNS (brain, brain stem, and spinal cord), altering both perception of and emotional response to pain through an unknown mechanism.

INDICATIONS & DOSAGE

Mild to moderate pain –
Adults: 65 mg (hydrochloride) P.O. q 4 hours p.r.n.
Mild to moderate pain –
Adults: 100 mg (napsylate) P.O. q 4 hours p.r.n.

ADVERSE REACTIONS

Common reactions are in italics; life-threatening reactions are in bold italics.
CNS: *dizziness,* headache, sedation, euphoria, paradoxical excitement, insomnia.
GI: nausea, vomiting, constipation.
Other: ***respiratory depression,*** psychological and physical dependence.

INTERACTIONS

Alcohol, CNS depressants: additive effects. Use together cautiously.

NURSING CONSIDERATIONS

- *Contraindicated* in patients with hypersensitivity to the drug or other opiate analgesics.
- *Use cautiously* in patients with hepatic or renal disease, emotional instability, or a history of drug abuse.
- Respiratory depression, hypotension, profound sedation, and coma may result if used in excessive doses or with other CNS depressants. Studies have shown that propoxyphene-containing products alone or in combination with other drugs are a major cause of drug-related overdose and death. Warn patient not to exceed recommended dosage.
- Not to be prescribed for maintenance purposes in narcotic addiction.
- Warn ambulatory patient to avoid hazardous activities that require mental alertness or physical coordination until CNS effects of the drug are known.
- Do not use caffeine or amphetamines to treat overdose; may cause fatal seizures. Use narcotic antagonist instead.
- May cause false decreases in urinary steroid excretion tests.
- 65 mg propoxyphene hydrochloride equals 100 mg propoxyphene napsylate.
- Can be considered a mild narcotic analgesic, but pain relief is equivalent to aspirin. Tolerance and physical dependence have been observed. Used with aspirin or acetaminophen to maximize analgesia.
- To minimize GI upset, advise patient to take drug with food or milk.
- Advise patient to limit alcohol intake when taking this drug.

sufentanil citrate

Sufenta
Controlled Substance Schedule II

Pregnancy Risk Category: C (D for prolonged use or use of high doses at term)

HOW SUPPLIED

Injection: 50 mcg/ml

*Liquid form contains alcohol. **May contain tartrazine.

MECHANISM OF ACTION
Binds with opiate receptors at many sites in the CNS (brain, brain stem, and spinal cord), altering both perception of and emotional response to pain through an unknown mechanism.

INDICATIONS & DOSAGE
Adjunct to general anesthetic –
Adults: 1 to 8 mcg/kg I.V. administered with nitrous oxide/oxygen.
As a primary anesthetic –
Adults: 8 to 30 mcg/kg I.V. administered with 100% oxygen and a muscle relaxant.

ADVERSE REACTIONS
Common reactions are in italics; life-threatening reactions are in bold italics.
CNS: chills.
CV: *hypotension,* hypertension, bradycardia, tachycardia.
GI: nausea, vomiting.
Skin: itching.
Other: ***chest wall rigidity,*** intraoperative muscle movement, ***respiratory depression.***

INTERACTIONS
Alcohol, CNS depressants: additive effects. Use together cautiously.

NURSING CONSIDERATIONS
- *Contraindicated* in patients with hypersensitivity to the drug or other opiate analgesics.
- *Use cautiously* in head injury; pulmonary, hepatic, or renal disease; or decreased respiratory reserve.
- **I.V. use:** Should be administered only by persons specifically trained in the use of I.V. anesthetics.
- When used at doses over 8 mcg/kg, postoperative mechanical ventilation and observation are essential because of prolonged respiratory depression.
- Keep narcotic antagonist (naloxone) and resuscitative equipment available when giving drug.
- Monitor respirations of neonates exposed to the drug during labor.
- Because drug decreases both rate and depth of respirations, monitoring of arterial oxygen saturation may aid in assessing respiratory depression. Notify doctor if respirations decrease or rate falls below 12 breaths/minute.
- Dose should be reduced in elderly and debilitated patients.
- Monitor postoperative vital signs frequently, including circulatory and respiratory status and urinary function. Drug may cause respiratory depression, hypotension, urine retention, nausea, vomiting, ileus, or altered level of consciousness. Encourage turning, coughing, and deep breathing to prevent atelectasis.
- Has more rapid onset and shorter duration of action than fentanyl.
- High doses can produce muscle rigidity reversible by neuromuscular blockers; however, patient must be artificially ventilated.

28

Sedative-hypnotics

amobarbital
amobarbital sodium
aprobarbital
butabarbital sodium
chloral hydrate
estazolam
ethchlorvynol
flurazepam hydrochloride
glutethimide
methotrimeprazine hydrochloride
methyprylon
midazolam hydrochloride
pentobarbital
pentobarbital sodium
phenobarbital sodium
(See Chapter 29, ANTICONVULSANTS.)
quazepam
secobarbital sodium
temazepam
triazolam
zolpidem tartrate

COMBINATION PRODUCTS
TRI-BARBS CAPSULES: phenobarbital 32 mg, butabarbital sodium 32 mg, and secobarbital sodium 32 mg.
TUINAL 200 MG PULVULES: amobarbital sodium 100 mg and secobarbital sodium 100 mg.

---

amobarbital
Amytal

amobarbital sodium
Amytal Sodium

Controlled Substance Schedule II
Pregnancy Risk Category: B

HOW SUPPLIED
amobarbital
Tablets: 50 mg
amobarbital sodium
Capsules: 200 mg
Powder for injection: 500 mg

MECHANISM OF ACTION
Probably interferes with transmission of impulses from the thalamus to the cortex of the brain. A barbiturate.

INDICATIONS & DOSAGE
Sedation –
Adults: usually 50 mg P.O. b.i.d. or t.i.d.
Children: 3 to 6 mg/kg P.O. daily in four equally divided doses.
Insomnia –
Adults: 50 to 200 mg P.O. or deep I.M. h.s.; I.M. injection not to exceed 5 ml in any one site. Maximum dosage is 500 mg.
Children: 3 to 5 mg/kg deep I.M. h.s.; I.M. injection not to exceed 5 ml in any one site.
Preanesthetic sedation –
Adults and children: 200 mg P.O. or I.M. 1 to 2 hours before surgery.
Manic reactions, as an adjunct in psychotherapy, anticonvulsant –
Adults and children over 6 years: 65 to 500 mg slow I.V.; not to exceed 100 mg/minute. Maximum dose is 1 g.
Children under 6 years: 3 to 5 mg/kg slow I.V. or I.M.

ADVERSE REACTIONS
Common reactions are in italics; life-threatening reactions are in bold italics.
CNS: *drowsiness, lethargy, hangover,* paradoxical excitement.
GI: nausea, vomiting.
Skin: rash, urticaria.
Local: pain, irritation, sterile abscess at injection site.
Other: ***Stevens-Johnson syndrome, angioedema,*** exacerbation of porphyria.

*Liquid form contains alcohol. **May contain tartrazine.

INTERACTIONS

Alcohol or other CNS depressants, including narcotic analgesics: excessive CNS and respiratory depression. Use together cautiously.
Griseofulvin: decreased absorption of griseofulvin.
MAO inhibitors: inhibit metabolism of barbiturates; may cause prolonged CNS depression. Reduce barbiturate dosage.
Oral anticoagulants, estrogens and oral contraceptives, doxycycline, corticosteroids: amobarbital may enhance the metabolism of these drugs. Monitor for decreased effect.
Rifampin: may decrease barbiturate levels. Monitor for decreased effect.

NURSING CONSIDERATIONS

- *Contraindicated* in uncontrolled severe pain, respiratory disease with dyspnea or obstruction, hypersensitivity to barbiturates, previous addiction to sedatives, or porphyria.
- *Use cautiously* in hepatic or renal impairment.
- Elderly patients are more sensitive to the drug's adverse CNS effects. Assess mental status before and after initiating therapy.
- Use injection solution within 30 minutes after opening container to minimize deterioration. Don't use cloudy or precipitated solution. Don't shake solution; mix with sterile water only.
- **I.V. use:** Reserve I.V. injection for emergency treatment. Give under close supervision. Be prepared to give artificial respiration. Administer slowly I.V.; do not exceed 100 mg/ minute.
- Administer I.M. injection deeply. Superficial injection may cause pain, sterile abscess, and sloughing.
- Because barbiturates potentiate narcotics, reduce dose when giving during labor. Excessive dose may cause respiratory depression in neonate.
- Supervise walking; raise bed rails, especially for elderly patients.
- Long-term high dosage may cause drug dependence and severe withdrawal symptoms. Withdraw barbiturates gradually.
- Prevent hoarding or self-overdosing by patients who are depressed, suicidal, or drug-dependent or who have a history of drug abuse.
- Watch for signs of barbiturate toxicity: coma, pupillary constriction, cyanosis, clammy skin, and hypotension. Overdose can be fatal.
- Morning "hangover" common after hypnotic dose. Hypnotic doses suppress REM sleep. Patient may experience increased dreaming after drug is discontinued.
- Used in psychiatric settings as an "Amytal interview" to elicit information that patient can't or won't offer when fully conscious.
- Used in Wada testing to help determine language and memory function.
- I.V. administration of barbiturates may cause severe respiratory depression, laryngospasm, or hypotension. Have emergency resuscitation equipment readily available.
- Local tissue reactions and pain at the injection site have been noted with I.V. use. Assess patency of I.V. site before and during administration.
- Assess CBCs before and periodically during long-term therapy. Observe for signs of hematologic toxicity, such as easy bruising or bleeding, or signs of infection.
- Skin eruptions may precede potentially fatal reactions to barbiturate therapy. Discontinue drug when skin reactions occur. In some patients, high fever, stomatitis, headache, or rhinitis may precede skin reactions.

aprobarbital

Alurate*
Controlled Substance Schedule III
Pregnancy Risk Category: D

HOW SUPPLIED
Elixir: 40 mg/5 ml

MECHANISM OF ACTION
Probably interferes with transmission of impulses from the thalamus to the cortex of the brain. A barbiturate.

INDICATIONS & DOSAGE
Sedation –
Adults: 15 to 40 mg P.O. t.i.d. or q.i.d.; usual dose is 40 mg t.i.d.
Insomnia –
Adults: 40 to 160 mg P.O. h.s.

ADVERSE REACTIONS
Common reactions are in italics; life-threatening reactions are in bold italics.
CNS: *drowsiness, lethargy, hangover,* paradoxical excitement in elderly patients.
GI: nausea, vomiting.
Skin: rash, urticaria.
Other: ***Stevens-Johnson syndrome,*** angioedema, exacerbation of porphyria.

INTERACTIONS
Alcohol or other CNS depressants, including narcotic analgesics: excessive CNS and respiratory depression. Use together cautiously.
Griseofulvin: decreased absorption of griseofulvin.
MAO inhibitors: inhibit metabolism of barbiturates; may cause prolonged CNS depression. Reduce barbiturate dosage.
Oral anticoagulants, estrogens and oral contraceptives, doxycycline, corticosteroids: aprobarbital may enhance the metabolism of these drugs. Monitor for decreased effectiveness.
Rifampin: may decrease barbiturate levels. Monitor for decreased effect.

NURSING CONSIDERATIONS
- *Contraindicated* in uncontrolled severe pain, respiratory disease with dyspnea or obstruction, hypersensitivity to barbiturates, previous addiction to sedatives, or porphyria.
- *Use cautiously* in hepatic or renal impairment and in elderly patients.
- Warn patient to exercise caution when performing activities that require mental alertness or physical coordination. Supervise walking; raise bed rails, especially for elderly patients.
- Prolonged administration is not recommended. Drug loses efficacy in promoting sleep after 14 days of continued use. Long-term high dosage may cause drug dependence, and patient may experience withdrawal symptoms if drug is suddenly discontinued. Withdraw barbiturates gradually.
- Take precautions to prevent hoarding or self-overdosing by patients who are depressed, suicidal, or drug-dependent or who have a history of drug abuse.
- Watch for signs of barbiturate toxicity: coma, pupillary constriction, cyanosis, clammy skin, and hypotension. Overdose can be fatal.
- Morning "hangover" common after hypnotic dose.
- Hypnotic doses suppress REM sleep. Patient may experience increased dreaming after drug is discontinued.
- Women who use oral contraceptives should consider alternate birth control methods when taking this drug because it may enhance contraceptive hormone metabolism and decrease its effect.
- Skin eruptions may precede potentially fatal reactions to barbiturate therapy. Discontinue drug when skin reactions occur. In some patients, high fever, stomatitis, headache, or rhinitis may precede skin reactions.

butabarbital sodium

Barbased*, Butalan*, Buticaps, Butisol* **, Day-Barb†, Sarisol No. 2* **

Controlled Substance Schedule III

Pregnancy Risk Category: D

HOW SUPPLIED

Tablets: 15 mg, 30 mg, 50 mg, 100 mg
Capsules: 15 mg, 30 mg
Elixir: 30 mg/5 ml, 33.3 mg/5 ml

MECHANISM OF ACTION

Probably interferes with transmission of impulses from the thalamus to the cortex of the brain. A barbiturate.

INDICATIONS & DOSAGE

Sedation –
Adults: 15 to 30 mg P.O. t.i.d. or q.i.d.
Children: 6 mg/kg P.O. divided t.i.d. Dosage range 7.5 to 30 mg P.O. t.i.d.
Preoperatively –
Adults: 50 to 100 mg P.O. 60 to 90 minutes before surgery.
Insomnia –
Adults: 50 to 100 mg P.O. h.s.

ADVERSE REACTIONS

Common reactions are in italics; life-threatening reactions are in bold italics.
CNS: *drowsiness, lethargy, hangover,* paradoxical excitement in elderly patients.
GI: nausea, vomiting.
Skin: rash, urticaria.
Other: ***Stevens-Johnson syndrome, angioedema,*** exacerbation of porphyria.

INTERACTIONS

Alcohol or other CNS depressants, including narcotic analgesics: excessive CNS and respiratory depression. Use together cautiously.
Griseofulvin: decreased absorption of griseofulvin.
MAO inhibitors: inhibit the metabolism of barbiturates; may cause prolonged CNS depression. Reduce barbiturate dosage.
Oral anticoagulants, estrogens and oral contraceptives, doxycycline, corticosteroids: butabarbital may enhance the metabolism of these drugs. Monitor for decreased effect.
Rifampin: may decrease barbiturate levels. Monitor for decreased effect.

NURSING CONSIDERATIONS

- *Contraindicated* in uncontrolled severe pain, respiratory disease with dyspnea or obstruction, hypersensitivity to barbiturates, previous addiction to sedatives, or porphyria.
- *Use cautiously* in hepatic or renal impairment.
- Elderly patients are more sensitive to the drug's adverse CNS reactions. Assess mental status before and after initiating therapy.
- Advise caution with activities requiring mental alertness or physical coordination. Supervise walking; raise bed rails, especially for elderly patients.
- Prolonged administration is not recommended: drug loses its efficacy in promoting sleep after 14 days. A drug-free interval of at least 1 week is advised if continued treatment is appropriate.
- Long-term high dosage may cause drug dependence, and patient may experience withdrawal symptoms if drug is suddenly stopped. Withdraw barbiturates gradually.
- Take precautions to prevent hoarding or self-overdosing by patients who are depressed, suicidal, or drug-dependent or who have a history of drug abuse.
- Butisol sodium elixir is sugar-free.
- Watch for signs of barbiturate toxicity: coma, pupillary constriction, cyanosis, clammy skin, and hypotension. Overdose can be fatal.
- Skin eruptions may precede potentially fatal reactions to barbiturate

therapy. Discontinue drug when skin reactions occur. In some patients, high fever, stomatitis, headache, or rhinitis may precede skin reactions.
- Morning "hangover" common after hypnotic dose.
- Hypnotic doses suppress REM sleep. Patient may experience increased dreaming after drug is discontinued.
- Women who use oral contraceptives should consider alternate birth control methods when taking this drug because it may enhance contraceptive hormone metabolism and decrease its effect.

chloral hydrate

Aquachloral Supprettes, Noctec, Novochlorhydrate†
Controlled Substance Schedule IV

Pregnancy Risk Category: C

HOW SUPPLIED

Capsules: 250 mg, 500 mg
Syrup: 250 mg/5 ml, 500 mg/5 ml
Suppositories: 325 mg, 500 mg, 648 mg

MECHANISM OF ACTION

Unknown. Sedative effects may be caused by its primary metabolite, trichloroethanol.

INDICATIONS & DOSAGE

Sedation –
Adults: 250 mg P.O. or P.R. t.i.d. after meals.
Children: 8.3 mg/kg or 250 mg/m^2 P.O. or P.R. t.i.d. Maximum dosage is 500 mg t.i.d.
Insomnia –
Adults: 500 mg to 1 g P.O. or P.R. 15 to 30 minutes before bedtime.
Children: 50 mg/kg or 1.5 g/m^2 P.O. or P.R. 15 to 30 minutes before bedtime. Maximum single dose is 1 g.
Premedication for EEG –
Children: 20 to 25 mg/kg P.O. or P.R. Maximum single dose is 1 g.
Management of alcohol withdrawal symptoms –
Adults: 500 mg to 1 g P.O. or P.R. q 6 hours, not to exceed 2 g daily.

ADVERSE REACTIONS

Common reactions are in italics; life-threatening reactions are in bold italics.
Blood: eosinophilia.
CNS: *hangover, drowsiness,* nightmares, dizziness, ataxia, paradoxical excitement.
GI: *nausea,* vomiting, diarrhea, flatulence.
Skin: hypersensitivity reactions.

INTERACTIONS

Alcohol or other CNS depressants, including narcotic analgesics: excessive CNS depression or vasodilation reaction. Use together cautiously.
Furosemide I.V.: sweating, flushes, variable blood pressure, and uneasiness. Use together cautiously or use a different hypnotic drug.
Oral anticoagulants: increased risk of bleeding. Monitor patient closely.

NURSING CONSIDERATIONS

- *Contraindicated* in marked hepatic or renal impairment and hypersensitivity to chloral hydrate or trichloroacetic acid. Oral administration contraindicated in gastric disorders.
- *Use cautiously* in severe cardiac disease, mental depression, and suicidal tendencies.
- Prolonged administration is not recommended. Drug loses efficacy in promoting sleep after 14 days of continued use. Long-term use may cause drug dependence, and patient may experience withdrawal symptoms if drug is suddenly discontinued.
- Dilute or administer with liquid to minimize unpleasant taste and stomach irritation. Administer after meals.
- Note two strengths of oral liquid form. Double check dose, especially when administering to children. Fatal overdoses have occurred.

*Liquid form contains alcohol. **May contain tartrazine.

• Take precautions to prevent hoarding or self-overdosing by patients who are depressed, suicidal, or drug-dependent or who have a history of drug abuse.
• Advise caution with activities requiring mental alertness or physical coordination. Supervise walking; raise bed rails, especially for elderly patients.
• Large dosage may raise BUN levels.
• May interfere with fluorometric tests for urine catecholamines and Reddy-Jenkins-Thorn test for urine 17-hydroxycorticosteroids. Do not administer drug for 48 hours before fluorometric test. May also cause false-positive tests for urine glucose when using copper sulfate tests. Use glucose enzymatic tests instead.
• Aqueous solutions are incompatible with alkaline substances.
• Store in dark container; store suppositories in refrigerator.

estazolam

ProSom
Controlled Substance Schedule IV
Pregnancy Risk Category: X

HOW SUPPLIED

Tablets: 1 mg, 2 mg

MECHANISM OF ACTION

Acts on the limbic system and thalamus of the CNS by binding to specific benzodiazepine receptors.

INDICATIONS & DOSAGE

Adjunctive treatment of insomnia –
Adults: 1 mg P.O. h.s. Some patients may require 2 mg.
Elderly patients: 1 mg P.O. h.s. Use higher doses with extreme care. Frail elderly or debilitated patients may take 0.5 mg, but this low dose may be only marginally effective.

ADVERSE REACTIONS

Common reactions are in italics; life-threatening reactions are in bold italics.
CNS: fatigue, dizziness, *daytime drowsiness,* headache.

INTERACTIONS

Alcohol, CNS depressants including antihistamines, opiate analgesics, and other benzodiazepines: increased CNS depression. Avoid concomitant use.
Cimetidine, oral contraceptives, disulfiram, isoniazid: may impair the metabolism and clearance of benzodiazepines and prolong their plasma half-life. Monitor for increased CNS depression.
Rifampin, cigarette smoking: may increase metabolism and clearance and decrease plasma half-life. Monitor for decreased effectiveness.
Theophylline: pharmacologic antagonism. Monitor for decreased effectiveness.

NURSING CONSIDERATIONS

• *Contraindicated* in patients allergic to the drug or other benzodiazepines, in pregnant patients, and in patients with suspected or confirmed sleep apnea.
• *Use cautiously* in patients with hepatic, renal, or pulmonary disease.
• Consider the possibility of purposeful overdose by patients who are depressed, suicidal, or known users of illegal drugs. Closely monitor drug administration to prevent hoarding of doses.
• Warn patient that additive depressant effects can occur if alcohol is consumed on the day after use of the drug.
• Patients who receive prolonged treatment with benzodiazepines may experience withdrawal symptoms if the drug is suddenly discontinued (possibly after 6 weeks of continuous therapy).
• Hepatic and renal function and CBC

should be checked before and periodically during long-term therapy.
- Warn patient about dizziness and drowsiness. Tell him to avoid driving and other hazardous activities that require alertness until the adverse CNS effects of the drug are known. Supervise walking; raise bed rails, especially for elderly patients.
- Tell patient not to increase dosage of the drug but to inform the doctor if he feels that the drug is no longer effective.
- If estazolam overdose occurs, flumazenil (a specific benzodiazepine antagonist) may be useful. Know that the duration of action of flumazenil is shorter than that of estazolam, and resedation is possible.

ethchlorvynol

Placidyl**
Controlled Substance Schedule IV
Pregnancy Risk Category: C

HOW SUPPLIED
Capsules: 200 mg, 500 mg, 750 mg**

MECHANISM OF ACTION
Unknown.

INDICATIONS & DOSAGE
Sedation–
Adults: 100 to 200 mg P.O. b.i.d. or t.i.d.
Insomnia–
Adults: 500 mg to 1 g P.O. h.s. May repeat 100 to 200 mg if awakened in early morning.

ADVERSE REACTIONS
Common reactions are in italics; life-threatening reactions are in bold italics.
Blood: thrombocytopenia.
CNS: facial numbness, drowsiness, fatigue, nightmares, dizziness, residual sedation, muscular weakness, syncope, ataxia.
CV: hypotension.
EENT: unpleasant aftertaste, blurred vision.
GI: distress, nausea, vomiting.
Skin: rashes, urticaria.

INTERACTIONS
Alcohol or other CNS depressants, including narcotic analgesics, tricyclic antidepressants, and MAO inhibitors: excessive CNS depression. Use together cautiously.
Oral anticoagulants: ethchlorvynol may enhance the metabolism of coumarin derivatives, decreasing their effectiveness. Monitor closely.

NURSING CONSIDERATIONS
- *Contraindicated* in patients with hypersensitivity to the drug and in those with uncontrolled pain or porphyria.
- *Use cautiously* in hepatic or renal impairment; in elderly or debilitated patients; in mental depression with suicidal tendencies; and if patient has previously overreacted to barbiturates or alcohol.
- Give with milk or food to minimize transient dizziness or ataxia caused by rapid absorption.
- May cause dependence and severe withdrawal symptoms. Withdraw gradually.
- Take precautions to prevent hoarding or self-overdosing by patients who are depressed, suicidal, or drug-dependent or who have a history of drug abuse. Overdosage is very difficult to treat and has a high mortality.
- Watch for signs of toxicity, such as poor muscle coordination, confusion, hypothermia, speech or vision disturbances, tremor, and weakness.
- The 750-mg strength contains tartrazine dye. May cause allergic reactions in susceptible patients.
- Advise caution with hazardous activities requiring mental alertness or physical coordination. Supervise walking; raise bed rails, especially for elderly patients.
- Slight darkening of liquid from ex-

*Liquid form contains alcohol. **May contain tartrazine.

posure to air and light doesn't affect safety or potency, but store in tight, light-resistant container to avoid possible deterioration.
- Drug is effective for short-term use only; treatment period should not exceed 1 week.

flurazepam hydrochloride

Apo-Flurazepam†, Dalmane, Durapam, Novoflupam†, Sam-Pam†
Controlled Substance Schedule IV
Pregnancy Risk Category: D

HOW SUPPLIED
Capsules: 15 mg, 30 mg

MECHANISM OF ACTION
Acts on the limbic system, thalamus, and hypothalamus of the central nervous system to produce hypnotic effects. A benzodiazepine.

INDICATIONS & DOSAGE
Insomnia –
Adults: 15 to 30 mg P.O. h.s. May repeat dose once.
Adults over 65 years: 15 mg P.O. h.s.

ADVERSE REACTIONS
Common reactions are in italics; life-threatening reactions are in bold italics.
Blood: leukopenia, granulocytopenia.
CNS: *daytime sedation, dizziness, drowsiness, disturbed coordination,* lethargy, confusion, *headache.*
GI: nausea, vomiting, heartburn.
Metabolic: elevated liver enzymes.

INTERACTIONS
Alcohol or other CNS depressants, including narcotic analgesics: excessive CNS depression. Use together cautiously.
Cimetidine: increased sedation. Monitor carefully.

NURSING CONSIDERATIONS
- *Contraindicated* in patients with hypersensitivity to benzodiazepines.
- *Use cautiously* in patients with impaired hepatic or renal function, mental depression, suicidal tendencies, or history of drug abuse.
- May cause elevations in certain liver function tests (AST [SGOT], ALT [SGPT], total and direct bilirubin, and alkaline phosphatase). Hepatic and renal function and CBC should be checked before and periodically during long-term therapy.
- Elderly patients are more sensitive to the drug's adverse CNS reactions. Assess mental status before initiating therapy.
- Prevent hoarding or self-overdosing by patients who are depressed, suicidal, or drug-dependent or who have a history of drug abuse.
- Advise caution with hazardous activities requiring mental alertness or physical coordination. Supervise walking; raise bed rails, especially for elderly patients.
- Dependence is possible with long-term use.
- More effective on second, third, and fourth nights of use because active metabolite accumulates. Encourage patient to continue drug if it doesn't relieve insomnia the first night.
- If flurazepam overdose occurs, flumazenil (a specific benzodiazepine antagonist) may be useful. Know that the duration of action of flumazenil is shorter than that of flurazepam, and resedation is possible.

glutethimide

Doriden, Doriglute
Controlled Substance Schedule III
Pregnancy Risk Category: C

HOW SUPPLIED
Tablets: 250 mg, 500 mg
Capsules: 500 mg

MECHANISM OF ACTION
Unknown.

INDICATIONS & DOSAGE
Insomnia –
Adults: 250 to 500 mg P.O. h.s. May be repeated, but not less than 4 hours before intended awakening. Total daily dosage should not exceed 1 g.

ADVERSE REACTIONS
Common reactions are in italics; life-threatening reactions are in bold italics.
CNS: *residual sedation, dizziness, ataxia,* paradoxical excitation, headache, vertigo.
EENT: dry mouth, blurred vision.
GI: irritation, nausea.
GU: bladder atony.
Skin: rash, urticaria.

INTERACTIONS
Alcohol or other CNS depressants, including narcotic analgesics: excessive CNS depression. Use together cautiously.
Oral anticoagulants: glutethimide enhances the metabolism of coumarin derivatives. Monitor for decreased effect.

NURSING CONSIDERATIONS
• *Contraindicated* in patients with hypersensitivity to the drug and in patients with uncontrolled pain, severe renal impairment, or porphyria.
• *Use cautiously* in patients with mental depression, suicidal tendencies, history of drug abuse, and conditions that may be worsened by the drug's anticholinergic activity (prostatic hypertrophy, stenosing peptic ulcer, pyloroduodenal or bladder-neck obstruction, narrow-angle glaucoma, and cardiac arrhythmias).
• Drug is effective for short-term use only.
• Advise caution with activities requiring mental alertness or physical coordination. Supervise walking; raise bed rails, especially for elderly patients.
• Take precautions to prevent hoarding or self-overdosing by patients who are depressed, suicidal, or drug-dependent or who have a history of drug abuse.
• Abrupt withdrawal after long-term use may produce nausea, vomiting, nervousness, tremor, chills, fever, nightmares, insomnia, tachycardia, delirium, numbness of extremities, hallucinations, dysphagia, and seizures. Withdraw drug gradually.
• Assess patient for anticholinergic symptoms, including mydriasis, dry mouth, tachycardia, or urine retention.
• Monitor prothrombin times carefully when patient on glutethimide starts or ends anticoagulant therapy. Anticoagulant dose may need to be adjusted.
• Suppresses REM sleep, as do barbiturates. Patient may experience increased dreaming after drug is discontinued.
• May interfere with laboratory determinations of 17-hydroxycorticosteroids using the Glenn-Nelson technique.

methotrimeprazine hydrochloride (levomepromazine hydrochloride)
Levoprome, Nozinan†**

Pregnancy Risk Category: C

HOW SUPPLIED
Tablets: 2 mg†, 5 mg†, 25 mg†, 50 mg†
Oral solution: 40 mg/ml†
Drops: 40 mg/ml†
Injection: 20 mg/ml in 10-ml vials, 25 mg/ml†

MECHANISM OF ACTION
Acts on the limbic system, thalamus, and hypothalamus of the central ner-

*Liquid form contains alcohol. **May contain tartrazine.

vous system to produce hypnotic effects. A phenothiazine.

INDICATIONS & DOSAGE

Postoperative analgesia –
Adults and children over 12 years: initially, 2.5 to 7.5 mg I.M. q 4 to 6 hours, then adjust dose.
Preanesthetic medication –
Adults and children over 12 years: 2 to 20 mg I.M. 45 minutes to 3 hours before surgery.
Sedation, analgesia –
Adults and children over 12 years: 10 to 20 mg deep I.M. q 4 to 6 hours as required; or 6 to 25 mg P.O. daily in three divided doses with meals. For severe pain, dosage may be increased to 50 to 75 mg daily in two or three divided doses with meals.
Adults over 65 years: 5 to 10 mg I.M. q 4 to 6 hours.
Psychosis –
Adults: 6 to 25 mg P.O. daily in three divided doses with meals. Dosage may be gradually increased as needed and tolerated to 50 to 75 mg daily in two or three divided doses.
Sedation and analgesia during labor –
Adults: 15 to 20 mg I.M.

ADVERSE REACTIONS

Common reactions are in italics; life-threatening reactions are in bold italics.
Blood: ***agranulocytosis*** and other dyscrasias after long-term high dosage.
CNS: *fainting, weakness, dizziness,* drowsiness, excessive sedation, amnesia, disorientation, euphoria, headache, slurred speech.
CV: *orthostatic hypotension,* palpitations.
EENT: dry mouth, nasal congestion.
GI: nausea, vomiting, abdominal discomfort.
GU: difficulty urinating.
Local: *pain, inflammation, swelling at injection site.*

INTERACTIONS

All antihypertensive agents: increased orthostatic hypotension. Don't use together.
Epinephrine: methotrimeprazine reverses the effect of epinephrine on blood pressure, worsening hypotension. Don't use together.

NURSING CONSIDERATIONS

- *Contraindicated* in patients receiving concurrent antihypertensive drug therapy, including MAO inhibitors; in patients with a history of seizure disorders; in hypersensitivity to phenothiazines; in severe cardiac, hepatic, or renal disease; in previous overdose of CNS depressant; and in coma.
- *Use with extreme caution* in elderly or debilitated patients with cardiac disease or in any patient who may suffer serious consequences from a sudden drop in blood pressure.
- Because the injectable form contains sulfites, *use cautiously* in asthmatic patients or in patients with sulfite sensitivity.
- Use low initial dose in debilitated patients; increase gradually while frequently checking pulse rate, blood pressure, and circulation.
- Expect drop in blood pressure 10 to 20 minutes after I.M. injection. May last 4 to 12 hours.
- Keep patient in bed or closely supervised for 6 to 12 hours after each of the first several injections because orthostatic hypotension may occur. If hypotension is severe, combat with phenylephrine, methoxamine, or levarterenol. Don't use epinephrine because it may worsen hypotension.
- Because drowsiness and amnesia may occur, warn patient to avoid hazardous activities that require mental alertness or physical coordination.
- Assess patient for anticholinergic symptoms, including mydriasis, dry mouth, tachycardia, or urine retention.
- Don't use for longer than 30 days

except in terminal illness or when narcotics are contraindicated.
- In prolonged use, monitor liver function and blood studies periodically.
- Inject I.M. into large muscle masses. Rotate sites. Do not administer subcutaneously, as local irritation results. I.V. injection not recommended.
- May be mixed in same syringe with reduced dose of atropine and scopolamine. Do not mix with other drugs. Protect solution from light.
- If high oral doses (> 100 mg) are used, patient should be confined to bed for the first few days to prevent orthostatic hypotension.
- Rarely may cause neuroleptic malignant syndrome, with fever, leukocytosis, and dystonic reaction. Can be fatal if untreated.
- Methotrimeprazine interferes with provocative and blocking tests for pheochromocytoma because of its alpha-adrenergic antagonist effects.

methyprylon

Noludar
Controlled Substance Schedule III
Pregnancy Risk Category: B

HOW SUPPLIED

Tablets: 50 mg, 200 mg
Capsules: 300 mg

MECHANISM OF ACTION

Raises threshold of arousal centers in the brain stem.

INDICATIONS & DOSAGE

Insomnia –
Adults: 200 to 400 mg P.O. 15 minutes before bedtime.
Children over 3 months: 50 mg P.O. at bedtime, increased to 200 mg, if necessary. Maximum dosage is 400 mg daily.

ADVERSE REACTIONS

Common reactions are in italics; life-threatening reactions are in bold italics.
Blood: thrombocytopenic purpura, neutropenia, ***aplastic anemia***.
CNS: *morning drowsiness, dizziness,* headache, paradoxical excitation.
CV: hypotension.
GI: nausea, vomiting, diarrhea, esophagitis.
Skin: rash, pruritus.

INTERACTIONS

Alcohol or other CNS depressants, including narcotic analgesics: excessive CNS and respiratory depression. Use together cautiously.

NURSING CONSIDERATIONS

- *Contraindicated* in patients with hypersensitivity to the drug and in patients with intermittent porphyria.
- *Use cautiously* in renal or hepatic impairment.
- Periodic blood counts are advisable during repeated or long-term use.
- May cause drug dependence after long-term use. Withdrawal should be gradual and closely monitored.
- Take precautions to prevent hoarding or self-overdosing by patients who are depressed, suicidal, or drug-dependent or who have a history of drug abuse.
- Advise caution with hazardous activities requiring mental alertness or physical coordination. Supervise walking; raise bed rails, especially for elderly patients.
- Value of this drug as a sedative has not been established.
- Symptoms of overdosage include somnolence, confusion, constricted pupils, respiratory depression, hypotension, and coma. Hemodialysis is useful in severe intoxication.
- Suppresses REM sleep, as do barbiturates. Patient may experience increased dreaming after drug is discontinued.

midazolam hydrochloride

Versed

Controlled Substance Schedule IV

Pregnancy Risk Category: D

HOW SUPPLIED

Injection: 1 mg/ml, 5 mg/ml

MECHANISM OF ACTION

Depresses the CNS at the limbic and subcortical levels of the brain.

INDICATIONS & DOSAGE

Preoperative sedation (to induce sleepiness or drowsiness and relieve apprehension) –

Adults: 0.07 mg to 0.08 mg/kg I.M. approximately 1 hour before surgery. May be administered with atropine or scopolamine and reduced doses of narcotics.

Conscious sedation before short diagnostic or endoscopic procedures –

Adults: initially, 0.035 mg/kg slowly I.V.(not to exceed 2.5 mg). Dose is then titrated in small amounts to a total dosage of 0.1 mg/kg.

Induction of general anesthesia –

Adults: 0.3 to 0.35 mg/kg I.V. over 20 to 30 seconds. Additional increments of 25% of the initial dose may be needed to complete induction. Up to 0.6 mg/kg total dosage may be given.

ADVERSE REACTIONS

Common reactions are in italics; life-threatening reactions are in bold italics.

CNS: headache, oversedation, involuntary movements, combativeness.

CV: variations in blood pressure and pulse rate.

GI: nausea, vomiting, hiccups.

Local: pain and tenderness at injection site.

Other: decreased respiratory rate, apnea.

INTERACTIONS

CNS depressants: may increase the risk of apnea. Prepare to adjust drug dosage.

NURSING CONSIDERATIONS

- *Contraindicated* in acute narrow-angle glaucoma, shock, coma, or acute alcohol intoxication.
- *Use cautiously* in CHF, COPD, or renal disease and in elderly or debilitated patients.
- **I.V. use:** Before administering, have oxygen and resuscitation equipment available in case of severe respiratory depression. Excessive dosage or rapid infusion has been associated with respiratory arrest, particularly in elderly or debilitated patients. Administer slowly over at least 2 minutes, and wait at least 2 minutes when titrating doses to effect.
- When administering I.V., take care to avoid extravasation.
- Monitor blood pressure, heart rate and rhythm, respirations, airway integrity, and arterial oxygen saturation during procedure, especially in patients who have also been premedicated with narcotics.
- Midazolam has a beneficial amnestic effect, which diminishes patient's recall of perioperative events. This effect requires extra caution when teaching patients; written information, instruction of family members, and follow-up contact may be required to ensure that patient has adequate information.
- Advise caution with hazardous activities requiring mental alertness or physical coordination.
- When injecting I.M., give deep into a large muscle mass.
- May be mixed in the same syringe with morphine sulfate, meperidine, atropine sulfate, or scopolamine.
- If midazolam overdose occurs, flumazenil (a specific benzodiazepine antagonist) may be useful. Know that the duration of action of flumazenil is

shorter than that of midazolam, and resedation is possible.

pentobarbital
Nembutal* **

pentobarbital sodium
Nembutal Sodium*,
Novopentobarb†
Controlled Substance Schedule II
Pregnancy Risk Category: D

HOW SUPPLIED
pentobarbital
Elixir: 20 mg/5 ml
pentobarbital sodium
Capsules: 50 mg, 100 mg
Injection: 50 mg/ml
Suppositories: 30 mg, 60 mg, 120 mg, 200 mg

MECHANISM OF ACTION
Probably interferes with transmission of impulses from the thalamus to the cortex of the brain. A barbiturate.

INDICATIONS & DOSAGE
Sedation –
Adults: 20 to 40 mg P.O. b.i.d., t.i.d., or q.i.d.
Children: 6 mg/kg daily P.O. in divided doses.
Insomnia –
Adults: 100 to 200 mg P.O. h.s. or 150 to 200 mg deep I.M.; 100 mg initially, I.V., then additional doses up to 500 mg; 120 to 200 mg rectally.
Children: 3 to 5 mg/kg I.M. Maximum dosage is 100 mg. Rectal dosages are 2 months to 1 year, 30 mg; 1 to 4 years, 30 to 60 mg; 5 to 12 years, 60 mg; 12 to 14 years, 60 to 120 mg.
Preanesthetic medication –
Adults: 150 to 200 mg I.M. or P.O. in two divided doses.

ADVERSE REACTIONS
Common reactions are in italics; life-threatening reactions are in bold italics.
CNS: *drowsiness, lethargy, hangover,* paradoxical excitement in elderly patients.
GI: nausea, vomiting.
Skin: rash, urticaria.
Other: ***Stevens-Johnson syndrome, angioedema,*** exacerbation of porphyria.

INTERACTIONS
Alcohol or other CNS depressants, including narcotic analgesics: excessive CNS and respiratory depression. Use together cautiously.
Griseofulvin: decreased absorption of griseofulvin.
MAO inhibitors: inhibit metabolism of barbiturates; may cause prolonged CNS depression. Reduce barbiturate dosage.
Oral anticoagulants, estrogens and oral contraceptives, doxycycline, corticosteroids: pentobarbital may enhance the metabolism of these drugs. Monitor for decreased effect.
Rifampin: may decrease barbiturate levels. Monitor for decreased effect.

NURSING CONSIDERATIONS
- *Contraindicated* in uncontrolled severe pain, respiratory disease with dyspnea or obstruction, hypersensitivity to barbiturates, previous addiction to sedatives, or porphyria.
- *Use cautiously* in hepatic or renal impairment.
- Elderly patients are more sensitive to the drug's adverse CNS reactions. Assess mental status before initiating therapy.
- Use injection solution within 30 minutes after opening container to minimize deterioration. Don't use cloudy solution.
- **I.V. use:** I.V. injection should be reserved for emergency treatment and should be given under close supervision. Administer slowly at a rate not exceeding 50 mg/minute.
- I.V. administration of barbiturates may cause severe respiratory depression, laryngospasm, or hypotension.

*Liquid form contains alcohol. **May contain tartrazine.

Have emergency resuscitation equipment readily available.

- Parenteral solution is alkaline. Local tissue reactions and pain at the injection site have followed I.V. use. Avoid extravasation. Assess patency of I.V. site before and during administration.
- Administer I.M. injection deeply. Superficial injection may cause pain, sterile abscess, and sloughing.
- Do not mix in syringe or I.V. with other medications.
- Advise caution with activities requiring mental alertness or physical coordination. Supervise walking; raise bed rails, especially for elderly patients.
- Prolonged administration is not recommended. Drug loses efficacy in promoting sleep after 14 days of continued use. Long-term high dosage may cause drug dependence, and patient may experience withdrawal symptoms if drug is suddenly discontinued. Withdraw barbiturates gradually.
- Take precautions to prevent hoarding or self-overdosing by patients who are depressed, suicidal, or drug-dependent or who have a history of drug abuse.
- No analgesic effect. May cause restlessness or delirium in presence of pain.
- Watch for signs of barbiturate toxicity: coma, pupillary constriction, cyanosis, clammy skin, and hypotension. Overdose can be fatal.
- Skin eruptions may precede potentially fatal reactions to barbiturate therapy. Discontinue drug when skin reactions occur. In some patients, high fever, stomatitis, headache, or rhinitis may precede skin reactions.
- To ensure accurate dosage, don't divide suppositories.
- Morning "hangover" common after hypnotic dose.
- Hypnotic doses suppress REM sleep. Patient may experience increased dreaming after drug is discontinued.

quazepam

Doral

Controlled Substance Schedule IV

Pregnancy Risk Category: X

HOW SUPPLIED

Tablets: 7.5 mg, 15 mg

MECHANISM OF ACTION

Acts on the limbic system and thalamus of the CNS by binding to specific benzodiazepine receptors.

INDICATIONS & DOSAGE

Insomnia –

Adults: 15 mg P.O. h.s. Some patients may respond to lower doses. Decrease dosage in elderly patients to 7.5 mg P.O. h.s. after 2 days of therapy.

ADVERSE REACTIONS

Common reactions are in italics; life-threatening reactions are in bold italics.

CNS: *fatigue, dizziness, daytime drowsiness, headache.*

INTERACTIONS

Alcohol or other CNS depressants, including antihistamines, opiate analgesics, and other benzodiazepines: increased CNS depression.

NURSING CONSIDERATIONS

- *Contraindicated* in patients allergic to the drug or other benzodiazepines, in pregnant patients, and in patients with suspected or established sleep apnea.
- *Use cautiously* in patients with hepatic, renal, or respiratory disease and in elderly patients.
- Warn the patient about the possible additive depressant effects that can occur with alcohol consumption. Additive effects can occur if alcohol is

consumed on the day after the use of quazepam.

- Patients who receive prolonged therapy with benzodiazepines may experience withdrawal symptoms if the drug is suddenly withdrawn (possibly after 6 weeks of continuous therapy).
- CBC should be checked before and periodically during long-term therapy. Observe for signs of hematologic toxicity, such as easy bruising or bleeding, or signs of infection.
- Take precautions to prevent hoarding or self-overdosing by patients who are depressed, suicidal, or known drug abusers.
- Supervise walking and use bed rails, especially for elderly patients. Warn patients to avoid driving and other hazardous activities that require alertness until CNS reactions to the drug are known.
- Warn patients not to increase the drug dosage but to inform the doctor if they feel that the drug is no longer effective.
- If quazepam overdose occurs, flumazenil (a specific benzodiazepine antagonist) may be useful. Know that the duration of action of flumazenil is shorter than that of quazepam, and resedation is possible.

secobarbital sodium

Novosecobarb†, Seconal Sodium
Controlled Substance Schedule II
Pregnancy Risk Category: D

HOW SUPPLIED

Tablets: 100 mg
Capsules: 50 mg, 100 mg
Injection: 50 mg/ml
Rectal injection: 50 mg/ml
Suppositories: 200 mg

MECHANISM OF ACTION

Probably interferes with transmission of impulses from the thalamus to the cortex of the brain. A barbiturate.

INDICATIONS & DOSAGE

Sedation, preoperatively –
Adults: 200 to 300 mg P.O. 1 to 2 hours before surgery.
Children: 50 to 100 mg P.O. or 4 to 5 mg/kg P.R. 1 to 2 hours before surgery.
Insomnia –
Adults: 100 to 200 mg P.O. or I.M.
Children: 3 to 5 mg/kg I.M., not to exceed 100 mg, with no more than 5 ml injected in any one site or 4 to 5 mg/kg P.R.
Acute tetanus seizure –
Adults and children: 5.5 mg/kg I.M. or slow I.V., repeated q 3 to 4 hours, if needed; I.V. injection rate not to exceed 50 mg/15 seconds.
Acute psychotic agitation –
Adults: 50 mg/minute I.V. up to 250 mg I.V. initially, additional doses given cautiously after 5 minutes if desired response is not obtained. Not to exceed 500 mg total.
Status epilepticus –
Adults and children: 250 to 350 mg I.M. or I.V.

ADVERSE REACTIONS

Common reactions are in italics; life-threatening reactions are in bold italics.
CNS: *drowsiness, lethargy, hangover,* paradoxical excitement in elderly patients.
GI: nausea, vomiting.
Skin: rash, urticaria.
Other: ***Stevens-Johnson syndrome, angioedema,*** exacerbation of porphyria.

INTERACTIONS

Alcohol or other CNS depressants, including narcotic analgesics: excessive CNS and respiratory depression. Use together cautiously.
Griseofulvin: decreased absorption of griseofulvin.
MAO inhibitors: inhibit metabolism of barbiturates; may cause prolonged CNS depression. Reduce barbiturate dosage.

*Liquid form contains alcohol. **May contain tartrazine.

Oral anticoagulants, estrogens and oral contraceptives, doxycycline, corticosteroids: secobarbital may enhance the metabolism of these drugs. Monitor for decreased effect.
Rifampin: may decrease barbiturate levels. Monitor for decreased effect.

NURSING CONSIDERATIONS

- *Contraindicated* in uncontrolled severe pain, respiratory disease with dyspnea or obstruction, hypersensitivity to barbiturates, previous addiction to sedatives, or porphyria.
- *Use cautiously* in hepatic or renal impairment and in pregnant women with toxemia or history of bleeding.
- If used in the management of seizures, appropriate seizure precautions should be taken.
- Elderly patients are more sensitive to the drug's adverse CNS reactions. Assess mental status before initiating therapy.
- Use injection solution within 30 minutes after opening container to minimize deterioration. Don't use cloudy solution.
- **I.V. use:** I.V. injection should be reserved for emergency treatment and should be given under close supervision. Administer slowly at a rate not exceeding 50 mg/15 seconds.
- I.V. administration of barbiturates may cause severe respiratory depression, laryngospasm, or hypotension. Have emergency resuscitation equipment readily available.
- Local tissue reactions and pain at the injection site have been noted with I.V. use. Assess patency of I.V. site before and during administration.
- Give I.M. injection deeply. Superficial injection may cause pain, sterile abscess, and sloughing.
- Because barbiturates potentiate narcotics, reduce dose when giving during labor. Excessive dose may cause respiratory depression in neonate.
- Advise caution with activities requiring mental alertness or physical coordination. Supervise walking; raise bed rails, especially for elderly patients.
- May cause drug dependence and severe withdrawal symptoms. Withdraw barbiturates gradually.
- Take precautions to prevent hoarding or self-overdosing by patients who are depressed, suicidal, or drug-dependent or who have a history of drug abuse.
- In renal insufficiency, use sterile drug reconstituted with sterile water for injection. Avoid commercial solution containing polyethylene glycol; it may irritate kidneys.
- Secobarbital in polyethylene glycol must be refrigerated.
- Secobarbital sodium injection not compatible with lactated Ringer's solution.
- Sterile secobarbital sodium compatible with Ringer's injection and normal saline solution. Don't mix with acidic solutions.
- To reconstitute, rotate ampule. Do not shake.
- Watch for signs of barbiturate toxicity: coma, pupillary construction, cyanosis, clammy skin, and hypotension. Overdose can be fatal.
- Morning "hangover" common after hypnotic dose.
- Hypnotic doses suppress REM sleep. Patient may experience increased dreaming after drug is discontinued.
- Prolonged administration is not recommended. Drug loses efficacy in promoting sleep after 14 days of continued use. Long-term high dosage may cause drug dependence, and patient may experience withdrawal symptoms if drug is suddenly stopped. Withdraw barbiturates gradually.
- Skin eruptions may precede potentially fatal reactions to barbiturate therapy. Discontinue drug when skin reactions occur. In some patients,

high fever, stomatitis, headache, or rhinitis may precede skin reactions.

temazepam

Restoril, Temaze‡
Controlled Substance Schedule IV
Pregnancy Risk Category: X

HOW SUPPLIED
Capsules: 15 mg, 30 mg

MECHANISM OF ACTION
Acts on the limbic system, thalamus, and hypothalamus of the CNS to produce hypnotic effects. A benzodiazepine.

INDICATIONS & DOSAGE
Insomnia –
Adults: 15 to 30 mg P.O. h.s.
Adults over 65 years: 15 mg P.O. h.s.

ADVERSE REACTIONS
Common reactions are in italics; life-threatening reactions are in bold italics.
CNS: *drowsiness, dizziness, lethargy,* disturbed coordination, daytime sedation, confusion.
GI: anorexia, diarrhea.

INTERACTIONS
Alcohol or CNS depressants, including narcotic analgesics: increased CNS depression. Use together cautiously.

NURSING CONSIDERATIONS
- *Use cautiously* in impaired hepatic or renal function, mental depression, suicidal tendencies, and history of drug abuse. Also use cautiously and in low end of dosage range in elderly or debilitated patients.
- Elderly patients are more sensitive to the drug's adverse CNS reactions. Assess mental status before initiating therapy.
- Take precautions to prevent hoarding or self-overdosing by patients who are depressed, suicidal, or drug-dependent or who have a history of drug abuse.
- Warn about increased depressant effects of alcohol and against hazardous activity requiring alertness or physical coordination.
- Supervise walking; raise bed rails, especially for elderly patients.
- May cause less residual sedation ("hangover") the next day than flurazepam and diazepam. Relatively short-acting.
- Onset of action may take as long as 2 to 2½ hours.
- If temazepam overdose occurs, flumazenil (a specific benzodiazepine antagonist) may be useful. Know that the duration of action of flumazenil is shorter than that of temazepam, and resedation is possible.

triazolam

Halcion
Controlled Substance Schedule IV
Pregnancy Risk Category: X

HOW SUPPLIED
Tablets: 0.125 mg, 0.25 mg

MECHANISM OF ACTION
Acts on the limbic system, thalamus, and hypothalamus of the CNS to produce hypnotic effects. A benzodiazepine.

INDICATIONS & DOSAGE
Insomnia –
Adults: 0.125 to 0.25 mg P.O. h.s.
Adults over 65: 0.125 mg P.O. h.s.; increase as needed to 0.25 mg P.O. h.s.

ADVERSE REACTIONS
Common reactions are in italics; life-threatening reactions are in bold italics.
CNS: *drowsiness, dizziness, headache,* rebound insomnia, amnesia, light-headedness, lack of coordination, mental confusion, depression.
GI: nausea, vomiting.

INTERACTIONS

Alcohol or other CNS depressants, including narcotic analgesics: excessive CNS depression. Use together cautiously.

Cimetidine, erythromycin: may cause prolonged triazolam blood levels. Monitor for increased sedation.

NURSING CONSIDERATIONS

- *Contraindicated* in patients with hypersensitivity to benzodiazepines.
- *Use cautiously* in impaired hepatic or renal function, mental depression, suicidal tendencies, or history of drug abuse.
- Elderly patients are more sensitive to the drug's adverse CNS reactions. Assess mental status before initiating therapy.
- Drug should be used in the lowest effective dose for very short duration (5 to 7 days).
- Take precautions to prevent hoarding or self-overdosing by patients who are depressed, suicidal, or drug-dependent or who have a history of drug abuse.
- Advise caution with hazardous activities requiring mental alertness or physical coordination. Supervise walking; raise bed rails, especially for elderly patients.
- Dependence is possible with long-term use.
- Triazolam is a benzodiazepine compound with similarities to flurazepam. However, it is very short-acting and therefore has less tendency to cause morning drowsiness.
- Faster acting than temazepam, another benzodiazepine derivative.
- Warn patient not to take more than the prescribed amount since overdosage can occur at a total daily dose of 2 mg (or four times the highest recommended amount).
- Tell patient that rebound insomnia may develop for one or two nights after stopping therapy.
- Because of numerous reports of adverse CNS reactions, triazolam has been withdrawn from several foreign markets. An FDA panel recently reviewed the safety and efficacy of the drug; it is currently still available in the United States.
- If triazolam overdose occurs, flumazenil (a specific benzodiazepine antagonist) may be useful. Know that the duration of action of flumazenil is shorter than that of triazolam, and resedation is possible.

zolpidem tartrate

Ambien

Controlled Substance Schedule IV

Pregnancy Risk Category: B

HOW SUPPLIED

Tablets: 5 mg, 10 mg

MECHANISM OF ACTION

Although zolpidem interacts with one of three identified GABA-benzodiazepine (gamma-aminobutyric acid-benzodiazepine) receptor complexes, it's not a benzodiazepine. It exhibits hypnotic activity, but no muscle relaxant or anticonvulsant properties.

INDICATIONS & DOSAGE

Short-term management of insomnia –
Adults: 10 mg P.O. immediately before bedtime.
Elderly or debilitated patients; patients with hepatic insufficiency: 5 mg P.O. immediately before bedtime.

Maximum daily dose is 10 mg.

ADVERSE REACTIONS

Common reactions are in italics; life-threatening reactions are in bold italics.
CNS: daytime drowsiness, light-headedness, abnormal dreams, amnesia, dizziness, headache, hangover effect, sleep disorder.
EENT: sinusitis, pharyngitis.
GI: nausea, vomiting, diarrhea, dry mouth.
Other: back or chest pain, influenza-

like symptoms, allergy, rash, palpitations.

INTERACTIONS
Alcohol, CNS depressants: enhanced CNS depression. Avoid concomitant use.

NURSING CONSIDERATIONS
- *Contraindicated* in patients with hypersensitivity to the drug.
- *Use cautiously* in patients with compromised respiratory status because hypnotics may depress respiratory drive and in patients with depression or a history of alcohol or drug abuse.
- Hypnotics should be used only for short-term management of insomnia, usually 7 to 10 days. Persistent insomnia may indicate a primary psychiatric or medical disorder. Patient should be reevaluated if drug is taken for more than 2 to 3 weeks. Usually, prescriptions for this drug should provide a maximum of 1 month's supply.
- Because most adverse reactions are dose-related, the smallest effective dose should be used in all patients, but especially in elderly and debilitated patients.
- Hypnotics may uncover underlying psychiatric illness. Patient may display abnormal thinking or behavior, such as aggression or assertiveness, because drug decreases inhibition similarly to alcohol or other CNS depressants. Other behavioral changes may include agitation, depersonalization, hallucinations, amnesia, worsening depression, and suicidal thinking. It's unknown if these symptoms are drug-related. Careful and immediate evaluation is necessary.
- Although abrupt discontinuation of hypnotics after prolonged therapy is commonly associated with withdrawal syndrome, there's no clear evidence of such a syndrome after abrupt termination of zolpidem therapy.
- Take precautions to prevent hoarding or self-overdosing by patients who are depressed, suicidal, or drug-dependent or who have a history of drug abuse.
- Zolpidem overdose may be treated with flumazenil, a specific benzodiazepine antagonist; however, because the mean elimination half-life of zolpidem, (2½ hours), is longer than that of flumazenil, repeated doses of flumazenil may be necessary.
- Supervise walking; raise bed rails, especially for elderly patients.
- Food decreases drug's absorption. For faster onset of sleep, instruct patient not to take drug with or immediately after meals.

29
Anticonvulsants

acetazolamide sodium
(See Chapter 60, DIURETICS.)
carbamazepine
clonazepam
diazepam
(See Chapter 31, ANTIANXIETY AGENTS.)
ethosuximide
ethotoin
magnesium sulfate
mephenytoin
mephobarbital
methsuximide
paramethadione
phenacemide
phenobarbital
phenobarbital sodium
phensuximide
phenytoin
phenytoin sodium
phenytoin sodium (extended)
phenytoin sodium (prompt)
primidone
trimethadione
valproate sodium
valproic acid
divalproex sodium

COMBINATION PRODUCTS
DILANTIN WITH PHENOBARBITAL: phenytoin sodium 100 mg and phenobarbital 16 mg; phenytoin sodium 100 mg and phenobarbital 32 mg.

carbamazepine
Apo-Carbamazepine†, Epitol, Mazepine†, Tegretol, Tegretol CR†, Teril‡
Pregnancy Risk Category: C

HOW SUPPLIED
Tablets: 200 mg
Tablets (chewable): 100 mg
Oral suspension: 100 mg/5 ml

MECHANISM OF ACTION
Stabilizes neuronal membranes and limits seizure activity by either increasing efflux or decreasing influx of sodium ions across cell membranes in the motor cortex during generation of nerve impulses.

INDICATIONS & DOSAGE
Generalized tonic-clonic and complex-partial seizures, mixed seizure patterns –
Adults and children over 12 years: initially, 200 mg P.O. b.i.d. May increase by 200 mg P.O. daily, in divided doses at 6- to 8-hour intervals. Adjust to minimum effective level when control achieved.
Children under 12 years: 10 to 20 mg/kg P.O. daily in two to four divided doses.
Trigeminal neuralgia –
Adults: initially, 100 mg P.O. b.i.d. with meals. Increase by 100 mg q 12 hours until pain is relieved. Don't exceed 1.2 g daily. Maintenance dose is 200 to 400 mg P.O. b.i.d.

ADVERSE REACTIONS
Common reactions are in italics; life-threatening reactions are in bold italics.
Blood: ***aplastic anemia, agranulocytosis,*** eosinophilia, leukocytosis, ***thrombocytopenia.***
CNS: dizziness, *vertigo, drowsiness,* fatigue, *ataxia,* ***worsening of seizures.***
CV: ***CHF,*** hypertension, hypotension, aggravation of coronary artery disease.
EENT: conjunctivitis, dry mouth and pharynx, blurred vision, diplopia, nystagmus.
GI: *nausea,* vomiting, abdominal pain, diarrhea, anorexia, *stomatitis,* glossitis.

†Available in Canada only. ‡Available in Australia only. ◇Available OTC.

GU: urinary frequency, urine retention, impotence, albuminuria, glycosuria, elevated BUN.
Hepatic: abnormal liver function tests, ***hepatitis.***
Metabolic: water intoxication.
Skin: *rash,* urticaria, erythema multiforme, ***Stevens-Johnson syndrome.***
Other: diaphoresis, fever, chills, pulmonary hypersensitivity.

INTERACTIONS

Lithium: increased CNS toxicity of lithium. Avoid concomitant use.
Phenytoin, primidone, phenobarbital, nicotinic acid: may decrease carbamazepine levels. Monitor for decreased effect.
Phenytoin, warfarin, doxycycline, theophylline, haloperidol: carbamazepine may decrease blood levels of these drugs. Monitor for decreased effect.
Propoxyphene, troleandomycin, erythromycin, isoniazid, verapamil: may increase carbamazepine blood levels. Use cautiously.

NURSING CONSIDERATIONS

• *Contraindicated* in patients with bone marrow suppression or hypersensitivity to carbamazepine or tricyclic antidepressants and in patients who have taken an MAO inhibitor within 14 days of therapy.
• *Use cautiously* in cardiac, renal, or hepatic damage and increased intraocular pressure. Also use cautiously in children with mixed seizure disorders because they may experience an increased incidence of seizures (usually atypical absence or generalized seizures).
• When used in the management of seizures, institute appropriate seizure precautions.
• Tell patient to keep tablets in their original container, tightly closed and away from moisture. Some formulations may harden when exposed to excess moisture, resulting in decreased bioavailability and loss of seizure control.
• Shake oral suspension well before measuring dose.
• When administering by nasogastric tube, mix dose with an equal volume of water, 0.9% sodium chloride solution, or dextrose 5% in water. Flush tube with 100 ml of diluent after administering dose.
• Not effective in treating absence seizures.
• Warn patient to avoid hazardous activities that require alertness and good psychomotor coordination until CNS effects of the drug are known.
• May cause mild to moderate dizziness and drowsiness when first taken. Effect usually disappears within 3 to 4 days. Should be taken three times a day, when possible, to provide consistent blood levels.
• Observe for signs of anorexia or subtle appetite changes, which may indicate excessive blood levels.
• Never discontinue the drug suddenly when treating seizures or status epilepticus. Notify doctor immediately if adverse reactions occur.
• Obtain baseline determinations of urinalysis, BUN, liver function, CBC, platelet and reticulocyte counts, and serum iron levels. Then, periodic monitoring is recommended.
• Periodic eye examinations are recommended.
• Tell patient to notify doctor immediately if fever, sore throat, mouth ulcers, or easy bruising or bleeding occur.
• Therapeutic carbamazepine blood level is 3 to 9 mcg/ml.
• Monitor blood levels and effects closely. Ask patient when last dose of medication was taken to approximately evaluate blood levels.
• When used for trigeminal neuralgia, an attempt should be made every 3 months to decrease dosage or withdraw drug.

*Liquid form contains alcohol. **May contain tartrazine.

• Adverse reactions may be minimized by increasing dosage gradually.
• An alternative to lithium in treatment of some affective disorders.
• Patient may take with food to minimize GI distress.

clonazepam

Klonopin, Rivotril
Controlled Substance Schedule IV
Pregnancy Risk Category: C

HOW SUPPLIED
Tablets: 0.5 mg, 1 mg, 2 mg
Drops: 2.5 mg/ml‡
Injection: 1 mg/ml‡

MECHANISM OF ACTION
Appears to act on the limbic system, thalamus, and hypothalamus to produce anticonvulsant effects. A benzodiazepine.

INDICATIONS & DOSAGE
Lennox-Gastaut syndrome and atypical absence seizures; akinetic and myoclonic seizures –
Adults: initial dosage should not exceed 1.5 mg P.O. daily in three divided doses. May be increased by 0.5 to 1 mg q 3 days until seizures are controlled. If given in unequal doses, the largest dose should be given h.s. Maximum recommended daily dosage is 20 mg.
Children up to 10 years or 30 kg: 0.01 to 0.03 mg/kg P.O. daily (not to exceed 0.05 mg/kg daily), divided q 8 hours. Increase dosage by 0.25 to 0.5 mg q third day to a maximum maintenance dosage of 0.1 to 0.2 mg/kg daily.
Status epilepticus (where parenteral form is available) –
Adults: 1 mg by slow I.V. infusion.
Children: 0.5 mg by slow I.V. infusion.

ADVERSE REACTIONS
Common reactions are in italics; life-threatening reactions are in bold italics.
Blood: leukopenia, thrombocytopenia, eosinophilia.
CNS: *drowsiness, ataxia, behavioral disturbances (especially in children),* slurred speech, tremor, confusion.
EENT: *increased salivation,* diplopia, nystagmus, abnormal eye movements.
GI: constipation, gastritis, change in appetite, nausea, abnormal thirst, sore gums.
GU: dysuria, enuresis, nocturia, urinary retention.
Skin: rash.
Other: ***respiratory depression.***

INTERACTIONS
Alcohol, CNS depressants: increased CNS depression. Monitor closely.

NURSING CONSIDERATIONS
• *Contraindicated* in hepatic disease; chlordiazepoxide, diazepam, or other benzodiazepine sensitivity; or acute narrow-angle glaucoma.
• *Use cautiously* in patients with mixed seizure types because drug may precipitate generalized tonic-clonic seizures and in those with chronic respiratory disease, impaired renal function, and open-angle glaucoma.
• Therapeutic blood level is 20 to 80 ng/ml.
• Elderly patients are more sensitive to the drug's CNS effects.
• Warn patient to avoid activities that require alertness and good psychomotor coordination until CNS effects of the drug are known.
• Never withdraw drug suddenly. Call doctor at once if adverse reactions develop.
• Obtain periodic CBC and liver function tests.
• Monitor patient for oversedation.
• Withdrawal symptoms similar to those of barbiturates.
• Clonazepam may interfere with

children's attentiveness in school. Instruct parents to monitor child's school performance.
• **I.V. use:** Administer by slow infusion.

ethosuximide
Zarontin
Pregnancy Risk Category: C

HOW SUPPLIED
Capsules: 250 mg
Syrup: 250 mg/5 ml

MECHANISM OF ACTION
Increases seizure threshold. Reduces the paroxysmal spike-and-wave pattern of absence seizures by depressing nerve transmission in the motor cortex. A succinimide derivative.

INDICATIONS & DOSAGE
Absence seizure –
Adults and children over 6 years: initially, 250 mg P.O. b.i.d. May increase by 250 mg q 4 to 7 days up to 1.5 g daily.
Children 3 to 6 years: 250 mg P.O. daily or 125 mg P.O. b.i.d. May increase by 250 mg q 4 to 7 days up to 1.5 g daily.

ADVERSE REACTIONS
Common reactions are in italics; life-threatening reactions are in bold italics.
Blood: leukopenia, eosinophilia, ***agranulocytosis,*** pancytopenia, ***aplastic anemia.***
CNS: *drowsiness,* headache, *fatigue, dizziness,* ataxia, irritability, hiccups, *euphoria, lethargy.*
EENT: myopia.
GI: *nausea, vomiting,* diarrhea, gum hypertrophy, weight loss, cramps, tongue swelling, *anorexia, epigastric and abdominal pain.*
GU: vaginal bleeding.
Skin: urticaria, pruritic and erythematous rashes, hirsutism.

INTERACTIONS
None significant.

NURSING CONSIDERATIONS
• *Contraindicated* in hypersensitivity to succinimide derivatives.
• *Use cautiously* in hepatic or renal disease.
• Never withdraw drug suddenly. Abrupt withdrawal may precipitate absence seizures. Call doctor immediately if adverse reactions develop.
• Warn patient to avoid activities that require alertness and good psychomotor coordination until CNS effects of the drug are known.
• Obtain CBC every 3 to 6 months.
• Therapeutic blood levels are 40 to 80 mcg/ml.
• May increase frequency of generalized tonic-clonic seizures when used alone in patients who have mixed types of seizures.
• May cause positive direct Coombs' test.
• Currently the drug of choice for treating absence seizures.
• Patient may take with food to minimize GI distress.

ethotoin
Peganone
Pregnancy Risk Category: D

HOW SUPPLIED
Tablets: 250 mg, 500 mg

MECHANISM OF ACTION
Stabilizes neuronal membranes and limits seizure activity by either increasing efflux or decreasing influx of sodium ions across cell membranes in the motor cortex during generation of nerve impulses. Hydantoin derivative.

INDICATIONS & DOSAGE
Generalized tonic-clonic or complex-partial seizures –
Adults: initially, 250 mg P.O. q.i.d.

*Liquid form contains alcohol. **May contain tartrazine.

after meals. May increase slowly over several days to 3 g daily divided q.i.d.
Children: initially, 250 mg P.O. b.i.d. May increase up to 250 mg P.O. q.i.d.

ADVERSE REACTIONS
Common reactions are in italics; life-threatening reactions are in bold italics.
Blood: thrombocytopenia, leukopenia, ***agranulocytosis, pancytopenia,*** megaloblastic anemia.
CNS: fatigue, insomnia, dizziness, headache, numbness.
CV: chest pain.
EENT: diplopia, nystagmus.
GI: *nausea, vomiting, diarrhea,* gingival hyperplasia (rare).
Skin: rash.
Other: fever, lymphadenopathy.

INTERACTIONS
Alcohol, folic acid: monitor for decreased ethotoin activity.
Oral anticoagulants, antihistamines, chloramphenicol, cimetidine, diazepam, diazoxide, disulfiram, isoniazid, phenylbutazone, salicylates, sulfamethizole, valproate: monitor for increased ethotoin activity and toxicity.
Phenacemide: paranoia. Use together cautiously.

NURSING CONSIDERATIONS
- *Contraindicated* in hydantoin hypersensitivity or hepatic or hematologic disorders.
- *Use cautiously* in patients receiving other hydantoin derivatives.
- Never withdraw drug suddenly. Call doctor at once if adverse reactions develop.
- Warn patient to avoid activities that require alertness and good psychomotor coordination until CNS effects of the drug are known.
- Obtain CBC and urinalysis when therapy starts and periodically thereafter. Also, periodically monitor liver function tests on long-term use.
- Give after meals. Schedule doses as evenly as possible over 24 hours.
- Discontinue drug if lymphadenopathy or lupus-like syndrome (fever, bruising, and sore throat) develops.
- Heavy use of alcohol may diminish benefits of drug.
- Hydantoin derivative of choice in young adults who are prone to gingival hyperplasia caused by phenytoin. Otherwise, infrequently used in the treatment of epilepsy.
- Ethotoin generally produces milder adverse reactions than phenytoin; however, the large doses required to maintain its therapeutic effect frequently cause GI distress.

magnesium sulfate

Pregnancy Risk Category: B

HOW SUPPLIED
Injection: 10% (0.8 mEq/ml), 12.5% (1 mEq/ml), 25% (2 mEq/ml), 50% (4 mEq/ml)

MECHANISM OF ACTION
May decrease acetylcholine released by nerve impulses, but its anticonvulsant mechanism is unknown.

INDICATIONS & DOSAGE
Hypomagnesemic seizures –
Adults: 1 to 2 g (as 10% solution) I.V. over 15 minutes, then 1 g I.M. q 4 to 6 hours, based on patient response and blood magnesium levels.
Seizures secondary to hypomagnesemia in acute nephritis –
Children: 0.2 ml/kg of 50% solution I.M. q 4 to 6 hours, p.r.n. or 100 mg/kg of 10% solution I.V. very slowly. Titrate dosage according to blood magnesium levels and seizure response.
Prevention or control of seizures in preeclampsia or eclampsia –
Women: initially, 4 g I.V. in 250 ml dextrose 5% in water and 4 g deep I.M. each buttock; then 4 g deep I.M.

into alternate buttock q 4 hours, p.r.n. Alternatively, 4 g I.V. loading dose followed by 1 to 4 g hourly as an I.V. infusion.
Management of paroxysmal atrial tachycardia –
Adults: 3 to 4 g I.V. over 30 seconds.
Management of life-threatening ventricular arrhythmias, such as sustained ventricular tachycardia or torsades de pointes –
Adults: 2 to 6 g I.V. over several minutes, followed by a continuous infusion of 3 to 20 mg/minute for 5 to 48 hours. Dosage and duration of therapy depend on patient response and serum magnesium levels.

ADVERSE REACTIONS
Common reactions are in italics; life-threatening reactions are in bold italics.
CNS: *sweating,* drowsiness, *depressed reflexes,* flaccid paralysis, hypothermia.
CV: *hypotension, flushing,* ***circulatory collapse,*** depressed cardiac function, ***heart block.***
Other: ***respiratory paralysis,*** hypocalcemia.

INTERACTIONS
Anesthetics, CNS depressants: may cause additive CNS depression. Use cautiously.
Neuromuscular blocking agents: may cause increased neuromuscular blockade. Use cautiously.

NURSING CONSIDERATIONS
- *Use cautiously* in patients with arrhythmias, impaired renal function, myocardial damage, and heart block and in women in labor.
- Drug can decrease the frequency and force of uterine contractions. Has been used as a tocolytic agent (suppresses uterine contractions) to inhibit premature labor.
- If used to treat seizures, institute appropriate seizure precautions.
- Keep I.V. calcium gluconate available to reverse magnesium intoxication; however, use cautiously in patients undergoing digitalization because of danger of arrhythmias.
- **I.V. use:** Monitor vital signs every 15 minutes when giving drug I.V.
- Watch for respiratory depression and signs of heart block. Respirations should be approximately 16 breaths/minute before each dose given.
- Monitor intake and output. Urine output should be 100 ml or more in 4-hour period before each dose.
- Check blood magnesium levels after repeated doses. Disappearance of knee-jerk and patellar reflexes is a sign of pending magnesium toxicity.
- Maximum infusion rate is 150 mg/minute. Rapid drip will induce uncomfortable feeling of heat.
- Especially when given I.V. to toxemic mothers within 24 hours before delivery, observe neonates for signs of magnesium toxicity, including neuromuscular or respiratory depression.
- Signs of hypermagnesemia begin to appear at blood levels of 4 mEq/liter.

mephenytoin
Mesantoin

Pregnancy Risk Category: C

HOW SUPPLIED
Tablets: 100 mg

MECHANISM OF ACTION
Stabilizes neuronal membranes and limits seizure activity by either increasing efflux or decreasing influx of sodium ions across cell membranes in the motor cortex during generation of nerve impulses. Hydantoin derivative.

INDICATIONS & DOSAGE
Generalized tonic-clonic or complex-partial seizures –
Adults: 50 to 100 mg P.O. daily. May increase by 50 to 100 mg at weekly intervals up to 200 mg P.O. t.i.d.
Children: initially, 50 to 100 mg P.O.

*Liquid form contains alcohol. **May contain tartrazine.

daily or 100 to 450 mg/m² P.O. daily in three divided doses. May increase slowly by 50 to 100 mg at weekly intervals up to 200 mg P.O. t.i.d., divided q 8 hours. Dosage must be adjusted individually.

ADVERSE REACTIONS
Common reactions are in italics; life-threatening reactions are in bold italics.
Blood: ***leukopenia, neutropenia, agranulocytosis, thrombocytopenia, pancytopenia,*** eosinophilia.
CNS: ataxia, *drowsiness,* fatigue, irritability, choreiform movements, depression, tremor, sleeplessness, dizziness (usually transient).
EENT: conjunctivitis, diplopia, nystagmus.
GI: gingival hyperplasia, nausea and vomiting (with prolonged use).
Skin: *rashes,* ***exfoliative dermatitis.***
Other: hypertrichosis, edema, dysarthria, lymphadenopathy, polyarthropathy, ***pulmonary fibrosis,*** photosensitivity.

INTERACTIONS
Alcohol, folic acid: monitor for decreased mephenytoin activity.
Oral anticoagulants, antihistamines, chloramphenicol, cimetidine, diazepam, diazoxide, disulfiram, isoniazid, phenylbutazone, salicylates, sulfamethizole, valproate: monitor for increased mephenytoin activity and toxicity.

NURSING CONSIDERATIONS
- *Contraindicated* in hydantoin hypersensitivity.
- *Use cautiously* in patients receiving other hydantoin derivatives.
- Periodically monitor liver function studies with long-term use. Check baseline CBC and platelet count and periodically thereafter. Discontinue drug if neutrophil count becomes less than 1,600/mm³.
- Never withdraw drug suddenly. Call doctor if adverse reactions develop.
- Therapeutic blood level of mephenytoin and its active metabolite is 25 to 40 mcg/ml.
- Heavy use of alcohol may diminish benefit of drug.
- Potentially life-threatening blood dyscrasias limit this drug's usefulness.
- Tell patient to notify doctor if fever, sore throat, bleeding, or rash occurs.
- Warn patient to avoid activities that require alertness and good psychomotor coordination until CNS effects of the drug are known.

mephobarbital
Mebaral
Controlled Substance Schedule IV
Pregnancy Risk Category: D

HOW SUPPLIED
Tablets: 32 mg, 50 mg, 100 mg

MECHANISM OF ACTION
Depresses monosynaptic and polysynaptic transmission in the CNS and increases the threshold for seizure activity in the motor cortex. A barbiturate.

INDICATIONS & DOSAGE
Generalized tonic-clonic or absence seizures –
Adults: 400 to 600 mg P.O. daily or in divided doses.
Children: 6 to 12 mg/kg P.O. daily, divided q 6 to 8 hours (smaller doses are given initially and increased over 4 to 5 days as needed).

ADVERSE REACTIONS
Common reactions are in italics; life-threatening reactions are in bold italics.
Blood: megaloblastic anemia, ***agranulocytosis,*** thrombocytopenia.
CNS: *dizziness,* headache, *hangover,* confusion, paradoxical excitation, exacerbation of existing pain, drowsiness.
CV: hypotension, bradycardia.

GI: nausea, vomiting, epigastric pain.
Skin: urticaria, morbilliform rash, blisters, purpura, ***erythema multiforme.***
Other: allergic reactions (facial edema).

INTERACTIONS
Alcohol and other CNS depressants, including narcotic analgesics: excessive CNS depression. Use cautiously.
Griseofulvin: decreased absorption of griseofulvin.
MAO inhibitors: potentiated barbiturate effect. Monitor patient for increased CNS and respiratory depression.
Oral anticoagulants, estrogens and oral contraceptives, doxycycline, corticosteroids: mephobarbital may enhance the metabolism of these drugs. Monitor for decreased effect.
Rifampin: may decrease barbiturate levels. Monitor for decreased effect.

NURSING CONSIDERATIONS
- *Contraindicated* in barbiturate hypersensitivity, porphyria, or respiratory disease with dyspnea or obstruction.
- *Use cautiously* in hepatic, renal, cardiac, or respiratory function impairment; myasthenia gravis; and myxedema.
- Never withdraw drug suddenly. Call doctor at once if adverse reactions develop.
- Warn patient to avoid activities that require alertness and good psychomotor coordination until CNS effects of drug are known.
- Store in light-resistant container.
- In adults, give total or largest dose at night if seizures occur then.
- Three-quarters of drug is metabolized to phenobarbital; therapeutic blood levels as phenobarbital are 15 to 40 mcg/ml.
- Periodically monitor CBC, BUN, and creatinine.
- Women who use oral contraceptives should consider alternate birth control methods when receiving this drug because it may enhance contraceptive hormone metabolism and decrease its effectiveness.
- Suppresses REM sleep, as do other barbiturates. When drug is discontinued, patient may experience increased dreaming.

methsuximide
Celontin
Pregnancy Risk Category: C

HOW SUPPLIED
Capsules: 150 mg, 300 mg

MECHANISM OF ACTION
Increases seizure threshold. Reduces the paroxysmal spike-and-wave pattern of absence seizures by depressing nerve transmission in the motor cortex. A succinimide derivative.

INDICATIONS & DOSAGE
Refractory absence seizures –
Adults and children: initially, 300 mg P.O. daily. May increase by 300 mg weekly. Maximum daily dosage is 1.2 g in divided doses.

ADVERSE REACTIONS
Common reactions are in italics; life-threatening reactions are in bold italics.
Blood: eosinophilia, ***leukopenia,*** monocytosis, ***pancytopenia.***
CNS: *drowsiness, ataxia, dizziness,* irritability, nervousness, headache, insomnia, confusion, depression, aggressiveness.
EENT: blurred vision, photophobia, periorbital edema.
GI: *nausea, vomiting, anorexia,* diarrhea, weight loss, abdominal or epigastric pain.
Skin: urticaria, pruritic and erythematous rashes.

*Liquid form contains alcohol. **May contain tartrazine.

INTERACTIONS
None significant.

NURSING CONSIDERATIONS
- *Contraindicated* in hypersensitivity to succinimide derivatives.
- *Use cautiously* in hepatic or renal dysfunction.
- Never change or withdraw drug suddenly. Abrupt withdrawal may precipitate absence seizures. Call doctor immediately if adverse reactions develop.
- Warn patient to avoid activities that require alertness and good psychomotor coordination until CNS effects of the drug are known.
- Obtain CBC, urinalysis, and liver function tests periodically.
- Tell patient to call doctor promptly if lupus-like syndrome develops.
- May color urine pink or brown.
- Not as popular an anticonvulsant as ethosuximide.

paramethadione
Paradione* **
Pregnancy Risk Category: D

HOW SUPPLIED
Capsules: 150 mg, 300 mg
Oral solution: 300 mg/ml (65% alcohol) with dropper

MECHANISM OF ACTION
Raises the threshold for cortical seizures but does not modify seizure pattern. Decreases projection of focal activity and reduces both repetitive spinal-cord transmission and spike-and-wave patterns of absence (petit mal) seizures.

INDICATIONS & DOSAGE
Refractory absence seizures –
Adults: initially, 300 mg P.O. t.i.d. May increase by 300 mg weekly, up to 600 mg q.i.d., if needed.
Children over 6 years: 0.9 g P.O. daily in divided doses t.i.d. or q.i.d.
Children 2 to 6 years: 0.6 g P.O. daily in divided doses t.i.d. or q.i.d.
Children under 2 years: 0.3 g P.O. daily in divided doses b.i.d.

ADVERSE REACTIONS
Common reactions are in italics; life-threatening reactions are in bold italics.
Blood: ***neutropenia, leukopenia,*** eosinophilia, ***thrombocytopenia, pancytopenia, agranulocytosis, hypoplastic and aplastic anemia.***
CNS: *drowsiness,* fatigue, vertigo, headache, paresthesias, irritability.
CV: hypertension, hypotension.
EENT: hemeralopia, photophobia, diplopia, epistaxis, retinal hemorrhage.
GI: nausea, vomiting, abdominal pain, weight loss, bleeding gums.
GU: albuminuria, vaginal bleeding.
Hepatic: abnormal liver function tests.
Skin: acneiform or morbilliform rash, ***exfoliative dermatitis, erythema multiforme,*** petechiae, alopecia.
Other: lymphadenopathy, lupus erythematosus.

INTERACTIONS
None significant.

NURSING CONSIDERATIONS
- *Contraindicated* in renal and hepatic dysfunction or severe blood dyscrasia.
- *Use cautiously* in retinal or optic nerve diseases.
- Nausea, dizziness, and visual disturbances can be signs of overdosage. Patient should call doctor at once if these signs appear.
- Never withdraw drug suddenly. Call doctor at once if adverse reactions develop.
- Discontinue drug if scotomata or signs of hepatitis, systemic lupus erythematosus, lymphadenopathy, skin rash, nephrosis, hair loss, or generalized tonic-clonic seizures appear.
- Tell patient to report sore throat, fe-

ver, malaise, bruises, petechiae, or epistaxis to doctor immediately. Advise patient to wear dark glasses if photosensitivity occurs. Warn him not to drive car or operate machinery until CNS effects of the drug are known.
• Obtain liver function studies and urinalysis before therapy; then monthly.
• Dilute oral solution with water before giving because it contains 65% alcohol.
• Give drug with food or milk to minimize GI upset.
• Monitor CBC. Discontinue drug if neutrophil count falls below 2,500/mm³.

phenacemide

Phenurone

Pregnancy Risk Category: D

HOW SUPPLIED

Tablets: 500 mg

MECHANISM OF ACTION

Stabilizes neuronal membranes and limits seizure activity by either increasing efflux or decreasing influx of sodium ions across cell membranes in the motor cortex during generation of nerve impulses. Hydantoin derivative.

INDICATIONS & DOSAGE

Refractory, complex-partial, generalized tonic-clonic, absence, and atypical absence seizures –
Adults: 500 mg P.O. t.i.d. May increase by 500 mg weekly up to 5 g daily, p.r.n.
Children 5 to 10 years: 250 mg P.O. t.i.d. May increase by 250 mg weekly, up to 1.5 g daily, p.r.n.

ADVERSE REACTIONS

Common reactions are in italics; life-threatening reactions are in bold italics.
Blood: *aplastic anemia, agranulocytosis,* leukopenia.
CNS: drowsiness, dizziness, insomnia, headaches, paresthesias, *depression, suicidal tendencies,* aggressiveness.
GI: anorexia, weight loss.
GU: nephritis with marked albuminuria.
Hepatic: hepatitis, jaundice.
Skin: rashes.

INTERACTIONS

Ethotoin: paranoia. Use together cautiously.
Other anticonvulsants: enhanced risk of toxicity.

NURSING CONSIDERATIONS

• *Contraindicated* in patients with preexisting personality disturbances or in patients achieving satisfactory seizure control with other anticonvulsants.
• *Use cautiously* in patients with hepatic dysfunction or history of allergy, and when a hydantoin derivative is used concomitantly.
• Extremely toxic. Use drug only when other anticonvulsants are ineffective.
• Obtain liver function tests, CBCs, and urinalyses before and at monthly intervals during therapy.
• Tell patient to report sore throat or fever to doctor immediately.
• Warn patient to avoid activities that require alertness or good psychomotor coordination until CNS effects of the drug are known.
• Never withdraw drug suddenly. Call doctor at once if adverse reactions develop.
• Tell patient's family to watch for personality or psychological changes and report them to doctor at once.
• When phenacemide replaces another anticonvulsant, phenacemide dosage should be increased slowly while the dosage of the drug being discontinued is decreased slowly to maintain adequate seizure control.
• Notify doctor if patient develops jaundice or other signs of hepatitis,

abnormal urinary findings, or WBC count below 4,000/mm³.

phenobarbital (phenobarbitone)

Barbita, Gardenal†, Luminal†, Solfoton

phenobarbital sodium (phenobarbitone sodium)

Luminal Sodium†

Controlled Substance Schedule IV
Pregnancy Risk Category: D

HOW SUPPLIED

Tablets: 8 mg, 15 mg, 16 mg, 30 mg, 32 mg, 60 mg, 65 mg, 100 mg
Capsules: 16 mg
Oral solution: 15 mg/5 ml, 20 mg/5 ml
Elixir: 20 mg/5 ml
Injection: 30 mg/ml, 60 mg/ml, 65 mg/ml, 130 mg/ml
Powder for injection: 120 mg/ampule

MECHANISM OF ACTION

Depresses monosynaptic and polysynaptic transmission in the CNS and increases the threshold for seizure activity in the motor cortex. As a sedative, probably interferes with transmission of impulses from the thalamus to the cortex of the brain. A barbiturate.

INDICATIONS & DOSAGE

All forms of epilepsy, febrile seizures in children –
Adults: 100 to 200 mg P.O. daily, divided t.i.d. or given as single dosage h.s.
Children: 4 to 6 mg/kg P.O. daily, usually divided q 12 hours. It can, however, be administered once daily, usually h.s.
Status epilepticus –
Adults: 10 mg/kg as I.V. infusion no faster than 50 mg/minute. May give up to 20 mg/kg total. Administer in acute care or emergency area only.
Children: 5 to 10 mg/kg I.V. May repeat q 10 to 15 minutes up to total of 20 mg/kg. I.V. injection rate should not exceed 50 mg/minute.
Sedation –
Adults: 30 to 120 mg P.O. daily in two or three divided doses.
Children: 6 mg/kg P.O. divided t.i.d.
Insomnia –
Adults: 100 to 320 mg P.O. or I.M.
Children: 3 to 6 mg/kg.
Preoperative sedation –
Adults: 100 to 200 mg I.M. 60 to 90 minutes before surgery.
Children: 16 to 100 mg I.M. 60 to 90 minutes before surgery.
Hyperbilirubinemia –
Neonates: 7 mg/kg daily P.O. from first to fifth day of life; or 5 mg/kg daily I.M. on first day, repeated P.O. on second to seventh days.
Chronic cholestasis –
Adults: 90 to 180 mg P.O. daily in two or three divided doses.
Children under 12 years: 3 to 12 mg/kg daily P.O. in two or three divided doses.

ADVERSE REACTIONS

Common reactions are in italics; life-threatening reactions are in bold italics.
CNS: *drowsiness, lethargy, hangover,* paradoxical excitement in elderly patients.
GI: nausea, vomiting.
Skin: rash, ***Stevens-Johnson syndrome,*** urticaria.
Local: pain, swelling, thrombophlebitis, necrosis, nerve injury.
Other: ***angioedema.***

INTERACTIONS

Alcohol and other CNS depressants, including narcotic analgesics: excessive CNS depression. Use cautiously.
Diazepam: increased effects of both drugs. Use together cautiously.
Griseofulvin: decreased absorption of griseofulvin.
MAO inhibitors: potentiated barbitu-

†Available in Canada only. ‡Available in Australia only. ◇Available OTC.

rate effect. Monitor for increased CNS and respiratory depression.
Oral anticoagulants, estrogens and oral contraceptives, doxycycline, corticosteroids: may enhance the metabolism of these drugs. Monitor for decreased effect.
Primidone: monitor for excessive phenobarbital blood levels.
Rifampin: may decrease barbiturate levels. Monitor for decreased effect.
Valproic acid: increased phenobarbital levels. Monitor for toxicity.

NURSING CONSIDERATIONS

- *Contraindicated* in barbiturate hypersensitivity, porphyria, hepatic dysfunction, respiratory disease with dyspnea or obstruction, and nephritis; and in breast-feeding women.
- *Use cautiously* in hyperthyroidism, diabetes mellitus, and anemia and in elderly or debilitated patients.
- Elderly patients are more sensitive to the drug's effects.
- **I.V. use:** I.V. injection should be reserved for emergency treatment and should be given slowly under close supervision. Monitor respirations closely. When administering I.V., do not give more than 60 mg/minute. Have resuscitation equipment readily available.
- Give I.M. injection deeply. Superficial injection may cause pain, sterile abscess, and tissue sloughing.
- Do not use injectable solution if it contains a precipitate.
- Do not mix parenteral form with acidic solutions; precipitation may result.
- Watch for signs of barbiturate toxicity: coma, asthmatic breathing, cyanosis, clammy skin, and hypotension. Overdose can be fatal.
- Warn patient to avoid activities that require alertness and good psychomotor coordination until CNS effects of the drug are known.
- Don't stop drug abruptly. Call doctor immediately if adverse reactions develop.
- Full therapeutic effects not seen for 2 to 3 weeks, except when loading dose is used.
- Therapeutic blood levels are 15 to 40 mcg/ml.
- Make sure patient is aware that phenobarbital is available in different milligram strengths and sizes.

phensuximide

Milontin

Pregnancy Risk Category: D

HOW SUPPLIED

Capsules: 500 mg

MECHANISM OF ACTION

Increases seizure threshold. Reduces the paroxysmal spike-and-wave pattern of absence seizures by depressing nerve transmission in the motor cortex. A succinimide derivative.

INDICATIONS & DOSAGE

Absence seizures –
Adults and children: 500 mg to 1 g P.O. b.i.d. to t.i.d.

ADVERSE REACTIONS

Common reactions are in italics; life-threatening reactions are in bold italics.
Blood: transient leukopenia, ***pancytopenia, agranulocytosis.***
CNS: muscular weakness, *drowsiness,* dizziness, ataxia, headache.
GI: nausea, vomiting, anorexia.
GU: urinary frequency, renal damage, hematuria.
Skin: pruritus, eruptions, erythema.
Other: lupus-like syndrome.

INTERACTIONS

None significant.

NURSING CONSIDERATIONS

- *Contraindicated* in hypersensitivity to succinimide derivatives.

- *Use cautiously* in patients with hepatic or renal disease.
- Never withdraw drug suddenly. Abrupt withdrawal may precipitate absence seizures. Call doctor immediately if adverse reactions develop.
- Warn patient to avoid hazardous activities that require alertness and good coordination until CNS effects of the drug are known.
- Obtain CBC every 3 to 4 months; urinalysis and liver function tests every 6 months.
- Tell patient to report lupus-like symptoms immediately.
- May color urine pink or red to reddish brown.
- Therapeutic blood level 40 to 80 mcg/ml.
- May increase incidence of generalized tonic-clonic seizures if used alone to treat patients with mixed seizure types.

phenytoin (diphenylhydantoin)

Dilantin, Dilantin Infatabs, Dilantin-30 Pediatric, Dilantin-125

phenytoin sodium

Dilantin

phenytoin sodium (extended)

Dilantin Kapseals

phenytoin sodium (prompt)

Diphenylan

Pregnancy Risk Category: D

HOW SUPPLIED

phenytoin
Tablets (chewable): 50 mg
Oral suspension: 30 mg/5 ml, 125 mg/5 ml
phenytoin sodium
Capsules: 30 mg (27.6-mg base), 100 mg (92-mg base)
Injection: 50 mg/ml (46-mg base)
phenytoin sodium (extended)
Capsules: 30 mg (27.6-mg base), 100 mg (92-mg base)
phenytoin sodium (prompt)
Capsules: 30 mg (27.6-mg base), 100 mg (92 mg-base)

MECHANISM OF ACTION

Stabilizes neuronal membranes and limits seizure activity by either increasing efflux or decreasing influx of sodium ions across cell membranes in the motor cortex during generation of nerve impulses. Produces antiarrhythmic effect by normalizing sodium influx to Purkinje's fibers when used to treat digitalis-induced arrhythmias. A hydantoin derivative.

INDICATIONS & DOSAGE

Generalized tonic-clonic seizures, status epilepticus, nonepileptic seizures (post-head trauma, Reye's syndrome) –
Adults: loading dose is 900 mg to 1.5 g I.V. at 50 mg/minute or P.O. divided t.i.d., then start maintenance dosage of 300 mg P.O. daily (extended only) or divided t.i.d. (extended or prompt).
Children: loading dose is 15 mg/kg I.V. at 50 mg/minute or P.O. divided q 8 to 12 hours, then start maintenance dosage of 5 to 7 mg/kg P.O. or I.V. daily, divided q 12 hours.
If patient has not received phenytoin previously or has no detectable blood level, use loading dose –
Adults: 900 mg to 1.5 g I.V. divided into t.i.d. at 50 mg/minute. Do not exceed 500 mg each dose.
Children: 15 mg/kg I.V. at 50 mg/minute.
If patient has been receiving phenytoin but has missed one or more doses and has subtherapeutic levels –
Adults: 100 to 300 mg I.V. at 50 mg/minute.
Children: 5 to 7 mg/kg I.V. at 50 mg/minute. May repeat lower dose in 30 minutes if needed.

Neuritic pain (migraine, trigeminal neuralgia, Bell's palsy) –
Adults: 200 to 400 mg P.O. daily.
Ventricular arrhythmias unresponsive to lidocaine or procainamide; supraventricular and ventricular arrhythmias induced by cardiac glycosides –
Adults: loading dose is 1 g P.O. divided over first 24 hours, followed by 500 mg daily for 2 days, then maintenance dose of 300 mg P.O. daily; 250 mg I.V. over 5 minutes until arrhythmias subside, adverse reactions develop, or 1 g has been given. Infusion rate should never exceed 50 mg/minute (slow I.V. push).
Alternate method: 100 mg I.V. q 15 minutes until adverse reactions develop, arrhythmias are controlled, or 1 g has been given. May also administer entire loading dose of 1 g I.V. slowly at 25 mg/minute. Can be diluted in normal saline solution. I.M. dose not recommended because of pain and erratic absorption.
Children: 3 to 8 mg/kg P.O. or slow I.V. daily or 250 mg/m^2 daily given as single dose or in two divided doses.

ADVERSE REACTIONS

Common reactions are in italics; life-threatening reactions are in bold italics.
Blood: ***thrombocytopenia, leukopenia, agranulocytosis, pancytopenia,*** macrocytosis, megaloblastic anemia.
CNS: *ataxia, slurred speech, confusion,* dizziness, insomnia, nervousness, twitching, headache.
CV: hypotension, ***ventricular fibrillation.***
EENT: *nystagmus, diplopia,* blurred vision.
GI: *nausea, vomiting, gingival hyperplasia (especially children).*
Hepatic: ***toxic hepatitis.***
Skin: scarlatiniform or morbilliform rash; bullous, *exfoliative,* or purpuric dermatitis; ***Stevens-Johnson syndrome;*** lupus erythematosus; *hirsutism;* ***toxic epidermal necrolysis;*** photosensitivity.
Local: pain, necrosis, and inflammation at injection site; purple glove syndrome.
Other: periarteritis nodosa, lymphadenopathy, hyperglycemia, osteomalacia, hypertrichosis.

INTERACTIONS

Alcohol, dexamethasone, folic acid: monitor for decreased phenytoin activity.
Oral anticoagulants, antihistamines, amiodarone, chloramphenicol, cimetidine, cycloserine, diazepam, diazoxide, disulfiram, influenza vaccine, isoniazid, phenylbutazone, salicylates, sulfamethizole, valproate: monitor for increased phenytoin activity and toxicity.
Oral tube feedings with Osmolite or Isocal: may interfere with absorption of oral phenytoin. Schedule feedings as far as possible from drug administration.

NURSING CONSIDERATIONS

- *Contraindicated* in phenacemide or hydantoin hypersensitivity, bradycardia, SA and AV block, or Stokes-Adams syndrome.
- *Use cautiously* in hepatic or renal dysfunction, hypotension, myocardial insufficiency, and respiratory depression; in elderly or debilitated patients; and in patients receiving other hydantoin derivatives.
- Elderly patients tend to metabolize phenytoin slowly. Therefore, they may require lower dosages.
- If used to treat seizures, institute appropriate seizure precautions.
- Phenytoin requirements usually increase during pregnancy. Monitor serum levels closely.
- Don't withdraw drug suddenly. Call doctor at once if adverse reactions develop.
- Warn patient to avoid hazardous activities that require alertness and good

*Liquid form contains alcohol. **May contain tartrazine.

psychomotor coordination until CNS effects of the drug are known.
• **I.V. use:** Don't mix drug with dextrose 5% in water because it will precipitate. Clear I.V. tubing first with normal saline solution. Never use cloudy solution. May mix with normal saline solution if necessary and give as an infusion. Administer infusion over 30 to 60 minutes, when possible. Infusion must begin within 1 hour after preparation and should run through an in-line filter. Discard 4 hours after preparation. Preferably, administer slowly (50 mg/minute) as an I.V. bolus.
• Check patency of I.V. catheter before administering. Extravasation has caused severe local tissue damage.
• Check vital signs, especially ECG and blood pressure, during I.V. administration.
• Avoid administering I.V. push phenytoin into veins in the back of the hand to avoid discoloration known as purple glove syndrome. Inject into larger veins or central venous catheter if available.
• Do not give I.M. unless dosage adjustments are made. Drug may precipitate at injection site, cause pain, and be erratically absorbed.
• Obtain CBC and serum calcium levels every 6 months, and periodically monitor hepatic function. Doctor may order folic acid and vitamin B_{12} if megaloblastic anemia is evident.
• Drug may color urine pink, red, or reddish-brown.
• Tell patient to carry identification stating that he's taking phenytoin.
• Stress importance of good oral hygiene and regular dental examinations. Gingivectomy may be necessary periodically if dental hygiene is poor.
• Drug should be discontinued if rash appears. If rash is scarlet or measles-like, drug may be resumed after rash clears. If rash reappears, therapy should be discontinued. If rash is exfoliative, purpuric, or bullous, don't resume drug.
• Use only clear solution for injection. Slight yellow color acceptable. Don't refrigerate.
• Divided doses given with or after meals may decrease GI adverse reactions.
• Shake suspension well before each dose. Use solid forms (tablets or capsules) if possible.
• Therapeutic phenytoin blood level is 10 to 20 mcg/ml.
• Heavy use of alcohol may diminish benefits of drug.
• Phenytoin levels may be decreased in mononucleosis. Monitor for increased seizure activity.
• Dilantin brand and Bolar generic capsules are the only oral forms that can be given once daily. Toxic levels may result if any other brand is given once daily. Dilantin brand tablets and oral suspension should not be taken once daily.
• Advise patient not to change brands or dosage forms once stabilized on therapy.
• Suspension available as 30 mg/5 ml or 125 mg/5 ml. Read label carefully.
• Therapy with phenytoin may cause laboratory test interferences, including reduced serum protein-bound iodine and free thyroxine levels without clinical signs of hypothyroidism; a slight decrease in urinary 17-hydroxysteroid and 17-ketosteroid levels; increased urinary 6-ß hydroxycortisol excretion and serum levels of alkaline phosphatase or γ-glutamyltransferase; and decreased values for dexamethasone suppression or metyrapone tests.

primidone

Apo-Primidone†, Myidone, Mysoline, Sertan†

Pregnancy Risk Category: D

HOW SUPPLIED
Tablets: 50 mg, 250 mg
Oral suspension: 250 mg/5 ml

MECHANISM OF ACTION
Unknown, but some activity may be caused by phenobarbital, which is an active metabolite.

INDICATIONS & DOSAGE
Generalized tonic-clonic seizures, complex-partial seizures –
Adults and children over 8 years: 250 mg P.O. daily. Increase by 250 mg weekly, up to maximum of 2 g daily, divided q.i.d.
Children under 8 years: 125 mg P.O. daily. Increase by 125 mg weekly, up to maximum of 1 g daily, divided q.i.d.

ADVERSE REACTIONS
Common reactions are in italics; life-threatening reactions are in bold italics.
Blood: leukopenia, eosinophilia.
CNS: *drowsiness, ataxia,* emotional disturbances, vertigo, hyperirritability, fatigue.
EENT: *diplopia,* nystagmus, edema of the eyelids.
GI: anorexia, *nausea, vomiting.*
GU: impotence, polyuria.
Skin: morbilliform rash, alopecia.
Other: edema, thirst.

INTERACTIONS
Carbamazepine: increased primidone levels. Observe for toxicity.
Phenytoin: stimulated conversion of primidone to phenobarbital. Observe for increased phenobarbital effect.

NURSING CONSIDERATIONS
- *Contraindicated* in phenobarbital hypersensitivity or porphyria.
- Don't withdraw drug suddenly. Call doctor if adverse reactions develop.
- Warn patient to avoid hazardous activities that require alertness and good psychomotor coordination until CNS effects of the drug are known. Full therapeutic response may take 2 weeks or more.
- Therapeutic blood level of primidone is 5 to 12 mcg/ml. Therapeutic blood level of phenobarbital is 15 to 40 mcg/ml.
- CBC and routine blood chemistry should be done every 6 months.
- Partially converted to phenobarbital; use cautiously with phenobarbital.
- Shake liquid suspension well.

trimethadione
Tridione

Pregnancy Risk Category: D

HOW SUPPLIED
Capsules: 150 mg, 300 mg
Oral solution: 40 mg/ml

MECHANISM OF ACTION
Raises the threshold for cortical seizure but does not modify seizure pattern. Decreases projection of focal activity and reduces both repetitive spinal-cord transmission and spike-and-wave patterns of absence (petit mal) seizures. An oxazolidinedione derivative.

INDICATIONS & DOSAGE
Refractory absence seizures –
Adults and children over 13 years: initially, 300 mg P.O. t.i.d. May increase by 300 mg weekly up to 600 mg P.O. q.i.d.
Children: 13 mg/kg P.O. t.i.d. or 335 mg/m² P.O. t.i.d.; alternatively, give according to age.
Children under 2 years: 100 mg P.O. t.i.d.
Children 2 to 6 years: 200 mg P.O. t.i.d.
Children 6 to 13 years: 300 mg P.O. t.i.d.

ADVERSE REACTIONS
Common reactions are in italics; life-threatening reactions are in bold italics.
Blood: ***neutropenia, leukopenia,*** eo-

*Liquid form contains alcohol. **May contain tartrazine.

sinophilia, ***thrombocytopenia, pancytopenia, agranulocytosis, hypoplastic and aplastic anemia.***
CNS: *drowsiness,* fatigue, *malaise,* insomnia, dizziness, headache, paresthesias, irritability.
CV: hypertension, hypotension.
EENT: *hemeralopia,* diplopia, photophobia, epistaxis, retinal hemorrhage.
GI: nausea, vomiting, anorexia, abdominal pain, bleeding gums.
GU: nephrosis, albuminuria, vaginal bleeding.
Hepatic: abnormal liver function tests.
Skin: acneiform and morbilliform rash, ***exfoliative dermatitis, erythema multiforme,*** petechiae, alopecia.
Other: lymphadenopathy, systemic lupus-like syndrome, myasthenia-like syndrome.

INTERACTIONS
None significant.

NURSING CONSIDERATIONS
- *Contraindicated* in paramethadione and trimethadione hypersensitivity, severe blood dyscrasia, or hepatic dysfunction.
- *Use with extreme caution* in retinal and optic nerve diseases.
- Don't withdraw drug suddenly. Abrupt withdrawal may precipitate absence seizures. Call doctor immediately if adverse reactions develop.
- Check CBC, hepatic function, and urinalysis before starting therapy and monthly thereafter. Drug should be stopped if neutrophil count falls below 2,500/mm^3.
- Watch for impending toxicity; may precipitate tonic-clonic seizure.
- Warn patient to report skin rash, alopecia, sore throat, fever, bruises, or epistaxis to doctor immediately.
- Warn patient to avoid activities requiring alertness and good psychomotor coordination until CNS effects of the drug are known.
- Suggest sunglasses if vision blurs in bright light. Notify doctor.
- If scotomata or rash develops, drug should be discontinued.
- May increase risk of tonic-clonic seizures if used alone to treat patients who have mixed types of seizures.
- Has been largely replaced by succinimide derivatives.

valproate sodium
Depakene Syrup, Epilim‡, Myproic Acid Syrup

valproic acid
Dalpro, Depa, Depakene, Myproic Acid

divalproex sodium
Depakote, Epival†, Valcote‡
Pregnancy Risk Category: D

HOW SUPPLIED
valproate sodium
Syrup: 250 mg/ml‡
valproic acid
Tablets (enteric-coated): 200 mg‡, 500 mg‡
Crushable tablets: 100 mg‡
Capsules: 250 mg
Syrup: 200 mg/5 ml‡
divalproex sodium
Tablets (enteric-coated): 125 mg, 250 mg, 500 mg

MECHANISM OF ACTION
Increases brain levels of gamma-aminobutyric acid, which transmits inhibitory nerve impulses in the CNS.

INDICATIONS & DOSAGE
Simple and complex absence seizures, mixed seizure types (including absence seizures), investigationally in generalized, tonic-clonic seizures –
Adults and children: initially, 15 mg/kg P.O. daily divided b.i.d. or t.i.d.; then may increase by 5 to 10

mg/kg daily at weekly intervals up to maximum of 60 mg/kg daily, divided b.i.d. or t.i.d.

ADVERSE REACTIONS

Because drug usually used in combination with other anticonvulsants, adverse reactions reported may not be caused by valproic acid alone.

Common reactions are in italics; life-threatening reactions are in bold italics.

Blood: inhibited platelet aggregation, thrombocytopenia, increased bleeding time.

CNS: *sedation,* emotional upset, depression, psychosis, aggression, hyperactivity, behavioral deterioration, muscle weakness, tremor.

EENT: stomatitis.

GI: *nausea, vomiting,* indigestion, diarrhea, abdominal cramps, constipation, increased appetite and weight gain, *anorexia, **pancreatitis**. (Note:* lower incidence of GI effects with divalproex.)

Hepatic: *elevated enzymes, **toxic hepatitis**.*

Metabolic: *elevated serum ammonia.*

Other: alopecia.

INTERACTIONS

Antacids, aspirin: May cause valproic acid toxicity. Use together cautiously and monitor blood levels.

Phenobarbital: increased phenobarbital levels.

Phenytoin: increased or decreased phenytoin levels.

NURSING CONSIDERATIONS

- *Contraindicated* in hepatic dysfunction.
- *Use cautiously* in children under 2 years; in children with congenital metabolic disorders or mental retardation; in patients with organic brain disease; and in those taking multiple anticonvulsants.
- Tell patient not to discontinue the drug suddenly. Call doctor at once if adverse reactions develop.
- Obtain liver function studies, platelet counts, and prothrombin time before starting drug and periodically thereafter.
- Serious or fatal hepatotoxicity may follow nonspecific symptoms, such as malaise, fever, and lethargy.
- Warn patient to avoid activities that require alertness and good psychomotor coordination until CNS effects of the drug are known.
- May give drug with food or milk to reduce adverse GI reactions. Advise against chewing capsules; causes irritation of mouth and throat.
- May need to reduce dosage if tremors occur.
- May produce false-positive test results for ketones in urine.
- Available as tasty red syrup. Keep out of reach of children.
- Syrup is more rapidly absorbed. Peak effect within 15 minutes.
- Syrup shouldn't be mixed with carbonated beverages; may be irritating to mouth and throat.
- Don't administer syrup to patients who need sodium restriction. Check with doctor.
- Valproic acid has been used investigationally to prevent recurrent febrile seizures in children.

*Liquid form contains alcohol. **May contain tartrazine.

30

Antidepressants

amitriptyline hydrochloride
amoxapine
bupropion hydrochloride
clomipramine hydrochloride
desipramine hydrochloride
doxepin hydrochloride
fluoxetine hydrochloride
imipramine hydrochloride
imipramine pamoate
isocarboxazid
maprotiline hydrochloride
nortriptyline hydrochloride
paroxetine hydrochloride
phenelzine sulfate
protriptyline hydrochloride
sertraline hydrochloride
tranylcypromine sulfate
trazodone hydrochloride
trimipramine maleate

COMBINATION PRODUCTS

ETRAFON 2-10: perphenazine 2 mg and amitriptyline hydrochloride 10 mg.
ETRAFON: perphenazine 2 mg and amitriptyline hydrochloride 25 mg.
ETRAFON-A: perphenazine 4 mg and amitriptyline hydrochloride 10 mg.
ETRAFON-FORTE: perphenazine 4 mg and amitriptyline hydrochloride 25 mg.
LIMBITROL 5-12.5: chlordiazepoxide 5 mg and amitriptyline hydrochloride 12.5 mg.
LIMBITROL 10-25: chlordiazepoxide 10 mg and amitriptyline hydrochloride 25 mg.
TRIAVIL 2-10, TRIAVIL 4-10, TRIAVIL 2-25, TRIAVIL 4-25 are products identical to the Etrafon products listed above. Triavil is also available as TRIAVIL 4-50 (perphenazine 4 mg and amitriptyline hydrochloride 50 mg).

amitriptyline hydrochloride

Amitril, Apo-Amitriptyline†, Elavil, Emitrip, Endep, Enovil, Laroxyl‡, Levate†, Meravil†, Novo-Triptyn†

Pregnancy Risk Category: D

HOW SUPPLIED

Tablets: 10 mg, 25 mg, 50 mg, 75 mg, 100 mg, 150 mg
Injection: 10 mg/ml

MECHANISM OF ACTION

A tricyclic antidepressant (TCA) that increases the amount of norepinephrine or serotonin, or both, in the CNS by blocking their reuptake by the presynaptic neurons. This allows these neurotransmitters to accumulate.

INDICATIONS & DOSAGE

Treatment of depression –
Adults: 50 to 100 mg P.O. h.s., increasing to 200 mg daily; maximum dosage is 300 mg daily if needed; or 20 to 30 mg I.M. q.i.d. Alternatively, the entire dosage can be given at bedtime.
Elderly patients and adolescents: 30 mg P.O. daily in divided doses. May be increased to 150 mg.

ADVERSE REACTIONS

Common reactions are in italics; life-threatening reactions are in bold italics.
CNS: *drowsiness, dizziness,* excitation, tremors, weakness, confusion, headache, nervousness, EEG alterations, seizures, extrapyramidal reactions.
CV: *orthostatic hypotension, tachycardia, ECG changes,* hypertension.
EENT: *blurred vision,* tinnitus, mydriasis.
GI: *dry mouth, constipation,* nausea, vomiting, anorexia, paralytic ileus.

GU: *urine retention.*
Skin: rash, urticaria, photosensitivity.
Other: *sweating,* allergy.
After abrupt withdrawal of long-term therapy: nausea, headache, malaise. (Does not indicate addiction.)

INTERACTIONS

Barbiturates: decrease TCA blood levels. Monitor for decreased antidepressant effect.
Cimetidine, methylphenidate: increases TCA blood levels. Monitor for enhanced antidepressant effect.
Epinephrine, norepinephrine: increase hypertensive effect. Use with caution.
MAO inhibitors: may cause severe excitation, hyperpyrexia, or seizures, usually with high dosage. Use together cautiously.

NURSING CONSIDERATIONS

• *Contraindicated* during acute recovery phase of myocardial infarction, in patients with history of seizure disorders, and in prostatic hypertrophy.
• *Use cautiously* in patients who are suicide risks; in patients with urine retention, narrow-angle glaucoma, increased intraocular pressure, cardiovascular disease, impaired hepatic function, or hyperthyroidism; and in patients receiving thyroid medications, electroshock therapy, or elective surgery.
• Reduce dosage in elderly or debilitated persons and adolescents.
• Do not withdraw drug abruptly.
• If psychotic signs increase, dosage should be reduced. Record mood changes. Watch for suicidal tendencies. Allow minimum supply of tablets to lessen suicide risk.
• Warn patient to avoid activities that require alertness and good psychomotor coordination until CNS effects of the drug are known. Drowsiness and dizziness usually subside after first few weeks.
• Whenever possible, patient should take full dose at bedtime. Warn patient about the possibility of morning orthostatic hypotension.
• Has strong anticholinergic effects; one of the most sedating TCAs. Avoid combining with alcohol or other depressants.
• Dry mouth may be relieved with sugarless hard candy or gum. Saliva substitutes may be necessary.
• Check for urine retention and constipation. Increase fluids to lessen constipation. Suggest stool softener or high-fiber diet, if needed.
• Expect delay of 2 weeks or more before noticeable effect. Full effect may take 4 weeks or more.
• Advise the patient not to take any other drugs (prescription or OTC) without first consulting the doctor.
• Because hypertensive episodes have occurred during surgery in patients receiving TCAs, these drugs should be discontinued several days before surgery.
• Some patients may experience photosensitivity reactions. Advise patient to use a sunscreen, wear protective clothing, and avoid prolonged exposure to strong sunlight.
• Has been used to treat intractable hiccups, chronic severe pain, and patients with eating disorders (bulimia or anorexia nervosa). Dosage is highly variable and individualized.

amoxapine

Asendin

Pregnancy Risk Category: C

HOW SUPPLIED

Tablets: 25 mg, 50 mg, 100 mg, 150 mg

MECHANISM OF ACTION

A tricyclic antidepressant (TCA) that increases the amount of norepineph-

*Liquid form contains alcohol. **May contain tartrazine.

rine or serotonin, or both, in the CNS by blocking their reuptake by the presynaptic neurons. This allows these neurotransmitters to accumulate.

INDICATIONS & DOSAGE

Treatment of depression –
Adults: initial dose 50 mg P.O. t.i.d. May increase to 100 mg t.i.d. on third day of treatment. Increases above 300 mg daily should be made only if 300 mg daily has been ineffective during a trial period of at least 2 weeks. When effective dosage is established, entire dosage (not exceeding 300 mg) may be given at bedtime. Maximum dosage is 600 mg in hospitalized patients.

ADVERSE REACTIONS

Common reactions are in italics; life-threatening reactions are in bold italics.
CNS: *drowsiness, dizziness,* excitation, tremors, weakness, confusion, headache, nervousness, *tardive dyskinesia* (especially in elderly women); EEG changes, ***seizures,*** extrapyramidal reactions.
CV: *orthostatic hypotension, tachycardia, ECG changes,* hypertension.
EENT: *blurred vision,* tinnitus, mydriasis.
GI: *dry mouth, constipation,* nausea, vomiting, anorexia, paralytic ileus.
GU: *urine retention; acute renal failure (with overdose).*
Skin: rash, urticaria, photosensitivity.
Other: *sweating;* weight gain and craving for sweets; allergy; rarely, ***neuroleptic malignant syndrome*** (high fever, tachycardia, tachypnea, profuse diaphoresis).
After abrupt withdrawal of long-term therapy: nausea, headache, malaise. (Does not indicate addiction.)

INTERACTIONS

Barbiturates: decrease TCA blood levels. Monitor for decreased antidepressant effect.
Cimetidine: may increase amoxapine serum levels. Monitor for increased adverse effects.
Epinephrine, norepinephrine: increase hypertensive effect. Use with caution.
MAO inhibitors: may cause severe excitation, hyperpyrexia, or seizures, usually with high dose. Use together cautiously.
Methylphenidate: increases TCA blood levels. Monitor for enhanced antidepressant effect.

NURSING CONSIDERATIONS

- *Contraindicated* in acute recovery phase of myocardial infarction, in patients with history of seizure disorders, and in prostatic hypertrophy.
- *Use cautiously* in patients who are suicide risks; in urine retention, narrow-angle glaucoma, increased intraocular pressure, cardiovascular disease, impaired hepatic function, or hyperthyroidism; and in patients receiving thyroid medications, electroshock therapy, or elective surgery.
- Whenever possible, patient should take full dose at bedtime.
- Monitor for signs and symptoms of tardive dyskinesia, especially in elderly women.
- Reduce dosage in elderly or debilitated persons and adolescents.
- Do not withdraw drug abruptly.
- If psychotic signs increase, reduce dosage. Record mood changes. Watch for suicidal tendencies. Allow minimum supply of tablets to lessen suicide risk.
- Expect delay of 2 weeks or more before noticeable effect. Full effect may take 4 weeks or more.
- Check for urine retention and constipation. Increase fluids to lessen constipation. Suggest stool softener, if needed.
- Warn patient to avoid activities that require alertness and good psychomotor coordination until CNS effects of the drug are known. Drowsiness and

dizziness usually subside after first few weeks.

- Dry mouth may be relieved with sugarless hard candy or gum. Saliva substitutes may be necessary.
- Because hypertensive episodes have occurred during surgery in patients receiving TCAs, these drugs should be discontinued several days before surgery.
- Some patients may experience photosensitivity reactions. Advise patient to use a sunscreen, wear protective clothing, and avoid prolonged exposure to strong sunlight.
- Amoxapine therapy has been associated with neuroleptic malignant syndrome, a rare but life-threatening syndrome usually seen with phenothiazines. Discontinue drug immediately and institute appropriate therapy if symptoms occur.

bupropion hydrochloride

Wellbutrin

Pregnancy Risk Category: B

HOW SUPPLIED

Tablets: 75 mg, 100 mg

MECHANISM OF ACTION

Unknown. Bupropion is not a tricyclic antidepressant, does not inhibit MAO, and is a weak inhibitor of norepinephrine, dopamine, and serotonin reuptake.

INDICATIONS & DOSAGE

Treatment of depression –

Adults: initially, 100 mg P.O. b.i.d. If necessary, dosage is increased after 3 days to the usual dose of 100 mg P.O. t.i.d. If there is no response after several weeks of therapy, dosage may be increased to 150 mg t.i.d.

ADVERSE REACTIONS

Common reactions are in italics; life-threatening reactions are in bold italics.

CNS: *headache,* akathisia, ***seizures,*** *agitation,* anxiety, *confusion,* decreased libido, delusions, euphoria, hostility, impaired sleep quality, insomnia, sedation, sensory disturbance, tremor.

CV: ***arrhythmias,*** hypertension, hypotension, palpitations, syncope, tachycardia.

GI: appetite increase, constipation, dyspepsia, nausea, vomiting, dry mouth.

GU: impotence, menstrual complaints, urinary frequency.

Skin: pruritus, rash, cutaneous temperature disturbance.

Other: arthritis, fever and chills, excessive sweating, auditory disturbance, gustatory disturbance, blurred vision.

INTERACTIONS

Levodopa, phenothiazines, MAO inhibitors, or tricyclic antidepressants; or recent and rapid withdrawal of benzodiazepines: increased risk of adverse reactions, including seizures.

NURSING CONSIDERATIONS

- *Contraindicated* in patients who are allergic to the drug; in patients who have taken MAO inhibitors within the previous 14 days; and in those with seizure disorders. About 0.4% of patients treated at doses up to 450 mg/day may experience seizures. If dosage is increased to 600 mg/day, the incidence of seizures increases about tenfold. Risk of seizure may be minimized by not exceeding 450 mg/day and by administering the daily dose in three to four equally divided doses. Also contraindicated in patients with a history of bulimia or anorexia nervosa because of a higher incidence of seizures in these patients. Studies have also shown that patients who experience seizures often have predisposing factors, including history of head trauma or prior seizures, or CNS tumors, or they may be taking a drug that lowers the seizure threshold.

• Animal data suggest that bupropion may induce drug metabolizing enzymes, decreasing the effectiveness of other drugs taken concomitantly.
• Many patients experience a period of increased restlessness, especially at initiation of therapy. This may include agitation, insomnia, and anxiety. In clinical studies, some patients required sedative-hypnotic agents; about 2% had to discontinue the drug.
• Antidepressants can cause manic episodes during the depressed phase of bipolar manic depression.
• Clinical trials revealed that 28% of the patients experienced a 5 lb or greater weight loss. This drug effect should be considered if weight loss is a major factor in the patient's depressive illness.
• Advise patients to take the drug regularly as scheduled, and to take each day's dosage in three divided doses to minimize the risk of seizures.
• Patients should be advised to avoid alcohol use, since it may contribute to the development of seizures.
• Advise the patient to avoid hazardous activities that require alertness, including operating heavy machinery or driving a car, until the CNS effects of the drug are known.
• Warn patients not to take any other medications, including OTC medications, without first checking with their doctors.

clomipramine hydrochloride
Anafranil

Pregnancy Risk Category: C

HOW SUPPLIED
Capsules: 25 mg, 50 mg, 75 mg

MECHANISM OF ACTION
A tricyclic antidepressant (TCA). Mechanism is unknown; selectively inhibits reuptake of serotonin.

INDICATIONS & DOSAGE
Treatment of obsessive-compulsive disorder –

Adults: initially, 25 mg P.O. daily in divided doses with meals, gradually increasing to 100 mg daily during first 2 weeks. Maximum dosage, 250 mg/day in divided doses with meals. After titration, total daily dose may be given h.s.

Children and adolescents: initially, 25 mg P.O. daily, gradually increased to daily maximum of 3 mg/kg or 100 mg P.O., whichever is smaller; given in divided doses with meals during first 2 weeks. Maximum daily dosage is 3 mg/kg or 200 mg, whichever is smaller; may be given h.s. after titration.

Maintenance dosage in children, adolescents, and adults is the lowest effective dose h.s. Periodic reassessment and adjustment are necessary.

ADVERSE REACTIONS
Common reactions are in italics; life-threatening reactions are in bold italics.

CNS: *somnolence, tremor, dizziness,* headache, insomnia, *libido change, nervousness, myoclonus, increased appetite, fatigue, EEG changes,* ***seizures,*** extrapyramidal reactions.

CV: postural hypotension, palpitations, tachycardia.

EENT: otitis media (children), *abnormal vision,* laryngitis, pharyngitis, rhinitis.

GI: *dry mouth, constipation, nausea, dyspepsia,* diarrhea, *anorexia,* abdominal pain, *nausea.*

GU: *micturition disorder,* urinary tract infection, dysmenorrhea, *ejaculation failure,* impotence.

Skin: *increased sweating,* rash, pruritus, photosensitivity.

Other: myalgia, weight gain

INTERACTIONS
Barbiturates: decrease TCA blood levels. Monitor for decreased antidepressant effect.

Epinephrine, norepinephrine: increase hypertensive effect. Use with caution.
MAO inhibitors: hyperpyretic crisis, seizures, coma, death may result. Alcohol, barbiturates, other CNS depressants: exaggerated response.
Methylphenidate: increases TCA blood levels. Monitor for enhanced antidepressant effect.

NURSING CONSIDERATIONS

- *Contraindicated* during acute recovery period after MI.
- *Use cautiously* in patients with history of seizure disorder; in brain damage of varying etiology; in patients who are receiving other seizure threshold-lowering drugs; in patients at risk for suicide; in patients who are hyperthyroid or are receiving thyroid medication; in those with urine retention, narrow-angle glaucoma, increased intraocular pressure, cardiovascular disease, or impaired hepatic function; and in patients with tumors of the adrenal medulla or who are receiving electroshock therapy or elective surgery.
- Warn patients to avoid hazardous activities requiring alertness and good psychomotor coordination, especially during titration. Daytime sedation, dizziness may occur.
- Avoid combining with other depressants or alcohol.
- Dry mouth may be relieved with sugarless candy or gum. Saliva substitutes may also be used.
- Monitor for urine retention and constipation. Increase fluids to lessen constipation. Suggest stool softener or high-fiber diet as needed.
- Total daily dose may be taken at bedtime after titration. During titration, dose may be divided and given with meals to minimize GI effects.
- Do not withdraw drug abruptly.
- Because hypertensive episodes have occurred during surgery in patients receiving TCAs, these drugs should be discontinued several days before surgery.
- Some patients may experience photosensitivity reactions. Advise patient to use a sunscreen, wear protective clothing, and avoid prolonged exposure to strong sunlight.

desipramine hydrochloride

Norpramin**, Pertofran‡, Pertofrane

Pregnancy Risk Category: C

HOW SUPPLIED

Tablets: 10 mg, 25 mg, 50 mg, 75 mg, 100 mg, 150 mg
Capsules: 25 mg, 50 mg

MECHANISM OF ACTION

A tricyclic antidepressant (TCA) that increases the amount of norepinephrine or serotonin, or both, in the CNS by blocking their reuptake by the presynaptic neurons. This allows these neurotransmitters to accumulate.

INDICATIONS & DOSAGE

Treatment of depression –
Adults: 75 to 150 mg P.O. daily in divided doses, increasing to maximum of 300 mg daily. Alternatively, the entire dosage can be given at bedtime.
Elderly and adolescents: 25 to 50 mg P.O. daily, increasing gradually to maximum of 100 mg daily.

ADVERSE REACTIONS

Common reactions are in italics; life-threatening reactions are in bold italics.
CNS: *drowsiness, dizziness,* excitation, tremors, weakness, confusion, headache, nervousness, EEG changes, ***seizures,*** extrapyramidal reactions.
CV: orthostatic hypotension, *tachycardia, ECG changes,* hypertension.
EENT: *blurred vision,* tinnitus, mydriasis.
GI: *dry mouth, constipation,* nausea, vomiting, anorexia, paralytic ileus.
GU: *urine retention.*

*Liquid form contains alcohol. **May contain tartrazine.

Skin: rash, urticaria, photosensitivity.
Other: *sweating,* allergy.
After abrupt withdrawal of long-term therapy: nausea, headache, malaise. (Does not indicate addiction.)

INTERACTIONS

Barbiturates: decrease TCA blood levels. Monitor for decreased antidepressant effect.
Cimetidine: may increase desipramine serum levels. Monitor for increased adverse reactions.
Epinephrine, norepinephrine: increase hypertensive effect. Use with caution.
MAO inhibitors: may cause severe excitation, hyperpyrexia, or seizures, usually with high dose. Use together cautiously.
Methylphenidate: increases TCA blood levels. Monitor for enhanced antidepressant effect.

NURSING CONSIDERATIONS

- *Contraindicated* during acute recovery phase of myocardial infarction, in patients with history of seizure disorders, and in prostatic hypertrophy.
- *Use cautiously* in cardiovascular disease, urine retention, narrow-angle glaucoma, thyroid disease, blood dyscrasias, or hepatic dysfunction; in patients who are suicide risks; and in those receiving electroshock therapy, thyroid drugs, or elective surgery.
- Reduce dosage in elderly or debilitated persons and adolescents.
- Do not withdraw drug abruptly.
- If psychotic signs increase, dosage should be decreased. Record mood changes. Watch for suicidal tendencies. To lessen suicide risk, allow minimum supply of tablets.
- Drug has low potential for anticholinergic effects and is a metabolite of imipramine; it produces less sedation than amitriptyline or doxepin and does not usually cause orthostatic hypotension. Alcohol may antagonize effects of desipramine.
- Because desipramine produces less tachycardia and other anticholinergic effects than other TCAs, it is often prescribed for cardiac patients.
- Check for urine retention and constipation. Increase fluids to lessen constipation. Suggest stool softener and high-fiber diet, if needed.
- Warn patient to avoid hazardous activities that require alertness and good psychomotor coordination until CNS effects of the drug are known. Drowsiness and dizziness usually subside after a few weeks.
- Expect delay of 2 weeks or more before noticeable effect; 4 weeks or more before full effect.
- Whenever possible, patient should take full dose at bedtime.
- Dry mouth may be relieved with sugarless hard candy or gum. Saliva substitutes may be necessary.
- Advise patient not to take any other drugs (prescription or OTC) without first consulting the doctor.
- Because hypertensive episodes have occurred during surgery in patients receiving TCAs, these drugs should be discontinued several days before surgery.
- Some patients may experience photosensitivity reactions. Advise patient to use a sunscreen, wear protective clothing, and avoid prolonged exposure to strong sunlight.

doxepin hydrochloride

Adapin**, Deptran‡, Sinequan, Triadapin†

Pregnancy Risk Category: C

HOW SUPPLIED

Tablets: 10 mg, 25 mg, 50 mg, 75 mg, 100 mg, 150 mg
Capsules: 10 mg‡, 25 mg‡
Oral concentrate: 10 mg/ml

MECHANISM OF ACTION
A tricyclic antidepressant (TCA) that increases the amount of norepinephrine or serotonin, or both, in the CNS by blocking their reuptake by the presynaptic neurons. This allows these neurotransmitters to accumulate.

INDICATIONS & DOSAGE
Treatment of depression –
Adults: initially, 50 to 75 mg P.O. daily in divided doses, to maximum of 300 mg daily. Alternatively, entire dosage may be given at bedtime.

ADVERSE REACTIONS
Common reactions are in italics; life-threatening reactions are in bold italics.
CNS: *drowsiness, dizziness,* excitation, tremors, weakness, confusion, headache, nervousness, EEG changes, ***seizures,*** extrapyramidal reactions.
CV: *orthostatic hypotension, tachycardia, ECG changes,* hypertension.
EENT: *blurred vision,* tinnitus, glossitis, mydriasis.
GI: *dry mouth, constipation,* nausea, vomiting, anorexia, paralytic ileus.
GU: *urine retention.*
Skin: rash, urticaria, photosensitivity.
Other: *sweating,* allergy.
After abrupt withdrawal of long-term therapy: nausea, headache, malaise. (Does not indicate addiction.)

INTERACTIONS
Barbiturates: decrease TCA blood levels. Monitor for decreased antidepressant effect.
Cimetidine: may increase doxepin serum levels. Monitor for increased adverse reactions.
MAO inhibitors: may cause severe excitation, hyperpyrexia, or seizures, usually with high dose. Use together cautiously.
Methylphenidate: increases TCA blood levels. Monitor for enhanced antidepressant effect.

NURSING CONSIDERATIONS
- *Contraindicated* in patients with narrow-angle glaucoma, prostatic hypertrophy, or history of seizures or during the acute recovery phase of MI.
- *Use cautiously* in patients with urine retention or thyroid, cardiovascular, or hepatic disease and in patients at risk for suicide.
- Whenever possible, patient should take full dose at bedtime. Warn patient about the possibility of morning orthostatic hypotension.
- Reduce dose in elderly or debilitated patients, adolescents, and those receiving other medications (especially anticholinergics).
- Dilute oral concentrate with 120 ml water, milk, or juice (orange, grapefruit, tomato, prune, or pineapple). Incompatible with carbonated beverages.
- If psychotic symptoms increase, dosage should be decreased. Record mood changes. Watch for suicidal tendencies.
- Warn patient to avoid hazardous activities that require alertness and good psychomotor coordination until CNS effects of the drug are known. Drowsiness and dizziness usually subside after a few weeks.
- Expect delay of 2 weeks or more before noticeable effect; 4 weeks or more before full effect.
- Has strong anticholinergic effects; one of the most sedating TCAs. Avoid combining with alcohol or other depressants.
- Dry mouth may be relieved with sugarless hard candy or gum. Saliva substitutes may be necessary.
- Check for urine retention and constipation. Increase fluids to lessen constipation. Suggest stool softener or a high-fiber diet, if needed.
- Advise patient not to take any other drugs (OTC or prescription) without first consulting the doctor.
- Well tolerated by elderly patients.

*Liquid form contains alcohol. **May contain tartrazine.

• May be useful for chronic, severe neurogenic pain.
• Because hypertensive episodes have occurred during surgery in patients receiving TCAs, these drugs should be discontinued several days before surgery.
• Some patients may experience photosensitivity reactions. Advise patient to use a sunscreen, wear protective clothing, and avoid prolonged exposure to strong sunlight.

fluoxetine hydrochloride

Prozac

Pregnancy Risk Category: B

HOW SUPPLIED

Pulvules: 20 mg
Oral solution: 20 mg/5 ml

MECHANISM OF ACTION

Inhibits the CNS neuronal uptake of serotonin. Not a tricyclic derivative; considered an atypical antidepressant.

INDICATIONS & DOSAGE

Short-term management of depressive illness –
Adults: initially, 20 mg P.O. in the morning; dosage increased according to patient response. May be given b.i.d. in the morning and at noon. Maximum dosage is 80 mg/day.

ADVERSE REACTIONS

Common reactions are in italics; life-threatening reactions are in bold italics.
CNS: *nervousness, anxiety, insomnia, headache, drowsiness, tremor, dizziness,* abnormal dreams.
CV: palpitations, flushing, bradycardia, ***arrhythmias***.
EENT: flu-like syndrome, nasal congestion, upper respiratory infection, pharyngitis, cough, sinusitis, visual disturbances, tinnitus, respiratory distress.
GI: *nausea, diarrhea, dry mouth, anorexia, dyspepsia,* constipation, abdominal pain, vomiting, taste change, flatulence, increased appetite.
GU: sexual dysfunction, urine retention.
Other: muscle pain, *weight loss, rash, pruritus, urticaria, asthenia,* edema, lymphadenopathy.

INTERACTIONS

Diazepam: half-life may be prolonged.
Drugs highly bound to plasma proteins (warfarin, digitoxin) can displace drug and cause toxic effects.
Insulin, oral antidiabetic agents: fluoxetine alters blood glucose levels and may alter requirements for antidiabetic medication. Adjust dosage as ordered.
Tricyclic antidepressants: risk of increased adverse CNS effects. Avoid concomitant use.
Tryptophan: agitation, GI distress, and restlessness.

NURSING CONSIDERATIONS

• *Contraindicated* in patients with hypersensitivity to the drug and in patients taking MAO inhibitors within 14 days of starting therapy.
• *Use cautiously* in patients at high risk for suicide and in patients with a history of hepatic, renal, or cardiovascular disease; diabetes mellitus; or a history of seizures.
• Because fluoxetine commonly causes nervousness and insomnia, patient should avoid taking drug in the afternoon to prevent sleep disturbances.
• Less sedating than other antidepressants, but may cause dizziness or drowsiness in some patients. Warn patient to avoid driving or other hazardous activities that require alertness until CNS effects of the drug are known.
• Elderly or debilitated patients and patients with renal or hepatic dysfunction may require lower dosages or less frequent dosing.
• Fluoxetine and its active metabolite have a long elimination half-life.

Clinical effects of dosage changes may not be evident for weeks; full antidepressant effects may not appear for 4 or more weeks of treatment.
- Advise patient not to take any other drugs (OTC or prescription) without consulting the doctor.
- Rashes or pruritus, which usually occur early in therapy, may respond to antihistamines or topical corticosteroids.

imipramine hydrochloride

Apo-Imipramine†, Imiprin‡, Impril†, Janimine**, Novo-Pramine†, Tipramine, Tofranil**

imipramine pamoate

Tofranil-PM**

Pregnancy Risk Category: D

HOW SUPPLIED

hydrochloride
Tablets: 10 mg, 25 mg, 50 mg
Injection: 12.5 mg/ml
pamoate
Capsules: 75 mg, 100 mg, 125 mg, 150 mg

MECHANISM OF ACTION

A tricyclic antidepressant (TCA) that increases the amount of norepinephrine or serotonin, or both, in the CNS by blocking their reuptake by the presynaptic neurons. This action allows these neurotransmitters to accumulate.

INDICATIONS & DOSAGE

Treatment of depression –
Adults: 75 to 100 mg P.O. or I.M. daily in divided doses, with 25- to 50-mg increments up to 200 mg. (I.M. route rarely used). Maximum dosage is 300 mg daily. Alternatively, entire dosage may be given at bedtime (using pamoate salt).
Childhood enuresis –
Children 6 years and over: 25 mg P.O. 1 hour before bedtime. If no response within 1 week, increase to 50 mg if the child is under 12 years; increase to 75 mg for children 12 years and over. In either case, do not exceed 2.5 mg/kg/day.

ADVERSE REACTIONS

Common reactions are in italics; life-threatening reactions are in bold italics.
CNS: *drowsiness, dizziness,* excitation, tremors, weakness, confusion, headache, nervousness, EEG changes, ***seizures,*** extrapyramidal reactions.
CV: *orthostatic hypotension, tachycardia, ECG changes,* hypertension.
EENT: *blurred vision,* tinnitus, mydriasis.
GI: *dry mouth, constipation,* nausea, vomiting, anorexia, paralytic ileus.
GU: *urine retention.*
Skin: rash, urticaria, photosensitivity.
Other: *sweating,* allergy.
After abrupt withdrawal of long-term therapy: nausea, headache, malaise. (Does not indicate addiction.)

INTERACTIONS

Barbiturates: decrease TCA blood levels. Monitor for decreased antidepressant effect.
Cimetidine: may increase imipramine serum levels. Monitor for increased adverse reactions.
Epinephrine, norepinephrine: increase hypertensive effect. Use with caution.
MAO inhibitors: may cause severe excitation, hyperpyrexia, or seizures, usually with high dose. Use together cautiously.
Methylphenidate: increases TCA blood levels. Monitor for enhanced antidepressant effect.

NURSING CONSIDERATIONS

- *Contraindicated* during acute recovery phase of MI, in prostatic hypertrophy, and in patients with history of seizure disorders.

*Liquid form contains alcohol. **May contain tartrazine.

• *Use with extreme caution* in cardiovascular disease, urine retention, narrow-angle glaucoma or increased intraocular pressure, thyroid disease, blood dyscrasias, or impaired hepatic function; in patients who are at risk for suicide; and in those receiving electroshock therapy, thyroid medication, or elective surgery. Injectable form contains sulfites, which may precipitate allergic reactions in certain individuals with hypersensitivity.
• Reduce dosage in elderly or debilitated persons, adolescents, and patients with aggravated psychotic symptoms.
• Do not withdraw drug abruptly.
• If psychotic signs increase, dosage should be reduced. Record mood changes. Watch for suicidal tendencies. To lessen suicide risk, allow minimum supply of tablets.
• Check for urine retention and constipation. Increase fluids to lessen constipation. Suggest stool softener, if needed.
• Warn patient to avoid hazardous activities that require alertness and good psychomotor coordination until CNS effects of the drug are known. Drowsiness and dizziness usually subside after a few weeks.
• Expect delay of 2 weeks or more before noticeable effect; 4 weeks or more before full effect.
• Dry mouth may be relieved with sugarless hard candy or gum. Saliva substitutes may be necessary.
• Avoid combining with alcohol or other depressants.
• Advise patient not to take any other drugs (prescription or OTC) without first consulting the doctor.
• Imipramine has a high potential for inducing orthostatic hypotension. Whenever possible, patient should take full dose at bedtime. Warn patient about the possibility of morning orthostatic hypotension.
• May be useful for chronic, severe neurogenic pain.
• When treating enuresis, it may be more effective to divide dosage and administer the first dose earlier in the day (such as late afternoon) if the child is an "early night" bedwetter.
• To prevent relapse in children receiving the drug for enuresis, withdraw dosage gradually.
• Because hypertensive episodes have occurred during surgery in patients receiving TCAs, these drugs should be discontinued several days before surgery.
• Some patients may experience photosensitivity reactions. Advise patient to use a sunscreen, wear protective clothing, and avoid prolonged exposure to strong sunlight.

isocarboxazid

Marplan

Pregnancy Risk Category: C

HOW SUPPLIED

Tablets: 10 mg

MECHANISM OF ACTION

An MAO inhibitor that promotes accumulation of neurotransmitters by inhibiting MAO.

INDICATIONS & DOSAGE

Treatment of depression –
Adults: 30 mg P.O. daily in divided doses. Reduce to 10 to 20 mg daily when condition improves. Not recommended for children under 16 years.

ADVERSE REACTIONS

Common reactions are in italics; life-threatening reactions are in bold italics.
CNS: *dizziness,* vertigo, weakness, headache, overactivity, hyperreflexia, tremors, muscle twitching, mania, *insomnia,* confusion, memory impairment, fatigue.
CV: *orthostatic hypotension,* ***arrhythmias,*** paradoxical hypertension.
EENT: blurred vision.

GI: dry mouth, *anorexia,* nausea, diarrhea, constipation.
Skin: rash.
Other: peripheral edema, sweating, weight changes, altered libido.

INTERACTIONS

Alcohol, barbiturates, and other sedatives; narcotics; dextromethorphan; TCAs: unpredictable interaction. Use with caution and in reduced dosage.
Amphetamines, antihistamines, ephedrine, levodopa, meperidine, metaraminol, methotrimeprazine, methylphenidate, phenylephrine, phenylpropanolamine, sympathomimetics: pressor effects of these drugs are enhanced by isocarboxazid. Avoid concomitant use.
Insulin, oral hypoglycemic agents: isocarboxazid may alter requirements for antidiabetic medications.

NURSING CONSIDERATIONS

• *Contraindicated* in elderly or debilitated patients; severe hepatic or renal impairment; CHF; pheochromocytoma; hypertensive, cardiovascular, or cerebrovascular disease; severe or frequent headaches; with foods containing tryptophan or tyramine; during therapy with other MAO inhibitors (including phenelzine, tranylcypromine) or within 10 days of such therapy; and within 10 days of elective surgery requiring general anesthetic, cocaine, or local anesthetic containing sympathomimetic vasoconstrictors.
• *Use cautiously* with other psychotropic drugs or with spinal anesthetic; in hyperactive, agitated, or schizophrenic patients; in patients at risk for suicide; and in patients with Parkinson's disease, diabetes, or seizure disorders.
• Avoid combining with alcohol or other depressant.
• Because MAO inhibitors may alleviate chest pain in patients with angina, warn such patients to moderate activities and avoid overexertion.
• If patient develops symptoms of overdosage (palpitations, frequent headaches, or severe orthostatic hypotension), hold dose and notify doctor.
• Monitor closely for suicidal tendencies.
• Dosage is usually reduced to maintenance level as soon as possible.
• Do not withdraw drug abruptly.
• Weigh patient biweekly. Teach patient how to check for edema and urine retention.
• Warn patient to avoid foods high in tyramine or tryptophan (aged cheese, Chianti wine, beer, avocados, chicken livers, chocolate, bananas, soy sauce, meat tenderizers, salami, bologna) and large amounts of caffeine.
• Warn patient not to take any other medications (prescription or OTC) without first checking with the doctor. Severe adverse effects can occur if MAO inhibitors are taken with OTC cold, hay fever, or diet preparations.
• Monitor blood pressure and heart rate. Incidence of orthostatic hypotension is high. Supervise walking. Tell patient to get out of bed slowly, sitting up first for 1 minute.
• Have phentolamine (Regitine) available to counteract severe hypertension.
• Continue precautions 10 days after discontinuation of the drug because it has long-lasting effects.
• Expect delay of 2 weeks or more before noticeable effect; 4 weeks or more for full effect.
• Obtain baseline blood pressure readings, CBC, and liver function tests before beginning therapy, and continue to monitor throughout treatment.
• In most patients, MAO inhibitors should be discontinued 14 days before elective surgery to avoid drug interactions that may occur during anesthetic procedure.

maprotiline hydrochloride
Ludiomil

Pregnancy Risk Category: B

HOW SUPPLIED
Tablets: 25 mg, 50 mg, 75 mg

MECHANISM OF ACTION
A tricyclic antidepressant (TCA) that increases the amount of norepinephrine or serotonin, or both, in the CNS by blocking their reuptake by the presynaptic neurons. This allows these neurotransmitters to accumulate.

INDICATIONS & DOSAGE
Treatment of depression–
Adults: initial dose of 75 mg P.O. daily for patients with mild to moderate depression. The dosage may be increased as required to a dose of 150 mg daily. Maximum dosage is 225 mg in patients who are not hospitalized. Severely depressed, hospitalized patients may receive up to 300 mg daily.

ADVERSE REACTIONS
Common reactions are in italics; life-threatening reactions are in bold italics.
CNS: *drowsiness, dizziness,* excitation, ***seizures,*** tremor, weakness, confusion, headache, nervousness, extrapyramidal reactions.
CV: *orthostatic hypotension, tachycardia, ECG changes.*
EENT: *blurred vision,* tinnitus, mydriasis.
GI: *dry mouth, constipation,* nausea, vomiting, anorexia, paralytic ileus.
GU: *urine retention.*
Skin: rash, urticaria, photosensitivity.
Other: *sweating,* allergy.
After abrupt withdrawal of long-term therapy: nausea, headache, malaise. (Does not indicate addiction.)

INTERACTIONS
Barbiturates: decrease maprotiline blood levels. Monitor for decreased antidepressant effect.
Cimetidine: may increase maprotiline serum levels. Monitor for increased adverse reactions.
Epinephrine, norepinephrine: increase hypertensive effect. Use with caution.
MAO inhibitors: may cause severe excitation, hyperpyrexia, or seizures, usually with high dose. Use together cautiously.
Methylphenidate: increases maprotiline blood levels. Monitor for enhanced antidepressant effect.

NURSING CONSIDERATIONS
- *Contraindicated* during acute recovery phase of myocardial infarction and in prostatic hypertrophy.
- *Use cautiously* in CV disease, urine retention, narrow-angle glaucoma, thyroid disease or medication, blood dyscrasias, and impaired hepatic function; in patients with a history of seizures; in patients who are at risk for suicide; and in those receiving electroshock therapy or elective surgery.
- Reduce dosage in elderly or debilitated persons and adolescents.
- Expect delay of 2 weeks or more before noticeable effect; 4 weeks or more before full effect.
- Do not withdraw drug abruptly.
- If psychotic signs increase, reduce dosage. Record mood changes. Monitor closely for suicidal tendencies. To lessen suicide risk, allow minimum supply of tablets.
- Check for urine retention and constipation. Increase fluids to lessen constipation. Suggest stool softener, if needed.
- Warn patient to avoid hazardous activities that require alertness and good psychomotor coordination until CNS effects of the drug are known. Drows-

iness and dizziness usually subside after a few weeks.

- Dry mouth may be relieved with sugarless hard candy or gum, but maprotiline usually has a low potential for inducing anticholinergic effects. Saliva substitutes may be necessary.
- Whenever possible, patient should take full dose at bedtime.
- Advise patient not to take any other medication (prescription or OTC) without first checking with the doctor.
- Because hypertensive episodes have occurred during surgery in patients receiving TCAs, these drugs should be discontinued several days before surgery.
- Some patients may experience photosensitivity reactions. Advise patient to use a sunscreen, wear protective clothing, and avoid prolonged exposure to strong sunlight.

nortriptyline hydrochloride

Aventyl*, Pamelor*

Pregnancy Risk Category: D

HOW SUPPLIED

Capsules: 10 mg, 25 mg, 50 mg, 75 mg
Oral solution: 10 mg/5 ml (4% alcohol)

MECHANISM OF ACTION

A tricyclic antidepressant (TCA) that increases the amount of norepinephrine or serotonin, or both, in the CNS by blocking their reuptake by the presynaptic neurons. This allows these neurotransmitters to accumulate.

INDICATIONS & DOSAGE

Treatment of depression –
Adults: 25 mg P.O. t.i.d. or q.i.d., gradually increasing to maximum of 150 mg daily. Alternatively, entire dose may be given h.s.

ADVERSE REACTIONS

Common reactions are in italics; life-threatening reactions are in bold italics.
CNS: *drowsiness, dizziness,* excitation, ***seizures,*** tremor, weakness, confusion, headache, nervousness, EEG changes, extrapyramidal reactions.
CV: *tachycardia, ECG changes,* hypertension.
EENT: *blurred vision,* tinnitus, mydriasis.
GI: *dry mouth, constipation,* nausea, vomiting, anorexia, paralytic ileus.
GU: *urine retention.*
Skin: rash, urticaria, photosensitivity.
Other: *sweating,* allergy.
After abrupt withdrawal of long-term therapy: nausea, headache, malaise. (Does not indicate addiction.)

INTERACTIONS

Barbiturates: decrease TCA blood levels. Monitor for decreased antidepressant effect.
Cimetidine: may increase nortriptyline serum levels. Monitor for increased adverse reactions.
Epinephrine, norepinephrine: increase hypertensive effect. Use with caution.
MAO inhibitors: may cause severe excitation, hyperpyrexia, or seizures, usually with high dose. Use together cautiously.
Methylphenidate: increases TCA blood levels. Monitor for enhanced antidepressant effect.

NURSING CONSIDERATIONS

- *Contraindicated* during acute recovery phase of myocardial infarction, in prostatic hypertrophy, and in patients with history of seizure disorders.
- *Use cautiously* in CV disease, urine retention, glaucoma, thyroid disease, impaired hepatic function, or blood dyscrasias; in patients who are at risk for suicide; or in those receiving elec-

*Liquid form contains alcohol. **May contain tartrazine.

troshock therapy, thyroid medication, or elective surgery.
• Drug is a TCA, similar in anticholinergic effects to other cyclics. Has low potential for orthostatic hypotension. Avoid combining with alcohol or other depressants.
• Dry mouth may be relieved with sugarless hard candy or gum. Saliva substitutes may be necessary.
• Check for urine retention and constipation. Increase fluids to lessen constipation. Suggest stool softener, if needed.
• Reduce dosage in elderly or debilitated persons and adolescents.
• Do not withdraw drug abruptly.
• If psychotic signs increase, dosage should be reduced. Record mood changes. Watch for suicidal tendencies. To lessen suicide risk, allow minimum tablet supply.
• Warn patient to avoid hazardous activities that require alertness and good psychomotor coordination until CNS effects of the drug are known. Drowsiness and dizziness usually subside after a few weeks.
• Expect delay of 2 weeks or more before noticeable effect; 4 weeks or more before full effect.
• Advise patient not to use other drugs (prescription or OTC) without first consulting the doctor.
• Whenever possible, patient should take full dose at bedtime.
• Because hypertensive episodes have occurred during surgery in patients receiving TCAs, these drugs should be discontinued several days before surgery.
• Some patients may experience photosensitivity reactions. Advise patient to use a sunscreen, wear protective clothing, and avoid prolonged exposure to strong sunlight.

paroxetine hydrochloride

Paxil

Pregnancy Risk Category: B

HOW SUPPLIED

Tablets: 20 mg, 30 mg

MECHANISM OF ACTION

Blocks the reuptake of serotonin (5-hydroxytryptamine; 5-HT) into nerve terminals within the CNS.

INDICATIONS & DOSAGE

Depression–
Adults: initially, 20 mg P.O. daily, preferably in the morning. As indicated, increase dosage in 10-mg/day increments, at 1-week intervals, to a maximum of 50 mg daily.
Elderly or debilitated patients; patients with severe hepatic or renal disease: initially, 10 mg P.O. daily, preferably in the morning. As indicated, increase dosage in 10-mg/day increments, at 1-week intervals, to a maximum of 40 mg daily.

ADVERSE REACTIONS

Common reactions are in italics; life-threatening reactions are in bold italics.
CNS: blurred vision, *somnolence, dizziness, insomnia, tremor, nervousness,* anxiety, paresthesia, decreased libido.
CV: palpitations, vasodilation, postural hypotension.
EENT: lump or tightness in throat.
GI: *nausea, dry mouth, constipation, diarrhea, decreased appetite,* flatulence, vomiting, dyspepsia, increased appetite.
GU: *ejaculatory disturbances, male genital disorders* (including anorgasmy, erectile difficulties, delayed ejaculation or orgasm, impotence, and sexual dysfunction), urinary frequency, urinary disorder, female genital disorder (including anorgasmy, difficulty with orgasm).
Skin: *sweating,* rash.

Other: *asthenia,* hyponatremia, myopathy, myalgia, myasthenia, taste perversion.

INTERACTIONS

Cimetidine: decreased hepatic metabolism of paroxetine, leading to risk of toxicity. Dosage adjustments may be necessary.
Digoxin: paroxetine may decrease digoxin levels. Monitor closely.
MAO inhibitors: concomitant use may increase risk of serious, sometimes fatal, adverse reactions. Don't administer paroxetine with or within 14 days of discontinuing MAO inhibitor therapy. Allow at least 2 weeks after discontinuing paroxetine before starting treatment with an MAO inhibitor.
Phenobarbital, phenytoin: possible altered pharmacokinetics of both drugs. Dosage adjustments may be necessary.
Procyclidine: paroxetine may increase procyclidine levels. Monitor for excessive anticholinergic effects.
Tryptophan: may increase incidence of adverse reactions, such as sweating, headache, nausea, and dizziness. Avoid concomitant use.
Warfarin: increased risk of bleeding. Avoid concomitant use.

NURSING CONSIDERATIONS

- *Contraindicated* in patients taking MAO inhibitors.
- *Use cautiously* in patients with a history of seizure disorders or mania; hepatic or renal impairment; or severe, concomitant systemic illness.
- Several cases of hyponatremia have been reported, usually in elderly patients; some were taking diuretics or were otherwise volume depleted. Therefore, use cautiously in patients at risk for volume depletion and monitor appropriately.
- Because drug is excreted in breast milk, also use cautiously in breast-feeding women.
- Because the potential for suicide is inherent in depressed patients, closely supervise high-risk patients during initial drug therapy. Such patients should receive prescriptions for a limited number of tablets, as appropriate, to reduce the risk of overdose.
- Expect a delay before maximum clinical benefits of drug are seen. Typically, full effects of antidepressant therapy are usually seen after 4 weeks or more of therapy.
- It's unknown how long a patient should continue antidepressant therapy. Most clinicians treat acute episodes of depressive illness with several months of sustained pharmacologic therapy. Clinical trials with paroxetine have demonstrated clinical efficacy for periods of 1 year at average doses of 30 mg daily.
- Overdosage is usually associated with nausea, vomiting, drowsiness, sinus tachycardia, and dilated pupils. There is no specific antidote for the drug, and forced diuresis, dialysis, hemoperfusion, or exchange transfusion is believed to be of little benefit. Establish and maintain an airway, and perform gastric evacuation. Activated charcoal (20 to 30 g) may be administered every 4 to 6 hours for the first 24 to 48 hours after ingestion. Provide supportive care with frequent monitoring of vital signs.
- Warn patient to avoid activities that require alertness and good psychomotor coordination until adverse CNS effects of the drug are known.

phenelzine sulfate

Nardil

Pregnancy Risk Category: C

HOW SUPPLIED

Tablets: 15 mg

MECHANISM OF ACTION

An MAO inhibitor that promotes accumulation of neurotransmitters by inhibiting MAO.

*Liquid form contains alcohol. **May contain tartrazine.

INDICATIONS & DOSAGE
Treatment of depression –
Adults: 45 mg P.O. daily in divided doses, increasing rapidly to 60 mg daily. Then dosage can usually be reduced to 15 mg daily. Maximum is 90 mg daily.

ADVERSE REACTIONS
Common reactions are in italics; life-threatening reactions are in bold italics.
CNS: *dizziness,* vertigo, headache, overactivity, hyperreflexia, tremors, muscle twitching, mania, jitters, *insomnia,* confusion, memory impairment, drowsiness, weakness, fatigue.
CV: paradoxical hypertension, *orthostatic hypotension,* ***arrhythmias.***
GI: dry mouth, *anorexia,* nausea, constipation.
Other: peripheral edema, sweating, weight changes.

INTERACTIONS
Alcohol, barbiturates, and other sedatives; narcotics; dextromethorphan; tricyclic antidepressants: unpredictable interaction. Use with caution and in reduced dosage.
Amphetamines, antihistamines, ephedrine, levodopa, meperidine, metaraminol, methotrimeprazine, methylphenidate, phenylephrine, phenylpropanolamine, sympathomimetics: enhance pressor effects. Avoid concomitant use.
Insulin, oral hypoglycemic agents: phenelzine may alter requirements for antidiabetic medications.

NURSING CONSIDERATIONS
- *Contraindicated* in elderly or debilitated patients and in hepatic impairment, CHF, pheochromocytoma, hypertension, cardiovascular or cerebrovascular disease, or severe or frequent headaches. Also contraindicated with foods containing tryptophan (broad beans) or tyramine; during therapy with other MAO inhibitors (isocarboxazid, tranylcypromine) or within 10 days of such therapy; within 10 days of elective surgery requiring general anesthetic, cocaine, or local anesthetic containing sympathomimetic vasoconstrictors; and in hyperactive, agitated, or schizophrenic patients.
- *Use cautiously* with antihypertensive agents containing thiazide diuretics, with spinal anesthetics, and in patients at risk for suicide or with diabetes, seizure disorders, or Parkinson's disease.
- Avoid combining with alcohol or other depressant.
- Because MAO inhibitors may alleviate chest pain in patients with angina, warn such patients to moderate activities to prevent overexertion.
- If patient develops symptoms of overdose (severe hypotension, palpitations, or frequent headaches), hold dose and notify doctor.
- Monitor closely for suicidal tendencies.
- Dosage is usually reduced to maintenance level as soon as possible.
- Store drug in tight container, away from heat and light.
- Have phentolamine (Regitine) available to combat severe hypertension.
- Warn patient to avoid foods high in tyramine or tryptophan (aged cheese, Chianti wine, beer, avocados, chicken livers, chocolate, bananas, soy sauce, meat tenderizers, salami, bologna) and large amounts of caffeine.
- Warn patient not to take any other medications (prescription or OTC) without first checking with the doctor. Severe adverse effects can occur if MAO inhibitors are taken with OTC cold, hay fever, or diet preparations.
- Monitor blood pressure and heart rate. Incidence of orthostatic hypotension is high. Supervise walking. Tell patient to get out of bed slowly, sitting up first for 1 minute.
- Continue precautions 10 days after stopping drug because it has long-lasting effects.
- Expect delay of 2 weeks or more be-

fore noticeable effect; 4 weeks or more before full effect.
• Obtain baseline blood pressure readings, CBC, and liver function tests before therapy, and continue to monitor throughout treatment.
• In most patients, MAO inhibitors should be discontinued 14 days before elective surgery to avoid drug interactions that may occur during the anesthetic procedure.

protriptyline hydrochloride

Triptil†, Vivactil

Pregnancy Risk Category: C

HOW SUPPLIED

Tablets: 5 mg, 10 mg

MECHANISM OF ACTION

A tricyclic antidepressant (TCA) that increases the amount of norepinephrine or serotonin, or both, in the CNS by blocking their reuptake by the presynaptic neurons. This allows these neurotransmitters to accumulate.

INDICATIONS & DOSAGE

Treatment of depression –
Adults: 15 to 40 mg P.O. daily in divided doses, increasing gradually to maximum of 60 mg daily.

ADVERSE REACTIONS

Common reactions are in italics; life-threatening reactions are in bold italics.
CNS: excitation, ***seizures,*** tremor, weakness, confusion, headache, nervousness, EEG changes, extrapyramidal reactions.
CV: *tachycardia, ECG changes,* orthostatic hypotension, hypertension.
EENT: *blurred vision,* tinnitus, mydriasis.
GI: *dry mouth, constipation,* nausea, vomiting, anorexia, paralytic ileus.
GU: *urine retention.*
Skin: rash, urticaria, photosensitivity.
Other: *sweating,* allergy.
After abrupt withdrawal of long-term therapy: nausea, headache, malaise. (Does not indicate addiction.)

INTERACTIONS

Barbiturates: decrease TCA blood levels. Monitor for decreased antidepressant effect.
Cimetidine: may increase protriptyline serum levels. Monitor for increased adverse reactions.
Epinephrine, norepinephrine: increase hypertensive effect. Use with caution.
MAO inhibitors: may cause severe excitation, hyperpyrexia, or seizures, and death, usually with high dose. Use together cautiously.
Methylphenidate: increases TCA blood levels. Monitor for enhanced antidepressant effect.

NURSING CONSIDERATIONS

• *Contraindicated* during acute recovery phase of MI, in prostatic hypertrophy, and in patients with seizure disorders.
• *Use cautiously* in elderly patients and in CV disease, urine retention, increased intraocular tension, thyroid disease, or blood dyscrasias; in patients at risk for suicide; and in those receiving electroshock therapy, thyroid drugs, or elective surgery.
• Protriptyline has high anticholinergic effects. Dry mouth may be relieved with sugarless hard candy or gum, or saliva substitutes if necessary.
• Check for urine retention and constipation. Increase fluids to lessen constipation. Suggest stool softener or high-fiber diet, if needed.
• Protriptyline has low potential for producing orthostatic hypotension and is the least sedating of the TCAs. It may even have amphetamine-like effects. Avoid late-day dosing to prevent insomnia.

*Liquid form contains alcohol. **May contain tartrazine.

- Reduce dosage in elderly or debilitated patients and adolescents.
- Do not withdraw drug abruptly.
- Watch for increased psychotic signs, anxiety, agitation, or CV reactions; dosage should be reduced if they occur. Record mood changes. Watch for suicidal tendencies. To lessen suicide risk, allow minimum supply of tablets.
- Expect delay of 2 weeks or more before noticeable effect; 4 weeks or more before full effect.
- Warn patient not to use other drugs without first consulting the doctor. Avoid combining with alcohol or other depressants.
- Used investigationally to treat obstructive sleep apnea.
- Because hypertensive episodes have occurred during surgery in patients receiving TCAs, these drugs should be discontinued several days before surgery.
- Some patients may experience photosensitivity reactions. Advise patient to use a sunscreen, wear protective clothing, and avoid prolonged exposure to strong sunlight.

sertraline hydrochloride

Zoloft

Pregnancy Risk Category: B

HOW SUPPLIED

Tablets: 50 mg, 100 mg

MECHANISM OF ACTION

An antidepressant that is chemically unrelated to tricyclic, tetracyclic, or any other currently available agents. Probably acts by blocking the reuptake of serotonin (5-hydroxytryptamine; 5-HT) into presynaptic neurons in the CNS, prolonging the action of 5-HT.

INDICATIONS & DOSAGE

Depression, obsessive-compulsive disorder –

Adults: 50 mg P.O. daily. Adjust dosage as needed and tolerated; clinical trials involved dosage of 50 to 200 mg daily. Dosage adjustments should be made at intervals of no less than 1 week.

ADVERSE REACTIONS

Common reactions are in italics; life-threatening reactions are in bold italics.

CNS: *headache, tremor, dizziness, insomnia, somnolence,* syncope, paresthesia, hypoesthesia, hyperesthesia, twitching, hypertonia, confusion, ataxia, abnormal coordination or gait, nystagmus, vertigo, hyperkinesia, hypokinesia, mania.

CV: palpitations, chest pain, postural hypotension, hypertension, hypotension, edema, peripheral ischemia, tachycardia.

GI: *dry mouth, nausea, diarrhea, loose stools, dyspepsia,* vomiting, flatulence, anorexia, abdominal pain, increased appetite, dysphagia.

GU: male sexual dysfunction.

Skin: rash, acne, alopecia, pruritus, erythematous or maculopapular rash, dry skin.

Other: *increased sweating,* cold or clammy skin, flushing, myalgia.

INTERACTIONS

Diazepam, tolbutamide: sertraline decreases clearance of these drugs. Clinical significance is unknown; however, monitor patient for increased drug effects.

MAO inhibitors: may cause serious mental status changes, hyperthermia, autonomic instability, rapid fluctuations of vital signs, delirium, coma, and death. Do not administer sertraline with or within 14 days after discontinuing an MAO inhibitor; also, allow 14 days after discontinuing sertraline before starting an MAO inhibitor.

Warfarin, other highly protein-bound drugs: interactions may occur, increasing the plasma levels of sertraline or of the other highly bound drug.

Small (8%) increases in prothrombin time have been seen with concomitant use of warfarin. Monitor closely.

NURSING CONSIDERATIONS

- *Contraindicated* in patients with hypersensitivity to the drug and within 14 days of taking an MAO inhibitor.
- *Use cautiously* in patients with hepatic impairment because drug is extensively metabolized in the liver; in patients with seizure disorders; in those with a history of drug abuse, and in suicidal ideation.
- Because drug is highly bound to plasma proteins (98%), use cautiously with other drugs that are also highly protein-bound, such as warfarin.
- Administer once daily, either in the morning or evening. May administer with or without food.
- Because of the inherent risk of suicide in depressed patients, provide close supervision during initiation of drug therapy. Prescriptions for the drug should limit the supply of tablets to reduce the risk of overdose.
- Mania or hypomania occurred in a few patients (0.4%) in clinical trials. Like other antidepressants, the drug can activate mania in patients with major affective disorders.
- Small changes in several laboratory values have been noted in patients taking sertraline: increases in serum cholesterol and triglyceride levels and decreases in uric acid concentrations. Elevations in serum transaminases (AST [SGOT], ALT [SGPT]) have occurred, usually within the first 9 weeks of therapy; values returned to normal after discontinuing drug. Clinical significance is unknown.
- Patients who improve during the first 8 weeks of therapy will probably continue to respond to the drug; however, information is limited about use for longer than 16 weeks. Periodically monitor effectiveness during prolonged use. It is unknown if periodic dosage adjustments are necessary to maintain effectiveness.
- Although problems have not been reported to date, advise patient to use caution when performing hazardous tasks that require alertness, such as driving a car or operating heavy machinery, and to avoid use of alcohol while taking this drug. Drugs that influence the CNS may impair judgment.
- Caution patient to check with the doctor or pharmacist before taking any OTC medications.

tranylcypromine sulfate

Parnate

Pregnancy Risk Category: C

HOW SUPPLIED

Tablets: 10 mg

MECHANISM OF ACTION

An MAO inhibitor that promotes accumulation of neurotransmitters by inhibiting MAO.

INDICATIONS & DOSAGE

Treatment of depression –

Adults: 10 mg P.O. b.i.d. Increase to maximum of 30 mg daily, if necessary, after 2 weeks. Not recommended for children under 16 years.

ADVERSE REACTIONS

Common reactions are in italics; life-threatening reactions are in bold italics.

CNS: *dizziness,* vertigo, headache, overactivity, hyperreflexia, tremors, muscle twitching, mania, jitters, confusion, memory impairment, fatigue.
CV: *orthostatic hypotension,* ***arrhythmias,*** paradoxical hypertension.
EENT: blurred vision.
GI: dry mouth, *anorexia,* nausea, diarrhea, constipation, abdominal pain.
GU: impotence.
Skin: rash.

Other: peripheral edema, sweating, weight changes, chills, altered libido.

INTERACTIONS

Alcohol, barbiturates, and other sedatives; narcotics; dextromethorphan; tricyclic antidepressants: use with caution and in reduced dosage.
Amphetamines, antihistamines, ephedrine, levodopa, meperidine, metaraminol, methotrimeprazine, methylphenidate, phenylephrine, phenylpropanolamine, sympathomimetics: pressor effects of these drugs are enhanced by tranylcypromine. Avoid concomitant use.
Insulin, oral hypoglycemic agents: tranylcypromine may alter requirements of antidiabetic medications.

NURSING CONSIDERATIONS

- *Contraindicated* in severe hepatic or renal impairment; CHF; pheochromocytoma, hypertension, or cardiovascular or cerebrovascular disease; severe or frequent headaches; in patients taking antihypertensives or diuretics; in elderly or debilitated patients; in patients for whom close supervision is not possible; and in hyperactive, agitated, or schizophrenic patients. Also contraindicated with foods containing tryptophan or tyramine; during therapy with other MAO inhibitors (phenelzine, isocarboxazid) or within 7 days of such therapy; and within 7 days of elective surgery requiring general anesthetic, cocaine, or local anesthetic containing sympathomimetic vasoconstrictors.
- *Use cautiously* with antiparkinsonian drugs or spinal anesthetics; in renal disease, diabetes, seizure disorder, Parkinson's disease, and hyperthyroidism; and in those at risk for suicide.
- MAO inhibitor most often reported to cause hypertensive crisis with high-tyramine ingestion.
- Avoid combining with alcohol or other depressants.
- Because MAO inhibitors may alleviate chest pain in patients with angina, warn such patients to moderate activities to avoid overexertion.
- Obtain baseline blood pressure readings, CBC, and liver function tests before beginning therapy, and monitor throughout treatment.
- If patient develops symptoms of overdose (palpitations, severe hypotension, or frequent headaches), hold dose and notify doctor.
- Watch for suicidal tendencies.
- Dosage is usually reduced to maintenance level as soon as possible.
- Do not withdraw drug abruptly.
- Have phentolamine (Regitine) available to combat severe hypertension.
- Warn patient to avoid foods high in tyramine or tryptophan (aged cheese, Chianti wine, beer, avocados, chicken livers, chocolate, bananas, soy sauce, meat tenderizers, salami, bologna) and large amounts of caffeine.
- Warn patient not to take any other medications (prescription or OTC) without first checking with the doctor. Severe effects can occur if MAO inhibitors are taken with OTC cold, hay fever, or diet preparations.
- To prevent dizziness resulting from orthostatic hypotension, tell patient to get out of bed slowly, sitting up for 1 minute.
- Continue precautions for 7 days after stopping drug; effects last that long.
- Expect delay of 2 weeks or more before noticeable effect; 4 weeks or more before full effect.
- In most patients, MAO inhibitors should be discontinued 14 days before elective surgery to avoid drug interactions that may occur during the anesthetic procedure.

trazodone hydrochloride

Desyrel, Trazon, Trialodine
Pregnancy Risk Category: C

HOW SUPPLIED
Tablets: 50 mg, 100 mg, 150 mg

MECHANISM OF ACTION
Inhibits serotonin uptake in the brain. Not a tricyclic derivative; considered an atypical antidepressant.

INDICATIONS & DOSAGE
Treatment of depression –
Adults: initial dosage is 150 mg P.O. daily in divided doses, which can be increased by 50 mg daily q 3 to 4 days. Average dosage ranges from 150 mg to 400 mg daily. Maximum dosage is 600 mg.

ADVERSE REACTIONS
Common reactions are in italics; life-threatening reactions are in bold italics.
CNS: *drowsiness, dizziness,* nervousness, fatigue, confusion, tremors, weakness.
CV: orthostatic hypotension, tachycardia.
EENT: blurred vision, tinnitus.
GI: dry mouth, constipation, nausea, vomiting, anorexia.
GU: urine retention, priapism possibly leading to impotence.
Skin: rash, urticaria.
Other: sweating.

INTERACTIONS
Alcohol, CNS depressants: enhanced CNS depression.
Antihypertensives: added hypotensive effect of trazodone. Antihypertensive dosage may have to be decreased.
Digoxin, phenytoin: trazodone may increase serum levels of these drugs. Monitor for toxicity.
MAO inhibitors: No clinical experience. Use together very cautiously.

NURSING CONSIDERATIONS
- *Contraindicated* during initial recovery phase of myocardial infarction. Avoid concurrent administration with electroshock therapy. Drug may be discontinued before surgery.
- *Use cautiously* in cardiac disease, in suicidal patients, and in patients receiving CNS depressants.
- Priapism is a potential problem in men taking trazodone. Be sure to note if patient complains of prolonged and painful erections. May need surgical intervention.
- Watch for suicidal tendencies and record mood changes. Allow minimum amount of tablets to lessen suicide risk.
- Teach family how to recognize signs of suicidal tendency or ideation.
- Warn patient to avoid activities that require alertness until CNS effects of the drug are known. Drowsiness and dizziness usually subside after the first few weeks.
- Administer after meals or a light snack for optimal absorption and to decrease incidence of dizziness.
- Anticholinergic and adverse cardiac effects are minimal.
- Full effect may take 4 weeks or more.

trimipramine maleate
Apo-Trimip†, Surmontil
Pregnancy Risk Category: C

HOW SUPPLIED
Tablets: 25 mg‡
Capsules: 25 mg, 50 mg, 100 mg

MECHANISM OF ACTION
A tricyclic antidepressant (TCA) that increases the amount of norepinephrine or serotonin, or both, in the CNS by blocking their reuptake by the presynaptic neurons. This allows these neurotransmitters to accumulate.

INDICATIONS & DOSAGE
Treatment of depression –
Adults: 75 mg P.O. daily in divided doses, increased to 200 mg daily. Dosages over 300 mg daily not recommended.
Enuresis –

Children over 6 years: initial dosage 25 mg P.O. 1 hour before bedtime; if no response, increase dosage to 50 mg in children under 12 years, and to 75 mg in children over 12 years.

ADVERSE REACTIONS
Common reactions are in italics; life-threatening reactions are in bold italics.
CNS: *drowsiness, dizziness,* excitation, tremors, weakness, confusion, headache, nervousness, EEG changes, ***seizures,*** extrapyramidal reactions.
CV: *orthostatic hypotension, tachycardia, ECG changes,* hypertension.
EENT: *blurred vision,* tinnitus, mydriasis.
GI: *dry mouth, constipation,* nausea, vomiting, anorexia, paralytic ileus.
GU: *urine retention.*
Skin: rash, urticaria, photosensitivity.
Other: *sweating,* allergy.
After abrupt withdrawal of long-term therapy: nausea, headache, malaise. (Does not indicate addiction.)

INTERACTIONS
Barbiturates: decrease TCA blood levels. Monitor for decreased antidepressant effect.
Cimetidine: may increase trimipramine serum levels. Monitor for increased adverse reactions.
Epinephrine, norepinephrine: increase hypertensive effect. Use with caution.
MAO inhibitors: may cause severe excitation, hyperpyrexia, or seizures, usually with high dose. Use together cautiously.
Methylphenidate: increases TCA blood levels. Monitor for enhanced antidepressant effects.

NURSING CONSIDERATIONS
- *Contraindicated* during acute recovery phase of myocardial infarction; in patients with prostatic hypertrophy, seizure disorders, and suicidal ideation; and in those receiving electroshock therapy, thyroid drugs, or elective surgery.
- *Use with extreme caution* in CV disease, urine retention, narrow-angle glaucoma or increased intraocular pressure, thyroid disease, blood dyscrasia, or impaired hepatic function.
- Dry mouth may be relieved with sugarless hard candy or gum. Saliva substitutes may be necessary.
- Check for urine retention and constipation. Increase fluids to lessen constipation or suggest stool softener.
- Reduce dosage in elderly or debilitated persons and adolescents.
- Do not withdraw drug abruptly.
- Watch for increased psychotic signs; dosage should be reduced if they occur. Record mood changes. Watch for suicidal tendencies. Allow only minimum supply of tablets to lessen suicide risk.
- Warn patient to avoid hazardous activities that require alertness and good psychomotor coordination until CNS effects of the drug are known. Drowsiness and dizziness usually subside after a few weeks.
- Don't combine with alcohol or other depressants.
- Full effect may take 4 weeks or more.
- Effectiveness in enuresis may decrease over time.
- To avoid daytime sedation, patient should take full dose at bedtime if possible. Warn patient about possible morning orthostatic hypotension.
- Because hypertensive episodes have occurred during surgery in patients receiving TCAs, these drugs should be discontinued several days before surgery.
- Some patients may experience photosensitivity reactions. Advise patient to use a sunscreen, wear protective clothing, and avoid prolonged exposure to strong sunlight.

31
Antianxiety agents

alprazolam
buspirone hydrochloride
chlordiazepoxide
chlordiazepoxide hydrochloride
clorazepate dipotassium
diazepam
halazepam
hydroxyzine hydrochloride
hydroxyzine pamoate
lorazepam
meprobamate
oxazepam
prazepam

COMBINATION PRODUCTS
DEPROL**: meprobamate 400 mg and benactyzine hydrochloride 1 mg.
EQUAGESIC: meprobamate 200 mg and aspirin 325 mg.
LIBRAX CAPSULES: chlordiazepoxide hydrochloride 5 mg and clidinium bromide 2.5 mg.
LIMBITROL 5-12.5: chlordiazepoxide 5 mg and amitriptyline hydrochloride 12.5 mg.
LIMBITROL 10-25: chlordiazepoxide 10 mg and amitriptyline hydrochloride 25 mg.
MENRIUM 5-2: chlordiazepoxide 5 mg and esterified estrogens 0.2 mg.
MENRIUM 5-4: chlordiazepoxide 5 mg and esterified estrogens 0.4 mg.
MENRIUM 10-4: chlordiazepoxide 10 mg and esterified estrogens 0.4 mg.
MILPREM-200: meprobamate 200 mg and conjugated estrogens 0.45 mg.
MILPREM-400: meprobamate 400 mg and conjugated estrogens 0.45 mg.
PMB 200: meprobamate 200 mg and conjugated estrogens 0.45 mg.
PMB 400: meprobamate 400 mg and conjugated estrogens 0.45 mg.

alprazolam
Xanax
Controlled Substance Schedule IV
Pregnancy Risk Category: D

HOW SUPPLIED
Tablets: 0.25 mg, 0.5 mg, 1 mg, 2 mg

MECHANISM OF ACTION
Depresses the CNS at the limbic and subcortical levels of the brain.

INDICATIONS & DOSAGE
Anxiety and tension –
Adults: usual starting dose is 0.25 to 0.5 mg P.O. t.i.d. Maximum total daily dosage is 4 mg in divided doses. In elderly or debilitated patients, usual starting dose is 0.25 mg b.i.d. or t.i.d.

ADVERSE REACTIONS
Common reactions are in italics; life-threatening reactions are in bold italics.
CNS: *drowsiness, light-headedness,* headache, confusion, hostility.
CV: transient hypotension, tachycardia.
EENT: dry mouth.
GI: nausea, vomiting, constipation, discomfort.

INTERACTIONS
Alcohol, other CNS depressants: increased CNS depression. Avoid concomitant use.
Cigarette smoking: increased clearance of benzodiazepines. Monitor for lack of effect.
Cimetidine: increased sedation. Monitor carefully.
Digoxin: benzodiazepines may increase serum levels of digoxin, increasing risk of toxicity. Monitor closely.

*Liquid form contains alcohol. **May contain tartrazine.

Tricyclic antidepressants: increased plasma levels of tricyclic antidepressants. Monitor for toxicity.

NURSING CONSIDERATIONS

• *Contraindicated* in acute narrow-angle glaucoma, psychoses, or anxiety-free psychiatric disorders.
• *Use cautiously* in patients with hepatic or renal disease and in elderly or debilitated patients.
• Reduce dosage in elderly or debilitated patients because they may be more susceptible to the adverse CNS effects of the drug.
• Do not withdraw drug abruptly after long-term use. Withdrawal symptoms may occur. Abuse or addiction is possible.
• Warn patient not to combine drug with alcohol or other depressants and also to avoid hazardous activities that require alertness and psychomotor coordination until CNS effects are known.
• Caution patient against giving medication to others.
• Drug should not be prescribed for everyday stress or for long-term use (more than 4 months).
• Warn patient not to increase dosage or discontinue drug without doctor's approval.
• Alprazolam is the first triazolobenzodiazepine. It's more rapidly metabolized and excreted than most of the other benzodiazepines and has a lower incidence of lethargy than other drugs of this class.
• May also be effective for treatment of depression.
• Periodic hepatic, renal, and hematopoietic function studies should be performed in patients receiving repeated or prolonged therapy.
• If alprazolam overdose occurs, flumazenil (a specific benzodiazepine antagonist) may be useful. Know that the duration of action of alprazolam is longer than that of flumazenil, and resedation is possible.

buspirone hydrochloride

BuSpar

Pregnancy Risk Category: B

HOW SUPPLIED

Tablets: 5 mg, 10 mg

MECHANISM OF ACTION

Unknown. However, the drug may inhibit neuronal firing and reduce 5-HT turnover in cortical, amygdaloid, and septohippocampal tissue.

INDICATIONS & DOSAGE

Management of anxiety disorders; short-term relief of anxiety –
Adults: initially, 5 mg P.O. t.i.d. Dosage may be increased at 3-day intervals. Usual maintenance dosage is 20 to 30 mg daily in divided doses.

ADVERSE REACTIONS

Common reactions are in italics; life-threatening reactions are in bold italics.
CNS: *dizziness, drowsiness,* nervousness, insomnia, headache.
GI: nausea, dry mouth, diarrhea.
Other: fatigue.

INTERACTIONS

Alcohol, other CNS depressants: increased CNS depression. Avoid concomitant use.
MAO inhibitors: may elevate blood pressure.

NURSING CONSIDERATIONS

• *Contraindicated in* patients with hypersensitivity to the drug.
• *Use cautiously* in patients with hepatic or renal failure.
• Although buspirone is less sedating than other anxiolytics and does not produce any serious functional impairment, CNS effects in an individual patient may be unpredictable. Therefore, warn patients to avoid hazardous activities that require alertness and neuromuscular coordination until CNS effects of the drug are known.

• Unlike the benzodiazepines, buspirone is not an effective anticonvulsant or skeletal muscle relaxant. Its use is limited to the treatment of anxiety.
• Tell patient to take drug with food.
• Before initiating buspirone therapy in patients already being treated with benzodiazepines, warn them against stopping the benzodiazepine abruptly. Abrupt discontinuation may cause a benzodiazepine withdrawal reaction.
• Signs of improvement with buspirone are usually evident within 7 to 10 days; optimal results are achieved after 3 to 4 weeks of therapy.
• This drug has shown no potential for abuse and has not been classified as a controlled substance. However, it is not recommended for use to relieve everyday stress.

chlordiazepoxide

Libritabs

chlordiazepoxide hydrochloride

Apo-Chlordiazepoxide†, Librium, Lipoxide, Medilium†, Mitran, Novopoxide†, Reposans, Sereen, Solium†

Controlled Substance Schedule IV
Pregnancy Risk Category: D

HOW SUPPLIED

chlordiazepoxide
Tablets: 5 mg, 10 mg, 25 mg
chlordiazepoxide hydrochloride
Capsules: 5 mg, 10 mg, 25 mg
Powder for injection: 100 mg/ampule

MECHANISM OF ACTION

Depresses the CNS at the limbic and subcortical levels of the brain.

INDICATIONS & DOSAGE

Mild to moderate anxiety and tension –
Adults: 5 to 10 mg P.O. t.i.d. or q.i.d.
Children over 6 years: 5 mg P.O. b.i.d. to q.i.d. Maximum dosage is 10 mg P.O. b.i.d. to t.i.d.
Severe anxiety and tension –
Adults: 20 to 25 mg P.O. t.i.d. or q.i.d.
Withdrawal symptoms of acute alcoholism –
Adults: 50 to 100 mg P.O., I.M., or I.V. Maximum dosage is 300 mg daily.
Preoperative apprehension and anxiety –
Adults: 5 to 10 mg P.O. t.i.d. or q.i.d. on day preceding surgery; or 50 to 100 mg I.M. 1 hour before surgery.

Note: Parenteral form not recommended in children under 12 years.

ADVERSE REACTIONS

Common reactions are in italics; life-threatening reactions are in bold italics.
CNS: *drowsiness, lethargy, hangover,* fainting.
CV: transient hypotension.
GI: nausea, vomiting, abdominal discomfort.
Local: *thrombophlebitis, swelling, pain at injection site.*

INTERACTIONS

Alcohol, other CNS depressants: increased CNS depression. Avoid concomitant use.
Cigarette smoking: increased clearance of benzodiazepines. Monitor for lack of effect.
Cimetidine: increased sedation. Monitor carefully.
Digoxin: increased serum digoxin levels and risk of toxicity. Monitor closely.

NURSING CONSIDERATIONS

• *Contraindicated* in patients with hypersensitivity to the drug and in those with acute narrow-angle glaucoma, psychoses, or anxiety-free psychiatric disorders.
• *Use cautiously* in mental depression, psychiatric disturbances, blood dyscrasias, porphyria, hepatic or

*Liquid form contains alcohol. **May contain tartrazine.

renal disease, or in those undergoing anticoagulant therapy.

- Dosage should be reduced in elderly or debilitated patients.
- Possibility of abuse and addiction. Do not withdraw drug abruptly after long-term administration; withdrawal symptoms may occur.
- Warn patient to avoid hazardous activities that require alertness and good psychomotor coordination until CNS effects of the drug are known.
- Warn patient not to combine drug with alcohol or other depressants.
- Package recommends I.M. use only, but this drug may be given I.V.
- Injectable form (as hydrochloride) comes as two ampules – diluent and powdered drug. Read directions carefully. For I.M. use, add 2 ml of diluent to powder and agitate gently until clear. Use immediately. I.M. form may be erratically absorbed.
- **I.V. use:** Use 5 ml of saline injection or sterile water for injection as diluent; do not give packaged diluent I.V. Give slowly over 1 minute.
- Be sure that equipment and personnel needed for emergency airway management are available when giving drug I.V. Monitor respirations every 5 to 15 minutes and before each repeated I.V. dose.
- If chlordiazepoxide overdose occurs, flumazenil (a specific benzodiazepine antagonist) may be useful. Know that the duration of action of chlordiazepoxide is longer than that of flumazenil, and resedation is possible.
- Keep powder away from light and store in the refrigerator; mix just before use; discard remainder.
- Do not mix injectable form with any other parenteral drug.
- Caution patient against giving medication to others.
- Drug should not be prescribed regularly for everyday stress.
- May cause false-positive reaction in the Gravindex pregnancy test. May also interfere with certain tests for urine 17-ketosteroids.
- Periodic hepatic, renal, and hematopoietic function studies should be performed in patients receiving repeated or prolonged therapy.

clorazepate dipotassium

Gen-Xene, Novoclopate†, Tranxene, Tranxene-SD, Tranxene-T-Tab

Controlled Substance Schedule IV

Pregnancy Risk Category: C

HOW SUPPLIED

Tablets: 3.75 mg, 7.5 mg, 11.25 mg, 15 mg, 22.5 mg
Capsules: 3.75 mg, 7.5 mg, 15 mg

MECHANISM OF ACTION

Depresses the CNS at the limbic and subcortical levels of the brain. As an anticonvulsant, suppresses the spread of seizure activity produced by epileptogenic foci in the cortex, thalamus, and limbic structures.

INDICATIONS & DOSAGE

Acute alcohol withdrawal –
Adults: Day 1 – 30 mg P.O. initially, followed by 30 to 60 mg P.O. in divided doses; Day 2 – 45 to 90 mg P.O. in divided doses; Day 3 – 22.5 to 45 mg P.O. in divided doses; Day 4 – 15 to 30 mg P.O. in divided doses; gradually reduce daily dosage to 7.5 to 15 mg.

Anxiety –
Adults: 15 to 60 mg P.O. daily.

As an adjunct in seizure disorder –
Adults and children over 12 years: Maximum recommended initial dosage is 7.5 mg P.O. t.i.d. Dosage increases should be no greater than 7.5 mg/week. Maximum daily dosage should not exceed 90 mg daily.
Children between 9 and 12 years: Maximum recommended initial dosage is 7.5 mg P.O. b.i.d. Dosage increases should be no greater than 7.5

mg/week. Maximum daily dosage should not exceed 60 mg/day.

ADVERSE REACTIONS

Common reactions are in italics; life-threatening reactions are in bold italics.
CNS: *drowsiness, lethargy, hangover,* fainting.
CV: transient hypotension.
GI: nausea, vomiting, abdominal discomfort.

INTERACTIONS

Alcohol, other CNS depressants: increased CNS depression. Avoid concomitant use.
Cigarette smoking: increased clearance of benzodiazepines. Monitor for lack of effect.
Cimetidine: increased sedation. Monitor carefully.
Digoxin: benzodiazepines may increase serum levels of digoxin, increasing risk of toxicity. Monitor closely.

NURSING CONSIDERATIONS

- *Contraindicated* in acute narrow-angle glaucoma, depressive neuroses, and psychotic reactions and in children under 18 years.
- *Use cautiously* when hepatic or renal damage is present.
- Dosage should be reduced in elderly or debilitated patients.
- Possibility of abuse and addiction exists. Do not withdraw drug abruptly after prolonged use; withdrawal symptoms may occur.
- Warn patient to avoid activities requiring alertness and good psychomotor coordination until CNS effects of the drug are known.
- Warn patient not to combine drug with alcohol or other depressants.
- Suggest sugarless chewing gum or hard candy to relieve dry mouth.
- Caution patient against giving medication to others.
- Drug should not be prescribed regularly for everyday stress.
- Periodic hepatic, renal, and hematopoietic function studies should be performed in patients receiving repeated or prolonged therapy.
- If clorazepate overdose occurs, flumazenil (a specific benzodiazepine antagonist) may be useful. Know that the duration of action of clorazepate is longer than that of flumazenil, and resedation is possible.

diazepam

Apo-Diazepam†, Diazemuls†, Diazepam Intensol, E-Pam†, Meval†, Novodipam†, Q-Pam, Rival†, Valium, Valrelease, Vasepam, Vivol†, Zetran
Controlled Substance Schedule IV
Pregnancy Risk Category: D

HOW SUPPLIED

Tablets: 2 mg, 5 mg, 10 mg
Capsules (extended-release): 15 mg
Oral solution: 5 mg/5 ml, 5 mg/ml
Injection: 5 mg/ml
Sterile emulsion for injection: 5 mg/ml†

MECHANISM OF ACTION

Depresses the CNS at the limbic and subcortical levels of the brain. As an anticonvulsant, suppresses the spread of seizure activity produced by epileptogenic foci in the cortex, thalamus, and limbic structures.

INDICATIONS & DOSAGE

Tension, anxiety, adjunct in seizure disorders or skeletal muscle spasm –
Adults: 2 to 10 mg P.O. t.i.d. or q.i.d. Or, 15 to 30 mg of extended-release capsule once daily.
Children over 6 months: 1 to 2.5 mg P.O. t.i.d. or q.i.d.
Tension, anxiety, muscle spasm, endoscopic procedures, seizures –
Adults: 5 to 10 mg I.V. initially, up to 30 mg in 1 hour or possibly more for cardioversion or status epilepticus, depending on response.

*Liquid form contains alcohol. **May contain tartrazine.

Children 5 years and older: 1 mg I.V. or I.M. slowly q 2 to 5 minutes to maximum of 10 mg. Repeat q 2 to 4 hours.
Children 30 days to 5 years: 0.2 to 0.5 mg I.V. or I.M. slowly q 2 to 5 minutes to maximum of 5 mg. Repeat q 2 to 4 hours.
Tetanic muscle spasms –
Children over 5 years: 5 to 10 mg I.M. or I.V. q 3 to 4 hours, p.r.n.
Infants over 30 days: 1 to 2 mg I.M. or I.V. q 3 to 4 hours, p.r.n.
Status epilepticus –
Adults: 5 to 20 mg slow I.V. push 2 to 5 mg/minute; may repeat q 5 to 10 minutes up to maximum total dose of 60 mg. Use 2 to 5 mg in elderly or debilitated patients. May repeat therapy in 20 to 30 minutes with caution if seizures recur.
Children: 0.1 to 0.3 mg/kg slow I.V. push (1 mg/minute over 3 minutes). May repeat q 15 minutes for 2 doses. Maximum single dose in children under 5 years is 5 mg; in children over 5 years, 10 mg.

ADVERSE REACTIONS

Common reactions are in italics; life-threatening reactions are in bold italics.
CNS: *drowsiness, lethargy, hangover, ataxia,* fainting, slurred speech, tremor.
CV: transient hypotension, bradycardia, ***cardiovascular collapse.***
EENT: diplopia, blurred vision, nystagmus.
GI: nausea, vomiting, abdominal discomfort.
Skin: rash, urticaria.
Local: desquamation, *pain, phlebitis at injection site.*
Other: respiratory depression.

INTERACTIONS

Alcohol, other CNS depressants: increased CNS depression. Avoid concomitant use.
Cigarette smoking: increased clearance of benzodiazepines. Monitor for lack of effect.
Cimetidine: increased sedation. Monitor carefully.
Digoxin: benzodiazepines may increase serum levels of digoxin, increasing risk of toxicity. Monitor closely.
Phenobarbital: increased effects of both drugs. Use together cautiously.

NURSING CONSIDERATIONS

- *Contraindicated* in shock, coma, acute alcohol intoxication, acute narrow-angle glaucoma, psychoses, myasthenia gravis; in oral form for children under 6 months.
- *Use cautiously* in blood dyscrasia, hepatic or renal damage, depression, open-angle glaucoma; in elderly and debilitated patients; and in those with limited pulmonary reserve.
- Dosage should be reduced in elderly or debilitated patients because they may be more susceptible to the adverse CNS effects of the drug.
- Whenever oral concentrate solution is used, the dose should be diluted just before administering. Use water, juice, or carbonated beverages, or mix with semisolid food such as applesauce or pudding.
- Possibility of abuse and addiction exists. Do not withdraw drug abruptly after long-term use; withdrawal symptoms may occur.
- Monitor CBC and hepatic and renal function during long-term use.
- Warn patient to avoid activities that require alertness and good psychomotor coordination until CNS effects of the drug are known.
- Warn patient not to combine drug with alcohol or other depressants.
- Do not mix injectable form with other drugs because diazepam is incompatible with most drugs.
- **I.V. use:** Give I.V. slowly, at rate not exceeding 5 mg/minute. When injecting I.V., best to administer directly into the vein. If this is not pos-

sible, inject slowly through the infusion tubing as close as possible to the vein insertion site. Watch daily for phlebitis at injection site.
- Avoid extravasation. Do not inject into small veins.
- There is considerable controversy about the use of diluted diazepam solutions for continuous I.V. infusion because of its low aqueous solubility. Under certain conditions, it may be compatible with 0.9% sodium chloride or lactated Ringer's injection, but the solution may not be stable. Consult hospital pharmacy.
- Monitor respirations every 5 to 15 minutes and before each repeated I.V. dose. Have emergency resuscitation equipment and oxygen at bedside.
- If diazepam overdose occurs, flumazenil (a specific benzodiazepine antagonist) may be useful. Know that the duration of action of diazepam is longer than that of flumazenil, and resedation is possible.
- I.V. route is more reliable; I.M. administration is not recommended because absorption is variable and injection is painful (because the solution is highly alkaline).
- Drug of choice (I.V. form) for status epilepticus.
- Seizures may recur within 20 to 30 minutes of initial control, because of redistribution of the drug.
- Continuous infusions of 1 to 10 mg hourly have been used to prevent seizure recurrence.
- Do not store diazepam in plastic syringes.
- Caution patient against giving medication to others.
- Drug should not be prescribed regularly for everyday stress.
- Periodic hepatic, renal, and hematopoietic function studies should be performed in patients receiving repeated or prolonged therapy.

halazepam

Paxipam

Controlled Substance Schedule IV

Pregnancy Risk Category: D

HOW SUPPLIED

Tablets: 20 mg, 40 mg

MECHANISM OF ACTION

Depresses the CNS at the limbic and subcortical levels of the brain.

INDICATIONS & DOSAGE

Relief of anxiety and tension –
Adults: Usual dose is 20 to 40 mg P.O. t.i.d. or q.i.d. Optimal daily dosage is generally 80 to 160 mg. Daily dosages up to 600 mg have been given. In elderly or debilitated patients, initial dosage is 20 mg once or twice daily.

ADVERSE REACTIONS

Common reactions are in italics; life-threatening reactions are in bold italics.
CNS: *drowsiness, lethargy, hangover,* fainting.
CV: transient hypotension.
EENT: dry mouth.
GI: nausea and vomiting, discomfort.

INTERACTIONS

Alcohol, other CNS depressants: increased CNS depression. Avoid concomitant use.
Cigarette smoking: increased clearance of benzodiazepines. Monitor for lack of effect.
Cimetidine: possible increased sedation. Monitor carefully.
Digoxin: benzodiazepines may increase serum levels of digoxin, increasing risk of toxicity. Monitor closely.

NURSING CONSIDERATIONS

- *Contraindicated* in patients with hypersensitivity to the drug and in patients with acute narrow-angle glau-

coma, psychoses, or anxiety-free psychiatric disorders.
- *Use cautiously* in hepatic or renal impairment.
- Reduce dosage in elderly or debilitated patients.
- Possibility of abuse and addiction exists. Do not withdraw drug abruptly after long-term use; withdrawal symptoms may occur.
- Warn patient not to combine drug with alcohol or other depressants, and to avoid hazardous activities that require alertness and psychomotor coordination until CNS effects are known.
- Caution patient against giving medication to others.
- Periodic hepatic, renal, and hematopoietic function studies should be performed in patients receiving repeated or prolonged therapy.
- Drug should not be prescribed for everyday stress or for long-term use (more than 4 months).
- If halazepam overdose occurs, flumazenil (a specific benzodiazepine antagonist) may be useful. Know that the duration of action of halazepam is longer than that of flumazenil, and resedation is possible.

hydroxyzine hydrochloride (hydroxyzine embonate)

Anxanil, Apo-Hydroxyzine†, Atarax*, Atozine, Durrax, E-Vista, Hydroxacen, Hyzine-50, Multipax†, Novohydroxyzin†, Quiess, Vistacon, Vistaject, Vistaquel, Vistaril, Vistazine

hydroxyzine pamoate

Hy-Pam, Vamate, Vistaril

Pregnancy Risk Category: C

HOW SUPPLIED

hydrochloride
Tablets: 10 mg, 25 mg, 50 mg, 100 mg
Capsules: 10 mg†‡, 25 mg†‡, 50 mg†‡
Syrup: 10 mg/5 ml
Injection: 25 mg/ml, 50 mg/ml

pamoate
Capsules: 25 mg, 50 mg, 100 mg
Oral suspension: 25 mg/5 ml

MECHANISM OF ACTION

A piperazine antihistamine. Depresses the CNS at the limbic and subcortical levels of the brain.

INDICATIONS & DOSAGE

Anxiety and tension –
Adults: 25 to 100 mg P.O. t.i.d. or q.i.d.
Anxiety, tension, hyperkinesia –
Children 6 years and over: 50 to 100 mg P.O. daily in divided doses.
Children under 6 years: 50 mg P.O. daily in divided doses.
Preoperative and postoperative adjunctive therapy –
Adults: 25 to 100 mg I.M. q 4 to 6 hours.
Children: 1.1 mg/kg I.M. q 4 to 6 hours.
Rashes, pruritus –
Adults: 25 mg P.O. t.i.d. or q.i.d.
Children 6 years and over: 50 to 100 mg P.O. daily in divided doses.
Children under 6 years: 50 mg P.O. daily in divided doses.

ADVERSE REACTIONS

Common reactions are in italics; life-threatening reactions are in bold italics.
CNS: *drowsiness,* involuntary motor activity.
GI: *dry mouth.*
Local: marked discomfort at site of I.M. injection.

INTERACTIONS

Alcohol, other CNS depressants: increased CNS depression. Avoid concomitant use.

NURSING CONSIDERATIONS

- *Contraindicated* in patients with hypersensitivity to the drug, in patients in shock or comatose states, and during acute asthmatic attacks.
- *Use cautiously* in patients with an-

gle-closure glaucoma, prostatic hypertrophy, COPD, asthma, hyperthyroidism, or cardiovascular disease.
• Dosage should be reduced in elderly or debilitated patients.
• Warn patient to avoid hazardous activities that require alertness and good psychomotor coordination until CNS effects of the drug are known.
• Warn patient not to combine drug with alcohol or other depressants.
• Observe for excessive sedation due to potentiation with other CNS drugs.
• Used perioperatively as an antiemetic and anxiolytic. Its sedative and antihistamine properties make it especially useful to treat pruritus that prevents sleep.
• Used in psychogenically induced allergic conditions, such as chronic urticaria and pruritus.
• Parenteral form (hydroxyzine hydrochloride) for I.M. use only. Never administer I.V. (Z-track injection is preferred.)
• Aspirate injection carefully to prevent inadvertent intravascular injection. Inject deep into a large muscle.
• Suggest sugarless hard candy or gum to relieve dry mouth.
• Hydroxyzine may cause false elevations of urine 17-hydroxycorticosteroids, depending on test method used.

lorazepam

Alzapam, Apo-Lorazepam†, Ativan, Loraz, Novolorazem†
Controlled Substance Schedule IV

Pregnancy Risk Category: D

HOW SUPPLIED

Tablets: 0.5 mg, 1 mg, 2 mg
Tablets (sublingual): 1 mg†, 2 mg†
Injection: 2 mg/ml, 4 mg/ml

MECHANISM OF ACTION

Depresses the CNS at the limbic and subcortical levels of the brain.

INDICATIONS & DOSAGE

Anxiety, tension, agitation, irritability, especially in anxiety neuroses or organic (especially GI or CV) disorders –
Adults: 2 to 6 mg P.O. daily in divided doses. Maximum dosage is 10 mg daily.
Insomnia –
Adults: 2 to 4 mg P.O. h.s.
Premedication before operative procedure –
Adults: 0.05 mg/kg I.M. or slow I.V. injection (< 2 mg/minute). Total dose should not exceed 4 mg.

ADVERSE REACTIONS

Common reactions are in italics; life-threatening reactions are in bold italics.
CNS: *drowsiness, lethargy, hangover,* fainting.
CV: transient hypotension.
GI: dry mouth, abdominal discomfort.

INTERACTIONS

Alcohol, other CNS depressants: increased CNS depression. Avoid concomitant use.
Cigarette smoking: increased clearance of benzodiazepines. Monitor for lack of effect.
Digoxin: benzodiazepines may increase serum levels of digoxin, increasing risk of toxicity. Monitor closely.

NURSING CONSIDERATIONS

• *Contraindicated* in acute narrow-angle glaucoma, psychoses, or mental depression.
• *Use cautiously* in organic brain syndrome, myasthenia gravis, and pulmonary, renal, or hepatic impairment.
• Dosage should be reduced in elderly or debilitated patients. Preoperative I.V. dose should not exceed 2 mg in patients over 50.
• Possibility of abuse and addiction exists. Do not withdraw drug abruptly after long-term use; withdrawal symptoms may occur.

• When administering I.M., inject deep into muscle mass. Don't dilute.
• **I.V. use:** Give I.V. slowly, at rate not exceeding 2 mg/minute. Dilute with an equal volume of sterile water for injection, 0.9% sodium chloride injection, or dextrose 5% injection.
• Monitor respirations every 5 to 15 minutes and before each repeated I.V. dose. Have emergency resuscitation equipment and oxygen at bedside.
• If lorazepam overdose occurs, flumazenil (a specific benzodiazepine antagonist) may be useful. Know that the duration of action of lorazepam is longer than that of flumazenil, and resedation is possible.
• Store parenteral form in refrigerator to prolong shelf life.
• Used as a premedication before surgery, lorazepam provides substantial preoperative amnesia. Therefore, patient teaching requires extra care to ensure adequate recall. Provide written materials or inform a family member if possible.
• Warn patient to avoid hazardous activities that require alertness or good psychomotor coordination until CNS effects of the drug are known.
• Warn patient not to combine drug with alcohol or other depressants.
• Caution patient against giving medication to others.
• Drug should not be prescribed regularly for everyday stress.
• Fewer cumulative effects than other benzodiazepines, due to short half-life.
• Periodic hepatic, renal, and hematopoietic function studies should be performed in patients receiving repeated or prolonged therapy.

meprobamate

Apo-Meprobamate†, Equanil**, Meditran, Meprospan, Miltown, Neuramate, Novo-Mepro†, Sedabamate, Tranmep
Controlled Substance Schedule IV
Pregnancy Risk Category: D

HOW SUPPLIED

Tablets: 200 mg, 400 mg, 600 mg
Capsules: 200 mg, 400 mg
Capsules (sustained-release): 200 mg, 400 mg

MECHANISM OF ACTION

Depresses the CNS at the limbic and subcortical levels of the brain.

INDICATIONS & DOSAGE

Anxiety and tension –
Adults: 1.2 to 1.6 g P.O. in three or four equally divided doses. Maximum dosage is 2.4 g daily.
Children 6 to 12 years: 100 to 200 mg P.O. b.i.d. or t.i.d. Not recommended for children under 6 years.

ADVERSE REACTIONS

Common reactions are in italics; life-threatening reactions are in bold italics.
Blood: ***thrombocytopenia, leukopenia,*** eosinophilia.
CNS: *drowsiness,* ataxia, dizziness, slurred speech, headache, vertigo.
CV: palpitation, tachycardia, hypotension.
GI: anorexia, nausea, vomiting, diarrhea, stomatitis.
Skin: pruritus, urticaria, erythematous maculopapular rash.

INTERACTIONS

Alcohol, other CNS depressants: increased CNS depression. Avoid concomitant use.

NURSING CONSIDERATIONS

• *Contraindicated* in patients with hypersensitivity to meprobamate, carisoprodol, mebutamate, tybamate, and carbromal and in renal insufficiency or porphyria.

- *Use cautiously* in patients with impaired hepatic or renal function, seizure disorders, or suicidal tendencies and in patients with a history of aspirin hypersensitivity.
- Dosage should be reduced in elderly or debilitated patients.
- Possibility of abuse and addiction exists with long-term use. Meprobamate should not be used for everyday stress. Withdraw drug gradually (over 2 weeks) or withdrawal symptoms may occur, including severe generalized tonic-clonic seizures.
- Warn patient to avoid hazardous activities that require alertness or good psychomotor coordination until CNS effects of the drug are known.
- Warn patient not to combine drug with alcohol or other depressants.
- Give drug with meals to reduce GI distress.
- Therapeutic blood levels 0.5 to 2 mg/100 ml; levels above 20 mg/100 ml may cause coma and death.
- Periodic evaluation of CBC and renal and hepatic function tests are indicated in patients receiving high doses.
- Tell patient to report any unusual bruising or bleeding, fever, or sore throat. These symptoms may indicate serious hematologic toxicity.
- Meprobamate may interfere with certain laboratory tests for urinary 17-ketogenic steroids and 17-hydroxycorticosteroids.

oxazepam

Apo-Oxazepam†, Novoxapam†, Ox-Pam†, Serax**, Zapex†
Controlled Substance Schedule IV
Pregnancy Risk Category: C

HOW SUPPLIED

Tablets: 10 mg, 15 mg, 30 mg
Capsules: 10 mg, 15 mg, 30 mg

MECHANISM OF ACTION

Depresses the CNS at the limbic and subcortical levels of the brain.

INDICATIONS & DOSAGE

Alcohol withdrawal –
Adults: 15 to 30 mg P.O. t.i.d. or q.i.d.
Severe anxiety –
Adults: 15 to 30 mg P.O. t.i.d. or q.i.d.
Tension, mild to moderate anxiety –
Adults: 10 to 15 mg P.O. t.i.d. or q.i.d.

ADVERSE REACTIONS

Common reactions are in italics; life-threatening reactions are in bold italics.
Blood: ***leukopenia (rare).***
CNS: *drowsiness, lethargy, hangover,* fainting.
CV: transient hypotension.
GI: nausea, vomiting, abdominal discomfort.
Metabolic: ***hepatic dysfunction.***

INTERACTIONS

Alcohol, other CNS depressants: increased CNS depression. Avoid concomitant use.
Cigarette smoking: increased clearance of benzodiazepines. Monitor for lack of effect.
Digoxin: benzodiazepines may increase serum levels of digoxin, increasing risk of toxicity. Monitor closely.

NURSING CONSIDERATIONS

- *Contraindicated* in patients with hypersensitivity to the drug and in those with acute narrow-angle glaucoma, depression, or psychoses.
- *Use cautiously* in patients with history of convulsive disorders, drug allergies, blood dyscrasias, renal disease, and depression.
- Dose should be reduced in elderly or debilitated patients.
- Possibility of abuse and addiction

*Liquid form contains alcohol. **May contain tartrazine.

exists. Don't stop drug abruptly; withdrawal symptoms may occur.
- Warn patient to avoid hazardous activities that require alertness or good psychomotor coordination until CNS effects of the drug are known.
- Warn patient not to combine drug with alcohol or other depressants.
- Fewer cumulative effects than many other benzodiazepines due to short half-life.
- Periodic hepatic, renal, and hematopoietic function studies should be performed in patients receiving repeated or prolonged therapy.
- If oxazepam overdose occurs, flumazenil (a specific benzodiazepine antagonist) may be useful. Know that the duration of action of oxazepam is longer than that of flumazenil, and resedation is possible.

prazepam

Centrax

Controlled Substance Schedule IV

Pregnancy Risk Category: C

HOW SUPPLIED
Tablets: 10 mg
Capsules: 5 mg, 10 mg, 20 mg

MECHANISM OF ACTION
Depresses the CNS at the limbic and subcortical levels of the brain.

INDICATIONS & DOSAGE
Anxiety–
Adults: 20 to 60 mg P.O. daily in divided dose, or 20 mg h.s.

ADVERSE REACTIONS
Common reactions are in italics; life-threatening reactions are in bold italics.
CNS: *drowsiness, lethargy, hangover,* dizziness, ataxia, fainting.
CV: transient hypotension.
GI: dry mouth, nausea, vomiting, abdominal discomfort.
Skin: rash.

INTERACTIONS
Alcohol, other CNS depressants: increased CNS depression. Avoid concomitant use.
Cigarette smoking: increased clearance of benzodiazepines. Monitor for lack of effect.
Cimetidine: increased sedation. Monitor carefully.
Digoxin: benzodiazepines may increase serum levels of digoxin, increasing risk of toxicity. Monitor closely.

NURSING CONSIDERATIONS
- *Contraindicated* in acute narrow-angle glaucoma, psychoses, or anxiety-free psychiatric disorders.
- *Use cautiously* in renal or hepatic impairment.
- Dosage should be reduced in elderly or debilitated patients.
- Possibility of abuse and addiction exists. Don't stop drug abruptly: withdrawal symptoms may occur.
- Warn patient to avoid activities that require alertness until CNS effects of the drug are known.
- Prazepam should not be prescribed for everyday stress.
- Periodic hepatic, renal, and hematopoietic function studies should be performed in patients receiving repeated or prolonged therapy.
- If prazepam overdose occurs, flumazenil (a specific benzodiazepine antagonist) may be useful. Know that the duration of action of prazepam is longer than that of flumazenil, and resedation is possible.

32

Antipsychotics

acetophenazine maleate
chlorpromazine hydrochloride
chlorprothixene
clozapine
fluphenazine decanoate
fluphenazine enanthate
fluphenazine hydrochloride
haloperidol
haloperidol decanoate
haloperidol lactate
loxapine hydrochloride
loxapine succinate
mesoridazine besylate
molindone hydrochloride
perphenazine
pimozide
prochlorperazine
(See Chapter 49, ANTIEMETICS.)
promazine hydrochloride
thioridazine hydrochloride
thiothixene
thiothixene hydrochloride
trifluoperazine hydrochloride

COMBINATION PRODUCTS
ETRAFON 2-10: perphenazine 2 mg and amitriptyline hydrochloride 10 mg.
ETRAFON-A: perphenazine 2 mg and amitriptyline hydrochloride 25 mg.
ETRAFON-FORTE: perphenazine 4 mg and amitriptyline hydrochloride 25 mg.
TRIAVIL 2-10, TRIAVIL 4-10, TRIAVIL 2-25 are identical to Etrafon products above; TRIAVIL 4-50: perphenazine 4 mg and amitriptyline hydrochloride 50 mg.

acetophenazine maleate
Tindal

Pregnancy Risk Category: C

HOW SUPPLIED
Tablets: 20 mg

MECHANISM OF ACTION
Blocks postsynaptic dopamine receptors in the brain. A piperazine phenothiazine.

INDICATIONS & DOSAGE
Psychotic disorders –
Adults: initially, 20 mg P.O. t.i.d. or q.i.d. Daily dosage ranges from 40 to 80 mg in outpatients, or 80 to 120 mg in hospitalized patients, but in severe psychotic states up to 600 mg daily has been safely administered. Smallest effective dosage should be used at all times.

ADVERSE REACTIONS
Common reactions are in italics; life-threatening reactions are in bold italics.
Blood: transient leukopenia, *agranulocytosis.*
CNS: *extrapyramidal reactions (high incidence), tardive dyskinesia,* sedation (low incidence), pseudoparkinsonism, EEG changes, dizziness.
CV: *orthostatic hypotension,* tachycardia, ECG changes.
EENT: ocular changes, *blurred vision.*
GI: *dry mouth, constipation.*
GU: *urine retention,* dark urine, menstrual irregularities, gynecomastia, inhibited ejaculation.
Hepatic: cholestatic jaundice, abnormal liver function tests.
Metabolic: hyperprolactinemia.
Skin: *mild photosensitivity,* dermal allergic reactions.
Other: weight gain; increased appetite; rarely, ***neuroleptic malignant syndrome*** (fever, tachycardia, tachypnea, profuse diaphoresis).
After abrupt withdrawal of long-term therapy: gastritis, nausea, vomiting, dizziness, tremors, feeling of

*Liquid form contains alcohol. **May contain tartrazine.

warmth or cold, sweating, tachycardia, headache, insomnia.

INTERACTIONS

Alcohol, other CNS depressants: increased CNS depression. Avoid concomitant use.
Antacids: inhibit absorption of oral phenothiazines. Separate antacid and phenothiazine doses by at least 2 hours.
Barbiturates: may decrease phenothiazine effect. Observe patient.

NURSING CONSIDERATIONS

- *Contraindicated* in CNS depression, bone marrow suppression, subcortical damage, and coma, with use of spinal or epidural anesthetic or adrenergic blockers.
- *Use cautiously* with other CNS depressants and anticholinergics; in elderly or debilitated patients; and in hepatic disease, arteriosclerosis or cardiovascular disease (may cause sudden drop in blood pressure), exposure to extreme heat or cold (including antipyretic therapy), respiratory disorders, hypocalcemia, seizure disorders (may lower seizure threshold), severe reactions to insulin or electroshock therapy, suspected brain tumor or intestinal obstruction, glaucoma, or prostatic hypertrophy.
- Tardive dyskinesia may occur after prolonged use. It may not appear until months or years later and may disappear spontaneously or persist for life despite discontinuation of drug.
- Acute dystonic reactions may be treated with I.V. diphenhydramine.
- Neuroleptic malignant syndrome is rare, but frequently fatal. It is not necessarily related to length of drug use or type of neuroleptic, but over 60% of affected patients are men. Watch for symptoms.
- Hold dose and notify doctor if patient develops symptoms of blood dyscrasias (fever, sore throat, infection, cellulitis, weakness), persistent (longer than a few hours) extrapyramidal reactions, or any such reaction during pregnancy.
- Dose of 20 mg is therapeutic equivalent of 100 mg chlorpromazine.
- Monitor therapy by weekly bilirubin tests during first month; periodic blood tests (CBC and liver function); and ophthalmic tests (long-term use).
- Have patient report urine retention or constipation.
- Tell patient to use sunscreening agents and protective clothing to avoid photosensitivity reactions.
- Tell patient that the drug may discolor the urine.
- Warn against activities requiring alertness or good psychomotor coordination until CNS effects of the drug are known.
- Obtain baseline measures of blood pressure before starting therapy and monitor routinely. Watch for orthostatic hypotension. Advise patient to get up slowly.
- Dry mouth may be relieved with sugarless gum, sour hard candy, or rinsing with mouthwash.
- Do not withdraw drug abruptly unless required by severe adverse reactions.
- Patient on maintenance may take medication at bedtime to facilitate sleep and decrease sedation during daytime.

chlorpromazine hydrochloride

Chlorpromanyl†, Largactil†‡, Novo-Chlorpromazine†, Protran‡, Thorazine, Thor-Pram

Pregnancy Risk Category: C

HOW SUPPLIED

Tablets: 10 mg, 25 mg, 50 mg, 100 mg, 200 mg
Capsules (sustained-release): 30 mg, 75 mg, 150 mg, 200 mg, 300 mg
Oral concentrate: 30 mg/ml, 100 mg/ml

Syrup: 10 mg/5ml
Injection: 25 mg/ml
Suppositories: 25 mg, 100 mg

MECHANISM OF ACTION

Blocks postsynaptic dopamine receptors in the brain. As an antiemetic, inhibits the medullary chemoreceptor trigger zone. Aliphatic phenothiazine.

INDICATIONS & DOSAGE

Intractable hiccups –
Adults: 25 to 50 mg P.O. or I.M. t.i.d. or q.i.d.
Mild alcohol withdrawal, acute intermittent porphyria, and tetanus –
Adults: 25 to 50 mg I.M. t.i.d. or q.i.d.
Psychosis –
Adults: initially, 30 to 75 mg P.O. daily in two to four divided doses. Increase dosage by 20 to 50 mg twice weekly until symptoms are controlled. Up to 800 mg daily may be required in some patients. Or give 25 to 50 mg I.M. q 1 to 4 hours p.r.n. Switch to oral therapy as soon as possible.
Children: 0.25 mg/kg P.O. q 4 to 6 hours; or 0.25 mg/kg I.M. q 6 to 8 hours; or 0.5 mg/kg rectally q 6 to 8 hours. Maximum I.M. dose is 40 mg in children under 5 years, and 75 mg in children 5 to 12 years.
Nausea and vomiting –
Adults: 10 to 25 mg P.O. or I.M. q 4 to 6 hours, p.r.n.; or 50 to 100 mg rectally q 6 to 8 hours, p.r.n.
Children: 0.25 mg/kg P.O. q 4 to 6 hours; or 0.25 mg/kg I.M. q 6 to 8 hours; or 0.5 mg/kg rectally q 6 to 8 hours.

ADVERSE REACTIONS

Common reactions are in italics; life-threatening reactions are in bold italics.
Blood: transient leukopenia, ***agranulocytosis.***
CNS: *extrapyramidal reactions (moderate incidence), sedation (high incidence), tardive dyskinesia,* pseudoparkinsonism, EEG changes, dizziness.
CV: *orthostatic hypotension,* tachycardia, ECG changes.
EENT: ocular changes, *blurred vision.*
GI: *dry mouth, constipation.*
GU: *urine retention,* dark urine, menstrual irregularities, gynecomastia, inhibited ejaculation.
Hepatic: cholestatic jaundice, abnormal liver function tests.
Metabolic: hyperprolactinemia.
Skin: *mild photosensitivity,* dermal allergic reactions.
Local: *pain on I.M. injection,* sterile abscess.
Other: weight gain; increased appetite; rarely, ***neuroleptic malignant syndrome*** (fever, tachycardia, tachypnea, profuse diaphoresis).
After abrupt withdrawal of long-term therapy: gastritis, nausea, vomiting, dizziness, tremors, feeling of warmth or cold, sweating, tachycardia, headache, insomnia.

INTERACTIONS

Alcohol, other CNS depressants: increased CNS depression. Avoid concomitant use.
Antacids: inhibit absorption of oral phenothiazines. Separate antacid and phenothiazine doses by at least 2 hours.
Anticholinergics (including antidepressant and antiparkinsonian agents): increased anticholinergic activity, aggravated parkinsonian symptoms. Use with caution.
Barbiturates, lithium: may decrease phenothiazine effect. Observe patient.
Centrally acting antihypertensive agents: decreased antihypertensive effect.
Lithium: possible decreased response to chlorpromazine. Observe patient.
Oral anticoagulants: decreased anticoagulant effect.

*Liquid form contains alcohol. **May contain tartrazine.

Propranolol: increased levels of both propranolol and chlorpromazine.

NURSING CONSIDERATIONS

- *Contraindicated* in CNS depression, bone marrow suppresion, subcortical damage, Reye's syndrome, and coma; also contraindicated with use of spinal or epidural anesthetic, or adrenergic blocking agents.
- *Use cautiously* with other CNS depressants, anticholinergics; in elderly or debilitated patients; in hepatic disease, arteriosclerosis or CV disease (may cause sudden drop in blood pressure), exposure to extreme heat or cold (including antipyretic therapy), respiratory disorders, hypocalcemia, seizure disorders (may lower seizure threshold), severe reactions to insulin or electroshock therapy, suspected brain tumor or intestinal obstruction, glaucoma, or prostatic hypertrophy; and in acutely ill or dehydrated children. Use parenteral form cautiously in asthmatics and in patients allergic to sulfites.
- Tardive dyskinesia may occur after prolonged use. It may not appear until months or years later and may disappear spontaneously or persist for life despite discontinuation of drug.
- Neuroleptic malignant syndrome is rare, but frequently fatal. It is not necessarily related to length of drug use or type of neuroleptic, but over 60% of affected patients are men. Watch for symptoms.
- Acute dystonic reactions may be treated with I.V. diphenhydramine.
- Hold dose and notify doctor if patient develops jaundice, symptoms of blood dyscrasia (fever, sore throat, infection, cellulitis, weakness), persistent (longer than a few hours) extrapyramidal reactions, or any such reaction in pregnancy or in children.
- Monitor therapy by weekly bilirubin tests during first month; periodic blood tests (CBC and liver function); and ophthalmic tests (long-term use).
- Have patient report urine retention or constipation.
- Tell patient that the drug may discolor the urine.
- Tell patient to use sunscreening agents and protective clothing to avoid photosensitivity reactions. Chlorpromazine causes higher incidence of photosensitivity than any other drug in its class.
- Warn against activities that require alertness or good psychomotor coordination until CNS effects of the drug are known. Drowsiness and dizziness usually subside after first few weeks.
- Obtain baseline measures of blood pressure before starting therapy and monitor regularly. Watch for orthostatic hypotension, especially with parenteral administration. Monitor blood pressure before and after I.M. administration. Keep patient supine for 1 hour afterward. Advise patient to get up slowly.
- Give deep I.M. only in upper outer quadrant of buttocks. Massage slowly afterward to prevent sterile abscess. Injection stings.
- Liquid (oral) and parenteral forms of drug can cause contact dermatitis. If susceptible, wear gloves when preparing solutions of this drug, and prevent any contact with skin and clothing.
- Protect liquid concentrate from light. Dilute with fruit juice, milk, or semisolid food just before administration.
- Slight yellowing of injection or concentrate is common; does not affect potency. Discard markedly discolored solutions.
- Do not withdraw drug abruptly unless required by severe adverse reactions.
- Dry mouth may be relieved by sugarless gum, sour hard candy, or rinsing with mouthwash.

chlorprothixene

Taractan**, Tarasan†

Pregnancy Risk Category: C

HOW SUPPLIED

Tablets: 10 mg, 25 mg, 50 mg, 100 mg
Oral concentrate: 100 mg/5 ml (fruit)
Injection: 12.5 mg/ml

MECHANISM OF ACTION

Blocks postsynaptic dopamine receptors in the brain. A thioxanthene.

INDICATIONS & DOSAGE

Psychotic disorders –
Adults: initially, 10 mg P.O. t.i.d. or q.i.d. Increase gradually to maximum of 600 mg daily.
Children over 6 years: 10 to 25 mg P.O. t.i.d. or q.i.d.
Agitation of severe neurosis, depression, schizophrenia –
Adults: 25 to 50 mg P.O. or I.M. t.i.d. or q.i.d. Increase as needed up to maximum of 600 mg.

ADVERSE REACTIONS

Common reactions are in italics; life-threatening reactions are in bold italics.
Blood: transient leukopenia, ***agranulocytosis.***
CNS: extrapyramidal reactions (low incidence), tardive dyskinesia, *sedation,* pseudoparkinsonism, EEG changes, dizziness.
CV: *orthostatic hypotension,* tachycardia, ECG changes.
EENT: ocular changes, *blurred vision.*
GI: *dry mouth, constipation.*
GU: *urine retention,* dark urine, menstrual irregularities, gynecomastia, inhibited ejaculation.
Hepatic: cholestatic jaundice, abnormal liver function tests.
Metabolic: hyperprolactinemia.
Skin: *mild photosensitivity,* dermal allergic reactions.
Local: pain on I.M. injection, sterile abscess.
Other: weight gain; increased appetite; rarely, ***neuroleptic malignant syndrome*** (fever, tachycardia, tachypnea, profuse diaphoresis).
After abrupt withdrawal of long-term therapy: gastritis, nausea, vomiting, dizziness, tremors, feeling of warmth or cold, sweating, tachycardia, headache, insomnia.

INTERACTIONS

Alcohol, other CNS depressants: increased CNS depression. Avoid concomitant use.
Anticholinergics: potentiated central anticholinergic effects.
Centrally acting antihypertensives: decreased antihypertensive effect.

NURSING CONSIDERATIONS

- *Contraindicated* in coma, CNS depression, bone marrow suppression, circulatory collapse, CHF, cardiac decompensation, coronary artery or cerebrovascular disorders, subcortical damage; with use of spinal or epidural anesthetic, or adrenergic blocking agents.
- *Use cautiously* with other CNS depressants, anticholinergics; in elderly or debilitated patients; in hepatic or renal disease, arteriosclerosis or CV disease (may cause sudden drop in blood pressure), exposure to extreme heat or cold (including antipyretic therapy), respiratory disorders, hypocalcemia, seizure disorders (may lower seizure threshold), severe reactions to insulin or electroshock therapy, suspected brain tumor or intestinal obstruction, glaucoma, or prostatic hypertrophy; and in acutely ill or dehydrated children.
- Tardive dyskinesia may occur after prolonged use. It may not appear until months or years later and may disappear spontaneously or persist for life despite discontinuation of drug.
- Neuroleptic malignant syndrome is

*Liquid form contains alcohol. **May contain tartrazine.

rare, but frequently fatal. It is not necessarily related to length of drug use or type of neuroleptic, but over 60% of affected patients are men. Watch for symptoms.
- Acute dystonic reactions may be treated with I.V. diphenhydramine.
- Hold dose and notify doctor if patient develops symptoms of blood dyscrasias (fever, sore throat, infection, cellulitis, weakness), jaundice, persistent (longer than a few hours) extrapyramidal reactions, or any such reactions in children.
- Monitor therapy by weekly bilirubin tests during first month; periodic blood tests (CBC and liver function) before and during therapy; and ophthalmic tests (long-term therapy).
- Have patient report urine retention or constipation.
- Tell patient to use sunscreen and protective clothing to avoid photosensitivity reactions.
- Warn against activities that require alertness or good psychomotor coordination until CNS effects of the drug are known. Drowsiness and dizziness usually subside after first few weeks.
- Obtain baseline measures of blood pressure before starting therapy and monitor regularly. Watch for orthostatic hypotension, especially with parenteral administration, since adrenergic blockage is high. Keep patient in a supine position for 1 hour afterward. Advise patient to change positions slowly.
- Give deep I.M. only in upper outer quadrant of buttocks or midlateral thigh. Massage slowly afterward to prevent sterile abscess. Injection stings.
- Dilute liquid concentrate with fruit juice, milk, or semisolid food just before administration.
- Protect medication from light. Slight yellowing of injection or concentrate is common; does not affect potency. Discard markedly discolored solutions.
- Do not withdraw drug abruptly unless required by severe adverse reactions.
- Prevent contact dermatitis by keeping drug off patient's skin and clothes. Wear gloves when preparing liquid forms of the drug.
- Dry mouth may be relieved by sugarless gum, sour hard candy, or rinsing with mouthwash.
- Dose of 100 mg is the therapeutic equivalent of 100 mg chlorpromazine.

clozapine

Clozaril

Pregnancy Risk Category: B

HOW SUPPLIED

Tablets: 25 mg, 100 mg

MECHANISM OF ACTION

Binds to dopamine receptors (both D-1 and D-2) within the limbic system of the CNS. It also may interfere with adrenergic, cholinergic, histaminergic, and serotoninergic receptors.

INDICATIONS & DOSAGE

Treatment of schizophrenia in severely ill patients unresponsive to other therapies –

Adults: initially, 25 mg P.O. q.i.d. or b.i.d., titrated upward at 25 to 50 mg daily (if tolerated) to a daily dosage of 300 to 450 mg daily by the end of 2 weeks. Individual dosage is based on clinical response, patient tolerance, and adverse reactions. Subsequent dosage should not be increased more than once or twice weekly, and should not exceed 100 mg. Many patients respond to doses of 300 to 600 mg daily, but some may require as much as 900 mg daily. Do not exceed 900 mg/day.

ADVERSE REACTIONS

Common reactions are in italics; life-threatening reactions are in bold italics.

Blood: leukopenia, granulocytopenia, agranulocytosis.

CNS: *drowsiness, sedation, seizures, dizziness,* syncope, vertigo, headache, tremor, disturbed sleep or nightmares, restlessness, hypokinesia or akinesia, agitation, rigidity, akathisia, confusion, fatigue, insomnia, hyperkinesia, weakness, lethargy, ataxia, slurred speech, depression, myoclonia, anxiety.
CV: *tachycardia, hypotension,* hypertension, chest pain, ECG changes.
GI: *constipation,* nausea, vomiting, *salivation, dry mouth,* heartburn, constipation.
GU: urinary abnormalities, incontinence, abnormal ejaculation, urinary frequency or urgency, urine retention.
Other: fever, muscle pain or spasm, muscle weakness, weight gain, rash.

INTERACTIONS
Anticholinergics: may potentiate the anticholinergic effects of clozapine.
Antihypertensives: hypotensive effects may be potentiated by clozapine.
Bone marrow suppressant drugs: potentially increased bone marrow toxicity.
Psychoactive drugs: possible additive effects. Use together cautiously.
Warfarin, digoxin, and other highly protein bound drugs: increased serum levels of these drugs may occur. Monitor closely for adverse reactions.

NURSING CONSIDERATIONS
• *Contraindicated* in patients with a history of clozapine-induced agranulocytosis or severe granulocytopenia; in patients with a WBC count below 3,500/mm³; in patients with severe CNS depression or coma; in patients who are taking other drugs that suppress bone marrow function; and in those with myelosuppressive disorders.
• *Use cautiously* in patients with prostatic hypertrophy or glaucoma because clozapine has potent anticholinergic effects.
• Seizures may occur, especially in patients receiving high doses of the drug. Patients should avoid hazardous activities that require alertness and good coordination, such as driving, swimming, or climbing, while taking the drug.
• Clozapine carries a significant risk of agranulocytosis (early trials estimate the incidence at 1.3%). If possible, patients should receive at least two trials of a standard antipsychotic drug therapy before clozapine therapy is initiated. Baseline WBC and differential counts are required before therapy; WBC counts must be monitored weekly and for at least 4 weeks after clozapine therapy is discontinued.
• Clozapine should only be given when there is assurance of weekly testing of WBC counts. Blood tests should be performed once a week, and no more than a 1-week supply of drug is distributed.
• If WBC count drops below 3,500/mm³ after initiating therapy or exhibits a substantial drop from baseline, monitor patient closely for signs of infection. If WBC count is 3,000 to 3,500/mm³ and granulocyte count is above 1,500/mm³, perform twice weekly WBC and differential counts. If WBC count drops below 3,000/mm³ and granulocyte count drops below 1,500/mm³, therapy should be interrupted and the patient monitored for signs of infection. Therapy may be cautiously restarted if WBC count returns above 3,000/mm³ and granulocyte count returns above 1,500/mm³, but twice weekly monitoring of WBC and differential counts should occur until the WBC count exceeds 3,500/mm³.
• If the WBC count drops below 2,000/mm³ and granulocyte count drops below 1,000/mm³, the patient may require protective isolation. If the patient develops infection, prepare cultures according to policy and administer antibiotics, as ordered. Some clinicians may perform bone

marrow aspiration to assess bone marrow function. In such patients, future clozapine therapy is contraindicated.
• If clozapine therapy must be discontinued, the drug is usually withdrawn gradually (over a 1- to 2-week period). However, changes in the patient's medical condition (including the development of leukopenia) may require abrupt discontinuation of the drug. Monitor closely for the recurrence of psychotic symptoms.
• If therapy is reinstated in patients withdrawn from the drug, the usual guidelines for dosage build-up should be followed. However, reexposure of the patient to this drug may increase the severity and risk of adverse reactions. If therapy was terminated for WBC counts below 2,000/mm^3 or granulocyte counts below 1,000/mm^3, the drug should not be continued.
• Patients should be warned about the risk of agranulocytosis. They should know that the drug is available only through a special monitoring program that will require weekly blood tests to monitor for agranulocytosis. Advise the patient to report flu-like symptoms, fever, sore throat, lethargy, malaise, or other signs of infection.
• Some patients experience transient fevers (temperature > 100.4° F, or 38° C), especially in the first 3 weeks of therapy. Monitor patients closely.
• Advise patients to check with the doctor before taking any OTC drugs or alcohol.
• Recommend ice chips or sugarless candy or gum to help relieve dry mouth.
• Patients should rise slowly to avoid orthostatic hypotension.

fluphenazine decanoate
Modecate Decanoate†‡, Prolixin Decanoate

fluphenazine enanthate
Moditen Enanthate†, Prolixin Enanthate

fluphenazine hydrochloride
Anatensol‡*, Apo-Fluphenazine†, Moditen HCl†, Moditen HCl-HP†, Permitil* **, Prolixin* **

Pregnancy Risk Category: C

HOW SUPPLIED
decanoate
Depot injection: 25 mg/ml
enanthate
Depot injection: 25 mg/ml
hydrochloride
Tablets: 1 mg, 2.5 mg, 5 mg, 10 mg
Oral concentrate: 5 mg/ml (contains 14% alcohol)
Elixir: 2.5 mg/5 ml (with 14% alcohol)
I.M. injection: 2.5 mg/ml

MECHANISM OF ACTION
Blocks postsynaptic dopamine receptors in the brain. A piperazine phenothiazine.

INDICATIONS & DOSAGE
Psychotic disorders –
Adults: initially, 0.5 to 10 mg (fluphenazine hydrochloride) P.O. daily in divided doses q 6 to 8 hours; may increase cautiously to 20 mg. Higher doses (50 to 100 mg) have been given. Maintenance dosage is 1 to 5 mg P.O. daily. I.M. doses are ⅓ to ½ oral doses. Lower dosages for geriatric patients (1 to 2.5 mg daily).
Children: 0.25 to 3.5 mg fluphenazine hydrochloride P.O. daily in divided doses q 4 to 6 hours; or ⅓ to ½ of oral dose I.M.; maximum dosage is 10 mg daily.
Adults and children over 12 years: 12.5 to 25 mg of long-acting esters (fluphenazine decanoate and enanthate) I.M. or S.C. q 1 to 6 weeks. Maintenance dosage is 25 to 100 mg, p.r.n.

ADVERSE REACTIONS

Common reactions are in italics; life-threatening reactions are in bold italics.

Blood: transient leukopenia, ***agranulocytosis.***

CNS: *extrapyramidal reactions (high incidence), tardive dyskinesia,* sedation (low incidence), pseudoparkinsonism, EEG changes, dizziness.

CV: *orthostatic hypotension,* tachycardia, ECG changes.

EENT: ocular changes, *blurred vision.*

GI: *dry mouth, constipation.*

GU: *urine retention,* dark urine, menstrual irregularities, gynecomastia, inhibited ejaculation.

Hepatic: cholestatic jaundice, abnormal liver function tests.

Metabolic: hyperprolactinemia.

Skin: *mild photosensitivity,* dermal allergic reactions.

Other: weight gain; increased appetite; rarely, ***neuroleptic malignant syndrome*** (fever, tachycardia, tachypnea, profuse diaphoresis).

After abrupt withdrawal of long-term therapy: gastritis, nausea, vomiting, dizziness, tremors, feeling of warmth or cold, sweating, tachycardia, headache, insomnia.

INTERACTIONS

Alcohol, other CNS depressants: increased CNS depression. Avoid concomitant use.

Antacids: inhibit absorption of oral phenothiazines. Separate antacid and phenothiazine doses by at least 2 hours.

Barbiturates, lithium: may decrease phenothiazine effect. Observe patient.

Centrally acting antihypertensives: decreased antihypertensive effect.

NURSING CONSIDERATIONS

- *Contraindicated* in coma, CNS depression, bone marrow suppression or other blood dyscrasia, subcortical damage, hepatic damage, renal insufficiency; and with use of spinal or epidural anesthetic, or adrenergic blocking agents.
- *Use cautiously* with other CNS depressants, anticholinergics; in elderly or debilitated patients; in acutely ill or dehydrated children; and in hepatic disease; pheochromocytoma; arteriosclerotic, cerebrovascular, or CV disease (may cause sudden drop in blood pressure); peptic ulcer; exposure to extreme heat or cold (including antipyretic therapy); respiratory disorders, hypocalcemia; seizure disorders (may lower seizure threshold); severe reactions to insulin or electroshock therapy; suspected brain tumor; or intestinal obstruction; glaucoma; or prostatic hypertrophy. Use parenteral form cautiously in asthmatic patients and patients allergic to sulfites.
- For long-acting forms (decanoate and enanthate), which are oil preparations, use a dry needle of at least 21 gauge. Allow 24 to 96 hours for onset of action. Note and report adverse adverse reactions in patients taking the long-acting drug forms.
- Tardive dyskinesia may occur after prolonged use. It may not appear until months or years later and may disappear spontaneously or persist for life despite discontinuation of drug.
- Neuroleptic malignant syndrome is rare, but frequently fatal. It is not necessarily related to length of drug use or type of neuroleptic, but over 60% of affected patients are men. Watch for symptoms.
- Acute dystonic reactions may be treated with I.V. diphenhydramine.
- Hold dose and notify doctor if patient develops symptoms of blood dyscrasia (fever, sore throat, infection, cellulitis, weakness), persistent (longer than a few hours) extrapyramidal reactions, or any such reactions in pregnancy or in children.
- Monitor therapy by weekly bilirubin tests during first month; periodic blood tests (CBC and liver function);

*Liquid form contains alcohol. **May contain tartrazine.

periodic renal function and ophthalmic tests (long-term use).
- Have patient report urine retention or constipation.
- Tell patient that the drug may discolor the urine.
- Tell patient to use sunscreening agents and protective clothing to avoid photosensitivity reactions.
- Warn against activities that require alertness and good psychomotor coordination until CNS effects of the drug are known. Drowsiness and dizziness usually subside after first few weeks.
- Decanoate and enanthate may be given subcutaneously.
- Liquid (oral) and parenteral forms can cause contact dermatitis. If susceptible, wear gloves when preparing solutions of this drug, and prevent any contact with skin and clothing.
- Dilute liquid concentrate with water, fruit juice, milk, or semisolid food just before administration.
- Protect medication from light. Slight yellowing of injection or concentrate is common; does not affect potency. Discard markedly discolored solutions.
- Dry mouth may be relieved by sugarless gum, sour hard candy, or rinsing with mouthwash.
- Do not withdraw drug abruptly unless required by severe adverse reactions.
- Dose of 2 mg is therapeutic equivalent of 100 mg chlorpromazine.
- Note that Prolixin Concentrate and Permitil Concentrate are 10 times more concentrated than Prolixin Elixir (5 mg/ml vs. 0.5 mg/ml).

haloperidol
Apo-Haloperidol†, Haldol**, Halperon, Novoperidol†, Peridol†, Serenace‡

haloperidol decanoate
Haldol Decanoate, Haldol LA†

haloperidol lactate
Haldol

Pregnancy Risk Category: C

HOW SUPPLIED
haloperidol
Tablets: 0.5 mg, 1 mg, 2 mg, 5 mg, 10 mg, 20 mg
haloperidol decanoate
Injection: 50 mg/ml
haloperidol lactate
Oral concentrate: 2 mg/ml
Injection: 5 mg/ml

MECHANISM OF ACTION
Blocks postsynaptic dopamine receptors in the brain. A butyrophenone.

INDICATIONS & DOSAGE
Psychotic disorders –
Adults: dosage varies for each patient. Initial range is 0.5 to 5 mg P.O. b.i.d. or t.i.d.; or 2 to 5 mg I.M. q 4 to 8 hours, increasing rapidly if necessary for prompt control. Maximum dosage is 100 mg P.O. daily. Doses over 100 mg have been used for patients with severely resistant conditions.
Chronic psychotic patients who require prolonged therapy –
Adults: 50 to 100 mg I.M. haloperidol decanoate q 4 weeks.
Control of tics, vocal utterances in Gilles de la Tourette's syndrome –
Adults: 0.5 to 5 mg P.O. b.i.d. or t.i.d., increasing p.r.n.

ADVERSE REACTIONS
Common reactions are in italics; life-threatening reactions are in bold italics.
Blood: transient leukopenia and leukocytosis.
CNS: *high incidence of severe extrapyramidal reactions, tardive dyskinesia,* low incidence of sedation.
CV: low incidence of cardiovascular effects with therapeutic dosages.
EENT: *blurred vision, dry mouth.*
GU: urine retention, menstrual irregularities, gynecomastia.

Skin: rash.
Other: rarely, ***neuroleptic malignant syndrome*** (fever, tachycardia, tachypnea, profuse diaphoresis).

INTERACTIONS
Alcohol, other CNS depressants: increased CNS depression. Avoid concomitant use.
Lithium: lethargy and confusion with high doses. Observe patient.
Methyldopa: possible symptoms of dementia. Observe patient.

NURSING CONSIDERATIONS
• *Contraindicated* in parkinsonism, coma, or CNS depression.
• *Use cautiously* in elderly and debilitated patients; in severe CV disorders, allergies, glaucoma, urine retention; and in conjunction with anticonvulsant, anticoagulant, antiparkinsonian, or lithium medications.
• Tardive dyskinesia may occur after prolonged use. It may not appear until months or years later and may disappear spontaneously or persist for life despite discontinuation of drug.
• Neuroleptic malignant syndrome is rare, but frequently fatal. It is not necessarily related to length of drug use or type of neuroleptic, but over 60% of affected patients are men. Watch for symptoms.
• Acute dystonic reactions may be treated with I.V. diphenhydramine.
• Elderly patients usually require lower initial doses and a more gradual dosage titration.
• Haloperidol is the least sedating of the antipsychotic agents. However, warn patient against activities that require alertness and good psychomotor coordination until CNS effects of the drug are known. Drowsiness and dizziness usually subside after a few weeks.
• Protect medication from light. Slight yellowing of injection or concentrate is common; does not affect potency. Discard markedly discolored solutions.
• Do not withdraw drug abruptly unless required by severe adverse reactions.
• Dry mouth may be relieved by sugarless gum, sour hard candy, and rinsing with mouthwash.
• Dose of 2 mg is therapeutic equivalent of 100 mg chlorpromazine.
• Especially useful for agitation associated with senile dementia.
• When changing from tablets to decanoate injection, patient should receive 10 to 15 times the oral dose once a month (maximum 100 mg).
• Don't administer the decanoate form I.V.

loxapine hydrochloride
Loxapac†, Loxitane C, Loxitane I.M.

loxapine succinate
Loxapac†, Loxitane
Pregnancy Risk Category: C

HOW SUPPLIED
Capsules: 5 mg, 10 mg, 25 mg, 50 mg
Oral concentrate: 25 mg/ml
Injection: 50 mg/ml

MECHANISM OF ACTION
Blocks postsynaptic dopamine receptors in the brain. A dibenzoxazepine.

INDICATIONS & DOSAGE
Psychotic disorders –
Adults: 10 mg P.O. or I.M. b.i.d. to q.i.d., rapidly increasing to 60 to 100 mg P.O. daily for most patients; dosage varies from patient to patient.

ADVERSE REACTIONS
Common reactions are in italics; life-threatening reactions are in bold italics.
Blood: transient leukopenia.
CNS: *extrapyramidal reactions (moderate incidence), sedation (moderate incidence), tardive dyskinesia,* pseu-

*Liquid form contains alcohol. **May contain tartrazine.

doparkinsonism, EEG changes, dizziness.
CV: *orthostatic hypotension,* tachycardia, ECG changes.
EENT: *blurred vision.*
GI: *dry mouth, constipation.*
GU: *urine retention,* dark urine, menstrual irregularities, gynecomastia.
Skin: *mild photosensitivity,* dermal allergic reactions.
Other: weight gain; increased appetite; rarely, ***neuroleptic malignant syndrome*** (fever, tachycardia, tachypnea, profuse diaphoresis).

INTERACTIONS
Alcohol, other CNS depressants: increased CNS depression. Avoid concomitant use.

NURSING CONSIDERATIONS
- *Contraindicated* in coma, severe CNS depression, or drug-induced depressed states.
- *Use cautiously* in seizure disorder, CV disorders, glaucoma, urine retention, suspected intestinal obstruction or brain tumor, and renal damage.
- Tardive dyskinesia may occur after prolonged use. It may not appear until months or years later and may disappear spontaneously or persist for life despite discontinuation of drug.
- Neuroleptic malignant syndrome is rare, but frequently fatal. It is not necessarily related to length of drug use or type of neuroleptic, but over 60% of affected patients are men. Watch for symptoms.
- Acute dystonic reactions may be treated with I.V. diphenhydramine.
- Warn against activities that require alertness and good psychomotor coordination until CNS effects of the drug are known. Drowsiness and dizziness usually subside after first few weeks.
- Obtain baseline measures of blood pressure before starting therapy and monitor regularly. Advise patient to get up slowly to avoid orthostatic hypotension.
- Dilute liquid concentrate with orange or grapefruit juice just before giving.
- Dry mouth may be relieved by sugarless gum, sour hard candy, or rinsing with mouthwash.
- Periodic eye examinations are recommended.
- Tricyclic dibenzoxazepine; the only dibenzoxazepine derivative.
- Dose of 10 mg is therapeutic equivalent of 100 mg chlorpromazine.

mesoridazine besylate
Serentil* **

Pregnancy Risk Category: C

HOW SUPPLIED
Tablets: 10 mg, 25 mg, 50 mg, 100 mg
Oral concentrate: 25 mg/ml (0.6% alcohol)
Injection: 25 mg/ml

MECHANISM OF ACTION
Blocks postsynaptic dopamine receptors in the brain. It is a piperidine phenothiazine and the major sulfoxide metabolite of thioridazine.

INDICATIONS & DOSAGE
Alcoholism –
Adults and children over 12 years: 25 mg P.O. b.i.d. up to maximum of 200 mg daily.
Behavioral problems associated with chronic brain syndrome –
Adults and children over 12 years: 25 mg P.O. t.i.d. up to maximum of 300 mg daily.
Psychoneurotic manifestations (anxiety) –
Adults and children over 12 years: 10 mg P.O. t.i.d. up to maximum of 150 mg daily.
Schizophrenia –
Adults and children over 12 years: initially, 50 mg P.O. t.i.d. or 25 mg I.M. repeated in 30 to 60 minutes, p.r.n.

ADVERSE REACTIONS

Common reactions are in italics; life-threatening reactions are in bold italics.

Blood: transient leukopenia, ***agranulocytosis.***

CNS: extrapyramidal reactions (low incidence), *tardive dyskinesia, sedation (high incidence),* EEG changes, dizziness.

CV: *orthostatic hypotension,* tachycardia, ECG changes.

EENT: *ocular changes, blurred vision,* pigmentary retinopathy.

GI: *dry mouth, constipation.*

GU: *urine retention,* dark urine, menstrual irregularities, gynecomastia, inhibited ejaculation.

Hepatic: cholestatic jaundice, abnormal liver function tests.

Metabolic: hyperprolactinemia.

Skin: *mild photosensitivity,* dermal allergic reactions.

Local: pain at I.M. injection site, sterile abscess.

Other: weight gain; increased appetite; rarely, ***neuroleptic malignant syndrome*** (fever, tachycardia, tachypnea, profuse diaphoresis).

After abrupt withdrawal of long-term therapy: gastritis, nausea, vomiting, dizziness, tremors, feeling of warmth or cold, sweating, tachycardia, headache, insomnia.

INTERACTIONS

Alcohol, other CNS depressants: increased CNS depression. Avoid concomitant use.

Antacids: inhibit absorption of oral phenothiazines. Separate antacid and phenothiazine doses by at least 2 hours.

Barbiturates: may decrease phenothiazine effect. Observe patient.

NURSING CONSIDERATIONS

- *Contraindicated* in coma, CNS depression, bone marrow suppression, subcortical damage, and with use of spinal or epidural anesthetic or adrenergic blocking agents.
- *Use cautiously* with other CNS depressants, anticholinergics; in elderly or debilitated patients; in acutely ill or dehydrated children; and in hepatic disease, arteriosclerosis or CV disease (may cause sudden drop in blood pressure), exposure to extreme heat or cold (including antipyretic therapy), respiratory disorders, hypocalcemia, seizure disorders, severe reactions to insulin or electroshock therapy, suspected brain tumor or intestinal obstruction, glaucoma, and prostatic hypertrophy.
- Tardive dyskinesia may occur after prolonged use. It may not appear until months or years later and may disappear spontaneously or persist for life despite discontinuation of drug.
- Neuroleptic malignant syndrome is rare, but frequently fatal. It is not necessarily related to length of drug use or type of neuroleptic, but over 60% of affected patients are men. Watch for symptoms.
- Acute dystonic reactions may be treated with I.V. diphenhydramine.
- Hold dose and notify doctor if patient develops jaundice, symptoms of blood dyscrasias (fever, sore throat, infection, cellulitis, weakness), persistent (longer than a few hours) extrapyramidal reactions, or any such reactions in pregnancy or in children.
- Monitor therapy by weekly bilirubin tests during first month; periodic blood tests (CBC and liver function); and ophthalmic tests (long-term use).
- Have patient report urine retention or constipation.
- Tell patient that the drug may discolor the urine.
- Tell patient to use sunscreening agents and protective clothing to avoid photosensitivity reactions.
- Warn against activities that require alertness and good psychomotor coordination until CNS effects of the drug are known. Drowsiness and dizziness usually subside after a few weeks.
- Obtain baseline measures of blood

*Liquid form contains alcohol. **May contain tartrazine.

pressure before starting therapy and monitor regularly. Watch for orthostatic hypotension, especially with parenteral administration. Advise patient to change positions slowly.

- Give deep I.M. only in upper outer quadrant of buttocks. Massage slowly afterward to prevent sterile abscess. Injection may sting.
- Protect medication from light. Slight yellowing of injection or concentrate is common; does not affect potency. Discard markedly discolored solutions.
- Liquid (oral) and parenteral forms may cause contact dermatitis. If susceptible, wear gloves when preparing solutions of this drug, and prevent contact with skin and clothing.
- Dry mouth may be relieved with sugarless gum, sour hard candy, or rinsing with mouthwash.
- Do not withdraw drug abruptly unless required by severe adverse reactions.
- Dose of 50 mg is therapeutic equivalent of 100 mg chlorpromazine.

molindone hydrochloride

Moban

Pregnancy Risk Category: C

HOW SUPPLIED

Tablets: 5 mg, 10 mg, 25 mg, 50 mg, 100 mg
Oral solution: 20 mg/ml

MECHANISM OF ACTION

Blocks postsynaptic dopamine receptors in the brain. A dihydroindolone.

INDICATIONS & DOSAGE

Psychotic disorders –
Adults: 50 to 75 mg P.O. daily, increasing to maximum of 225 mg daily. Doses up to 400 mg may be required.

ADVERSE REACTIONS

Common reactions are in italics; life-threatening reactions are in bold italics.
Blood: transient leukopenia.
CNS: *extrapyramidal reactions (moderate incidence), tardive dyskinesia, sedation (moderate incidence),* pseudoparkinsonism, EEG changes, dizziness.
CV: *orthostatic hypotension,* tachycardia, ECG changes.
EENT: *blurred vision.*
GI: *dry mouth, constipation.*
GU: *urine retention,* dark urine, menstrual irregularities, gynecomastia, inhibited ejaculation.
Hepatic: cholestatic jaundice, abnormal liver function tests.
Metabolic: hyperprolactinemia.
Skin: *mild photosensitivity,* dermal allergic reactions.
Other: rarely, ***neuroleptic malignant syndrome*** (fever, tachycardia, tachypnea, profuse diaphoresis).

INTERACTIONS

Alcohol, other CNS depressants: increased CNS depression. Avoid concomitant use.

NURSING CONSIDERATIONS

- *Contraindicated* in coma or severe CNS depression.
- *Use cautiously* when increased physical activity would be harmful, as this agent increases activity; in seizures (may lower seizure threshold), suicide risk, suspected brain tumor, or intestinal obstruction.
- Tardive dyskinesia may occur after prolonged use. It may not appear until months or years later and may disappear spontaneously or persist for life despite discontinuation of drug.
- Neuroleptic malignant syndrome is rare, but frequently fatal. It is not necessarily related to length of drug use or type of neuroleptic, but over 60% of affected patients are men. Watch for symptoms.

• Acute dystonic reactions may be treated with I.V. diphenhydramine.
• Warn against activities that require alertness or good psychomotor coordination until CNS effects of the drug are known. Drowsiness and dizziness usually subside after first few weeks.
• Dry mouth may be relieved with sugarless gum, sour hard candy, or rinsing with mouthwash.
• Drug is the only dihydroindolone derivative.
• Dose of 10 mg is therapeutic equivalent of 100 mg chlorpromazine.
• May be administered in a single daily dose.

perphenazine

Apo-Perphenazine†, Phenazine†, Trilafon
Pregnancy Risk Category: C

HOW SUPPLIED
Tablets: 2 mg, 4 mg, 8 mg, 16 mg
Repetabs (sustained-release): 8 mg
Oral concentrate: 16 mg/5ml
Injection: 5 mg/ml

MECHANISM OF ACTION
Blocks postsynaptic dopamine receptors in the brain. As an antiemetic, inhibits the medullary chemoreceptor trigger zone.

INDICATIONS & DOSAGE
Hospitalized psychiatric patients –
Adults: initially, 8 to 16 mg P.O. b.i.d., t.i.d., or q.i.d., increasing to 64 mg daily.
Children over 12 years: 6 to 12 mg P.O. daily in divided doses.
Mental disturbances, acute alcoholism, nausea, vomiting, hiccups –
Adults and children over 12 years: 5 to 10 mg I.M., p.r.n. Maximum 15 mg daily in ambulatory patients, 30 mg daily in hospitalized patients.

ADVERSE REACTIONS
Common reactions are in italics; life-threatening reactions are in bold italics.
Blood: transient leukopenia, ***agranulocytosis.***
CNS: *extrapyramidal reactions (high incidence), tardive dyskinesia,* sedation (low incidence), pseudoparkinsonism, EEG changes, dizziness.
CV: *orthostatic hypotension,* tachycardia, ECG changes.
EENT: ocular changes, *blurred vision.*
GI: *dry mouth, constipation.*
GU: *urine retention,* dark urine, menstrual irregularities, gynecomastia, inhibited ejaculation.
Hepatic: cholestatic jaundice, abnormal liver function tests.
Metabolic: hyperprolactinemia.
Skin: *mild photosensitivity,* dermal allergic reactions.
Local: pain at I.M. injection site, sterile abscess.
Other: weight gain; increased appetite; rarely, ***neuroleptic malignant syndrome*** (fever, tachycardia, tachypnea, profuse diaphoresis).
After abrupt withdrawal of long-term therapy: gastritis, nausea, vomiting, dizziness, tremors, feeling of warmth or cold, sweating, tachycardia, headache, insomnia.

INTERACTIONS
Alcohol, other CNS depressants: increased CNS depression. Avoid concomitant use.
Antacids: inhibit absorption of oral phenothiazines. Separate antacid and phenothiazine doses by at least 2 hours.
Barbiturates: may decrease phenothiazine effect. Observe patient.

NURSING CONSIDERATIONS
• *Contraindicated* in coma, CNS depression, bone marrow suppression, subcortical damage, use of spinal or epidural anesthetic or adrenergic blocking agents.

*Liquid form contains alcohol. **May contain tartrazine.

• *Use cautiously* with other CNS depressants, anticholinergics; in elderly or debilitated patients; in acutely ill or dehydrated children; and in hepatic disease, arteriosclerosis or CV disease (may cause sudden drop in blood pressure), exposure to extreme heat or cold (including antipyretic therapy), respiratory disorders, hypocalcemia, seizure disorders (may lower seizure threshold), severe reactions to insulin or electroshock therapy, suspected brain tumor or intestinal obstruction, glaucoma, prostatic hypertrophy.
• Tardive dyskinesia may occur after prolonged use. It may not appear until months or years later and may disappear spontaneously or persist for life despite discontinuation of drug.
• Neuroleptic malignant syndrome is rare, but frequently fatal. It is not necessarily related to length of drug use or type of neuroleptic, but over 60% of affected patients are men. Watch for symptoms.
• Acute dystonic reactions may be treated with I.V. diphenhydramine.
• Hold dose and notify doctor if patient develops jaundice, symptoms of blood dyscrasias (fever, sore throat, infection, cellulitis, weakness), persistent (longer than a few hours) extrapyramidal reactions, or any such reactions in pregnancy or in children.
• Monitor therapy by weekly bilirubin tests during first month; periodic blood tests (CBC and liver function); and ophthalmic tests (long-term use).
• Have patient report urine retention or constipation.
• Tell patient to use sunscreening agents and protective clothing to avoid photosensitivity reactions.
• Warn against activities that require alertness or good psychomotor coordination until CNS effects of the drug are known. Drowsiness and dizziness usually subside after a few weeks.
• Obtain baseline measures of blood pressure before starting therapy and monitor regularly. Watch for orthostatic hypotension, especially with parenteral administration. Keep patient supine for 1 hour afterward. Advise patient to change positions slowly.
• Give deep I.M. only in upper outer quadrant of buttocks. Massage slowly afterward to prevent sterile abscess. Injection may sting.
• Do not withdraw drug abruptly unless required by severe adverse reactions.
• Protect drug from light. Slight yellowing of injection or concentrate is common; does not affect potency. Discard markedly discolored solutions.
• Prevent contact dermatitis by keeping drug off patient's skin and clothes. Wear gloves when preparing liquid forms of the drug.
• Dilute liquid concentrate with fruit juice, milk, carbonated beverage, or semisolid food just before giving. Exceptions: Oral concentrate causes turbidity or precipitation in colas, black coffee, grape or apple juice, or tea. Do not mix with these liquids.
• Dry mouth may be relieved with sugarless gum, sour hard candy, or rinsing with mouthwash.
• Dose of 8 mg is therapeutic equivalent of 100 mg chlorpromazine.

pimozide
Orap

Pregnancy Risk Category: C

HOW SUPPLIED
Tablets: 2 mg

MECHANISM OF ACTION
Blocks dopaminergic receptors.

INDICATIONS & DOSAGE
Suppression of severe motor and phonic tics in patients with Tourette's disorder–
Adults and children over 12 years: initially, 1 to 2 mg P.O. daily in di-

vided doses. Then, increase dosage every other day. Maintenance dosage ranges from 7 to 16 mg daily.

ADVERSE REACTIONS
Common reactions are in italics; life-threatening reactions are in bold italics.
CNS: *parkinsonian-like symptoms,* other extrapyramidal symptoms (dystonia, akathisia, hyperreflexia, opisthotonus, oculogyric crisis), *tardive dyskinesia, sedation.*
CV: *ECG changes (prolonged Q-T interval),* hypotension.
EENT: visual disturbances.
GI: *dry mouth, constipation.*
GU: impotence.
Other: rarely, ***neuroleptic malignant syndrome*** (fever, tachycardia, tachypnea, profuse diaphoresis), muscle tightness.

INTERACTIONS
Alcohol, other CNS depressants: increased CNS depression.
Phenothiazines, tricyclic antidepressants, antiarrhythmics: increased incidence of ECG abnormalities.

NURSING CONSIDERATIONS
• *Contraindicated* in congenital long Q-T syndrome or history of cardiac arrhythmias, severe toxic CNS depression, or in coma.
• *Use cautiously* in hepatic or renal dysfunction, glaucoma, and prostatic hypertrophy.
• Tardive dyskinesia may occur after prolonged use. It may not appear until months or years later and may disappear spontaneously or persist for life despite discontinuation of drug.
• Neuroleptic malignant syndrome is rare, but frequently fatal. It is not necessarily related to length of drug use or type of neuroleptic, but over 60% of affected patients are men. Watch for symptoms.
• Acute dystonic reactions may be treated with I.V. diphenhydramine.
• Pimozide is not recommended for treatment of simple tics except those associated with Tourette's disorder. Don't use in drug-induced motor and phonic tics.
• Avoid concurrent administration of other drugs that prolong the Q-T interval, such as antiarrhythmic agents.
• Perform an ECG before treatment begins and periodically thereafter. Monitor for prolonged Q-T interval.
• Monitor patients who are also taking anticonvulsants for increased seizure activity. Pimozide may lower the seizure threshold.
• Because pimozide may cause serious adverse effects, the patient and his family should be thoroughly informed before deciding whether he should take the drug. Pimozide is indicated only in patients who have failed to respond satisfactorily to standard treatment.
• Warn patient not to stop taking drug abruptly and not to exceed prescribed dose.
• Tell patient to use sugarless hard candy, gum, and liquids, as needed, to relieve dry mouth.

promazine hydrochloride
Sparine**

Pregnancy Risk Category: C

HOW SUPPLIED
Tablets: 25 mg, 50 mg, 100 mg
Syrup: 10 mg/5 ml
Injection: 25 mg/ml, 50 mg/ml

MECHANISM OF ACTION
Blocks postsynaptic dopamine receptors in the brain. An aliphatic phenothiazine.

INDICATIONS & DOSAGE
Psychosis –
Adults: 10 to 200 mg P.O. or I.M. q 4 to 6 hours, up to 1 g daily. I.V. dose in concentrations no greater than 25 mg/ml for acutely agitated patients. Initial

*Liquid form contains alcohol. **May contain tartrazine.

dose is 50 to 150 mg; repeat within 5 to 10 minutes if necessary.
Children over 12 years: 10 to 25 mg P.O. or I.M. q 4 to 6 hours.

ADVERSE REACTIONS
Common reactions are in italics; life-threatening reactions are in bold italics.
Blood: transient leukopenia, ***agranulocytosis.***
CNS: *extrapyramidal reactions (moderate incidence), tardive dyskinesia, sedation (high incidence),* pseudoparkinsonism, EEG changes, dizziness.
CV: *orthostatic hypotension,* tachycardia, ECG changes.
EENT: ocular changes, *blurred vision.*
GI: *dry mouth, constipation.*
GU: *urine retention,* dark urine, menstrual irregularities, gynecomastia, inhibited ejaculation.
Hepatic: cholestatic jaundice, abnormal liver function tests.
Metabolic: hyperprolactinemia.
Skin: *mild photosensitivity,* dermal allergic reactions.
Local: pain at I.M. injection site, sterile abscess.
Other: weight gain; increased appetite; rarely, ***neuroleptic malignant syndrome*** (fever, tachycardia, tachypnea, profuse diaphoresis).
After abrupt withdrawal of long-term therapy: gastritis, nausea, vomiting, dizziness, tremors, feeling of warmth or cold, sweating, tachycardia, headache, insomnia.

INTERACTIONS
Alcohol, other CNS depressants: increased CNS depression. Avoid concomitant use.
Antacids: inhibit absorption of oral phenothiazines. Separate antacid and phenothiazine doses by at least 2 hours.
Anticholinergics (including antidepressant and antiparkinsonian agents): increased anticholinergic activity, aggravated parkinsonian symptoms. Use with caution.
Barbiturates, lithium: may decrease phenothiazine effect. Observe patient.
Centrally acting antihypertensives: decreased antihypertensive effect.
Oral anticoagulants: decreased effectiveness.
Propranolol: increased serum levels of propranolol and promazine.

NURSING CONSIDERATIONS
- *Contraindicated* in coma, CNS depression, bone marrow suppression, subcortical damage, and with use of spinal or epidural anesthetic or adrenergic blocking agents.
- *Use cautiously* with other CNS depressants, anticholinergics; in elderly or debilitated patients; in hepatic disease, arteriosclerosis or CV disease (may cause sudden drop in blood pressure), exposure to extreme heat or cold (including antipyretic therapy), respiratory disorders, hypocalcemia, seizure disorders (may lower seizure threshold), severe reactions to insulin or electroshock therapy, suspected brain tumor or intestinal obstruction, glaucoma, prostatic hypertrophy; and in acutely ill or dehydrated children.
- Tardive dyskinesia may occur after prolonged use. It may not appear until months or years later and may disappear spontaneously or persist for life despite discontinuation of drug.
- Neuroleptic malignant syndrome is rare, but frequently fatal. It is not necessarily related to length of drug use or type of neuroleptic, but over 60% of affected patients are men. Watch for symptoms.
- Acute dystonic reactions may be treated with I.V. diphenhydramine.
- Hold dose and notify doctor if patient develops jaundice, symptoms of blood dyscrasias (fever, sore throat, infection, cellulitis, weakness), persistent (longer than a few hours) ex-

trapyramidal reactions, or such reactions during pregnancy or in children.

- Monitor therapy by weekly bilirubin tests during first month; periodic blood tests (CBC and liver function); and ophthalmic tests (long-term use).
- Have patient report urine retention or constipation.
- Tell patient to use sunscreen and protective clothing to avoid photosensitivity reactions.
- Warn against activities that require alertness or good psychomotor coordination until CNS effects of the drug are known. Drowsiness and dizziness usually subside after a few weeks.
- Monitor blood pressure with patient lying and standing before starting therapy, and routinely throughout course of treatment.
- Watch for orthostatic hypotension, especially with parenteral administration. Keep patient supine for 1 hour afterward. Advise patient to change positions slowly.
- Give deep I.M. only in upper outer quadrant of buttocks. Massage slowly afterward to prevent sterile abscess. Injection may sting.
- Protect drug from light. Slight yellowing of injection or concentrate is common; does not affect potency. Discard markedly discolored solutions.
- Prevent contact dermatitis by keeping drug off patient's skin and clothes. Wear gloves when preparing liquid forms of the drug.
- Dilute liquid concentrate with fruit juice, milk, semisolid food, or chocolate-flavored drinks just before giving. For best taste, use at least 10 ml diluent per 25 mg drug.
- Do not withdraw drug abruptly unless required by severe adverse reactions.
- Dry mouth may be relieved with sugarless gum, sour hard candy, or rinsing with mouthwash.

thioridazine hydrochloride

Aldazine‡, Apo-Thioridazine†, Mellaril*, Mellaril-S, Novoridazine†, PMS Thioridazine†

Pregnancy Risk Category: C

HOW SUPPLIED

Tablets: 10 mg, 15 mg, 25 mg, 50 mg, 100 mg, 150 mg, 200 mg
Oral suspension: 25 mg/5 ml, 100 mg/5 ml
Oral concentrate: 30 mg/ml, 100 mg/ml (3% to 4.2% alcohol)
Syrup: 10 mg/5 ml

MECHANISM OF ACTION

Blocks postsynaptic dopamine receptors in the brain. A piperidine phenothiazine.

INDICATIONS & DOSAGE

Psychosis –
Adults: initially, 25 to 100 mg P.O. t.i.d., with gradual increments up to 800 mg daily in divided doses, if needed. Dosage varies.
Adults over 65 years: initial dose, 25 mg P.O. t.i.d.
Depressive neurosis, alcohol withdrawal, dementia in geriatric patients, behavioral problems in children –
Adults: initially, 25 mg P.O. t.i.d. Maintenance dosage is 20 to 200 mg daily.
Children over 2 years: 0.5 to 3 mg/kg P.O. daily in divided doses.

ADVERSE REACTIONS

Common reactions are in italics; life-threatening reactions are in bold italics.
Blood: transient leukopenia, ***agranulocytosis.***
CNS: extrapyramidal reactions (low incidence), *tardive dyskinesia, sedation (high incidence),* EEG changes, dizziness.
CV: *orthostatic hypotension,* tachycardia, ECG changes.

EENT: *ocular changes, blurred vision,* pigmentary retinopathy.
GI: *dry mouth, constipation.*
GU: *urine retention,* dark urine, menstrual irregularities, gynecomastia, inhibited ejaculation.
Hepatic: cholestatic jaundice.
Metabolic: hyperprolactinemia.
Skin: *mild photosensitivity,* dermal allergic reactions.
Other: weight gain; increased appetite; rarely, ***neuroleptic malignant syndrome*** (fever, tachycardia, tachypnea, profuse diaphoresis).
After abrupt withdrawal of long-term therapy: gastritis, nausea, vomiting, dizziness, tremors, feeling of warmth or cold, sweating, tachycardia, headache, insomnia.

INTERACTIONS

Alcohol, other CNS depressants: increased CNS depression. Avoid concomitant use.
Antacids: inhibit absorption of oral phenothiazines. Separate antacid and phenothiazine doses by at least 2 hours.
Barbiturates, lithium: may decrease phenothiazine effect. Observe patient.
Centrally acting antihypertensives: decreased antihypertensive effect.

NURSING CONSIDERATIONS

- *Contraindicated* in coma, CNS depression, bone marrow suppression, hypertensive or hypotensive cardiac disease, subcortical damage, and with use of spinal or epidural anesthetic or adrenergic blocking agents.
- *Use cautiously* with other CNS depressants, anticholinergics; in elderly or debilitated patients; in hepatic disease, arteriosclerosis or CV disease (may cause sudden drop in blood pressure), exposure to extreme heat or cold (including antipyretic therapy), respiratory disorders, hypocalcemia, seizure disorders, severe reactions to insulin or electroshock therapy, suspected brain tumor or intestinal obstruction, glaucoma, or prostatic hypertrophy; and in acutely ill or dehydrated children.
- Tardive dyskinesia may occur after prolonged use. It may not appear until months or years later and may disappear spontaneously or persist for life despite discontinuation of drug.
- Neuroleptic malignant syndrome is rare, but frequently fatal. It is not necessarily related to length of drug use or type of neuroleptic, but over 60% of affected patients are men. Watch for symptoms.
- Acute dystonic reactions may be treated with I.V. diphenhydramine.
- Hold dose and notify doctor if patient develops jaundice, symptoms of blood dyscrasias (fever, sore throat, infection, cellulitis, weakness), persistent (longer than a few hours) extrapyramidal reactions, or such reactions during pregnancy or in children.
- Monitor therapy by weekly bilirubin tests during first month; periodic blood tests (CBC and liver function); and ophthalmic tests (long-term therapy).
- Have patient report urine retention or constipation.
- Tell patient that drug may discolor the urine.
- Tell patient to watch for and notify doctor of blurred vision.
- Tell patient to use sunscreen and protective clothing to avoid photosensitivity reactions.
- Warn against activities that require alertness or good psychomotor coordination until CNS effects of the drug are known. Drowsiness and dizziness usually subside after a few weeks.
- Watch for orthostatic hypotension, especially with parenteral administration. Advise patient to change positions slowly.
- Prevent contact dermatitis by keeping drug off patient's skin and clothes. Wear gloves when preparing liquid forms of the drug.

• Caution: Note different concentrations of liquid formulations.
• Not available in injectable form. Mesoridazine is prescribed when parenteral use of a thioridazine-like drug is desirable.
• Dilute liquid concentrate with water or fruit juice just before giving. Avoid contact with skin because contact dermatitis has been reported.
• Be sure to shake suspension well before using.
• Do not withdraw abruptly unless required by severe adverse reactions.
• Dry mouth may be relieved with sugarless gum, sour hard candy, or rinsing with mouthwash.
• Dose of 100 mg is the therapeutic equivalent of 100 mg chlorpromazine.
• Dosage above 800 mg may be associated with ocular toxicity (pigmentary retinopathy).

thiothixene
Navane

thiothixene hydrochloride
Navane*

Pregnancy Risk Category: C

HOW SUPPLIED
thiothixene
Capsules: 1 mg, 2 mg, 5 mg, 10 mg, 20 mg
thiothixene hydrochloride
Oral concentrate: 5 mg/ml (7% alcohol)
Injection: 2 mg, 5 mg/ml

MECHANISM OF ACTION
Blocks postsynaptic dopamine receptors in the brain. A thioxanthene.

INDICATIONS & DOSAGE
Acute agitation –
Adults: 4 mg I.M. b.i.d. to q.i.d. Maximum dosage is 30 mg daily I.M. Change to P.O. as soon as possible.
Mild to moderate psychosis –
Adults: initially, 2 mg P.O. t.i.d. May increase gradually to 15 mg daily.
Severe psychosis –
Adults: initially, 5 mg P.O. b.i.d. May increase gradually to 15 to 30 mg daily. Maximum recommended daily dose is 60 mg. Not recommended in children under 12 years.

ADVERSE REACTIONS
Common reactions are in italics; life-threatening reactions are in bold italics.
Blood: transient leukopenia, ***agranulocytosis.***
CNS: *extrapyramidal reactions (high incidence), tardive dyskinesia,* sedation (low incidence), pseudoparkinsonism, EEG changes, dizziness.
CV: *orthostatic hypotension,* tachycardia, ECG changes.
EENT: ocular changes, *blurred vision.*
GI: *dry mouth, constipation.*
GU: *urine retention,* dark urine, menstrual irregularities, gynecomastia, inhibited ejaculation.
Hepatic: cholestatic jaundice.
Metabolic: hyperprolactinemia.
Skin: *mild photosensitivity,* dermal allergic reactions.
Local: pain at I.M. injection site, sterile abscess.
Other: weight gain; increased appetite; rarely, ***neuroleptic malignant syndrome*** (fever, tachycardia, tachypnea, profuse diaphoresis).
After abrupt withdrawal of long-term therapy: gastritis, nausea, vomiting, dizziness, tremors, feeling of warmth or cold, sweating, tachycardia, headache, insomnia.

INTERACTIONS
Alcohol, other CNS depressants: increased CNS depression. Avoid concomitant use.

NURSING CONSIDERATIONS
• *Contraindicated* in convulsive seizures, circulatory collapse, coma,

*Liquid form contains alcohol. **May contain tartrazine.

CNS depression, blood dyscrasia, bone marrow suppression, alcohol withdrawal, akathisia or restlessness, subcortical damage, and with use of spinal or epidural anesthetic or adrenergic blocking agents.

• *Use cautiously* with other CNS depressants, anticholinergics; in elderly or debilitated patients; and in hepatic disease, arteriosclerosis or CV disease (may cause sudden drop in blood pressure), exposure to extreme heat or cold (including antipyretic therapy) or undue sunlight, respiratory disorders, hypocalcemia, severe reactions to insulin or electroshock therapy, suspected brain tumor or intestinal obstruction, glaucoma, and prostatic hypertrophy.

• Tardive dyskinesia may occur after prolonged use. It may not appear until months or years later and may disappear spontaneously or persist for life despite discontinuation of drug.

• Neuroleptic malignant syndrome is rare, but frequently fatal. It is not necessarily related to length of drug use or type of neuroleptic, but over 60% of affected patients are men. Watch for symptoms.

• Acute dystonic reactions may be treated with I.V. diphenhydramine.

• Hold dose and notify doctor if patient develops jaundice, symptoms of blood dyscrasias (fever, sore throat, infection, cellulitis, weakness), persistent (longer than a few hours) extrapyramidal reactions, or any such reactions during pregnancy.

• Monitor therapy by weekly bilirubin tests during first month; periodic blood tests (CBC and liver function); and ophthalmic tests (long-term use).

• Have patient report urine retention or constipation.

• Tell patient to use sunscreen and protective clothing to avoid photosensitivity reactions.

• Warn against activities that require alertness or good psychomotor coordination until CNS effects of the drug are known. Drowsiness and dizziness usually subside after a few weeks.

• Watch for orthostatic hypotension, especially with parenteral administration. Keep patient in a supine position for 1 hour afterward. Advise patient to change positions slowly.

• Give I.M. only in upper outer quadrant of buttocks or midlateral thigh. Massage slowly afterward to prevent sterile abscess. Injection may sting.

• I.M. form must be stored in refrigerator.

• Slight yellowing of injection or concentrate is common; does not affect potency. Discard markedly discolored solutions.

• Prevent contact dermatitis by keeping drug off patient's skin and clothes. Wear gloves when preparing liquid forms of the drug.

• Dilute liquid concentrate with fruit juice, milk, or semisolid food just before giving.

• Do not withdraw abruptly unless required by severe adverse reactions.

• Dry mouth may be relieved with sugarless gum, sour hard candy, or rinsing with mouthwash.

• Dose of 4 mg is therapeutic equivalent of 100 mg chlorpromazine.

trifluoperazine hydrochloride

Apo-Trifluoperazine†, Calmazine‡, Novo-Flurazine†, Solazine†, Stelazine, Suprazine, Terfluzine†

Pregnancy Risk Category: C

HOW SUPPLIED

Tablets (regular and film-coated): 1 mg, 2 mg, 5 mg, 10 mg
Oral concentrate: 10 mg/ml
Injection: 2 mg/ml

MECHANISM OF ACTION

Blocks postsynaptic dopamine receptors in the brain. A piperazine phenothiazine.

INDICATIONS & DOSAGE
Anxiety states –
Adults: 1 to 2 mg P.O. b.i.d.
Schizophrenia and other psychotic disorders –
Adults: *outpatients* – 1 to 2 mg P.O. b.i.d., up to 4 mg daily; *hospitalized* – 2 to 5 mg P.O. b.i.d.; may gradually increase to 40 mg daily. 1 to 2 mg I.M. q 4 to 6 hours, p.r.n.
Children 6 to 12 years (hospitalized or under close supervision): 1 mg P.O. daily or b.i.d.; may increase gradually to 15 mg daily.

ADVERSE REACTIONS
Common reactions are in italics; life-threatening reactions are in bold italics.
Blood: transient leukopenia, ***agranulocytosis.***
CNS: *extrapyramidal reactions (high incidence), tardive dyskinesia,* sedation (low incidence), pseudoparkinsonism, EEG changes, dizziness.
CV: *orthostatic hypotension,* tachycardia, ECG changes.
EENT: ocular changes, *blurred vision.*
GI: *dry mouth, constipation.*
GU: *urine retention,* dark urine, menstrual irregularities, gynecomastia, inhibited ejaculation.
Hepatic: cholestatic jaundice.
Metabolic: hyperprolactinemia.
Skin: *mild photosensitivity,* dermal allergic reactions.
Local: pain at I.M. injection site, sterile abscess.
Other: weight gain; increased appetite; rarely, ***neuroleptic malignant syndrome*** (fever, tachycardia, tachypnea, profuse diaphoresis).
After abrupt withdrawal of long-term therapy: gastritis, nausea, vomiting, dizziness, tremors, feeling of warmth or cold, sweating, tachycardia, headache, insomnia.

INTERACTIONS
Alcohol, other CNS depressants: increased CNS depression. Avoid concomitant use.
Antacids: inhibit absorption of oral phenothiazines. Separate antacid and phenothiazine doses by at least 2 hours.
Barbiturates, lithium: may decrease phenothiazine effect. Observe patient.
Centrally acting antihypertensives: decreased antihypertensive effect.

NURSING CONSIDERATIONS
- *Contraindicated* in coma, CNS depression, bone marrow suppression, subcortical damage, and with use of spinal or epidural anesthetic or adrenergic blocking agents.
- *Use cautiously* with other CNS depressants, anticholinergics; in elderly or debilitated patients; in hepatic disease, arteriosclerosis or CV disease (may cause drop in blood pressure), exposure to extreme heat or cold (including antipyretic therapy), respiratory disorders, hypocalcemia, seizure disorders, severe reactions to insulin or electroshock therapy, suspected brain tumor or intestinal obstruction, glaucoma, or prostatic hypertrophy; and in acutely ill or dehydrated children.
- Tardive dyskinesia may occur after prolonged use. It may not appear until months or years later and may disappear spontaneously or persist for life despite discontinuation of drug.
- Neuroleptic malignant syndrome is rare, but frequently fatal. It is not necessarily related to length of drug use or type of neuroleptic, but over 60% of affected patients are men. Watch for symptoms.
- Acute dystonic reactions may be treated with I.V. diphenhydramine.
- Hold dose and notify doctor if patient develops jaundice, symptoms of blood dyscrasia (fever, sore throat, infection, cellulitis, weakness), persis-

tent (longer than a few hours) extrapyramidal reactions, or any such reactions during pregnancy or in children.

- Monitor therapy by weekly bilirubin tests during first month; periodic blood tests (CBC and liver function); and ophthalmic tests (long-term use).
- Have patient report urine retention or constipation.
- Tell patient to use sunscreen and protective clothing to avoid photosensitivity reactions.
- Warn against activities that require alertness or good psychomotor coordination until CNS effects of the drug are known. Drowsiness and dizziness usually subside after a few weeks.
- Watch for orthostatic hypotension, especially with parenteral administration. Keep patient supine for 1 hour afterward. Advise patient to change positions slowly.
- Give deep I.M. only in upper outer quadrant of buttocks. Massage slowly afterward to prevent sterile abscess. Injection may sting.
- Protect drug from light. Slight yellowing of injection or concentrate is common; does not affect potency. Discard markedly discolored solutions.
- Prevent contact dermatitis by keeping drug off patient's skin and clothes. Wear gloves when preparing liquid forms of the drug.
- Dilute liquid concentrate with 60 ml tomato or fruit juice, carbonated beverages, coffee, tea, milk, water, or semisolid food just before giving.
- Do not withdraw abruptly unless required by severe adverse reactions.
- Dry mouth may be relieved with sugarless gum, sour hard candy, or rinsing with mouthwash.
- Drug is a prototype piperazine phenothiazine.
- Dose of 5 mg is therapeutic equivalent of 100 mg chlorpromazine.

33

Miscellaneous psychotherapeutics

lithium carbonate
lithium citrate

COMBINATION PRODUCTS
None.

lithium carbonate

Camcolit‡, Carbolith†, Duralith†, Eskalith, Eskalith CR, Lithane**, Lithicarb‡, Lithizine†, Lithobid, Lithonate, Lithotabs, Priadel‡

lithium citrate

Cibalith-S*

Pregnancy Risk Category: D

HOW SUPPLIED
carbonate
Tablets: 250 mg‡, 300 mg (300 mg = 8.12 mEq lithium)
Tablets (sustained-release): 300 mg, 400 mg‡, 450 mg
Capsules: 300 mg
citrate
Syrup (sugarless): 300 mg/5 ml (0.3% alcohol)

MECHANISM OF ACTION
Alters chemical transmitters in the CNS, possibly by interfering with ionic pump mechanisms in brain cells. Its exact mechanism of action in mania, however, is unknown.

INDICATIONS & DOSAGE
Prevention or control of mania –
Adults: 300 to 600 mg P.O. up to q.i.d., increasing on the basis of blood levels to achieve optimal dosage. Recommended therapeutic lithium blood levels: 1 to 1.5 mEq/liter for acute mania; 0.6 to 1.2 mEq/liter for maintenance therapy; and 2 mEq/liter as maximum.

Note: 5 ml lithium citrate (liquid) contains 8 mEq lithium equal to 300 mg lithium carbonate.

ADVERSE REACTIONS
Common reactions are in italics; life-threatening reactions are in bold italics.
Blood: *leukocytosis of 14,000 to 18,000/mm³ (reversible).*
CNS: tremors, drowsiness, headache, confusion, restlessness, dizziness, psychomotor retardation, stupor, lethargy, ***coma,*** blackouts, epileptiform seizures, EEG changes, worsened organic brain syndrome, impaired speech, ataxia, muscle weakness, incoordination, hyperexcitability.
CV: *reversible ECG changes,* ***arrhythmias,*** hypotension, peripheral circulatory collapse, allergic vasculitis, ankle and wrist edema.
EENT: tinnitus, impaired vision.
GI: nausea, vomiting, anorexia, diarrhea, dry mouth, *thirst,* metallic taste.
GU: *polyuria,* glycosuria, incontinence, renal toxicity with long-term use.
Metabolic: transient hyperglycemia, goiter, hypothyroidism (lowered T_3, T_4, and protein-bound iodine, but elevated ^{131}I uptake), hyponatremia.
Skin: pruritus, rash, diminished or lost sensation, drying and thinning of hair.

INTERACTIONS
Aminophylline, sodium bicarbonate, and sodium chloride: ingestion of these salts increases lithium excretion. Avoid salt loads and monitor lithium levels.
Carbamazepine, probenecid, indomethacin, methyldopa and piroxicam: increased effect of lithium. Monitor for lithium toxicity.
Diuretics: increased reabsorption of

*Liquid form contains alcohol. **May contain tartrazine.

lithium by kidneys, with possible toxic effect. Use with extreme caution, and monitor lithium and electrolyte levels (especially sodium).
Haloperidol and thioridazine: encephalopathic syndrome (lethargy, tremors, extrapyramidal symptoms). Watch for syndrome, and stop drug if it occurs.
Neuromuscular blockers: lithium may cause prolonged paralysis or weakness. Monitor patient closely.
Thyroid hormones: lithium may induce hypothyroidism.

NURSING CONSIDERATIONS

- *Contraindicated* if therapy cannot be closely monitored.
- *Use cautiously* with haloperidol, other antipsychotics, neuromuscular blockers, and diuretics; in elderly or debilitated patients; and in thyroid disease, seizure disorder, renal or cardiovascular disease, brain damage, severe debilitation or dehydration, and sodium depletion.
- Monitor baseline ECG, thyroid, and renal studies, and electrolyte levels. Monitor lithium blood levels 8 to 12 hours after first dose, usually before morning dose, two or three times weekly first month, then weekly to monthly on maintenance.
- Determination of lithium blood concentration is crucial to the safe use of the drug. Shouldn't be used in patients who can't have regular lithium blood level checks.
- Explain to patient that lithium has a narrow therapeutic margin of safety. A blood level that is even slightly too high can be dangerous.
- When blood levels of lithium are below 1.5 mEq/liter, adverse reactions usually remain mild.
- Expect delay of 1 to 3 weeks before drug's beneficial effects are noticed.
- Check fluid intake and output, especially when surgery is scheduled.
- May alter glucose tolerance in diabetics. Monitor blood glucose closely.
- Warn patient and family to watch for signs of toxicity (diarrhea, vomiting, drowsiness, muscular weakness, ataxia) and to expect transient nausea, polyuria, thirst, and discomfort during first few days. Patient should withhold one dose and call doctor if toxic symptoms appear, but not stop drug abruptly.
- Weigh patient daily; check for signs of edema or sudden weight gain.
- Adjust fluid and salt ingestion to compensate if excessive loss occurs through protracted sweating or diarrhea. Under normal conditions, patients should have fluid intake of 2,500 to 3,000 ml daily and a balanced diet with adequate salt intake.
- Have outpatient follow-up of thyroid and renal functions every 6 to 12 months. Palpate thyroid to check for enlargement.
- Patient should carry identification/instruction card (available from pharmacy) with toxicity and emergency information.
- Warn ambulatory patient to avoid hazardous activities that require alertness and good psychomotor coordination until CNS effects of the drug are known.
- Administer with plenty of water, and after meals to minimize GI upset.
- Check urine for specific gravity and report level below 1.005, which may indicate diabetes insipidus syndrome.
- Tell patient not to switch brands of lithium or to take other drugs (prescription or OTC) without doctor's guidance.
- Investigationally used to increase white cells in patients undergoing cancer chemotherapy.
- Also used investigationally for treatment of cluster headaches, aggression, organic brain syndrome, and tardive dyskinesia. Has been used to treat SIADH.

34

Cerebral stimulants

amphetamine sulfate
benzphetamine hydrochloride
caffeine
dextroamphetamine sulfate
diethylpropion hydrochloride
fenfluramine hydrochloride
mazindol
methamphetamine hydrochloride
methylphenidate hydrochloride
pemoline
phendimetrazine tartrate
phentermine hydrochloride

COMBINATION PRODUCTS

BIPHETAMINE 12½: dextroamphetamine 6.25 mg and amphetamine 6.25 mg.
BIPHETAMINE 20: dextroamphetamine 10 mg and amphetamine 10 mg.

amphetamine sulfate

Controlled Substance Schedule II
Pregnancy Risk Category: C

HOW SUPPLIED

Tablets: 5 mg, 10 mg
Capsules: 5 mg, 10 mg

MECHANISM OF ACTION

Main site of activity appears to be the cerebral cortex and the reticular activating system. Promotes nerve impulse transmission by releasing stored norepinephrine from nerve terminals in the brain. In children with hyperkinesia, amphetamines have a paradoxical calming effect.

INDICATIONS & DOSAGE

Attention deficit disorder with hyperactivity (ADDH) –
Children 6 years and older: 5 mg P.O. daily, with 5-mg increments weekly, p.r.n.
Children 3 to 5 years: 2.5 mg P.O. daily, with 2.5-mg increments weekly, p.r.n.
Narcolepsy –
Adults: 5 to 60 mg P.O. daily in divided doses.
Children over 12 years: 10 mg P.O. daily, with 10-mg increments weekly, p.r.n.
Children 6 to 12 years: 5 mg P.O. daily, with 5-mg increments weekly, p.r.n.
Short-term adjunct in exogenous obesity –
Adults: single 10- or 15-mg long-acting capsule daily, or 2 if needed, up to 30 mg daily; or 5 to 30 mg daily in divided doses 30 to 60 minutes before meals. Not recommended for children under 12 years.

ADVERSE REACTIONS

Common reactions are in italics; life-threatening reactions are in bold italics.
CNS: *restlessness,* tremor, *hyperactivity, talkativeness, insomnia,* irritability, dizziness, headache, chills, overstimulation, dysphoria.
CV: *tachycardia, palpitations,* hypertension, hypotension.
GI: nausea, vomiting, cramps, dry mouth, diarrhea, constipation, metallic taste, anorexia, weight loss.
Other: urticaria, impotence, altered libido.

INTERACTIONS

Ammonium chloride, ascorbic acid: observe for decreased amphetamine effect.
Antacids, sodium bicarbonate, acetazolamide: increased renal reabsorption. Monitor for enhanced effect.
MAO inhibitors: severe hypertension; possible hypertensive crisis. Don't use together or within 14 days after an

MAO inhibitor has been discontinued.
Phenothiazines, haloperidol: observe for decreased amphetamine effect.

NURSING CONSIDERATIONS

- *Contraindicated* in symptomatic CV diseases, hyperthyroidism, nephritis, angina pectoris, moderate to severe hypertension, parkinsonism due to arteriosclerosis, certain types of glaucoma, advanced arteriosclerosis, in agitated states, or patients with history of drug abuse.
- *Use cautiously* in diabetes mellitus; in elderly, debilitated, or hyperexcitable patients; and in children with Tourette's disorder.
- Psychic dependence may occur, especially in patients with history of drug addiction. Avoid prolonged administration. When used long-term, lower dosage gradually to prevent acute rebound depression.
- Not recommended for first-line treatment of obesity. Use as an anorexigenic agent is prohibited in some states.
- When used for obesity, make sure patient is also on a weight-reduction program. Give drug 30 to 60 minutes before meals. Monitor dietary intake. Do calorie counts, if necessary.
- Fatigue may result as drug effects wear off. Patient will need more rest.
- Tell patient to avoid drinks containing caffeine, which increase the effects of amphetamines and related amines.
- Have patient report signs of excessive stimulation.
- Urine acidification enhances renal excretion; urine alkalinization enhances renal reabsorption and recycling.
- When tolerance to anorexigenic effect develops, dosage should not be increased, but drug discontinued.
- Should not be used to combat fatigue.
- Warn patient to avoid activities that require alertness or good psychomotor coordination until CNS effects of the drug are known.
- May alter daily insulin needs in patients with diabetes. Monitor blood and urine sugars.
- Use as analeptic is usually discouraged, since CNS stimulation superimposed on CNS depression can lead to neuronal instability and seizures.
- May reverse beneficial effect of antihypertensives. Monitor blood pressure.
- Give at least 6 hours before bedtime to avoid sleep interference.

benzphetamine hydrochloride

Didrex**
Controlled Substance Schedule III
Pregnancy Risk Category: X

HOW SUPPLIED
Tablets: 25 mg, 50 mg

MECHANISM OF ACTION
Main site of activity appears to be the cerebral cortex and the reticular activating system. Promotes nerve impulse transmission by releasing stored norepinephrine from nerve terminals in the brain.

INDICATIONS & DOSAGE
Short-term adjunct in exogenous obesity –
Adults: 25 to 50 mg P.O. daily, b.i.d., or t.i.d.

ADVERSE REACTIONS
Common reactions are in italics; life-threatening reactions are in bold italics.
CNS: *restlessness,* tremor, *hyperactivity, talkativeness, insomnia,* irritability, dizziness, headache, chills, overstimulation, dysphoria.
CV: *tachycardia, palpitations,* hypertension, hypotension.
GI: nausea, vomiting, cramps, dry

mouth, diarrhea, constipation, metallic taste, anorexia, weight loss.
Skin: urticaria.
Other: impotence, altered libido.

INTERACTIONS
Antacids, sodium bicarbonate, acetazolamide: increased renal reabsorption. Monitor for enhanced effects.
Ammonium chloride, ascorbic acid: observe for decreased benzphetamine effects.
MAO inhibitors: severe hypertension; possible hypertensive crisis. Don't use together or within 14 days after MAO inhibitor has been discontinued.
Phenothiazines, haloperidol: observe for decreased benzphetamine effects.

NURSING CONSIDERATIONS
- *Contraindicated* in symptomatic CV diseases, hyperthyroidism, nephritis, angina pectoris, moderate to severe hypertension, parkinsonism due to arteriosclerosis, certain types of glaucoma, advanced arteriosclerosis, agitated states, or patients with history of drug abuse.
- *Use cautiously* in diabetes mellitus and in elderly, debilitated, or hyperexcitable patients.
- Psychic dependence or habituation may occur, especially in patients with history of drug addiction. Avoid prolonged administration. When used long-term, lower dosage gradually to prevent acute rebound depression.
- Use in conjunction with weight-reduction program. Monitor dietary intake. Do calorie counts, if necessary. Give 30 to 60 minutes before meals.
- Fatigue may result as drug effects wear off. Patient will need more rest.
- Tell patient to avoid drinks containing caffeine, which increase the effects of amphetamines and related amines.
- Have patient report signs of excessive stimulation.
- Urine acidification enhances renal excretion; urine alkalinization enhances renal reabsorption and recycling.
- When tolerance to anorexigenic effect develops, dosage should not be increased, but drug discontinued.
- Warn patient to avoid activities that require alertness or good psychomotor coordination until CNS effects of the drug are known.
- May alter daily insulin needs in patients with diabetes. Monitor blood and urine sugars.
- Give at least 6 hours before bedtime to avoid sleep interference.

caffeine

Caffedrine◇, Dexitac◇, No Doz◇, Quick Pep◇, Tirend◇, Vivarin◇
Pregnancy Risk Category: B

HOW SUPPLIED
Tablets: 100 mg◇, 150 mg◇, 200 mg◇
Capsules (timed-release): 200 mg◇, 250 mg◇
Injection: caffeine (125 mg/ml) with sodium benzoate (125 mg/ml)

MECHANISM OF ACTION
Inhibits phosphodiesterase, the enzyme that degrades cyclic adenosine monophosphate.

INDICATIONS & DOSAGE
CNS stimulant –
Adults: 100 to 200 mg anhydrous caffeine P.O.
Neonatal apnea –
Neonates: 5 to 10 mg/kg P.O., I.M., or I.V. as a loading dose, then 2.5 to 5 mg. P.O., I.M., or I.V. daily, according to patient tolerance and serum caffeine levels (therapeutic range is 5 to 20 mcg/ml).

ADVERSE REACTIONS
Common reactions are in italics; life-threatening reactions are in bold italics.
Blood: hyperglycemia.
CNS: *stimulation, insomnia,* restless-

ness, nervousness, mild delirium, headache, excitement, agitation, muscle tremors, twitches.
CV: *tachycardia.*
GI: nausea, vomiting.
GU: *diuresis.*
Skin: hyperesthesia.

INTERACTIONS
Theophylline, beta-adrenergic agonists: Excessive CNS stimulation.

NURSING CONSIDERATIONS
- *Contraindicated* in gastric or duodenal ulcer, arrhythmias, or post-MI.
- Caffeine-containing beverages should be restricted in patients who experience palpitations.
- Tolerance or psychological dependence may develop.
- Be alert for signs of overdose: GI pain, mild delirium, insomnia, diuresis, dehydration, and fever. Treat with short-acting barbiturates, gastric emesis, or lavage.
- Single dose should not exceed 1 g.
- Caffeine content in cola beverages, 17 to 55 mg/180 ml; tea, 40 to 100 mg/180 ml; instant coffee, 60 to 180 mg/180 ml; brewed coffee, 100 to 150 mg/180 ml; decaffeinated coffee, 1 to 6 mg/180 ml.
- Caffeine does not reverse alcohol intoxication or CNS depressant effects of alcohol. Overvigorous therapy with caffeine may aggravate depression in an already depressed patient.
- Sudden discontinuation of caffeine may cause headache and irritability.
- Caffeine is included in many OTC analgesic preparations. There's conflicting evidence regarding whether it increases pain relief.
- Treatment of neonatal apnea is an unlabeled indication. Solution may have to be made in pharmacy because most commercially available parenteral caffeine injections contain sodium benzoate, a preservative that may cause kernicterus in neonates.
- Used experimentally to treat certain types of vascular headaches.

dextroamphetamine sulfate
Dexedrine* **, Ferndex, Oxydess II, Robese, Spancap #1
Controlled Substance Schedule II
Pregnancy Risk Category: C

HOW SUPPLIED
Tablets: 5 mg, 10 mg
Capsules (sustained-release): 5 mg, 10 mg, 15 mg
Elixir: 5 mg/5 ml

MECHANISM OF ACTION
Main site of activity appears to be the cerebral cortex and the reticular activating system. Promotes nerve impulse transmission by releasing stored norepinephrine from nerve terminals in the brain. In children with hyperkinesia, amphetamines have a paradoxical calming effect.

INDICATIONS & DOSAGE
Narcolepsy –
Adults: 5 to 60 mg P.O. daily in divided doses.
Children over 12 years: 10 mg P.O. daily, with 10-mg increments weekly, p.r.n.
Children 6 to 12 years: 5 mg P.O. daily, with 5-mg increments weekly, p.r.n.
Short-term adjunct in exogenous obesity –
Adults: single 10- to 15-mg long-acting capsule, up to 30 mg daily; or in divided doses, 5 to 10 mg half hour before meals.
Attention deficit disorders with hyperactivity (ADDH) –
Children 6 years and older: 5 mg P.O. once daily or b.i.d., with 5-mg increments weekly, p.r.n.
Children 3 to 5 years: 2.5 mg P.O. daily, with 2.5-mg increments weekly, p.r.n.

ADVERSE REACTIONS

Common reactions are in italics; life-threatening reactions are in bold italics.

CNS: *restlessness,* tremor, *hyperactivity, talkativeness, insomnia,* irritability, dizziness, headache, chills, overstimulation, dysphoria.

CV: *tachycardia, palpitations,* hypertension, hypotension.

GI: nausea, vomiting, cramps, dry mouth, diarrhea, constipation, metallic taste, anorexia, weight loss.

Skin: urticaria.

Other: impotence, altered libido.

INTERACTIONS

Ammonium chloride, ascorbic acid: observe for decreased amphetamine effects.

Antacids, sodium bicarbonate, acetazolamide: increased renal reabsorption. Monitor for enhanced amphetamine effects.

MAO inhibitors: severe hypertension; possible hypertensive crisis. Don't use together or within 14 days after MAO inhibitor has been discontinued.

Phenothiazines, haloperidol: observe for decreased amphetamine effects.

NURSING CONSIDERATIONS

- *Contraindicated* in hyperthyroidism, nephritis, severe hypertension, angina pectoris or other severe CV disease, some types of glaucoma, or history of drug abuse.
- *Use cautiously* in diabetes mellitus; in elderly, debilitated, or hyperexcitable patients; and in children with Tourette's disorder.
- Psychic dependence or habituation may occur, especially in patients with history of drug addiction. Avoid prolonged administration. When used long-term, lower dosage gradually to prevent acute rebound depression.
- Not recommended for first-line treatment of obesity. Use as an anorexigenic agent is prohibited in some states.
- When used for obesity, be sure patient is also on a weight-reduction program. Give 30 to 60 minutes before meals. Avoid giving within 6 hours of bedtime.
- Fatigue may result as drug effects wear off. Patient will need more rest.
- Tell patient to avoid drinks containing caffeine, which increase the effects of amphetamines and related amines.
- Have patient report signs of excessive stimulation.
- Urine acidification enhances renal excretion; urine alkalinization enhances renal reabsorption and recycling.
- When tolerance to anorexigenic effect develops, dosage should not be increased, but drug discontinued.
- Should not be used to prevent fatigue.
- Warn patient to avoid activities that require alertness or good psychomotor coordination until CNS effects of the drug are known.
- May alter daily insulin needs in patients with diabetes. Monitor blood and urine sugars.
- Use as analeptic is usually discouraged, since CNS stimulation superimposed on CNS depression can lead to neuronal instability and seizures.
- Give at least 6 hours before bedtime to avoid sleep interference.

diethylpropion hydrochloride

Nobesine†, Propion†, Tenuate, Tenuate Dospan, Tepanil, Tepanil Ten-Tab

Controlled Substance Schedule IV

Pregnancy Risk Category: B

HOW SUPPLIED

Tablets: 25 mg

Tablets (controlled-release): 75 mg

MECHANISM OF ACTION
Main site of activity appears to be the cerebral cortex and the reticular activating system. Promotes nerve impulse transmission by releasing stored norepinephrine from nerve terminals in the brain.

INDICATIONS & DOSAGE
Short-term adjunct in exogenous obesity –
Adults: 25 mg P.O. before meals, t.i.d.; or 75 mg controlled-release tablet P.O. in mid-morning.

ADVERSE REACTIONS
Common reactions are in italics; life-threatening reactions are in bold italics.
CNS: headache, *nervousness,* dizziness.
CV: *tachycardia, palpitations,* rise in blood pressure.
EENT: blurred vision.
GI: nausea, abdominal cramps, dry mouth, diarrhea, constipation.
Skin: urticaria.
Other: impotence, altered libido, menstrual changes.

INTERACTIONS
MAO inhibitors: hypertension; possible hypertensive crisis. Don't use together or within 14 days after MAO inhibitor has been discontinued.

NURSING CONSIDERATIONS
- *Contraindicated* in hyperthyroidism, hypertension, angina pectoris, severe CV disease, glaucoma, or history of drug abuse.
- *Use cautiously* in seizure disorder, diabetes mellitus, and hyperexcitability states.
- May alter insulin requirements. Monitor blood and urine sugars.
- When tolerance to anorexigenic effect develops, dosage should not be increased, but drug discontinued.
- Habituation or psychic dependence may occur.
- Be sure patient is also on a weight-reduction program.
- Can be used to stop nighttime eating. Rarely causes insomnia.
- Fatigue may result as drug effects wear off. Patient will need more rest.
- Tell patient to avoid drinks containing caffeine, which increase the effects of amphetamines and related amines.
- Have patient report signs of excessive stimulation.
- Urine acidification enhances renal excretion; urine alkalinization enhances renal reabsorption and recycling.
- Use as analeptic is usually discouraged, since CNS stimulation superimposed on CNS depression can lead to neuronal instability and seizures.
- Give at least 6 hours before bedtime to avoid sleep interference.

fenfluramine hydrochloride
Ponderal†, Ponderal Pacaps†, Ponderax‡, Ponderax Pacaps‡, Pondimin, Pondimin Extentabs
Controlled Substance Schedule IV
Pregnancy Risk Category: C

HOW SUPPLIED
Tablets: 20 mg, 40 mg
Capsules (sustained-release): 60 mg†‡

MECHANISM OF ACTION
Stimulates ventromedial nucleus of the hypothalamus. May also affect serotonin metabolism.

INDICATIONS & DOSAGE
Short-term adjunct in exogenous obesity –
Adults: initially, 20 mg P.O. t.i.d. before meals. Maximum dosage is 40 mg t.i.d. Adjust dosage according to patient's response.

ADVERSE REACTIONS
Common reactions are in italics; life-threatening reactions are in bold italics.
CNS: *drowsiness,* dizziness, incoordination, headache, euphoria or depression, anxiety, *insomnia,* weakness, fatigue, agitation.
CV: *palpitations,* hypotension, hypertension, chest pain.
EENT: eye irritation, blurred vision.
GI: *diarrhea, dry mouth,* nausea, vomiting, abdominal pain, constipation.
GU: dysuria, increased urinary frequency, impotence.
Skin: rashes, urticaria, burning sensation.
Other: sweating, chills, fever, increased libido.

INTERACTIONS
Alcohol, CNS depressants: enhanced CNS depression.
Centrally acting antihypertensives: decreased antihypertensive effect.
MAO inhibitors: severe hypertension; possible hypertensive crisis. Don't use together or within 14 days after an MAO inhibitor has been discontinued.

NURSING CONSIDERATIONS
- *Contraindicated* in glaucoma, hypersensitivity to sympathomimetic amines, symptomatic cardiovascular disease, alcoholism, or history of drug abuse.
- *Use cautiously* in hypertension, history of mental depression, and diabetes mellitus.
- Because of possible hypoglycemia, patients with diabetes may have altered insulin or sulfonylurea requirements. Monitor blood and urine sugars.
- Differs pharmacologically from amphetamines in that it produces CNS depression more often than stimulation.
- Have patient report signs of excessive sedation, depression, or excessive stimulation. Closely monitor blood pressure.
- Be sure patient is on a weight-reduction program.
- Tolerance or dependence may occur. Avoid prolonged administration.
- Fenfluramine should not be discontinued abruptly; may precipitate an acute depressive reaction.
- Has been proven effective for treating autistic children.

mazindol
Mazanor, Sanorex
Controlled Substance Schedule IV
Pregnancy Risk Category: C

HOW SUPPLIED
Tablets: 1 mg, 2 mg

MECHANISM OF ACTION
Inhibits neuronal uptake of norepinephrine and dopamine.

INDICATIONS & DOSAGE
Short-term adjunct in exogenous obesity–
Adults: 1 mg P.O. t.i.d. 1 hour before meals, or 2 mg daily 1 hour before lunch. Use lowest effective dosage.

ADVERSE REACTIONS
Common reactions are in italics; life-threatening reactions are in bold italics.
CNS: *nervousness,* restlessness, dizziness, *insomnia,* dysphoria, headache, depression, drowsiness, weakness, tremor.
CV: *palpitations, tachycardia.*
GI: dry mouth, nausea, constipation, diarrhea, unpleasant taste.
GU: difficulty initiating micturition, impotence.
Skin: rash, clamminess, pallor.
Other: shivering, excessive sweating, altered libido.

INTERACTIONS
Centrally acting antihypertensives: decreased antihypertensive effect.

MAO inhibitors: severe hypertension; possible hypertensive crisis. Don't use together or within 14 days after an MAO inhibitor has been discontinued.

NURSING CONSIDERATIONS

- *Contraindicated* in glaucoma, CV disease including arrhythmias, agitated states, or history of drug abuse.
- *Use cautiously* in diabetes mellitus, hypertension, and hyperexcitability states.
- Warn patient to avoid activities that require alertness or good psychomotor coordination until CNS effects of the drug are known.
- Fatigue may result as drug effects wear off. Patient will need more rest.
- Tell patient to avoid drinks containing caffeine, which increase the effects of amphetamines and related amines.
- Have patient report signs of excessive stimulation.
- Tolerance or dependence may develop. Avoid prolonged use.
- Be sure patient is also on a weight-reduction program.
- May alter insulin needs in patients with diabetes. Monitor blood and urine sugars.
- Give at least 6 hours before bedtime to avoid sleep interference.

methamphetamine hydrochloride

Desoxyn, Desoxyn Gradumet
Controlled Substance Schedule II
Pregnancy Risk Category: C

HOW SUPPLIED
Tablets: 5 mg, 10 mg
Tablets (long-acting): 5 mg, 10 mg, 15 mg

MECHANISM OF ACTION
Main site of activity appears to be the cerebral cortex and the reticular activating system. Promotes nerve impulse transmission by releasing stored norepinephrine from nerve terminals in the brain. In children with hyperkinesia, amphetamines have a paradoxical calming effect.

INDICATIONS & DOSAGE
Attention deficit disorder with hyperactivity (ADDH)–
Children 6 years and older: 2.5 to 5 mg P.O. once daily or b.i.d., with 5-mg increments weekly, p.r.n. Usual effective dosage is 20 to 25 mg daily.
Short-term adjunct in exogenous obesity–
Adults: 2.5 to 5 mg P.O. once to t.i.d. 30 minutes before meals; or 1 long-acting 5- to 15-mg tablet daily before breakfast.

ADVERSE REACTIONS
Common reactions are in italics; life-threatening reactions are in bold italics.
CNS: *nervousness, insomnia,* irritability, *talkativeness,* dizziness, headache, hyperexcitability, tremor.
CV: hypertension, hypotension, *tachycardia, palpitations,* cardiac arrhythmias.
EENT: blurred vision, mydriasis.
GI: nausea, vomiting, abdominal cramps, diarrhea, constipation, dry mouth, anorexia, metallic taste.
Skin: urticaria.
Other: impotence, altered libido.

INTERACTIONS
Ammonium chloride, ascorbic acid: observe for decreased amphetamine effects.
Antacids, sodium bicarbonate, acetazolamide: increased renal reabsorption. Monitor for enhanced effects.
MAO inhibitors: severe hypertension; possible hypertensive crisis. Don't use together or within 14 days after an MAO inhibitor has been discontinued.
Phenothiazines, haloperidol: observe for decreased amphetamine effects.

NURSING CONSIDERATIONS

- *Contraindicated* in hypertension, hyperthyroidism, nephritis, angina pectoris or other severe CV disease, glaucoma, parkinsonism due to arteriosclerosis, agitated states, or history of drug abuse
- *Use cautiously* in diabetes mellitus; in patients who are elderly, debilitated, asthenic, psychopathic, or who have a history of suicidal or homicidal tendencies; and in children with Tourette's disorder.
- Warn that potential for abuse is high. Should not be used to prevent fatigue.
- May alter insulin needs in patients with diabetes. Monitor blood and urine sugars.
- Not recommended for first-line treatment of obesity. Use as an anorexigenic agent is prohibited in some states.
- When used for obesity, be sure patient is on a weight-reduction program.
- Tell patient to avoid drinks containing caffeine, which increase the effects of amphetamines and related amines.
- Have patient report signs of excessive stimulation.
- Urine acidification enhances renal excretion; urine alkalinization enhances renal reabsorption and recycling.
- When tolerance to anorexigenic effect develops, dosage should not be increased, but drug discontinued.
- Warn patient to avoid activities that require alertness or good psychomotor coordination until CNS effects of the drug are known.
- Give at least 6 hours before bedtime to avoid sleep interference.
- Never crush sustained-release tablets.

methylphenidate hydrochloride

Ritalin, Ritalin-SR

Controlled Substance Schedule II

Pregnancy Risk Category: C

HOW SUPPLIED

Tablets: 5 mg, 10 mg, 20 mg
Tablets (sustained-release): 20 mg

MECHANISM OF ACTION

Main site of activity appears to be the cerebral cortex and the reticular activating system. Promotes nerve impulse transmission by releasing stored norepinephrine from nerve terminals in the brain. In children with hyperkinesia, amphetamines have a paradoxical calming effect.

INDICATIONS & DOSAGE

Attention deficit disorder with hyperactivity (ADDH) –
Children 6 years and older: initial dose 5 to 10 mg P.O. daily before breakfast and lunch, with 5- to 10-mg increments weekly as needed, up to 60 mg daily.
Narcolepsy –
Adults: 10 mg P.O. b.i.d. or t.i.d. half hour before meals. Dosage varies with patient needs. Dosage range is 5 to 50 mg daily.

ADVERSE REACTIONS

Common reactions are in italics; life-threatening reactions are in bold italics.
Blood: thrombocytopenia.
CNS: *nervousness, insomnia,* dizziness, headache, akathisia, dyskinesia, *Tourette's disorder.*
CV: *palpitations,* angina, *tachycardia,* changes in blood pressure and pulse rate.
EENT: difficulty with accommodation and blurring of vision.
GI: nausea, dry throat, abdominal pain, anorexia, weight loss.
Skin: rash, urticaria, ***exfoliative der-***

*Liquid form contains alcohol. **May contain tartrazine.

matitis, erythema multiforme, thrombocytopenic purpura.
Other: growth suppression.

INTERACTIONS
Anticonvulsants, tricyclic antidepressants, oral anticoagulants: methylphenidate may increase plasma levels of these drugs and enhance their pharmacologic effects.
Centrally acting antihypertensives: decreased antihypertensive effect.
MAO inhibitors: severe hypertension; possible hypertensive crisis. Don't use together or within 14 days after an MAO inhibitor has been discontinued.

NURSING CONSIDERATIONS
- *Contraindicated* in symptomatic cardiac disease; hyperthyroidism; moderate to severe hypertension; angina pectoris; advanced arteriosclerosis; severe depression of either endogenous or exogenous form; glaucoma; parkinsonism; history of drug abuse or dependency; or history of marked anxiety, tension, or agitation.
- *Use cautiously* in elderly, debilitated, or hyperexcitable patients, and those with history of CV disease, diabetes, or seizures.
- May precipitate Tourette's disorder in children. Monitor especially at start of therapy.
- Closely monitor blood pressure. Observe for signs of excessive stimulation.
- Should not be used to prevent fatigue.
- Observe for interactions, as treatment of other disease states may be affected. May alter daily insulin needs in patients with diabetes. Monitor blood and urine sugars. May decrease seizure threshold in patients with seizure disorders.
- Drug of choice for ADDH. Usually stopped after puberty.
- Periodic CBC, differential, and platelet counts advised with long-term use.
- Tolerance or psychic dependence may develop, especially in patients with history of drug addiction. Avoid long-term use because of high abuse potential. After long-term use, lower dosage gradually to prevent acute rebound depression.
- Fatigue may result as drug effects wear off. Patient will need more rest.
- Tell patient to avoid drinks containing caffeine, which increase the effects of amphetamines and related amines.
- Warn patient to avoid activities that require alertness or good psychomotor coordination until CNS effects of the drug are known.
- Monitor height and weight in children on prolonged therapy because drug has been associated with growth suppression. Recent evidence suggests it may delay "growth spurt," but children will attain normal height when drug is discontinued.
- Now available in a sustained-release form (duration, 6 to 8 hours). Warn patient against chewing these tablets.
- Give at least 6 hours before bedtime to prevent insomnia. Administer after meals to reduce appetite-suppressive effects.

pemoline
Cylert, Cylert Chewable
Controlled Substance Schedule IV

Pregnancy Risk Category: B

HOW SUPPLIED
Tablets: 18.75 mg, 37.5 mg, 75 mg
Tablets (chewable and containing povidine): 37.5 mg

MECHANISM OF ACTION
Main site of activity appears to be the cerebral cortex and the reticular activating system. Promotes nerve impulse transmission by releasing stored

norepinephrine from nerve terminals in the brain.

INDICATIONS & DOSAGE
Attention deficit disorder with hyperactivity (ADDH) –
Children 6 years and older: initially, 37.5 mg P.O. given in the morning. Daily dose can be raised by 18.75 mg weekly. Effective dosage range is 56.25 to 75 mg daily; maximum dosage is 112.5 mg daily.

ADVERSE REACTIONS
Common reactions are in italics; life-threatening reactions are in bold italics.
CNS: *insomnia,* malaise, irritability, fatigue, mild depression, dizziness, headache, drowsiness, hallucinations, nervousness (large doses), ***seizures,*** *Tourette's disorder,* psychosis.
CV: *tachycardia (large doses).*
GI: anorexia, abdominal pain, nausea, diarrhea.
Hepatic: elevated liver enzymes.
Skin: rash.

INTERACTIONS
Insulin, oral hypoglycemics: pemoline may alter requirements of antidiabetic agents.

NURSING CONSIDERATIONS
- *Contraindicated* in patients with hepatic dysfunction, and in children under 6 years.
- *Use cautiously* in patients with impaired renal function or a history of Tourette's disorder. Drug may accumulate.
- May precipitate Tourette's disorder in children. Monitor especially at start of therapy.
- Closely monitor patients on long-term therapy for possible blood or hepatic function abnormalities and for growth suppression.
- Structurally dissimilar to amphetamines or methylphenidate. However, may produce similar adverse reactions, including lowered seizure threshold. Also, has a greater potential for drug abuse and dependence than previously thought.
- Therapeutic effects may not be evident for up to 3 to 4 weeks.
- Give at least 6 hours before bedtime to avoid sleep interference.

phendimetrazine tartrate

Adipost, Adphen, Anorex, Bacarate, Bontril PDM, Bontril Slow Release, Dyrexan OD, Melfiat, Metra, Obalan, Obeval, Phenazine-35, Phenzine, Plegine, Prelu-2, Slyn-LL, Sprx-105, Statobex**, Trimtabs, Trimstat, Wehless, Weightrol, X-Trozine, X-Trozine LA
Controlled Substance Schedule IV
Pregnancy Risk Category: C

HOW SUPPLIED
Tablets: 35 mg
Capsules: 35 mg
Capsules (sustained-release): 105 mg

MECHANISM OF ACTION
Main site of activity appears to be the cerebral cortex and the reticular activating system. Promotes nerve impulse transmission by releasing stored norepinephrine from nerve terminals in the brain.

INDICATIONS & DOSAGE
Short-term adjunct in exogenous obesity –
Adults: 35 mg P.O. b.i.d. to t.i.d. 1 hour before meals. Maximum dosage is 70 mg t.i.d. Use lowest effective dosage. Adjust dose to individual response.

ADVERSE REACTIONS
Common reactions are in italics; life-threatening reactions are in bold italics.
CNS: *nervousness,* dizziness, *insomnia,* tremor, headache.
CV: *tachycardia, palpitations,* rise in blood pressure.

*Liquid form contains alcohol. **May contain tartrazine.

EENT: blurred vision
GI: dry mouth, nausea, abdominal cramps, diarrhea, constipation.
GU: dysuria.

INTERACTIONS
Ammonium chloride, ascorbic acid: observe for decreased phendimetrazine effects.
Antacids, sodium bicarbonate, acetazolamide: increased renal reabsorption. Monitor for enhanced effects.
MAO inhibitors: severe hypertension; possible hypertensive crisis. Don't use together or within 14 days after an MAO inhibitor has been discontinued.
Phenothiazines, haloperidol: observe for decreased effect.

NURSING CONSIDERATIONS
- *Contraindicated* in hyperthyroidism, hypertension, angina pectoris or other severe CV disease, or glaucoma.
- *Use cautiously* in hyperexcitability states or with history of drug addiction.
- Warn patient to avoid activities that require alertness or good psychomotor coordination until CNS effects of the drug are known.
- Be sure patient is following weight-reduction program.
- Tolerance or dependence can develop. Not advised for prolonged use.
- Fatigue may result as drug effects wear off. Patient will need more rest.
- Tell patient to avoid drinks containing caffeine, which increase the effects of amphetamines and related amines.
- Have patient report signs of excessive stimulation.
- Urine acidification enhances renal excretion; urine alkalinization enhances renal reabsorption and recycling.
- May alter daily insulin needs in patients with diabetes. Monitor blood and urine glucose levels.
- Give at least 6 hours before bedtime to avoid sleep interference.

phentermine hydrochloride
Adipex-P, Dapex, Duromine‡, Fastin, Ionamin, Obe-Nix, Obephen, Obermine, Obestin, Oby-Trim, Parmine, Phentrol, Span R/D, Teramine, Unifast
Controlled Substance Schedule IV
Pregnancy Risk Category: C

HOW SUPPLIED
Tablets and capsules: 8 mg, 15 mg, 18.75 mg, 30 mg, 37.5 mg
Capsules (resin complex, sustained-release): 15 mg, 30 mg

MECHANISM OF ACTION
Main site of activity appears to be the cerebral cortex and the reticular activating system. Promotes nerve impulse transmission by releasing stored norepinephrine from nerve terminals in the brain.

INDICATIONS & DOSAGE
Short-term adjunct in exogenous obesity –
Adults: 8 mg P.O. t.i.d. half hour before meals; or 15 to 30 mg daily before breakfast (resin complex).

ADVERSE REACTIONS
Common reactions are in italics; life-threatening reactions are in bold italics.
CNS: *nervousness,* dizziness, *insomnia.*
CV: *palpitations, tachycardia,* increased blood pressure.
GI: dry mouth, unpleasant taste, nausea, constipation, diarrhea.
Skin: urticaria.
Other: altered libido, impotence.

INTERACTIONS
Ammonium chloride, ascorbic acid: observe for decreased phentermine effects.
Antacids, sodium bicarbonate, acet-

azolamide: increased renal reabsorption. Monitor for enhanced effects.
MAO inhibitors: severe hypertension; possible hypertensive crisis. Don't use together or within 14 days after an MAO inhibitor has been discontinued.
Phenothiazines, haloperidol: observe for decreased effects.

NURSING CONSIDERATIONS

- *Contraindicated* in hyperthyroidism, hypertension, angina pectoris or other severe CV disease, or glaucoma.
- *Use cautiously* in hyperexcitability states or history of drug addiction.
- Tolerance or dependence may develop. Avoid prolonged administration.
- Use with weight-reduction program. Give 30 minutes before meals.
- Fatigue may result as drug effects wear off. Patient will need more rest.
- Tell patient to avoid drinks containing caffeine, which increase the effects of amphetamines and related amines.
- Have patient report signs of excessive stimulation.
- Urine acidification enhances renal excretion; urine alkalinization enhances renal reabsorption and recycling.
- Give at least 6 hours before bedtime to avoid sleep interference.

*Liquid form contains alcohol. **May contain tartrazine.

35

Antiparkinsonian agents

amantadine hydrochloride
(See Chapter 17, ANTIVIRALS.)
benztropine mesylate
biperiden hydrochloride
biperiden lactate
bromocriptine mesylate
carbidopa-levodopa
levodopa
pergolide mesylate
procyclidine hydrochloride
selegiline hydrochloride
trihexyphenidyl hydrochloride

COMBINATION PRODUCTS
None.

benztropine mesylate

Apo-Benztropine†, Bensylate†, Cogentin, PMS Benztropine†

Pregnancy Risk Category: C

HOW SUPPLIED
Tablets: 0.5 mg, 1 mg, 2 mg
Injection: 1 mg/ml in 2-ml ampules

MECHANISM OF ACTION
Blocks central cholinergic receptors, helping to balance cholinergic activity in the basal ganglia.

INDICATIONS & DOSAGE
Acute dystonic reaction –
Adults: 1 to 2 mg I.V. or I.M. followed by 1 to 2 mg P.O. b.i.d. to prevent recurrence.
Parkinsonism –
Adults: 0.5 to 6 mg P.O. daily. Initial dose is 0.5 mg to 1 mg. Increase 0.5 mg q 5 to 6 days. Adjust dosage to meet individual requirements. Usual dose is 1 to 2 mg per day.

ADVERSE REACTIONS
Common reactions are in italics; life-threatening reactions are in bold italics.
CNS: disorientation, restlessness, irritability, incoherence, hallucinations, headache, sedation, depression, muscular weakness.
CV: palpitations, tachycardia, paradoxical bradycardia.
EENT: dilated pupils, blurred vision, photophobia, difficulty swallowing.
GI: *constipation, dry mouth,* nausea, vomiting, epigastric distress.
GU: urinary hesitancy, urine retention.
Skin: warming, dry, flushing.
Some adverse reactions may be due to pending atropine-like toxicity and are dose related.

INTERACTIONS
Amantadine, phenothiazines, tricyclic antidepressants: additive anticholinergic adverse reactions, such as confusion and hallucinations. Reduce dosage before administering amantadine.

NURSING CONSIDERATIONS
- *Contraindicated* in narrow-angle glaucoma.
- *Use cautiously* in prostatic hypertrophy, tendency to tachycardia, and in elderly or debilitated patients; produces atropine-like adverse reactions and may aggravate tardive dyskinesia.
- Monitor vital signs carefully. Watch closely for adverse reactions, especially in elderly or debilitated patients. Call doctor promptly.
- Never discontinue this drug abruptly. Dosage must be reduced gradually.
- Warn patient to avoid activities that require alertness until CNS effects of the drug are known. If patient is to receive single daily dose, give at bedtime.

• Explain that drug may take 2 to 3 days to exert full effect.
• **I.V. use:** rarely used because of small difference in onset as compared to I.M. route.
• Advise patient to report signs of urinary hesitancy or urine retention.
• Watch for intermittent constipation, distention, abdominal pain; may be onset of paralytic ileus.
• Relieve dry mouth with cool drinks, ice chips, sugarless gum or hard candy.
• To help prevent GI distress, administer after meals.
• Advise patient to limit activities during hot weather because drug-induced anhydrosis may result in hyperthermia.

biperiden hydrochloride
Akineton

biperiden lactate
Akineton Lactate

Pregnancy Risk Category: C

HOW SUPPLIED
Tablets: 2 mg
Injection: 5 mg/ml in 1-ml ampules

MECHANISM OF ACTION
Blocks central cholinergic receptors, helping to balance cholinergic activity in the basal ganglia.

INDICATIONS & DOSAGE
Extrapyramidal disorders –
Adults: 2 to 6 mg P.O. daily, b.i.d., or t.i.d., depending on severity. Usual dose is 2 mg daily, or 2 mg I.M. or I.V. q half hour, not to exceed 4 doses or 8 mg total daily.
Parkinsonism –
Adults: 2 mg P.O. t.i.d. to q.i.d. Some patients may require as much as 16 mg per day.

ADVERSE REACTIONS
Common reactions are in italics; life-threatening reactions are in bold italics.
CNS: disorientation, euphoria, restlessness, irritability, incoherence, dizziness, increased tremor.
CV: transient postural hypotension (with parenteral use).
EENT: blurred vision.
GI: *constipation, dry mouth,* nausea, vomiting, epigastric distress.
GU: urinary hesitancy, urine retention.

Adverse reactions are dose-related and may resemble atropine toxicity.

INTERACTIONS
Phenothiazines, tricyclic antidepressants: excessive CNS anticholinergic effects.

NURSING CONSIDERATIONS
• *Use cautiously* in prostatism, cardiac arrhythmias, narrow-angle glaucoma, and seizure disorder.
• Monitor vital signs carefully. Watch closely for adverse reactions, especially in elderly or debilitated patients. Call doctor promptly.
• Give oral doses with or after meals to decrease GI adverse reactions.
• When giving parenterally, keep patient in a supine position. Parenteral administration may cause transient postural hypotension and coordination disturbances.
• **I.V. use:** Administer very slowly.
• Because of possible dizziness, help patient when he gets out of bed.
• Tolerance may develop, requiring increased dosage.
• In severe parkinsonism, tremors may increase as spasticity is relieved.
• Warn patient to avoid activities that require alertness until CNS effects of the drug are known.
• Advise patient to report signs of urinary hesitancy or urine retention.
• Relieve dry mouth with cool drinks, ice chips, sugarless gum, or hard candy.

bromocriptine mesylate

Parlodel

Pregnancy Risk Category: C

HOW SUPPLIED

Tablets: 2.5 mg
Capsules: 5 mg

MECHANISM OF ACTION

Inhibits secretion of prolactin. It acts as a dopamine-receptor agonist by activating postsynaptic dopamine receptors.

INDICATIONS & DOSAGE

To treat amenorrhea and galactorrhea associated with hyperprolactinemia; treatment of female infertility –
Women: 1.25 to 2.5 mg P.O. daily. Increase dosage by 2.5 mg daily at 3- to 7-day intervals until desired effect is achieved. Safety and efficacy of doses greater than 100 mg daily have not been established.
Prevention of postpartum lactation –
Women: 2.5 mg P.O. b.i.d. with meals for 14 days. Treatment may be extended for up to 21 days, if necessary.
Treatment of Parkinson's disease –
Adults: 1.25 mg P.O. b.i.d. with meals. Dosage may be increased q 14 to 28 days, up to 100 mg daily.
Treatment of acromegaly –
Adults: 1.25 to 2.5 mg P.O. for 3 days. An additional 1.25 to 2.5 mg may be added q 3 to 7 days until patient receives therapeutic benefit.

ADVERSE REACTIONS

Common reactions are in italics; life-threatening reactions are in bold italics.
CNS: confusion, hallucinations, uncontrolled body movements, *dizziness, headache,* fatigue, mania, delusions, nervousness, insomnia, depression.
CV: *hypotension,* syncope.
EENT: nasal congestion, tinnitus, blurred vision.
GI: *nausea,* vomiting, *abdominal cramps,* constipation, diarrhea.
GU: urine retention, urinary frequency.
Other: ***pulmonary infiltration and pleural effusion,*** coolness and pallor of fingers and toes.

INTERACTIONS

Antihypertensive drugs: increased hypotensive effects. Adjust dosage of antihypertensive agent.
Haloperidol, loxapine, phenothiazines, methyldopa, metoclopramide, MAO inhibitors, reserpine: may interfere with bromocriptine's effects.
Levodopa: additive effects. Adjust dosage of levodopa.
Oral contraceptives, estrogens, progestins: interfere with effects of bromocriptine. Concurrent use not recommended.

NURSING CONSIDERATIONS

- *Contraindicated* in hypersensitivity to ergot derivatives.
- *Use cautiously* in preexisting psychiatric disorders.
- Patient should be examined carefully for pituitary tumor (Forbes-Albright syndrome). Use of bromocriptine will not affect tumor size although it may alleviate amenorrhea or galactorrhea.
- May lead to early postpartum conception. Test for pregnancy every 4 weeks or whenever period is missed after menses are reinitiated.
- Advise patient to use contraceptive methods other than oral contraceptives during treatment.
- Baseline and periodic evaluations of cardiac, hepatic, renal, and hematopoietic function are recommended during prolonged therapy.
- Patients with impaired renal function may require dosage adjustments.
- Incidence of adverse reactions is high, particularly at beginning of therapy. Orthostatic hypotension is common. Adverse reactions can be

minimized by gradually titrating doses to effective levels. Advise patients to avoid dizziness and fainting by rising slowly to an upright position and avoiding sudden position changes.

- Monitor blood pressure closely in women who receive bromocriptine for suppression of postpartum lactation. In such patients, transient hypotension is common; however, hypertension, seizures, and stroke have also been reported.
- Incidence of adverse reactions is high (about 68%); however, most are mild to moderate, and only 6% of patients discontinue drug for this reason. Nausea is the most common adverse reaction.
- Recurrence rates when used to treat amenorrhea or galactorrhea associated with hyperprolactinemia are high (from 70% to 80%).
- Advise the patient that it may take 6 to 8 weeks or longer for menses to be reinstated and galactorrhea to be suppressed.
- Patient may experience mild to moderate rebound breast secretion, congestion, or engorgement when therapy is discontinued.
- Should be given with meals.
- When used to treat Parkinson's disease, bromocriptine is usually given in addition to either levodopa alone or levodopa-carbidopa combination (Sinemet).
- Adverse reactions are more frequent when drug is used for Parkinson's disease.

carbidopa-levodopa

Sinemet, Sinemet CR

Pregnancy Risk Category: C

HOW SUPPLIED

Tablets: carbidopa 10 mg with levodopa 100 mg (Sinemet 10-100), carbidopa 25 mg with levodopa 100 mg (Sinemet 25-100), carbidopa 25 mg with levodopa 250 mg (Sinemet 25-250)

Tablets (sustained-release): carbidopa 50 mg with levodopa 200 mg (Sinemet CR)

MECHANISM OF ACTION

Levodopa is decarboxylated to dopamine, countering the depletion of striatal dopamine in extrapyramidal centers. Carbidopa inhibits the peripheral decarboxylation of levodopa without affecting levodopa's metabolism within the CNS. Therefore, more levodopa is available to be decarboxylated to dopamine in the brain.

INDICATIONS & DOSAGE

Treatment of idiopathic Parkinson's disease, postencephalitic parkinsonism, and symptomatic parkinsonism resulting from carbon monoxide or manganese intoxication –

Adults: 3 to 6 tablets of 25 mg carbidopa/250 mg levodopa daily given in divided doses. Do not exceed 8 tablets of 25 mg carbidopa/250 mg levodopa daily. Optimum daily dosage must be determined by careful titration for each patient.

Patients treated with conventional tablets may receive sustained-release preparation; dosage is calculated on current levodopa intake. Initially, give Sinemet CR equal to 10% more levodopa per day; increase as needed and tolerated to 30% more levodopa per day. Administer in divided doses at intervals of 4 to 8 hours.

ADVERSE REACTIONS

Common reactions are in italics; life-threatening reactions are in bold italics.

Blood: ***hemolytic anemia.***

CNS: *choreiform, dystonic, dyskinetic movements; involuntary grimacing, head movements, myoclonic body jerks, ataxia,* tremors, muscle twitching; bradykinetic episodes; psychiatric disturbances, memory loss, nervousness, anxiety, disturbing dreams, euphoria, malaise, fatigue; severe depression, suicidal tendencies, demen-

*Liquid form contains alcohol. **May contain tartrazine.

tia, delirium, hallucinations (may necessitate reduction or withdrawal of drug).
CV: *orthostatic hypotension, **cardiac irregularities**,* flushing, hypertension, phlebitis.
EENT: blepharospasm, blurred vision, diplopia, mydriasis or miosis, widening of palpebral fissures, activation of latent Horner's syndrome, oculogyric crises, nasal discharge.
GI: *nausea, vomiting, anorexia,* weight loss may occur at start of therapy; constipation; flatulence; diarrhea; *epigastric pain;* hiccups; sialorrhea; *dry mouth;* bitter taste.
GU: urinary frequency, urine retention, urinary incontinence, darkened urine, excessive and inappropriate sexual behavior, priapism.
Hepatic: hepatotoxicity.
Other: dark perspiration, hyperventilation.

INTERACTIONS

Antihypertensives: additive hypotensive effects.
Papaverine, phenothiazines and other antipsychotics, phenytoin: may antagonize antiparkinsonian actions. Use together cautiously.
Sympathomimetics: increased risk of cardiac arrhythmias.

NURSING CONSIDERATIONS

- *Contraindicated* in narrow-angle glaucoma, melanoma, or undiagnosed skin lesions.
- *Use cautiously* in cardiovascular, renal, hepatic, and pulmonary disorders; in history of peptic ulcer; psychiatric illness; MI with residual arrhythmias; bronchial asthma, emphysema; and endocrine disease.
- Carefully monitor patients also receiving antihypertensive medication, hypoglycemic agents. Discontinue MAO inhibitors at least 2 weeks before therapy is begun.
- Dosage is adjusted according to patient's response and tolerance to drug. Therapeutic and adverse reactions occur more rapidly with levodopa-carbidopa than with levodopa alone. Observe and monitor vital signs, especially while dosage is being adjusted; report significant changes.
- Instruct patient to report adverse reactions and therapeutic effects.
- Warn patient of possible dizziness and orthostatic hypotension, especially at start of therapy. Patient should change position slowly and dangle legs before getting out of bed. Elastic stockings may control this adverse reaction in some patients.
- Muscle twitching and blepharospasm (twitching of eyelids) may be an early sign of drug overdosage; report immediately.
- Patients on long-term therapy should be tested regularly for diabetes and acromegaly; hepatic, renal, and hematopoietic function studies should be repeated periodically.
- If patient is being treated with levodopa, discontinue at least 8 hours before starting levodopa-carbidopa.
- This combination drug usually reduces the amount of levodopa needed by 75%, thereby reducing the incidence of adverse reactions.
- Pyridoxine (vitamin B_6) does not reverse the beneficial effects of Sinemet. Multivitamins can be taken without fear of losing control of symptoms.
- If therapy is interrupted temporarily, the usual daily dosage may be given as soon as patient resumes oral medication.
- The different ratios of carbidopa: levodopa facilitate dosage adjustments. At least 70 mg of the carbidopa component should be given daily to effectively block peripheral dopa decarboxylase.
- Carbidopa (Lodosyn) as a single agent is available from Merck Sharp & Dohme on doctor's request.
- Warn patient and his family not to

increase dosage without doctor's order.

• Assess patient for signs and symptoms of GI intolerance. To minimize GI upset, tell him to take drug with food.

• Laboratory test interferences have been reported, including false-positive increases in levels of uric acid, urine ketones, catecholamines, and vanillylmandelic acid, depending on reagent and test method used.

• False-positive tests for urine glucose can occur if reagents using copper sulfate are used; false-negative results can occur with tests that use glucose enzymatic methods. An accurate measure can be obtained if the paper strip is only partially immersed in the urine sample. Urine will migrate up the strip, as with an ascending chromatographic system. Read only the top of the strip.

levodopa

Dopar, Larodopa, Levopa

Pregnancy Risk Category: C

HOW SUPPLIED

Tablets: 100 mg, 250 mg, 500 mg
Capsules: 100 mg, 250 mg, 500 mg

MECHANISM OF ACTION

Levodopa is decarboxylated to dopamine, countering the depletion of striatal dopamine in extrapyramidal centers, which is thought to produce parkinsonism.

INDICATIONS & DOSAGE

Treatment of idiopathic parkinsonism, postencephalitic parkinsonism, and symptomatic parkinsonism after carbon monoxide or manganese intoxication; or in association with cerebral arteriosclerosis –

Adults and children over 12 years: initially, 0.5 to 1 g P.O. daily, given b.i.d., t.i.d., or q.i.d. with food; increase by no more than 0.75 g daily q 3 to 7 days, until usual maximum of 8 g is reached. Carefully adjust dosage to individual requirements, tolerance, and response. Higher dosage requires close supervision.

ADVERSE REACTIONS

Common reactions are in italics; life-threatening reactions are in bold italics.

Blood: ***hemolytic anemia,*** leukopenia.

CNS: *aggressive behavior, choreiform, dystonic, and dyskinetic movements, involuntary grimacing, head movements, myoclonic body jerks, ataxia, tremors, muscle twitching, bradykinetic episode, psychiatric disturbances, memory loss, mood changes, nervousness, anxiety, disturbing dreams, euphoria, malaise, fatigue, severe depression, suicidal tendencies, dementia, delirium, hallucinations (may necessitate reduction or withdrawal of drug).*

CV: *orthostatic hypotension,* cardiac irregularities, flushing, hypertension, phlebitis.

EENT: blepharospasm, blurred vision, diplopia, mydriasis or miosis, widening of palpebral fissures, activation of latent Horner's syndrome, oculogyric crises, nasal discharge.

GI: *nausea, vomiting, anorexia,* weight loss may occur at start of therapy, constipation, flatulence, diarrhea, epigastric pain, hiccups, sialorrhea, dry mouth, bitter taste.

GU: urinary frequency, retention, incontinence; darkened urine; excessive and inappropriate sexual behavior; priapism.

Hepatic: hepatotoxicity.

Other: dark perspiration, hyperventilation.

INTERACTIONS

Antacids: increased absorption of levodopa.

Antihypertensives: additive hypertensive effect.

*Liquid form contains alcohol. **May contain tartrazine.

High-protein foods: decreased absorption of levodopa.
Metoclopramide: accelerated gastric emptying of levodopa.
Papaverine, phenothiazines and other antipsychotics, phenytoin: watch for decreased levodopa effect.
Pyridoxine: reduced efficacy of levodopa. Examine vitamin preparations and nutritional supplements for content of vitamin B_6 (pyridoxine).
Sympathomimetics: increased risk of cardiac arrhythmias.

NURSING CONSIDERATIONS

- *Contraindicated* in narrow-angle glaucoma, melanoma, or undiagnosed skin lesions.
- *Use cautiously* in cardiovascular, renal, hepatic, and pulmonary disorders; peptic ulcer; psychiatric illness; myocardial infarction with residual arrhythmias; bronchial asthma; emphysema; and endocrine disease.
- Carefully monitor patients also receiving antihypertensive medication and hypoglycemic agents. Stop MAO inhibitors at least 2 weeks before therapy is begun.
- Adjust dosage according to patient's response and tolerance. Observe and monitor vital signs, especially while adjusting dose. Report significant changes.
- Instruct patient to report adverse reactions and therapeutic effects.
- Warn patient of possible dizziness and orthostatic hypotension, especially at start of therapy. Patient should change position slowly and dangle legs before getting out of bed. Elastic stockings may control this adverse reaction in some patients.
- Muscle twitching and blepharospasm (twitching of eyelids) may be early signs of drug overdosage; report immediately.
- Patients receiving long-term treatment should be tested regularly for diabetes and acromegaly and should have periodic tests of renal, hepatic, and hematopoietic function.
- Advise patient and family that multivitamin preparations, fortified cereals, and certain OTC medications may contain pyridoxine (vitamin B_6), which can block the effects of levodopa.
- If therapy is interrupted for a long time, drug should be adjusted gradually to previous level.
- Therapeutic response usually occurs following each dose and disappears within 5 hours but varies considerably.
- Patient who must undergo surgery should continue levodopa as long as oral intake is permitted, generally 6 to 24 hours before surgery. Drug should be resumed as soon as patient is able to take oral medication.
- Protect from heat, light, and moisture. If preparation darkens, it has lost potency and should be discarded.
- Coombs' test occasionally becomes positive during extended use. Expect uric acid elevations with colorimetric method but not with uricase method.
- Alkaline phosphatase, AST (SGOT), ALT (SGPT), lactate dehydrogenase, bilirubin, BUN, and protein-bound iodine show transient elevations in patients receiving levodopa; WBC, hemoglobin, and hematocrit show occasional reduction.
- A doctor-supervised period of drug discontinuance (called a drug holiday) may reestablish the effectiveness of a lower dosage regimen.
- Combination of levodopa-carbidopa usually reduces amount of levodopa needed by 75%, thereby reducing incidence of adverse reactions.
- Tablets may be crushed and mixed with applesauce or baby food fruits for patients who have difficulty swallowing pills.
- Warn patient and family not to increase dosage without the doctor's orders (they may be tempted to do this as disease symptoms of parkinsonism

progress). Daily dosage should not exceed 8 g.

- Assess patient for signs and symptoms of GI intolerance. To minimize GI upset, tell him to take the drug with food.
- Laboratory test interferences have been reported, including false-positive increases in levels of uric acid, urine ketones, catecholamines, and vanillylmandelic acid, depending on reagent and test method used.
- False-positive tests for urine glucose can occur if reagents using copper sulfate are used; false-negative results can occur with tests that use glucose enzymatic methods. An accurate measure can be obtained if the paper strip is only partially immersed in the urine sample. Urine will migrate up the strip, as with an ascending chromatographic system. Read only the top of the strip.

pergolide mesylate

Permax

Pregnancy Risk Category: B

HOW SUPPLIED

Tablets: 0.05 mg, 0.25 mg, 1 mg

MECHANISM OF ACTION

Directly stimulates dopamine receptors in the nigrostriatal system.

INDICATIONS & DOSAGE

Adjunctive treatment to carbidopa-levodopa in the management of the symptoms associated with Parkinson's disease –

Adults: initially, 0.05 mg P.O. daily for the first 2 days. Gradually increase dosage by 0.1 to 0.15 mg every third day over the next 12 days of therapy. Subsequent dosage can be increased by 0.25 mg every third day until optimum response is seen. The drug is usually administered in divided doses t.i.d. Gradual reductions in carbidopa-levodopa dosage may be made during dosage titration.

ADVERSE REACTIONS

Common reactions are in italics; life-threatening reactions are in bold italics.

CNS: headache, asthenia, *dyskinesia, dizziness, hallucinations,* dystonia, confusion, *somnolescence,* insomnia, anxiety, depression, tremor, abnormal dreams, personality disorder, psychosis, abnormal gait, akathisia, extrapyramidal syndrome, incoordination, paresthesias, akinesia, hypertonia, neuralgia, speech disorder.

CV: *orthostatic hypotension,* vasodilation, palpitations, hypotension, syncope, hypertension, ***arrhythmias, myocardial infarction.***

EENT: *rhinitis,* epistaxis, abnormal vision, diplopia, eye disorder.

GI: abdominal pain, *nausea, constipation,* diarrhea, dyspepsia, anorexia, vomiting, dry mouth, taste alteration.

GU: urinary frequency, urinary tract infection, hematuria.

Skin: rash, sweating.

Other: accident or injury; chest, neck, and back pain; flu-like syndrome; chills; infection; facial, peripheral, or generalized edema; weight gain; arthralgia; bursitis; myalgia; twitching.

Note: The above adverse reactions, although not always attributable to the drug, occurred in > 1% of the study population.

INTERACTIONS

Phenothiazines, butyrophenones, thioxanthines, metoclopramide, and other drugs that are dopamine antagonists: may antagonize the effects of pergolide.

NURSING CONSIDERATIONS

- *Contraindicated* in patients allergic to the drug or to ergot alkaloids. Symptomatic orthostatic or sustained hypotension may occur in some pa-

tients, especially at the start of therapy.
• Hallucinations may occur in some patients. Tolerance to this adverse reaction was not seen in early clinical trials.
• In premarketing trials, over 140 of approximately 2,300 patients died while taking pergolide. However, the drug did not appear to be responsible for these deaths because these patients were elderly, ill, and at high risk for death.
• In early clinical trials, 27% of the patients who attempted pergolide therapy did not finish the trial because of adverse reactions (primarily hallucinations and confusion). Inform patients of the potential adverse reactions. Warn them to avoid activities that could expose them to injury as a result of orthostatic hypotension and syncope.

procyclidine hydrochloride

Kemadrin, PMS Procyclidine†, Procyclid†

Pregnancy Risk Category: C

HOW SUPPLIED
Tablets: 5 mg

MECHANISM OF ACTION
Blocks central cholinergic receptors, helping to balance cholinergic activity in the basal ganglia.

INDICATIONS & DOSAGE
Parkinsonism, muscle rigidity –
Adults: initially, 2 to 2.5 mg P.O. t.i.d., after meals. Increase gradually as needed. Usual dosage range is 20 to 30 mg/day, but some patients may require up to 60 mg daily.

Also used to relieve extrapyramidal dysfunction that accompanies treatment with phenothiazines and rauwolfia derivatives. Also controls excessive salivation from neuroleptic medications.

ADVERSE REACTIONS
Common reactions are in italics; life-threatening reactions are in bold italics.
CNS: light-headedness, giddiness.
EENT: blurred vision, mydriasis.
GI: *constipation, dry mouth,* nausea, vomiting, epigastric distress.
Skin: rash.
Other: muscle weakness.

INTERACTIONS
None significant.

NURSING CONSIDERATIONS
• *Contraindicated* in narrow-angle glaucoma.
• *Use cautiously* in tachycardia, hypotension, urine retention, and prostatic hypertrophy.
• Watch closely for mental confusion, disorientation, agitation, hallucinations, and psychotic symptoms, especially in the elderly. Call doctor promptly if these occur.
• In severe parkinsonism, tremors may increase as spasticity is relieved.
• Give after meals to minimize GI distress.
• Warn patient to avoid activities that require alertness until CNS effects of the drug are known.
• Relieve dry mouth with cool drinks, ice chips, sugarless gum, or hard candy.

selegiline hydrochloride (L-deprenyl hydrochloride)

Eldepryl

Pregnancy Risk Category: C

HOW SUPPLIED
Tablets: 5 mg

MECHANISM OF ACTION
Probably acts by selectively inhibiting MAO type B (found mostly in the brain). At higher-than-recommended doses, it is a nonselective inhibitor of MAO, including MAO type A (found in the GI tract). It also may directly

increase dopaminergic activity by decreasing the reuptake of dopamine into nerve cells. It has pharmacologically active metabolites (amphetamine and methamphetamine) that may contribute to this effect.

INDICATIONS & DOSAGE
Adjunctive treatment to carbidopa-levodopa in the management of the symptoms associated with Parkinson's disease –
Adults: 10 mg P.O. daily, taken as 5 mg at breakfast and 5 mg at lunch. After 2 or 3 days of therapy, begin gradual decrease of carbidopa-levodopa dosage.

ADVERSE REACTIONS
Common reactions are in italics; life-threatening reactions are in bold italics.
CNS: *dizziness,* increased tremor, chorea, loss of balance, restlessness, blepharospasm, increased bradykinesia, facial grimace, stiff neck, dyskinesia, involuntary movements, increased apraxia, behavioral changes, tiredness, headache.
CV: orthostatic hypotension, hypertension, hypotension, ***arrhythmias,*** palpitations, new or increased anginal pain, tachycardia, peripheral edema, syncope.
GI: *nausea,* vomiting, constipation, weight loss, anorexia or poor appetite, dysphagia, diarrhea, heartburn, dry mouth, taste alteration.
GU: slow urination, transient nocturia, prostatic hypertrophy, urinary hesitancy, urinary frequency, urine retention, sexual dysfunction.
Skin: rash, hair loss, sweating.
Other: malaise.

INTERACTIONS
Adrenergic agents: possible increased pressor response, particularly in patients that have taken an overdose of selegiline.

NURSING CONSIDERATIONS
- *Contraindicated* in patients with hypersensitivity to the drug.
- Warn patients to move about cautiously at the start of therapy because they may experience dizziness and risk falling.
- Some patients experience increased adverse reactions associated with levodopa (including muscle twitches) and require reduction of carbidopa-levodopa dosage. Such patients commonly reduce carbidopa-levodopa dosage by 10% to 30%.
- Because the drug is an MAO inhibitor, patients should be told about the possibility of an interaction with tyramine-containing foods. They should immediately report any signs or symptoms of hypertension, including severe headache. However, at recommended dosage, there is no evidence that this interaction occurs because, at 10 mg daily, the drug inhibits only MAO type B. No dietary restrictions appear necessary if the patient does not exceed the recommended dose.
- Advise patient not to take more than 10 mg daily, because there is no evidence that a greater amount improves efficacy and it may increase adverse reactions.

trihexyphenidyl hydrochloride
Aparkane†, Apo-Trihex†, Artane*, Artane Sequels, Novohexidyl†, Trihexane, Trihexy-2, Trihexy-5

Pregnancy Risk Category: C

HOW SUPPLIED
Tablets: 2 mg, 5 mg
Capsules (sustained-release): 5 mg
Elixir: 2 mg/5 ml

MECHANISM OF ACTION
Blocks central cholinergic receptors, helping to balance cholinergic activity in the basal ganglia.

*Liquid form contains alcohol. **May contain tartrazine.

INDICATIONS & DOSAGE

Drug-induced parkinsonism –

Adults: 1 mg P.O. 1st day, 2 mg 2nd day, then increases by 2 mg q 3 to 5 days until total of 6 to 10 mg is given daily. Usually given t.i.d. with meals and, if needed, q.i.d. (last dose should be before bedtime) or may switch to extended-release form b.i.d. Postencephalitic parkinsonism may require 12 to 15 mg total daily dosage.

ADVERSE REACTIONS

Common reactions are in italics; life-threatening reactions are in bold italics.

CNS: nervousness, dizziness, headache, restlessness, agitation, hallucinations, euphoria, delusion, amnesia.

CV: tachycardia.

EENT: blurred vision, mydriasis, increased intraocular pressure.

GI: constipation, *dry mouth, nausea.*

GU: urinary hesitancy, urine retention.

Adverse reactions are dose-related.

INTERACTIONS

Amantadine: additive anticholinergic adverse reactions, such as confusion and hallucinations. Reduce dosage before administering amantadine.

NURSING CONSIDERATIONS

- *Use cautiously* in patients with narrow-angle glaucoma; cardiac, hepatic, or renal disorders; hypertension; obstructive disease of the GI and GU tracts; possible prostatic hypertrophy; patients over 60 years; and those with arteriosclerosis or history of drug hypersensitivities. Adverse reactions are usually mild and transient.
- Warn patient to avoid activities that require alertness until CNS effects of the drug are known.
- Causes nausea if given before meals.
- Relieve dry mouth with cool drinks, ice chips, sugarless gum, or hard candy.
- Patient may develop a tolerance to this drug, so dosage may need to be gradually increased.
- Advise patient to report signs of urinary hesitancy or urine retention.
- Gonioscopic evaluation and close monitoring of intraocular pressure is advised, especially in patients over 40 years.

36

Cholinergics (parasympathomimetics)

ambenonium chloride
bethanechol chloride
edrophonium chloride
neostigmine bromide
neostigmine methylsulfate
physostigmine salicylate
pyridostigmine bromide

COMBINATION PRODUCTS
None.

ambenonium chloride
Mytelase

Pregnancy Risk Category: C

HOW SUPPLIED
Tablets: 10 mg

MECHANISM OF ACTION
Inhibits the destruction of acetylcholine released from the parasympathetic and somatic efferent nerves. Acetylcholine accumulates, promoting increased stimulation of the receptor.

INDICATIONS & DOSAGE
Symptomatic treatment of myasthenia gravis in patients who cannot take neostigmine bromide or pyridostigmine bromide –
Adults: dosage must be individualized for each patient, but usually ranges from 5 to 25 mg P.O. t.i.d. to q.i.d. Starting dose usually is 5 mg P.O. t.i.d. to q.i.d. Increase gradually and adjust at 1- to 2-day intervals to avoid drug accumulation and overdosage. Usual dosage range is 15 to 100 mg daily, but some patients may require as much as 75 mg two to four times a day.

ADVERSE REACTIONS
Common reactions are in italics; life-threatening reactions are in bold italics.
CNS: headache, dizziness, muscle weakness, incoordination, ***seizures,*** mental confusion, jitters, sweating.
CV: bradycardia, hypotension.
EENT: miosis, blurred vision.
GI: *nausea, vomiting, diarrhea, abdominal cramps,* increased salivation.
GU: urinary frequency, incontinence.
Other: ***bronchospasm,*** *muscle cramps,* ***bronchoconstriction,*** increased bronchial secretions, ***respiratory paralysis.***

INTERACTIONS
Aminoglycosides, anesthetics, atropine, corticosteroids, magnesium, procainamide, quinidine: may impair drug effect. Observe for lack of drug effect.
Mecamylamine, other ganglionic blockers: increased toxicity. Avoid concomitant use.

NURSING CONSIDERATIONS
- *Contraindicated* in mechanical obstruction of intestine or urinary tract, bradycardia, or hypotension.
- *Use with extreme caution* in bronchial asthma.
- Use cautiously in epilepsy, recent coronary occlusion, vagotonia, hyperthyroidism, cardiac arrhythmias, and peptic ulcer.
- Avoid large dose in patients with decreased GI motility or megacolon.
- Discontinue all other cholinergics before administering this drug.
- Watch patient very closely for adverse reactions, particularly if total dosage is greater than 200 mg daily. Adverse reactions may indicate drug toxicity. Notify doctor immediately if they develop.

• Monitor and document vital signs frequently, being especially careful to check respirations. Always have atropine injection readily available and be prepared to give atropine 0.5 mg subcutaneously or slow I.V. push as ordered, and provide respiratory support as needed.
• Administer each dose exactly as ordered, on time. Amount and frequency of dosage should vary with patient's activity level. The doctor will probably order larger doses to be given when patient is fatigued, for example, in the afternoon and at mealtime.
• If muscle weakness is severe, doctor must determine if this is caused by drug toxicity or exacerbation of myasthenia gravis. A test dose of edrophonium I.V. will aggravate drug-induced weakness but will temporarily relieve weakness that results from the disease.
• Weakness occurring 30 to 60 minutes after taking dose is a warning sign of drug toxicity. Notify doctor immediately.
• Observe and record the patient's variations in muscle strength. Show him how to do it himself.
• When given for myasthenia gravis, explain to patient that this drug will relieve symptoms of ptosis, double vision, difficulty in chewing and swallowing, and trunk and limb weakness. Stress the importance of taking this drug exactly as ordered. Explain to patient and his family that he may have to take this drug for the rest of his life. Teach them about the disease and the drug's effect on symptoms.
• Patient may develop resistance to drug.
• Seek approval when indicated for hospitalized patient to have bedside supply of tablets to take himself. Patients with long-standing disease often insist on this.
• Give with milk or food to produce fewer muscarinic adverse reactions.
• Advise patient to wear identification tag indicating he has myasthenia gravis.

bethanechol chloride

Duvoid, Myotonachol, Urabeth, Urecholine, Urocarb Liquid‡, Urocarb Tablets‡

Pregnancy Risk Category: C

HOW SUPPLIED

Tablets: 5 mg, 10 mg, 25 mg, 50 mg
Liquid: 1 mg/5 ml‡
Injection: 5 mg/ml

MECHANISM OF ACTION

Binds to cholinergic (muscarinic) receptors, mimicking the action of acetylcholine.

INDICATIONS & DOSAGE

Acute postoperative and postpartum nonobstructive (functional) urine retention, neurogenic atony of urinary bladder with retention, abdominal distention, megacolon, or reflux esophagitis caused by low esophageal sphincter pressure –
Adults: 10 to 30 mg P.O. b.i.d. to q.i.d. Or, 2.5 to 10 mg S.C. Never give I.M. or I.V. When used for urine retention, some patients may require 50 to 100 mg P.O. per dose. Use such doses with extreme caution.

Test dose is 2.5 mg S.C. repeated at 15- to 30-minute intervals to total of 4 doses to determine the minimal effective dose; then use minimal effective dose q 6 to 8 hours. All doses must be adjusted individually.

ADVERSE REACTIONS

Common reactions are in italics; life-threatening reactions are in bold italics.
Dose-related:
CNS: headache, malaise.
CV: bradycardia, hypotension, ***cardiac arrest,*** reflex tachycardia.
EENT: lacrimation, miosis.
GI: *abdominal cramps, diarrhea,* sal-

ivation, nausea, vomiting, belching, borborygmus, esophageal spasms.
GU: urinary urgency.
Skin: flushing, sweating.
Other: ***bronchoconstriction,*** increased bronchial secretions.

INTERACTIONS
Atropine, anticholinergic agents, procainamide, quinidine: may reverse cholinergic effects. Observe for lack of drug effect.
Cholinergic agonists, anticholinergic agents: may cause additive effects, or increase toxicity. Avoid concomitant use.
Ganglionic blockers: may cause hypotension. Avoid concomitant use.

NURSING CONSIDERATIONS
- *Contraindicated* in patients with uncertain strength or integrity of bladder wall; when increased muscular activity of GI or urinary tract is harmful; in mechanical obstructions of GI or urinary tract; in hyperthyroidism, peptic ulcer, latent or active bronchial asthma, cardiac or coronary artery disease, vagotonia, epilepsy, Parkinson's disease, bradycardia, chronic obstructive pulmonary disease, hypotension.
- *Use cautiously* in hypertension, vasomotor instability, peritonitis, and other acute inflammatory conditions of GI tract.
- *Never* give I.M. or I.V.; could cause circulatory collapse, hypotension, severe abdominal cramping, bloody diarrhea, shock, or cardiac arrest.
- Should stop all other cholinergics before giving this drug.
- Watch closely for adverse reactions that may indicate drug toxicity, especially with S.C. administration.
- Monitor vital signs frequently, being especially careful to check respirations. Always have atropine injection readily available and be prepared to give atropine 0.5 mg S.C. or slow I.V. push as ordered, and provide respiratory support if needed.
- If used to treat urine retention, make sure bedpan is readily available. Monitor intake and output.
- When used to prevent abdominal distention and GI distress, the doctor may also order a rectal tube inserted to help passage of gas.
- Poor and variable oral absorption requires larger oral doses. Oral and S.C. doses are *not* interchangeable.
- Drug usually effective 5 to 15 minutes after injection and 30 to 90 minutes after oral use.
- Give on empty stomach; if taken after meals, may cause nausea and vomiting.
- Bethanechol increases pancreatic secretion, raising serum levels of amylase and lipase. Because drug causes a spasm in the sphincter of Oddi, it may raise serum bilirubin and AST (SGOT) levels and increase sulfobromophthalein retention.

edrophonium chloride
Enlon, Reversol, Tensilon
Pregnancy Risk Category: C

HOW SUPPLIED
Injection: 10 mg/ml in 1-ml ampules or 10-ml vials

MECHANISM OF ACTION
Inhibits the destruction of acetylcholine released from the parasympathetic and somatic efferent nerves. Acetylcholine accumulates, promoting increased stimulation of the receptor. Edrophonium has a very short duration of action.

INDICATIONS & DOSAGE
As a curare antagonist (to reverse neuromuscular blocking action) –
Adults: 10 mg I.V. given over 30 to 45 seconds. Dose may be repeated as necessary to 40 mg maximum dosage.

Larger dosages may potentiate rather than antagonize effect of curare.
Diagnostic aid in myasthenia gravis (Tensilon test) –
Adults: 1 to 2 mg I.V. within 15 to 30 seconds, then 8 mg if no response (increase in muscular strength). Alternatively, give 10 mg I.M. If a cholinergic reaction occurs, give 2 mg I.M. 30 minutes later to rule out a false-negative response.
Children over 34 kg: 2 mg I.V. If no response within 45 seconds, give 1 mg q 45 seconds to maximum of 10 mg. Alternatively, give 5 mg I.M.
Children up to 34 kg: 1 mg I.V. If no response within 45 seconds, give 1 mg q 45 seconds to maximum of 5 mg. Alternatively, give 2 mg I.M.
Infants: 0.5 mg to 1 mg I.M. or S.C.
To differentiate myasthenic crisis from cholinergic crisis –
Adults: 1 mg I.V. If no response in 1 minute, repeat dose once. Increased muscular strength confirms myasthenic crisis; no increase or exaggerated weakness confirms cholinergic crisis.
Paroxysmal supraventricular tachycardia –
Adults: 5 to 10 mg I.V. given over 1 minute or less. Alternatively, give a test dose of 2 mg I.V., followed by 2 mg every minute for a total of 10 mg I.V. If heart rate decreases, infuse at 0.25 mg/minute; increase as needed to a maximum of 2 mg/minute.
Children: 2 mg I.V. Administer slowly.

ADVERSE REACTIONS

Common reactions are in italics; life-threatening reactions are in bold italics.
CNS: ***seizures,*** weakness, dysarthria, dysphagia, sweating.
CV: hypotension, bradycardia, AV block.
EENT: excessive lacrimation, diplopia, miosis, conjunctival hyperemia.
GI: nausea, vomiting, *diarrhea, abdominal cramps,* excessive salivation.
GU: urinary frequency, incontinence.
Respiratory: ***paralysis, bronchospasm, laryngospasm,*** increased bronchial secretions.
Other: muscle cramps, muscle fasciculation.

INTERACTIONS

Aminoglycosides, anesthetics: prolonged or enhanced muscle weakness. Monitor closely.
Digitalis glycosides: may increase the heart's sensitivity to edrophonium. Use together cautiously.
Procainamide, quinidine: may reverse cholinergic effects. Observe for lack of drug effect.

NURSING CONSIDERATIONS

- *Contraindicated* in mechanical obstruction of intestine or urinary tract, bradycardia, or hypotension.
- *Use cautiously* in hyperthyroidism, cardiac disease, peptic ulcer, and bronchial asthma.
- Should stop all other cholinergics before giving this drug.
- Watch closely for adverse reactions; may indicate toxicity.
- Monitor vital signs frequently, being especially careful to check respirations. Always have atropine injection readily available and be prepared to give atropine 0.5 mg subcutaneously or slow I.V. push as ordered, and provide respiratory support as needed.
- **I.V. use:** For easier parenteral administration, use a tuberculin syringe with an I.V. needle. When giving drug to differentiate myasthenic crisis from cholinergic crisis, observe patient's muscle strength closely.
- Continuous I.V. infusions have been used to control atrial tachycardia or supraventricular tachycardia associated with Wolff-Parkinson-White syndrome that is unresponsive to digitalis glycosides.

• Edrophonium not effective against muscle relaxation induced by decamethonium bromide and succinylcholine chloride.
• This cholinergic has the most rapid onset but shortest duration; therefore, not used for treatment of myasthenia gravis.
• I.M. route may be used in children because of difficulty with I.V. route: for children under 34 kg, inject 2 mg I.M.; children over 34 kg, 5 mg I.M. Expect same reactions as with I.V. test, but these appear after 2- to 10-minute delay.

neostigmine bromide
Prostigmin Bromide

neostigmine methylsulfate
Prostigmin

Pregnancy Risk Category: C

HOW SUPPLIED
Tablets: 15 mg
Injection: 0.25 mg/ml, 0.5 mg/ml, 1 mg/ml

MECHANISM OF ACTION
Inhibits the destruction of acetylcholine released from the parasympathetic and somatic efferent nerves. Acetylcholine accumulates, promoting increased stimulation of the receptor.

INDICATIONS & DOSAGE
Antidote for nondepolarizing neuromuscular blocking agents –
Adults: 0.5 to 2 mg I.V. slowly. Repeat p.r.n. to a total of 5 mg. Give 0.6 to 1.2 mg atropine sulfate I.V. before antidote dose.
Postoperative abdominal distention and bladder atony –
Adults: 0.5 to 1 mg I.M. or S.C. q 4 to 6 hours.
Postoperative ileus –
Adults: 0.25 to 1 mg I.M. or S.C. q 4 to 6 hours.
Diagnosis of myasthenia gravis –
Adults: 0.022 mg/kg I.M. 30 minutes after 0.4 to 0.6 mg of atropine sulfate.
Children: 0.025 to 0.04 mg/kg. I.M. after 0.11 mg/kg atropine sulfate S.C.
Treatment of myasthenia gravis –
Adults: 15 to 30 mg P.O. t.i.d. (range is 15 to 375 mg daily); or 0.5 to 2 mg S.C., I.M., or I.V. q 1 to 3 hours. Dosage must be individualized, depending on response and tolerance of adverse reactions. Therapy may be required day and night.
Children: 7.5 to 15 mg P.O. t.i.d. to q.i.d.

Note: 1:1,000 solution of injectable solution contains 1 mg/ml; 1:2,000 solution contains 0.5 mg/ml.

ADVERSE REACTIONS
Common reactions are in italics; life-threatening reactions are in bold italics.
CNS: dizziness, muscle weakness, mental confusion, jitters, sweating.
CV: bradycardia, hypotension.
EENT: blurred vision, lacrimation, miosis.
GI: *nausea, vomiting, diarrhea, abdominal cramps,* excessive salivation.
GU: urinary frequency.
Respiratory: ***depression, bronchospasm, bronchoconstriction.***
Skin: rash (bromide).
Other: *muscle cramps,* muscle fasciculations.

INTERACTIONS
Atropine, anticholinergic agents, procainamide, aminoglycosides, quinidine: may reverse cholinergic effect on muscle. Observe for lack of drug effect.

NURSING CONSIDERATIONS
• *Contraindicated* in hypersensitivity to cholinergics or to bromide, mechanical obstruction of the intestine or urinary tract, bradycardia, or hypotension.
• *Use with extreme caution* in bronchial asthma. *Use cautiously* in sei-

zure disorders, recent coronary occlusion, peritonitis, vagotonia, hyperthyroidism, cardiac arrhythmias, and peptic ulcer.
• Should stop all other cholinergics before giving this drug.
• Monitor vital signs frequently, being especially careful to check respirations. Have atropine injection readily available and be prepared to give as ordered, and provide respiratory support as needed.
• Difficult to judge optimum dosage. Monitor and document patient's response after each dose. Observe closely for improvement in strength, vision, and ptosis 45 to 60 minutes after each dose. Show patient how to observe and record variations in muscle strength.
• When using for myasthenia gravis, explain that this drug will relieve ptosis, double vision, difficulty in chewing and swallowing, trunk and limb weakness. Stress importance of taking drug exactly as ordered. Explain that drug may have to be taken for life.
• In myasthenia gravis, schedule the dose before periods of fatigue. For example, if patient has dysphagia, schedule dose 30 minutes before each meal.
• When used to prevent abdominal distention and GI distress, the doctor may order a rectal tube inserted to help passage of gas.
• Patients sometimes develop a resistance to neostigmine.
• If muscle weakness is severe, doctor determines if it is caused by drug-induced toxicity or exacerbation of myasthenia gravis. Test dose of edrophonium I.V. will aggravate drug-induced weakness but will temporarily relieve weakness caused by disease.
• Hospitalized patient with long-standing myasthenia may request bedside supply of tablets. This will enable patient to take each dose precisely as ordered. Seek approval for self-medication program according to hospital policy, but continue to oversee medication regimen.
• GI adverse reactions may be reduced by taking drug with milk or food.
• Advise patient to wear an identification tag indicating that he has myasthenia gravis.
• I.M. neostigmine may be used instead of edrophonium to diagnose myasthenia gravis. May be preferable to edrophonium when limb weakness is the only symptom.

physostigmine salicylate (eserine)

Antilirium

Pregnancy Risk Category: C

HOW SUPPLIED

Injection: 1 mg/ml

MECHANISM OF ACTION

Inhibits the destruction of acetylcholine released from the parasympathetic and somatic efferent nerves. Acetylcholine accumulates, promoting increased stimulation of the receptor.

INDICATIONS & DOSAGE

To reverse the CNS toxicity associated with tricyclic antidepressant and anticholinergic poisoning–

Adults: 0.5 to 2 mg I.M. or I.V. (1 mg/minute I.V.) repeated every 20 minutes as necessary if life-threatening signs recur (coma, seizures, arrhythmias). Additional doses of 1 to 4 mg I.M. or I.V. every 30 to 60 minutes may be given.

Children: 0.02 mg/kg I.M. or I.V. Repeat every 5 to 10 minutes until response is obtained. Maximum dose to 2 mg.

ADVERSE REACTIONS

Common reactions are in italics; life-threatening reactions are in bold italics.

CNS: ***seizures,*** hallucinations, mus-

cular twitching, muscle weakness, ataxia, *restlessness, excitability, sweating.*
CV: irregular pulse, palpitations.
EENT: miosis.
GI: nausea, vomiting, epigastric pain, *diarrhea, excessive salivation.*
Other: ***bronchospasm,*** bronchial constriction, dyspnea.

INTERACTIONS
Atropine, anticholinergic agents, procainamide, quinidine: may reverse cholinergic effects. Observe for lack of drug effect.

NURSING CONSIDERATIONS
- *Contraindicated* in patients with mechanical obstruction of intestine or urogenital tract, bronchial asthma, gangrene, diabetes, CV disease, or vagotonia.
- *Use cautiously* in patients with bradycardia, hypotension, seizure disorder, Parkinson's disease, hyperthyroidism, and peptic ulcer.
- Watch closely for adverse reactions, particularly CNS disturbances. Use side rails if patient becomes restless or hallucinates. Adverse reactions may indicate drug toxicity.
- Monitor vital signs frequently, being especially careful to check respirations. Position patient to make breathing easier. Always have atropine injection readily available and be prepared to give atropine 0.5 mg subcutaneously or slow I.V. push as ordered, and provide respiratory support as needed. Best administered in presence of doctor.
- Use only clear solution. Darkening may indicate loss of potency.
- **I.V. use:** Give I.V. at controlled rate; use slow, direct injection at no more than 1 mg/minute.
- Only cholinergic that crosses blood-brain barrier; therefore the only one useful for treating CNS effects of anticholinergic or tricyclic antidepressant toxicity.
- Effectiveness often immediate and dramatic but may be transient and may require repeat dose.
- Is used investigationally to improve cognitive function in patients with Alzheimer's disease. Investigators have used 0.5 mg P.O. q 2 hours, increasing to 2 to 2.5 mg P.O. q 2 hours, 6 or 7 times a day. Maximum dose is 16 mg/day.

pyridostigmine bromide

Mestinon*, Mestinon Supraspan†, Mestinon Timespan, Regonol

Pregnancy Risk Category: C

HOW SUPPLIED
Tablets: 60 mg
Tablets (timed-release): 180 mg
Syrup: 60 mg/5 ml
Injection: 5 mg/ml in 2-ml ampules or 5-ml vials

MECHANISM OF ACTION
Inhibits the destruction of acetylcholine released from the parasympathetic and somatic efferent nerves. Acetylcholine accumulates, promoting increased stimulation of the receptor.

INDICATIONS & DOSAGE
Antidote for nondepolarizing neuromuscular blocking agents –
Adults: 10 to 20 mg I.V. preceded by atropine sulfate 0.6 to 1.2 mg I.V.
Myasthenia gravis –
Adults: 60 to 120 mg P.O. q 3 or 4 hours. Usual dosage is 600 mg daily but higher dosage may be needed (up to 1,500 mg daily). Give 1/30 of oral dose I.M. or I.V. Dosage must be adjusted for each patient, depending on response and tolerance of adverse reactions. Alternatively, may give 180 to 540 mg timed-release tablets (1 to 3 tablets) b.i.d., with at least 6 hours between doses.

*Liquid form contains alcohol. **May contain tartrazine.

ADVERSE REACTIONS
Common reactions are in italics; life-threatening reactions are in bold italics.
CNS: headache (with high doses), weakness, sweating, ***seizures.***
CV: bradycardia, hypotension.
EENT: miosis.
GI: abdominal cramps, nausea, vomiting, diarrhea, excessive salivation.
Skin: rash.
Local: thrombophlebitis.
Other: ***bronchospasm, bronchoconstriction,*** increased bronchial secretions, muscle cramps, muscle fasciculations.

INTERACTIONS
Aminoglycosides, anesthetics: may decrease response to pyridostigmine. Use together cautiously.
Atropine, anticholinergic agents, procainamide, quinidine: may reverse cholinergic effects. Observe for lack of drug effect.

NURSING CONSIDERATIONS
- *Contraindicated* in mechanical obstruction of intestine or urinary tract, bradycardia, or hypotension. Use with extreme caution in bronchial asthma.
- *Use cautiously* in epilepsy, recent coronary occlusion, vagotonia, hyperthyroidism, cardiac arrhythmias, and peptic ulcer. Avoid large doses in decreased GI motility.
- Difficult to judge optimum dosage. Monitor and document patient's response after each dose.
- Should stop all other cholinergics before giving this drug.
- **I.V. use:** Administer I.V. injection very slowly, no faster than 1 mg/minute. If I.V. administration is too rapid, bradycardia and seizures may result. Monitor vital signs frequently, and check respirations carefully. Position patient to ease breathing. Have atropine injection readily available and be prepared to give as ordered; provide respiratory support as needed.
- If muscle weakness is severe, doctor determines if it is caused by drug-induced toxicity or exacerbation of myasthenia gravis. Test dose of edrophonium I.V. will aggravate drug-induced weakness but will temporarily relieve weakness caused by disease.
- When using for myasthenia gravis, stress importance of taking drug exactly as ordered, on time, in evenly spaced doses. If doctor has ordered extended-release tablets, explain how these work. Patient must take them at the same time each day, at least 6 hours apart. Explain that he may have to take this drug for life.
- Has longest duration of the cholinergics used for myasthenia gravis.
- Used by the oral route in the treatment of senility associated with Alzheimer's disease.
- Don't crush the timed-release (Timespan or Supraspan) tablets.
- Available as a syrup for patients who have difficulty swallowing. Syrup is very sweet; give over ice chips if patient can't tolerate flavor.
- Store tablets in a tightly capped bottle, away from moisture.

37

Anticholinergics

anisotropine methylbromide
atropine sulfate
(See Chapter 20, ANTIARRHYTHMICS.)
belladonna leaf
clidinium bromide
dicyclomine hydrochloride
glycopyrrolate
hexocyclium methylsulfate
hyoscyamine
hyoscyamine sulfate
isopropamide iodide
levorotatory alkaloids of belladonna
mepenzolate bromide
methantheline bromide
methscopolamine bromide
oxyphencyclimine hydrochloride
propantheline bromide
scopolamine
scopolamine butylbromide
scopolamine hydrobromide

COMBINATION PRODUCTS

BAND O SUPPRETTES NO. 15A: alkaloids of belladonna leaf 0.21 mg and powdered opium 30 mg.
BAND O SUPPRETTES NO. 16A: alkaloids of belladonna leaf 0.21 mg and powdered opium 60 mg.
BARBIDONNA ELIXIR*: atropine sulfate 0.034 mg/5 ml, phenobarbital 21.6 mg/5 ml, hyoscyamine hydrobromide or sulfate 0.174 mg/5 ml, scopolamine hydrobromide 0.01 mg/5 ml, and alcohol 15%.
BARBIDONNA TABLETS: atropine sulfate 0.025 mg, scopolamine hydrobromide 0.0074 mg, hyoscyamine hydrobromide or sulfate 0.1286 mg, and phenobarbital 16 mg.
BARBIDONNA NO. 2 TABLETS: atropine sulfate 0.025 mg, scopolamine hydrobromide 0.0074 mg, hyoscyamine hydrobromide or sulfate 0.1286 mg, and phenobarbital 32 mg.
BELLADENAL TABLETS: L-alkaloids of belladonna 0.25 mg and phenobarbital 50 mg.
CHARDONNA-2: belladonna extract 15 mg and phenobarbital 15 mg.
DONNATAL ELIXIR*: atropine sulfate 0.0194 mg/5 ml, scopolamine hydrobromide 0.0065 mg/5 ml, alcohol 23%, hyoscyamine hydrobromide or sulfate 0.1037 mg/5 ml, and phenobarbital 16 mg/5 ml.
DONNATAL EXTENTABS: atropine sulfate 0.0582 mg, scopolamine hydrobromide 0.0195 mg, hyoscyamine sulfate 0.3111 mg, and phenobarbital 48.6 mg.
DONNATAL TABLETS AND CAPSULES: atropine sulfate 0.0194 mg, scopolamine hydrobromide 0.0065 mg, hyoscyamine hydrobromide or sulfate 0.1037 mg, and phenobarbital 16 mg.
DONNATAL NO. 2 TABLETS: atropine sulfate 0.0194 mg, scopolamine hydrobromide 0.0065 mg, hyoscyamine hydrobromide or sulfate 0.1037 mg, and phenobarbital 32.4 mg.
KINESED TABLETS: atropine sulfate 0.02 mg, scopolamine hydrobromide 0.007 mg, hyoscyamine hydrobromide or sulfate 0.1 mg, and phenobarbital 16 mg.
LIBRAX CAPSULES: clidinium bromide 2.5 mg and chlordiazepoxide hydrochloride 5 mg.
ROBINUL FORTE TABLETS: glycopyrrolate 2 mg and phenobarbital 16.2 mg.
ROBINUL TABLETS: glycopyrrolate 1 mg and phenobarbital 16.2 mg.
VISTRAX 10 TABLETS: oxyphencyclimine hydrochloride 10 mg and hydroxyzine hydrochloride 25 mg.

*Liquid form contains alcohol. **May contain tartrazine.

anisotropine methylbromide

Valpin 50

Pregnancy Risk Category: C

HOW SUPPLIED

Tablets: 50 mg

MECHANISM OF ACTION

Competitively blocks acetylcholine, which decreases GI motility and inhibits gastric acid secretion.

INDICATIONS & DOSAGE

Adjunctive treatment of peptic ulcer– **Adults:** 50 mg P.O. t.i.d. To be effective, should be titrated to individual patient's needs.

ADVERSE REACTIONS

Common reactions are in italics; life-threatening reactions are in bold italics.

CNS: headache, insomnia, drowsiness, dizziness, *confusion or excitement in elderly patients,* nervousness, weakness.

CV: *palpitations,* tachycardia.

EENT: *blurred vision,* mydriasis, increased ocular tension, cycloplegia, photophobia.

GI: *dry mouth,* dysphagia, heartburn, loss of taste, nausea, vomiting, *paralytic ileus, constipation.*

GU: *urinary hesitancy, urine retention,* impotence.

Skin: urticaria, decreased sweating and possible anhidrosis, other dermal manifestations.

Other: fever, allergic reactions.

Overdosage may cause curare-like symptoms.

INTERACTIONS

Amantadine, antihistamines, antiparkinsonian agents, disopyramide, glutethimide, meperidine, phenothiazines, procainamide quinidine: additive adverse effects. Avoid concomitant use.

Ketoconazole: anisotropine may interfere with absorption of ketoconazole. Avoid concomitant use.

Methotrimeprazine: possible extrapyramidal symptoms. Avoid concomitant use.

NURSING CONSIDERATIONS

- *Contraindicated* in narrow-angle glaucoma, obstructive uropathy, obstructive disease of the GI tract, severe ulcerative colitis, myasthenia gravis, hypersensitivity to anticholinergics, paralytic ileus, intestinal atony, unstable cardiovascular status in acute hemorrhage, or toxic megacolon.
- *Use cautiously* in autonomic neuropathy, hyperthyroidism, coronary artery disease, cardiac arrhythmias, CHF, hypertension, hiatal hernia associated with reflux esophagitis, hepatic or renal disease, and ulcerative colitis, or in patients over 40 years because of increased incidence of glaucoma. Also *use cautiously* in hot or humid environments. Drug-induced heatstroke can develop.
- Give 30 minutes to 1 hour before meals.
- Administer smaller doses to elderly patients.
- Monitor patient's vital signs and urine output carefully.
- Instruct patient to avoid driving and other hazardous activities if he is drowsy, dizzy, or has blurred vision; to drink plenty of fluids to help prevent constipation; to report any skin rash or local eruption.
- Gum or sugarless hard candy may relieve dry mouth.

belladonna leaf

(used to prepare extract and tincture)

Belladonna Tincture USP*

Pregnancy Risk Category: C

HOW SUPPLIED
Tablets: 15 mg
Oral solution: 27 to 33 mg belladonna alkaloids/100 ml in 67% alcohol solution

MECHANISM OF ACTION
Competitively blocks acetylcholine, which decreases GI motility and inhibits gastric acid secretion.

INDICATIONS & DOSAGE
Adjunctive therapy for peptic ulcer, irritable bowel syndrome, functional gastrointestinal disorders, and neurogenic bowel disturbances –
Adults: 15 mg P.O. t.i.d. or q.i.d. of the extract; 0.3 to 1 ml t.i.d. or q.i.d. of tincture.
Children: 0.1 ml/kg or 2.5 ml/m^2 tincture P.O. t.i.d. to q.i.d. Total dose should not exceed 3.5 ml/day.

ADVERSE REACTIONS
Common reactions are in italics; life-threatening reactions are in bold italics.
CNS: headache, insomnia, drowsiness, dizziness, *confusion or excitement in elderly patients,* nervousness, weakness.
CV: *palpitations,* tachycardia.
EENT: *blurred vision,* mydriasis, increased ocular tension, cycloplegia, photophobia.
GI: *dry mouth,* dysphagia, heartburn, loss of taste, *constipation,* nausea, vomiting.
GU: *urinary hesitancy, urine retention,* impotence.
Skin: urticaria, decreased sweating or possible anhidrosis, other dermal manifestations.
Other: fever, allergic reactions.
Overdosage may cause curare-like symptoms.

INTERACTIONS
Amantadine, antihistamines, antiparkinsonian agents, disopyramide, glutethimide, meperidine, phenothiazines, procainamide, quinidine: additive adverse effects. Avoid concomitant use.
Ketoconazole: anticholinergics may interfere with ketoconazole absorption. Avoid concomitant use.
Methotrimeprazine: anticholinergics may enhance risk of extrapyramidal reactions. Avoid concomitant use.

NURSING CONSIDERATIONS
- *Contraindicated* in narrow-angle glaucoma, obstructive uropathy, obstructive disease of GI tract, severe ulcerative colitis, myasthenia gravis, hypersensitivity to anticholinergics, paralytic ileus, intestinal atony, unstable cardiovascular status in acute hemorrhage, or toxic megacolon.
- *Use cautiously* in autonomic neuropathy, hyperthyroidism, coronary artery disease, cardiac arrhythmias, CHF, hypertension, hiatal hernia associated with reflux esophagitis, hepatic or renal disease, and ulcerative colitis, or in patients over 40 years because of increased incidence of glaucoma. Also *use cautiously* in hot or humid environments. Drug-induced heatstroke can develop.
- Give 30 minutes to 1 hour before meals and at bedtime. Bedtime dose can be larger and should be given at least 2 hours after last meal of day.
- Administer smaller doses to elderly patients.
- Monitor patient's vital signs and urine output carefully.
- Instruct patient to avoid driving and other hazardous activities if he is drowsy, dizzy, or has blurred vision; to drink plenty of fluids to help prevent constipation; to report any skin rash or local eruption.
- Gum or sugarless hard candy may relieve dry mouth.

clidinium bromide
Quarzan

Pregnancy Risk Category: C

HOW SUPPLIED
Capsules: 2.5 mg, 5 mg

MECHANISM OF ACTION
Competitively blocks acetylcholine, which decreases GI motility and inhibits gastric acid secretion.

INDICATIONS & DOSAGE
Adjunctive therapy for peptic ulcers – Dosage should be individualized according to severity of symptoms and occurrence of adverse reactions.
Elderly or debilitated patients: 2.5 to 5 mg P.O. t.i.d. or q.i.d. before meals and h.s.

ADVERSE REACTIONS
Common reactions are in italics; life-threatening reactions are in bold italics.
CNS: headache, insomnia, drowsiness, dizziness, *confusion or excitement in elderly patients,* nervousness, weakness.
CV: *palpitations,* tachycardia.
EENT: *blurred vision,* mydriasis, increased ocular tension, cycloplegia, photophobia.
GI: *dry mouth,* dysphagia, heartburn, loss of taste, nausea, vomiting, *paralytic ileus, constipation.*
GU: *urinary hesitancy, urine retention,* impotence.
Skin: urticaria, decreased sweating or possible anhidrosis, other dermal manifestations.
Other: fever, allergic reactions.

Overdosage may cause curare-like symptoms.

INTERACTIONS
Amantadine, antihistamines, antiparkinsonian agents, disopyramide, glutethimide, meperidine, phenothiazines, procainamide, quinidine: additive adverse effects. Avoid concomitant use.
Ketoconazole: anticholinergics may interfere with ketoconazole absorption. Avoid concomitant use.
Methotrimeprazine: anticholinergics may enhance risk of extrapyramidal reactions. Avoid concomitant use.

NURSING CONSIDERATIONS
- *Contraindicated* in narrow-angle glaucoma, obstructive uropathy, obstructive disease of GI tract, severe ulcerative colitis, myasthenia gravis, hypersensitivity to anticholinergics, paralytic ileus, intestinal atony, unstable cardiovascular status in acute hemorrhage, or toxic megacolon.
- *Use cautiously* in autonomic neuropathy, hyperthyroidism, coronary artery disease, cardiac arrhythmias, CHF, hypertension, hiatal hernia associated with reflux esophagitis, hepatic or renal disease, and ulcerative colitis, or in patients over 40 years, because of increased incidence of glaucoma. Also use cautiously in hot or humid environments. Drug-induced heatstroke may develop.
- Give 30 minutes to 1 hour before meals and at bedtime. Bedtime dose can be larger and should be given at least 2 hours after last meal of day.
- Monitor patient's vital signs and urine output carefully.
- Instruct patient to avoid driving and other hazardous activities if he is drowsy, dizzy, or has blurred vision; to drink plenty of fluids to help prevent constipation; and to report any rash or skin eruption.
- Gum or sugarless hard candy may relieve dry mouth.
- Dysphagia may cause aspiration.
- There is no conclusive evidence that clidinium aids in healing, decreases recurrence of, or prevents complications of peptic ulcers.

dicyclomine hydrochloride

Antispas, Bemote, Bentyl, Bentylol†, Byclomine, Dibent, Di-Cyclonex, Dilomine, Di-Spaz, Formulex†, Lomine†, Merbentyl‡, Neoquess Injection, Or-Tyl, Spasmoban†, Spasmoject, Viscerol†

Pregnancy Risk Category: B

HOW SUPPLIED

Tablets: 10 mg‡, 20 mg
Capsules: 10 mg, 20 mg
Syrup: 5 mg/5 ml‡, 10 mg/5 ml
Injection: 10 mg/ml

MECHANISM OF ACTION

Exerts a nonspecific, direct spasmolytic action on smooth muscle. Also possesses local anesthetic properties that may be partly responsible for spasmolysis.

INDICATIONS & DOSAGE

Adjunctive therapy for peptic ulcers and other functional GI disorders – **Adults:** 10 to 20 mg P.O. t.i.d. or q.i.d.; 20 mg I.M. q 6 hours.

Always adjust dosage according to patient's needs and response. Doses up to 40 mg P.O. q.i.d. have been used, but safety and efficacy of their dosage for more than 2 weeks has not been established.

ADVERSE REACTIONS

Common reactions are in italics; life-threatening reactions are in bold italics.
CNS: *headache,* insomnia, drowsiness, *dizziness.*
CV: *palpitations,* tachycardia.
GI: nausea, *constipation,* vomiting, *paralytic ileus.*
GU: *urinary hesitancy, urine retention, impotence.*
Skin: urticaria, decreased sweating or possible anhidrosis, other dermal manifestations.
Other: fever, allergic reactions.

Overdosage may cause curare-like symptoms.

INTERACTIONS

Amantadine, antihistamines, antiparkinsonian agents, disopyramide, glutethimide, meperidine, phenothiazines, procainamide, quinidine: additive adverse effects. Avoid concomitant use.
Ketoconazole: anticholinergics may interfere with ketoconazole absorption. Avoid concomitant use.
Methotrimeprazine: anticholinergics may enhance risk of extrapyramidal reactions. Avoid concomitant use.

NURSING CONSIDERATIONS

- *Contraindicated* in obstructive uropathy, obstructive disease of GI tract, severe ulcerative colitis, myasthenia gravis, hypersensitivity to anticholinergics, paralytic ileus, intestinal atony, unstable cardiovascular status in acute hemorrhage, or toxic megacolon.
- *Use cautiously* in autonomic neuropathy, narrow-angle glaucoma, hyperthyroidism, coronary artery disease, cardiac arrhythmias, CHF, hypertension, hiatal hernia associated with reflux esophagitis, hepatic or renal disease, and ulcerative colitis. Also use cautiously in hot or humid environments. Drug-induced heatstroke can develop.
- Give 30 minutes to 1 hour before meals and at bedtime. Bedtime dose can be larger and should be given at least 2 hours after last meal of day.
- Monitor patient's vital signs and urine output carefully.
- Instruct patient to avoid driving and other hazardous activities if he is drowsy, dizzy, or has blurred vision; to drink plenty of fluids to help prevent constipation; and to report any rash or skin eruption.
- Gum or sugarless hard candy may relieve dry mouth.
- A synthetic tertiary derivative that

may have fewer atropine-like adverse reactions.
• Not for I.V. use.

glycopyrrolate
Robinul, Robinul Forte
Pregnancy Risk Category: B

HOW SUPPLIED
Tablets: 1 mg, 2 mg
Injection: 0.2 mg/ml

MECHANISM OF ACTION
Inhibits cholinergic (muscarinic) actions of acetylcholine on autonomic effectors innervated by postganglionic cholinergic nerves.

INDICATIONS & DOSAGE
To reverse neuromuscular blockade –
Adults: 0.2 mg I.V. for each 1 mg neostigmine or 5 mg of pyridostigmine. May be given I.V. without dilution or may be added to dextrose injection and given by infusion.
Preoperatively to diminish secretions and block cardiac vagal reflexes –
Adults: 0.002 mg/lb of body weight I.M. 30 to 60 minutes before anesthesia.
Children 2 years and older: 0.0044 mg/kg I.M. 30 to 60 minutes before anesthesia.
Children under 2 years: 0.0088 mg/kg I.M. 30 minutes before anesthesia.
Adjunctive therapy in peptic ulcers and other GI disorders –
Adults: 1 to 2 mg P.O. t.i.d. or 0.1 mg I.M. t.i.d. or q.i.d. Dosage must be individualized. Maximum P.O. dose is 8 mg/day.

ADVERSE REACTIONS
Common reactions are in italics; life-threatening reactions are in bold italics.
CNS: disorientation, irritability, incoherence, weakness, nervousness, drowsiness, dizziness, headache.
CV: palpitations, tachycardia, paradoxical bradycardia.
EENT: *dilated pupils, blurred vision,* photophobia, increased intraocular pressure, difficulty swallowing.
GI: *constipation, dry mouth,* nausea, vomiting, epigastric distress.
GU: *urinary hesitancy, urine retention,* impotence.
Skin: urticaria, decreased sweating or anhidrosis, other dermal manifestations.
Local: burning at injection site.
Other: bronchial plugging, fever.

INTERACTIONS
Amantadine, antihistamines, antiparkinsonian agents, disopyramide, glutethimide, meperidine, phenothiazines, procainamide, quinidine: additive adverse effects. Avoid concomitant use.
Ketoconazole: anticholinergics may interfere with ketoconazole absorption. Avoid concomitant use.
Methotrimeprazine: anticholinergics may enhance risk of extrapyramidal reactions. Avoid concomitant use.

NURSING CONSIDERATIONS
• *Contraindicated* in narrow-angle glaucoma, obstructive uropathy, obstructive disease of the GI tract, myasthenia gravis, paralytic ileus, intestinal atony, unstable cardiovascular status in acute hemorrhage, or toxic megacolon.
• *Use cautiously* in patients with autonomic neuropathy, hyperthyroidism, coronary artery disease, cardiac arrhythmias, CHF, hypertension, hiatal hernia associated with reflux esophagitis, hepatic or renal disease, and ulcerative colitis; and in patients over 40 years because of increased incidence of glaucoma. Use with caution in hot or humid environments. Drug-induced heatstroke possible.
• Check all dosages carefully. Even slight overdose could lead to toxicity.
• **I.V. use:** Don't mix with I.V. solution containing sodum bicarbonate or alkaline solutions with a pH > 6.

• Monitor vital signs carefully. Watch closely for adverse reactions, especially in elderly or debilitated patients. Call doctor promptly.
• Advise patient to report signs of urinary hesitancy or urine retention.
• Warn patient to avoid activities that require alertness until CNS effects of the drug are known.
• Administer 30 minutes to 1 hour before meals.
• Administer smaller doses to elderly patients.

hexocyclium methylsulfate

Tral Filmtabs**

Pregnancy Risk Category: C

HOW SUPPLIED

Tablets: 25 mg

MECHANISM OF ACTION

Competitively blocks acetylcholine, which decreases GI motility and inhibits gastric acid secretion.

INDICATIONS & DOSAGE

Adjunctive therapy in peptic ulcer and other GI disorders –

Adults: 25 mg P.O. q.i.d. before meals and h.s.

ADVERSE REACTIONS

Common reactions are in italics; life-threatening reactions are in bold italics.

CNS: headache, insomnia, drowsiness, dizziness, *confusion or excitement in elderly patients,* nervousness, weakness.

CV: *palpitations,* tachycardia.

EENT: *blurred vision,* mydriasis, increased ocular tension, cycloplegia, photophobia.

GI: *dry mouth,* dysphagia, heartburn, loss of taste, nausea, *constipation,* vomiting, *paralytic ileus.*

GU: *urinary hesitancy, urine retention,* impotence.

Skin: urticaria, decreased sweating or possible anhidrosis, other dermal manifestations.

Other: fever, allergic reactions.

Overdosage may cause curare-like symptoms.

INTERACTIONS

Amantadine, antihistamines, antiparkinsonian agents, disopyramide, glutethimide, meperidine, phenothiazines, procainamide, quinidine: additive adverse effects. Avoid concomitant use.

Ketoconazole: anticholinergics may interfere with ketoconazole absorption. Avoid concomitant use.

Methotrimeprazine: anticholinergics may enhance risk of extrapyramidal reactions. Avoid concomitant use.

NURSING CONSIDERATIONS

• *Contraindicated* in narrow-angle glaucoma, obstructive uropathy, obstructive disease of GI tract, severe ulcerative colitis, myasthenia gravis, hypersensitivity to anticholinergics, paralytic ileus, intestinal atony, unstable cardiovascular status in acute hemorrhage, or toxic megacolon.
• *Use cautiously* in autonomic neuropathy, hyperthyroidism, coronary artery disease, cardiac arrhythmias, CHF, hypertension, hiatal hernia associated with reflux esophagitis, hepatic or renal disease, and ulcerative colitis, or in patients over 40 years because of increased incidence of glaucoma. Also use cautiously in hot or humid environments. Drug-induced heatstroke can develop.
• Give 30 minutes to 1 hour before meals and at bedtime. Bedtime dose can be larger and should be given at least 2 hours after last meal of day.
• Monitor patient's vital signs and urine output carefully.
• Instruct patient to avoid driving and other hazardous activities if he is drowsy, dizzy, or has blurred vision; to drink plenty of fluids to help pre-

*Liquid form contains alcohol. **May contain tartrazine.

vent constipation; and to report any rash or skin eruption.

- Gum or sugarless hard candy may relieve dry mouth.

hyoscyamine
Cystospaz

hyoscyamine sulfate
Anaspaz, Cystospaz, Cystospaz-M, Levsin*, Levsinex Timecaps, Neoquess

Pregnancy Risk Category: C

HOW SUPPLIED
hyoscyamine
Tablets: 150 mcg
hyoscyamine sulfate
Tablets: 125 mcg, 130 mcg, 150 mcg
Capsules (timed-release): 375 mcg
Elixir: 125 mcg/5 ml
Oral solution: 125 mg/ml
Injection: 500 mcg/ml

MECHANISM OF ACTION
Competitively blocks acetylcholine, which decreases GI motility and inhibits gastric acid secretion.

INDICATIONS & DOSAGE
Treatment of GI tract disorders caused by spasm; adjunctive therapy for peptic ulcers –
Adults: 0.125 to 0.25 mg P.O. or sublingually t.i.d. or q.i.d. before meals and h.s.; sustained-release form 0.375 mg P.O. q 8 hours; or 0.25 to 0.5 mg (1 or 2 ml) I.M., I.V., or S.C. b.i.d. to q.i.d. (Substitute oral medication when symptoms are controlled.)
Children 2 to 10 years: half of adult dose P.O., not to exceed 1.5 mg daily.

ADVERSE REACTIONS
Common reactions are in italics; life-threatening reactions are in bold italics.
CNS: headache, insomnia, drowsiness, dizziness, *confusion or excitement in elderly patients,* nervousness, weakness.
CV: *palpitations,* tachycardia.
EENT: *blurred vision,* mydriasis, increased ocular tension, cycloplegia, photophobia.
GI: *dry mouth,* dysphagia, *constipation,* heartburn, loss of taste, nausea, vomiting, *paralytic ileus.*
GU: *urinary hesitancy, urine retention,* impotence.
Skin: urticaria, decreased sweating or possible anhidrosis, other dermal manifestations.
Other: fever, allergic reactions.

Overdosage may cause curare-like symptoms.

INTERACTIONS
Amantadine, antihistamines, antiparkinsonian agents, disopyramide, glutethimide, meperidine, phenothiazines, procainamide, quinidine: additive adverse effects. Avoid concomitant use.
Ketoconazole: anticholinergics may interfere with ketoconazole absorption. Avoid concomitant use.
Methotrimeprazine: anticholinergics may enhance risk of extrapyramidal reactions. Avoid concomitant use.

NURSING CONSIDERATIONS
- *Contraindicated* in narrow-angle glaucoma, obstructive uropathy, obstructive disease of GI tract, severe ulcerative colitis, myasthenia gravis, hypersensitivity to anticholinergics, paralytic ileus, intestinal atony, unstable cardiovascular status in acute hemorrhage, or toxic megacolon.
- *Use cautiously* in autonomic neuropathy, hyperthyroidism, coronary artery disease, cardiac arrhythmias, CHF, hypertension, hiatal hernia associated with reflux esophagitis, hepatic or renal disease, and ulcerative colitis, or in patients over 40 years, because of the increased incidence of glaucoma. Also use cautiously in hot

or humid environments. Drug-induced heatstroke can develop.
• Injection contains sodium metabisulfite which may cause allergic reaction in certain individuals.
• Give 30 minutes to 1 hour before meals and at bedtime. Bedtime dose can be larger and should be given at least 2 hours after the last meal of the day.
• Monitor patient's vital signs and urine output carefully.
• Instruct patient to avoid driving and other hazardous activities if he is drowsy, dizzy, or has blurred vision; to drink plenty of fluids to help prevent constipation; and to report any rash or skin eruption.
• Gum or sugarless hard candy may relieve dry mouth.

isopropamide iodide

Darbid, Tyrimide‡

Pregnancy Risk Category: C

HOW SUPPLIED

Tablets: 5 mg

MECHANISM OF ACTION

Competitively blocks acetylcholine, resulting in decreased GI motility and reduced gastric acid secretion.

INDICATIONS & DOSAGE

Adjunctive therapy for peptic ulcer, irritable bowel syndrome –
Adults and children over 12 years: 5 mg P.O. q 12 hours. Some patients may require 10 mg or more b.i.d.

Dosage should be individualized to patient's need.

ADVERSE REACTIONS

Common reactions are in italics; life-threatening reactions are in bold italics.
CNS: headache, insomnia, drowsiness, dizziness, *confusion or excitement in elderly patients,* nervousness, weakness.
CV: *palpitations,* tachycardia.
EENT: *blurred vision,* mydriasis, increased ocular tension, cycloplegia, photophobia.
GI: *dry mouth,* dysphagia, heartburn, loss of taste, nausea, vomiting, *constipation, paralytic ileus.*
GU: *urinary hesitancy, urine retention,* impotence.
Skin: urticaria, decreased sweating or possible anhidrosis, other dermal manifestations, iodine skin rash.
Other: fever, allergic reactions.

Overdosage may cause curare-like symptoms.

INTERACTIONS

Amantadine, antihistamines, antiparkinsonian agents, disopyramide, glutethimide, meperidine, phenothiazines, procainamide, quinidine: additive adverse effects. Avoid concomitant use.
Ketoconazole: anticholinergics may interfere with ketoconazole absorption. Avoid concomitant use.
Methotrimeprazine: anticholinergics may enhance risk of extrapyramidal reactions. Avoid concomitant use.

NURSING CONSIDERATIONS

• *Contraindicated* in hypersensitivity to iodine, narrow-angle glaucoma, obstructive uropathy, obstructive disease of GI tract, severe ulcerative colitis, myasthenia gravis, hypersensitivity to anticholinergics, paralytic ileus, intestinal atony, unstable cardiovascular status in acute hemorrhage, or toxic megacolon.
• *Use cautiously* in autonomic neuropathy, hyperthyroidism, coronary artery disease, cardiac arrhythmias, CHF, hypertension, hiatal hernia associated with reflux esophagitis, hepatic or renal disease, and ulcerative colitis, or in patients over 40 years because of increased incidence of glaucoma. Also use cautiously in hot or humid environments. Drug-induced heatstroke can develop.
• Give 30 minutes to 1 hour before

meals and at bedtime. Bedtime dose can be larger and should be given at least 2 hours after the last meal of the day.

- Monitor patient's vital signs and urine output carefully.
- Instruct patient to avoid driving and other hazardous activities if he is drowsy, dizzy, or has blurred vision; to drink plenty of fluids to help prevent constipation; and to report any rash or skin eruption.
- Gum or sugarless hard candy may relieve dry mouth.
- Single dose produces 10- to 12-hour antisecretory effect and GI antispasmodic effect.
- Because isopropamide interferes with the 24-hour ^{131}I uptake test and may interfere with determinations of protein-bound iodine, discontinue it 1 week before thyroid function tests.

levorotatory alkaloids of belladonna

Bellafoline

Pregnancy Risk Category: C

HOW SUPPLIED

Tablets: 0.25 mg

MECHANISM OF ACTION

Competitively blocks acetylcholine, which decreases GI motility and inhibits gastric acid secretion.

INDICATIONS & DOSAGE

Adjunctive therapy for peptic ulcer, irritable bowel syndrome, and functional GI disorders –

Adults: 0.25 to 0.5 mg P.O. t.i.d.

Children over 6 years: 0.125 to 0.25 mg P.O. t.i.d.

ADVERSE REACTIONS

Common reactions are in italics; life-threatening reactions are in bold italics.

CNS: headache, insomnia, drowsiness, dizziness, *confusion or excitement in elderly patients,* nervousness, weakness.

CV: *palpitations,* tachycardia.

EENT: *blurred vision,* mydriasis, increased ocular tension, cycloplegia, photophobia.

GI: *dry mouth,* dysphagia, heartburn, loss of taste, *constipation, paralytic ileus.*

GU: *urinary hesitancy, urine retention,* impotence.

Skin: urticaria, decreased sweating or possible anhidrosis, other dermal manifestations.

Other: fever, allergic reactions.

Overdosage may cause curare-like symptoms.

INTERACTIONS

Amantadine, antihistamines, antiparkinsonian agents, disopyramide, glutethimide, meperidine, phenothiazines, procainamide, quinidine: additive adverse effects. Avoid concomitant use.

Ketoconazole: anticholinergics may interfere with ketoconazole absorption. Avoid concomitant use.

Methotrimeprazine: anticholinergics may enhance risk of extrapyramidal reactions. Avoid concomitant use.

NURSING CONSIDERATIONS

- *Contraindicated* in narrow-angle glaucoma, obstructive uropathy, obstructive disease of GI tract, severe ulcerative colitis, myasthenia gravis, hypersensitivity to anticholinergics, paralytic ileus, intestinal atony, unstable cardiovascular status in acute hemorrhage, or toxic megacolon.
- *Use cautiously* in autonomic neuropathy, hyperthyroidism, coronary artery disease, cardiac arrhythmias, CHF, hypertension, hiatal hernia associated with reflux esophagitis, hepatic or renal disease, and ulcerative colitis, or in patients over 40 years because of increased incidence of glaucoma. Also use cautiously in hot or

humid environments. Drug-induced heatstroke can develop.
- Administer 30 minutes to 1 hour before meals.
- Monitor patient's vital signs and urine output carefully.
- Instruct patient to avoid driving and other hazardous activities if he is drowsy, dizzy, or has blurred vision; to drink plenty of fluids to help prevent constipation; to report any rash or skin eruption.
- Gum or sugarless hard candy may relieve dry mouth.

mepenzolate bromide
Cantil**

Pregnancy Risk Category: C

HOW SUPPLIED
Tablets: 25 mg

MECHANISM OF ACTION
Competitively blocks acetylcholine, which decreases GI motility and inhibits gastric acid secretion.

INDICATIONS & DOSAGE
Adjunctive therapy in treating peptic ulcer, irritable bowel syndrome, and neurologic bowel disturbances –
Adults: 25 to 50 mg P.O. t.i.d. to q.i.d. with meals and h.s. Adjust dosage to individual patient's needs.

ADVERSE REACTIONS
Common reactions are in italics; life-threatening reactions are in bold italics.
CNS: headache, insomnia, drowsiness, dizziness, *confusion or excitement in elderly patients,* nervousness, weakness.
CV: *palpitations,* tachycardia.
EENT: *blurred vision,* mydriasis, increased ocular tension, cycloplegia, photophobia.
GI: *dry mouth,* dysphagia, heartburn, loss of taste, nausea, *constipation,* vomiting, *paralytic ileus.*
GU: *urinary hesitancy, urine retention,* impotence.
Skin: urticaria, decreased sweating or possible anhidrosis, other dermal manifestations.
Other: fever, allergic reactions.
Overdosage may cause curare-like symptoms.

INTERACTIONS
Amantadine, antihistamines, antiparkinsonian agents, disopyramide, glutethimide, meperidine, phenothiazines, procainamide, quinidine: additive adverse effects. Avoid concomitant use.
Ketoconazole: anticholinergics may interfere with ketoconazole absorption. Avoid concomitant use.
Methotrimeprazine: anticholinergics may enhance risk of extrapyramidal reactions. Avoid concomitant use.

NURSING CONSIDERATIONS
- *Contraindicated* in narrow-angle glaucoma, obstructive uropathy, obstructive disease of GI tract, severe ulcerative colitis, myasthenia gravis, hypersensitivity to anticholinergics, paralytic ileus, intestinal atony, unstable cardiovascular status in acute hemorrhage, or toxic megacolon. Contains tartrazine, which may precipitate an allergic reaction in certain hypersensitive individuals, especially those with a history of sensitivity to aspirin.
- *Use cautiously* in autonomic neuropathy, hyperthyroidism, coronary artery disease, cardiac arrhythmias, CHF, hypertension, hiatal hernia associated with reflux esophagitis, hepatic or renal disease, and ulcerative colitis, or in patients over 40 years, because of increased incidence of glaucoma. Also use cautiously in hot or humid environments. Drug-induced heatstroke can develop.
- Give with meals and at bedtime.
- Monitor patient's vital signs and urine output carefully.

*Liquid form contains alcohol. **May contain tartrazine.

• Instruct patient to avoid driving and other hazardous activities if he is drowsy, dizzy, or has blurred vision; to drink plenty of fluids to help prevent constipation; and to report any rash or skin eruption.
• Gum or sugarless hard candy may relieve dry mouth.

methantheline bromide
Banthine

Pregnancy Risk Category: C

HOW SUPPLIED
Tablets: 50 mg

MECHANISM OF ACTION
Competitively blocks acetylcholine, which decreases GI motility and inhibits gastric acid secretion.

INDICATIONS & DOSAGE
Adjunctive therapy in peptic ulcer, pylorospasm, spastic colon, biliary dyskinesia, pancreatitis, and certain forms of gastritis –
Adults: 50 to 100 mg P.O. q 6 hours.
Children over 1 year: 12.5 to 50 mg P.O. q.i.d.
Children under 1 year: 12.5 to 25 mg P.O. q.i.d.
Neonates: 12.5 mg P.O. b.i.d. to t.i.d.

ADVERSE REACTIONS
Common reactions are in italics; life-threatening reactions are in bold italics.
CNS: headache, insomnia, drowsiness, dizziness, *confusion or excitement in elderly patients,* nervousness, weakness.
CV: *palpitations,* tachycardia.
EENT: *blurred vision,* mydriasis, increased ocular tension, cycloplegia, photophobia.
GI: *dry mouth,* dysphagia, *constipation,* heartburn, loss of taste, nausea, vomiting, *paralytic ileus.*
GU: *urinary hesitancy, urine retention,* impotence.
Skin: urticaria, decreased sweating or possible anhidrosis, other dermal manifestations.
Other: fever, allergic reactions.

Overdosage may cause curare-like symptoms.

INTERACTIONS
Amantadine, antihistamines, antiparkinsonian agents, disopyramide, glutethimide, meperidine, phenothiazines, procainamide, quinidine: additive adverse effects. Avoid concomitant use.
Ketoconazole: anticholinergics may interfere with ketoconazole absorption. Avoid concomitant use.
Methotrimeprazine: anticholinergics may enhance risk of extrapyramidal reactions. Avoid concomitant use.

NURSING CONSIDERATIONS
• *Contraindicated* in narrow-angle glaucoma, obstructive uropathy, obstructive disease of GI tract, severe ulcerative colitis, myasthenia gravis, hypersensitivity to anticholinergics, paralytic ileus, intestinal atony, unstable cardiovascular status in acute hemorrhage, or toxic megacolon.
• *Use cautiously* in autonomic neuropathy, hyperthyroidism, coronary artery disease, cardiac arrhythmias, CHF, hypertension, hiatal hernia associated with reflux esophagitis, hepatic or renal disease, and ulcerative colitis, or in patients over 40 years because of the increased incidence of glaucoma. Also use cautiously in hot or humid environments. Drug-induced heatstroke can develop.
• Give 30 minutes to 1 hour before meals and at bedtime. Bedtime dose can be larger and should be given at least 2 hours after the last meal of the day.
• If patient is also taking antihistamines, he may experience increased dryness of mouth.
• Monitor patient's vital signs and urine output carefully.

• Instruct patient to avoid driving and other hazardous activities if he is drowsy, dizzy, or has blurred vision; to drink plenty of fluids to help prevent constipation; and to report any rash or skin eruption.
• Gum or sugarless hard candy may relieve dry mouth.
• Therapeutic effects appear in 30 to 45 minutes; persist for 4 to 6 hours after oral administration.

methscopolamine bromide

Pamine

Pregnancy Risk Category: C

HOW SUPPLIED

Tablets: 2.5 mg

MECHANISM OF ACTION

Competitively blocks acetylcholine, which decreases GI motility and inhibits gastric acid secretion.

INDICATIONS & DOSAGE

Adjunctive therapy in peptic ulcer –
Adults: 2.5 to 5 mg P.O. half hour before meals and h.s.
Children: 0.2 mg/kg P.O. q.i.d.

ADVERSE REACTIONS

Common reactions are in italics; life-threatening reactions are in bold italics.
CNS: headache, insomnia, dizziness, *confusion or excitement in elderly patients,* nervousness, weakness.
CV: *palpitations,* tachycardia.
EENT: *blurred vision,* mydriasis, increased ocular tension, cycloplegia, photophobia.
GI: *dry mouth,* dysphagia, *constipation,* heartburn, loss of taste, nausea, vomiting, *paralytic ileus.*
GU: *urinary hesitancy, urine retention,* impotence.
Skin: urticaria, decreased sweating or possible anhidrosis, other dermal manifestations.
Other: fever, allergic reactions.

Overdosage may cause curare-like symptoms.

INTERACTIONS

Amantadine, antihistamines, antiparkinsonian agents, disopyramide, glutethimide, meperidine, phenothiazines, procainamide, quinidine: additive adverse effects. Avoid concomitant use.
Ketoconazole: anticholinergics may interfere with ketoconazole absorption. Avoid concomitant use.
Methotrimeprazine: anticholinergics may enhance risk of extrapyramidal reactions. Avoid concomitant use.

NURSING CONSIDERATIONS

• *Contraindicated* in narrow-angle glaucoma, obstructive uropathy, obstructive disease of GI tract, severe ulcerative colitis, myasthenia gravis, hypersensitivity to anticholinergics, paralytic ileus, intestinal atony, unstable cardiovascular status in acute hemorrhage, or toxic megacolon.
• *Use cautiously* in autonomic neuropathy, hyperthyroidism, coronary artery disease, cardiac arrhythmias, CHF, hypertension, hiatal hernia associated with reflux esophagitis, hepatic or renal disease, and ulcerative colitis, or in patients over 40 years because of increased incidence of glaucoma. Also use cautiously in hot or humid environments. Drug-induced heatstroke can develop.
• Give 30 minutes to 1 hour before meals and at bedtime. Bedtime dose can be larger and should be given at least 2 hours after the last meal of the day.
• Monitor patient's vital signs and urine output carefully.
• Instruct patient to avoid driving and other hazardous activities if he is drowsy, dizzy, or has blurred vision; to drink plenty of fluids to help prevent constipation; and to report any rash or skin eruption.

• Gum or sugarless hard candy may relieve dry mouth.

oxyphencyclimine hydrochloride

Daricon

Pregnancy Risk Category: C

HOW SUPPLIED

Tablets: 10 mg

MECHANISM OF ACTION

Exerts a nonspecific, direct spasmolytic action on smooth muscle. Also possesses local anesthetic properties that may be partly responsible for spasmolysis.

INDICATIONS & DOSAGE

Adjunctive treatment of peptic ulcer—
Adults: 10 mg P.O. b.i.d. in the morning and at bedtime, or 5 mg b.i.d. or t.i.d.

ADVERSE REACTIONS

Common reactions are in italics; life-threatening reactions are in bold italics.
CNS: *headache,* insomnia, drowsiness, *dizziness.*
CV: *palpitations,* tachycardia.
EENT: *blurred vision,* mydriasis, increased ocular tension, cycloplegia, photophobia.
GI: *constipation,* nausea, vomiting, *paralytic ileus.*
GU: *urinary hesitancy, urine retention, impotence.*
Skin: urticaria, decreased sweating or possible anhidrosis, other dermal manifestations.
Other: fever, allergic reactions.

Overdosage may cause curare-like symptoms.

INTERACTIONS

Amantadine, antihistamines, antiparkinsonian agents, disopyramide, glutethimide, meperidine, phenothiazines, procainamide, quinidine: additive adverse effects. Avoid concomitant use.
Ketoconazole: anticholinergics may interfere with ketoconazole absorption. Avoid concomitant use.
Methotrimeprazine: anticholinergics may enhance risk of extrapyramidal reactions. Avoid concomitant use.

NURSING CONSIDERATIONS

• *Contraindicated* in narrow-angle glaucoma, obstructive uropathy, obstructive disease of GI tract, severe ulcerative colitis, myasthenia gravis, hypersensitivity to anticholinergics, paralytic ileus, intestinal atony, unstable cardiovascular status in acute hemorrhage, or toxic megacolon.
• *Use cautiously* in autonomic neuropathy, hyperthyroidism, coronary artery disease, cardiac arrhythmias, CHF, hypertension, hiatal hernia associated with reflux esophagitis, hepatic or renal disease, and ulcerative colitis, or in patients over 40 years because of increased incidence of glaucoma. Also use cautiously in hot or humid environments. Drug-induced heatstroke can develop.
• Give 30 minutes to 1 hour before breakfast and at bedtime.
• Monitor patient's vital signs and urine output carefully.
• Instruct patient to avoid driving and other hazardous activities if he is drowsy, dizzy, or has blurred vision; to drink plenty of fluids to help prevent constipation; and to report any rash or skin eruption.
• Gum or sugarless hard candy may relieve dry mouth.
• A synthetic tertiary derivative that may have fewer atropine-like adverse reactions.

propantheline bromide

Norpanth, Pantheline‡, Pro-Banthine, Propanthel†

Pregnancy Risk Category: C

†Available in Canada only. ‡Available in Australia only. ◊Available OTC.

HOW SUPPLIED
Tablets: 7.5 mg, 15 mg

MECHANISM OF ACTION
Competitively blocks acetylcholine, which decreases GI motility and inhibits gastric acid secretion.

INDICATIONS & DOSAGE
Adjunctive treatment of peptic ulcer, irritable bowel syndrome, and other GI disorders; to reduce duodenal motility during diagnostic radiologic procedures –
Adults: 15 mg P.O. t.i.d. before meals, and 30 mg h.s. up to 60 mg q.i.d. For elderly patients, 7.5 mg P.O. t.i.d. before meals.

ADVERSE REACTIONS
Common reactions are in italics; life-threatening reactions are in bold italics.
CNS: headache, insomnia, drowsiness, dizziness, *confusion or excitement in elderly patients,* nervousness, weakness.
CV: *palpitations,* tachycardia.
EENT: *blurred vision,* mydriasis, increased ocular tension, cycloplegia, photophobia.
GI: *dry mouth,* dysphagia, constipation, heartburn, loss of taste, nausea, vomiting, paralytic ileus.
GU: *urinary hesitancy, urine retention,* impotence.
Skin: urticaria, decreased sweating or possible anhidrosis, other dermal manifestations.
Other: fever, allergic reactions.

Overdosage may cause curare-like symptoms.

INTERACTIONS
Amantadine, antihistamines, antiparkinsonian agents, disopyramide, glutethimide, meperidine, phenothiazines, procainamide, quinidine: additive adverse effects. Avoid concomitant use.
Ketoconazole: anticholinergics may interfere with ketoconazole absorption. Avoid concomitant use.
Methotrimeprazine: anticholinergics may enhance risk of extrapyramidal reactions. Avoid concomitant use.

NURSING CONSIDERATIONS
- *Contraindicated* in narrow-angle glaucoma, obstructive uropathy, obstructive disease of GI tract, severe ulcerative colitis, myasthenia gravis, hypersensitivity to anticholinergics, paralytic ileus, intestinal atony, unstable cardiovascular status in acute hemorrhage, or toxic megacolon.
- *Use cautiously* in autonomic neuropathy, hyperthyroidism, coronary artery disease, cardiac arrhythmias, congestive heart failure, hypertension, hiatal hernia associated with reflux esophagitis, hepatic or renal disease, and ulcerative colitis, or in patients over 40 years because of the increased incidence of glaucoma. Also use cautiously in hot or humid environments. Drug-induced heatstroke can develop.
- Give 30 minutes to 1 hour before meals and at bedtime. Bedtime dose can be larger and should be given at least 2 hours after the last meal of the day.
- Monitor patient's vital signs and urine output carefully.
- Instruct patient to avoid driving and other hazardous activities if he is drowsy, dizzy, or has blurred vision; to drink plenty of fluids to help prevent constipation; and to report any rash or skin eruption.
- Gum or sugarless hard candy may relieve dry mouth.

scopolamine (hyoscine)
Transderm-Scōp, Transderm-V†

scopolamine butylbromide (hyoscine butylbromide)
Buscopan†‡

scopolamine hydrobromide (hyoscine hydrobromide)

Pregnancy Risk Category: C

HOW SUPPLIED

scopolamine
Transdermal patch: 1.5 mg
scopolamine butylbromide
Capsules: 0.25 mg
scopolamine hydrobromide
Injection: 0.3, 0.4, 0.5, 0.6, and 1 mg/ml in 1-ml vials and ampules; 0.86 mg/ml in 0.5-ml ampules

MECHANISM OF ACTION

Inhibits muscarinic actions of acetylcholine on autonomic effectors innervated by postganglionic cholinergic neurons. May also affect neural pathways originating in the labyrinth to inhibit nausea and vomiting.

INDICATIONS & DOSAGE

Postencephalitic parkinsonism and other spastic states –
Adults: 0.5 to 1 mg P.O. t.i.d. to q.i.d.; 0.3 to 0.6 mg S.C., I.M., or I.V. (with suitable dilution) t.i.d. to q.i.d.
Children: 0.006 mg/kg P.O. or S.C. t.i.d. to q.i.d.; or 0.2 mg/m^2.
Preoperatively to reduce secretions and block cardiac vagal reflexes –
Adults: 0.4 to 0.6 mg S.C. 30 to 60 minutes before induction of anesthesia.
Prevention of nausea and vomiting associated with motion sickness –
Adults: one Transderm-Scōp or Transderm-V patch (a circular flat unit) programmed to deliver 0.5 mg scopolamine daily over 3 days (72 hours), applied to the skin behind the ear several hours before the antiemetic is required.

Not recommended for children.

ADVERSE REACTIONS

Common reactions are in italics; life-threatening reactions are in bold italics.
CNS: disorientation, restlessness, irritability, dizziness, drowsiness, headache.
CV: palpitations, tachycardia, paradoxical bradycardia.
EENT: dilated pupils, blurred vision, photophobia, increased intraocular pressure, difficulty swallowing.
GI: *constipation, dry mouth, nausea, vomiting, epigastric distress.*
GU: urinary hesitancy, urine retention.
Skin: rash, flushing, dryness.
Other: bronchial plugging, fever, depressed respirations.

Adverse reactions may be caused by pending atropine-like toxicity and are dose related. Individual tolerance varies greatly.

INTERACTIONS

Alcohol, CNS depressants: increased CNS depression.
Centrally acting anticholinergics (tricyclic antidepressants, phenothiazines): increased CNS adverse reactions.
Digoxin: increased digoxin levels.

NURSING CONSIDERATIONS

- *Contraindicated* in narrow-angle glaucoma, obstructive uropathy, obstructive disease of the GI tract, asthma, chronic pulmonary disease, myasthenia gravis, paralytic ileus, intestinal atony, unstable cardiovascular status in acute hemorrhage, or toxic megacolon.
- *Use cautiously* in patients with autonomic neuropathy, hyperthyroidism, coronary artery disease, cardiac arrhythmias, CHF, hypertension, hiatal hernia associated with reflux esophagitis, hepatic or renal disease, ulcerative colitis; in patients over 40 years because of the increased incidence of glaucoma; and in children under 6 years. Also use cautiously in hot or humid environments. Drug-induced heatstroke possible.
- Some patients become temporarily excited or disoriented. Symptoms dis-

appear when sedative effect is complete. Raise side rails as a precaution.
• In therapeutic doses, scopolamine may produce amnesia, drowsiness, and euphoria. These effects are desirable when used as an adjunct to anesthesia. May need to reorient patient.
• Warn patient against driving and other activities that require alertness until CNS effects of the drug are known.
• Sugarless gum or hard candy may be helpful in minimizing dry mouth.
• Advise patient to report signs of urinary hesitancy or urine retention.
• Tolerance may develop when given over a long period of time.
• Many of the adverse reactions (such as dry mouth, constipation) are an expected extension of the drug's pharmacologic activity.
• To determine m² for dosage calculation in children, use a nomogram.
• **I.V. use:** Intermittent and continuous infusions are not recommended. For direct injection, dilute with sterile water for injection and inject diluted drug at ordered rate through patent I.V. line. Protect I.V. solutions from freezing and light and store at room temperature.
• Transdermal method of administration releases a controlled therapeutic amount of scopolamine. Transderm-Scōp is effective if applied 2 to 3 hours before experiencing motion, but more effective if used 12 hours before. Therefore, advise patient to apply patch the night before a planned trip.
• A patient brochure is available with the transdermal product; tell patient to request it from the pharmacist.
• Wash and dry hands thoroughly before applying the transdermal patch on dry skin behind the ear. After removing the system, discard it, then wash both the hands and application site thoroughly.
• If the patch becomes displaced, remove and replace it with another patch on a fresh skin site in the postauricular area.
• Caution patient to wash hands after applying transdermal patch, particularly before touching eye. May cause pupil to dilate.

*Liquid form contains alcohol. **May contain tartrazine.

38

Adrenergics (sympathomimetics)

dobutamine hydrochloride
dopamine hydrochloride
mephentermine sulfate
metaraminol bitartrate
norepinephrine injection
phenylephrine hydrochloride
pseudoephedrine hydrochloride
pseudoephedrine sulfate

COMBINATION PRODUCTS

ENTEX: phenylephrine hydrochloride 5 mg, phenylpropanolamine hydrochloride 45 mg, guaifenesin 400 mg.
ENTEX LIQUID: phenylephrine hydrochloride 5 mg/5 ml, phenylpropanolamine hydrochloride 20 mg/5 ml, guaifenesin 100 mg/5 ml (alcohol 5%).

dobutamine hydrochloride

Dobutrex

Pregnancy Risk Category: C

HOW SUPPLIED

Injection: 12.5 mg/ml in 20-ml vials (parenteral)

MECHANISM OF ACTION

An analog of isoproterenol that directly stimulates $beta_1$ receptors of the heart to increase myocardial contractility and stroke volume, resulting in increased cardiac output.

INDICATIONS & DOSAGE

Refractory heart failure and as adjunct in cardiac surgery –
Adults: 2.5 to 10 mcg/kg/minute as an I.V. infusion. Rarely, infusion rates up to 40 mcg/kg/minute may be needed.

ADVERSE REACTIONS

Common reactions are in italics; life-threatening reactions are in bold italics.
CNS: headache.
CV: *increased heart rate,* ***hypertension, premature ventricular contractions,*** angina, nonspecific chest pain.
GI: nausea, vomiting.
Other: shortness of breath.

INTERACTIONS

Beta blockers: may antagonize dobutamine effects. Do not use together.
General anesthetics: greater incidence of ventricular arrhythmias.

NURSING CONSIDERATIONS

- *Contraindicated* in idiopathic hypertrophic subaortic stenosis and in patients with hypersensitivity to the drug or any component of the formulation. Contains sulfites, which may cause an allergic response in sensitive patients.
- *Use cautiously* in patients with a history of hypertension. Drug may precipitate an exaggerated pressor response.
- Because drug increases AV conduction, patients with atrial fibrillation may develop a rapid ventricular rate. Administer a digitalis glycoside before dobutamine as ordered.
- A unique agent. Increases contractility of failing heart without inducing marked tachycardia, except at high doses.
- Hypovolemia should be corrected with plasma volume expanders before initiating therapy with dobutamine.
- Often used with nitroprusside for additive effects.
- ECG, blood pressure, pulmonary wedge pressure, and cardiac output should be monitored continuously. Also monitor urine output.
- Monitor serum electrolytes. Drug may lower serum potassium levels.
- **I.V. use:** Administer using a central venous catheter or large peripheral

vein. Titrate infusion according to doctor's orders and patient's condition. Use an infusion pump.

- Concentrate for injection must be diluted before administration. Compatible solutions include dextrose 5% in water, 0.45% sodium chloride injection, 0.9% sodium chloride injection, and lactated Ringer's injection. The contents of one vial (250 mg) diluted with 1,000 ml of solution yields a concentration of 250 mcg/ml; diluted with 500 ml, a concentration of 500 mcg/ml; diluted with 250 ml, a concentration of 1,000 mcg/ml. Maximum concentration should not exceed 5 mg/ml.
- Incompatible with alkaline solutions. Do not mix with sodium bicarbonate injection. Infusions for up to 72 hours produce no more adverse effects than shorter infusions.
- Avoid extravasation, which may cause an inflammatory response. Change I.V. sites regularly to avoid phlebitis.
- I.V. solutions remain stable for 24 hours.
- Oxidation of drug may slightly discolor admixtures containing dobutamine. This does not indicate a significant loss of potency.

dopamine hydrochloride

Intropin, Revimine†‡

Pregnancy Risk Category: C

HOW SUPPLIED

Injection: 40 mg/ml, 80 mg/ml, 160 mg/ml parenteral concentrate for injection for I.V. infusion; 0.8 mg/ml (200 or 400 mg) in dextrose 5%; 1.6 mg/ml (400 or 800 mg) in dextrose 5%, 3.2 mg/ml (800 mg) in dextrose 5% parenteral injection for I.V. infusion.

MECHANISM OF ACTION

Stimulates dopaminergic, beta-adrenergic, and alpha-adrenergic receptors of the sympathetic nervous system.

INDICATIONS & DOSAGE

To treat shock and correct hemodynamic imbalances; to improve perfusion to vital organs; to increase cardiac output; to correct hypotension; to treat acute renal failure –

Adults: 2 to 5 mcg/kg/minute I.V. infusion, up to 50 mcg/kg/minute. Titrate the dosage to the desired hemodynamic or renal response.

ADVERSE REACTIONS

Common reactions are in italics; life-threatening reactions are in bold italics.

CNS: headache.

CV: ***arrhythmias,*** ectopic beats, tachycardia, anginal pain, palpitations, *hypotension.* Less frequently, bradycardia, widening of QRS complex, conduction disturbances, vasoconstriction.

GI: nausea, vomiting.

Local: necrosis and tissue sloughing with extravasation.

Other: piloerection, dyspnea.

INTERACTIONS

Beta blockers: may antagonize dopamine's effects.

Ergot alkaloids: extreme elevations in blood pressure. Don't use together.

Inhalational anesthetics: increased risk of arrhythmias or hypertension. Monitor closely.

MAO inhibitors: may cause hypertensive crisis. Avoid if possible.

Phenytoin: may lower blood pressure of dopamine-stabilized patients. Monitor carefully.

NURSING CONSIDERATIONS

- *Contraindicated* in uncorrected tachyarrhythmias, pheochromocytoma, or ventricular fibrillation. *Use cautiously* in patients with occlusive vascular disease, cold injuries, dia-

betic endarteritis, and arterial embolism; also, in pregnant patients and those taking MAO inhibitors.
• Not a substitute for blood or fluid volume deficit. Volume deficit should be replaced before vasopressors are administered.
• During infusion, frequently monitor ECG, blood pressure, cardiac output, central venous pressure, pulmonary capillary wedge pressure, pulse rate, urine output, and color and temperature of extremities. Titrate infusion rate according to findings and doctor's guidelines. Use a continuous infusion pump to regulate flow rate.
• Observe patient closely for adverse effects. If adverse effects develop, dosage may need to be adjusted or discontinued.
• If a disproportionate rise in the diastolic pressure (a marked decrease in pulse pressure) is observed in patients receiving dopamine, decrease infusion rate and observe carefully for further evidence of predominant vasoconstrictor activity, unless such an effect is desired.
• Patient response depends upon dosage and pharmacologic effect. Doses of 0.5 to 2 mcg/kg/minute predominantly stimulate dopamine receptors and produce vasodilation of the renal vasculature. Doses of 2 to 10 mcg/kg/minute stimulate beta-adrenergic receptors. Higher doses also stimulate alpha-adrenergic receptors.
• Most patients satisfactorily maintained on less than 20 mcg/kg/minute.
• If doses exceed 50 mcg/kg/minute, check urine output often. If urine flow decreases without hypotension, consider reducing dose.
• If drug is stopped, watch closely for sudden drop in blood pressure. Drug should be tapered slowly to evaluate stability of blood pressure.
• **I.V. use:** Use a central line or a large vein, such as in the antecubital fossa, to minimize risk of extravasation. Watch infusion site carefully for signs of extravasation; if it occurs, stop infusion immediately and call doctor. Extravasation may require treatment by infiltration of the area with 5 to 10 mg phentolamine and 10 to 15 ml 0.9% sodium chloride solution. Don't mix with alkaline solutions. Use dextrose 5% in water (D_5W), 0.9% sodium chloride solution, or a combination of D_5W and 0.9% sodium chloride solution. Mix just before use.
• Do not mix other drugs in I.V. container with dopamine. Do not give alkaline drugs (for example, sodium bicarbonate, phenytoin sodium) through I.V. line containing dopamine.
• Dopamine solutions deteriorate after 24 hours. Discard at that time or earlier if solution is discolored.
• Acidosis decreases effectiveness of dopamine.

mephentermine sulfate
Wyamine

Pregnancy Risk Category: C

HOW SUPPLIED
Injection: 15 mg/ml, 30 mg/ml

MECHANISM OF ACTION
Indirectly stimulates beta- and alpha-adrenergic receptors by releasing norepinephrine.

INDICATIONS & DOSAGE
Hypotension following spinal anesthesia –
Adults: 30 to 45 mg I.V. in a single injection, then 30 mg I.V. repeated p.r.n. Maintenance of blood pressure: continuous I.V. infusion of 0.1% solution of mephentermine in dextrose 5% in water.
Children: 0.4 mg/kg I.M. or I.V.
Hypotension following spinal anesthesia during obstetric procedures –
Adults: initially 15 mg I.V. p.r.n.
Prevention of hypotension during spinal anesthesia –

Adults: 30 to 45 mg I.M. 10 to 20 minutes before anesthesia.

ADVERSE REACTIONS

Common reactions are in italics; life-threatening reactions are in bold italics.

CNS: euphoria, nervousness, anxiety, tremor, incoherence, drowsiness, ***seizures,*** visual hallucinations (with large doses).

CV: ***arrhythmias, marked elevation of blood pressure (with large doses).***

INTERACTIONS

Antihypertensives, guanethidine, phenothiazines, reserpine, nitrates: decreased effects of these adrenergic blocking agents.

Beta-adrenergic blocking agents, rauwolfia alkaloids: mutual inhibition of therapeutic effects.

CNS stimulants, mazindol, methylphenidate, sympathomimetics: increased CNS stimulation.

Digitalis glycosides, levodopa, inhalation anesthetics: increased risk of cardiac arrhythmias.

Ergot alkaloids, oxytocin: enhanced vasoconstriction.

MAO inhibitors: may cause severe hypertension (hypertensive crisis) or arrhythmias. Don't use together.

Thyroid hormones: enhanced risk of coronary insufficiency.

Tricyclic antidepressants, maprotiline: decreased pressure of mephentermine.

NURSING CONSIDERATIONS

- *Contraindicated* in concealed hemorrhage or hypotension from hemorrhage, except in emergencies; also in patients receiving phenothiazines, or who have received MAO inhibitors within 2 weeks.
- *Use cautiously* in arteriosclerosis, cardiovascular disease, hyperthyroidism, hypertension, and chronic illness.
- Not a substitute for blood or fluid volume deficit. If deficit exists, it should be replaced before vasopressors are administered.
- Observe patient closely for adverse effects. If adverse effects develop, dosage may need to be adjusted or discontinued.
- I.M. route may be used since drug is not irritating to tissue.
- **I.V. use:** Administer at 1 to 5 mg/minute. Can be given undiluted; I.V. drug is not irritating to tissue, and extravasation is not dangerous. To prepare 0.1% I.V. solution, add 16.6 ml mephentermine (30 mg/ml) to 500 ml dextrose 5% in water.
- Don't mix with I.V. hydralazine or epinephrine, which are physically incompatible with mephentermine.
- During infusion, check blood pressure every 2 minutes until stabilized; then every 10 to 15 minutes.
- Monitor blood pressure until stable, even after discontinuing drug. During infusion, frequently monitor ECG, blood pressure, cardiac output, central venous pressure, pulmonary capillary wedge pressure, pulse rate, urine output, and color and temperature of extremities. Titrate infusion rate according to findings and doctor's guidelines. Use a continuous infusion pump to regulate flow rate.
- May increase uterine contractions during third trimester of pregnancy.
- Hypercapnia, hypoxia, acidosis may reduce effectiveness or increase adverse effects. Identify and correct before and during administration.

metaraminol bitartrate

Aramine

Pregnancy Risk Category: D

HOW SUPPLIED

Injection: 10 mg/ml

MECHANISM OF ACTION

Predominantly stimulates alpha-adrenergic receptors within the sympathetic nervous system.

INDICATIONS & DOSAGE
Prevention of hypotension –
Adults: 2 to 10 mg I.M. or S.C.
Severe shock –
Adults: 0.5 to 5 mg direct I.V. followed by I.V. infusion.
Treatment of hypotension caused by shock –
Adults: 15 to 100 mg in 500 ml 0.9% sodium chloride solution or dextrose 5% in water I.V. infusion. Adjust rate to maintain blood pressure.
All indications –
Children: 0.01 mg/kg as single I.V. injection; 1 mg/25 ml dextrose 5% in water as I.V. infusion. Adjust rate to maintain blood pressure in normal range. 0.1 mg/kg I.M. as single dose, p.r.n. Allow at least 10 minutes to elapse before increasing dose because maximum effect is not immediately apparent.

ADVERSE REACTIONS
Common reactions are in italics; life-threatening reactions are in bold italics.
CNS: apprehension, restlessness, dizziness, headache, tremor, weakness; with excessive use, ***seizures***.
CV: hypertension; hypotension; precordial pain; palpitations; ***arrhythmias,*** including sinus or ***ventricular tachycardia;*** bradycardia; premature supraventricular contractions; atrioventricular dissociation.
GI: nausea, vomiting..
GU: decreased urine output.
Metabolic: hyperglycemia.
Skin: flushing, pallor, sweating.
Local: abscess, necrosis, and sloughing upon extravasation.
Other: ***metabolic acidosis in hypovolemia,*** *increased body temperature,* ***respiratory distress***.

INTERACTIONS
General anesthetics: increased risk of adverse cardiac effects. Monitor closely.
MAO inhibitors: may cause severe hypertension (hypertensive crisis). Don't use together.

NURSING CONSIDERATIONS
- *Contraindicated* in peripheral or mesenteric thrombosis, pulmonary edema, hypercarbia, or acidosis; also during anesthesia with cyclopropane and halogenated hydrocarbon anesthetics.
- *Use cautiously* in hypertension, thyroid disease, diabetes, cirrhosis, malaria, or sulfite sensitivity, and in patients receiving digitalis.
- Not a substitute for blood or fluid volume deficit. Volume deficit should be replaced before vasopressors are administered.
- Keep solution in light-resistant container, away from heat.
- **I.V. use:** Use a central venous catheter or large veins, such as in the antecubital fossa, to minimize risk of extravasation. Use a continuous infusion pump to regulate infusion flow rate and a piggyback setup so I.V. can continue if this drug is stopped. Watch infusion site carefully for signs of extravasation. If it occurs, stop infusion immediately and call doctor.
- During infusion, check blood pressure every 5 minutes until stabilized; then every 15 minutes. Monitor ECG, blood pressure, cardiac output, central venous pressure, pulmonary capillary wedge pressure, pulse rate, urine output, and extremity color and temperature often during infusion. Titrate infusion rate according to findings, using doctor's guidelines. Use a continuous infusion pump to regulate flow rate.
- When discontinuing therapy with this drug, slow infusion rate gradually. Continue monitoring vital signs, watching for possible severe drop in blood pressure. Keep equipment nearby to start drug again, if necessary. Pressor therapy should not be reinstated until the systolic blood pressure falls below 70 to 80 mm Hg.

• Observe patient closely for adverse effects. If adverse effects develop, dosage may need to be adjusted or discontinued.
• Blood pressure should be raised to slightly less than the patient's normal level. Be careful to avoid excessive blood pressure response. Headache may be a symptom of hypertension. Rapidly induced hypertensive response can cause acute pulmonary edema, arrhythmias, and cardiac arrest.
• Because of prolonged action, a cumulative effect is possible. With an excessive vasopressor response, elevated blood pressure may persist after the drug is stopped.
• Urine output may decrease initially, then increase as blood pressure reaches normal level. Report persistent decreased urine output.
• Keep emergency drugs on hand to reverse effects of metaraminol: atropine for reflex bradycardia; phentolamine to decrease vasopressor effects; and propranolol for arrhythmias.
• Closely monitor patients with diabetes. Adjustment in insulin dose may be needed.
• Metaraminol should not be mixed with other drugs.

norepinephrine injection (levarterenol bitartrate)

Levophed

Pregnancy Risk Category: D

HOW SUPPLIED

Injection: 1 mg/ml

MECHANISM OF ACTION

Stimulates alpha- and $beta_1$-adrenergic receptors within the sympathetic nervous system.

INDICATIONS & DOSAGE

To restore blood pressure in acute hypotensive states –

Adults: initially, 8 to 12 mcg/minute I.V. infusion, then adjust to maintain normal blood pressure. Average maintenance dosage is 2 to 4 mcg/minute.
Children: 2 mcg/m^2/minute I.V. infusion; adjust dosage based upon patient response.

ADVERSE REACTIONS

Common reactions are in italics; life-threatening reactions are in bold italics.
CNS: *headache,* anxiety, weakness, dizziness, tremor, restlessness, insomnia.
CV: bradycardia, ***severe hypertension,*** marked increase in peripheral resistance, decreased cardiac output, ***arrhythmias, ventricular tachycardia, fibrillation,*** bigeminal rhythm, atrioventricular dissociation, precordial pain.
GU: decreased urine output.
Metabolic: metabolic acidosis, hyperglycemia, increased glycogenolysis.
Local: irritation with extravasation.
Other: fever, respiratory difficulty.

INTERACTIONS

Alpha-adrenergic blocking agents: may antagonize drug effects.
Antihistamine, ergot alkaloids, guanethidine, methyldopa: when given with sympathomimetics, may cause severe hypertension (hypertensive crisis). Don't give together.
Inhalational anesthetics: increased risk of arrhythmias. Monitor closely.
MAO inhibitors: increased risk of hypertensive crisis.

NURSING CONSIDERATIONS

• *Contraindicated* in mesenteric or peripheral vascular thrombosis, pregnancy, profound hypoxia, hypercarbia, hypotension from blood volume deficits; and during cyclopropane and halothane anesthesia.
• *Use with extreme caution* in patients receiving MAO inhibitors or tricyclic antidepressants. *Use cautiously* in hypertension, hyperthyroidism, severe

cardiac disease, and sulfite sensitivity.

- Not a substitute for blood or fluid volume deficit. Volume deficit should be replaced before vasopressors are administered.
- Norepinephrine solutions deteriorate after 24 hours.
- **I.V. use:** Use a central venous catheter or a large vein, as in the antecubital fossa, to minimize risk of extravasation. Administer in dextrose 5% in 0.9% sodium chloride injection; 0.9% sodium chloride injection alone is not recommended. Use a continuous infusion pump to regulate infusion flow rate and a piggyback setup so I.V. can continue if norepinephrine is discontinued.
- Check site frequently for signs of extravasation. If it occurs, stop infusion immediately and call doctor. He may want to counteract the effect by infiltrating area with 5 to 10 mg phentolamine and 10 to 15 ml normal saline solution. Also check for blanching along course of infused vein; may progress to superficial sloughing.
- Never leave patient unattended during infusion. During infusion, check blood pressure every 2 minutes until stabilized; then every 5 minutes.
- During infusion, frequently monitor ECG, blood pressure, cardiac output, central venous pressure, pulmonary capillary wedge pressure, pulse rate, urine output, and color and temperature of extremities. Titrate infusion rate according to findings and doctor's guidelines. Use a continuous infusion pump to regulate flow rate. In previously hypertensive patients, blood pressure should be raised no higher than 40 mm Hg below preexisting systolic pressure.
- If prolonged I.V. therapy is necessary, change injection site frequently.
- When stopping drug, slow infusion rate gradually. Monitor vital signs, even after drug is stopped. Watch for severe drop in blood pressure.
- Report decreased urine output to doctor immediately.
- Keep emergency drugs on hand to reverse effects of norepinephrine: atropine for reflex bradycardia; phentolamine for increased vasopressor effects; and propranolol for arrhythmias.

phenylephrine hydrochloride

Neo-Synephrine

Pregnancy Risk Category: C

HOW SUPPLIED

Injection: 10 mg/ml

MECHANISM OF ACTION

Predominantly stimulates alpha-adrenergic receptors in the sympathetic nervous system.

INDICATIONS & DOSAGE

Hypotensive emergencies during spinal anesthesia –
Adults: initially, 0.2 mg I.V., then subsequent doses of 0.1 to 0.2 mg.
Maintenance of blood pressure during spinal or inhalation anesthesia –
Adults: 2 to 3 mg S.C. or I.M. 3 or 4 minutes before anesthesia.
Children: 0.04 mg to 0.088 mg/kg S.C. or I.M.
Mild to moderate hypotension –
Adults: 2 to 5 mg S.C. or I.M.; repeat in 1 to 2 hours as needed and tolerated. Initial dose should not exceed 5 mg. Alternatively, give 0.1 to 0.5 mg I.V., not to be repeated more often than 10 to 15 minutes.
Children: 0.1 mg/kg I.M. or S.C.; repeat in 1 to 2 hours as needed and tolerated.
Paroxysmal supraventricular tachycardia –
Adults: initially, 0.5 mg rapid I.V.; subsequent doses should not exceed the preceding dose by more than 0.1 to 0.2 mg and should not exceed 1 mg.

Prolongation of spinal anesthesia –
Adults: 2 to 5 mg added to anesthetic solution.
Severe hypotension and shock (including drug-induced) –
Adults: 10 mg in 250 ml to 500 ml dextrose 5% in water or 0.9% sodium chloride injection. Start 100 to 180 mcg/minute I.V. infusion, then decrease to a maintenance infusion of 40 to 60 mcg/minute when blood pressure stabilizes.
Vasoconstrictor for regional anesthesia –
Adults: 1 mg phenylephrine added to 20 ml local anesthetic.

ADVERSE REACTIONS
Common reactions are in italics; life-threatening reactions are in bold italics.
CNS: *headache, restlessness, lightheadedness, weakness.*
CV: palpitations, bradycardia, ***arrhythmias,*** hypertension, anginal pain.
EENT: blurred vision.
Skin: goose bumps, feeling of coolness.
Local: tissue sloughing with extravasation.
Other: tachyphylaxis may occur with continued use.

INTERACTIONS
MAO inhibitors: may cause severe hypertension (hypertensive crisis). Don't use together.
Oxytocics, tricyclic antidepressants: increased pressor response. Observe patient.

NURSING CONSIDERATIONS
- *Contraindicated* in narrow-angle glaucoma, hypotension, ventricular tachycardia, severe coronary disease, or cardiovascular disease (including myocardial infarction), and in patients who are taking MAO inhibitors or tricyclic antidepressants.
- *Use with extreme caution* in patients with heart disease, hyperthyroidism, diabetes, severe atherosclerosis, bradycardia, partial heart block, myocardial disease, sulfite sensitivity, and in elderly patients.
- Longer acting than ephedrine and epinephrine.
- Causes little or no CNS stimulation.
- Monitor blood pressure frequently. Avoid excessive rise in blood pressure. Maintain blood pressure at slightly below the patient's normal level. In previously normotensive patients, maintain systolic blood pressure at 80 to 100 mm Hg; in previously hypertensive patients, maintain systolic blood pressure at 30 to 40 mm Hg below their usual level.
- May reverse severe increase in blood pressure with phentolamine.
- **I.V. use:** Use a central venous catheter or a large vein, as in the antecubital fossa, to minimize risk of extravasation. Use a continuous infusion pump to regulate infusion flow rate.
- With prolonged I.V. infusions, avoid abrupt withdrawal. During infusion, frequently monitor ECG, blood pressure, cardiac output, central venous pressure, pulmonary capillary wedge pressure, pulse rate, urine output, and color and temperature of extremities. Titrate infusion rate according to findings and doctor's guidelines. Use a continuous infusion pump to regulate flow rate.

pseudoephedrine hydrochloride

Cenafed◇, Children's Sudafed Liquid◇, Decofed◇, Dorcol Children's Decongestant◇, Eltor†◇, Genaphed◇, Halofed◇, NeoFed◇, Ornex Cold†◇, Pediacare Infant's Oral Decongestant Drops◇, Pseudofrin†◇, Pseudogest◇, Robidrine◇, Sinufed◇, Sudafed◇, Sudafed 12-Hour◇, Sudrin◇, Sufedrin◇

*Liquid form contains alcohol. **May contain tartrazine.

pseudoephedrine sulfate

Afrinol Repetabs

Pregnancy Risk Category: C

HOW SUPPLIED

Tablets: 30 mg◇, 60 mg◇
Tablets (extended-release): 120 mg◇
Capsules (extended-release): 120 mg
Oral solution: 15 mg/5 ml◇, 30 mg/5 ml◇, 7.5 mg/0.8 ml◇

MECHANISM OF ACTION

Stimulates alpha-adrenergic receptors in the respiratory tract, producing vasoconstriction.

INDICATIONS & DOSAGE

Nasal and eustachian tube decongestant –
Adults: 60 mg P.O. q 4 hours. Maximum dosage is 240 mg daily.
Children 6 to 12 years: 30 mg P.O. q 4 to 6 hours. Maximum dosage is 120 mg daily.
Children 2 to 6 years: 15 mg P.O. q 4 hours. Maximum dosage is 60 mg/day.
Extended-release tablets:
Adults and children over 12 years: 120 mg P.O. q 12 hours. This form is contraindicated for children under 12 years.
Relief of nasal congestion –
Adults: 120 mg q 12 hours.

ADVERSE REACTIONS

Common reactions are in italics; life-threatening reactions are in bold italics.
CNS: *anxiety,* transient stimulation, tremors, dizziness, headache, insomnia, *nervousness.*
CV: arrhythmias, *palpitations,* tachycardia.
EENT: dry mouth.
GI: anorexia, nausea, vomiting.
GU: difficulty in urinating.
Skin: pallor.

INTERACTIONS

Antihypertensives: hypotensive effect may be attenuated.
MAO inhibitors: may cause severe hypertension (hypertensive crisis). Don't use together.

NURSING CONSIDERATIONS

- *Contraindicated* in severe hypertension or severe coronary artery disease; in patients receiving MAO inhibitors; and in breast-feeding women.
- *Use cautiously* in hypertension, cardiac disease, diabetes, glaucoma, hyperthyroidism, and prostatic hypertrophy.
- Elderly patients are more sensitive to the drug's effects.
- Tell patient to stop drug if he becomes unusually restless and to notify doctor promptly.
- Warn against using OTC products containing other sympathomimetics.
- Tell patient not to take drug within 2 hours of bedtime because it can cause insomnia.
- Tell patient to relieve dry mouth with sugarless gum or hard candy.
- Do not crush or break extended-release dosage forms.

39

Adrenergic blockers (sympatholytics)

dihydroergotamine mesylate
ergotamine tartrate
methysergide maleate
phenoxybenzamine hydrochloride
(See Chapter 22, ANTIHYPERTENSIVES.)
propranolol hydrochloride
(See Chapter 21, ANTIANGINALS.)

COMBINATION PRODUCTS
BELLERGAL-S**, BEL-PHEN-ERGOT S, PHENERBEL-S: ergotamine tartrate 0.6 mg, levorotatory belladonna alkaloids 0.2 mg, and phenobarbital 40 mg.
CAFERGOT, ERCAF, LANATRATE, WIGRAINE: ergotamine tartrate 1 mg and caffeine 100 mg.
CAFERGOT SUPPOSITORIES: ergotamine tartrate 2 mg and caffeine 100 mg.
CAFERGOT-PB SUPPOSITORIES: ergotamine tartrate 2 mg, caffeine 100 mg, levorotatory belladonna alkaloids 0.25 mg and pentobarbital 60 mg.
ERGO-CAFF PB: ergotamine tartrate 1 mg, belladonna alkaloids 0.125 mg, caffeine 100 mg, and pentobarbital sodium 30 mg.
HYDERGINE: dihydroergocornine mesylate 0.167 mg, dihydroergocristine mesylate 0.167 mg, and dihydroergocryptine mesylate 0.167 mg.
MIGRAL: ergotamine tartrate 1 mg, caffeine 50 mg, and cyclizine hydrochloride 25 mg.
WIGRAINE SUPPOSITORIES: ergotamine tartrate 2 mg and caffeine 100 mg.

dihydroergotamine mesylate

D.H.E. 45, Dihydergot‡

Pregnancy Risk Category: X

HOW SUPPLIED
Injection: 1 mg/ml

MECHANISM OF ACTION
Inhibits the effects of epinephrine, norepinephrine, and other sympathomimetic amines. Also has antiserotonin effects.

INDICATIONS & DOSAGE
Vascular or migraine headache –
Adults: 1 mg I.M. or I.V. May repeat q 1 to 2 hours, p.r.n., up to total of 2 mg I.V. or 3 mg I.M. per attack. Maximum weekly dosage is 6 mg.

ADVERSE REACTIONS
Common reactions are in italics; life-threatening reactions are in bold italics.
CV: numbness and tingling in fingers and toes, transient tachycardia or bradycardia, precordial distress and pain, increased arterial pressure.
GI: nausea, vomiting.
Skin: itching.
Other: weakness in legs, muscle pains in extremities, localized edema.

INTERACTIONS
Erythromycin, troleandomycin, other macrolides: may cause symptoms of ergot toxicity. Vasopressors (nitroprusside, nifedipine, or prazosin) may be ordered to treat such an attack. Monitor closely.
Propranolol and other beta blockers: blocked natural pathway for vasodilation in patients receiving ergot alkaloids and thus could result in excessive vasoconstriction. Watch closely if drugs are used together.

NURSING CONSIDERATIONS
• *Contraindicated* in pregnancy and in peripheral and occlusive vascular disease, coronary artery disease, hyper-

*Liquid form contains alcohol. **May contain tartrazine.

tension, hepatic or renal dysfunction, sepsis.
- Avoid prolonged administration; don't exceed recommended dosage.
- Tell patient to report any feeling of coldness in extremities or tingling of fingers and toes from vasoconstriction. Severe vasoconstriction may result in tissue damage. Keep extremities warm and administer vasodilators (such as nitroprusside) as ordered.
- Most effective when used at first sign of migraine or soon after onset. Provide a quiet, low-light environment to help patient relax.
- Help patient evaluate underlying causes of stress.
- **I.V. use:** Continuous and intermittent infusion are not recommended. Directly inject the solution into the vein over 3 minutes.
- Protect ampules from heat and light. Discard if solution is discolored.
- Best results are obtained by adjusting the dose to most effective, minimal dose.
- Ergotamine rebound, or an increase in frequency and duration of headache, may occur when the drug is stopped.
- For short-term use only.

ergotamine tartrate

Ergomar, Ergostat, Gynergen†, Medihaler-Ergotamine

Pregnancy Risk Category: X

HOW SUPPLIED
Tablets: 1 mg†
Tablets (sublingual): 2 mg
Aerosol inhaler: 360 mcg/metered spray†
Suppositories: 2 mg

MECHANISM OF ACTION
Inhibits the effects of epinephrine, norepinephrine, and other sympathomimetic amines. Also has antiserotonin effects.

INDICATIONS & DOSAGE
Vascular or migraine headache –
Adults: initially, 2 mg P.O. or S.L., then 1 to 2 mg P.O. q hour or S.L. q ½ hour, to maximum of 6 mg daily and 10 mg weekly. Alternatively, use aerosol inhaler: 1 spray (360 mcg) initially, repeated every 5 minutes p.r.n. to a maximum of 6 sprays (2.16 mg) per 24 hours or 15 sprays (5.4 mg) per week.

Patient may also use rectal suppositories. Initially, 2 mg rectally at the onset of the attack, repeated in 1 hour p.r.n. Maximum dose is 2 suppositories per attack or 5 suppositories per week.

ADVERSE REACTIONS
Common reactions are in italics; life-threatening reactions are in bold italics.
CV: numbness and tingling in fingers and toes, transient tachycardia or bradycardia, precordial distress and pain, increased arterial pressure, angina pectoris.
GI: nausea, vomiting, diarrhea, abdominal cramps.
Skin: itching.
Other: weakness in legs, muscle pains in extremities, localized edema.

INTERACTIONS
Erythromycin, troleandomycin, other macrolides: may cause symptoms of ergot toxicity. Vasopressors (nitroprusside, nifedipine, or prazosin) may be ordered to treat such an attack. Monitor closely.
Propranolol and other beta blockers: blocked natural pathway for vasodilation in patients receiving ergot alkaloids and thus could result in excessive vasoconstriction. Watch closely if drugs are used together.

NURSING CONSIDERATIONS
- *Contraindicated* in pregnancy and in peripheral and occlusive vascular diseases, coronary artery disease, hyper-

tension, hepatic or renal dysfunction, sepsis.
- Avoid prolonged administration; don't exceed recommended dosage.
- Most effective when used during prodromal stage of headache or as soon as possible after onset.
- Provide a quiet, low-light environment to help patient relax.
- Help patient evaluate underlying causes of physical or emotional stress, which may precipitate attacks.
- Prolonged exposure to cold weather should be avoided whenever possible. Cold may increase many of the adverse reactions.
- Instruct patient on long-term therapy to check for and report feeling of coldness in extremities or tingling of fingers and toes due to vasoconstriction. Severe vasoconstriction may result in tissue damage.
- Store drug in light-resistant container.
- Sublingual tablet is preferred during early stage of attack because of its rapid absorption.
- Warn patient not to increase dosage without first consulting the doctor.
- Obtain an accurate dietary history from patient to determine if a relationship exists between certain foods and onset of headache.
- Ergotamine rebound, or an increase in frequency and duration of headache, may occur if the drug is stopped.
- Instruct patient how to use the inhaler correctly.

methysergide maleate

Deseril‡, Sansert**

Pregnancy Risk Category: C

HOW SUPPLIED

Tablets: 1 mg‡, 2 mg

MECHANISM OF ACTION

Specifically blocks serotonin (a neurotransmitter) in the peripheral nervous system. In the CNS, the drug acts as a serotonin agonist.

INDICATIONS & DOSAGE

Prevention of frequent, severe, uncontrollable, or disabling migraine or vascular headache –

Adults: 4 to 8 mg P.O. daily with meals.

To control diarrhea caused by carcinoid disease –

Adults: initially, 2 mg P.O. t.i.d., increased p.r.n. to 4 to 16 mg t.i.d.

ADVERSE REACTIONS

Common reactions are in italics; life-threatening reactions are in bold italics.

Blood: neutropenia, eosinophilia.

CNS: insomnia, drowsiness, *euphoria, vertigo,* ataxia, *light-headedness,* hyperesthesia, weakness, hallucinations or feelings of dissociation.

CV: ***fibrotic thickening of cardiac valves and aorta, inferior vena cava, and common iliac branches (retroperitoneal fibrosis);*** vasoconstriction, causing chest pain, abdominal pain, vascular insufficiency of lower limbs; cold, numb, painful extremities with or without paresthesias and diminished or absent pulses; postural hypotension; tachycardia; peripheral edema; murmurs; bruits.

EENT: nasal stuffiness.

GI: nausea, vomiting, diarrhea, constipation, epigastric pain.

Skin: hair loss, dermatitis, sweating, flushing, rash.

Other: ***pulmonary fibrosis,*** causing dyspnea, tightness and pain in chest, pleural friction rubs and effusion, arthralgia, myalgia.

INTERACTIONS

None significant.

NURSING CONSIDERATIONS

- *Contraindicated* in severe hypertension, arteriosclerosis, peripheral vascular insufficiency, renal or hepatic disease, severe coronary artery dis-

*Liquid form contains alcohol. **May contain tartrazine.

eases, thromboembolic disorders, phlebitis or cellulitis of lower limbs, fibrotic processes, valvular heart disease; and in debilitated patients. Use cautiously in peptic ulcers or suspected coronary artery disease. ECG and cardiac status evaluation advisable before giving to patients over 40 years.

- GI effects may be prevented by gradual introduction of medication and by administering with meals.
- Obtain laboratory studies of cardiac and renal function, blood count, and sedimentation rate before and during therapy.
- Drug may be gradually withdrawn every 6 months; then restart after at least 3 or 4 weeks.
- Tell patient not to stop drug abruptly; may cause rebound headaches. Stop gradually over 2 to 3 weeks.
- Patient should keep daily weight record and report unusually rapid weight gain. Teach him to check for peripheral edema. Explain and suggest low-salt diet if necessary.
- Give drug for 3 weeks before evaluating effectiveness.
- Tell patient to report to doctor promptly if he experiences cold, numb, or painful hands and feet; leg cramps when walking; pelvic, chest, or flank pain.
- Not for treatment of migraine or vascular headache in progress or for treatment of tension (muscle contraction) headaches.
- Indicated only for patients who are unresponsive to other drugs and who can be kept under close medical supervision.

40

Skeletal muscle relaxants

baclofen
carisoprodol
chlorphenesin carbamate
chlorzoxazone
cyclobenzaprine
dantrolene sodium
methocarbamol
orphenadrine citrate

COMBINATION PRODUCTS
BLANEX: chlorzoxazone 250 mg and acetaminophen 300 mg.
CHLOROFON-F: chlorzoxazone 250 mg and acetaminophen 300 mg.
CHLORZONE FORTE: chlorzoxazone 250 mg and acetaminophen 300 mg.
LOBAC: chlorzoxazone 250 mg and acetaminophen 300 mg.
MUS-LAX: chlorzoxazone 250 mg and acetaminophen 300 mg.
NORGESIC: orphenadrine citrate 25 mg, aspirin 385 mg, and caffeine 30 mg.
NORGESIC FORTE: orphenadrine citrate 50 mg, aspirin 770 mg, and caffeine 60 mg.
PARACET FORTE: chlorzoxazone 250 mg and acetaminophen 300 mg.
POLYFLEX: chlorzoxazone 250 mg and acetaminophen 300 mg.
ROBAXISAL: methocarbamol 400 mg and aspirin 325 mg.
SKELEX: chlorzoxazone 250 mg and acetaminophen 300 mg.
SOMA COMPOUND: carisoprodol 200 mg and aspirin 325 mg.
SOMA COMPOUND WITH CODEINE: carisoprodol 200 mg, aspirin 325 mg, caffeine 32 mg, and codeine phosphate 16 mg.
ZOXAPHEN: chlorzoxazone 250 mg and acetaminophen 300 mg.

baclofen
Lioresal, Lioresal DS

Pregnancy Risk Category: C

HOW SUPPLIED
Tablets: 10 mg, 20 mg, 25 mg‡
Intrathecal injection: 500 mcg/ml, 2,000 mcg/ml

MECHANISM OF ACTION
Reduces transmission of impulses from the spinal cord to skeletal muscle.

INDICATIONS & DOSAGE
Spasticity in multiple sclerosis, spinal cord injury –
Adults: initially, 5 mg P.O. t.i.d. for 3 days, 10 mg t.i.d. for 3 days, 15 mg t.i.d. for 3 days, 20 mg t.i.d. for 3 days. Increase according to response up to maximum of 80 mg daily.
Management of severe spasticity in patients who don't respond to or can't tolerate oral baclofen therapy –
Screening phase –
Adults: After a test dose to check responsiveness, drug will be administered by an implantable infusion pump. The test dose is 1 ml of a 50-mcg/ml dilution administered into the intrathecal space by barbotage over 1 minute or more. Significantly decreased severity or frequency of muscle spasm or reduced muscle tone should be evident within 4 to 8 hours. If the response is inadequate, a second screening dose of 75 mcg/1.5 ml should be given 24 hours after the first. If response is still inadequate, a final test dose of 100 mcg/2 ml may be given 24 hours later. Patients unresponsive to the 100-mcg dose shouldn't be considered candidates for the implantable pump.

*Liquid form contains alcohol. **May contain tartrazine.

Maintenance therapy –
Adults: titrate initial dosage based on the screening dose that elicited an adequate response. Double this effective dose and administer over 24 hours. However, if the screening dose efficacy was maintained for 12 hours or more, don't double the dose. After the first 24 hours, increase the dose slowly as needed and tolerated by 10% to 30% daily. During prolonged maintenance therapy, daily dose may be increased by 10% to 40% if needed; if the patient experiences adverse effects, dosage may be decreased by 10% to 20%. Maintenance dosages have ranged from 12 mcg to 1,500 mcg daily; however, experience with dosages over 1,000 mcg daily is limited. Most patients need 300 to 800 mcg daily.

ADVERSE REACTIONS
Common reactions are in italics; life-threatening reactions are in bold italics.
CNS: *drowsiness, dizziness,* headache, *weakness, fatigue,* confusion, insomnia, dysarthria, ***seizures.***
CV: hypotension.
EENT: nasal congestion, blurred vision.
GI: *nausea,* constipation.
GU: urinary frequency.
Hepatic: increased AST (SGOT) and alkaline phosphatase.
Metabolic: hyperglycemia.
Skin: rash, pruritus.
Other: ankle edema, excessive perspiration, weight gain.

INTERACTIONS
Alcohol, CNS depressants: increased CNS depression. Avoid concomitant use.

NURSING CONSIDERATIONS
- *Contraindicated* in patients with hypersensitivity to the drug. Orally administered drug shouldn't be used to treat muscle spasm caused by rheumatic disorders, cerebral palsy, Parkinson's disease, or CVA because efficacy hasn't been established. Don't administer intrathecal injection by I.V., I.M., S.C., or epidural route.
- *Use cautiously* in patients with impaired renal function or seizure disorder or when spasticity is used to maintain motor function.
- Give oral form with meals or milk to prevent GI distress.
- Amount of relief determines if dosage (and drowsiness) can be reduced.
- Tell patient to avoid activities that require alertness until CNS effects of the drug are known. Drowsiness is usually transient.
- Watch for increased incidence of seizures in epileptics.
- Watch for sensitivity reactions, such as fever, skin eruptions, and respiratory distress.
- Advise patient to follow doctor's orders regarding rest and physical therapy.
- Don't withdraw abruptly after long-term use unless required by severe adverse reactions; may precipitate hallucinations or rebound spasticity.
- Treatment of oral overdosage is supportive only; don't induce emesis or use a respiratory stimulant in obtunded patients.
- Limited experience with long-term intrathecal use suggests that about 10% of patients may develop tolerance to the drug. In some cases, this may be treated by hospitalizing the patient and slowly withdrawing the drug over a 2-week period.
- Used investigationally for treatment of unstable bladder.

carisoprodol
Rela, Sodol, Soma, Soprodol, Soridol

Pregnancy Risk Category: C

HOW SUPPLIED
Tablets: 350 mg

MECHANISM OF ACTION
Precise mechanism unknown; reduces transmission of impulses from the spinal cord to skeletal muscle.

INDICATIONS & DOSAGE
As an adjunct in acute, painful musculoskeletal conditions –
Adults and children over 12 years: 350 mg P.O. t.i.d. and h.s.
Not recommended for children under 12 years.

ADVERSE REACTIONS
Common reactions are in italics; life-threatening reactions are in bold italics.
CNS: *drowsiness, dizziness,* vertigo, ataxia, tremor, agitation, irritability, headache, depressive reactions, insomnia.
CV: orthostatic hypotension, tachycardia, facial flushing.
GI: nausea, vomiting, hiccups, increased bowel activity, epigastric distress.
Skin: rash, ***erythema multiforme,*** pruritus.
Other: asthmatic episodes, fever, angioneurotic edema, ***anaphylaxis.***

INTERACTIONS
Alcohol, CNS depressants: increased CNS depression. Avoid concomitant use.

NURSING CONSIDERATIONS
- *Contraindicated* in hypersensitivity to related compounds (e.g., meprobamate, tybamate) or intermittent porphyria.
- *Use cautiously* in impaired hepatic or renal function.
- Watch for idiosyncratic reactions after first to fourth dose (weakness, ataxia, visual and speech difficulties, fever, skin eruptions, and mental changes) or severe reactions, including bronchospasm, hypotension, and anaphylactic shock. Withhold dose and notify doctor immediately of any unusual reactions.
- Record amount of relief to determine whether dosage can be reduced.
- Warn patient to avoid activities that require alertness until CNS effects of the drug are known. Drowsiness is transient.
- Avoid combining with alcohol or other depressants.
- Advise patient to follow doctor's orders regarding rest and physical therapy.
- Do not stop drug abruptly; mild withdrawal effects, such as insomnia, headache, nausea, and abdominal cramps, may result.

chlorphenesin carbamate
Maolate**

Pregnancy Risk Category: C

HOW SUPPLIED
Tablets: 400 mg

MECHANISM OF ACTION
Precise mechanism unknown; reduces transmission of impulses from the spinal cord to skeletal muscle.

INDICATIONS & DOSAGE
As an adjunct in short-term, acute, painful musculoskeletal conditions –
Adults: initial dose is 800 mg P.O. t.i.d. Maintenance dose is 400 mg P.O. q.i.d. for maximum of 8 weeks.
Trigeminal neuralgia –
Adults: 400 mg P.O. t.i.d. Usually given upon awakening, at noon, and h.s.

ADVERSE REACTIONS
Common reactions are in italics; life-threatening reactions are in bold italics.
Blood: thrombocytopenia, leukopenia, ***agranulocytosis.***
CNS: *drowsiness, dizziness,* confusion, headache, weakness. Dose-related adverse reactions include paradoxical stimulation, agitation, insomnia, nervousness, headache.
GI: *nausea, GI distress.*

*Liquid form contains alcohol. **May contain tartrazine.

Other: *anaphylaxis.*

INTERACTIONS
Alcohol and CNS depressants: increased CNS depression. Avoid concomitant use.

NURSING CONSIDERATIONS
- *Use cautiously* in hepatic disease or impaired renal function, and in patients hypersensitive to aspirin.
- Safe use for periods over 8 weeks not established.
- Take with meals or milk to prevent GI distress.
- Amount of relief determines if dosage (and drowsiness) can be reduced.
- Watch for sensitivity reactions, such as fever, skin eruptions, and respiratory distress. Withhold dose and notify doctor of unusual reactions.
- Monitor CBC and platelet studies in patients on long-term therapy. Watch for unusual bleeding and infections that may indicate blood dyscrasia.
- Tell patient to avoid activities that require mental alertness until adverse CNS effects of the drug are known.

chlorzoxazone
Paraflex, Parafon Forte DSC, Strifon Forte DSC

Pregnancy Risk Category: C

HOW SUPPLIED
Tablets: 250 mg
Caplets: 500 mg

MECHANISM OF ACTION
Precise mechanism unknown; reduces transmission of impulses from the spinal cord to skeletal muscle.

INDICATIONS & DOSAGE
As an adjunct in acute, painful musculoskeletal conditions –
Adults: 250 to 750 mg P.O. t.i.d. or q.i.d.
Children: 20 mg/kg P.O. daily in divided doses t.i.d. or q.i.d.

ADVERSE REACTIONS
Common reactions are in italics; life-threatening reactions are in bold italics.
Blood: anemia, granulocytopenia.
CNS: *drowsiness, dizziness, lightheadedness,* malaise, headache, overstimulation.
GI: anorexia, nausea, vomiting, heartburn, abdominal distress, constipation, diarrhea.
GU: urine discoloration (orange or purple-red).
Hepatic: hepatic dysfunction.
Skin: urticaria, redness, itching, petechiae, bruising.

INTERACTIONS
Alcohol and CNS depressants: increased CNS depression. Avoid concomitant use.

NURSING CONSIDERATIONS
- *Contraindicated* in impaired hepatic function. *Use cautiously* in history of drug allergies.
- Amount of relief determines if dosage (and drowsiness) can be reduced.
- Watch for signs of hepatic dysfunction. Withhold dose and notify doctor.
- Warn patient to avoid activities that require alertness until CNS effects of the drug are known.
- Avoid combining with alcohol or other depressants.
- Tell patient that the drug may discolor urine orange or purple-red.
- Advise patient to follow doctor's orders regarding physical activity.
- Give with meals or milk to prevent GI distress.

cyclobenzaprine
Flexeril

Pregnancy Risk Category: B

HOW SUPPLIED
Tablets: 10 mg

MECHANISM OF ACTION
Precise mechanism unknown; reduces transmission of impulses from the spinal cord to skeletal muscle.

INDICATIONS & DOSAGE
Short-term treatment of muscle spasm –
Adults: 10 mg P.O. t.i.d. for 7 days. Maximum dosage is 60 mg daily for 2 to 3 weeks.

ADVERSE REACTIONS
Common reactions are in italics; life-threatening reactions are in bold italics.
CNS: *drowsiness,* euphoria, weakness, headache, insomnia, nightmares, paresthesias, dizziness, depression, visual disturbances, ***precipitation of seizures.***
CV: tachycardia.
EENT: blurred vision, dry mouth.
GI: abdominal pain, dyspepsia, peculiar taste, constipation.
GU: urine retention.
Skin: rash, urticaria, pruritus.
Other: in high doses, watch for adverse reactions like those of other tricyclic drugs.

INTERACTIONS
Alcohol, CNS depressants: may cause additive CNS depression. Avoid concomitant use.
MAO inhibitors: can exacerbate CNS depression or anticholinergic effects. Don't give within 14 days after discontinuing MAO inhibitors.

NURSING CONSIDERATIONS
- *Contraindicated* in patients who have received MAO inhibitors within 14 days; during acute recovery phase of myocardial infarction; in heart block, arrhythmias, conduction disturbances, or CHF.
- *Use cautiously* in urine retention, narrow-angle glaucoma, increased intraocular pressure, CV disease, impaired hepatic function, and seizures; and in elderly or debilitated patients.
- Nausea, headache, and malaise may occur if drug is stopped abruptly after long-term use.
- Watch for symptoms of overdose, including possible cardiotoxicity. Notify doctor immediately and have physostigmine available.
- Advise patient to report urinary hesitancy or urine retention. If constipation is a problem, increase fluid intake and suggest a stool softener.
- Warn patient to avoid activities that require alertness until CNS effects of the drug are known.
- Tell patient that dry mouth may be relieved with sugarless candy or gum.

dantrolene sodium
Dantrium, Dantrium I.V.

Pregnancy Risk Category: C

HOW SUPPLIED
Capsules: 25 mg, 50 mg, 100 mg
Injection: 20 mg/vial

MECHANISM OF ACTION
Acts directly on skeletal muscle to interfere with intracellular calcium movement.

INDICATIONS & DOSAGE
Spasticity and sequelae secondary to severe chronic disorders (multiple sclerosis, cerebral palsy, spinal cord injury, stroke) –
Adults: 25 mg P.O. daily. Increase gradually in increments of 25 mg at 4- to 7-day intervals, up to 100 mg b.i.d. to q.i.d., to maximum of 400 mg daily.
Children: 1 mg/kg daily P.O. b.i.d. to q.i.d. Increase gradually as needed by 1 mg/kg daily to maximum of 100 mg q.i.d.
Management of malignant hyperthermia –
Adults and children: 1 mg/kg I.V. initially; may repeat dose up to cumulative dose of 10 mg/kg.
Prevention or attenuation of malignant

hyperthermia in susceptible patients who require surgery –
Adults: 4 to 8 mg/kg P.O. daily given in three to four divided doses for 1 to 2 days before procedure. Administer final dose 3 to 4 hours before procedure.
Prevention of recurrence of malignant hyperthermia –
Adults: 4 to 8 mg/kg/day P.O. given in four divided doses for up to 3 days following hyperthermic crisis.

ADVERSE REACTIONS

Common reactions are in italics; life-threatening reactions are in bold italics.
CNS: *muscle weakness, drowsiness,* dizziness, light-headedness, malaise, headache, confusion, nervousness, insomnia, ***precipitation of seizures.***
CV: tachycardia, blood pressure changes.
EENT: excessive tearing, visual disturbances.
GI: anorexia, constipation, cramping, dysphagia, metallic taste, severe diarrhea.
GU: urinary frequency, incontinence, nocturia, dysuria, crystalluria, difficulty achieving erection.
Hepatic: hepatitis.
Skin: eczematous eruption, pruritus, urticaria, photosensitivity.
Other: abnormal hair growth, drooling, sweating, pleural effusion, myalgia, chills, fever.

INTERACTIONS

Alcohol, CNS depressants: increased CNS depression. Avoid concomitant use.
Verapamil (I.V.): may result in cardiovascular collapse. Stop drug before administering I.V. dantrolene.

NURSING CONSIDERATIONS

- *Contraindicated* when spasticity is used to maintain motor function; for spasms in rheumatic disorders; in patients with active hepatic disease; and during breast-feeding.
- *Use cautiously* in severely impaired cardiac or pulmonary function or preexisting hepatic disease; in women; and in those over 35 years.
- Safety and efficacy in long-term use not established. Do not give more than 45 days if no benefits are obtained.
- Some patients may experience difficulty swallowing during therapy. Tell patient to use caution when eating to avoid choking.
- Give with meals or milk to prevent GI distress.
- Prepare oral suspension for single dose by dissolving capsule contents in juice or other suitable liquid. For multiple doses, use acid vehicle, such as citric acid in USP syrup; refrigerate. Use within several days.
- Amount of relief determines if dosage (and drowsiness) can be reduced.
- Liver function tests should be performed at the beginning of therapy.
- Watch for hepatitis (fever and jaundice), severe diarrhea, severe weakness, or sensitivity reactions (fever and skin eruptions). Withhold dose and notify doctor.
- Warn patient to avoid driving and other hazardous activities until CNS effects of the drug are known.
- Tell patient to avoid photosensitivity reactions by using sunscreen and protective clothing; to report abdominal discomfort or GI problems immediately; and to follow doctor's orders regarding rest and physical therapy.
- **I.V. use:** Administer as soon as malignant hyperthermia reaction is recognized. Reconstitute each vial by adding 60 ml of sterile water for injection and shaking vial until clear. Don't use a diluent that contains a bacteriostatic agent. Protect contents from light and use within 6 hours. Be careful to avoid extravasation.
- Has been used to treat neuroleptic malignant syndrome.

methocarbamol

Delaxin, Marbaxin-750, Robaxin, Robomol-500, Robomol-750

Pregnancy Risk Category: C

HOW SUPPLIED

Tablets: 500 mg, 750 mg
Injection: 100 mg/ml

MECHANISM OF ACTION

Precise mechanism unknown; reduces transmission of impulses from the spinal cord to skeletal muscle.

INDICATIONS & DOSAGE

As an adjunct in acute, painful musculoskeletal conditions –
Adults: 1.5 g P.O. q.i.d. for 2 to 3 days, then 1 g P.O. q.i.d., or not more than 500 mg (5 ml) I.M. into each gluteal region. May repeat q 8 hours. Or 1 to 3 g daily (10 to 30 ml) I.V. directly into vein at 3 ml/minute, or 10 ml may be added to no more than 250 ml of dextrose 5% in water or normal saline solution. Maximum dosage is 3 g daily.
Supportive therapy in tetanus management –
Adults: 1 to 2 g into tubing of running I.V. or 1 to 3 g in infusion bottle q 6 hours.
Children: 15 mg/kg I.V. q 6 hours.

ADVERSE REACTIONS

Common reactions are in italics; life-threatening reactions are in bold italics.
Blood: hemolysis, decreased hemoglobin (I.V. only).
CNS: drowsiness, dizziness, lightheadedness, headache, syncope, mild muscular incoordination (I.M. or I.V. only), ***seizures*** (I.V. only).
CV: hypotension, bradycardia (I.M. or I.V. only).
GI: nausea, anorexia, GI upset, metallic taste.
GU: hematuria (I.V. only), discoloration of urine.
Skin: urticaria, pruritus, rash.
Local: thrombophlebitis, extravasation (I.V. only).
Other: fever, flushing, ***anaphylactic reactions*** (I.M. or I.V. only).

INTERACTIONS

Alcohol and CNS depressants: increased CNS depression. Avoid concomitant use.

NURSING CONSIDERATIONS

- *Contraindicated* in impaired renal function (injectable form), myasthenia gravis, epilepsy (injectable form); in children under 12 years (except in tetanus); and in patients receiving anticholinesterase agents.
- **I.V. use:** Infuse slowly; maximum rate is 300 mg (3 ml)/minute. Drug irritates veins. It may cause phlebitis, aggravate seizures, and cause fainting if injected rapidly. Make sure patient remains in a supine position during infusion. Because drug is an irritant, avoid extravasation.
- Give I.M. deeply, only into upper outer quadrant of buttocks, with maximum of 5 ml in each buttock.
- Do not give subcutaneously.
- In tetanus management, use methocarbamol with tetanus antitoxin, penicillin, tracheotomy, and aggressive supportive care. Long course of I.V. methocarbamol required.
- Watch for orthostatic hypotension, especially with parenteral administration. Keep patient supine for 15 minutes afterward, and supervise ambulation. Advise patient to get up slowly.
- Watch for sensitivity reactions, such as fever and skin eruptions.
- Have epinephrine, antihistamines, and corticosteroids available.
- Warn patient to avoid activities that require alertness until CNS effects of the drug are known.
- Avoid combining with alcohol or other depressants.
- Advise patient to follow doctor's orders regarding physical activity.

• Tell patient urine may turn green, black, or brown.
• Give tablets with meals or milk to prevent GI distress.
• Prepare liquid by crushing tablets into water or saline solution. Give through nasogastric tube.
• Obtain CBC periodically during prolonged therapy.
• May interfere with urine tests for 5-hydroxyindoleacetic acid (5-HIAA) and vanillylmandelic acid (VMA).

orphenadrine citrate

Banflex, Flexoject, Flexon, K-Flex, Marflex, Myolin, Neocyten, Noradex, Norflex, O-Flex, Orflagen, Orphenate

Pregnancy Risk Category: C

HOW SUPPLIED

Tablets: 100 mg
Tablets (sustained-release): 100 mg
Injection: 30 mg/ml

MECHANISM OF ACTION

Precise mechanism unknown; reduces transmission of impulses from the spinal cord to skeletal muscle. May also block central cholinergic receptors in the cerebrum or medulla.

INDICATIONS & DOSAGE

Adjunctive treatment in painful, acute musculoskeletal conditions –
Adults: 100 mg P.O. b.i.d., or 60 mg I.V. or I.M. q 12 hours, p.r.n. For maintenance, switch to oral therapy beginning 12 hours after last parenteral dose.

ADVERSE REACTIONS

Common reactions are in italics; life-threatening reactions are in bold italics.
Blood: *aplastic anemia.*
CNS: disorientation, restlessness, irritability, weakness, *drowsiness,* headache, dizziness.
CV: palpitations, tachycardia.
EENT: dilated pupils, blurred vision, difficulty swallowing.
GI: constipation, *dry mouth,* nausea, vomiting, paralytic ileus, epigastric distress.
GU: urinary hesitancy or urine retention.

INTERACTIONS

Alcohol, other CNS depressants: increased CNS depression. Avoid concomitant use.

NURSING CONSIDERATIONS

• *Contraindicated* in narrow-angle glaucoma; prostatic hypertrophy; pyloric, duodenal, or bladder-neck obstruction; myasthenia gravis; tachycardia; severe hepatic or renal disease; or ulcerative colitis.
• *Use cautiously* in elderly or debilitated patients with cardiac disease, arrhythmias, sulfite sensitivity, and those exposed to high temperatures.
• Check all dosages carefully. Even a slight overdose can lead to toxicity. Early signs are excessive dry mouth, dilated pupils, blurred vision, skin flushing, and fever.
• Monitor vital signs carefully.
• **I.V. use:** Inject the drug over approximately 5 minutes while patient is supine. Wait 5 to 10 minutes and then help patient to sit up.
• When given I.V., may cause paradoxical initial bradycardia. Usually disappears in 2 minutes.
• Have patient report urinary hesitancy and urine retention. Have patient void before taking the drug.
• Relieve dry mouth with cool drinks, sugarless gum, or hard candy.
• Monitor CBC, hepatic function, and urinalysis in patients receiving long-term therapy.
• Advise patients to avoid tasks that require alertness until CNS effects of the drug are known.

41

Neuromuscular blockers

atracurium besylate
doxacurium chloride
gallamine triethiodide
metocurine iodide
mivacurium chloride
pancuronium bromide
pipecuronium bromide
succinylcholine chloride
tubocurarine chloride
vecuronium bromide

COMBINATION PRODUCTS
None.

atracurium besylate

Tracrium
Pregnancy Risk Category: C

HOW SUPPLIED
Injection: 10 mg/ml

MECHANISM OF ACTION
Prevents acetylcholine from binding to the receptors on the muscle end plate, thus blocking depolarization. Nondepolarizing agent.

INDICATIONS & DOSAGE
Adjunct to general anesthesia, to facilitate endotracheal intubation and to provide skeletal muscle relaxation during surgery or mechanical ventilation–
Dose depends on anesthetic used, individual needs, and response. Doses are representative and must be adjusted.
Adults and children over 2 years: 0.4 to 0.5 mg/kg by I.V. bolus. Maintenance dose of 0.08 to 0.10 mg/kg within 20 to 45 minutes of initial dose should be administered during prolonged surgical procedures. Maintenance doses may be administered q 12 to 25 minutes in patients receiving balanced anesthesia. For prolonged procedures, a constant infusion of 5 to 9 mcg/kg/minute may be used.
Children 1 month to 2 years: initial dose, 0.3 to 0.4 mg/kg. Frequent maintenance doses may be needed.

ADVERSE REACTIONS
Common reactions are in italics; life-threatening reactions are in bold italics.
CV: bradycardia, hypotension.
Skin: skin flush, erythema, pruritus, urticaria.
Other: ***prolonged dose-related apnea,*** wheezing, increased bronchial secretions.

INTERACTIONS
Aminoglycoside antibiotics (including amikacin, gentamicin, kanamycin, neomycin, streptomycin); polymyxin antibiotics (polymyxin B sulfate, colistin); clindamycin; quinidine; general anesthetics such as halothane, enflurane, and isoflurane: potentiated neuromuscular blockade, leading to increased skeletal muscle relaxation and possible respiratory paralysis. Use cautiously during surgical and postoperative periods.
Lithium, narcotic analgesics: potentiated neuromuscular blockade, leading to increased skeletal muscle relaxation and possible respiratory paralysis. Use with extreme caution and reduce dose of atracurium.

NURSING CONSIDERATIONS
- *Contraindicated* in patients with hypersensitivity to the drug.
- *Use cautiously* in patients with CV disease, severe electrolyte disorders, bronchogenic carcinoma, hepatic or pulmonary impairment, and neuromuscular diseases and in elderly or debilitated patients.

*Liquid form contains alcohol. **May contain tartrazine.

• This drug should be used only under direct medical supervision by personnel skilled in the use of neuromuscular blockers and techniques for maintaining a patent airway. It shouldn't be used unless facilities and equipment for mechanical ventilation, oxygen therapy, and intubation and an antagonist are within reach.
• Keep airway clear. Have emergency respiratory support equipment (endotracheal equipment, ventilator, oxygen, atropine, edrophonium, neostigmine, and epinephrine) on hand.
• Know that neuromuscular blockers don't obtund consciousness or alter the pain threshold. Sedatives or general anesthetics should be given before neuromuscular blockers are administered.
• A nerve stimulator and train-of-four monitoring are recommended to confirm antagonism of neuromuscular blockade and recovery of muscle strength. Before attempting pharmacologic reversal with neostigmine, some evidence of spontaneous recovery (T_4:T_1 ratio > 0 or T_1 > 10% of control) should be seen.
• Prior administration of succinylcholine doesn't prolong duration of action, but it quickens onset and may deepen neuromuscular blockade.
• Atracurium facilitates intubation within 2 to 2½ minutes. The duration of effect is 20 to 35 minutes.
• Once spontaneous recovery starts, atracurium-induced neuromuscular blockade may be reversed with an anticholinesterase agent (such as neostigmine or edrophonium). Usually administered together with an anticholinergic (such as atropine).
• Don't administer by I.M. injection.
• Don't mix with alkaline solutions such as barbiturates (precipitate may form).
• Monitor respirations closely until patient is fully recovered from neuromuscular blockade, as evidenced by tests of muscle strength (hand grip, head lift, and ability to cough).
• Atracurium has a longer duration of action than succinylcholine and a shorter duration of action than *d*-tubocurarine or pancuronium.

doxacurium chloride
Nuromax

Pregnancy Risk Category: C

HOW SUPPLIED
Injection: 1 mg/ml

MECHANISM OF ACTION
A nondepolarizing muscle relaxant that competes with acetylcholine for receptor sites at the motor end plate. Because this action may be antagonized by cholinesterase inhibitors, doxacurium is considered a competitive antagonist.

INDICATIONS & DOSAGE
To provide skeletal muscle relaxation during surgery as an adjunct to general anesthesia –

Adults: dosage is highly individualized. Note that all times of onset and duration of neuromuscular blockade are averages and considerable individual variation is normal. Reportedly, 0.05 mg/kg rapidly I.V. produces adequate conditions for endotracheal intubation in 5 minutes in about 90% of patients when used as part of a thiopental-narcotic induction technique. Lower doses may require longer delay before intubation is possible. Neuromuscular blockade at this dose will last for an average of 100 minutes.

Children over 2 years: an initial dose of 0.03 mg/kg I.V. administered during halothane anesthesia produces effective blockade in 7 minutes with duration of 30 minutes. Under the same conditions, 0.05 mg/kg produces a blockade in 4 minutes with duration of 45 minutes.

Maintenance of neuromuscular blockade during long procedures –
Adults and children: after initial dose of 0.5 mg/kg I.V., maintenance doses of 0.005 and 0.01 mg/kg will prolong neuromuscular blockade for an average of 30 minutes. Children usually require more frequent administration of maintenance doses.

ADVERSE REACTIONS

Common reactions are in italics; life-threatening reactions are in bold italics.
Respiratory: dyspnea, respiratory depression, ***respiratory insufficiency or apnea.***
Other: prolonged muscle weakness.

INTERACTIONS

Alkaline solutions (such as barbiturate solutions): physically incompatible; may form precipitate. Do not administer through the same I.V. line.
Aminoglycosides (kanamycin, neomycin, streptomycin, dihydrostreptomycin, and gentamicin), bacitracin, colistin, polymyxin B, colistimethate, and tetracyclines: increased muscle weakness. Use together cautiously.
Magnesium salts: may enhance neuromuscular blockade. Monitor for excessive weakness.
Phenytoin, carbamazepine: may prolong the time to maximal block or shorten the duration of block with neuromuscular blocking agents.
Quinidine, inhalational anesthetics: may enhance the activity (or prolonged action) of nondepolarizing neuromuscular blocking agents.

NURSING CONSIDERATIONS

- *Contraindicated* in patients hypersensitive to the drug. Do not use in neonates. The drug contains benzyl alcohol, which has been associated with fatalities in newborns.
- Because of the lack of data supporting safety, this drug is not recommended for use in patients requiring prolonged mechanical ventilation in the intensive care unit. It is not recommended for use before or after nondepolarizing neuromuscular blocking agents. It is also not recommended for use during cesarean section because safety of the neonate has not been established and because this drug's long duration of action exceeds the duration of the procedure.
- *Use cautiously,* possibly at reduced dosage, in debilitated patients, in patients with metastatic cancer, severe electrolyte disturbances, or neuromuscular diseases; and in patients in whom potentiation or difficulty in reversal of neuromuscular blockade is anticipated. Patients with myasthenia gravis or myasthenic syndrome (Eaton-Lambert syndrome) are particularly sensitive to the effects of nondepolarizing relaxants. Shorter-acting agents are recommended for use in such patients.
- Note that higher initial doses may be required in patients with severe burns and in some patients with severe liver disease. Higher doses (0.8 mg/kg) will produce intubating conditions more rapidly (4 minutes), with neuromuscular blockade for 160 minutes or more. Consequently, these higher doses should be reserved for long procedures. Administration during steady-state anesthesia with enflurane, halothane, or isoflurane may allow 33% reduction of the dose.
- The drug is not metabolized; it is excreted in the urine and bile. Therefore, patients with renal or hepatic insufficiency may require dosage adjustment.
- Dosage should be adjusted to ideal body weight in obese patients (patients 30% or more above their ideal weight) to avoid prolonged neuromuscular blockade.
- This drug should be used only under direct medical supervision by personnel familiar with the use of neuromuscular blocking agents and techniques involved in maintaining a patent air-

way. It should not be used unless facilities and equipment for mechanical ventilation, oxygen therapy, and intubation and an antagonist are within reach.

• A nerve stimulator and train-of-four monitoring are recommended to document antagonism of neuromuscular blockade and recovery of muscle strength. Before attempting pharmacologic reversal with neostigmine, some evidence of spontaneous recovery (T_4:T_1 ratio > 0 or T_1 > 10% of control) should be evident.

• Experimental evidence suggests that acid-base and electrolyte balance may influence the actions of nondepolarizing neuromuscular blockers. Alkalosis may counteract the paralysis and acidosis may enhance it.

• Because the drug has minimal vagolytic action, bradycardia during anesthesia may be common.

• Monitor respirations closely until patient is fully recovered from neuromuscular blockade as evidenced by tests of muscle strength (hand grip, head lift, and ability to cough).

• Note that doxacurium has no effect on consciousness or pain threshold. To avoid distress to the patient, this drug should not be administered until the patient's consciousness is obtunded by the general anesthetic.

• **I.V. use:** Drug is compatible with dextrose 5% in water, 0.9% sodium chloride injection, dextrose 5% in 0.9% sodium chloride injection, lactated Ringer's injection, and dextrose 5% in lactated Ringer's injection. Diluted solutions are stable for 24 hours at room temperature; however, because reconstitution dilutes the preservative, there is an increased risk of contamination. The manufacturer recommends that the product be administered immediately after reconstitution. Unused solutions should be discarded after 8 hours.

• When diluted as directed, doxacurium is compatible with alfentanil, fentanyl, and sufentanil.

gallamine triethiodide
Flaxedil

Pregnancy Risk Category: C

HOW SUPPLIED
Injection: 20 mg/ml

MECHANISM OF ACTION
Prevents acetylcholine from binding to the receptors on the muscle end plate, thus blocking depolarization. Nondepolarizing agent.

INDICATIONS & DOSAGE
Adjunct to anesthesia to induce skeletal muscle relaxation; facilitate intubation, reduction of fractures and dislocations; lessen muscle contractions in pharmacologically or electrically induced seizures; assist with mechanical ventilation –

Dosage depends on anesthetic used, individual needs, and response. Dosages are representative and must be adjusted.

Adults and children over 1 month: initially, 1 mg/kg I.V. to maximum of 100 mg, regardless of patient's weight; then 0.5 mg to 1 mg/kg q 30 to 40 minutes.

Children under 1 month but over 5 kg (11 lb): initially, 0.25 to 0.75 mg/kg I.V., then may give additional doses of 0.1 to 0.5 mg/kg q 30 to 40 minutes.

ADVERSE REACTIONS
Common reactions are in italics; life-threatening reactions are in bold italics.

CV: tachycardia.

Other: ***respiratory paralysis, dose-related prolonged apnea,*** residual muscle weakness, increased oropharyngeal secretions, allergic or idiosyncratic hypersensitivity reactions.

†Available in Canada only. ‡Available in Australia only. ◇Available OTC.

INTERACTIONS

Aminoglycoside antibiotics (amikacin, gentamicin, kanamycin, neomycin, streptomycin); polymyxin antibiotics (polymyxin B sulfate, colistin); clindamycin; quinidine; general anesthetics (such as halothane, enflurane, isoflurane: potentiated neuromuscular blockade, leading to increased skeletal muscle relaxation and possible respiratory paralysis. Monitor closely.
Narcotic analgesics, I.V. diazepam: potentiated neuromuscular blockade, leading to increased skeletal muscle relaxation and possible respiratory paralysis. Use with extreme caution, and reduce dose of gallamine.

NURSING CONSIDERATIONS

- *Contraindicated* in patients with hypersensitivity to iodides, impaired renal function, myasthenia gravis; patients in shock; and patients in whom tachycardia may be hazardous.
- *Use cautiously* in elderly or debilitated patients; in hepatic or pulmonary impairment, respiratory depression, myasthenic syndrome of lung cancer or bronchogenic carcinoma, dehydration, thyroid disorders, collagen diseases, porphyria, and electrolyte disturbances; in patients sensitive to sulfites; and in patients undergoing cesarean section.
- **I.V. use:** Give I.V. slowly (over 30 to 90 seconds).
- Protect drug from light or excessive heat; use only fresh solutions.
- Do not mix solution with meperidine or barbiturate solutions.
- This drug should be used only under direct medical supervision by personnel skilled in the use of neuromuscular blockers and techniques for maintaining a patent airway. It should not be used unless facilities and equipment for artificial respiration, mechanical ventilation, oxygen therapy, and intubation and an antagonist are within reach.
- Keep airway clear. Have emergency respiratory support equipment (endotracheal equipment, ventilator, oxygen, atropine, edrophonium, neostigmine, and epinephrine) on hand.
- Know that neuromuscular blockers do not obtund consciousness or alter the pain threshold. Patients should receive sedatives or general anesthetics before neuromuscular blockers are administered.
- A nerve stimulator and train-of-four monitoring are recommended to confirm antagonism of neuromuscular blockade and recovery of muscle strength. Before attempting pharmacologic reversal, some evidence of spontaneous recovery (T_4:T_1 ratio > 0 or T_1 > 10% of control) should be seen. Reversal agents, such as neostigmine, are usually administered with an anticholinergic (such as atropine or glycopyrrolate).
- Monitor baseline electrolyte determinations (electrolyte imbalance can potentiate neuromuscular effects).
- May be preferred for patients with bradycardia.
- Take vital signs every 15 minutes, especially for developing tachycardia. Notify doctor immediately of significant changes.
- Monitor respirations closely until patient is fully recovered from neuromuscular blockade, as evidenced by tests of muscle strength (hand grip, head lift, and ability to cough).

metocurine iodide

Metubine

Pregnancy Risk Category: C

HOW SUPPLIED

Injection: 2 mg/ml

MECHANISM OF ACTION

Prevents acetylcholine from binding to the receptors on the muscle end plate, thus blocking depolarization. Nondepolarizing agent.

INDICATIONS & DOSAGE

Adjunct to anesthesia to induce skeletal muscle relaxation; facilitate intubation, reduction of fractures and dislocations –

Dosage depends on anesthetic used, individual needs, and response. Dosages are representative and must be adjusted. Administer as sustained injection over 30 to 60 seconds.

Adults: given cyclopropane: 2 to 4 mg I.V. (2.68 mg average).

Given ether: 1.5 to 3 mg I.V. (2.1 mg average).

Given nitrous oxide: 4 to 7 mg I.V. (4.79 mg average). Supplemental injections of 0.5 to 1 mg in 25 to 90 minutes, repeated p.r.n.

Lessen muscle contractions in pharmacologically or electrically induced eizures –

Adults: 1.75 to 5.5 mg I.V.

ADVERSE REACTIONS

Common reactions are in italics; life-threatening reactions are in bold italics.

CV: hypotension secondary to histamine release, ganglionic blockade in rapid dose or overdose.

Other: ***dose-related prolonged apnea,*** residual muscle weakness, increased oropharyngeal secretions, allergic or idiosyncratic hypersensitivity reactions, ***bronchospasm.***

INTERACTIONS

Aminoglycoside antibiotics (including amikacin, gentamicin, kanamycin, neomycin, streptomycin); polymyxin antibiotics (polymyxin B sulfate, colistin); clindamycin; quinidine; general anesthetics (such as halothane, enflurane, isoflurane), furosemide, thiazide diuretics, and beta-adrenergic blocking agents: potentiated neuromuscular blockade, leading to increased skeletal muscle relaxation and possible respiratory paralysis. Use cautiously during surgical and postoperative periods.

Narcotic analgesics: potentiated neuromuscular blockade, leading to increased skeletal muscle relaxation and possible respiratory paralysis. Use with extreme caution, and reduce dose of metocurine iodide.

NURSING CONSIDERATIONS

- *Contraindicated* in patients with hypersensitivity to iodides or in whom histamine release is a hazard (asthmatic or atopic patients).
- *Use cautiously* in elderly or debilitated patients; and in renal, hepatic, or pulmonary impairment, respiratory depression, myasthenia gravis, myasthenic syndrome of lung cancer or bronchogenic carcinoma, dehydration, thyroid disorders, collagen diseases, porphyria, electrolyte disturbances, hyperthermia, and (in large doses) cesarean section.
- I.M. administration is not recommended.
- Metocurine should only be used by personnel skilled in airway management.
- Keep airway clear. Have emergency respiratory support equipment (endotracheal equipment, ventilator, oxygen, atropine, edrophonium, epinephrine, and neostigmine) on hand.
- Know that neuromuscular blockers do not obtund consciousness or alter the pain threshold. Patients should receive sedatives or general anesthetics before neuromuscular blockers are administered.
- A nerve stimulator and train-of-four monitoring are recommended to document antagonism of neuromuscular blockade and recovery of muscle strength. Before attempting pharmacologic reversal with neostigmine, some evidence of spontaneous recovery (T_4:T_1 ratio > 0 or T_1 > 10% of control) should be seen. Once spontaneous recovery starts, metocurine-induced neuromuscular blockade may be reversed with an anticholinesterase agent (such as neostigmine or edro-

phonium). Usually administered with an anticholinergic (such as atropine).
• Dose of 1 mg is the therapeutic equivalent of 3 mg *d*-tubocurarine chloride.
• Monitor baseline electrolyte determinations (electrolyte imbalance, especially potassium, calcium, and magnesium, can potentiate neuromuscular effects) and vital signs, especially respiration.
• Measure intake and output (renal dysfunction prolongs duration of action, since drug is mainly unchanged before excretion).
• Monitor respirations closely until patient is fully recovered from neuromuscular blockade, as evidenced by tests of muscle strength (hand grip, head lift, and ability to cough).
• Store solution away from heat, sunlight; do not mix with barbiturates (precipitate will form). Use fresh solutions only.

mivacurium chloride

Mivacron

Pregnancy Risk Category: C

HOW SUPPLIED

Injection: 2 mg/ml in 5-ml and 10-ml vials
Infusion: 0.5 mg/ml in 50 ml dextrose 5% in water (D_5W)

MECHANISM OF ACTION

A nondepolarizing muscle relaxant that competes with acetylcholine for receptor sites at the motor end plate. Because this action may be antagonized by cholinesterase inhibitors, mivacurium is considered a competitive antagonist. The drug is a mixture of three stereoisomers, each possessing neuromuscular blocking activity.

INDICATIONS & DOSAGE

As an adjunct to general anesthesia, to facilitate endotracheal intubation and to relax skeletal muscles during surgery or mechanical ventilation – **Adults:** dosage is highly individualized. Note that all times of onset and duration of neuromuscular blockade are averages and considerable individual variation is normal. Usually, 0.15 mg/kg I.V. push over 5 to 15 seconds provides adequate muscle relaxation within 2½ minutes for endotracheal intubation. Supplemental doses of 0.1 mg/kg I.V. q 15 minutes is usually sufficient to maintain muscle relaxation.

Alternatively, maintain neuromuscular blockade with a continuous infusion of 4 mcg/kg/minute begun simultaneously with the initial dose, or 9 to 10 mcg/kg/minute started after evidence of spontaneous recovery from the initial dose. When used with isoflurane or enflurane anesthesia, dosage is usually reduced about 25%.
Children 2 to 12 years: 0.20 mg/kg I.V. push administered over 5 to 15 seconds. Neuromuscular blockade is usually evident in less than 2 minutes. Maintenance doses are generally required more frequently in children.

Alternatively, maintain neuromuscular blockade with a continuous infusion titrated to effect. Most children respond to 5 to 31 mcg/kg/minute (average 14 mcg/kg/minute).

ADVERSE REACTIONS

Common reactions are in italics; life-threatening reactions are in bold italics.
CNS: dizziness.
CV: *flushing,* hypotension, tachycardia, bradycardia, arrhythmias.
Respiratory: ***bronchospasm,*** wheezing, ***respiratory insufficiency or apnea.***
Skin: rash, urticaria, erythema.
Other: prolonged muscle weakness, phlebitis, muscle spasms.

INTERACTIONS

Alkaline solutions (such as barbiturate solutions): physically incompatible;

*Liquid form contains alcohol. **May contain tartrazine.

may form precipitate. Do not administer through the same I.V. line.
Aminoglycosides (kanamycin, neomycin, streptomycin, and gentamicin), bacitracin, colistin, polymyxin B, colistimethate, and tetracyclines: increased muscle weakness. Use together cautiously.
Magnesium salts: may enhance neuromuscular blockade. Monitor for excessive weakness.
Phenytoin, carbamazepine: may prolong the time to maximal blockade or shorten the duration of blockade with neuromuscular blockers.
Quinidine, inhalational anesthetics (especially isoflurane or enflurane): may enhance the activity (or prolonged action) of nondepolarizing neuromuscular blockers. Monitor for excessive weakness.

NURSING CONSIDERATIONS

- *Contraindicated* in patients with hypersensitivity to the drug.
- *Use cautiously* in patients with significant CV disease and in patients who may be adversely affected by the release of histamine (such as asthmatics). To avoid hypotension, the initial dose of the drug should be lower or the drug should be given over longer periods of time (60 seconds).
- Also use cautiously, possibly at reduced dosage, in debilitated patients, in patients with metastatic cancer, severe electrolyte disturbances, or neuromuscular diseases; and in those in whom potentiation or difficulty in reversal of neuromuscular blockade is anticipated. Patients with myasthenia gravis or myasthenic syndrome (Eaton-Lambert syndrome) are particularly sensitive to the effects of nondepolarizing relaxants. Test doses of 0.015 to 0.020 mg/kg may be used to assess the patient's sensitivity to the drug.
- Drug should be used only under direct medical supervision by personnel familiar with the use of neuromuscular blockers and techniques involved in maintaining a patent airway. It should not be used unless facilities and equipment for artificial respiration, mechanical ventilation, oxygen therapy, intubation, and an antagonist are within reach.
- Drug is metabolized to inactive compounds by plasma pseudocholinesterase. Use very cautiously, if at all, in patients who are homozygous for the atypical plasma pseudocholinesterase gene.
- Like other neuromuscular blockers, dosage requirements for children are higher on a mg/kg basis than those for adults. Onset and recovery of neuromuscular blockade occur more rapidly in children.
- The duration of the drug effect is increased about 150% in patients with end-stage renal disease and 300% in patients with hepatic dysfunction.
- Patients with severe burns are known to develop resistance to nondepolarizing neuromuscular blockers; however, they may also have reduced plasma pseudocholinesterase activity. Administer a test dose to assess the patient's sensitivity to the drug.
- Dosage should be adjusted to ideal body weight in obese patients (patients 30% or more above their ideal weight) because they may experience prolonged neuromuscular blockade.
- A nerve stimulator and train-of-four monitoring are recommended to document antagonism of neuromuscular blockade and recovery of muscle strength. Before attempting pharmacologic reversal with neostigmine or edrophonium, some signs of spontaneous recovery should be evident.
- Experimental evidence suggests that acid-base and electrolyte balance may influence the actions of nondepolarizing neuromuscular blockers. Alkalosis may counteract the paralysis; acidosis may enhance it.
- Monitor respirations closely until patient is fully recovered from neuro-

muscular blockade as evidenced by tests of muscle strength (hand grip, head lift, and ability to cough).

- Note that mivacurium, like other neuromuscular blockers, has no effect on consciousness or pain threshold. To avoid distress to the patient, this drug should not be administered until the patient's consciousness is obtunded by the general anesthetic.
- **I.V. use:** When administered I.V. push to adults who are receiving anesthetic combinations of nitrous oxide and opiates, neuromuscular blockade usually lasts 15 to 20 minutes; most patients recover 95% of their muscle strength in 25 to 30 minutes.
- Drug is compatible with D_5W, 0.9% sodium chloride injection, dextrose 5% in 0.9% sodium chloride injection, lactated Ringer's injection, and dextrose 5% in lactated Ringer's injection. Diluted solutions are stable for 24 hours at room temperature.
- When diluted as directed, mivacurium is compatible with alfentanil, fentanyl, sufentanil, droperidol, and midazolam.
- Drug is also available as premixed infusion in D_5W. After removing the protective outer wrap, check container for minor leaks by squeezing the bag before administering. Do not add any other drugs to the container, and do not use the container in series connections.

pancuronium bromide

Pavulon

Pregnancy Risk Category: C

HOW SUPPLIED

Injection: 1 mg/ml, 2 mg/ml

MECHANISM OF ACTION

Prevents acetylcholine from binding to the receptors on the muscle end plate, thus blocking depolarization. Nondepolarizing agent.

INDICATIONS & DOSAGE

Adjunct to anesthesia to induce skeletal muscle relaxation; facilitate intubation; lessen muscle contractions in pharmacologically or electrically induced seizures; assist with mechanical ventilation –

Dosage depends on anesthetic used, individual needs, and response. Dosages are representative and must be adjusted.

Adults: initially, 0.04 to 0.1 mg/kg I.V.; then 0.01 mg/kg q 30 to 60 minutes.

Children over 10 years: initially, 0.04 to 0.1 mg/kg I.V., then 1/5 initial dose q 30 to 60 minutes.

ADVERSE REACTIONS

Common reactions are in italics; life-threatening reactions are in bold italics.

CV: tachycardia, increased blood pressure.

Skin: transient rashes.

Local: burning sensation.

Other: excessive sweating and salivation, ***prolonged dose-related apnea,*** wheezing, residual muscle weakness, allergic or idiosyncratic hypersensitivity reactions.

INTERACTIONS

Aminoglycoside antibiotics (including amikacin, gentamicin, kanamycin, neomycin, streptomycin); polymyxin antibiotics (polymyxin B sulfate, colistin); clindamycin; quinidine; general anesthetics (such as halothane, enflurane, isoflurane): potentiated neuromuscular blockade, leading to increased skeletal muscle relaxation and possible respiratory paralysis. Use cautiously during surgical and postoperative periods.

Lithium, narcotic analgesics: potentiated neuromuscular blockade, leading to increased skeletal muscle relaxation and possible respiratory paralysis. Use with extreme caution, and reduce dose of pancuronium.

*Liquid form contains alcohol. **May contain tartrazine.

NURSING CONSIDERATIONS

- *Contraindicated* in hypersensitivity to bromides; preexisting tachycardia; and in patients for whom even a minor increase in heart rate is undesirable.
- *Use cautiously* in elderly or debilitated patients; renal, hepatic, or pulmonary impairment; respiratory depression; myasthenia gravis; myasthenic syndrome of lung cancer or bronchogenic carcinoma; dehydration; thyroid disorders; collagen diseases; porphyria; electrolyte disturbances; hyperthermia; toxemic states; and (in large doses) cesarean section.
- Pancuronium should be used only by personnel experienced in airway management.
- Have emergency respiratory support equipment (endotracheal equipment, ventilator, oxygen, atropine, edrophonium, epinephrine, and neostigmine) on hand.
- Know that neuromuscular blockers do not obtund consciousness or alter the pain threshold. Patients should receive sedatives or general anesthetics before neuromuscular blockers are administered.
- Drug does not cause histamine release or hypotension, but may raise heart rate and blood pressure.
- Dose of 1 mg is the approximate therapeutic equivalent of 5 mg *d*-tubocurarine chloride.
- Monitor baseline electrolyte determinations (electrolyte imbalance can potentiate neuromuscular effects) and vital signs (watch respiration and heart rate closely).
- Measure intake and output (renal dysfunction may prolong duration of action, since 25% of the drug is unchanged before excretion).
- A nerve stimulator and train-of-four monitoring are recommended to confirm antagonism of neuromuscular blockade and recovery of muscle strength. Before attempting pharmacologic reversal with neostigmine, some evidence of spontaneous recovery (T_4:T_1 ratio > 0 or T_1 > 10% of control) should be seen.
- Once spontaneous recovery starts, pancuronium-induced neuromuscular blockade may be reversed with an anticholinesterase agent (such as neostigmine or edrophonium). Usually administered with an anticholinergic (such as atropine).
- Monitor respirations closely until patient is fully recovered from neuromuscular blockade, as evidenced by tests of muscle strength (hand grip, head lift, and ability to cough).
- Allow succinylcholine effects to subside before giving pancuronium.
- **I.V. use:** Do not mix with barbiturate solutions (precipitate will form); use only fresh solutions.
- Store in refrigerator. Do not store in plastic containers or syringes, although plastic syringes may be used for administration.

pipecuronium bromide

Arduan

Pregnancy Risk Category: C

HOW SUPPLIED

Powder for injection: 10 mg/vial

MECHANISM OF ACTION

A nondepolarizing muscle relaxant that competes with acetylcholine for receptor sites at the motor end-plate. Because this action may be antagonized by cholinesterase inhibitors, pipecuronium is considered a competitive antagonist.

INDICATIONS & DOSAGE

To provide skeletal muscle relaxation during surgery as a adjunct to general anesthesia –

Adults and children: dosage is highly individualized. The following doses may serve as a guide for use in nonobese patients with normal renal function. Initially, 70 to 85 mcg/kg I.V. provides conditions considered

†Available in Canada only. ‡Available in Australia only. ◊Available OTC.

ideal for endotracheal intubation and maintains paralysis for 1 to 2 hours. If succinylcholine is used for endotracheal intubation, initial doses of 50 mcg/kg I.V. provide good relaxation for 45 minutes or more. Maintenance doses of 10 to 15 mcg/kg provide relaxation for about 50 minutes.

ADVERSE REACTIONS

Common reactions are in italics; life-threatening reactions are in bold italics.

CV: hypotension, bradycardia, hypertension, myocardial ischemia, *CVA,* thrombosis, atrial fibrillation, ***ventricular extrasystole.***

GU: anuria.

Metabolic: increased creatinine levels.

Respiratory: dyspnea, respiratory depression, ***respiratory insufficiency or apnea.***

Other: prolonged muscle weakness.

INTERACTIONS

Aminoglycosides (kanamycin, neomycin, streptomycin, dihydrostreptomycin, and gentamicin), bacitracin, colistin, polymyxin B, colistimethate, and tetracyclines: increased muscle weakness. Use together cautiously.

Magnesium salts: may enhance neuromuscular blockade. Monitor for excessive weakness.

Quinidine, inhalational anesthetics: enhanced activity (or prolonged action) of nondepolarizing neuromuscular blocking agents.

NURSING CONSIDERATIONS

- *Contraindicated* in patients with hypersensitivity to the drug.
- This drug should be used only under direct medical supervision by persons familiar with the use of neuromuscular blockers and techniques involved in maintaining a patent airway. Drug should not be used unless facilities and equipment for artificial respiration, mechanical ventilation, oxygen therapy, intubation, and an antagonist are within reach.
- Because of the lack of data supporting safety, this drug is not recommended for use in patients requiring prolonged mechanical ventilation in the intensive care unit. It is not recommended before or after other nondepolarizing neuromuscular blockers. It is also not recommended for use during cesarean section because safety of the neonate has not been established and because this drug's long duration of action exceeds the duration of the procedure.
- Know that neuromuscular blockers do not obtund consciousness or alter the pain threshold. Patients should receive sedatives or general anesthetics before neuromuscular blockers are administered.
- Pipecuronium may be administered after succinylcholine when the latter is used to facilitate intubation. However, there is no evidence to support the safe use of pipecuronium before succinylcholine to decrease adverse effects of the latter drug.
- Because the drug is excreted by the kidneys, use with caution in patients with renal failure. No information is available regarding the use of the drug in patients with hepatic disease.
- Patients with myasthenia gravis or myasthenic syndrome (Eaton-Lambert syndrome) are particularly sensitive to the effects of nondepolarizing relaxants. Shorter-acting agents are recommended for use in such patients.
- Not recommended for use in neonates and infants younger than 3 months. Limited evidence suggests that infants and children (1 to 14 years) under balanced anesthesia or halothane anesthesia may be less sensitive than adults.
- Dosage should be adjusted to ideal body weight in obese patients. (30% or more over their ideal weight) because prolonged neuromuscular

blockade has been reported in such patients.
• Because the drug has minimal vagolytic action, bradycardia during anesthesia may be common.
• A nerve stimulator and train-of-four monitoring are recommended to document antagonism of neuromuscular blockade and recovery of muscle strength. Before attempting pharmacologic reversal with neostigmine, some evidence of spontaneous recovery (T_4:T_1 ratio > 0 or T_1 > 10% of control) should be evident.
• Experimental evidence suggests that acid-base and electrolyte balance may influence the actions of nondepolarizing neuromuscular blocking agents. Alkalosis may counteract the paralysis and acidosis may enhance it.
• Because of its prolonged duration of action, pipecuronium is recommended only for procedures that take 90 minutes or longer.
• Monitor respirations closely until patient is fully recovered from neuromuscular blockade, as evidenced by tests of muscle strength (hand grip, head lift, and ability to cough).
• **I.V. use:** Reconstitute with 10 ml solution before use to yield a solution of 1 mg/ml. Large volumes of diluent or addition of the drug to a hanging I.V. solution is not recommended.
• After reconstitution with sterile water for injection or other compatible I.V. solutions (such as 0.9% sodium chloride injection, dextrose 5% in water, lactated Ringer's injection, dextrose 5% in saline), the drug is stable for 24 hours if refrigerated.
• After reconstitution with any solution other than bacteriostatic water for injection, discard unused drug.
• After reconstitution with bacteriostatic water for injection, the drug is stable for 5 days at room temperature or in the refrigerator. Note that bacteriostatic water contains benzyl alcohol and is not intended for use in neonates.
• Store the powder at room temperature or in the refrigerator (36° to 86° F [2° to 30° C]).

succinylcholine chloride (suxamethonium chloride)

Anectine, Anectine Flo-Pack, Quelicin, Scoline‡, Sucostrin
Pregnancy Risk Category: C

HOW SUPPLIED
Injection: 20 mg/ml, 50 mg/ml, 100 mg/ml; 100 mg/vial, 500 mg/vial, 1 g/vial

MECHANISM OF ACTION
Prolongs depolarization of the muscle end plate. Depolarizing agent.

INDICATIONS & DOSAGE
Adjunct to anesthesia to induce skeletal muscle relaxation; facilitate intubation and assist with mechanical ventilation or orthopedic manipulations (drug of choice); lessen muscle contractions in pharmacologically or electrically induced seizures –
Dosage depends on anesthetic used, individual needs, and response. Dosages are representative and must be adjusted.
Adults: 25 to 75 mg I.V., then 2.5 mg/minute, p.r.n., or 2.5 mg/kg I.M. up to maximum of 150 mg I.M. in deltoid muscle.
Children: 1 to 2 mg/kg I.M. or I.V. Maximum I.M. dosage is 150 mg. (Children may be less sensitive to succinylcholine than adults.)

ADVERSE REACTIONS
Common reactions are in italics; life-threatening reactions are in bold italics.
CV: bradycardia, tachycardia, hypertension, hypotension, ***arrhythmias.***
EENT: increased intraocular pressure.
Other: ***prolonged respiratory depression, apnea, malignant hyperthermia,*** muscle fasciculation, *postoper-*

ative muscle pain, myoglobinemia, excessive salivation, allergic or idiosyncratic hypersensitivity reactions.

INTERACTIONS

Aminoglycoside antibiotics (including amikacin, gentamicin, kanamycin, neomycin, streptomycin); polymyxin antibiotics (polymyxin B sulfate, colistin); cholinesterase inhibitors (such as neostigmine, pyridostigmine, edrophonium, physostigmine, or echothiophate); general anesthetics (such as halothane, enflurane, isoflurane): potentiated neuromuscular blockade, leading to increased skeletal muscle relaxation and possible respiratory paralysis. Use cautiously during surgical and postoperative periods.

Digitalis glycosides: possible cardiac arrhythmias. Use together cautiously.

Magnesium sulfate (parenterally): potentiated neuromuscular blockade, increased skeletal muscle relaxation, and possible respiratory paralysis. Use with caution, preferably with reduced doses.

MAO inhibitors, lithium, cyclophosphamide: prolonged apnea. Use with caution.

Narcotic analgesics, methotrimeprazine: potentiated neuromuscular blockade, leading to increased skeletal muscle relaxation and possible respiratory paralysis. Use with extreme caution.

NURSING CONSIDERATIONS

- *Contraindicated* in abnormally low plasma pseudocholinesterase.
- *Use cautiously* in elderly or debilitated patients; patients with personal or family history of malignant hypertension or hyperthermia; hepatic, renal, or pulmonary impairment; and in respiratory depression, severe burns or trauma, electrolyte imbalances, quinidine or digitalis therapy, hyperkalemia, paraplegia, spinal neuraxis injury, degenerative or dystrophic neuromuscular disease, myasthenia gravis, myasthenic syndrome of lung cancer or bronchogenic carcinoma, dehydration, thyroid disorders, collagen diseases, porphyria, fractures, muscle spasms, glaucoma, eye surgery or penetrating eye wounds, pheochromocytoma, and (in large doses) cesarean section.
- Succinylcholine should be used only by personnel experienced in airway management.
- Keep airway clear. Have emergency respiratory support equipment (endotracheal equipment, ventilator, oxygen, atropine, and epinephrine) on hand.
- Unlike nondepolarizing agents, neostigmine or edrophonium may worsen neuromuscular blockade. Don't use reversing agents.
- Know that neuromuscular blockers do not obtund consciousness or alter the pain threshold. Patients should receive sedatives or general anesthetics before neuromuscular blockers are administered.
- Drug of choice for short procedures (less than 3 minutes) and for orthopedic manipulations; use caution in fractures or dislocations.
- Duration of action prolonged to 20 minutes by continuous I.V. infusion.
- Repeated or continuous infusions of succinylcholine alone not advised; may cause reduced response or prolonged muscle relaxation and apnea.
- Monitor baseline electrolyte determinations and vital signs (check respiration every 5 to 10 minutes during infusion).
- Reassure patient that postoperative stiffness is normal and will soon subside.
- **I.V. use:** Give test dose (10 mg I.M. or I.V.) after patient has been anesthetized. Normal response (no respiratory depression or transient depression for up to 5 minutes) indicates drug may be given. Do not give if patient develops respiratory paralysis sufficient to permit endotracheal intu-

*Liquid form contains alcohol. **May contain tartrazine.

bation. (Recovery within 30 to 60 minutes.)
- Store injectable form in refrigerator. Store powder form at room temperature, tightly closed. Use immediately after reconstitution. Do not mix with alkaline solutions (thiopental sodium, sodium bicarbonate, barbiturates).
- Monitor respirations closely until patient is fully recovered from neuromuscular blockade, as evidenced by tests of muscle strength (hand grip, head lift, and ability to cough).
- If given I.M., give deep I.M., preferably high into the deltoid muscle.

tubocurarine chloride

Tubarine†

Pregnancy Risk Category: C

HOW SUPPLIED
Injection: 3 mg (20 units)/ml; 10 mg/ml‡

MECHANISM OF ACTION
Prevents acetylcholine from binding to the receptors on the muscle end plate, thus blocking depolarization. Nondepolarizing agent.

INDICATIONS & DOSAGE
Adjunct to anesthesia to induce skeletal muscle relaxation; facilitate intubation, orthopedic manipulations –
Dosage depends on anesthetic used, individual needs, and response. Dosages listed are representative and must be adjusted.
Adults: 1 unit/kg or 0.15 mg/kg I.V. slowly over 60 to 90 seconds. Average, initially, 40 to 60 units I.V. May give 20 to 30 units in 3 to 5 minutes. For longer procedures, give 20 units, p.r.n.
Children: 1 unit/kg or 0.15 mg/kg.
Assist with mechanical ventilation –
Adults and children: initially, 0.0165 mg/kg I.V. (average 1 mg or 7 units), then adjust subsequent doses to patient's response.
Lessen muscle contractions in pharmacologically or electrically induced seizures –
Adults and children: 1 unit/kg or 0.15 mg/kg slowly over 60 to 90 seconds. Initial dose is 20 units (3 mg) less than calculated dose.

ADVERSE REACTIONS
Common reactions are in italics; life-threatening reactions are in bold italics.
CV: hypotension, circulatory depression.
Other: profound and prolonged muscle relaxation, ***respiratory depression or apnea,*** hypersensitivity, idiosyncrasy, residual muscle weakness, increased salivation, ***bronchospasm.***

INTERACTIONS
Aminoglycoside antibiotics (including amikacin, gentamicin, kanamycin, neomycin, streptomycin); polymyxin antibiotics (polymyxin B sulfate, colistin); general anesthetics (such as halothane, enflurane, isoflurane): potentiated neuromuscular blockade, leading to increased skeletal muscle relaxation and possible respiratory paralysis. Use cautiously during surgical and postoperative periods.
Quinidine: prolonged neuromuscular blockade. Use together with caution. Monitor closely.
Thiazide diuretics, furosemide, ethacrynic acid, amphotericin B, propranolol, methotrimeprazine, narcotic analgesics: potentiated neuromuscular blockade, leading to increased respiratory paralysis. Use with extreme caution during surgical and postoperative periods.

NURSING CONSIDERATIONS
- *Contraindicated* in patients for whom histamine release is a hazard (asthmatics).
- *Use cautiously* in elderly or debilitated patients; in hepatic or pulmo-

nary impairment, respiratory depression, myasthenia gravis, myasthenic syndrome of lung cancer or bronchogenic carcinoma, dehydration, thyroid disorders, collagen diseases, porphyria, electrolyte disturbances, fractures, muscle spasms, and (in large doses) cesarean section. Contains benzyl alcohol, which should not be used in neonates.

- Tubocurarine should be used only by personnel experienced in airway management.
- Keep airway clear. Have emergency respiratory support equipment (endotracheal equipment, ventilator, oxygen, atropine, edrophonium, epinephrine, and neostigmine) on hand.
- Know that neuromuscular blockers do not obtund consciousness or alter the pain threshold. Patients should receive sedatives or general anesthetics before neuromuscular blockers are administered.
- Allow succinylcholine effects to subside before giving tubocurarine.
- Monitor baseline electrolyte determinations (electrolyte imbalance can potentiate neuromuscular blocking effects).
- A nerve stimulator and train-of-four monitoring are recommended to confirm antagonism of neuromuscular blockade and recovery of muscle strength. Before attempting pharmacologic reversal with neostigmine, some evidence of spontaneous recovery (T_4:T_1 ratio > 0 or T_1 > 10% of control) should be seen. Once spontaneous recovery starts, tubocurarine-induced neuromuscular blockade may be reversed with an anticholinesterase agent (such as neostigmine or edrophonium). Usually administered with an anticholinergic (such as atropine).
- Monitor respirations closely until patient is fully recovered from neuromuscular blockade, as evidenced by tests of muscle strength (hand grip, head lift, and ability to cough).
- Check vital signs every 15 minutes. Notify doctor at once of changes.
- Measure intake and output (renal dysfunction prolongs duration of action, since much of drug is unchanged before excretion).
- **I.V. use:** Give I.V. slowly (60 to 90 seconds).
- Do not mix with barbiturates (precipitate will form). Use only fresh solutions and discard if discolored.
- Give deep I.M. in deltoid muscle.

vecuronium bromide

Norcuron

Pregnancy Risk Category: C

HOW SUPPLIED

Injection: 10 mg/vial

MECHANISM OF ACTION

Prevents acetylcholine from binding to the receptors on the muscle end plate, thus blocking depolarization. Nondepolarizing agent.

INDICATIONS & DOSAGE

Adjunct to general anesthesia, to facilitate endotracheal intubation and to provide skeletal muscle relaxation during surgery or mechanical ventilation –

Dosage depends on anesthetic used, individual needs, and response. Dosages are representative and must be adjusted.

Adults and children over 9 years: Initially, 0.08 to 0.10 mg/kg I.V. bolus. Maintenance doses of 0.010 to 0.015 mg/kg within 25 to 40 minutes of initial dose should be administered during prolonged surgical procedures. Maintenance doses may be given q 12 to 15 minutes in patients receiving balanced anesthesia.

Children under 9 years: may require a slightly higher initial dose and may also require supplementation slightly more often than adults. Alternatively, drug may be given by continuous I.V.

*Liquid form contains alcohol. **May contain tartrazine.

infusion of 1 mcg/kg/minute initially, than 0.8 to 1.2 mcg/kg/minute.

ADVERSE REACTIONS

Common reactions are in italics; life-threatening reactions are in bold italics.

CV: transient increases in heart rate.

Local: redness, itching, induration.

Other: ***prolonged dose-related apnea.***

INTERACTIONS

Aminoglycoside antibiotics (including amikacin, gentamicin, kanamycin, neomycin, streptomycin); polymyxin antibiotics (polymyxin B sulfate, colistin); clindamycin; quinidine; general anesthetics (such as halothane, enflurane, isoflurane): potentiated neuromuscular blockade, leading to increased skeletal muscle relaxation and possible respiratory paralysis. Use cautiously during surgical and postoperative periods.

Narcotic analgesics: potentiated neuromuscular blockade, leading to increased skeletal muscle relaxation and possible respiratory paralysis. Use with extreme caution, and reduce dose of vecuronium.

NURSING CONSIDERATIONS

- *Contraindicated* in hypersensitivity to bromides. *Use cautiously* in altered circulation time from cardiovascular disease, old age, and edematous states; in hepatic disease; in severe obesity; in bronchogenic carcinoma; and in neuromuscular disease.
- Vecuronium should be used only by personnel experienced in airway management.
- Keep airway clear. Have emergency respiratory support equipment (endotracheal equipment, ventilator, oxygen, atropine, edrophonium, epinephrine, and neostigmine) on hand.
- Know that neuromuscular blockers do not obtund consciousness or alter the pain threshold. Patients should receive sedatives or general anesthetics before neuromuscular blockers are administered.
- Unlike other nondepolarizing neuromuscular blockers, vecuronium has no effect on cardiovascular system. Also, the drug causes no histamine release and therefore no histamine-related hypersensitivity reactions, such as bronchospasm, hypotension, or tachycardia.
- The drug is well tolerated in renal failure.
- Prior administration of succinylcholine may enhance the neuromuscular blocking effect and duration of action.
- Vecuronium provides conditions for intubation within 3 minutes. The duration of effect is 25 to 40 minutes.
- A nerve stimulator and train-of-four monitoring are recommended to confirm antagonism of neuromuscular blockade and recovery of muscle strength. Before attempting pharmacologic reversal with neostigmine, some evidence of spontaneous recovery (T_4:T_1 ratio > 0 or $T_1 > 10\%$ of control) should be seen. Once spontaneous recovery starts, vecuronium-induced neuromuscular blockade may be reversed with an anticholinesterase agent (such as neostigmine or edrophonium). Usually administered with an anticholinergic (such as atropine).
- Monitor respirations closely until patient is fully recovered from neuromuscular blockade, as evidenced by tests of muscle strength (hand grip, head lift, and ability to cough).
- Store reconstituted solution in refrigerator. Discard after 24 hours.

42

Antihistamines

astemizole
azatadine maleate
brompheniramine maleate
chlorpheniramine maleate
clemastine fumarate
cyproheptadine hydrochloride
dexchlorpheniramine maleate
diphenhydramine hydrochloride
loratadine
methdilazine hydrochloride
promethazine hydrochloride
terfenadine
trimeprazine tartrate
tripelennamine citrate
tripelennamine hydrochloride
triprolidine hydrochloride

COMBINATION PRODUCTS

ALLEREST TABLETS◇: phenylpropanolamine hydrochloride 18.7 mg and chlorpheniramine maleate 2 mg.
ALLERGESIC: phenylpropanolamine hydrochloride 18.7 mg and chlorpheniramine maleate 2 mg.
BROMFED-AT: brompheniramine maleate 2 mg, dextromethorphan hydrobromide 10 mg, and pseudoephedrine hydrochloride 30 mg/5 ml.
CHLOR-TRIMETON DECONGESTANT◇: chlorpheniramine maleate 4 mg and pseudoephedrine sulfate 60 mg.
CHLOR-TRIMETON DECONGESTANT REPETABS◇: chlorpheniramine maleate 8 mg and pseudoephedrine sulfate 120 mg.
CODIMAL DH*: hydrocodone bitartrate 1.66 mg, phenylephrine hydrochloride 5 mg, pyrilamine maleate 8.33 mg, potassium guaiacolsulfonate 83.3 mg, sodium citrate 216 mg, and citric acid 50 mg.
CONDRIN-LA: phenylpropanolamine hydrochloride 75 mg and chlorpheniramine maleate 12 mg.
CONTAC CAPSULES◇: phenylpropanolamine 75 mg and chlorpheniramine maleate 8 mg.
CONTAC 12-HOUR CAPLETS◇: phenylpropanolamine 75 mg and chlorpheniramine maleate 12 mg.
CORICIDIN TABLETS◇: chlorpheniramine maleate 2 mg and acetaminophen 325 mg.
DECONADE: phenylpropanolamine hydrochloride 75 mg and chlorpheniramine maleate 12 mg.
DECONAMINE: pseudoephedrine hydrochloride 60 mg and chlorpheniramine maleate 4 mg.
DIMETAPP EXTENTABS: brompheniramine maleate 12 mg, and phenylpropanolamine hydrochloride 75 mg.
DISOPHROL CHRONOTABS◇: dexbrompheniramine maleate 6 mg and pseudoephedrine sulfate 120 mg.
DRIXORAL◇: dexbrompheniramine maleate 6 mg and pseudoephedrine sulfate 120 mg.
DRIZE: phenylpropanolamine hydrochloride 75 mg and chlorpheniramine maleate 12 mg.
FEDAHIST: pseudoephedrine hydrochloride 60 mg and chlorpheniramine maleate 4 mg.
HISTABID DURACAPS: phenylpropanolamine 75 mg and chlorpheniramine maleate 8 mg.
HISTASPAN-D: chlorpheniramine maleate 8 mg, phenylephrine hydrochloride 20 mg, and methscopolamine nitrate 2.5 mg.
NALDECON: phenylephrine hydrochloride 10 mg, phenylpropanolamine hydrochloride 40 mg, phenyltoloxamine citrate 15 mg, and chlorpheniramine maleate 5 mg.
NEOTEP-GRANUCAPS: chlorpheniramine maleate 9 mg and phenylephrine hydrochloride 21 mg.
NOLAMINE: chlorpheniramine maleate 4 mg, phenindamine tartrate 24

*Liquid form contains alcohol. **May contain tartrazine.

mg, and phenylpropanolamine hydrochloride 50 mg.
NOVAFED A: pseudoephedrine hydrochloride 120 mg and chlorpheniramine maleate 8 mg.
NOVAHISTINE ELIXIR◇*: phenylephrine 5 mg, chlorpheniramine maleate 2 mg, and alcohol 5%/5 ml.
ORAHIST: phenylpropanolamine hydrochloride 75 mg and chlorpheniramine maleate 12 mg.
ORNADE SPANSULES: phenylpropanolamine hydrochloride 75 mg and chlorpheniramine maleate 12 mg.
RHINEX D-LAY: acetaminophen 300 mg, salicylamide 300 mg, phenylpropanolamine hydrochloride 60 mg, and chlorpheniramine maleate 4 mg.
RONDEC: carbinoxamine maleate 4 mg and pseudoephedrine hydrochloride 60 mg.
SELDANE-D: terfenadine 60 mg and pseudoephedrine hydrochloride 120 mg.
SUDAFED PLUS◇: pseudoephedrine hydrochloride 60 mg and chlorpheniramine maleate 4 mg.
TAVIST-D◇: clemastine fumarate 1.34 mg and phenylpropanolamine 75 mg.
TRIAMINIC-12: phenylpropanolamine hydrochloride 75 mg and chlorpheniramine maleate 12 mg.
TRIAMINIC EXTENDED-RELEASE TABLETS†: phenylpropanolamine hydrochloride 50 mg, pheniramine maleate 25 mg, and pyrilamine maleate 25 mg.
TRINALIN REPETABS: azatadine maleate 1 mg and pseudoephedrine sulfate 120 mg.

astemizole

Hismanal

Pregnancy Risk Category: C

HOW SUPPLIED

Tablets: 10 mg
Oral suspension: 2 mg/ml*‡

MECHANISM OF ACTION

Blocks the effects of histamine at H_1 receptors. Astemizole is a nonsedating antihistamine because its chemical structure prevents entry into the CNS.

INDICATIONS AND DOSAGE

Relief of symptoms associated with chronic idiopathic urticaria and seasonal allergic rhinitis –
Adults and children over 12 years: 10 mg P.O. daily. A loading dose may be given in order to achieve steady-state plasma levels quickly. Begin therapy at 30 mg on the first day, followed by 20 mg on the second day, and 10 mg daily thereafter.

ADVERSE REACTIONS

Common reactions are in italics; life-threatening reactions are in bold italics.
CV: arrhythmias (with overdose).
CNS: headache, nervousness, dizziness, drowsiness.
EENT: dry mouth, pharyngitis, conjunctivitis.
GI: nausea, diarrhea, abdominal pain, increased appetite.
Other: arthralgia, weight gain, cholestatic jaundice.

INTERACTIONS

Itraconazole, ketoconazole, or macrolide antibiotics such as erythromycin: risk of serious adverse cardiac reactions. Don't use together.

NURSING CONSIDERATIONS

- *Contraindicated* in patients with hypersensitivity to astemizole and in those taking the antifungal agents itraconazole or ketoconazole or the macrolide antibiotics azithromycin, clarithromycin, erythromycin, or troleandomycin.
- Be sure the patient understands that this drug should only be taken once a day. If symptoms persist or worsen, he should contact the doctor. He should not increase the dose, because

†Available in Canada only. ‡Available in Australia only. ◇Available OTC.

high doses may increase risk of cardiac arrhythmias.
• *Use cautiously* in patients with hepatic or renal disease. Astemizole is not believed to be dialyzable.
• Instruct patient to take this drug on an empty stomach at least 2 hours after a meal and to avoid eating for at least 1 hour after dosing.
• Because of its potential for anticholinergic effects, also use cautiously in patients with lower respiratory diseases (including asthma) because drying effects can increase the risk of bronchial mucus plug formation.
• Warn patient not to increase dosage without consulting the doctor.
• Warn patient to stop taking drug 4 days before allergy skin tests to preserve accuracy of tests.

azatadine maleate

Optimine, Zadine‡

Pregnancy Risk Category: B

HOW SUPPLIED

Tablets: 1 mg
Syrup: 0.5 mg/5 ml‡

MECHANISM OF ACTION

Competes with histamine for H_1-receptor sites on effector cells. Prevents but does not reverse histamine-mediated responses.

INDICATIONS & DOSAGE

Rhinitis, allergy symptoms, chronic urticaria –
Adults: 1 to 2 mg P.O. b.i.d. Maximum dosage is 4 mg daily.

Not intended for children under 12 years.

ADVERSE REACTIONS

Common reactions are in italics; life-threatening reactions are in bold italics.
Blood: thrombocytopenia.
CNS: (especially in elderly patients) *drowsiness, dizziness,* vertigo, disturbed coordination.
CV: hypotension, palpitations.
GI: anorexia, nausea, vomiting, *dry mouth and throat,* epigastric distress.
GU: urine retention.
Skin: urticaria, rash.
Other: thick bronchial secretions.

INTERACTIONS

CNS depressants: increased sedation. Use together cautiously.
MAO inhibitors: increased anticholinergic effects. Don't use together.

NURSING CONSIDERATIONS

• *Contraindicated* in acute asthmatic attacks.
• *Use cautiously* in elderly patients and in increased intraocular pressure, hyperthyroidism, cardiovascular or renal disease, hypertension, bronchial asthma, urine retention, prostatic hypertrophy, bladder-neck obstruction, and stenosing peptic ulcers.
• Warn patient against drinking alcoholic beverages during therapy and against activities that require alertness until CNS response to drug is determined.
• Reduce GI distress by giving with food or milk.
• Coffee or tea may reduce drowsiness. Sugarless gum or sour hard candy, or ice chips may relieve dry mouth.
• If tolerance develops, another antihistamine may be substituted.
• Warn patient to stop taking drug 4 days before allergy skin tests to preserve accuracy of tests.
• Monitor blood counts during long-term therapy; watch for signs of blood dyscrasia.
• Antihistamines are not recommended for use by women who are breast-feeding because small amounts of drug are excreted in breast milk.

brompheniramine maleate

Brombay◇, Bromphen*◇, Chlorphed◇, Codimal-A, Conjec-B◇, Cophene-B, Dehist, Diamine TD, Dimetane*◇, Dimetane Extentabs◇, Dimetane-Ten◇, Histaject Modified, Nasahist B, ND-Stat Revised, Oraminic II, Sinusol-B, Veltane

Pregnancy Risk Category: C

HOW SUPPLIED

Tablets: 4 mg◇
Tablets (timed-release): 8 mg◇, 12 mg◇
Elixir: 2 mg/5 ml*◇
Injection: 10 mg/ml

MECHANISM OF ACTION

Competes with histamine for H_1-receptor sites on effector cells. Prevents but does not reverse histamine-mediated responses.

INDICATIONS & DOSAGE

Rhinitis, allergy symptoms –
Adults: 4 to 8 mg P.O. t.i.d. or q.i.d.; or (timed-release) 8 to 12 mg P.O. b.i.d. or t.i.d.; or 5 to 20 mg q 6 to 12 hours I.M., I.V., or S.C. Maximum dosage is 40 mg daily.
Children over 6 years: 2 to 4 mg P.O. t.i.d. or q.i.d.; or (timed-release) 8 to 12 mg q 12 hours; or 0.5 mg/kg I.M., I.V., or S.C. daily divided t.i.d. or q.i.d.
Children under 6 years: 0.5 mg/kg P.O., I.M., I.V., or S.C. daily divided t.i.d. or q.i.d.

Note: Children under 12 years should use only as directed by a doctor.

ADVERSE REACTIONS

Common reactions are in italics; life-threatening reactions are in bold italics.
Blood: thrombocytopenia, ***agranulocytosis.***
CNS: (especially in elderly patients) dizziness, tremors, irritability, insomnia, *drowsiness, stimulation.*
CV: hypotension, palpitations.
GI: anorexia, nausea, vomiting, *dry mouth and throat.*
GU: urine retention.
Skin: urticaria, rash.
After parenteral administration: local reaction, sweating, syncope.

INTERACTIONS

CNS depressants: increased sedation. Use together cautiously.
MAO inhibitors: increased anticholinergic effects. Don't use together.

NURSING CONSIDERATIONS

- *Contraindicated* in acute asthmatic attacks.
- *Use cautiously* in elderly patients, breast-feeding women, and in patients with increased intraocular pressure, hyperthyroidism, cardiovascular or renal disease, hypertension, bronchial asthma, urine retention, prostatic hypertrophy, bladder-neck obstruction, and stenosing peptic ulcers.
- Warn patient against drinking alcohol during therapy and against activities that require alertness until adverse CNS effects are known.
- Reduce GI distress by giving with food or milk.
- Causes less drowsiness than some other antihistamines.
- Coffee or tea may reduce drowsiness. Sugarless gum or sour hard candy, or ice chips may relieve dry mouth.
- If tolerance develops, another antihistamine may be substituted.
- Warn patient to stop taking drug 4 days before allergy skin tests to preserve accuracy of tests.
- **I.V. use:** Injectable form containing 10 mg/ml can be given diluted or undiluted very slowly I.V. The 100 mg/ml injection should not be given I.V.
- Monitor blood count during long-term therapy; observe for signs of blood dyscrasia.

• Antihistamines are not recommended for use by women who are breast-feeding because small amounts of drug are excreted in breast milk.

chlorpheniramine maleate

Aller-Chlor*◇, Allergex‡, Chlo-Amine◇, Chlor-100◇, Chlorate◇, Chlor-Niramine◇, Chlor-Pro, Chlor-Pro 10, Chlorspan-12, Chlortab-4, Chlortab-8, Chlor-Trimeton*◇, Chlor-Trimeton Repetabs◇, Chlor-Tripolon†◇, Genallerate◇, Novopheniram‡◇, Pfeiffer's Allergy◇, Phenetron*, Piriton‡, Pyranistan◇, Telachlor, Teldrin◇, Trymegen◇

Pregnancy Risk Category: B

HOW SUPPLIED

Tablets: 4 mg◇
Tablets (chewable): 2 mg◇
Tablets (timed-release): 8 mg◇, 12 mg◇
Capsules (timed-release): 8 mg◇, 12 mg◇
Syrup: 2 mg/5 ml*◇
Injection: 10 mg/ml, 100 mg/ml

MECHANISM OF ACTION

Competes with histamine for H_1-receptor sites on effector cells. Prevents but does not reverse histamine-mediated responses.

INDICATIONS & DOSAGE

Rhinitis, allergy symptoms –
Adults: 4 mg P.O. q 4 to 6 hours, not to exceed 24 mg/day; or (timed-release) 8 mg P.O. every 12 hours; or 5 to 40 mg I.M., I.V., or S.C. daily. Give I.V. injection over 1 minute.
Children 6 to 12 years: 2 mg P.O. q 4 to 6 hours, not to exceed 12 mg/day. Alternatively, may give 8 mg (timed-release) at bedtime.
Children 2 to 6 years: 1 mg P.O. q 4 to 6 hours.

Note: Children under 12 years should use only as directed by a doctor.

ADVERSE REACTIONS

Common reactions are in italics; life-threatening reactions are in bold italics.
CNS: *stimulation,* sedation, *drowsiness* (especially in elderly patients), excitability (in children).
CV: hypotension, palpitations.
GI: epigastric distress, *dry mouth.*
GU: urine retention.
Skin: rash, urticaria.
Other: thick bronchial secretions.
After parenteral administration: local stinging, burning sensation, pallor, weak pulse, transient hypotension.

INTERACTIONS

CNS depressants: increased sedation. Use together cautiously.
MAO inhibitors: increased anticholinergic effects. Don't use together.

NURSING CONSIDERATIONS

• *Contraindicated* in acute asthmatic attacks.
• *Use cautiously* in elderly patients and in increased intraocular pressure, hyperthyroidism, cardiovascular or renal disease, hypertension, bronchial asthma, urine retention, prostatic hypertrophy, bladder-neck obstruction, and stenosing peptic ulcers.
• Warn patient against drinking alcoholic beverages and using other CNS depressants during therapy and against driving or other activities that require alertness until CNS response to drug is determined.
• Available as nonprescription item for self-medication by adults.
• Coffee or tea may reduce drowsiness. Sugarless gum or sour hard candy, or ice chips may relieve dry mouth.
• If tolerance develops, another antihistamine may be substituted.
• Warn patient to stop taking drug 4 days before allergy skin tests to preserve accuracy of tests.

*Liquid form contains alcohol. **May contain tartrazine.

• **I.V. use:** Only injectable forms *without* preservatives can be given I.V. Give *slowly*.
• If symptoms occur during or after parenteral dose, discontinue drug. Notify doctor.
• Because of the potential risk to the infant, antihistamines are not recommended for use by women who are breast-feeding because small amounts of drug are excreted in breast milk.

clemastine fumarate

Tavist-1◇

Pregnancy Risk Category: C

HOW SUPPLIED
Tablets: 1.34 mg

MECHANISM OF ACTION
Competes with histamine for H_1-receptor sites on effector cells. Prevents but does not reverse histamine-mediated responses.

INDICATIONS & DOSAGE
Rhinitis, allergy symptoms –
Adults and children 12 years and over: 1.34 mg P.O. q 12 hours.
Note: Children under 12 years should use only as directed by a doctor.

ADVERSE REACTIONS
Common reactions are in italics; life-threatening reactions are in bold italics.
Blood: hemolytic anemia, thrombocytopenia, ***agranulocytosis.***
CNS: (especially in elderly patients) *sedation, drowsiness.*
CV: hypotension, palpitations, tachycardia.
GI: epigastric distress, anorexia, nausea, vomiting, constipation, *dry mouth.*
GU: urine retention.
Skin: rash, urticaria.
Other: thick bronchial secretions.

INTERACTIONS
CNS depressants: increased sedation. Use together cautiously.
MAO inhibitors: Increased anticholinergic effects. Don't use together.

NURSING CONSIDERATIONS
• *Contraindicated* in acute asthmatic attacks.
• *Use cautiously* in elderly patients and in increased intraocular pressure, hyperthyroidism, cardiovascular or renal disease, hypertension, bronchial asthma, urine retention, prostatic hypertrophy, bladder-neck obstruction, and stenosing peptic ulcers.
• Warn patient against drinking alcoholic beverages during therapy and against driving or other activities that require alertness until CNS response to drug is determined.
• Coffee or tea may reduce drowsiness. Sugarless gum or sour hard candy, or ice chips may relieve dry mouth.
• If tolerance develops, another antihistamine may be substituted.
• Warn patient to stop taking drug 4 days before allergy skin tests to preserve accuracy of tests.
• Monitor blood counts during long-term therapy; observe for signs of blood dyscrasia.
• Antihistamines are not recommended for use by women who are breast-feeding because small amounts of drug are excreted in breast milk.

cyproheptadine hydrochloride

Periactin

Pregnancy Risk Category: B

HOW SUPPLIED
Tablets: 4 mg
Syrup: 2 mg/5 ml

MECHANISM OF ACTION
Competes with histamine for H_1-receptor sites on effector cells. Prevents

but does not reverse histamine-mediated responses.

INDICATIONS & DOSAGE

Allergy symptoms, pruritus –
Adults: 4 mg P.O. t.i.d. or q.i.d. Maximum dosage is 0.5 mg/kg daily.
Children 7 to 14 years: 4 mg P.O. b.i.d. or t.i.d. Maximum dosage is 16 mg daily.
Children 2 to 6 years: 2 mg P.O. b.i.d. or t.i.d. Maximum dosage is 12 mg daily.

Note: Children under 14 years should use only as directed by a doctor.

ADVERSE REACTIONS

Common reactions are in italics; life-threatening reactions are in bold italics.
CNS: (especially in elderly patients) *drowsiness,* dizziness, headache, fatigue.
GI: nausea, vomiting, epigastric distress, *dry mouth.*
GU: urine retention.
Skin: rash.
Other: weight gain.

INTERACTIONS

CNS depressants: increased sedation. Use together cautiously.
MAO inhibitors: increased anticholinergic effects. Don't use together.

NURSING CONSIDERATIONS

- *Contraindicated* in acute asthmatic attacks.
- *Use cautiously* in elderly patients and in increased intraocular pressure, hyperthyroidism, cardiovascular or renal disease, hypertension, bronchial asthma, urine retention, prostatic hypertrophy, bladder-neck obstruction, and stenosing peptic ulcers.
- Warn patient against drinking alcoholic beverages during therapy and against driving or other activities that require alertness until CNS response to drug is determined.
- Reduce GI distress by giving with food or milk.
- Coffee or tea may reduce drowsiness. Sugarless gum or sour hard candy, or ice chips may relieve dry mouth.
- If tolerance develops, another antihistamine may be substituted.
- Warn patient to stop taking drug 4 days before allergy skin tests to preserve accuracy of tests.
- Antihistamines are not recommended for use by women who are breast-feeding because small amounts of drug are excreted in breast milk.

dexchlorpheniramine maleate

Dexchlor, Poladex TD, Polaramine*, Polaramine Repetabs, Polargen

Pregnancy Risk Category: B

HOW SUPPLIED

Tablets: 2 mg
Tablets (timed-release): 4 mg, 6 mg
Syrup: 2 mg/5 ml*

MECHANISM OF ACTION

Competes with histamine for H_1-receptor sites on effector cells. Prevents but does not reverse histamine-mediated responses.

INDICATIONS & DOSAGE

Rhinitis, allergy symptoms, contact dermatitis, pruritus –
Adults: 2 mg P.O. q 4 to 6 hours, not to exceed 12 mg/day; or (timed-release) 4 to 6 mg b.i.d. or t.i.d.
Children 6 to 12 years: 1 mg P.O. q 4 to 6 hours, not to exceed 6 mg/day; or 4 mg (timed-release tablet) at bedtime.
Children 2 to 6 years: 0.5 mg P.O. q 4 to 6 hours, not to exceed 3 mg/day.

Note: Children under 6 years should use only as directed by a doc-

*Liquid form contains alcohol. **May contain tartrazine.

tor. Do not use timed-release tablets for children younger than 6 years.

ADVERSE REACTIONS
Common reactions are in italics; life-threatening reactions are in bold italics.
CNS: (especially in elderly patients) *drowsiness,* dizziness, *stimulation.*
GI: nausea, *dry mouth.*
GU: polyuria, dysuria, urine retention.

INTERACTIONS
CNS depressants: increased sedation. Use together cautiously.
MAO inhibitors: increased anticholinergic effects. Don't use together.

NURSING CONSIDERATIONS
• *Contraindicated* in acute asthmatic attacks.
• *Use cautiously* in elderly patients and in increased intraocular pressure, hyperthyroidism, cardiovascular or renal disease, hypertension, bronchial asthma, urine retention, prostatic hypertrophy, bladder-neck obstruction, and stenosing peptic ulcers.
• Warn patient against drinking alcoholic beverages during therapy and against driving or other activities that require alertness until CNS response to drug is determined.
• Coffee or tea may reduce drowsiness. Sugarless gum or sour hard candy, or ice chips may relieve dry mouth.
• If tolerance develops, another antihistamine may be substituted.
• Warn patient to stop taking drug 4 days before allergy skin tests to preserve accuracy of tests.
• Antihistamines are not recommended for use by women who are breast-feeding because small amounts of drug are excreted in breast milk.

diphenhydramine hydrochloride

Allerdryl†◊, AllerMax◊, Beldin*◊, Belix◊, Bena-D, Bena-D 50◊, Benadryl*◊, Benadryl Complete Allergy◊, Benahist 10, Benahist 50, Ben-Allergin-50, Benaphen◊, Benoject-10, Benoject-50, Benylin Cough*◊, Benylin Dietetic†, Benylin Expectorant†, Benylin Pediatric†, Bydramine Cough◊, Compoz Diahist◊, Dihydrex, Diphenacen-50, Diphenadryl◊, Diphen Cough*◊, Diphenhist◊, Dormarex 2◊, Fenylhist◊, Fynex◊, Hydramine*, Hydramyn, Hydril◊, Hyrexin-50, Insomnal†, Nervine Nighttime Sleep-Aid◊, Noradryl, Nordryl, Nytol with DPH◊, Sleep-Eze 3◊, Sominex◊, Sominex Liquid◊, Tusstat*◊, Twilite◊, Valdrene*◊, Wehdryl

Pregnancy Risk Category: B

HOW SUPPLIED
Tablets: 25 mg◊, 50 mg◊
Capsules: 25 mg◊, 50 mg◊
Elixir: 12.5 mg/5 ml (14% alcohol)*◊
Syrup: 12.5 mg/5 ml◊, 13.3 mg/5 ml (5% alcohol)◊
Injection: 10 mg/ml, 50 mg/ml

MECHANISM OF ACTION
Competes with histamine for H_1-receptor sites on effector cells. Prevents but does not reverse histamine-mediated responses, particularly histamine's effects on the smooth muscle of the bronchial tubes, GI tract, uterus, and blood vessels. Structurally related to local anesthetics, diphenhydramine provides local anesthesia by preventing initiation and transmission of nerve impulses. Also suppresses the cough reflex by a direct effect in the medulla of the brain.

INDICATIONS & DOSAGE
Rhinitis, allergy symptoms, motion sickness, Parkinson's disease –

Adults: 25 to 50 mg P.O. t.i.d. or q.i.d.; or 10 to 50 mg deep I.M. or I.V. Maximum I.M. or I.V. dosage is 400 mg daily.
Children under 12 years: 5 mg/kg daily P.O., deep I.M., or I.V. divided q.i.d. Maximum dosage is 300 mg daily.
Sedation –
Adults: 25 to 50 mg P.O., or deep I.M., p.r.n.
As a nighttime sleep aid –
Adults: 50 mg P.O. at bedtime.
Nonproductive cough –
Adults: 25 mg P.O. q 4 hours (not to exceed 150 mg daily).
Children 6 to 12 years: 12.5 mg P.O. q 4 hours (not to exceed 75 mg daily).
Children 2 to 6 years: 6.25 mg P.O. q 4 hours (not to exceed 37.5 mg daily).

Note: Children under 12 years should use only as directed by a doctor.

ADVERSE REACTIONS
Common reactions are in italics; life-threatening reactions are in bold italics.
CNS: (especially in elderly patients) *drowsiness,* confusion, insomnia, headache, vertigo.
CV: palpitations.
EENT: diplopia, nasal stuffiness.
GI: *nausea,* vomiting, diarrhea, *dry mouth,* constipation.
GU: dysuria, urine retention.
Skin: urticaria, photosensitivity.

INTERACTIONS
CNS depressants: increased sedation. Use together cautiously.
MAO inhibitors: increased anticholinergic effects. Don't use together.

NURSING CONSIDERATIONS
- *Contraindicated* in acute asthmatic attacks. *Use cautiously* in narrow-angle glaucoma, prostatic hypertrophy, pyloroduodenal and bladder-neck obstruction, and stenosing peptic ulcers; in newborns; and in asthmatic, hypertensive, or cardiac patients.
- Alternate injection sites to prevent irritation. Administer deep I.M. into large muscle.
- Warn patient against drinking alcoholic beverages during therapy and against driving or other hazardous activities until CNS response to drug is determined.
- Reduce GI distress by giving with food or milk.
- Coffee or tea may reduce drowsiness. Sugarless gum or sour hard candy, or ice chips may relieve dry mouth.
- If tolerance develops, another antihistamine may be substituted.
- For use to prevent motion sickness, instruct patient to take 30 minutes before travel.
- Warn patient to stop taking drug 4 days before allergy skin tests to preserve accuracy of tests.
- Used with epinephrine in anaphylaxis.
- One of most sedating antihistamines; often used as a hypnotic.
- Warn patient of possible photosensitivity. Advise use of a sunscreen.
- Antihistamines are not recommended for use by women who are breast-feeding because small amounts of drug are excreted in breast milk.

loratadine
Claritin

Pregnancy Risk Category: B

HOW SUPPLIED
Tablets: 10 mg

MECHANISM OF ACTION
Blocks the effects of histamine at H_1 receptors. Loratadine is a nonsedating antihistamine because its chemical structure prevents entry into the CNS.

*Liquid form contains alcohol. **May contain tartrazine.

INDICATIONS & DOSAGE
Symptomatic treatment of seasonal allergic rhinitis –
Adults and children 12 years and over: 10 mg P.O. daily. Patients with hepatic failure should start therapy with 10 mg every other day.

ADVERSE REACTIONS
Common reactions are in italics; life-threatening reactions are in bold italics.
CNS: headache, somnolence, fatigue.
GI: dry mouth.

INTERACTIONS
None reported.

NURSING CONSIDERATIONS
- *Contraindicated* in patients with hypersensitivity to the drug.
- *Use cautiously* and in lower dosages in patients with liver failure to prevent accumulation of drug and its active metabolites. Also *use cautiously* with drugs that are known to impair hepatic drug metabolism. Studies to rule out drug interactions have not been performed.
- Because trace amounts of drug are found in human breast milk, use cautiously in breast-feeding women.
- Although administration with food has been observed to cause only small changes in drug absorption, the manufacturer recommends that loratadine be taken on an empty stomach. Instruct patient to take drug at least 2 hours after a meal and to avoid eating for at least 1 hour after dosing.
- Be sure patient understands that drug should be taken only once daily. If symptoms persist or worsen, he should contact the doctor.
- Warn patient to stop taking drug 4 days before allergy skin tests to preserve accuracy of tests.

methdilazine hydrochloride
Dilosyn†, Tacaryl*
Pregnancy Risk Category: C

HOW SUPPLIED
Tablets: 8 mg
Tablets (chewable): 3.6 mg methdilazine (equal to 4 mg methdilazine hydrochloride)
Syrup: 4 mg/5 ml*

MECHANISM OF ACTION
Competes with histamine for H_1-receptor sites on effector cells. Prevents but does not reverse histamine-mediated responses.

INDICATIONS & DOSAGE
Allergic rhinitis; pruritus –
Adults: 8 mg P.O. b.i.d. to q.i.d. or (chewable tablets) 7.2 mg P.O. b.i.d. to q.i.d.
Children over 3 years: 4 mg P.O. b.i.d. to q.i.d. or (chewable tablets) 3.6 mg P.O. b.i.d. to q.i.d.

ADVERSE REACTIONS
Common reactions are in italics; life-threatening reactions are in bold italics.
CNS: (especially in elderly patients) *drowsiness,* dizziness, headache.
GI: nausea, *dry mouth and throat.*
GU: urine retention.
Hepatic: cholestatic jaundice.
Skin: rash.

INTERACTIONS
CNS depressants: increased sedation. Use together cautiously.
MAO inhibitors: increased anticholinergic effects. Don't use together.
Phenothiazines: increased effects. Don't use together.

NURSING CONSIDERATIONS
- *Contraindicated* in acute asthmatic attacks.
- *Use cautiously* in elderly or debilitated patients; acutely ill or dehydrated children; in patients with a his-

tory of seizures; in pulmonary, hepatic, or cardiovascular disease; and in asthma, hypertension, prostatic hypertrophy, bladder-neck obstruction, CNS depression, and stenosing peptic ulcers.

- Warn patient against drinking alcoholic beverages during therapy and against driving or other activities that require alertness until CNS response to drug is determined.
- Reduce GI distress by giving with food or milk.
- Coffee or tea may reduce drowsiness. Sugarless gum or sour hard candy, or ice chips may relieve dry mouth.
- If tolerance develops, another antihistamine may be substituted.
- Available as chewable tablet for children. Instruct child to chew completely and swallow promptly; may cause local anesthetic effect in mouth, which increases the risk of choking.
- Warn patient to stop taking drug 4 days before allergy skin tests to preserve accuracy of tests.
- Antihistamines are not recommended for use by women who are breast-feeding because small amounts of drug are excreted in breast milk.

promethazine hydrochloride

Anergan 25, Anergan 50, Histanil†, K-Phen, Mallergan, Pentazine, Phenameth, Phenazine 25, Phenazine 50, Phencen-50, Phenergan*, Phenergan-Fortis*, Phenergan-Plain*, Phenoject-50, PMS-Promethazine†, Pro-50, Prometh-25, Prometh-50, Promethegan, Prothazine‡*, Prothazine-25, Prothazine-50, Prothazine Plain, Remsed, V-Gan-25, V-Gan-50

Pregnancy Risk Category: C

HOW SUPPLIED

Tablets: 12.5 mg, 25 mg, 50 mg
Syrup: 5 mg/5 ml‡*, 6.25 mg/5 ml*, 10 mg/5 ml*, 25 mg/5 ml*
Injection: 25 mg/ml, 50 mg/ml
Suppositories: 12.5 mg, 25 mg, 50 mg

MECHANISM OF ACTION

Competes with histamine for H_1-receptor sites on effector cells. Prevents but does not reverse histamine-mediated responses.

INDICATIONS & DOSAGE

Motion sickness –
Adults: 25 mg P.O. b.i.d.
Children: 1 mg/kg P.O., I.M., or P.R. b.i.d.
Nausea –
Adults: 12.5 to 25 mg P.O., I.M., or P.R. q 4 to 6 hours, p.r.n.
Children: 1 mg/kg I.M. or P.R. q 4 to 6 hours, p.r.n.
Rhinitis, allergy symptoms –
Adults: 12.5 mg P.O. q.i.d.; or 25 mg P.O. h.s.
Children: 6.25 to 12.5 mg P.O. t.i.d. or 25 mg P.O. or P.R. h.s.
Sedation –
Adults: 25 to 50 mg P.O. or I.M. h.s. or p.r.n.
Children: 12.5 to 25 mg P.O., I.M., or P.R. h.s.
Routine preoperative or postoperative sedation or as an adjunct to analgesics –
Adults: 25 to 50 mg I.M., I.V., or P.O.
Children: 12.5 to 25 mg I.M., I.V., or P.O.

ADVERSE REACTIONS

Common reactions are in italics; life-threatening reactions are in bold italics.
Blood: leukopenia, ***agranulocytosis.***
CNS: (especially in elderly patients) *sedation,* confusion, restlessness, tremors, *drowsiness.*
CV: hypotension.
EENT: transient myopia, nasal congestion.

*Liquid form contains alcohol. **May contain tartrazine.

GI: anorexia, nausea, vomiting, constipation, *dry mouth.*
GU: urine retention.
Other: photosensitivity.

INTERACTIONS
Alcohol, CNS depressants: increased sedation. Use together cautiously.
Anticholinergics, tricyclic antidepressants, phenothiazines: increased effects. Don't give together.
MAO inhibitors: increased anticholinergic effects. Don't use together.
Levodopa: promethazine may decrease levodopa's antiparkinsonian action. Avoid concomitant use.
Lithium: promethazine may reduce GI absorption or enhance renal elimination of lithium. Avoid concomitant use.

NURSING CONSIDERATIONS
• *Contraindicated* in increased intraocular pressure, intestinal obstruction, prostatic hypertrophy, bladder-neck obstruction, seizure disorders, bone-marrow depression, coma, CNS depression, stenosing peptic ulcers, and in newborns and acutely ill or dehydrated children.
• *Use cautiously* in pulmonary, hepatic, or cardiovascular disease; asthma; hypertension; bone-marrow depression; elderly or debilitated patients; and in patients with a history of seizures.
• Warn patient against drinking alcoholic beverages during therapy and against driving or other activities that require alertness until CNS response to drug is determined.
• Reduce GI distress by giving with food or milk.
• Coffee or tea may reduce drowsiness. Sugarless gum or sour hard candy, or ice chips may relieve dry mouth.
• Warn patient to stop taking drug 4 days before allergy skin tests to preserve accuracy of tests.
• Pronounced sedative effect limits use in many ambulatory patients.
• May cause false-positive immunologic urine pregnancy test (Gravindex). Also may interfere with blood grouping in ABO system.
• When treating motion sickness, tell patient to take first dose 30 to 60 minutes before travel. On succeeding days of travel, he should take dose upon arising and with evening meal.
• Inject deep I.M. into large muscle mass. Don't administer S.C. Rotate injection sites.
• **I.V. use:** May be administered I.V., but don't give in a concentration greater than 25 mg/ml, nor at a rate exceeding 25 mg/minute. Shield I.V. infusion from direct light.
• Used as an adjunct to analgesics (usually to increase sedation), but promethazine has no analgesic activity.
• May be safely mixed with meperidine (Demerol) in the same syringe.
• Warn patient about possible photosensitivity and precautions to avoid it.
• If patient to scheduled for a myelogram, drug should be discontinued 48 hours before and not resumed until 24 hours after the procedure because of the risk of seizures.
• Antihistamines are not recommended for use by women who are breast-feeding because small amounts of drug are excreted in breast milk.

terfenadine
Seldane, Teldane‡

Pregnancy Risk Category: C

HOW SUPPLIED
Tablets: 60 mg

MECHANISM OF ACTION
Competes with histamine for H_1-receptor sites on effector cells. Prevents but does not reverse histamine-mediated responses.

INDICATIONS & DOSAGE
Rhinitis, allergy symptoms –
Adults and children over 12 years: 60 mg P.O. b.i.d.
Children 6 to 12 years: 30 to 60 mg P.O. b.i.d.
Children 3 to 5 years: 15 mg P.O. b.i.d.

ADVERSE REACTIONS
Common reactions are in italics; life-threatening reactions are in bold italics.
CNS: fatigue, dizziness, *headache,* sedation.
CV: ***arrhythmias*** (with overdose).
GI: abdominal distress, nausea.
EENT: dry throat and mouth, nasal stuffiness.
Other: alopecia, cholestatic jaundice.

INTERACTIONS
Cimetidine, ciprofloxacin, itraconazole, ketoconazole, macrolide antibiotics (erythromycin, troleandomycin): decreased hepatic metabolism of terfenadine, leading to increased serum levels and risk of serious arrhythmias. Avoid concomitant use.

NURSING CONSIDERATIONS
- *Contraindicated* in patients with hypersensitivity to terfenadine and in those taking the antifungal agents itraconazole or ketoconazole or the macrolide antibiotics.
- May cause a mild anticholinergic drying effect in patients with lower airway disease, such as asthma. Keep patients well hydrated.
- Instruct patients not to exceed prescribed dose. In the event of an overdose, monitor patient for arrhythmias.
- Does not cause the degree of drowsiness and sedation associated with other antihistamines because drug does not cross blood-brain barrier; its anticholinergic and antiserotonin effects are mild.
- Tablets must be broken for children's dosages.

trimeprazine tartrate
Panectyl†, Temaril*
Pregnancy Risk Category: C

HOW SUPPLIED
Tablets: 2.5 mg
Spansule capsules (sustained-release): 5 mg
Syrup: 2.5 mg/5 ml (5.7% alcohol)*

MECHANISM OF ACTION
Competes with histamine for H_1-receptor sites on effector cells. Prevents but does not reverse histamine-mediated responses.

INDICATIONS & DOSAGE
Pruritus –
Adults: 2.5 mg P.O. q.i.d.; or (timed-release) 5 mg P.O. b.i.d.
Children 3 to 12 years: 2.5 mg P.O. at bedtime or t.i.d., p.r.n.
Children 6 months to 3 years: 1.25 mg P.O. at bedtime or t.i.d., p.r.n.
Note: Children under 12 years should use only as directed by a doctor.

ADVERSE REACTIONS
Common reactions are in italics; life-threatening reactions are in bold italics.
Blood: ***agranulocytosis,*** leukopenia.
CNS: (especially in elderly patients) drowsiness, dizziness, confusion, headache, restlessness, tremors, irritability, insomnia; (in children) paradoxical excitation.
CV: hypotension, palpitations, tachycardia.
GI: anorexia, nausea, vomiting, *dry mouth and throat.*
GU: urinary frequency, urine retention.
Skin: urticaria, rash, *photosensitivity.*

INTERACTIONS
Alcohol, CNS depressants: increased sedation. Use together cautiously.
Anticholinergics, MAO inhibitors,

phenothiazines, tricyclic antidepressants: increased anticholinergic effect. Don't use together.
Levodopa: trimeprazine may block levodopa's antiparkinsonian effects. Don't use together.
Lithium: trimeprazine may decrease GI absorption and enhance renal excretion of lithium. Don't use together.

NURSING CONSIDERATIONS
- *Contraindicated* in acute asthmatic attacks.
- *Use cautiously* in pulmonary, hepatic, or cardiovascular disease; asthma; hypertension; narrow-angle glaucoma; intestinal obstruction; prostatic hypertrophy; bladder-neck obstruction; seizure disorder; bone-marrow depression; coma; CNS depression; stenosing peptic ulcers; in elderly or debilitated patients; and in acutely ill or dehydrated children.
- Warn patient against drinking alcoholic beverages during therapy and against driving or other activities that require alertness until CNS response to drug is determined.
- Reduce GI distress by giving with food or milk.
- Coffee or tea may reduce drowsiness. Sugarless gum or sour hard candy, or ice chips may relieve dry mouth.
- Warn patient to stop taking drug 4 days before allergy skin tests to preserve accuracy of tests.
- Monitor blood counts during long-term therapy.
- Warn patient about risk of photosensitivity. Recommend use of a sunscreen. If photosensitivity occurs, tell patient to stop taking the drug and call the doctor.
- If patient is scheduled for a myelogram, drug should be discontinued 48 hours before and not resumed until 24 hours after the procedure because of the risk of seizures.
- Antihistamines are not recommended for use by women who are breast-feeding because small amounts of drug are excreted in breast milk.

tripelennamine citrate
PBZ*

tripelennamine hydrochloride
PBZ, PBZ-SR, Pelamine, Pyribenzamine

Pregnancy Risk Category: B

HOW SUPPLIED
citrate
Elixir: 37.5 mg/5 ml (equivalent to 25 mg/5 ml tripelennamine hydrochloride)*
hydrochloride
Tablets: 25 mg, 50 mg
Tablets (sustained-release): 100 mg

MECHANISM OF ACTION
Competes with histamine for H_1-receptor sites on effector cells. Prevents but does not reverse histamine-mediated responses.

INDICATIONS & DOSAGE
Rhinitis, allergy symptoms –
Adults: 25 to 50 mg P.O. q 4 to 6 hours; or (timed-release) 100 mg b.i.d. or t.i.d. Maximum dosage is 600 mg daily.
Children: 5 mg/kg P.O. daily in four to six divided doses. Maximum dosage is 300 mg daily.

ADVERSE REACTIONS
Common reactions are in italics; life-threatening reactions are in bold italics.
CNS: (especially in elderly patients) *drowsiness,* dizziness, confusion, restlessness, tremors, irritability, insomnia.
CV: palpitations.
GI: anorexia, diarrhea or constipation, *nausea, vomiting, dry mouth.*
GU: urinary frequency, urine retention.
Skin: urticaria, rash.

Other: thick bronchial secretions.

INTERACTIONS

CNS depressants: increased sedation. Use together cautiously.
MAO inhibitors: increased anticholinergic effects. Don't use together.

NURSING CONSIDERATIONS

- *Contraindicated* in acute asthmatic attacks.
- *Use cautiously* in elderly patients, and in increased intraocular pressure, hyperthyroidism, CV or renal disease, hypertension, bronchial asthma, urine retention, prostatic hypertrophy, bladder-neck obstruction, and stenosing peptic ulcers.
- Warn patient against drinking alcoholic beverages during therapy and against driving or other activities that require alertness until CNS response to drug is determined.
- Reduce GI distress by giving with food or milk.
- Coffee or tea may reduce drowsiness. Sugarless gum or sour hard candy, or ice chips may relieve dry mouth.
- If tolerance develops, another antihistamine may be substituted.
- Warn patient to stop taking drug 4 days before allergy skin tests to preserve accuracy of tests.
- Antihistamines are not recommended for use by women who are breast-feeding because small amounts of drug are excreted in breast milk.

triprolidine hydrochloride

Actidil*◇, Myidyl

Pregnancy Risk Category: C

HOW SUPPLIED

Tablets: 2.5 mg◇
Syrup: 1.25 mg/5 ml◇

MECHANISM OF ACTION

Competes with histamine for H_1-receptor sites on effector cells. Prevents but does not reverse histamine-mediated responses.

INDICATIONS & DOSAGE

Colds and allergy symptoms –
Adults: 2.5 mg P.O. q 4 to 6 hours. Maximum dosage is 10 mg/day.
Children over 6 years: 1.25 mg P.O. q 4 to 6 hours. Maximum dosage is 5 mg/day.
Children 4 to 6 years: 0.9 mg P.O. q 4 to 6 hours. Maximum dosage is 3.75 mg/day.
Children 2 to 4 years: 0.6 mg P.O. q 4 to 6 hours. Maximum dosage is 2.5 mg/day.
Children 4 months to 2 years: 0.3 mg P.O. q 4 to 6 hours. Maximum dosage is 1.25 mg/day.

Note: Children under 12 years should use only as directed by a doctor.

ADVERSE REACTIONS

Common reactions are in italics; life-threatening reactions are in bold italics.
CNS: (especially in elderly patients) *drowsiness,* dizziness, confusion, restlessness, insomnia, *stimulation.*
GI: anorexia, diarrhea or constipation, nausea, vomiting, *dry mouth.*
GU: urinary frequency, urine retention.
Skin: urticaria, rash.

INTERACTIONS

CNS depressants: increased sedation.
MAO inhibitors: increased anticholinergic effects. Don't use together.

NURSING CONSIDERATIONS

- *Contraindicated* in acute asthma attacks.
- *Use cautiously* in elderly patients and in increased intraocular pressure, hyperthyroidism, cardiovascular or renal disease, hypertension, diabetes mellitus, bronchial asthma, urine retention, prostatic hypertrophy, bladder-neck obstruction, and stenosing peptic ulcers.

*Liquid form contains alcohol. **May contain tartrazine.

- Warn patient against drinking alcoholic beverages during therapy and against driving or other activities that require alertness until CNS response to drug is determined.
- Reduce GI distress by giving with food or milk.
- Coffee or tea may reduce drowsiness. Sugarless gum or sour hard candy, or ice chips may relieve dry mouth.
- Warn patient to stop taking drug 4 days before allergy skin tests to preserve accuracy of tests.
- Antihistamines are not recommended for use by women who are breast-feeding because small amounts of drug are excreted in breast milk.

43

Bronchodilators

albuterol
albulterol sulfate
aminophylline
atropine sulfate
(See Chapter 20, ANTIARRHYTHMICS.)
bitolterol mesylate
dyphylline
ephedrine hydrochloride
ephedrine sulfate
epinephrine
epinephrine bitartrate
epinephrine hydrochloride
ethylnorepinephrine hydrochloride
ipratropium bromide
isoetharine hydrochloride
isoetharine mesylate
isoproterenol
isoproterenol hydrochloride
isoproterenol sulfate
metaproterenol sulfate
oxtriphylline
pirbuterol
terbutaline sulfate
theophylline
theophylline sodium glycinate

COMBINATION PRODUCTS

Inhalants

DUO-MEDIHALER: isoproterenol hydrochloride 0.16 mg and phenylephrine bitartrate 0.24 mg per dose.

Oral bronchodilators

BRONCHIAL CAPSULES: 150 mg theophylline and 90 mg guaifenesin.
BRONCHOBID DURACAPS: theophylline 260 mg and ephedrine hydrochloride 35 mg.
BRONDECON TABLETS: 200 mg oxtriphylline and 100 mg guaifenesin.
DILOR-G TABLETS: 200 mg dyphylline and 200 mg guaifenesin.
DYFLEX-G TABLETS: 200 mg dyphylline and 200 mg guaifenesin.
DYLINE-GG TABLETS: 200 mg dyphylline and 200 mg guaifenesin.
ENTEX LA: phenylpropanolamine hydrochloride 75 mg and guaifenesin 400 mg.
GLYCERYL-T CAPSULES: 150 mg theophylline and 90 mg guaifenesin.
LANOPHYLLIN-GG CAPSULES: 150 mg theophylline and 90 mg guaifenesin.
MARAX*: theophylline 130 mg, ephedrine sulfate 25 mg, and hydroxyzine hydrochloride 10 mg.
NEOTHYLLINE-GG TABLETS: 200 mg dyphylline and 200 mg guaifenesin.
QUADRINAL: theophylline calcium salicylate 65 mg, ephedrine hydrochloride 24 mg, potassium iodide 320 mg, and phenobarbital 24 mg.
QUIBRON CAPSULES: 150 mg theophylline and 90 mg guaifenesin.
QUIBRON PLUS*: theophylline 150 mg, ephedrine hydrochloride 25 mg, guaifenesin 100 mg, and butabarbital 20 mg.
TEDRAL◊: theophylline 130 mg, ephedrine hydrochloride 24 mg, and phenobarbital 8 mg.
TEDRAL SA: theophylline 180 mg, ephedrine hydrochloride 48 mg, and phenobarbital 25 mg.
THALFED◊: theophylline 120 mg, ephedrine hydrochloride 25 mg, and phenobarbital 8 mg.

Decongestants

ACTIFED◊: pseudoephedrine hydrochloride 60 mg and triprolidine hydrochloride 2.5 mg.
CONGESPIRIN◊: phenylephrine hydrochloride 1.25 mg and acetaminophen 81 mg.
DRISTAN◊: phenylephrine hydrochloride 5 mg, chlorpheniramine maleate 2 mg, and acetaminophen 325 mg.
HISTASPAN-PLUS: phenylephrine hydrochloride 20 mg and chlorpheniramine maleate 8 mg.

*Liquid form contains alcohol. **May contain tartrazine.

NALDECON: phenylpropanolamine hydrochloride 40 mg, phenylephrine hydrochloride 10 mg, chlorpheniramine maleate 5 mg, and phenyltoloxamine citrate 15 mg.
ORNEX◇: phenylpropanolamine hydrochloride 18 mg and acetaminophen 325 mg.
PHENERGAN-D: pseudoephedrine hydrochloride 60 mg and promethazine hydrochloride 6.25 mg.

albuterol (salbutamol)

Proventil, Respolin‡

albuterol sulfate (salbutamol sulphate)

Proventil, Proventil Repetabs, Respolin Inhaler‡, Respolin Inhaler Solution‡, Ventolin Obstetric Injection‡

Pregnancy Risk Category: C

HOW SUPPLIED

albuterol
Aerosol inhaler: 90 mcg/metered spray, 100 mcg/metered spray‡
albuterol sulfate
Tablets: 2 mg, 4 mg
Tablets (extended-release): 4 mg
Syrup: 2 mg/5 ml
Aqueous solution (for respirator): 5 mg/ml‡
Injection: 1 mg/ml‡

MECHANISM OF ACTION

Relaxes bronchial and uterine smooth muscle by acting on $beta_2$-adrenergic receptors.

INDICATIONS & DOSAGE

Prevention and treatment of bronchospasm in patients with reversible obstructive airway disease –
Adults and children over 13 years: 1 to 2 inhalations q 4 to 6 hours. More frequent administration or a greater number of inhalations is not recommended.
Oral tablets – 2 to 4 mg t.i.d. or q.i.d. Maximum dosage is 8 mg q.i.d.
Extended-release tablets – 4 to 8 mg q 12 hours. Maximum dosage is 16 mg b.i.d.
Children 6 to 13 years: 2 mg (1 teaspoonful) P.O. t.i.d. or q.i.d.
Children 2 to 5 years: 0.1 mg/kg P.O. t.i.d., not to exceed 2 mg (1 teaspoonful) t.i.d.
Adults over 65 years: 2 mg P.O. t.i.d. or q.i.d.
To prevent exercise-induced asthma –
Adults: 2 inhalations 15 minutes before exercise.
Prevention of premature labor‡ –
Adults: initially, 10 mcg/minute by continuous I.V. infusion (use an infusion pump). Dosage should be increased in 10-minute intervals until the desired response is achieved.

ADVERSE REACTIONS

Common reactions are in italics; life-threatening reactions are in bold italics.
CNS: *tremor, nervousness,* dizziness, insomnia, headache.
CV: tachycardia, palpitations, hypertension.
EENT: drying and irritation of nose and throat (with inhaled form).
GI: heartburn, nausea, vomiting.
Other: muscle cramps, hypokalemia (with high doses).

INTERACTIONS

CNS stimulants: increased CNS stimulation. Avoid concomitant use.
Levodopa: risk of cardiac arrhythmias. Monitor closely.
MAO inhibitors, tricyclic antidepressants: increased adverse cardiovascular effects.
Propranolol and other beta blockers: mutual antagonism. Monitor patient carefully.

NURSING CONSIDERATIONS

- *Contraindicated in* patients with hypersensitivity to the drug or any component of the formulation.

†Available in Canada only. ‡Available in Australia only. ◇Available OTC.

• *Use cautiously* in cardiovascular disorders, including coronary insufficiency and hypertension; in hyperthyroidism or diabetes mellitus; and in patients who are unusually responsive to adrenergics.
• Warn patient about the possibility of paradoxical bronchospasm. If this occurs, the drug should be discontinued immediately.
• Patients may use tablets and aerosol concomitantly. Monitor closely for toxicity.
• Albuterol reportedly produces less cardiac stimulation than other sympathomimetics, especially isoproterenol.
• Aerosol form may be prescribed for use 15 minutes before exercise to prevent exercise-induced bronchospasm.
• Teach patient how to perform oral inhalation correctly. Give the following instructions for using a metered-dose inhaler:
  – Clear nasal passages and throat.
  – Breathe out, expelling as much air from lungs as possible.
  – Place mouthpiece well into mouth as dose from inhaler is released, and inhale deeply.
  – Hold breath for several seconds, remove mouthpiece, and exhale slowly.
• If more than one inhalation is ordered, the patient should wait at least 2 minutes before repeating the procedure for a second dose.
• Tell patient who is also using a steroid inhaler to use the bronchodilator first, then wait about 5 minutes before using the steroid. This allows the bronchodilator to open air passages for maximum effectiveness.
• When used to prevent premature labor, monitor maternal heart rate closely. It should not exceed 140 beats/minute.
• After uterine contractions have ceased, the drip rate of the drug should be maintained for 1 hour, then gradually tapered at 50% increments in six hourly intervals. Infusions should not continue for more than 48 hours. If therapy needs to continue over 48 hours, the doctor may prescribe 4 to 8 mg P.O. q.i.d.
• **I.V. use:** I.V. form (where available) may be used to prepare infusion using sodium chloride injection, glucose injection, or sodium chloride and glucose injection. The drug should never be administered without dilution. Do not mix with any other medication. Discard unused dilution after 24 hours.
• Pleasant-tasting syrup may be taken by children as young as age 2. Contains no alcohol or sugar.
• Store drug in light-resistant container.

aminophylline (theophylline ethylenediamine)

Aminophyllin, Cardophyllin‡, Corophyllin†, Phyllocontin, Somophyllin-DF

Pregnancy Risk Category: C

HOW SUPPLIED

Tablets: 100 mg, 200 mg
Tablets (controlled-release): 225 mg
Oral liquid: 105 mg/5 ml
Injection: 250 mg/10 ml, 500 mg/20 ml, 500 mg/2 ml, 100 mg/100 ml in 0.45% sodium chloride, 200 mg/100 ml in 0.45% sodium chloride
Rectal solution: 300 mg/5 ml
Rectal suppositories: 250 mg, 500 mg

MECHANISM OF ACTION

Inhibits phosphodiesterase, the enzyme that degrades cyclic AMP. Results in relaxation of smooth muscle of the bronchial airways and pulmonary blood vessels.

INDICATIONS & DOSAGE

Symptomatic relief of bronchospasm – **Patients not currently receiving theophylline who require rapid relief of**

symptoms: loading dose is 6 mg/kg (equivalent to 4.7 mg/kg anhydrous theophylline) I.V. slowly (less than or equal to 25 mg/minute), then maintenance infusion.
Adults (nonsmokers): 0.7 mg/kg/hour for 12 hours; then 0.5 mg/kg/hour.
Otherwise healthy adult smokers: 1 mg/kg/hour for 12 hours; then 0.8 mg/kg/hour.
Older patients and adults with cor pulmonale: 0.6 mg/kg/hour for 12 hours; then 0.3 mg/kg/hour.
Adults with CHF or liver disease: 0.5 mg/kg/hour for 12 hours; then 0.1 to 0.2 mg/kg/hour.
Children 9 to 16 years: 1 mg/kg/hour for 12 hours; then 0.8 mg/kg/hour.
Children 6 months to 9 years: 1.2 mg/kg/hour for 12 hours; then 1 mg/kg/hour.
Patients currently receiving theophylline: aminophylline infusions of 0.63 mg/kg (0.5 mg/kg anhydrous theophylline) will increase plasma levels of theophylline by 1 mcg/ml. Some clinicians recommend a dose of 3.1 mg/kg (2.5 mg/kg anhydrous theophylline) if no obvious signs of theophylline toxicity are present.
Chronic bronchial asthma –
Adults: 600 to 1,600 mg P.O. daily divided t.i.d. or q.i.d.
Children: 12 mg/kg P.O. daily divided t.i.d. or q.i.d.
Adjunctive treatment of neonatal apnea –
Neonates: 5.7 mg/kg I.V. as a loading dose, followed by 2.3 mg/kg/day I.V. in 2 or 3 divided doses.

ADVERSE REACTIONS

Common reactions are in italics; life-threatening reactions are in bold italics.
CNS: *nervousness, restlessness, dizziness,* headache, *insomnia,* light-headedness, ***seizures,*** muscle twitching.
CV: *palpitations, sinus tachycardia,* extrasystoles, flushing, marked hypotension, increase in respiratory rate.
GI: *nausea, vomiting, anorexia,* bitter aftertaste, dyspepsia, heavy feeling in stomach, diarrhea.
Skin: urticaria.
Local: rectal suppositories may cause irritation.

INTERACTIONS

Adenosine: decreased antiarrhythmic effectiveness. Higher doses of adenosine may be necessary.
Alkali-sensitive drugs: reduced activity. Do not add to I.V. fluids containing aminophylline.
Barbiturates, carbamazepine, nicotine, phenytoin, rifampin: enhanced metabolism and decreased theophylline blood levels. Monitor for decreased aminophylline effect.
Beta-adrenergic blockers: antagonism. Propranolol and nadolol, especially, may cause bronchospasm in sensitive patients. Use together cautiously.
Cimetidine, influenza virus vaccine, macrolide antibiotics (such as erythromycin), oral contraceptives, quinolone antibiotics (such as ciprofloxacin): decreased hepatic clearance of theophylline; elevated theophylline levels. Monitor for signs of toxicity.

NURSING CONSIDERATIONS

- *Contraindicated* in hypersensitivity to xanthine compounds (caffeine, theobromine) and in preexisting cardiac arrhythmias, especially tachyarrhythmias.
- *Use cautiously* in young children; in elderly patients with CHF or other cardiac or circulatory impairment, cor pulmonale, or hepatic disease; in active peptic ulcer, because drug may increase volume and acidity of gastric secretions; and in hyperthyroidism or diabetes mellitus.
- Individuals metabolize xanthines at different rates. Adjust dosage by monitoring response, tolerance, pulmonary function, and serum theophylline levels. Theophylline concentrations

should range from 10 to 20 mcg/ml; toxicity has been reported with levels above 20 mcg/ml.

- Plasma clearance may be decreased in patients with CHF, hepatic dysfunction, or pulmonary edema. Smokers show accelerated clearance. Dosage adjustments are necessary.
- **I.V. use:** I.V. drug administration can cause burning; dilute with 5% dextrose in water solution.
- Monitor vital signs; measure and record intake and output. Expected clinical effects include improvement in quality of pulse and respiration.
- Warn elderly patient of dizziness, a common adverse reaction at start of therapy.
- GI symptoms may be relieved by taking oral drug with full glass of water at meals, although food in stomach delays absorption. Enteric-coated tablets may also delay and impair absorption. No evidence that antacids reduce GI adverse reactions.
- Suppositories are slowly and erratically absorbed; retention enemas may be absorbed more rapidly. Rectally administered preparations can be given if patient cannot take drug orally. Schedule after evacuation, if possible; may be retained better if given before meal. Advise patient to remain recumbent 15 to 20 minutes after insertion.
- Question patient closely about other drugs used. Warn him that OTC remedies may contain ephedrine in combination with theophylline salts; excessive CNS stimulation may result. Tell him to check with doctor or pharmacist before taking *any* other medications.
- Before giving loading dose, check that patient has not had recent theophylline therapy.
- Supply instructions for home care and dosage schedule. Some patients may require an around-the-clock dosage schedule.
- Advise patient to avoid switching brand products without first checking with doctor.
- Warn patients with allergies that exposure to allergens may exacerbate bronchospasm.
- If patient experiences urticaria, he may still tolerate other theophylline preparations. Urticaria may be caused by the ethylene diamine salt.

bitolterol mesylate
Tornalate

Pregnancy Risk Category: C

HOW SUPPLIED
Aerosol inhaler: 370 mcg/metered spray

MECHANISM OF ACTION
Relaxes bronchial smooth muscle by acting on $beta_2$-adrenergic receptors.

INDICATIONS & DOSAGE
To prevent and treat bronchial asthma and bronchospasm –

Adults and children over 12 years: to treat bronchospasm, two inhalations at an interval of at least 1 to 3 minutes followed by a third inhalation, if needed. To prevent bronchospasm, the usual dose is two inhalations q 8 hours. In either case, dose should never exceed three inhalations q 6 hours or two inhalations q 4 hours.

ADVERSE REACTIONS
Common reactions are in italics; life-threatening reactions are in bold italics.

CNS: *tremors,* nervousness, headache, dizziness, light-headedness.
CV: palpitations, chest discomfort, tachycardia.
EENT: throat irritation, cough.
GI: nausea.
Other: dyspnea, *hypersensitivity*.

INTERACTIONS
None significant.

*Liquid form contains alcohol. **May contain tartrazine.

NURSING CONSIDERATIONS

- *Contraindicated* in patients with hypersensitivity to the drug.
- *Use cautiously* in ischemic heart disease or hypertension, hyperthyroidism, diabetes mellitus, cardiac arrhythmias, and seizure disorders.
- Monitor blood pressure regularly.
- Advise patients not to exceed recommended dosages. Too frequent use may cause tachycardia.
- Remind patients that beneficial effects last for up to 8 hours, longer than most other similar bronchodilators.
- Has rapid onset of action (about 3 to 4 minutes). Peak effect occurs in 30 to 60 minutes.
- Teach patient to perform oral inhalation correctly. Give the following instructions for using a metered-dose inhaler:
  - Clear nasal passages and throat.
  - Breathe out, expelling as much air from lungs as possible.
  - Place mouthpiece well into mouth as dose from inhaler is released, and inhale deeply.
  - Hold breath for several seconds, remove mouthpiece, and exhale slowly.
- If more than one inhalation is ordered, the patient should wait at least 2 minutes before repeating the procedure for a second dose.
- Tell patient who is also using a steroid inhaler to use the bronchodilator first, then wait about 5 minutes before using the steroid. This allows the bronchodilator to open air passages for maximum effectiveness.

dyphylline

Brophylline, Dilin, Dilor*, Dyflex, Dylline*, Emfabid, Lufyllin*, Protophylline†

Pregnancy Risk Category: C

HOW SUPPLIED

Tablets: 200 mg, 400 mg
Elixir: 100 mg/15 ml, 160 mg/15 ml*
Injection: 250 mg/ml

MECHANISM OF ACTION

Inhibits phosphodiesterase, the enzyme that degrades cyclic adenosine monophosphate. Results in relaxation of smooth muscle of the bronchial airways and pulmonary blood vessels.

INDICATIONS & DOSAGE

For relief of acute and chronic bronchial asthma and reversible bronchospasm associated with chronic bronchitis and emphysema –
Adults: 15 mg/kg P.O. q 6 hours. I.M. route is rarely used, but patients may receive 250 to 500 mg I.M. injected slowly at 6-hour intervals. Dosage should be decreased in renal insufficiency.

ADVERSE REACTIONS

Common reactions are in italics; life-threatening reactions are in bold italics.
CNS: *restlessness, dizziness,* headache, *insomnia,* light-headedness, ***seizures,*** muscle twitching.
CV: *palpitations, sinus tachycardia,* extrasystoles, flushing, marked hypotension, increase in respiratory rate.
GI: *nausea, vomiting, anorexia,* bitter aftertaste, dyspepsia, heavy feeling in stomach.
Skin: urticaria.

INTERACTIONS

Probenecid: increased serum dyphylline levels. Monitor for adverse effects.

NURSING CONSIDERATIONS

- *Contraindicated* in hypersensitivity to xanthine compounds (caffeine, theobromine) or preexisting cardiac arrhythmias, especially tachycardias.
- *Use cautiously* in young children; in elderly patients with CHF, any impaired cardiac or circulatory function,

cor pulmonale, renal or hepatic disease; and in peptic ulcer, hyperthyroidism, or diabetes mellitus.
• Do not administer I.V.
• Monitor vital signs; measure and record intake and output. Expected clinical effects include improvement in quality of pulse and respiration.
• Warn elderly patient of dizziness, a common adverse reaction at start of therapy.
• Gastric irritation may be relieved by taking oral drug after meals; there is no evidence that antacids reduce this adverse reaction. May produce less gastric discomfort than theophylline.
• Discard injectable dyphylline if precipitate is present. Protect from light.
• Question patient closely about other drugs used. Warn him that OTC remedies may contain ephedrine in combination with theophylline salts; excessive CNS stimulation may result. Tell him to check with doctor or pharmacist before taking *any* other medications.
• Supply instructions for home care and dosage schedule.

ephedrine hydrochloride

Fedrine†

ephedrine sulfate

Ephed II

Pregnancy Risk Category: C

HOW SUPPLIED
Tablets: 30 mg‡
Capsules: 25 mg, 50 mg
Capsules (extended-release): 15 mg, 30 mg, 60 mg
Oral solution: 11 mg/5 ml, 20 mg/5 ml
Injection: 5 mg/ml, 20 mg/ml, 25 mg/ml, 50 mg/ml (parenteral)

MECHANISM OF ACTION
Both a direct- and indirect-acting sympathomimetic that stimulates alpha- and beta-adrenergic receptors.

INDICATIONS & DOSAGE
To correct hypotensive states; to support ventricular rate in Adams-Stokes syndrome –
Adults: 25 to 50 mg I.M. or S.C., or 10 to 25 mg I.V. p.r.n. to maximum of 150 mg/24 hours.
Children: 3 mg/kg S.C. or I.V. daily, in four to six divided doses.
Bronchodilator or nasal decongestant –
Adults: 12.5 to 50 mg P.O. b.i.d., t.i.d., or q.i.d. Maximum dosage is 400 mg daily in six to eight divided doses.
Children: 2 to 3 mg/kg P.O. daily in four to six divided doses.

ADVERSE REACTIONS
Common reactions are in italics; life-threatening reactions are in bold italics.
CNS: *insomnia, nervousness,* dizziness, headache, muscle weakness, sweating, euphoria, confusion, delirium.
CV: *palpitations,* tachycardia, hypertension.
EENT: dryness of nose and throat.
GI: nausea, vomiting, anorexia.
GU: urine retention, painful urination due to visceral sphincter spasm.

INTERACTIONS
Acetazolamide: increased serum ephedrine levels. Monitor for toxicity.
Alpha-adrenergic blocking agents: unopposed beta-adrenergic effects, resulting in hypotension.
Antihypertensives: decreased effects.
Beta-adrenergic blocking agents: unopposed alpha-adrenergic effects, resulting in hypertension.
Digitalis glycosides, general anesthetics (halogenated hydrocarbons): increased risk of ventricular arrhythmias.

Ergot alkaloids: enhanced vasoconstrictor activity.
Guanadrel, guanethidine: enhanced pressor effects of ephedrine.
Levodopa: enhanced risk of ventricular arrhythmias.
MAO inhibitors and tricyclic antidepressants: when given with sympathomimetics, may cause severe hypertension (hypertensive crisis).
Methyldopa: may inhibit effects of ephedrine. Use together cautiously.

NURSING CONSIDERATIONS

- *Contraindicated* in porphyria, severe coronary artery disease, cardiac arrhythmias, narrow-angle glaucoma, or psychoneurosis; and in patients on MAO-inhibitor therapy.
- *Use cautiously* in elderly patients and those with hypertension, hyperthyroidism, nervous or excitable states, cardiovascular disease, and prostatic hypertrophy.
- Not a substitute for blood or fluid volume deficit. Volume deficit should be replaced before vasopressors are administered.
- **I.V. use:** Give I.V. injection slowly.
- Hypoxia, hypercapnia, and acidosis, which may reduce effectiveness or increase the incidence of adverse reactions, must be identified and corrected before or during ephedrine administration.
- Effectiveness decreases after 2 to 3 weeks. Then increased dosage may be needed. Tolerance develops, but drug is not known to cause addiction.
- To prevent insomnia, avoid giving within 2 hours before bedtime.
- Warn patient not to take OTC drugs that contain ephedrine without informing doctor.

epinephrine

Adrenalin◇, Bronkaid Mist◇, Bronkaid Mistometer†, Dysne-Inhal†, Primatene Mist Solution◇

epinephrine bitartrate

AsthmaHaler◇, Broniten Mist◇, Bronkaid Mist Suspension◇, Medihaler-Epi◇, Primatene Mist Suspension◇

epinephrine hydrochloride

Adrenalin Chloride◇, Epi-Pen, Epi-Pen Jr., Sus-Phrine

Pregnancy Risk Category: C

HOW SUPPLIED

Aerosol inhaler: 160 mcg◇, 200 mcg◇, 250 mcg/metered spray◇
Nebulizer inhaler: 1% (1:100)†◇, 1.25%†◇, 2.25%†◇
Injection: 0.01 mg/ml (1:100,000), 0.1 mg/ml (1:10,000), 0.5 mg/ml (1:2,000), 1 mg/ml (1:1,000) parenteral; 5 mg/ml (1:200) parenteral suspension

MECHANISM OF ACTION

Stimulates alpha- and beta-adrenergic receptors within the sympathetic nervous system.

INDICATIONS & DOSAGE

Bronchospasm, hypersensitivity reactions, anaphylaxis –
Adults: 0.1 to 0.5 ml of 1:1,000 S.C. or I.M. Repeat q 10 to 15 minutes, p.r.n. Or 0.1 to 0.25 ml 1:1,000 I.V.
Children: 0.01 ml (10 mcg) of 1:1,000/kg S.C. Repeat q 20 minutes to 4 hours, p.r.n.; 0.005 ml/kg of 1:200 (Sus-Phrine). Repeat q 8 to 12 hours, p.r.n.
Hemostasis –
Adults: 1:50,000 to 1:1,000, applied topically.
Acute asthmatic attacks (inhalation) –
Adults and children: 1 or 2 inhalations of 1:100 or 2.25% racemic, every 1 to 5 minutes until relief is obtained; 0.2 mg/dose usual content.
To prolong local anesthetic effect –
Adults and children: 0.2 to 0.4 ml of 1:1,000 intraspinal; 1:500,000 to 1:50,000 local mixed with local anesthetic.

To restore cardiac rhythm in cardiac arrest –
Adults: 0.5 to 1 mg I.V. or into endotracheal tube. May be given intracardiac if no I.V. route or intratracheal route available. Some clinicians advocate higher dose (up to 5 mg), especially in patients who don't respond to usual I.V dose. Following initial I.V. administration, may be infused I.V. at a rate of 1 to 4 mcg/minute.
Children: 10 mcg/kg I.V. or 5 to 10 mcg (0.05 to 0.1 ml of 1:10,000)/kg intracardiac.

Note: 1 mg = 1 ml of 1:1,000 or 10 ml of 1:10,000.

ADVERSE REACTIONS

Common reactions are in italics; life-threatening reactions are in bold italics.
CNS: *nervousness,* tremor, euphoria, anxiety, coldness of extremities, vertigo, *headache,* sweating, disorientation, agitation. In patients with Parkinson's disease, the drug increases rigidity and tremor.
CV: *palpitations;* widened pulse pressure; ***hypertension; tachycardia; ventricular fibrillation; CVA;*** anginal pain; ECG changes, including a decrease in the T wave amplitude.
Metabolic: hyperglycemia, glycosuria.
Other: pulmonary edema, dyspnea, pallor.

INTERACTIONS

Alpha-adrenergic blocking agents: hypotension due to unopposed beta-adrenergic effects.
Beta blockers, such as propranolol: vasoconstriction and reflex bradycardia. Monitor patient carefully.
Digitalis glycosides, general anesthetics (halogenated hydrocarbons): increased risk of ventricular arrhythmias.
Doxapram, mazindol, methylphenidate: enhanced CNS stimulation or pressor effects.
Ergot alkaloids: enhanced vasoconstrictor activity.
Guanadrel, guanethidine: enhanced pressor effects of epinephrine.
Levodopa: enhanced risk of cardiac arrhythmias.
MAO inhibitors: increased risk of hypertensive crisis.
Tricyclic antidepressants, antihistamines, thyroid hormones: when given with sympathomimetics, may cause severe adverse cardiac effects. Avoid giving together.

NURSING CONSIDERATIONS

- *Contraindicated* in narrow-angle glaucoma, shock (other than anaphylactic shock), organic brain damage, cardiac dilatation, or coronary insufficiency. Also contraindicated during general anesthesia with halogenated hydrocarbons or cyclopropane and in labor (may delay second stage).
- *Use with extreme caution* in long-standing bronchial asthma and emphysema who have developed degenerative heart disease. Also use cautiously in elderly patients, and those with hyperthyroidism, angina, hypertension, psychoneurosis, and diabetes.
- **I.V. use:** Don't mix with alkaline solutions. Use dextrose 5% in water, normal saline solution, or a combination of dextrose 5% in water and saline solution. Mix just before use.
- When administered I.V., monitor blood pressure, heart rate, and ECG when therapy is initiated and frequently thereafter.
- Epinephrine is rapidly destroyed by oxidizing agents, such as iodine, chromates, nitrates, nitrites, oxygen, and salts of easily reducible metals (such as iron).
- Epinephrine solutions deteriorate after 24 hours. Discard after that time or before if solution is discolored or contains precipitate. Keep solution in light-resistant container, and don't remove before use.
- Massage site after injection to

counteract possible vasoconstriction. Repeated local injection can cause necrosis at site from vasoconstriction.

- Avoid I.M. administration of oil injection into buttocks. Gas gangrene may occur because epinephrine reduces oxygen tension of the tissues, encouraging the growth of contaminating organisms.
- In the event of a sharp blood pressure rise, rapid-acting vasodilators, such as nitrites or alpha-adrenergic blocking agents, can be given to counteract the marked pressor effect of large doses of epinephrine.
- Observe patient closely for adverse reactions. If adverse reactions develop, dosage may need to be adjusted or discontinued.
- If patient has acute hypersensitivity reactions, it may be necessary to instruct him to self-inject epinephrine at home.
- Drug of choice in emergency treatment of acute anaphylactic reactions.
- Teach patient to perform oral inhalation correctly. Give the following instructions for using a metered-dose inhaler:
  - Clear nasal passages and throat.
  - Breathe out, expelling as much air from lungs as possible.
  - Place mouthpiece well into mouth as dose from inhaler is released, and inhale deeply.
  - Hold breath for several seconds, remove mouthpiece, and exhale slowly.
- If more than one inhalation is ordered, the patient should wait at least 2 minutes before repeating the procedure for a second dose.
- Tell patient who is also using a steroid inhaler to use the bronchodilator first, then wait about 5 minutes before using the steroid. This allows the bronchodilator to open air passages for maximum effectiveness.

ethylnorepinephrine hydrochloride

Bronkephrine

Pregnancy Risk Category: C

HOW SUPPLIED

Injection: 2 mg/ml

MECHANISM OF ACTION

Relaxes bronchial smooth muscle by acting on beta-adrenergic receptors.

INDICATIONS & DOSAGE

To relieve bronchospasm caused by asthma –

Adults: 0.6 to 2 mg S.C. or I.M.
Children: 0.2 to 1 mg S.C. or I.M.

ADVERSE REACTIONS

Common reactions are in italics; life-threatening reactions are in bold italics.
CNS: *headache,* dizziness.
CV: changes in blood pressure, *elevation in pulse rate,* palpitations.
GI: nausea.

INTERACTIONS

Beta blockers: mutual inhibition of clinical effects.
CNS stimulants, xanthine derivatives: enhanced CNS stimulation.
Digitalis glycosides, levodopa, halogenated inhalational anesthetics, cyclopropane: increased risk of cardiac arrhythmias. Monitor closely.
Nitrates, antihypertensives: decreased effects of these agents.
Rauwolfia alkaloids, sympathomimetics: enhanced effects.
Thyroid hormones: increased risk of coronary insufficiency.

NURSING CONSIDERATIONS

- *Contraindicated* in patients with hypersensitivity to the drug; in patients with tachyarrhythmias, tachycardia caused by digitalis toxicity, narrow-angle glaucoma, or shock; and in those receiving general anesthesia with cyclopropane or halogenated inhalational anesthetics.

• *Use cautiously* in cardiovascular disease or history of stroke.

• Safer than epinephrine for use in hypertensive or severely ill patients in whom significant pressor effects are undesirable.

• Valuable when used in children because of low incidence of adverse reactions; may be useful in diabetic asthmatics due to low glycogenolytic activity.

• Choose anatomic injection site carefully to avoid inadvertent intraneural or intravascular injection.

ipratropium bromide

Atrovent

Pregnancy Risk Category: B

HOW SUPPLIED

Inhaler: each metered dose supplies 18 mcg

Solution (for nebulizer): 0.025% (250 mcg/ml)‡

MECHANISM OF ACTION

Inhibits vagally mediated reflexes by antagonizing acetylcholine. An anticholinergic.

INDICATIONS & DOSAGE

Maintenance treatment of bronchospasm associated with chronic obstructive pulmonary disease –

Adults: 2 inhalations (26 mcg) q.i.d. Additional inhalations may be needed. However, total inhalations should not exceed 12 in 24 hours.

ADVERSE REACTIONS

Common reactions are in italics; life-threatening reactions are in bold italics.

CNS: nervousness, dizziness, headache.

CV: palpitations.

EENT: cough, blurred vision.

GI: nausea, GI distress, dry mouth.

Skin: rash.

INTERACTIONS

Anticholinergics: increased anticholinergic effects. Avoid concomitant use.

Cromolyn sodium: will form a precipitate if mixed in the same nebulizer. Don't use together.

NURSING CONSIDERATIONS

• *Contraindicated* in patients with hypersensitivity to the drug.

• *Use cautiously* in patients with narrow-angle glaucoma, prostatic hypertrophy, and bladder-neck obstruction.

• Warn patient that this drug is not effective in the treatment of acute episodes of bronchospasm where rapid response is required.

• Teach patient to perform oral inhalation correctly. Give the following instructions for using a metered-dose inhaler:
  – Clear nasal passages and throat.
  – Breathe out, expelling as much air from lungs as possible.
  – Place mouthpiece well into mouth as dose from inhaler is released, and inhale deeply.
  – Hold breath for several seconds, remove mouthpiece, and exhale slowly.

• If more than one inhalation is ordered, the patient should wait at least 2 minutes before repeating the procedure for a second dose.

• Tell patient who is also using a steroid inhaler to use ipratropium first, then wait about 5 minutes before using the steroid. This allows the bronchodilator to open air passages for maximum effectiveness.

• Tell patient to avoid accidentally spraying into eyes. Temporary blurring of vision may result.

• Ipratropium is the first anticholinergic bronchodilator available as an aerosol. Works by a different mechanism from either the adrenergics or theophylline compounds.

• Patient may experience a dry mouth or throat. Suggest using sugarless

*Liquid form contains alcohol. **May contain tartrazine.

hard candy or gum, or use a saliva substitute.

- If a dose in missed, take as soon as possible. If it's almost time for the next dose, skip the missed dose. Do not double-dose.

isoetharine hydrochloride

Arm-a-Med Isoetharine, Beta-2, Bisorine, Bronkosol, Dey-Dose Isoetharine, Dey-Dose Isoetharine S/F, Dey-Lute Isoetharine, Dispos-a-Med Isoetharine

isoetharine mesylate

Bronkometer

Pregnancy Risk Category: C

HOW SUPPLIED

Aerosol inhaler: 340 mcg/metered spray
Nebulizer inhaler: 0.062%, 0.08%, 0.1%, 0.125%, 0.14%, 0.167%, 0.17%, 0.2%, 0.25%, 0.5%, 1% solution

MECHANISM OF ACTION

Relaxes bronchial smooth muscle by acting on beta$_2$-adrenergic receptors.

INDICATIONS & DOSAGE

Bronchial asthma and reversible bronchospasm that may occur with bronchitis and emphysema –
Adults: (hydrochloride) administered by hand nebulizer, oxygen aerosolization, or IPPB.

Method	*Dose*	*Dilution*
Hand	3 to 7 inhalations	undiluted
Oxygen aerosolization	0.5 ml	1:3 with saline
IPPB	0.5 ml	1:3 with saline

Adults: (mesylate) 1 to 2 inhalations. Occasionally, more may be required.

ADVERSE REACTIONS

Common reactions are in italics; life-threatening reactions are in bold italics.

CNS: *tremor, headache,* dizziness, excitement.
CV: *palpitations,* increased heart rate.
GI: nausea, vomiting.

INTERACTIONS

Propranolol and other beta blockers: blocked bronchodilating effect of isoetharine. Monitor patient carefully if used together.
Digitalis glycosides, levodopa, halogenated inhalational anesthetics, cyclopropane: increased risk of cardiac arrhythmias. Monitor closely.

NURSING CONSIDERATIONS

- *Contraindicated* in patients with hypersensitivity to the drug; in patients with tachyarrhythmias, tachycardia caused by digitalis toxicity, narrow-angle glaucoma, or shock; and in those receiving general anesthesia with cyclopropane or halogenated inhalational anesthetics.
- *Use cautiously* in hyperthyroidism, hypertension, or coronary disease, and in patients with sensitivity to sympathomimetics.
- Excessive use can lead to decreased effectiveness.
- Monitor for severe paradoxical bronchoconstriction after excessive use. Discontinue immediately if bronchoconstriction occurs.
- Although isoetharine has minimal effects on the heart, use cautiously in patients receiving general anesthetics that sensitize the myocardium to sympathomimetic drugs.
- Teach patient to perform oral inhalation correctly. Give the following instructions for using a metered-dose inhaler:
  – Clear nasal passages and throat.
  – Breathe out, expelling as much air from lungs as possible.
  – Place mouthpiece well into mouth as dose from inhaler is released, and inhale deeply.
  – Hold breath for several seconds,

remove mouthpiece, and exhale slowly.

- If more than one inhalation is ordered, the patient should wait at least 2 minutes before repeating the procedure for a second dose.
- Tell patient who is also using a steroid inhaler to use the bronchodilator first, then wait about 5 minutes before using the steroid. This allows the bronchodilator to open air passages for maximum effectiveness.
- Due to oxidation of drug when diluted with water, pink sputum mimicking hemoptysis may occur after inhaling isoetharine solution. Tell patient not to be concerned.

isoproterenol

Aerolone, Dey-Dose Isoproterenol, Dispos-a-Med Isoproterenol, Isuprel, Vapo-Iso

isoproterenol hydrochloride

Isuprel, Isuprel Mistometer, Norisodrine Aerotrol

isoproterenol sulfate

Medihaler-Iso

Pregnancy Risk Category: C

HOW SUPPLIED

isoproterenol
Nebulizer inhaler: 0.25%, 0.5%, 1%
isoproterenol hydrochloride
Tablets (sublingual): 10 mg, 15 mg
Aerosol inhaler: 120 mcg or 131 mcg/metered spray
Injection: 200 mcg/ml
isoproterenol sulfate
Aerosol inhaler: 80 mcg/metered spray

MECHANISM OF ACTION

Relaxes bronchial smooth muscle by acting on $beta_2$-adrenergic receptors. As a cardiac stimulant, acts on $beta_1$-adrenergic receptors in the heart.

INDICATIONS & DOSAGE

Bronchial asthma and reversible bronchospasm –
Adults: 10 to 20 mg (hydrochloride) S.L. q 6 to 8 hours.
Children: 5 to 10 mg (hydrochloride) S.L. q 6 to 8 hours. Not recommended for children under 6 years.
Bronchospasm –
Adults and children: (sulfate) acute dyspneic episodes: 1 inhalation initially. May repeat if needed after 2 to 5 minutes.

Maintenance dosage is 1 to 2 inhalations q.i.d. to 6 times daily. May repeat once more 10 minutes after second dose. Not more than 3 doses should be administered for each attack.

Heart block and ventricular arrhythmias –
Adults: (hydrochloride) initially, 0.02 to 0.06 mg I.V. Subsequent doses 0.01 to 0.2 mg I.V. or 5 mcg/minute I.V.; or 0.2 mg I.M. initially, then 0.02 to 1 mg, p.r.n.
Children: (hydrochloride) may give half of initial adult dose.
Shock –
Adults and children: (hydrochloride) 0.5 to 5 mcg/minute by continuous I.V. infusion. Usual concentration is 1 mg (5 ml) in 500 ml dextrose 5% in water. Adjust rate according to heart rate, central venous pressure, blood pressure, and urine flow.

ADVERSE REACTIONS

Common reactions are in italics; life-threatening reactions are in bold italics.
CNS: *headache,* mild tremor, weakness, dizziness, nervousness, insomnia.
CV: *palpitations, tachycardia, anginal pain; blood pressure may rise and then fall.*
GI: nausea, vomiting.
Metabolic: hyperglycemia.
Other: sweating, flushing of face, ***bronchial edema and inflammation.***

*Liquid form contains alcohol. **May contain tartrazine.

INTERACTIONS

Epinephrine: increased risk of arrhythmias.
Propranolol and other beta blockers: blocked bronchodilating effect of isoproterenol. Monitor patient carefully if used together.

NURSING CONSIDERATIONS

- *Contraindicated* in tachycardia caused by digitalis intoxication; in preexisting arrhythmias, especially tachycardia, because chronotropic effect on the heart may aggravate such disorders; and in recent myocardial infarction.
- *Use cautiously* in coronary insufficiency, diabetes, or hyperthyroidism.
- Not a substitute for blood or fluid volume deficit. Volume deficit should be replaced before vasopressors are administered.
- If heart rate exceeds 110 beats/minute, it may be advisable to decrease infusion rate or temporarily stop infusion. Doses sufficient to increase the heart rate to more than 130 beats/minute may induce ventricular arrhythmias.
- If precordial distress or anginal pain occurs, stop drug immediately.
- **I.V. use:** When administering I.V. isoproterenol for shock, closely monitor blood pressure, central venous pressure, ECG, arterial blood gas measurements, and urine output. Carefully adjust infusion rate according to these measurements. Use a continuous infusion pump to regulate infusion flow rate.
- Oral and sublingual tablets are poorly and erratically absorbed.
- Teach patient how to take sublingual tablet properly. Tell him to hold tablet under tongue until it dissolves and is absorbed and not to swallow saliva until that time. Prolonged use of sublingual tablets can cause tooth decay. Instruct patient to rinse mouth with water between doses. Will also help prevent dryness of oropharynx.
- If possible, don't give at bedtime because it interrupts sleep patterns.
- This drug may cause a slight rise in systolic blood pressure and a slight to marked drop in diastolic blood pressure.
- Observe patient closely for adverse reactions. Dosage may need to be adjusted or discontinued.
- Tell patient to discontinue the drug if it causes an increase in chest tightness or dyspnea.
- Teach patient to perform oral inhalation correctly. Give the following instructions for using a metered-dose inhaler:
  - Clear nasal passages and throat.
  - Breathe out, expelling as much air from lungs as possible.
  - Place mouthpiece well into mouth as dose from inhaler is released, and inhale deeply.
  - Hold breath for several seconds, remove mouthpiece, and exhale slowly.
- If more than one inhalation is ordered, the patient should wait at least 2 minutes before repeating the procedure for a second dose.
- Tell patient who is also using a steroid inhaler to use the bronchodilator first, then wait about 5 minutes before using the steroid. This allows the bronchodilator to open air passages for maximum effectiveness.
- Instructions for metered powder nebulizer are the same, except that deep inhalation is not necessary.
- Patient may develop a tolerance to this drug. Warn against overuse.
- Warn patient using oral inhalant that drug may turn sputum and saliva pink.
- May aggravate ventilation perfusion abnormalities; even while ease of breathing is improved, arterial oxygen tension may fall paradoxically.
- If ordered via inhalation with oxygen, be sure oxygen concentration will not suppress respiratory drive.

• Discard inhalation solution if it is discolored or contains precipitate.

metaproterenol sulfate
Alupent, Arm-A-Med Metaproterenol, Dey-Dose Metaproterenol, Dey-Med Metaproterenol, Metaprel
Pregnancy Risk Category: C

HOW SUPPLIED
Tablets: 10 mg, 20 mg
Solution: 10 mg/5 ml
Aerosol inhaler: 0.65 mg/metered spray
Nebulizer inhaler: 0.6%, 5% solution

MECHANISM OF ACTION
Relaxes bronchial smooth muscle by acting on $beta_2$-adrenergic receptors.

INDICATIONS & DOSAGE
Acute episodes of bronchial asthma –
Adults and children: 2 to 3 inhalations. Should not repeat inhalations more often than q 3 to 4 hours. Should not exceed 12 inhalations daily.
Bronchial asthma and reversible bronchospasm –
Adults: 20 mg P.O. q 6 to 8 hours.
Children over 9 years or over 27 kg: 20 mg P.O. q 6 to 8 hours (0.4 mg to 0.9 mg/kg/dose t.i.d.).
Children 6 to 9 years or less than 27 kg: 10 mg P.O. q 6 to 8 hours (0.4 mg to 0.9 mg/kg/dose t.i.d.).

Not recommended for children under 6 years.

ADVERSE REACTIONS
Common reactions are in italics; life-threatening reactions are in bold italics.
CNS: nervousness, weakness, drowsiness, tremor.
CV: tachycardia, hypertension, palpitations; *with excessive use,* ***cardiac arrest.***
GI: vomiting, nausea, bad taste in mouth.
Other: paradoxical bronchiolar constriction with excessive use.

INTERACTIONS
Levodopa: risk of cardiac arrhythmias. Avoid concomitant use.
Propranolol and other beta blockers: blocked bronchodilating effect of metaproterenol. Monitor patient carefully if used together.

NURSING CONSIDERATIONS
• *Contraindicated* in tachycardia and arrhythmias associated with tachycardia. *Use cautiously* in hypertension, coronary artery disease, hyperthyroidism, and diabetes.
• Safe use of inhalant in children under 12 years not established.
• Teach patient how to administer metered dose correctly. Instructions: shake container; exhale through nose; administer aerosol while inhaling deeply on mouthpiece of inhaler; and hold breath for a few seconds, then exhale slowly. Allow 2 minutes between inhalations. Store drug in light-resistant container.
• Metaproterenol inhalations should precede steroid inhalations (when prescribed) by 10 to 15 minutes to maximize therapy.
• Warn patient about the possibility of paradoxical bronchospasm. If this occurs, the drug should be discontinued immediately.
• Patients may use tablets and aerosol concomitantly. Monitor closely for toxicity.
• Metaproterenol reportedly produces less cardiac stimulation than other sympathomimetics, especially isoproterenol.
• Inhalant solution can be administered by IPPB diluted in saline solution or via a hand nebulizer at full strength.
• Tell patient to notify doctor if no response is derived from dosage. Warn against changing dose without calling doctor.

- If more than one inhalation is ordered, the patient should wait at least 2 minutes before repeating the procedure for a second dose.
- Tell patient who is also using a steroid inhaler to use the bronchodilator first, then wait about 5 minutes before using the steroid. This allows the bronchodilator to open air passages for maximum effectiveness.

oxtriphylline (choline theophyllinate)

Choledyl*

Pregnancy Risk Category: C

HOW SUPPLIED

Tablets: 100 mg, 200 mg
Tablets (sustained-release): 400 mg, 600 mg
Elixir: 100 mg/5 ml
Syrup: 50 mg/5 ml

MECHANISM OF ACTION

Inhibits phosphodiesterase, the enzyme that degrades cyclic adenosine monophosphate. Results in relaxation of smooth muscle of the bronchial airways and pulmonary blood vessels.

INDICATIONS & DOSAGE

To relieve acute bronchial asthma and reversible bronchospasm associated with chronic bronchitis and emphysema –
Adults and children over 12 years: 200 mg P.O. q 6 hours; or 400 to 600 mg sustained-release form P.O. q 12 hours, then adjust dosage based upon serum theophylline levels.
Children 2 to 12 years: 4 mg/kg P.O. q 6 hours. Adjust as needed to maintain therapeutic levels of theophylline (10 to 20 mcg/ml).

ADVERSE REACTIONS

Common reactions are in italics; life-threatening reactions are in bold italics.
CNS: *restlessness, dizziness,* headache, *insomnia,* light-headedness, *seizures,* muscle twitching.
CV: *palpitations, sinus tachycardia,* extrasystoles, flushing, marked hypotension, increase in respiratory rate.
GI: *nausea, vomiting, anorexia,* bitter aftertaste, dyspepsia, heavy feeling in stomach.
Skin: urticaria.

INTERACTIONS

Adenosine: decreased antiarrhythmic effectiveness. Higher doses of adenosine may be necessary.
Barbiturates, carbamazepine, nicotine, phenytoin, rifampin: enhanced metabolism and decreased theophylline blood levels. Monitor for decreased effect.
Beta-adrenergic blockers: antagonism. Propranolol and nadolol, especially, may cause bronchospasms in sensitive patients. Use together cautiously.
Cimetidine, influenza virus vaccine, macrolide antibiotics (such as erythromycin), oral contraceptives, quinolone antibiotics (such as ciprofloxacin): decreased hepatic clearance of theophylline; elevated theophylline levels. Monitor for signs of toxicity.

NURSING CONSIDERATIONS

- *Contraindicated* in hypersensitivity to xanthines (caffeine, theobromine); preexisting cardiac arrhythmias, especially tachyarrhythmias.
- Monitor effectiveness of therapy by monitoring serum theophylline levels. Therapeutic levels are 10 to 20 mcg/ml, although some patients will respond at lower levels. Toxicity usually occurs with levels above 20 mcg/ml.
- Tell patient to report GI distress, palpitations, irritability, restlessness, nervousness, or insomnia; may indicate excessive CNS stimulation.
- Administer drug after meals and at bedtime.
- Store at 15° to 30° C (59° to 86° F).

Protect elixir from light and tablets from moisture.
• Equivalent to 64% anhydrous theophylline.
• Monitor therapy carefully. Individuals metabolize theophyllines at different rates. Dosage adjustments are necessary in the elderly, in patients with CHF, cor pulmonale, hepatic disease, and in smokers.
• Combination products that contain ephedrine are not recommended; excessive CNS stimulation may result (nervousness, tremors, akathisia).

pirbuterol

Maxair

Pregnancy Risk Category: C

HOW SUPPLIED
Inhaler: 0.2 mg/metered dose

MECHANISM OF ACTION
Relaxes bronchial smooth muscle by acting on beta$_2$-adrenergic receptors.

INDICATIONS AND DOSAGE
Prevention and reversal of bronchospasm, asthma –
Adults: 1 or 2 inhalations (0.2 to 0.4 mg) repeated q 4 to 6 hours. Not to exceed 12 inhalations daily.

ADVERSE REACTIONS
Common reactions are in italics; life-threatening reactions are in bold italics.
CNS: tremors, nervousness, dizziness, insomnia, headache.
CV: tachycardia, palpitations, increased blood pressure.
EENT: drying or irritation of throat.

INTERACTIONS
Propranolol and other beta-adrenergic blocking agents: decreased bronchodilating effects.

NURSING CONSIDERATIONS
• *Contraindicated* in hypersensitivity to pirbuterol or other adrenergics, and in patients with digitalis toxicity or cardiac arrhythmias associated with tachycardia.
• Tell patient to call the doctor if he experiences increased bronchospasm after using the drug.
• Teach patient to perform oral inhalation correctly. Give the following instructions for using a metered-dose inhaler:
  – Clear nasal passages and throat.
  – Breathe out, expelling as much air from lungs as possible.
  – Place mouthpiece well into mouth as dose from inhaler is released, and inhale deeply.
  – Hold breath for several seconds, remove mouthpiece, and exhale slowly.
• If more than one inhalation is ordered, the patient should wait at least 2 minutes before repeating the procedure for a second dose.
• Tell patient who is also using a steroid inhaler to use the bronchodilator first, then wait about 5 minutes before using the steroid. This allows the bronchodilator to open air passages for maximum effectiveness.
• Advise patient to seek medical attention if a previously effective dosage does not control symptoms because this may signify a worsening of the disease.

terbutaline sulfate

Brethaire, Brethine, Bricanyl

Pregnancy Risk Category: B

HOW SUPPLIED
Tablets: 2.5 mg, 5 mg
Aerosol inhaler: 200 mcg/metered spray
Injection: 1 mg/ml

MECHANISM OF ACTION
Relaxes bronchial smooth muscle by acting on beta$_2$-adrenergic receptors. Also relaxes uterine muscle.

*Liquid form contains alcohol. **May contain tartrazine.

INDICATIONS & DOSAGE

Relief of bronchospasm in patients with reversible obstructive airway disease –

Adults and children over 11 years: 2 inhalations separated by a 60-second interval, repeated q 4 to 6 hours. May also administer 2.5 to 5 mg P.O. q 8 hours or 0.25 mg S.C.

Treatment of premature labor –

Women: 0.01 mg/minute by I.V. infusion. Increase by 0.005 mg q 10 minutes up to 0.025 mg/minute or until contractions cease. Or, give 0.25 mg S.C. hourly until contractions cease. Maintenance dosage is 5 mg P.O. q 4 hours for 48 hours, then 5 mg q 6 hours.

ADVERSE REACTIONS

Common reactions are in italics; life-threatening reactions are in bold italics.

CNS: *nervousness, tremors, headache,* drowsiness, sweating.

CV: palpitations, increased heart rate.

EENT: drying and irritation of nose and throat (with inhaled form).

GI: vomiting, nausea.

Other: hypokalemia (with high doses).

INTERACTIONS

CNS stimulants: increased CNS stimulation. Avoid concomitant use.

Levodopa: increased risk of arrhythmia. Avoid concomitant use.

MAO inhibitors: when given with sympathomimetics, may cause severe hypertension (hypertensive crisis). Don't use together.

Propranolol and other beta blockers: blocked bronchodilating effects of terbutaline.

Digitalis glycosides, levodopa, halogenated inhalational anesthetics, cyclopropane: increased risk of cardiac arrhythmias. Monitor closely.

NURSING CONSIDERATIONS

- *Contraindicated* in patients with hypersensitivity to the drug; in patients with tachyarrhythmias, tachycardia caused by digitalis toxicity, narrow-angle glaucoma, or shock; and in those receiving general anesthesia with cyclopropane or halogenated inhalational anesthetics.
- *Use cautiously* in patients with diabetes, hypertension, hyperthyroidism, severe cardiac disease, and cardiac arrhythmias.
- Protect injection from light. Do not use if discolored.
- Make sure patient and his family understand why drug is necessary.
- Give S.C. injections in lateral deltoid area.
- Tolerance may develop with prolonged use.
- Warn patient about the possibility of paradoxical bronchospasm. If this occurs, the drug should be discontinued immediately.
- Patient may use tablets and aerosol concomitantly. Monitor closely for toxicity.
- Teach patient to perform oral inhalation correctly. Give the following instructions for using a metered-dose inhaler:
  - Clear nasal passages and throat.
  - Breathe out, expelling as much air from lungs as possible.
  - Place mouthpiece well into mouth as dose from inhaler is released, and inhale deeply.
  - Hold breath for several seconds, remove mouthpiece, and exhale slowly.
- If more than one inhalation is ordered, the patient should wait at least 2 minutes before repeating the procedure for a second dose.
- Tell patient who is also using a steroid inhaler to use the bronchodilator first, then wait about 5 minutes before using the steroid. This allows the bronchodilator to open air passages for maximum effectiveness.

• Although not approved by the FDA for treatment of preterm labor, it is considered very effective and is used in many hospitals. Monitor neonates for hypoglycemia.

theophylline

Immediate-release liquids: Accurbron*, Aerolate, Aquaphyllin, Asmalix*, Bronkodyl*, Elixicon, Elixomin*, Elixophyllin*, Lanophyllin*, Lixolin, Slo-Phyllin, Theolair, Theon*, Theophyl*
Immediate-release tablets and capsules: Bronkodyl, Elixophyllin, Nuelin‡, Slo-Phyllin, Somophyllin-T
Timed-release tablets: Constant-T, Duraphyl, Quibron-T/SR, Respbid, Sustaire, Theo-Dur, Theolair-SR, Theo-Time, Uniphyl
Timed-release capsules: Aerolate, Bronkodyl S-R, Elixophyllin SR, Lodrane, Nuelin-SR‡, Slo-bid Gyrocaps, Slo-Phyllin, Somophyllin-CRT, Theo-24, Theobid Duracaps, Theobid Jr., Theochron, Theo-Dur Sprinkle, Theophyl-SR, Theospan SR, Theovent Long-acting

theophylline sodium glycinate

Acet-Am†, Synophylate

Pregnancy Risk Category: C

HOW SUPPLIED

theophylline
Tablets: 100 mg, 125 mg, 200 mg, 225 mg, 250 mg, 300 mg
Tablets (chewable): 100 mg
Tablets (extended-release): 100 mg, 200 mg, 250 mg, 300 mg, 400 mg, 500 mg
Capsules: 50 mg, 100 mg, 200 mg, 250 mg
Capsules (extended-release): 50 mg, 60 mg, 65 mg, 75 mg, 100 mg, 125 mg, 130 mg, 200 mg, 250 mg, 260 mg, 300 mg
Elixir: 27 mg/5 ml, 50 mg/5 ml*
Oral solution: 27 mg/5 ml, 53 mg/5 ml
Oral suspension: 100 mg/5 ml
Syrup: 27 mg/5 ml, 50 mg/5 ml
Dextrose 5% injection: 200 mg in 50 ml or 100 ml; 400 mg in 100 ml, 250 ml, 500 ml, or 1,000 ml; 800 mg in 500 ml or 1,000 ml
theophylline sodium glycinate
Elixir: 110 mg/5 ml (equivalent to 55 mg anhydrous theophylline/5 ml)

MECHANISM OF ACTION

Inhibits phosphodiesterase, the enzyme that degrades cyclic adenosine monophosphate. Results in relaxation of smooth muscle of the bronchial airways and pulmonary blood vessels.

INDICATIONS & DOSAGE

Prophylaxis and symptomatic relief of bronchial asthma, bronchospasm of chronic bronchitis and emphysema –
Adults: 6 mg/kg P.O. followed by 2 to 3 mg/kg q 4 hours for 2 doses. Maintenance dosage is 1 to 3 mg/kg q 8 to 12 hours.
Children 9 to 16 years: 6 mg/kg P.O. followed by 3 mg/kg q 4 hours for 3 doses. Maintenance dosage is 3 mg/kg q 6 hours.
Children 6 months to 9 years: 6 mg/kg P.O. followed by 4 mg/kg q 4 hours for 3 doses. Maintenance dosage is 4 mg/kg q 6 hours.

Most oral timed-release forms are given q 8 to 12 hours. Several products, however, may be given q 24 hours.

Symptomatic relief of bronchial asthma, pulmonary emphysema, and chronic bronchitis –
Adults: 330 to 660 mg (sodium glycinate) P.O. q 6 to 8 hours, after meals.
Children over 12 years: 220 to 330 mg (sodium glycinate) P.O. q 6 to 8 hours.
Children 6 to 12 years: 330 mg (sodium glycinate) P.O. q 6 to 8 hours.
Children 3 to 6 years: 110 to 165 mg

*Liquid form contains alcohol. **May contain tartrazine.

(sodium glycinate) P.O. q 6 to 8 hours.
Children 1 to 3 years: 55 to 110 mg (sodium glycinate) P.O. q 6 to 8 hours.
Parenteral theophylline for patients not currently receiving theophylline –
Loading dose: 4.7 mg/kg I.V. slowly; then maintenance infusion.
Adults (nonsmokers): 0.55 mg/kg/hour for 12 hours, then 0.39 mg/kg/hour.
Otherwise-healthy adult smokers: 0.79 mg/kg/hour for 12 hours; then 0.63 mg/kg/hour.
Older adults with cor pulmonale: 0.47 mg/kg/hour for 12 hours; then 0.24 mg/kg/hour.
Adults with CHF or liver disease: 0.38 mg/kg/hour for 12 hours; then 0.08 to 0.16 mg/kg/hour.
Children 9 to 16 years: 0.79 mg/kg/hour for 12 hours; then 0.63 mg/kg/hour.
Children 6 months to 9 years: 0.95 mg/kg/hour for 12 hours; then 0.79 mg/kg/hour.

Switch to oral theophylline as soon as patient shows adequate improvement.
Symptomatic relief of bronchospasm in patients currently receiving theophylline –
Adults and children: each 0.5 mg/kg I.V. or P.O. (loading dose) will increase plasma levels by 1 mcg/ml. Ideally, dose is based upon current theophylline level. In emergency situations, some clinicians recommend a 2.5 mg/kg P.O. dose of rapidly absorbed form if no obvious signs of theophylline toxicity are present.
Adjunctive treatment of neonatal apnea –
Neonates: 5 mg/kg I.V. as a loading dose, followed by 2 mg/kg/day in two or three divided doses.

ADVERSE REACTIONS
Common reactions are in italics; life-threatening reactions are in bold italics.
CNS: *restlessness, dizziness,* headache, *insomnia,* light-headedness, *seizures,* muscle twitching.
CV: *palpitations, sinus tachycardia,* extrasystoles, flushing, marked hypotension, increase in respiratory rate.
GI: *nausea, vomiting, anorexia,* bitter aftertaste, dyspepsia, heavy feeling in stomach, diarrhea.
Skin: urticaria.

INTERACTIONS
Adenosine: decreased antiarrhythmic effectiveness. Higher doses of adenosine may be necessary.
Barbiturates, carbamazepine, nicotine, phenytoin, rifampin: enhanced metabolism and decreased theophylline blood levels. Monitor for decreased effect.
Beta-adrenergic blockers: antagonism. Propranolol and nadolol, especially, may cause bronchospasms in sensitive patients. Use together cautiously.
Cimetidine, influenza virus vaccine, macrolide antibiotics (such as erythromycin), oral contraceptives, quinolone antibiotics (such as ciprofloxacin): decreased hepatic clearance of theophylline; elevated theophylline levels. Monitor for signs of toxicity.

NURSING CONSIDERATIONS
- *Contraindicated* in hypersensitivity to xanthine compounds (caffeine, theobromine) and in preexisting cardiac arrhythmias, especially tachyarrhythmias.
- *Use cautiously* in young children; in elderly patients with CHF or other circulatory impairment, cor pulmonale, renal or hepatic disease; and in peptic ulcer, hyperthyroidism, or diabetes mellitus.
- Individuals metabolize xanthines at different rates; determine dosage by monitoring response, tolerance, pulmonary function, and serum theophylline levels. Serum theophylline concentrations should range from 10 to

20 mcg/ml; toxicity has been reported with levels above 20 mcg/ml.

- Monitor vital signs; measure and record intake and output. Expected clinical effects include improvement in quality of pulse and respiration.
- Warn elderly patients of dizziness, a common adverse reaction at start of therapy.
- GI symptoms may be relieved by taking oral drug with full glass of water after meals, although food in stomach delays absorption.
- Question patient closely about other drugs used. Warn him that OTC remedies may contain ephedrine in combination with theophylline salts; excessive CNS stimulation may result. Tell him to check with doctor or pharmacist before taking *any* other medications.
- Supply instructions for home care and dosage schedule.
- Daily dosage may need to be decreased in patients with CHF or hepatic disease, or in elderly patients, since metabolism and excretion may be decreased. Monitor carefully, using blood levels, observation, examination, and patient interview. Give drug around the clock, using sustained-release product at bedtime.
- Drug dosage may need to be increased in cigarette smokers and in habitual marijuana smokers because smoking causes the drug to be metabolized faster.
- Be careful not to confuse sustained-release dosage forms with standard-release dosage forms.
- Warn patient not to dissolve, crush, or chew slow-release products. Small children unable to swallow these can ingest (without chewing) the contents of bead-filled capsules sprinkled over soft food.
- Warn patients to take the drug regularly, as directed. Patients tend to want to take extra "breathing pills."
- Patients taking Theo-24 brand of theophylline should take it on an empty stomach because food accelerates the drug's absorption.
- **I.V. use:** Use infusion pump for continuous infusion.

*Liquid form contains alcohol. **May contain tartrazine.

44

Expectorants and antitussives

acetylcysteine
ammonium chloride
(See Chapter 62, ACIDIFIER AND ALKALINIZERS.)
benzonatate
codeine phosphate
(See Chapter 27, NARCOTIC AND OPIOID ANALGESICS.)
codeine sulfate
(See Chapter 27, NARCOTIC AND OPIOID ANALGESICS.)
dextromethorphan hydrobromide
diphenhydramine hydrochloride
(See Chapter 42, ANTIHISTAMINES.)
guaifenesin
hydromorphone hydrochloride
(See Chapter 27, NARCOTIC AND OPIOID ANALGESICS.)
potassium iodide
terpin hydrate

COMBINATION PRODUCTS

Preparations are available in the following combinations:

- expectorants with decongestants or antihistamines, or both
- antitussives with decongestants or antihistamines, or both
- expectorants and antitussives
- expectorants and antitussives with decongestants or antihistamines, or both.

acetylcysteine

Airbron†, Mucomyst, Mucosol, Parvolex†‡

Pregnancy Risk Category: B

HOW SUPPLIED

Solution: 10%, 20%
Injection: 200 mg/ml†‡

MECHANISM OF ACTION

A mucolytic, increases production of respiratory tract fluids to help liquefy and reduce the viscosity of tenacious secretions. Also restores liver stores of glutathione in the treatment of acetaminophen toxicity.

INDICATIONS & DOSAGE

Pneumonia, bronchitis, tuberculosis, cystic fibrosis, emphysema, atelectasis (adjunct), complications of thoracic surgery and CV surgery –
Adults and children: 1 to 2 ml 10% to 20% solution by direct instillation into trachea as often as every hour; or 3 to 5 ml 20% solution, or 6 to 10 ml 10% solution, by mouthpiece t.i.d. or q.i.d.
Acetaminophen toxicity –
Adults and children: 140 mg/kg P.O. initially, followed by 70 mg/kg q 4 hours for 17 doses (a total of 1,330 mg/kg). Alternatively, administer 300 mg/kg by I.V. infusion as follows: initially, give 150 mg/kg diluted in up to 200 ml of dextrose 5% in water (D_5W) and infuse over 15 minutes. Follow with a second infusion of 50 mg/kg diluted in 500 ml D_5W over 4 hours. Finally, give 100 mg/kg diluted in 1,000 ml D_5W and infuse over 16 hours.

ADVERSE REACTIONS

Common reactions are in italics; life-threatening reactions are in bold italics.
EENT: *rhinorrhea, hemoptysis.*
GI: *stomatitis, nausea, vomiting.*
Other: ***bronchospasm*** *(especially in asthmatics).*

INTERACTIONS

Activated charcoal: don't use together in treating acetaminophen toxicity. Limits acetylcysteine's effectiveness.

NURSING CONSIDERATIONS

- *Contraindicated* in patients with hypersensitivity to the drug.
- *Use cautiously* in asthma or severe respiratory insufficiency and in elderly or debilitated patients.
- May have a foul taste or smell that some patients find distressing.
- Use plastic, glass, stainless steel, or another nonreactive metal when administering by nebulization. Hand bulb nebulizers not recommended because output is too small and particle size too large.
- After opening, store in refrigerator; use within 96 hours.
- Incompatible with oxytetracycline, tetracycline, erythromycin lactobionate, amphotericin B, ampicillin, iodized oil, chymotrypsin, trypsin, and hydrogen peroxide. Administer separately.
- Monitor cough type and frequency. For maximum effect, instruct patient to clear his airway by coughing before aerosol administration.
- Acetylcysteine is administered for treatment of acetaminophen overdose within 24 hours after ingestion. Treatment should not be delayed for results of acetaminophen blood levels.
- When used orally to treat acetaminophen overdose, dilute oral doses with cola, fruit juice, or water before administering. Dilute the 20% solution to a concentration of 5% (add 3 ml diluent to each ml acetylcysteine). If patient vomits within 1 hour of administration of loading or maintenance dose, repeat dose.
- **I.V. use:** To prepare I.V. infusion, dilute calculated dose in D_5W. Dilute initial dose (150 mg/kg) in 200 ml D_5W and infuse over 15 minutes. Dilute second dose of 50 mg/kg in 500 ml D_5W and give over 4 hours. Dilute final dose of 100 mg/kg in 1,000 ml D_5W and infuse over 16 hours.

benzonatate

Tessalon

Pregnancy Risk Category: C

HOW SUPPLIED

Capsules: 100 mg

MECHANISM OF ACTION

Suppresses the cough reflex by direct action on the cough center in the medulla (brain). Also has local anesthetic action.

INDICATIONS & DOSAGE

Nonproductive cough–

Adults and children over 10 years: 100 mg P.O. t.i.d.; up to 600 mg daily.

Children under 10 years: 8 mg/kg P.O. in 3 to 6 divided doses.

ADVERSE REACTIONS

Common reactions are in italics; life-threatening reactions are in bold italics.

CNS: dizziness, drowsiness, headache.

EENT: nasal congestion, sensation of burning in eyes.

GI: nausea, constipation.

Skin: rash.

Other: chills.

INTERACTIONS

None significant.

NURSING CONSIDERATIONS

- *Contraindicated* in patients with hypersensitivity to the drug.
- Patient should not chew capsules or dissolve in mouth; local anesthesia will result. If capsules dissolve in mouth, CNS stimulation may cause restlessness, tremors, and possibly seizures.
- A nonnarcotic cough suppressant; don't use when cough is valuable as diagnostic sign or is beneficial (as after thoracic surgery).
- Monitor cough type and frequency.

• Use with percussion and chest vibration.
• Maintain fluid intake to help liquefy sputum.

dextromethorphan hydrobromide

Balminil D.M.◇, Benylin DM◇, Broncho-Grippol-DM†, Congespirin for Children◇, Cremacoat 1◇, Delsym◇, DM Cough*◇, Hold◇, Koffex†, Mediquell◇, Neo-DM†, Pediacare 1◇, Pertussin 8 Hour Cough Formula◇, Robidex†, Sedatuss†, St. Joseph for Children◇, Sucrets Cough Control Formula◇. More commonly available in combination products such as Contac Cough and Sore Throat Formula◇, Contact Cough Formula◇, Contac Jr. Children's Cold Medicine◇, Contac Nighttime Cold Medicine◇, Contac Severe Cold Formula Caplets◇, Novahistine DMX Liquid, Phenergan with Dextromethorphan*, Robitussin-DM*◇, Rondec-DM*◇, Triaminicol Multi-Symptom Cold◇, Trind-DM Liquid*◇

Pregnancy Risk Category: C

HOW SUPPLIED
Chewable pieces: 15 mg◇
Liquid (sustained-action): 30 mg/5 ml◇
Lozenges: 5 mg◇
Syrup: 5 mg/5 ml*◇, 7.5 mg/5 ml*◇, 10 mg/5 ml*◇, 15 mg/5 ml*◇

MECHANISM OF ACTION
Suppresses the cough reflex by direct action on the cough center in the medulla (brain).

INDICATIONS & DOSAGE
Nonproductive cough –
Adults: 10 to 20 mg P.O. q 4 hours, or 30 mg q 6 to 8 hours. Or the controlled-release liquid twice daily (60 mg b.i.d.). Maximum 120 mg daily.
Children 6 to 12 years: 5 to 10 mg P.O. q 4 hours, or 15 mg q 6 to 8 hours. Or the controlled-release liquid twice daily (30 mg b.i.d.). Maximum 60 mg daily.
Children 2 to 6 years: 2.5 to 5 mg P.O. q 4 hours, or 7.5 mg q 6 to 8 hours. Maximum 30 mg daily.

ADVERSE REACTIONS
Common reactions are in italics; life-threatening reactions are in bold italics.
CNS: drowsiness, dizziness.
GI: nausea, vomiting, stomach pain.

INTERACTIONS
MAO inhibitors: hypotension, coma, hyperpyrexia, and death have occurred. Do not use together.

NURSING CONSIDERATIONS
• *Contraindicated* in patients currently taking or within 2 weeks of discontinuing MAO inhibitors.
• Produces no analgesia or addiction and little or no CNS depression.
• An antitussive; don't use when cough is valuable diagnostic sign or beneficial (as after thoracic surgery).
• Use with percussion and chest vibration.
• Monitor cough type and frequency.
• Dose of 15 to 30 mg dextromethorphan is equivalent to 8 to 15 mg codeine as an antitussive.

guaifenesin (glyceryl guaiacolate)

Anti-Tuss*◇, Balminil Expectorant†, Baytussin◇, Breonesin◇, Colrex Expectorant*◇, Cremacoat 2◇, Gee-Gee◇, GG-CEN*◇, Glyate*◇, Glycotuss◇, Glytuss◇, Guiatuss*◇, Halotussin◇, Humibid L.A.◇, Hytuss◇, Hytuss-2X◇, Malotuss◇, Naldecon Senior EX◇, Neo-Spec†,

†Available in Canada only. ‡Available in Australia only. ◇Available OTC.

Nortussin◊, Resyl†◊, Robafen◊, Robitussin*◊, S-T Expectorant◊

Pregnancy Risk Category: C

HOW SUPPLIED
Tablets: 100 mg◊, 200 mg◊
Capsules: 200 mg◊
Syrup: 67 mg/5 ml*◊, 100 mg/5 ml*◊

MECHANISM OF ACTION
Increases production of respiratory tract fluids to help liquefy and reduce the viscosity of tenacious secretions.

INDICATIONS & DOSAGE
As expectorant –
Adults: 100 to 400 mg P.O. q 4 hours. Maximum 2,400 mg daily.
Children 6 to 12 years: 100 to 200 mg P.O. q 4 hours. Maximum 600 mg daily.
Children 2 to 5 years: 50 to 100 mg P.O. q 4 hours. Maximum 300 mg daily.

ADVERSE REACTIONS
Common reactions are in italics; life-threatening reactions are in bold italics.
CNS: drowsiness.
GI: stomach pain, diarrhea, vomiting and nausea occur with large doses.

INTERACTIONS
Heparin: increased risk of bleeding. Use together cautiously.

NURSING CONSIDERATIONS
- *Contraindicated* in patients with hypersensitivity to the drug.
- May interfere with certain laboratory tests for 5-hydroxyindoleacetic acid and vanillylmandelic acid.
- Drug is used to liquefy thick, tenacious sputum, but efficacy has not been established. Simply increasing fluid intake may prove beneficial. Tell patient to take each dose with a glass of water.
- Monitor cough type and frequency. Be sure patient understands that persistent cough may indicate a serious condition and that he should call the doctor if cough lasts longer than 1 week, recurs frequently, or is associated with high fever, rash, or severe headache.
- Encourage deep-breathing exercises.

potassium iodide

Pregnancy Risk Category: D

HOW SUPPLIED
Tablets (enteric-coated): 300 mg
Oral solution: 500 mg/15 ml
Saturated solution (SSKI): 1 g/ml
Strong iodine solution (Lugol's solution): iodine 50 mg/ml and potassium iodide 100 mg/ml
Syrup: 325 mg/5 ml

MECHANISM OF ACTION
Increases production of respiratory tract fluids to help liquefy and reduce the viscosity of thick secretions.

INDICATIONS & DOSAGE
As expectorant, chronic bronchitis, chronic pulmonary emphysema, bronchial asthma –
Adults: 0.3 to 0.6 ml P.O. q 4 to 6 hours.
Children: 0.25 to 0.5 ml P.O. of saturated solution (1 g/ml) b.i.d. to q.i.d.
Nuclear radiation protection –
Adults and children: 0.13 ml P.O. of SSKI immediately before or after initial exposure will block 90% of radioactive iodine. Same dose given 3 to 4 hours after exposure will provide 50% block. Should be administered for up to 10 days under medical supervision.
Infants under 1 year: ½ adult dose.

ADVERSE REACTIONS
Common reactions are in italics; life-threatening reactions are in bold italics.
GI: *nausea,* vomiting, *epigastric pain,* metallic taste.
Metabolic: goiter, hyperthyroid ade-

noma, hypothyroidism (with excessive use), collagen disease-like syndrome.
Skin: rash.
Other: drug fever.
Prolonged use: chronic iodine poisoning, soreness of mouth, coryza, sneezing, swelling of eyelids.

INTERACTIONS
Antithyroid medications, lithium carbonate: may potentiate the hypothyroid effect. Avoid concomitant use.

NURSING CONSIDERATIONS
- *Contraindicated* in iodine hypersensitivity, tuberculosis, hyperkalemia, acute bronchitis, hyperthyroidism.
- Maintain adequate fluid intake. Encourage patient to take each dose with a full glass of water to help liquefy secretions.
- Has strong, salty, metallic taste. Dilute with milk, fruit juice, or broth to reduce GI distress and disguise taste.
- Sudden withdrawal may precipitate thyroid storm.
- If skin rash appears, discontinue use. Contact doctor.
- Efficacy has not been established.

terpin hydrate*◊
Pregnancy Risk Category: C

HOW SUPPLIED
Elixir: 85 mg/5 ml (43% alcohol)*◊

MECHANISM OF ACTION
Increases production of respiratory tract fluids to help liquefy and reduce the viscosity of thick secretions.

INDICATIONS & DOSAGE
Excessive bronchial secretions –
Adults: 5 to 10 ml P.O. of elixir q 4 to 6 hours.

ADVERSE REACTIONS
Common reactions are in italics; life-threatening reactions are in bold italics.
GI: nausea, vomiting.

INTERACTIONS
None significant.

NURSING CONSIDERATIONS
- *Contraindicated* in peptic ulcer or severe diabetes mellitus.
- Don't give in large doses; *high alcoholic content of elixir* (86 proof).
- Monitor cough type and frequency.
- Efficacy as an expectorant has not been established.
- Contains alcohol. Drug should not be used during pregnancy. Consider risk and benefit in breast-feeding women.
- Tell patient to take each dose with a full glass of water to liquefy secretions.

45

Antacids, adsorbents, and antiflatulents

aluminum carbonate
aluminum hydroxide
aluminum phosphate
calcium carbonate
dihydroxyaluminum sodium carbonate
magaldrate
magnesium oxide
magnesium hydroxide
(See Chapter 48, LAXATIVES.)
simethicone
sodium bicarbonate
(See Chapter 62, ACIDIFIER AND ALKALINIZERS.)

COMBINATION PRODUCTS

ALKA-SELTZER, MEDI-SELTZER◇: sodium bicarbonate 1,916 mg, aspirin 325 mg, and citric acid 1,000 mg.
ALKA-SELTZER WITHOUT ASPIRIN◇: sodium bicarbonate 958 mg, citric acid 832 mg, and potassium bicarbonate 312 mg.
ALUDROX SUSPENSION◇: aluminum hydroxide 307 mg, magnesium hydroxide 103 mg.
CAMALOX TABLETS◇: aluminum hydroxide 225 mg, magnesium hydroxide 200 mg, and calcium carbonate 250 mg.
DELCID SUSPENSION◇: aluminum hydroxide 600 mg, magnesium hydroxide 665 mg.
DI-GEL LIQUID◇: aluminum hydroxide 200 mg, magnesium hydroxide 200 mg, simethicone 20 mg.
EXTRA STRENGTH MAALOX TABLETS◇: aluminum hydroxide 400 mg and magnesium hydroxide 400 mg.
FLATULEX: simethicone 80 mg and activated charcoal 250 mg.
GAVISCON◇: aluminum hydroxide 31.7 mg, magnesium carbonate 137 mg.
GELUSIL◇: aluminum hydroxide 200 mg, magnesium hydroxide 200 mg, simethicone 25 mg.
GELUSIL-II◇: aluminum hydroxide 400 mg, magnesium hydroxide 400 mg, simethicone 30 mg.
MAALOX NO. 1◇: aluminum hydroxide 200 mg and magnesium hydroxide 200 mg.
MAALOX PLUS TABLETS◇: aluminum hydroxide 200 mg, magnesium hydroxide 200 mg, simethicone 25 mg.
MAALOX TC TABLETS◇: aluminum hydroxide 600 mg, magnesium hydroxide 300 mg.
MAGNATRIL◇: aluminum hydroxide 260 mg, magnesium hydroxide 130 mg, and magnesium trisilicate 455 mg.
MYLANTA TABLETS◇: aluminum hydroxide 200 mg, magnesium hydroxide 200 mg, simethicone 20 mg.
MYLANTA-II TABLETS◇: aluminum hydroxide 400 mg, magnesium hydroxide 400 mg, simethicone 40 mg.
RIOPAN PLUS CHEW TABLETS◇: magaldrate 540 mg, simethicone 20 mg.
RIOPAN PLUS SUSPENSION◇: magaldrate 540 mg and simethicone 20 mg/5 ml.
SILAIN-GEL◇: aluminum hydroxide 282 mg, magnesium hydroxide 285 mg, simethicone 25 mg per 5 ml.
TITRALAC LIQUID◇: calcium carbonate 1,000 mg in glycine.
TITRALAC TABLETS◇: calcium carbonate 420 mg, glycine 150 mg.
UNIVOL†◇: aluminum hydroxide and magnesium carbonate co-dried gel 300 mg and magnesium hydroxide 100 mg.
WINGEL◇: aluminum hydroxide 180 mg, magnesium hydroxide 160 mg.

*Liquid form contains alcohol. **May contain tartrazine.

aluminum carbonate

Basaljel◊

Pregnancy Risk Category: C

HOW SUPPLIED

Tablets or capsules: aluminum hydroxide equivalent 500 mg◊

Oral suspension: aluminum hydroxide equivalent 400 mg/5 ml◊, 1 g/5 ml◊

MECHANISM OF ACTION

Reduces total acid load in the GI tract and elevates gastric pH to reduce pepsin activity. Also strengthens the gastric mucosal barrier and increases esophageal sphincter tone. An antacid.

INDICATIONS & DOSAGE

As antacid –

Adults: suspension: 5 to 10 ml P.O., p.r.n. Extra-strength suspension: 2.5 to 5 ml, p.r.n. Tablets: 1 to 2, p.r.n. Capsules: 1 to 2, p.r.n.

To prevent formation of urinary phosphate stones (with low-phosphate diet) –

Adults: suspension: 15 to 30 ml suspension in water or juice P.O. 1 hour after meals and h.s.; 5 to 15 ml extra-strength suspension in water or juice 1 hour after meals and h.s.; 2 to 6 tablets or capsules 1 hour after meals and h.s.

ADVERSE REACTIONS

Common reactions are in italics; life-threatening reactions are in bold italics.

GI: anorexia, *constipation,* intestinal obstruction.

Metabolic: hypophosphatemia.

INTERACTIONS

Allopurinol, antibiotics (including quinolones and tetracyclines), diflunisal, digoxin, iron, isoniazid, penicillamine, phenothiazines, quinidine: decreased pharmacologic effect because absorption may be impaired. Separate administration times.

NURSING CONSIDERATIONS

- *Use cautiously* in elderly patients, especially those with decreased GI motility (those receiving antidiarrheals, antispasmodics, or anticholinergics), dehydration, fluid restriction, chronic renal disease, and suspected intestinal obstruction.
- Record amount and consistency of stools. Manage constipation with laxatives or stool softeners; alternate with magnesium-containing antacids (if patient does not have renal disease).
- Shake suspension well; give with small amount of water or fruit juice to ensure passage to stomach. When administering through nasogastric tube, be sure tube is placed correctly and is patent; follow antacid with water to clear tube.
- Watch long-term high-dose use in patient on restricted sodium intake.
- Warn patient not to take aluminum carbonate indiscriminately and not to switch antacids without doctor's advice.
- Because it contains aluminum, it is used in renal failure to help control hyperphosphatemia. Binds phosphate in GI tract.
- Monitor serum phosphate.
- Watch for symptoms of hypophosphatemia with prolonged use (anorexia, malaise, muscle weakness); can also lead to resorption of calcium and bone demineralization.
- May cause enteric-coated drugs to be released prematurely in stomach. Separate doses by 1 hour.
- Basaljel liquid contains no sugar.

aluminum hydroxide

ALternaGEL◊, Alu-Cap◊, Alu-Tab◊, Amphojel◊, Amphotabs‡, Dialume◊, Nephrox◊

Pregnancy Risk Category: C

HOW SUPPLIED
Tablets: 300 mg◊, 600 mg◊
Capsules: 475 mg◊, 500 mg◊
Oral suspension: 320 mg/5 ml◊, 600 mg/5 ml◊

MECHANISM OF ACTION
Reduces total acid load in the GI tract and elevates gastric pH to reduce pepsin activity. Also strengthens the gastric mucosal barrier and increases esophageal sphincter tone. An antacid.

INDICATIONS & DOSAGE
Antacid –
Adults: 600 mg P.O. (5 to 10 ml of most products) 1 hour after meals and h.s.; 300- or 600-mg tablet, chewed before swallowing, taken with milk or water 5 to 6 times daily after meals and h.s.
Hyperphosphatemia in renal failure –
Adults: 500 mg to 2 g P.O. b.i.d. to q.i.d.

ADVERSE REACTIONS
Common reactions are in italics; life-threatening reactions are in bold italics.
GI: anorexia, *constipation,* intestinal obstruction.
Metabolic: hypophosphatemia.

INTERACTIONS
Allopurinol, antibiotics (including quinolones and tetracyclines), diflunisal, digoxin, iron, isoniazid, penicillamine, phenothiazines, quinidine: decreased pharmacologic effect because absorption may be impaired. Separate administration times.

NURSING CONSIDERATIONS
• *Use cautiously* in elderly patients, especially those with decreased GI motility (those receiving antidiarrheals, antispasmodics, or anticholinergics), dehydration, fluid restriction, chronic renal disease, and suspected intestinal obstruction.
• Record amount and consistency of stools. Manage constipation with laxatives or stool softeners; alternate with magnesium-containing antacids (if patient does not have renal disease).
• Shake suspension well; give with small amount of milk or water to assure passage to stomach. When administering through nasogastric tube, make sure tube is placed correctly and is patent. After instilling antacid, flush tube with water.
• Watch long-term high-dose use in patient on restricted sodium intake.
• Warn patient not to take aluminum hydroxide indiscriminately or switch antacids without doctor's advice.
• Because it contains aluminum, it is used in renal failure to help control hyperphosphatemia. Binds phosphate in the GI tract.
• Monitor serum phosphate.
• Watch for symptoms of hypophosphatemia with prolonged use (anorexia, malaise, and muscle weakness); can also lead to resorption of calcium and bone demineralization.
• May cause enteric-coated drugs to be released prematurely in stomach. Separate doses by 1 hour.

aluminum phosphate
Phosphaljel◊

Pregnancy Risk Category: C

HOW SUPPLIED
Oral suspension: 233 mg/5 ml◊

MECHANISM OF ACTION
Provides supplemental phosphate.

INDICATIONS & DOSAGE
To reduce fecal elimination of phosphorus –
Adults: 15 to 30 ml undiluted P.O. q 2 hours between meals and h.s.

ADVERSE REACTIONS
Common reactions are in italics; life-threatening reactions are in bold italics.

GI: *constipation,* intestinal obstruction.

INTERACTIONS

Ciprofloxacin, quinolone antibiotics, tetracyclines: decreased antibiotic effect. Separate administration times.

NURSING CONSIDERATIONS

- *Use cautiously* in elderly patients, especially those with decreased GI motility (those receiving antidiarrheals, antispasmodics, or anticholinergics), dehydration, fluid restriction, chronic renal disease, and suspected intestinal obstruction.
- Record amount and consistency of stools. Manage constipation with laxatives or stool softeners; alternate with magnesium-containing antacids (if patient does not have renal disease).
- Shake well; give alone or with small amount of milk or water. When administering through nasogastric tube, make sure tube is placed correctly and is patent; after instilling, flush tube with water to facilitate passage to stomach and maintain tube patency.
- Watch long-term high-dose use in patient on restricted sodium intake.
- Warn patient not to take aluminum phosphate indiscriminately and not to switch antacids without doctor's advice.
- This drug is a very weak antacid.
- Can reverse hypophosphatemia induced by aluminum hydroxide.
- May cause enteric-coated drugs to be released prematurely in stomach. Separate doses by 1 hour.
- Phosphaljel contains no sugar.

calcium carbonate

Alka-Mints◇, Amitone◇, Calcilac◇, Calcimax‡, Calglycine◇, Cal-Sup‡, Chooz◇, Dicarbosil◇, Effercal-600‡, Equilet◇, Genalac◇, Glycate◇, Gustalac◇, Mallamint◇, Pama No. 1◇, Rolaids Calcium Rich◇, Titracid◇, Titralac◇, Tums◇, Tums E-X◇, Tums Liquid Extra Strength◇

Pregnancy Risk Category: C

HOW SUPPLIED

Calcium carbonate contains 40% calcium; 20 mEq calcium/g.
Tablets◇*:* 350 mg, 420 mg, 500 mg, 650 mg, 750 mg, 850 mg, 1,250 mg‡
Oral suspension: 1 g/5 ml◇
Effervescent powder: 1,500 mg (600 g elemental calcium)/5 g◇

MECHANISM OF ACTION

Reduces total acid load in the GI tract and elevates gastric pH to reduce pepsin activity. Also strengthens the gastric mucosal barrier and increases esophageal sphincter tone. An antacid.

INDICATIONS & DOSAGE

Antacid, calcium supplement –
Adults: 1-g tablet, P.O. 4 to 6 times daily, chewed well and taken with water; or 1 g of suspension (5 ml of most products), 1 hour after meals and h.s.

ADVERSE REACTIONS

Common reactions are in italics; life-threatening reactions are in bold italics.
GI: *constipation,* gastric distention, flatulence, rebound hyperacidity, *nausea.*
Metabolic: *hypercalcemia, hypophosphatemia;* if taken with milk – milk-alkali syndrome.

INTERACTIONS

Allopurinol, antibiotics (including quinolones and tetracyclines), diflunisal, digoxin, iron, isoniazid, penicillamine, phenothiazines, quinidine: decreased pharmacologic effect because absorption may be impaired. Separate administration times.

NURSING CONSIDERATIONS

- *Contraindicated* in severe renal disease. *Use cautiously* in elderly patients, especially those with decreased GI motility (those receiving antidiarrheals, antispasmodics, or anticholinergics), dehydration, fluid restriction, chronic renal disease, and suspected intestinal obstruction.
- Do not administer with milk or other foods high in vitamin D. Can cause milk-alkali syndrome (headache, confusion, distaste for food, nausea, vomiting, hypercalcemia, hypercalciuria, calcinosis, and hypophosphatemia).
- Record amount and consistency of stools. Manage constipation with laxatives or stool softeners.
- Watch for symptoms of hypercalcemia (nausea, vomiting, headache, mental confusion, and anorexia).
- Monitor serum calcium, especially in mild renal impairment.
- Warn patient not to take calcium carbonate indiscriminately and not to switch antacids without doctor's advice.
- May cause enteric-coated tablets to be released prematurely in stomach. Separate doses by 1 hour.

dihydroxyaluminum sodium carbonate

Rolaids◇

Pregnancy Risk Category: C

HOW SUPPLIED

Tablets: 334 mg◇

MECHANISM OF ACTION

Reduces total acid load in the GI tract and elevates gastric pH to reduce pepsin activity. Also strengthens the gastric mucosal barrier and increases esophageal sphincter tone. An antacid.

INDICATIONS & DOSAGE

Antacid –

Adults: chew 1 to 2 tablets (334 to 668 mg), p.r.n.

ADVERSE REACTIONS

Common reactions are in italics; life-threatening reactions are in bold italics.

GI: anorexia, *constipation,* intestinal obstruction.

INTERACTIONS

Allopurinol, antibiotics (including quinolones and tetracyclines), diflunisal, digoxin, iron, isoniazid, penicillamine, phenothiazines, quinidine: decreased pharmacologic effect because absorption may be impaired. Separate administration times.

NURSING CONSIDERATIONS

- *Use cautiously* in elderly patients, especially those with decreased GI motility (those receiving antidiarrheals, antispasmodics, or anticholinergics), dehydration, fluid restriction, chronic renal disease, and suspected intestinal obstruction.
- Has high sodium content and may increase sodium and water retention.
- Record amount and consistency of stools. Manage constipation with laxatives or stool softeners; alternate with magnesium-containing antacids (if patient does not have renal disease).
- Watch long-term high-dose use in patient on restricted sodium intake.
- Warn patient not to take dihydroxyaluminum sodium carbonate indiscriminately.
- May cause enteric-coated drugs to be released prematurely in stomach. Separate doses by 1 hour.

magaldrate (aluminum-magnesium complex)

Antiflux†, Lowsium◇, Riopan◇

Pregnancy Risk Category: C

HOW SUPPLIED
Tablets: 480 mg◇
Tablets (chewable): 480 mg◇
Oral suspension: 540 mg/5 ml◇, 1,080 mg/5 ml◇

MECHANISM OF ACTION
Reduces total acid load in the GI tract and elevates gastric pH to reduce pepsin activity. Also strengthens the gastric mucosal barrier and increases esophageal sphincter tone. An antacid.

INDICATIONS & DOSAGE
Antacid –
Adults: suspension: 540 to 1,080 mg (5 to 10 ml) P.O. between meals and h.s. with water. Tablet: 480 to 960 mg (1 to 2 tablets) P.O. with water between meals and h.s. Chewable tablet: 480 to 960 mg (1 to 2 tablets) P.O. chewed before swallowing, between meals and h.s.

ADVERSE REACTIONS
Common reactions are in italics; life-threatening reactions are in bold italics.
GI: mild constipation or diarrhea.

INTERACTIONS
Allopurinol, antibiotics (including quinolones and tetracyclines), diflunisal, digoxin, iron, isoniazid, penicillamine, phenothiazines, quinidine: decreased pharmacologic effect because absorption may be impaired. Separate administration times.

NURSING CONSIDERATIONS
• *Contraindicated* in severe renal disease. *Use cautiously* in elderly patients, especially those with decreased GI motility (those receiving antidiarrheals, antispasmodics, or anticholinergics), dehydration, fluid restriction, and mild renal impairment.
• Record amount and consistency of stools.
• Shake suspension well; give with a little water to ensure passage to stomach. When giving through nasogastric tube, be sure tube is placed properly and is patent. After instilling, flush tube with water to ensure passage to stomach and maintain tube patency.
• Monitor serum magnesium in patients with mild renal impairment. Symptomatic hypermagnesemia usually occurs only in severe renal failure.
• Not usually used in renal failure (although it contains aluminum) to help control hypophosphatemia, because it contains magnesium, which may accumulate in renal failure.
• Good for patient on restricted sodium intake; very low sodium content.
• Warn patient not to take magaldrate indiscriminately and not to switch antacids without doctor's advice.
• May cause enteric-coated drugs to be released prematurely in stomach. Separate doses by 1 hour.

magnesium oxide
Mag-Ox 400◇, Maox◇, Par-Mag◇, Uro-Mag◇

Pregnancy Risk Category: C

HOW SUPPLIED
Tablets: 400 mg◇, 420 mg◇
Capsules: 140 mg◇
Oral suspension: 7.75%◇

MECHANISM OF ACTION
Reduces total acid load in the GI tract and elevates gastric pH to reduce pepsin activity. Also strengthens the gastric mucosal barrier and increases esophageal sphincter tone. An antacid.

INDICATIONS & DOSAGE
Antacid –
Adults: 140 mg P.O. with water or milk after meals and h.s.
Laxative –
Adults: 4 g P.O. with water or milk, usually h.s.

Oral replacement therapy in mild hypomagnesemia –
Adults: 400 mg to 840 mg P.O. daily. Monitor serum magnesium response.

ADVERSE REACTIONS
Common reactions are in italics; life-threatening reactions are in bold italics.
GI: *diarrhea,* nausea, abdominal pain.
Metabolic: hypermagnesemia.

INTERACTIONS
Allopurinol, antibiotics (including quinolones and tetracyclines), diflunisal, digoxin, iron, isoniazid, penicillamine, phenothiazines, quinidine: decreased pharmacologic effect because absorption may be impaired. Separate administration times.

NURSING CONSIDERATIONS
- *Contraindicated* in severe renal disease. *Use cautiously* in elderly patients, and in mild renal impairment.
- With prolonged use and some degree of renal impairment, watch for symptoms of hypermagnesemia (hypotension, nausea, vomiting, depressed reflexes, respiratory depression, and coma). Monitor serum magnesium.
- When used as laxative, do not give other oral drugs 1 to 2 hours before or after.
- If diarrhea occurs on antacid doses, suggest alternate preparation.
- Warn patient not to take magnesium oxide indiscriminately and not to switch antacid without doctor's advice.
- May cause enteric-coated drugs to be released prematurely in stomach. Separate doses by 1 hour.

simethicone
Extra Strength Gas-X◊, Gas-X◊, Mylicon-80◊, Mylicon-125◊, Ovol-40†, Ovol-80†, Phazyme◊, Phazyme 55◊, Phazyme 95◊, Phazyme 125◊, Silain◊

Pregnancy Risk Category: C

HOW SUPPLIED
Tablets◊: 40 mg, 50 mg, 60 mg, 80 mg, 95 mg, 125 mg
Capsules: 40 mg/0.6 ml◊

MECHANISM OF ACTION
By its defoaming action, disperses or prevents formation of mucus-surrounded gas pockets in the GI tract.

INDICATIONS & DOSAGE
Flatulence, functional gastric bloating –
Adults and children over 12 years: 40 to 125 mg after each meal and h.s.

ADVERSE REACTIONS
Common reactions are in italics; life-threatening reactions are in bold italics.
GI: expulsion of excessive liberated gas as belching, rectal flatus.

INTERACTIONS
None significant.

NURSING CONSIDERATIONS
- Warn patient not to take simethicone indiscriminately.
- Tell patient to chew tablet before swallowing.

*Liquid form contains alcohol. **May contain tartrazine.

46
Digestants

chenodiol
monoctanoin
pancreatin
pancrelipase
ursodiol

COMBINATION PRODUCTS
BILRON: bile salts 150 mg and iron 300 mg.
DONNAZYME TABLETS: pancreatin 300 mg, pepsin 150 mg, bile salts 150 mg, hyoscyamine sulfate 0.0518 mg, atropine sulfate 0.0097 mg, scopolamine hydrobromide 0.0033 mg, and phenobarbital 8.1 mg.
ENTOZYME TABLETS: pancreatin 300 mg, pepsin 250 mg, and bile salts 150 mg.
PANCREASE CAPSULES: lipase 4,000 units, protease 25,000 units, amylase 20,000 units, in enteric-coated microspheres.

chenodiol (chenodeoxycholic acid)
Chenix

Pregnancy Risk Category: X

HOW SUPPLIED
Tablets: 250 mg

MECHANISM OF ACTION
Suppresses hepatic synthesis of both cholesterol and cholic acid. These actions contribute to biliary cholesterol desaturation and gradual dissolution of gallstones.

INDICATIONS & DOSAGE
Dissolution of radiolucent cholesterol stones (gallstones) when systemic disease or age precludes surgery –
Adults: 250 mg P.O. b.i.d. for the first 2 weeks, followed, as tolerated, by weekly increases of 250 mg/day, up to 13 to 16 mg/kg/day for up to 24 months.

ADVERSE REACTIONS
Common reactions are in italics; life-threatening reactions are in bold italics.
GI: *diarrhea,* cramps, heartburn, constipation, nausea, vomiting, anorexia, epigastric distress.
Hepatic: reversible elevated hepatic enzymes, possible liver toxicity.

INTERACTIONS
Aluminum-containing antacids, cholestyramine, colestipol, estrogens, oral contraceptives, clofibrate: decreased chenodiol effect. Monitor patient carefully.

NURSING CONSIDERATIONS
- *Contraindicated* in known hepatocyte dysfunction; a gallbladder confirmed as nonvisualizing after two consecutive single doses of dye; radiopaque or radiolucent bile pigment stones; or gallstone complications or compelling reasons for gallbladder surgery, including unremitting acute cholecystitis, cholangitis, biliary obstruction, gallstone pancreatitis, or biliary GI fistula.
- Chenodiol treatment should be reserved for carefully selected patients.
- The drug is particularly effective in the dissolution of small, floatable gallstones.
- Monitor AST (SGOT) and ALT (SGPT) monthly for the first 3 months and thereafter every 3 months for duration of therapy.
- The final dosage shouldn't be less than 10 mg/kg/day; lower dosages are usually ineffective.
- Diarrhea occurs in 30% to 40% of all patients. Doctor may reduce dosage until diarrhea subsides. Antidi-

arrheals may also be prescribed. In some patients, however, persistent diarrhea will require discontinuation of chenodiol therapy.
- Monitor oral cholecystogram or ultrasonogram every 6 to 9 months to observe for gallstone dissolution. Periodic liver function tests are also recommended.
- Encourage compliance with the prescribed drug regimen and with scheduled follow-up appointments.
- Tell patient to report worsening symptoms immediately, for example, sudden right upper quadrant pain, nausea, and vomiting.

monoctanoin

Moctanin

Pregnancy Risk Category: C

HOW SUPPLIED

Infusion: 120-ml bottles

MECHANISM OF ACTION

Dissolves gallstones by rendering them more soluble.

INDICATIONS & DOSAGE

To solubilize cholesterol gallstones that are retained in the biliary tract after cholecystectomy –

Adults: Administered as a continuous infusion through a catheter inserted directly into the common bile duct via a T tube. Rate should not exceed 3 to 5 ml/hour at a pressure of 10 cm H_2O. Duration of infusion is 7 to 21 days.

ADVERSE REACTIONS

Common reactions are in italics; life-threatening reactions are in bold italics.

GI: *GI pain and discomfort, nausea, vomiting,* diarrhea, anorexia, indigestion.

Other: metabolic acidosis, fever.

INTERACTIONS

None reported.

NURSING CONSIDERATIONS

- *Contraindicated* in clinical jaundice, significant biliary tract infection, or a history of recent duodenal ulcer or jejunitis.
- Because impaired liver function may lead to metabolic acidosis during administration of this drug, routine liver function tests should be done before perfusion therapy begins.
- Monoctanoin should only be started by individuals experienced in infusion therapy.
- Not to be administered parenterally. For biliary tract infusion only.
- Pressure *must* be kept below 15 cm H_2O. Keeping the pressure at 10 cm H_2O will help minimize GI and biliary tract irritation.
- Use a peristaltic infusion pump to regulate the infusion. Outpatients may use a battery-operated portable pump.
- Warm the solution to 60° to 80° F (16° to 27° C) before perfusion. Temperature of the solution should not fall below 65° F (18° C) during administration.
- GI symptoms may be reduced by slowing the infusion rate or discontinuing the infusion during meals.

pancreatin

Dizymes Tablets◇, Hi-Vegi-Lip Tablets◇, Pancreatin Enseals◇, Pancreatin Tablets◇

Pregnancy Risk Category: C

HOW SUPPLIED

Dizymes

Tablets (enteric-coated): 250 mg pancreatin, 6,750 units lipase, 41,250 units protease, 43,750 units amylase◇

Hi-Vegi-Lip

Tablets (enteric-coated): 2,400 mg pancreatin, 12,000 units lipase, 60,000 units protease, and 60,000 units amylase◇

Pancreatin Enseals

Tablets (enteric-coated): 1,000 mg

pancreatin, 2,000 units lipase, 25,000 units protease, 25,000 units amylase◇

Pancreatin Tablets

Tablets (enteric-coated): 325 mg pancreatin, 650 units lipase, 8,125 units protease, 8,125 units amylase◇

MECHANISM OF ACTION

Replaces endogenous exocrine pancreatic enzymes and aids digestion of starches, fats, and proteins.

INDICATIONS & DOSAGE

Exocrine pancreatic secretion insufficiency, digestive aid in diseases associated with deficiency of pancreatic enzymes such as cystic fibrosis– **Adults and children:** 1 to 3 tablets P.O. with meals.

ADVERSE REACTIONS

Common reactions are in italics; life-threatening reactions are in bold italics.

GI: nausea, diarrhea with high doses.

Other: hyperuricosuria (with high doses).

INTERACTIONS

Antacids: may negate pancreatin's beneficial effect. Don't use together.

NURSING CONSIDERATIONS

- *Use cautiously* in patients who are hypersensitive to pork. Bovine preparations are available for these patients, but are less effective.
- Minimal USP standards dictate that each milligram of bovine or porcine pancreatin contains lipase 2 units, protease 25 units, and amylase 25 units.
- Balance fat, protein, and starch intake properly to avoid indigestion. Dosage varies according to degree of maldigestion and malabsorption, amount of fat in diet, and enzyme activity of individual preparations.
- Adequate replacement decreases number of bowel movements and improves stool consistency.
- Not effective in GI disorders unrelated to pancreatic enzyme deficiency.
- For infants, mix powder with applesauce and give with meals. Avoid inhalation of powder. Older children may swallow capsules with food.
- Enteric coating on some products may reduce availability of enzyme in upper portion of jejunum.
- Store in airtight containers at room temperature.
- Don't crush or chew enteric-coated dosage forms.

pancrelipase

Cotazym Capsules, Cotazym-S Capsules, Creon Capsules, Festal II Tablets◇, Ilozyme Tablets, Ku-Zyme HP Capsules, Pancrease Capsules, Pancrease MT4, Pancrease MT10, Pancrease MT16, Viokase Powder, Viokase Tablets

Pregnancy Risk Category: C

HOW SUPPLIED

Cotazym

Capsules: 8,000 units lipase, 30,000 units protease, 30,000 units amylase, 25 mg calcium carbonate

Cotazym-S

Capsules (enteric-coated spheres): 5,000 units lipase, 20,000 units protease, 20,000 units amylase

Creon

Capsules (enteric-coated microspheres): 8,000 units lipase, 13,000 units protease, 30,000 units amylase

Festal II

Tablets (enteric-coated): 6,000 units lipase, 20,000 units protease, 30,000 units amylase◇

Ilozyme

Tablets: 11,000 units lipase, 30,000 units protease, 30,000 units amylase

Ku-Zyme HP

Capsules: 8,000 units lipase, 30,000 units protease, 30,000 units amylase

Pancrease
Capsules (enteric-coated microspheres): 4,000 units lipase, 25,000 units protease, 20,000 units amylase
Pancrease MT4
Capsules (enteric-coated microtablets): 4,000 units lipase, 12,000 units protease, 30,000 units amylase
Pancrease MT10
Capsules (enteric-coated microtablets): 10,000 units lipase, 30,000 units protease, 30,000 units amylase
Pancrease MT16
Capsules (enteric-coated microtablets): 16,000 units lipase, 48,000 units protease, 48,000 units amylase
Viokase
Tablets: 8,000 units lipase, 30,000 units protease, 30,000 units amylase
Powder: 16,800 units lipase, 70,000 units protease, 70,000 units amylase

MECHANISM OF ACTION
Replaces endogenous exocrine pancreatic enzymes and aids digestion of starches, fats, and proteins.

INDICATIONS & DOSAGE
Dose must be titrated to patient's response. Exocrine pancreatic secretion insufficiency, cystic fibrosis in adults and children, steatorrhea and other disorders of fat metabolism secondary to insufficient pancreatic enzymes –
Adults and children: dosage ranges from 1 to 3 capsules or tablets P.O. before or with meals and 1 capsule or tablet with snack; or 1 to 2 powder packets before meals or snacks.

ADVERSE REACTIONS
Common reactions are in italics; life-threatening reactions are in bold italics.
GI: *nausea,* diarrhea with high doses.

INTERACTIONS
Antacids: may negate pancrelipase's beneficial effect. Don't use together.

NURSING CONSIDERATIONS
- *Contraindicated* in patients with severe pork hypersensitivity.
- Minimal USP standards dictate that each mg of pancrelipase contains 24 units lipase, 100 units protease, and 100 units amylase.
- Use only after confirmed diagnosis of exocrine pancreatic insufficiency. Not effective in GI disorders unrelated to enzyme deficiency.
- Lipase activity greater than with other pancreatic enzymes.
- For infants, mix powder with applesauce and give with meals. Avoid contact with or inhalation of powder because it may be very irritating. Older children may take capsules with food.
- Dosage varies with degree of maldigestion and malabsorption, amount of fat in diet, and enzyme activity of individual preparations.
- Adequate replacement decreases number of bowel movements and improves stool consistency.
- Enteric coating on some products may reduce availability of enzyme in upper portion of jejunum.
- Crushing or chewing of capsule interferes with the enteric coating.

ursodiol
Actigall
Pregnancy Risk Category: B

HOW SUPPLIED
Capsules: 300 mg

MECHANISM OF ACTION
A naturally occurring bile acid that suppresses hepatic synthesis and secretion of cholesterol as well as intestinal cholesterol absorption. After long-term administration, it can solubilize cholesterol from gallstones.

INDICATIONS & DOSAGE
Dissolution of gallstones less than 20 mm in diameter in patients who are

poor surgical candidates or refuse surgery –
Adults: 8 to 10 mg/kg P.O. daily in two or three divided doses. Most patients receive 300 mg P.O. b.i.d. Therapy is usually long-term, with ultrasound images of the gallbladder at 6 month intervals. If partial stone dissolution is not seen within 12 months, eventual success is unlikely. Safety of use for longer than 24 months has not been established.

ADVERSE REACTIONS
Common reactions are in italics; life-threatening reactions are in bold italics.
CNS: headache, fatigue, anxiety, depression, sleep disorders.
EENT: cough, rhinitis.
GI: nausea, vomiting, dyspepsia, metallic taste, abdominal pain, biliary pain, cholecystitis, diarrhea, constipation, stomatitis, flatulence.
Skin: pruritus, rash, dry skin, urticaria, itching, hair thinning.
Other: arthralgia, myalgia, back pain.

INTERACTIONS
Aluminum-containing antacids, cholestyramine, colestipol: bind ursodiol and prevent its absorption.
Estrogens, oral contraceptives, clofibrate: increase hepatic cholesterol secretion and may counteract the effects of ursodiol.

NURSING CONSIDERATIONS
- *Contraindicated* in patients with hypersensitivity to ursodiol or other bile acids. Also contraindicated in chronic liver disease, acute cholecystitis, cholangitis, biliary obstruction, gallstone pancreatitis, or biliary-GI fistulae.
- Ursodiol will not dissolve calcified cholesterol stones, radiolucent bile pigment stones, or radiopaque stones.
- Ursodiol therapy is long-term, requiring several months to produce an effect. The relapse rate after bile acid therapy may be as high as 50% after 5 years. Patients should be aware of alternative therapies, including 'watchful waiting' (no intervention) and cholecystectomy.
- Monitor liver function tests, including AST (SGOT) and ALT (SGPT) at the beginning of therapy, and after 1 month, 3 months and every 6 months while taking ursodiol. Abnormal tests may indicate a worsening of the disease. There is a theoretical risk of a hepatotoxic metabolite of ursodiol being formed in some patients.
- Ultrasound images of the gallbladder should be reviewed at least once every 6 months for the first year of therapy. Most patients who respond to ursodiol show significant improvement after 6 months of therapy.

47

Antidiarrheals

bismuth subgallate
bismuth subsalicylate
calcium polycarbophil
(See Chapter 48, LAXATIVES.)
difenoxin hydrochloride
diphenoxylate hydrochloride
kaolin and pectin mixtures
loperamide
octreotide acetate
opium tincture
opium tincture, camphorated

COMBINATION PRODUCTS

DONNAGEL-PG*: powdered opium 24 mg, kaolin 6 g, pectin 142.8 mg, hyoscyamine sulfate 0.1037 mg, atropine sulfate 0.0194 mg, scopolamine hydrobromide 0.0065 mg, and alcohol 5% in 30-ml suspension.
DONNAGEL SUSPENSION*: kaolin 6 g, pectin 142.8 mg, hyoscyamine sulfate 0.1037 mg, atropine sulfate 0.0194 mg, scopolamine hydrobromide 0.0065 mg, and alcohol 3.8% in 30-ml suspension.
PAREPECTOLIN*: opium 15 mg (equivalent to Paregoric 3.7 ml), kaolin 5.85 g, pectin 162 mg, and alcohol 0.69% in 30-ml suspension.

bismuth subgallate
Devrom◊

bismuth subsalicylate
Maximum Strength Pepto-Bismol Liquid◊, Pepto-Bismol◊

Pregnancy Risk Category: C (D in third trimester)

HOW SUPPLIED

subgallate
Tablets (chewable): 200 mg◊
subsalicylate
Tablets (chewable): 262 mg◊
Oral suspension: 262 mg/15 ml◊, 525 mg/15 ml◊

MECHANISM OF ACTION

Has a mild water-binding capacity; also may adsorb toxins and provide protective coating for mucosa.

INDICATIONS & DOSAGE

Mild, nonspecific diarrhea –
Adults: 1 to 2 tablets P.O. chewed or swallowed whole t.i.d. (subgallate).
Adults: 30 ml or 2 tablets P.O. q ½ to 1 hour up to a maximum of 8 doses and for no longer than 2 days (subsalicylate).
Children 9 to 12 years: 20 ml or 1 tablet P.O.
Children 6 to 9 years: 10 ml or ⅔ tablet P.O.
Children 3 to 6 years: 5 ml or ⅓ tablet P.O.
Prevention and treatment of traveler's diarrhea (turista) –
Adults: prophylactically, 60 ml (bismuth subsalicylate) P.O. q.i.d. during the first 2 weeks of travel. During acute illness, 30 to 60 ml P.O. q 30 minutes for a total of 8 doses. Alternatively, 2 tablets P.O. q.i.d. for up to 3 weeks.

ADVERSE REACTIONS

Common reactions are in italics; life-threatening reactions are in bold italics.
GI: temporary darkening of tongue and stools.
Other: salicylism (high doses).

INTERACTIONS

Aspirin, other salicylates: risk of salicylate toxicity. Monitor closely.
Oral anticoagulants, oral hypoglycemic agents: theoretical risk of increased effects of these agents follow-

*Liquid form contains alcohol. **May contain tartrazine.

ing high doses of bismuth subsalicylate. Monitor patient closely.
Probenecid: theoretical risk of decreased uricosuric effects following high doses of bismuth subsalicylate. Monitor patient closely.
Tetracycline: decreased tetracycline absorption if taken together. Separate administration times by at least 2 hours.

NURSING CONSIDERATIONS

- Warn patient that bismuth subsalicylate contains a large amount of salicylate (each tablet provides 102 mg salicylate; the regular strength liquid provides 130 mg/15 ml, and the extra strength liquid yields 230 mg/15 ml).
- *Use cautiously* in patients already taking aspirin. Discontinue if tinnitus occurs.
- Tell patient to call doctor if diarrhea persists for more than 2 days or is accompanied by high fever.
- Avoid use before GI radiologic procedures because bismuth is radiopaque and may interfere with X-rays.
- Consult with doctor before giving bismuth subsalicylate to children or teenagers during or after recovery from the flu or chicken pox.
- Instruct patient to chew tablets well. Liquid should be shaken well before measuring dose.
- Both the liquid and tablet forms of Pepto-Bismol are effective against traveler's diarrhea. Tablets may be more convenient to carry.
- Has been used investigationally to treat peptic ulcer disease, especially when ulcers are associated with *Helicobacter pylori* infection.

difenoxin hydrochloride

Lyspafen‡, Motofen

Pregnancy Risk Category: C

HOW SUPPLIED

Tablets: 0.5 mg (with atropine sulphate, 0.025 mg)‡, 1 mg (with atropine sulfate, 0.025 mg)

MECHANISM OF ACTION

Exerts a direct effect on the intestinal wall to slow motility.

INDICATIONS AND DOSAGE

Adjunct in acute nonspecific diarrhea, and acute exacerbations of chronic functional diarrhea –
Adults: initially, 2 mg P.O., then 1 mg P.O. after each loose bowel movement. Total dosage should not exceed 8 mg daily. Not recommended for use longer than 2 days.

ADVERSE REACTIONS

Common reactions are in italics; life-threatening reactions are in bold italics.
CNS: dizziness and light-headedness, drowsiness, headache, fatigue, nervousness, insomnia, confusion.
EENT: burning eyes, blurred vision.
GI: nausea, vomiting, dry mouth, epigastric distress, constipation.

INTERACTIONS

Alcohol, CNS depressants, tranquilizers, narcotics, barbiturates: enhanced CNS depression. Closely monitor patients.
MAO inhibitors: potential hypertensive crisis. Avoid concomitant use.

NURSING CONSIDERATIONS

- *Contraindicated* in patients with hypersensitivity to difenoxin or atropine, in children under 2 years, and in patients with diarrhea from pseudomembraneous colitis associated with antibiotics. Also contraindicated in patients with jaundice, or diarrhea from organisms that may penetrate the intestinal mucosa (including toxigenic *Escherichia coli, Salmonella,* or *Shigella*).
- Difenoxin is the principal metabolite of diphenoxylate (Lomotil) and is

chemically related to meperidine. Use cautiously in patients with a history of drug abuse, or in those currently receiving drugs with a high abuse potential.

- Atropine has been added to difenoxin to prevent abuse. The small dosage of atropine is unlikely to cause any significant clinical problems, but patients may experience dry mouth, tachycardia, urine retention, and flushing. Monitor for these effects.
- Advise patients to avoid hazardous activities that may require mental alertness, such as driving or operating heavy machinery, until the CNS effects of the drug are known.
- Monitor patients closely for fluid and electrolyte imbalance. Difenoxin-induced decreases in peristalsis may result in fluid retention in the colon, with subsequent dehydration and possibly delayed difenoxin intoxication.
- Advise patient to adhere to dosing schedule. Overdose with difenoxin may result in respiratory depression and coma. Encourage proper storage to keep drug out of children's reach.
- Patients who overdose with difenoxin should be observed for at least 48 hours. Respiratory depression may occur up to 30 hours after ingestion. Gastric lavage, establishment of a patent airway, and mechanically assisted ventilation are advised. Naloxone will reverse the respiratory depression. Because difenoxin has a longer duration of action than naloxone, repeated injections of naloxone will be necessary.

diphenoxylate hydrochloride

Diphenatol, Lofene, Logen, Lomanate, Lomotil*, Lonox, Lo-Trol, Low-Quel, Nor-Mil

Controlled Substance Schedule V

Pregnancy Risk Category: C

HOW SUPPLIED

Tablets: 2.5 mg (with atropine sulfate, 0.025 mg)
Liquid: 2.5 mg/5 ml (with atropine sulfate, 0.025 mg/5 ml)*

MECHANISM OF ACTION

Increases smooth muscle tone in the GI tract, inhibits motility and propulsion, and diminishes secretions.

INDICATIONS & DOSAGE

Acute, nonspecific diarrhea –
Adults: initially, 5 mg P.O. q.i.d., then adjust dosage.
Children 2 to 12 years: 0.3 to 0.4 mg/kg P.O. daily in 4 divided doses, using liquid form only. For maintenance, initial dose may be reduced by as much as 75%.

Don't use in children under 2 years.

ADVERSE REACTIONS

Common reactions are in italics; life-threatening reactions are in bold italics.
CNS: *sedation, dizziness,* headache, drowsiness, lethargy, restlessness, depression, euphoria.
CV: tachycardia.
EENT: mydriasis.
GI: *dry mouth,* nausea, vomiting, abdominal discomfort or distention, ***paralytic ileus,*** anorexia, fluid retention in bowel (may mask depletion of extracellular fluid and electrolytes, especially in young children treated for acute gastroenteritis).
GU: urine retention.
Skin: pruritus, giant urticaria, rash.
Other: possibly physical dependence in long-term use, ***angioedema, respiratory depression.***

INTERACTIONS

Alcohol, CNS depression, tranquilizers, narcotics, barbiturates: enhanced CNS depression. Closely monitor patients.
MAO inhibitors: potential hypertensive crisis. Avoid concomitant use.

*Liquid form contains alcohol. **May contain tartrazine.

NURSING CONSIDERATIONS

- *Contraindicated* in acute diarrhea resulting from poison until toxic material is eliminated from GI tract; acute diarrhea caused by organisms that penetrate intestinal mucosa; diarrhea resulting from antibiotic-induced pseudomembranous enterocolitis; and in jaundiced patients.
- *Use cautiously* in children, in hepatic disease, in narcotic dependence, in pregnant women, and in acute ulcerative colitis. Stop therapy immediately if abdominal distention or other signs of toxic megacolon develop.
- Advise patient to avoid hazardous activities such as driving until the adverse CNS effects of the drug are known.
- Risk of physical dependence increases with high dosage and long-term use. Atropine sulfate is included to discourage abuse.
- Not likely to be effective if there is no response within 48 hours.
- Patient should not use to treat acute diarrhea for longer than 2 days and should seek medical attention if diarrhea continues.
- Warn patient not to exceed recommended dosage. Naloxone may be used to treat respiratory depression resulting from overdose.
- Dehydration, especially in young children, may increase risk of delayed toxicity. Correct fluid and electrolyte disturbances before starting drug.
- Dose of 2.5 mg is as effective as 5 ml camphorated tincture of opium.
- Not indicated in treatment of antibiotic-induced diarrhea.

kaolin and pectin mixtures

Donnagel-MB*†, Kao-Con†, Kaopectate◇, Kaopectate Concentrate◇, Kao-tin◇, Kapectolin◇, K-P◇, K-Pek◇

Pregnancy Risk Category: C

HOW SUPPLIED

Oral suspension: 5.2 mg kaolin and 260 mg pectin per 30 ml◇ (K-P◇); 5.85 g kaolin and 130 mg pectin per 30 ml◇ (Kaopectate◇, Kao-tin◇, Kapectolin◇, K-Pek◇); 5.91 g kaolin and 132 mg pectin per 30 ml◇ (Kaopectate◇), 6 g kaolin and 130 mg pectin per 30 ml◇ (Kaopectate†◇); 6 g kaolin and 143 mg pectin per 30 ml◇, with 3.8% alcohol (Donnagel-MB*†); 8.7 g kaolin and 195 mg pectin per 30 ml◇ (Kaopectate Concentrate◇); 8.8 g kaolin and 195 mg pectin per 30 ml◇ (Kaopectate Concentrate†◇, Kao-Con†)

MECHANISM OF ACTION

Decrease the stool's fluid content, although *total* water loss seems to remain the same.

INDICATIONS & DOSAGE

Mild, nonspecific diarrhea—
Adults: 60 to 120 ml P.O. after each bowel movement.
Children over 12 years: 60 ml P.O. after each bowel movement.
Children 6 to 12 years: 30 to 60 ml P.O. after each bowel movement.
Children 3 to 6 years: 15 to 30 ml P.O. after each bowel movement.

ADVERSE REACTIONS

Common reactions are in italics; life-threatening reactions are in bold italics.
GI: drug absorbs nutrients, drugs, and enzymes; fecal impaction or ulceration in infants and elderly or debilitated patients after chronic use; constipation.

INTERACTIONS

Orally administered drugs: adsorption may occur. Separate administration times with other orally administered drugs.

NURSING CONSIDERATIONS

- *Contraindicated* in suspected obstructive bowel lesions.

†Available in Canada only. ‡Available in Australia only. ◇Available OTC.

- Don't use for more than 2 days.
- Don't use in place of specific therapy for underlying cause.
- May reduce absorption of other P.O. drugs, requiring dosage adjustments.
- It is a GI absorbent.

loperamide

Imodium, Imodium A-D◊

Pregnancy Risk Category: B

HOW SUPPLIED

Tablets: 2 mg
Capsules: 2 mg
Oral liquid: 1 mg/5 ml◊

MECHANISM OF ACTION

Inhibits peristaltic activity, prolonging transit of intestinal contents.

INDICATIONS & DOSAGE

Acute, nonspecific diarrhea –
Adults: initially, 4 mg P.O., then 2 mg after each unformed stool. Maximum 16 mg daily.
Children 8 to 12 years: 10 ml t.i.d. P.O. on first day. (Subsequent doses of 5 ml per 10 kg of body weight may be administered after each unformed stool.)
Children 5 to 8 years: 10 ml P.O. b.i.d. on first day.
Children 2 to 5 years: 5 ml P.O. t.i.d. on first day.
Chronic diarrhea –
Adults: initially, 4 mg P.O., then 2 mg after each unformed stool until diarrhea subsides. Adjust dosage to individual response.

ADVERSE REACTIONS

Common reactions are in italics; life-threatening reactions are in bold italics.
CNS: drowsiness, fatigue, dizziness.
GI: dry mouth; abdominal pain, distention, or discomfort; *constipation;* nausea; vomiting.
Skin: rash.

INTERACTIONS

None significant.

NURSING CONSIDERATIONS

- *Contraindicated* in acute diarrhea resulting from poison until toxic material is removed from GI tract, in acute diarrhea caused by organisms that penetrate intestinal mucosa, and when constipation must be avoided.
- *Use cautiously* in severe prostatic hypertrophy, hepatic disease, and history of narcotic dependence.
- Stop drug immediately if abdominal distention or other symptoms develop in acute colitis.
- In acute diarrhea, discontinue drug and seek medical attention if no improvement occurs within 48 hours; in chronic diarrhea, discontinue drug if no improvement occurs after giving 16 mg daily for at least 10 days.
- Warn patient not to exceed recommended dosage.
- Produces antidiarrheal action similar to diphenoxylate hydrochloride but without as many adverse CNS effects.

octreotide acetate

Sandostatin

Pregnancy Risk Category: B

HOW SUPPLIED

Injection: 0.05 mg, 0.1 mg, 0.5 mg

MECHANISM OF ACTION

Mimics the action of naturally occurring somatostatin.

INDICATIONS & DOSAGE

Symptomatic treatment of flushing and diarrhea associated with carcinoid tumors –
Adults: initially, 0.1 to 0.6 mg daily S.C. in two to four divided doses for the first 2 weeks of therapy (usual daily dosage is 0.3 mg). Subsequent dosage is based upon individual response.

Symptomatic treatment of watery diarrhea associated with vasoactive intestinal peptide secreting tumors (VIPomas) –
Adults: initially, 0.2 to 0.3 mg daily S.C. in two to four divided doses for the first 2 weeks of therapy. Subsequent dosage is based upon individual response, but usually will not exceed 0.45 mg daily.

ADVERSE REACTIONS
Common reactions are in italics; life-threatening reactions are in bold italics.
CNS: dizziness, light-headedness, fatigue.
GI: *nausea, diarrhea, abdominal pain or discomfort,* loose stools, vomiting, fat malabsorption.
Metabolic: hyperglycemia, hypoglycemia, hypothyroidism.
Skin: flushing, edema, wheal, erythema or pain at injection site.

INTERACTIONS
Cyclosporine: may decrease plasma levels of cyclosporine.

NURSING CONSIDERATIONS
- *Contraindicated* in patients with hypersensitivity to the drug or any of its components.
- Octreotide therapy may be associated with the development of cholelithiasis by either altering gallbladder motility or fat absorption. Monitor patient regularly for gallbladder disease, and tell patient to report any signs of abdominal discomfort.
- Half-life may be altered in patients in end-stage renal failure who are receiving dialysis.
- Baseline and periodic tests of thyroid function are advised because of the drug's metabolic effects.
- Laboratory tests that are frequently monitored during therapy include urine 5-hydroxyindole acetic acid (5-HIAA), plasma serotonin, and plasma substance P (for carcinoid tumors); plasma vasoactive intestinal peptide for VIPomas.
- Mild, transient hypoglycemia or hyperglycemia may occur during octreotide therapy. Monitor closely for symptoms of glucose imbalance during therapy.
- Insulin-dependent diabetic patients and patients receiving oral hypoglycemics (sulfonylureas) or oral diazoxide may require dosage adjustments during therapy.
- Octreotide therapy may alter fluid and electrolyte balance and may require adjustment of other drugs used to control symptoms of the disease (such as beta blockers).

opium tincture*
Controlled Substance Schedule II

opium tincture, camphorated* (paregoric)
Controlled Substance Schedule III

Pregnancy Risk Category: B (D for prolonged use or high doses at term)

HOW SUPPLIED
opium tincture
Oral solution: equivalent to morphine 10 mg/ml*
opium tincture, camphorated
Oral solution: Each 5 ml contains morphine, 2 mg; anise oil, 0.2 ml; benzoic acid, 20 mg; camphor, 20 mg; glycerin, 0.2 ml; and ethanol to make 5 ml

MECHANISM OF ACTION
Increases smooth muscle tone in the GI tract, inhibits motility and propulsion, and diminishes secretions.

INDICATIONS & DOSAGE
Acute, nonspecific diarrhea –
Adults: 0.6 ml opium tincture (range 0.3 to 1 ml) P.O. q.i.d. Maximum dosage 6 ml daily; or 5 to 10 ml cam-

phorated opium tincture daily b.i.d., t.i.d., or q.i.d. until diarrhea subsides.
Children: 0.25 to 0.5 ml/kg camphorated opium tincture P.O. daily, b.i.d., t.i.d., or q.i.d. until diarrhea subsides.

ADVERSE REACTIONS
Common reactions are in italics; life-threatening reactions are in bold italics.
GI: nausea, vomiting.
Other: physical dependence after long-term use.

INTERACTIONS
None significant.

NURSING CONSIDERATIONS
- *Contraindicated* in acute diarrhea resulting from poison until toxic material is removed from GI tract, and diarrhea caused by organisms that penetrate intestinal mucosa.
- *Use cautiously* in asthma, prostatic hypertrophy, hepatic disease, and narcotic dependence.
- Risk of physical dependence increases with long-term use.
- Don't use for more than 2 days.
- An effective and prompt-acting antidiarrheal; but unique because dosage can be adjusted precisely to patient's needs.
- Opium content of opium tincture 25 times greater than camphorated tincture of opium. Camphorated opium tincture is more dilute, and teaspoonful doses are easier to measure than dropper quantities of opium tincture.
- Milky fluid forms when camphorated opium tincture is added to water.
- Camphorated opium tincture 0.06 to 0.5 ml daily has been used to treat infants with mild narcotic physical dependence.
- Store in tightly capped, light-resistant container.
- Mix with sufficient water to ensure passage to stomach.
- Narcotic antagonist naloxone can reverse the respiratory depression resulting from overdose.

*Liquid form contains alcohol. **May contain tartrazine.

48

Laxatives

bisacodyl
calcium polycarbophil
cascara sagrada
cascara sagrada aromatic fluid extract
cascara sagrada fluid extract
castor oil
docusate calcium
docusate potassium
docusate sodium
glycerin
lactulose
magnesium citrate
magnesium hydroxide
magnesium sulfate
methylcellulose
mineral oil
phenolphthalein, white
phenolphthalein, yellow
polyethylene glycol-electrolyte solution
psyllium
senna
sodium phosphates

COMBINATION PRODUCTS

AGORAL◇: mineral oil 28% and white phenolphthalein 1.3% in emulsion, with tragacanth, agar, egg albumin, acacia, and glycerin.
DIALOSE-PLUS◇: docusate potassium 100 mg and casanthranol 30 mg.
DIOLAX◇: docusate sodium 100 mg and casanthranol 50 mg.
DOXIDAN◇: docusate calcium 60 mg and phenolphthalein 65 mg.
D-S-S PLUS◇: docusate sodium 100 mg and casanthranol 30 mg.
HALEY'S M-O◇: mineral oil (25%) and magnesium hydroxide.
KONDREMUL WITH CASCARA◇: heavy mineral oil 55%, cascara sagrada extract 660 mg/15 ml, and Irish moss as emulsifier.
KONDREMUL WITH PHENOLPHTHALEIN◇: heavy mineral oil 55%, white phenolphthalein 150 mg/15 ml, and Irish moss as emulsifier.
MODANE PLUS◇: docusate sodium 100 mg and phenolphthalein 60 mg.
PERI-COLACE◇ (capsules): docusate sodium 100 mg and casanthranol 30 mg.
PERI-COLACE◇ (syrup): docusate sodium 60 mg and casanthranol 30 mg/15 ml.
SENOKOT-S◇: docusate sodium 50 mg and standardized senna concentrate 187 mg.
UNILAX◇: docusate sodium 230 mg and yellow phenolphthalein 130 mg.

bisacodyl

Bisacolax†◇, Bisalax‡, Bisco-Lax**◇, Dacodyl◇, Deficol◇, Dulcolax◇, Durolax‡, Fleet Bisacodyl◇, Laxit†◇, Theralax◇

Pregnancy Risk Category: C

HOW SUPPLIED

Tablets (enteric-coated): 5 mg◇
Enema: 0.33 mg/dl◇, 10 mg/5 ml (microenema)‡
Powder for rectal solution (bisacodyl tannex): 1.5 mg bisacodyl and 2.5 g tannic acid
Suppositories: 5 mg◇, 10 mg◇

MECHANISM OF ACTION

Increases peristalsis by direct effect on the smooth muscle of the intestine. Thought either to irritate the musculature or to stimulate the colonic intramural plexus. Also promotes fluid accumulation in the colon and small intestine. A stimulant laxative.

INDICATIONS & DOSAGE

Chronic constipation; preparation for delivery, surgery, or rectal or bowel examination –

†Available in Canada only. ‡Available in Australia only. ◇Available OTC.

Adults: 10 to 15 mg P.O. in evening or before breakfast. Up to 30 mg may be used for thorough evacuation needed for examinations or surgery.
Children 6 years and older: 5 to 10 mg P.O.
Adults and children over 2 years: 10 mg rectally.
Children under 2 years: 5 mg rectally.

ADVERSE REACTIONS
Common reactions are in italics; life-threatening reactions are in bold italics.
CNS: muscle weakness in excessive use.
GI: *nausea, vomiting, abdominal cramps,* diarrhea with high doses, *burning sensation in rectum with suppositories.*
Metabolic: alkalosis, hypokalemia, tetany, protein-losing enteropathy in excessive use, fluid and electrolyte imbalance.
Other: laxative dependence in long-term or excessive use.

INTERACTIONS
None significant.

NURSING CONSIDERATIONS
- *Contraindicated* in patients with abdominal pain, nausea, vomiting, or other symptoms of appendicitis or acute surgical abdomen, or in rectal fissures or ulcerated hemorrhoids.
- Tell patient to swallow enteric-coated tablet whole to avoid GI irritation. Don't give within one hour of milk or antacid intake. Begins to act 6 to 12 hours after oral administration.
- Soft, formed stool usually produced 15 to 60 minutes after rectal administration. Time administration of drug so as not to interfere with scheduled activities or sleep.
- Tablets and suppositories may be used together to cleanse colon before and after surgery and before barium enema.
- Insert suppository as high as possible into the rectum, and try to position the suppository against the rectal wall. Avoid embedding within fecal material because this may delay the onset of action.
- Use for short-term treatment. A stimulant laxative, this type of laxative is most abused. Discourage excessive use.
- Before giving for constipation, determine if patient has adequate fluid intake, exercise, and diet. Tell him that dietary sources of bulk include bran and other cereals, fresh fruit, and vegetables.
- Store tablets and suppositories at temperature below 86° F (30° C).
- Tell patient to report adverse effects to the doctor.

calcium polycarbophil
Equalactin◊, FiberCon◊, Mitrolan◊

Pregnancy Risk Category: C

HOW SUPPLIED
Tablets: 500 mg◊ (FiberCon◊)
Tablets (chewable): 500 mg◊ (Equalactin◊, Mitrolan◊)

MECHANISM OF ACTION
Absorbs water and expands to increase bulk and moisture content of the stool. The increased bulk encourages peristalsis and bowel movement. A bulk-forming laxative. As an antidiarrheal, absorbs free fecal water, thereby producing formed stools.

INDICATIONS & DOSAGE
Constipation (Equalactin and Mitrolan must be chewed before swallowing) –
Adults: 1 g P.O. q.i.d. as required. Maximum 6 g in 24-hour period.
Children 6 to 12 years: 500 mg P.O. t.i.d. as required. Maximum 3 g in 24-hour period.
Children 2 to 6 years: 500 mg P.O. b.i.d. as required. Maximum 1.5 g in 24-hour period.

Diarrhea associated with irritable bowel syndrome, as well as acute nonspecific diarrhea (Mitrolan must be chewed before swallowing) –
Adults: 1 g P.O. q.i.d. as required. Maximum 6 g in 24-hour period.
Children 6 to 12 years 500 mg P.O. t.i.d. as required. Maximum 3 g in 24-hour period.
Children 2 to 6 years: 500 mg P.O. b.i.d. as required. Maximum 1.5 g in 24-hour period.

ADVERSE REACTIONS
Common reactions are in italics; life-threatening reactions are in bold italics.
GI: abdominal fullness and increased flatus, intestinal obstruction.
Other: laxative dependence in long-term or excessive use.

INTERACTIONS
None significant.

NURSING CONSIDERATIONS
- *Contraindicated* in signs of GI obstruction.
- Rectal bleeding or failure to respond to therapy may indicate need for surgery.
- Before giving for constipation, determine if patient has adequate fluid intake, exercise, and diet. Tell him that dietary sources of bulk include bran and other cereals, fresh fruit, and vegetables.
- Advise patient to chew the Equalactin or Mitrolan tablets thoroughly and drink a full glass of water with each dose. However, when used as an antidiarrheal, tell patient *not* to drink a glass of water.
- For episodes of severe diarrhea, the dose may be repeated every half hour, but maximum daily dosage should not be exceeded.

cascara sagrada ◇

cascara sagrada aromatic fluid extract* ◇

cascara sagrada fluid extract* ◇

Pregnancy Risk Category: C

HOW SUPPLIED
Tablets: 325 mg ◇
Aromatic fluid extract: 1 g/ml* ◇
Fluidextract: 1 g/ml* ◇

MECHANISM OF ACTION
Increases peristalsis by direct effect on the smooth muscle of the intestine. Thought either to irritate the musculature or to stimulate the colonic intramural plexus. Also promotes fluid accumulation in the colon and small intestine. A stimulant laxative.

INDICATIONS & DOSAGE
Acute constipation; preparation for bowel or rectal examination –
Adults: 325 mg cascara sagrada tablets P.O. h.s.; or 1 ml fluid extract daily; or 5 ml aromatic fluid extract daily.
Children 2 to 12 years: ½ adult dose.
Children under 2 years: ¼ adult dose.

ADVERSE REACTIONS
Common reactions are in italics; life-threatening reactions are in bold italics.
GI: *nausea;* vomiting; diarrhea; loss of normal bowel function with excessive use; *abdominal cramps,* especially in severe constipation; malabsorption of nutrients; "cathartic colon" (syndrome resembling ulcerative colitis radiologically and pathologically) after chronic misuse; discoloration of rectal mucosa after long-term use.
Metabolic: hypokalemia, protein enteropathy, electrolyte imbalance in excessive use.
Other: laxative dependence in long-term or excessive use.

INTERACTIONS
None significant.

NURSING CONSIDERATIONS
- *Contraindicated* in abdominal pain, nausea, vomiting, or other symptoms of appendicitis or acute surgical abdomen; acute surgical delirium, fecal impaction, intestinal obstruction or perforation. *Use cautiously* when rectal bleeding is present.
- Aromatic cascara fluid extract is less active and less bitter than nonaromatic fluid extract.
- Liquid preparations more reliable than solid dosage forms.
- Before giving for constipation, determine if patient has adequate fluid intake, exercise, and diet. Tell him that dietary sources of bulk include bran and other cereals, fresh fruit, and vegetables.
- May turn alkaline urine red-pink and acidic urine yellow-brown.
- Monitor serum electrolytes during prolonged use.
- Onset of action is 6 to 12 hours.

castor oil

Alphamul◇, Emulsoil◇, Fleet Flavored Castor Oil◇, Kellogg's Castor Oil◇, Minims Castor Oil‡◇, Neoloid◇, Purge◇

Pregnancy Risk Category: X

HOW SUPPLIED
Oral liquid◇: 36.4% (Neoloid◇), 60% (Alphamul◇), 67% (Fleet◇), 95% (Purge◇, Emulsoil◇), 100% (Kellogg's◇, Minims◇).

MECHANISM OF ACTION
Increases peristalsis by direct effect on the smooth muscle of the intestine. Thought either to irritate the musculature or to stimulate the colonic intramural plexus. Also promotes fluid accumulation in the colon and small intestine. A stimulant laxative.

INDICATIONS & DOSAGE
Preparation for rectal or bowel examination, or surgery; acute constipation (rarely) –
Adults: 15 to 60 ml P.O.
Children over 2 years: 5 to 15 ml P.O.
Children under 2 years: 1.25 to 7.5 ml P.O.
Infants: up to 4 ml P.O. Increased dose produces no greater effect.

ADVERSE REACTIONS
Common reactions are in italics; life-threatening reactions are in bold italics.
GI: *nausea;* vomiting; diarrhea; loss of normal bowel function with excessive use; *abdominal cramps,* especially in severe constipation; malabsorption of nutrients; "cathartic colon" (syndrome resembling ulcerative colitis radiologically and pathologically) in chronic misuse. May cause constipation after catharsis.
GU: pelvic congestion in menstruating women.
Metabolic: hypokalemia, protein-losing enteropathy, other electrolyte imbalance in excessive use.
Other: laxative dependence in long-term or excessive use.

INTERACTIONS
None significant.

NURSING CONSIDERATIONS
- *Contraindicated* in ulcerative bowel lesions; during menstruation; in abdominal pain, nausea, vomiting, or other symptoms of appendicitis or acute surgical abdomen; in anal or rectal fissures, fecal impaction, intestinal obstruction or perforation; and in pregnancy. *Use cautiously* in rectal bleeding.
- Failure to respond may indicate acute condition requiring surgery.
- Give with juice or carbonated beverage to mask oily taste. Patient should stir mixture and drink it promptly. Ice held in mouth before

*Liquid form contains alcohol. **May contain tartrazine.

taking drug will help prevent tasting it.

- Shake emulsion well. Store below 40° F (4.4° C). Don't freeze.
- Give on empty stomach for best results.
- Produces complete evacuation after 3 hours. Tell patient that after castor oil has emptied bowel he will not have bowel movement for 1 to 2 days.
- Time drug administration so that it doesn't interfere with scheduled activities or sleep.
- Monitor serum electrolytes during prolonged use.
- Generally used before diagnostic testing or therapy requiring thorough evacuation of GI tract.
- Use for short-term treatment. Not recommended for routine use; useful for acute constipation not responsive to milder laxatives.
- Before giving for constipation, determine if patient has adequate fluid intake, exercise, and diet. Tell him that dietary sources of bulk include bran and other cereals, fresh fruit, and vegetables.
- Increased intestinal motility lessens absorption of concomitantly administered P.O. drugs. Reschedule dose.
- Castor oil affects the small intestine. Regular use may cause excessive loss of water and salt.
- Castor oil emulsion is better tolerated but is more expensive.

docusate calcium (dioctyl calcium sulfosuccinate)

Pro-Cal-Sof◇, Surfak◇

docusate potassium (dioctyl potassium sulfosuccinate)

Dialose◇, Diocto-K◇, Kasof◇

docusate sodium (dioctyl sodium sulfosuccinate)

Afko-Lube◇, Colace◇, Coloxyl‡, Coloxyl Enema Concentrate‡, Diocto◇, Dioeze◇, Diosuccin◇, Dio-Sul◇, Disonate◇, Di-Sosul◇, DOK-250◇, DOK Liquid◇, Doss 300◇, Doxinate◇, D-S-S◇, Duosol◇, Genasoft◇, Laxinate 100◇, Modane Soft◇, Pro-Sof◇, Pro-Sof 250◇, Pro-Sof Liquid Concentrate◇, Regulax SS◇, Regutol◇, Stulex◇

Pregnancy Risk Category: C

HOW SUPPLIED

calcium
Capsules: 50 mg◇, 240 mg◇
potassium
Capsules: 100 mg◇, 240 mg◇
sodium
Tablets: 50 mg◇, 100 mg◇
Capsules◇*:* 50 mg, 60 mg, 100 mg, 240 mg, 250 mg, 300 mg
Oral liquid: 50 mg/ml◇
Syrup: 50 mg/15 ml◇, 60 mg/15 ml◇
Enema concentrate: 18 g/100 ml (must be diluted)‡

MECHANISM OF ACTION

Reduces surface tension of interfacing liquid contents of the bowel. This detergent activity promotes incorporation of additional liquid into the stool, forming a softer mass. A stool softener.

INDICATIONS & DOSAGE

Stool softener –
Adults and older children: 50 to 300 mg (docusate sodium) P.O. daily or 50 to 300 mg (docusate calcium and docusate potassium) P.O. daily until bowel movements are normal. Alternatively, give enema (where available). Dilute 1:24 with sterile water before administration, and give 100 to 150 ml (retention enema), 300 to 500 ml (evacuation enema), or 0.5 to 1.5 liters (flushing enema).

†Available in Canada only. ‡Available in Australia only. ◇Available OTC.

Children 6 to 12 years: 40 to 120 mg (docusate sodium) P.O. daily.
Children 3 to 6 years: 20 to 60 mg (docusate sodium) P.O. daily.
Children under 3 years: 10 to 40 mg (docusate sodium) P.O. daily.

Higher dosages are for initial therapy. Adjust dosage to individual response. Usual dosage in children and adults with minimal needs: 50 to 150 mg (docusate calcium) P.O. daily.

ADVERSE REACTIONS
Common reactions are in italics; life-threatening reactions are in bold italics.
EENT: throat irritation.
GI: bitter taste, mild abdominal cramping, diarrhea.
Other: laxative dependence in long-term or excessive use.

INTERACTIONS
Mineral oil: may increase mineral oil absorption and cause lipoid pneumonia. Don't administer together.

NURSING CONSIDERATIONS
- *Contraindicated* in patients with hypersensitivity to the drug and in those with intestinal obstruction, undiagnosed abdominal pain, vomiting or other signs of appendicitis, fecal impaction, or acute surgical abdomen.
- Should be used only occasionally. Don't use for more than 1 week without doctor's knowledge.
- Give liquid in milk, fruit juice, or infant formula to mask bitter taste.
- Not for use in treating existing constipation, but prevents constipation from developing.
- Laxative of choice in patients who should not strain during defecation, such as those recovering from myocardial infarction or rectal surgery; in disease of rectum and anus that makes passage of firm stool difficult; or in postpartum constipation.
- Acts within 24 to 48 hours to produce firm, semisolid stool.
- Instruct patient that dietary sources of bulk include bran and other cereals, fresh fruit, and vegetables.
- Doesn't stimulate intestinal peristaltic movements.
- Discontinue if severe cramping occurs.
- Store at 59° to 86° F (15° to 30° C). Protect liquid from light.
- Many doctors feel that the minimum effective dosage is 300 mg daily. A lower dosage may not produce satisfactory results.

glycerin
Fleet Babylax◊, Sani-Supp◊

Pregnancy Risk Category: C

HOW SUPPLIED
Enema (pediatric): 4 ml/applicator◊
Suppositories: adult, children, and infant sizes◊

MECHANISM OF ACTION
Draws water from the tissues into the feces and thus stimulates evacuation. A hyperosmolar laxative.

INDICATIONS & DOSAGE
Constipation –
Adults and children over 6 years: 3 g as a rectal suppository; or 5 to 15 ml as an enema.
Children under 6 years: 1 to 1.5 g as a rectal suppository; or 2 to 5 ml as an enema.

ADVERSE REACTIONS
Common reactions are in italics; life-threatening reactions are in bold italics.
GI: *cramping pain,* rectal discomfort, hyperemia of rectal mucosa.

INTERACTIONS
None significant.

NURSING CONSIDERATIONS
- *Contraindicated* in patients with hypersensitivity to the drug and in those with intestinal obstruction, undiagnosed abdominal pain, vomiting or

*Liquid form contains alcohol. **May contain tartrazine.

other signs of appendicitis, fecal impaction, or acute surgical abdomen.
- A hyperosmolar laxative used mainly to reestablish proper toilet habits in laxative-dependent patients.
- Must be retained for at least 15 minutes; usually acts within 1 hour. Entire suppository need not melt to be effective.

lactulose

Cephulac, Cholac, Chronulac, Constilac, Duphalac, Enulose, Lactulax†

Pregnancy Risk Category: B

HOW SUPPLIED

Syrup: 10 g/15 ml

MECHANISM OF ACTION

Produces an osmotic effect in the colon. Resultant distention promotes peristalsis. Also decreases blood ammonia, probably as a result of bacterial degradation, which decreases the pH of colon contents.

INDICATIONS & DOSAGE

Treatment of constipation –
Adults: 15 to 30 ml P.O. daily.
To prevent and treat portal-systemic encephalopathy, including hepatic precoma and coma in patients with severe hepatic disease –
Adults: initially, 20 to 30 g P.O. (30 to 45 ml) t.i.d. or q.i.d., until two or three soft stools are produced daily. Usual dosage is 60 to 100 g daily in divided doses. Can also be given by retention enema in at least 100 ml of fluid.

ADVERSE REACTIONS

Common reactions are in italics; life-threatening reactions are in bold italics.
GI: abdominal cramps, belching, diarrhea, gaseous distention, flatulence.
Metabolic: hypernatremia.

INTERACTIONS

Antibotics, orally administered Neomycin, antacids: decreased effectiveness of lactulose. Avoid concomitant use.

NURSING CONSIDERATIONS

- *Contraindicated* in low-galactose diet. *Use cautiously* in diabetes mellitus.
- Reduce dosage if diarrhea occurs. Replace fluid loss.
- Monitor serum sodium for possible hypernatremia, especially when giving in higher doses to treat hepatic encephalopathy.
- Minimize drug's sweet taste by diluting with water or fruit juice or giving with food.
- Store at room temperature, preferably below 86° F (30° C). Don't freeze.

magnesium citrate (citrate of magnesia)

Citroma◇, Citro-Nesia◇

magnesium hydroxide (milk of magnesia)

M.O.M.◇

magnesium sulfate (epsom salts)◇

Pregnancy Risk Category: B

HOW SUPPLIED

citrate
Oral solution: approximately 168 mEq magnesium/240 ml◇
hydroxide
Oral suspension: 7% to 8.5% (approximately 80 mEq magnesium/30 ml)◇
sulfate
Granules: approximately 40 mEq magnesium/5 g◇

MECHANISM OF ACTION

Produces an osmotic effect in the small intestine by drawing water into the intestinal lumen. A saline laxative.

INDICATIONS & DOSAGE
Constipation, to evacuate bowel before surgery –
Adults and children over 6 years: 15 g magnesium sulfate P.O. in glass of water; or 10 to 20 ml concentrated milk of magnesia P.O.; or 15 to 60 ml milk of magnesia P.O.; or 5 to 10 oz magnesium citrate h.s.
Children 2 to 6 years: 5 to 15 ml milk of magnesia P.O.
Antacid –
Adults: 5 to 15 ml milk of magnesia P.O. t.i.d. or q.i.d.

ADVERSE REACTIONS
Common reactions are in italics; life-threatening reactions are in bold italics.
GI: *abdominal cramping, nausea, diarrhea.*
Metabolic: fluid and electrolyte disturbances if used daily.
Other: laxative dependence in long-term or excessive use.

INTERACTIONS
None significant.

NURSING CONSIDERATIONS
- *Contraindicated* in abdominal pain, nausea, vomiting, or other symptoms of appendicitis or acute surgical abdomen; and in myocardial damage, heart block, imminent delivery, fecal impaction, rectal fissures, intestinal obstruction or perforation, or renal disease. *Use cautiously* in rectal bleeding.
- Shake suspension well; give with large amount of water when used as laxative. When administering through nasogastric tube, make sure tube is placed properly and is patent. After instilling, flush tube with water to ensure passage to stomach and maintain tube patency.
- For short-term therapy; don't use longer than 1 week.
- When used as laxative, don't give oral drugs 1 to 2 hours before or after administration.
- As a saline laxative, drug produces watery stool in 3 to 6 hours. Time drug administration so that it doesn't interfere with scheduled activities or sleep.
- Magnesium sulfate is more potent than other saline laxatives.
- Before giving for constipation, determine if patient has adequate fluid intake, exercise, and diet. Tell him that dietary sources of bulk include bran and other cereals, fresh fruit, and vegetables.
- Magnesium may accumulate in renal insufficiency.
- Chilling before use may make magnesium citrate more palatable.
- Monitor serum electrolytes during prolonged use.
- Frequent or prolonged use as a laxative may cause dependence.

methylcellulose
Citrucel◊, Cologel◊

Pregnancy Risk Category: C

HOW SUPPLIED
Powder: 2 g/heaping tablespoon◊
Tablets: 500 mg◊

MECHANISM OF ACTION
Absorbs water and expands to increase bulk and moisture content of the stool. The increased bulk encourages peristalsis and bowel movement. A bulk-forming laxative.

INDICATIONS & DOSAGE
Chronic constipation –
Adults: 1 heaping tablespoon in 8 ounces cold water daily to t.i.d.
Children 6 to 12 years: 1 level tablespoon in 4 ounces cold water daily to t.i.d.

ADVERSE REACTIONS
Common reactions are in italics; life-threatening reactions are in bold italics.
GI: *nausea,* vomiting, diarrhea (all after excessive use); esophageal, gastric, small intestinal, or colonic strictures when drug is chewed or taken in dry form; *abdominal cramps,* especially in severe constipation.
Other: laxative dependence in long-term or excessive use.

INTERACTIONS
None significant.

NURSING CONSIDERATIONS
- *Contraindicated* in abdominal pain, nausea, vomiting, or other symptoms of appendicitis or acute surgical abdomen; and in intestinal obstruction or ulceration, disabling adhesion, or difficulty swallowing.
- Laxative effect usually takes 12 to 24 hours, but may be delayed 3 days.
- Tell patient to take drug with at least 8 oz (240 ml) of pleasant-tasting liquid to mask grittiness.
- Especially useful in postpartum constipation, debilitated patients, chronic laxative abuse, irritable bowel syndrome, diverticular disease, colostomies, and to empty colon before barium enema examinations.
- Before giving for constipation, determine if patient has adequate fluid intake, exercise, and diet. Tell him that dietary sources of bulk include bran and other cereals, fresh fruit, and vegetables.
- Not absorbed systemically; nontoxic.

mineral oil (liquid petrolatum)

Agoral Plain◇, Fleet Mineral Oil◇, Kondremul Plain◇, Liqui-Doss◇, Milkinol◇, Neo-Cultol◇, Zymenol◇

Pregnancy Risk Category: C

HOW SUPPLIED
Emulsion: 50%◇
Jelly: 55%◇
Oral liquid: in pints, quarts, gallons◇

MECHANISM OF ACTION
Increases water retention in the stool by creating a barrier between colon wall and feces that prevents colonic reabsorption of fecal water. A lubricant laxative.

INDICATIONS & DOSAGE
Constipation; preparation for bowel studies or surgery –
Adults: 5 to 45 ml P.O. h.s.; or 120 ml enema.
Children: 5 to 20 ml P.O. h.s.; or 30 to 60 ml enema.

ADVERSE REACTIONS
Common reactions are in italics; life-threatening reactions are in bold italics.
GI: *nausea;* vomiting; diarrhea in excessive use; *abdominal cramps,* especially in severe constipation; decreased absorption of nutrients and fat-soluble vitamins, resulting in deficiency; and slowed healing after hemorrhoidectomy.
Other: laxative dependence in long-term or excessive use, pruritus, ***lipid pneumonitis.***

INTERACTIONS
Docusate salts: may increase mineral oil absorption and cause lipid pneumonia. Don't administer together.
Fat-soluble vitamins (A, D, E, K): absorption may be decreased after prolonged administration.

NURSING CONSIDERATIONS
- *Contraindicated* in abdominal pain, nausea, vomiting, or other symptoms of appendicitis or acute surgical abdomen; and in fecal impaction, or intestinal obstruction or perforation. Enema contraindicated in children under 2 years.
- *Use cautiously* in young children; in

elderly or debilitated patients because of susceptibility to lipid pneumonitis through aspiration, absorption, and transport from intestinal mucosa; and in rectal bleeding.
- Don't give drug with meals or immediately after, as it delays passage of food from stomach. More active on an empty stomach.
- To be taken only at bedtime. Warn patient not to take for more than 1 week.
- Give with fruit juices or carbonated drinks to disguise taste.
- Use when patient needs to ease the strain of evacuation.
- Warn patient of possible rectal leakage from excessive dosages so he can avoid soiling clothing.
- Before giving for constipation, determine if patient has adequate fluid intake, exercise, and diet. Tell him that dietary sources of bulk include bran and other cereals, fresh fruit, and vegetables.
- Onset of action is 6 to 8 hours.

phenolphthalein, white

Alophen Pills◇, Medilax◇, Modane◇, Modane Mild◇, Phenolax Wafers**◇, Prulet◇

phenolphthalein, yellow

Evac-U-Gen◇, Evac-U-Lax◇, Ex-Lax◇, Feen-A-Mint Gum◇, Lax-Pills◇

Pregnancy Risk Category: C

HOW SUPPLIED

phenolphthalein, white
Tablets: 60 mg◇
Tablets (chewable): 60 mg◇, 64.8 mg◇
phenolphthalein, yellow
Tablets (chewable): 80 mg◇, 90 mg◇, 97.2 mg◇
Chewing gum: 97.2 mg◇

MECHANISM OF ACTION

Increases peristalsis by direct effect on the smooth muscle of the intestine. Thought either to irritate the musculature or to stimulate the colonic intramural plexus. Also promotes fluid accumulation in the colon and small intestine. A stimulant laxative.

INDICATIONS & DOSAGE

Constipation –
Adults and children over 12 years: 30 to 270 mg P.O., preferably h.s.
Children 6 to 11 years: 30 to 60 mg P.O. h.s.
Children 2 to 5 years: 15 to 30 mg P.O. h.s.

ADVERSE REACTIONS

Common reactions are in italics; life-threatening reactions are in bold italics.
GI: diarrhea; *colic in large doses;* factitious nausea; vomiting; loss of normal bowel function in excessive use; *abdominal cramps,* especially in severe constipation; malabsorption of nutrients; "cathartic colon" (syndrome resembling ulcerative colitis radiologically and pathologically) in chronic misuse; reddish discoloration in alkaline feces or urine.
Skin: dermatitis, pruritus, rash, pigmentation.
Other: laxative dependence in long-term or excessive use, ***hypersensitivity.***

INTERACTIONS

None significant.

NURSING CONSIDERATIONS

- *Contraindicated* in abdominal pain, nausea, vomiting, or other symptoms of appendicitis or acute surgical abdomen; in fecal impaction, or intestinal obstruction or perforation. *Use cautiously* in rectal bleeding.
- Laxative effect may last up to 3 to 4 days.
- Produces semisolid stool within 6 to 8 hours. Time drug administration so

*Liquid form contains alcohol. **May contain tartrazine.

that it doesn't interfere with scheduled activities or sleep.
- Warn patient with rash to avoid sun and discontinue use. Don't use any other product containing phenolphthalein.
- Before giving for constipation, determine if patient has adequate fluid intake, exercise, and diet. Tell him that dietary sources of bulk include bran and other cereals, fresh fruit, and vegetables.
- May discolor alkaline urine red-pink and acidic urine yellow-brown.
- Drug is available in many dosage forms. Most popular OTC laxative.
- Children may mistake for candy. Keep out of reach.
- Yellow phenolphthalein is two to three times as potent as white phenolphthalein.

polyethylene glycol-electrolyte solution

CoLyte, Glycoprep‡, GoLYTELY

Pregnancy Risk Category: C

HOW SUPPLIED
Powder for oral solution: polyethylene glycol (PEG) 3350 (120 g), sodium sulfate (3.36 g), sodium chloride (2.92 g), potassium chloride (1.49 g) per 2 liters (CoLyte); PEG 3350 (60 g), sodium chloride (1.46 g), potassium chloride (745 mg), sodium bicarbonate (1.68 g), sodium sulfate (5.68 g) per liter (Glycoprep‡); PEG 3350 (236 g), sodium sulfate (22.74 g), sodium bicarbonate (6.74g), sodium chloride (5.86 g), potassium chloride (2.97 g), per 4.8 liter (GoLYTELY)

MECHANISM OF ACTION
PEG 3350, a nonabsorbable solution, acts as an osmotic agent. Using sodium sulfate as the major sodium source, sodium absorption is greatly reduced. The electrolyte concentration results in virtually no net absorption or secretion of ions.

INDICATIONS & DOSAGE
Bowel preparation before GI examination –

Adults: 240 ml P.O. q 10 minutes until 4 liters are consumed. Usually administered 4 hours before examination, allowing 3 hours for drinking and 1 hour for bowel evacuation.

ADVERSE REACTIONS
Common reactions are in italics; life-threatening reactions are in bold italics.

GI: *nausea, bloating, cramps, vomiting.*

INTERACTIONS
None significant.

NURSING CONSIDERATIONS
- *Contraindicated* in GI obstruction or perforation, gastric retention, toxic colitis, or megacolon.
- If administered to semiconscious patients or to patients with impaired gag reflex, take care to prevent aspiration.
- No major shifts in fluid and electrolytes have been reported.
- Orally administered solution induces a diarrhea (onset 30 to 60 minutes) which rapidly cleanses the bowel, usually within 4 hours. The solution may be administered in the early morning, if the patient is scheduled for a mid-morning exam.
- May be less useful as a preparation for barium enema, because it may interfere with the barium coating of the colonic mucosa. To avoid such interference, administer solution the evening before the examination.
- Patient should fast for 3 to 4 hours before taking the solution, and thereafter ingest only clear fluids until the examination is complete.
- Tap water may be used to reconstitute powder. Shake vigorously to ensure that all powder is dissolved. Re-

constituted solution may be refrigerated but should be used within 48 hours.

• Do not add flavoring or additional ingredients to the solution, and do not administer chilled solution. Hypothermia has been reported after ingestion of large amounts of chilled solution.

psyllium

Cillium◇, Konsyl◇, Metamucil◇, Metamucil Instant Mix◇, Metamucil Sugar Free◇, Naturacil◇, Perdiem Plain◇, Siblin◇, Syllact◇

Pregnancy Risk Category: C

HOW SUPPLIED

Chewable pieces: 1.7 g/piece◇
Effervescent powder: 3.4 g/packet◇, 3.7 g/packet◇
Granules: 2.5 g/tsp, 4.03 g/tsp◇
Powder: 3.3 g/tsp◇, 3.4 g/tsp◇, 3.5 g/tsp◇, 4.94 g/tsp◇
Wafers: 3.4 g/wafer◇

MECHANISM OF ACTION

Absorbs water and expands to increase bulk and moisture content of the stool. The increased bulk encourages peristalsis and bowel movement. A bulk-forming laxative.

INDICATIONS & DOSAGE

Constipation; bowel management–
Adults: 1 to 2 rounded teaspoonfuls P.O. in full glass of liquid daily, b.i.d. or t.i.d., followed by second glass of liquid; or 1 packet P.O. dissolved in water daily, b.i.d. or t.i.d.
Children over 6 years: 1 level teaspoonful P.O. in half a glass of liquid h.s.

ADVERSE REACTIONS

Common reactions are in italics; life-threatening reactions are in bold italics.
GI: nausea, vomiting, diarrhea, all after excessive use; esophageal, gastric, small intestinal, or colonic strictures when drug taken in dry form; abdominal cramps, especially in severe constipation.

INTERACTIONS

None significant.

NURSING CONSIDERATIONS

• *Contraindicated* in abdominal pain, nausea, vomiting, or other symptoms of appendicitis; and in intestinal obstruction or ulceration, disabling adhesion, or difficulty swallowing.
• In diabetic patients, use brand of psyllium that does not contain sugar. Check label.
• Mix with at least 8 oz (240 ml) of cold, pleasant-tasting liquid such as orange juice to mask grittiness, and stir only a few seconds. Patient should drink it immediately or mixture will congeal. Follow with additional glass of liquid.
• Before giving for constipation, determine if patient has adequate fluid intake, exercise, and diet. Tell him that dietary sources of bulk include bran and other cereals, fresh fruit, and vegetables.
• May reduce appetite if taken before meals.
• Laxative effect usually seen in 12 to 24 hours, but may be delayed 3 days.
• Not absorbed systemically; nontoxic. Especially useful in postpartum constipation, debilitated patients, chronic laxative abuse, irritable bowel syndrome, diverticular disease, and in combination with other laxatives to empty colon before barium enema examinations.

senna

Black-Draught◇, Senokot◇, X-Prep Liquid*◇

Pregnancy Risk Category: C

HOW SUPPLIED

Tablets: 187 mg◇, 217 mg◇, 600 mg◇
Granules: 326 mg/tsp◇, 1.65 g/½ tsp◇

*Liquid form contains alcohol. **May contain tartrazine.

Suppositories: 652 mg◇
Syrup: 218 mg/5 ml◇

MECHANISM OF ACTION
Increases peristalsis by direct effect on the smooth muscle of the intestine. Thought either to irritate the musculature or to stimulate the colonic intramural plexus. Also promotes fluid accumulation in the colon and small intestine. A stimulant laxative.

INDICATIONS & DOSAGE
Acute constipation, preparation for bowel or rectal examination –
Adults: Dosage range for Senokot: 1 to 8 tablets P.O.; ½ to 4 teaspoonfuls of granules added to liquid; 1 to 2 suppositories h.s.; 1 to 4 teaspoonfuls syrup h.s. Black-Draught: 2 tablets or ¼ to ½ level teaspoonfuls of granules mixed with water.
Children over 27 kg: half adult dose of tablets, granules, or syrup (except Black-Draught tablets and granules not recommended for children).
Children 1 month to 1 year: 1.25 to 2.5 ml Senokot syrup P.O. h.s.

X-Prep Liquid used solely as single dose for preradiographic bowel evacuation. Give 20 g powder dissolved in juice or 75 ml liquid between 2 p.m. and 4 p.m. on day before X-ray procedure. May be given in divided doses for elderly or debilitated patients.

ADVERSE REACTIONS
Common reactions are in italics; life-threatening reactions are in bold italics.
GI: *nausea;* vomiting; diarrhea; loss of normal bowel function in excessive use; *abdominal cramps,* especially in severe constipation; malabsorption of nutrients; "cathartic colon" (syndrome resembling ulcerative colitis radiologically) in chronic misuse; may cause constipation after catharsis; yellow, yellow-green cast to feces; diarrhea in nursing infants of mothers receiving senna; darkened pigmentation of rectal mucosa in long-term use, which is usually reversible within 4 to 12 months after stopping drug.
GU: red-pink discoloration in alkaline urine; yellow-brown color to acidic urine.
Metabolic: hypokalemia, protein-losing enteropathy, electrolyte imbalance with excessive use.
Other: laxative dependence in long-term or excessive use.

INTERACTIONS
None significant.

NURSING CONSIDERATIONS
- *Contraindicated* in ulcerative bowel lesions; in nausea, vomiting, abdominal pain, or other symptoms of appendicitis or acute surgical abdomen; fecal impaction; or intestinal obstruction or perforation.
- Use for short-term treatment.
- More potent than cascara sagrada. Acts in 6 to 10 hours. X-Prep Liquid gives thorough, strong bowel action beginning in 6 hours.
- Avoid exposing to excessive heat or light.
- Before giving for constipation, determine if patient has adequate fluid intake, exercise, and diet. Tell him that dietary sources of bulk include bran and other cereals, fresh fruit, and vegetables.
- After X-Prep Liquid is taken, diet should be confined to clear liquids.
- Senna is one of the most effective laxatives for counteracting constipation caused by narcotic analgesics.

sodium phosphates
Fleet Phospho-Soda◇

Pregnancy Risk Category: C

HOW SUPPLIED
Liquid: 2.4 g/5 ml sodium phosphate and 900 mg sodium biphosphate/5 ml◇
Enema: 160 mg/ml sodium phosphate and 60 mg/ml sodium biphosphate◇

MECHANISM OF ACTION
Produces an osmotic effect in the small intestine by drawing water into the intestinal lumen. A saline laxative.

INDICATIONS & DOSAGE
Constipation –
Adults: 20 to 30 ml solution mixed with 120 ml cold water P.O.; or 60 to 135 ml enema.
Children: 5 to 15 ml mixed with 120 ml P.O.; or 67.5 ml enema.

ADVERSE REACTIONS
Common reactions are in italics; life-threatening reactions are in bold italics.
GI: *abdominal cramping.*
Metabolic: fluid and electrolyte disturbances (hypernatremia, hyperphosphatemia) if used daily.
Other: laxative dependence in long-term or excessive use.

INTERACTIONS
None significant.

NURSING CONSIDERATIONS
- *Contraindicated* in abdominal pain, nausea, vomiting, or other symptoms of appendicitis or acute surgical abdomen; intestinal obstruction or perforation; edema; congestive heart failure; megacolon; impaired renal function; and in patients on salt-restricted diets.
- *Use cautiously* in patients with large hemorrhoids or anal excoriations.
- Available in oral and rectal forms.
- Before giving for constipation, determine if patient has adequate fluid intake, exercise, and diet. Tell him that dietary sources of bulk include bran and other cereals, fresh fruit, and vegetables.
- Saline laxative; up to 10% of sodium content may be absorbed.
- Enema form elicits response in 5 to 10 minutes.
- Used in preparation for barium enema, sigmoidoscopy, and for treatment of fecal impaction.
- Also prescribed to treat hypercalcemia or as a phosphate replacement.

*Liquid form contains alcohol. **May contain tartrazine.

49

Antiemetics

benzquinamide hydrochloride
buclizine hydrochloride
chlorpromazine hydrochloride
(See Chapter 32, ANTIPSYCHOTICS.)
cyclizine hydrochloride
cyclizine lactate
dimenhydrinate
diphenidol hydrochloride
dronabinol
meclizine hydrochloride
metoclopramide hydrochloride
ondansetron hydrochloride
perphenazine
(See Chapter 32, ANTIPSYCHOTICS.)
prochlorperazine
prochlorperazine edisylate
prochlorperazine maleate
promethazine hydrochloride
(See Chapter 42, ANTIHISTAMINES.)
scopolamine
(See Chapter 37, ANTICHOLINERGICS.)
thiethylperazine maleate
trimethobenzamide hydrochloride

COMBINATION PRODUCTS
None.

benzquinamide hydrochloride

Emete-Con

Pregnancy Risk Category: C

HOW SUPPLIED
Injection: 50 mg/vial

MECHANISM OF ACTION
Acts on the chemoreceptor trigger zone to inhibit nausea and vomiting.

INDICATIONS & DOSAGE
Nausea and vomiting associated with anesthesia and surgery –
Adults: 50 mg I.M. (0.5 mg/kg to 1 mg/kg). May repeat in 1 hour, and thereafter q 3 to 4 hours, p.r.n.; or 25 mg (0.2 mg/kg to 0.4 mg/kg) I.V. as single dose, administered slowly (25 mg/minute).

ADVERSE REACTIONS
Common reactions are in italics; life-threatening reactions are in bold italics.
CNS: *drowsiness,* fatigue, insomnia, restlessness, headache, excitation, tremors, twitching, dizziness.
CV: sudden rise in blood pressure and transient arrhythmias (premature atrial and ventricular contractions, atrial fibrillation) after I.V. administration; hypertension; hypotension.
EENT: dry mouth, salivation, blurred vision.
GI: anorexia, nausea.
Skin: urticaria, rash.
Other: muscle weakness, flushing, hiccups, sweating, chills, fever. May mask symptoms of ototoxicity, brain tumor, or intestinal obstruction.

INTERACTIONS
Alcohol, CNS depressants: enhanced CNS depression. Avoid concomitant use.

NURSING CONSIDERATIONS
- *Contraindicated* for I.V. use in cardiovascular disease and within 15 minutes of preanesthetic or cardiovascular drugs.
- Give I.M. injections in large muscle mass. Use deltoid area only if well developed. Be sure to aspirate syringe for I.M. injection to avoid inadvertent I.V. injection.
- **I.V. use:** Give I.V. dose slowly (25 mg/minute).
- Reconstituted solution is stable for 14 days at room temperature. Store dry powder and reconstituted solution in a light-resistant container.

• Precipitation occurs if reconstituted with 0.9% sodium chloride injection. Use bacteriostatic water for injection instead.
• Monitor blood pressure frequently.
• Excellent alternative if prochlorperazine (Compazine) is contraindicated.

buclizine hydrochloride
Bucladin-S**

Pregnancy Risk Category: C

HOW SUPPLIED
Tablets: 50 mg

MECHANISM OF ACTION
May affect neural pathways originating in the labyrinth to inhibit nausea and vomiting, but the exact mechanism of action is unknown.

INDICATIONS & DOSAGE
Motion sickness (prevention) –
Adults: 50 mg P.O. at least one half hour before beginning travel. If needed, may repeat another 50 mg P.O. after 4 to 6 hours.
Vertigo –
Adults: 50 mg P.O., up to 150 mg P.O. daily in severe cases. Maintenance dose is 50 mg b.i.d.

ADVERSE REACTIONS
Common reactions are in italics; life-threatening reactions are in bold italics.
CNS: *drowsiness,* headache, dizziness, jitters.
EENT: blurred vision, dry mouth.
GU: urine retention.
Other: may mask symptoms of ototoxicity, intestinal obstruction, or brain tumor.

INTERACTIONS
Alcohol, CNS depressants: additive CNS depression. Avoid concomitant use.

NURSING CONSIDERATIONS
• *Contraindicated* in patients with hypersensitivity to the drug.
• *Use cautiously* in patients with glaucoma, GU or GI obstruction, and in elderly males with possible prostatic hypertrophy.
• Warn patient against driving and other activities that require alertness until CNS effects of the drug are known.
• Tablets may be placed in mouth and allowed to dissolve without water. May also be chewed or swallowed whole.
• Classified as an antihistamine.

cyclizine hydrochloride
Marezine◇

cyclizine lactate
Marezine, Marzine†

Pregnancy Risk Category: B

HOW SUPPLIED
hydrochloride
Tablets: 50 mg◇
lactate
Injection: 50 mg/ml

MECHANISM OF ACTION
May affect neural pathways originating in the labyrinth to inhibit nausea and vomiting, but the exact mechanism of action is unknown.

INDICATIONS & DOSAGE
Motion sickness (prevention and treatment) –
Adults: 50 mg P.O. (hydrochloride) one half hour before travel, then q 4 to 6 hours, p.r.n., to maximum of 200 mg daily; or 50 mg I.M. (lactate) q 4 to 6 hours, p.r.n.
Postoperative vomiting (prevention) –
Adults: 50 mg I.M. (lactate) preoperatively or 20 to 30 minutes before expected termination of surgery; then postoperatively 50 mg I.M. (lactate) q 4 to 6 hours, p.r.n.

*Liquid form contains alcohol. **May contain tartrazine.

Motion sickness and postoperative vomiting –
Children 6 to 12 years: 3 mg/kg (lactate) I.M. divided t.i.d., or 25 mg (hydrochloride) P.O. q 4 to 6 hours p.r.n. to a maximum of 75 mg daily.

ADVERSE REACTIONS
Common reactions are in italics; life-threatening reactions are in bold italics.
CNS: *drowsiness,* dizziness, auditory and visual hallucinations.
CV: hypotension.
EENT: blurred vision, dry mouth.
GI: constipation.
GU: urine retention.
Other: may mask symptoms of ototoxicity, brain tumor, or intestinal obstruction.

INTERACTIONS
Alcohol, other CNS depressants: additive CNS depression. Avoid concomitant use.

NURSING CONSIDERATIONS
• *Contraindicated* in patients with hypersensitivity to the drug.
• *Use cautiously* in glaucoma, GU or GI obstruction, heart failure, and in elderly males with possible prostatic hypertrophy.
• Warn patient against driving and other activities that require alertness until CNS effects of the drug are known.
• Classified as an antihistamine.
• Store in cool place. When stored at room temperature, injection may turn slightly yellow, but this color change does not indicate loss of potency.

dimenhydrinate

Andrumin‡, Apo-Dimenhydrinate†, Calm X◇, Dimetabs, Dinate, Dommanate, Dramamine◇*, Dramamine Chewable◇**, Dramamine Liquid◇*, Dramanate, Dramilin, Dramocen, Dramoject, Dymenate, Gravol†, Hydrate, Marmine◇, Motion-Aid, Nauseatol†, Novodimenate†, PMS-Dimenhydrinate†, Reidamine, Tega-Vert◇, Travamine†, Travs‡, Triptone Caplets◇, Wehamine
Pregnancy Risk Category: B

HOW SUPPLIED
Tablets: 50 mg◇
Tablets (chewable): 50 mg◇
Capsules: 50 mg◇
Oral liquid: 12.5 mg/4 ml* ◇, 15.62 mg/5 ml
Injection: 50 mg/ml

MECHANISM OF ACTION
May affect neural pathways originating in the labyrinth to inhibit nausea and vomiting, but the exact mechanism of action is unknown. An antihistamine.

INDICATIONS & DOSAGE
Nausea, vomiting, dizziness of motion sickness (treatment and prevention) –
Adults: 50 mg P.O. q 4 hours, or 100 mg q 4 hours if drowsiness is not objectionable; or 50 mg I.M., p.r.n.; or 50 mg I.V. diluted in 10 ml sodium chloride solution, injected over 2 minutes. Maximum dose is 400 mg/day.
Children: 5 mg/kg P.O. or I.M., divided q.i.d. Maximum dosage is 300 mg daily. Don't use in children under 2 years.

ADVERSE REACTIONS
Common reactions are in italics; life-threatening reactions are in bold italics.
CNS: *drowsiness,* headache, incoordination, dizziness.
CV: palpitations, hypotension.

†Available in Canada only. ‡Available in Australia only. ◇Available OTC.

EENT: blurred vision, tinnitus, dry mouth and respiratory passages.
Other: may mask symptoms of ototoxicity, brain tumor, or intestinal obstruction.

INTERACTIONS
Alcohol, CNS depressants: additive CNS depression. Avoid concomitant use.

NURSING CONSIDERATIONS
- *Contraindicated* in patients with hypersensitivity to the drug.
- *Use cautiously* in seizures, narrow-angle glaucoma, and enlargement of prostate gland.
- Undiluted solution is irritating to veins; may cause sclerosis.
- Warn patient against driving and other activities that require alertness until CNS effects of the drug are known.
- May mask ototoxicity of aminoglycoside antibiotics.
- Avoid mixing parenteral preparation with other drugs; incompatible with many solutions.

diphenidol hydrochloride
Vontrol**

Pregnancy Risk Category: C

HOW SUPPLIED
Tablets: 25 mg

MECHANISM OF ACTION
Influences the chemoreceptor trigger zone to inhibit nausea and vomiting.

INDICATIONS & DOSAGE
Peripheral (labyrinthine) dizziness –
Adults: 25 to 50 mg P.O. q 4 hours, p.r.n.
Nausea and vomiting –
Adults: 25 to 50 mg P.O. q 4 hours, p.r.n.
Children over 23 kg: 0.88 mg/kg P.O. q 4 hours, not to exceed 5.5 mg/kg/24 hours. Usual dosage is 25 mg.

ADVERSE REACTIONS
Common reactions are in italics; life-threatening reactions are in bold italics.
CNS: *drowsiness,* dizziness, sleep disturbances, *confusion;* auditory and visual hallucinations, disorientation occur within 3 days of starting drug; subside within 3 days after stopping drug.
CV: transient hypotension.
GI: dry mouth, nausea, indigestion, heartburn.
Skin: urticaria.
Other: antiemetic effect may mask symptoms of ototoxicity, brain tumor, intestinal obstruction, or other conditions.

INTERACTIONS
None significant.

NURSING CONSIDERATIONS
- *Contraindicated* in anuria. *Use cautiously* in glaucoma, pyloric stenosis, pylorospasm, obstructive lesions of GI or GU tract, prostatic hypertrophy, or organic cardioaspasm.
- Used in Ménière's disease, following middle and inner ear surgery, labyrinthine disturbances, and to control nausea and vomiting associated with infectious diseases, cancers, radiation sickness, general anesthetics, and antineoplastic agents.
- Drug should be stopped if auditory or visual hallucinations or disorientation or confusion occurs.
- Closely supervise patient. Patients are usually hospitalized when receiving this drug. Monitor intake and output; report any changes.
- Treatment of toxicity is symptomatic and supportive.

dronabinol (tetrahydrocannabinol)
Marinol
Controlled Substance Schedule II

Pregnancy Risk Category: B

*Liquid form contains alcohol. **May contain tartrazine.

HOW SUPPLIED
Capsules: 2.5 mg, 5 mg, 10 mg

MECHANISM OF ACTION
A derivative of marijuana. Antiemetic and appetite stimulant effects are produced through an unknown action in the CNS.

INDICATIONS & DOSAGE
Treatment of nausea and vomiting associated with cancer chemotherapy –
Adults: 5 mg/m² P.O. 1 to 3 hours before administration of chemotherapy. Then give same dose q 2 to 4 hours after chemotherapy is administered for a total of four to six doses per day. Dosage may be increased in increments of 2.5 mg/m² to a maximum of 15 mg/m² per dose.
Treatment of anorexia and weight loss in patients with AIDS –
Adults: 2.5 mg P.O. b.i.d. before lunch and dinner.

ADVERSE REACTIONS
Common reactions are in italics; life-threatening reactions are in bold italics.
CNS: *dizziness, ataxia,* depersonalization, disorientation, hallucinations, headache, irritability, memory lapse, muddled thinking, paranoia, perceptual difficulties, weakness, paresthesias.
CV: tachycardia, orthostatic hypotension.
Other: *dry mouth,* visual distortions.

INTERACTIONS
Alcohol, CNS depressants, sedatives, psychotomimetic substances: additive effects. Don't use together.

NURSING CONSIDERATIONS
• *Contraindicated* for nausea and vomiting from any cause other than cancer chemotherapy, for anorexia and weight loss from any cause other than AIDS, and in patients with hypersensitivity to sesame oil.
• *Use cautiously* in elderly patients and those with hypertension, heart disease, and psychiatric illness.
• Warn patients against hazardous activities that require alertness until CNS effects of the drug are known.
• This drug is to be prescribed only for patients who have not responded satisfactorily to other antiemetics.
• Effects of this drug may persist for days after treatment ends. Duration of persistent effect varies greatly among patients. Therefore, patient should be supervised for untoward responses until it's certain that he's no longer experiencing the drug's effects.
• Dronabinol is the principal active substance present in *Cannabis sativa* (marijuana). Therefore, this can produce both physical and psychic dependence and has high potential for abuse.
• CNS effects are intensified at higher drug dosages.
• To prevent panic and anxiety, tell patients this drug may induce unusual changes in mood or other adverse behavioral effects.
• Impress upon family members that patient should be under supervision by a responsible person during and immediately after the treatment.

meclizine hydrochloride (meclozine hydrochloride)
Ancolan‡, Antivert, Antivert/25◊, Antivert/50, Bonamine†, Bonine◊, Dizmiss◊, Meni-D, Ru-Vert M

Pregnancy Risk Category: B

HOW SUPPLIED
Tablets: 12.5 mg, 25 mg◊, 50 mg
Tablets (chewable): 25 mg◊
Capsules: 15 mg, 25 mg, 30 mg

MECHANISM OF ACTION
May affect neural pathways originating in the labyrinth to inhibit nausea and vomiting, but the exact mechanism of action is unknown.

†Available in Canada only. ‡Available in Australia only. ◊Available OTC.

INDICATIONS & DOSAGE
Dizziness –
Adults: 25 to 100 mg P.O. daily in divided doses. Dosage varies with patient response.
Motion sickness –
Adults: 25 to 50 mg P.O. 1 hour before travel, repeated daily for duration of journey.

ADVERSE REACTIONS
Common reactions are in italics; life-threatening reactions are in bold italics.
CNS: *drowsiness,* fatigue.
EENT: dry mouth, blurred vision.
Other: may mask symptoms of ototoxicity, brain tumor, or intestinal obstruction.

INTERACTIONS
CNS depressants: increased drowsiness.

NURSING CONSIDERATIONS
• *Contraindicated* in patients with hypersensitivity to the drug.
• *Use cautiously* in glaucoma, GU or GI obstruction, and in elderly males with possible prostatic hypertrophy.
• Warn patient against driving and other hazardous activities that require alertness until CNS effects of the drug are known.
• This antihistamine has a slower onset and longer duration of action than other antihistamine antiemetics.

metoclopramide hydrochloride
Maxeran†, Maxolon‡, Maxolon High Dose‡, Reglan
Pregnancy Risk Category: B

HOW SUPPLIED
Tablets: 5 mg, 10 mg
Syrup: 5 mg/5 ml
Injection: 5 mg/ml

MECHANISM OF ACTION
Stimulates motility of the upper GI tract by increasing lower esophageal sphincter tone. Also blocks dopamine receptors at the chemoreceptor trigger zone.

INDICATIONS & DOSAGE
Preventing or reducing nausea and vomiting induced by cisplatin and other chemotherapy –
Adults: 2 mg/kg I.V. q 2 hours for 5 doses, beginning 30 minutes prior to cisplatin administration.
To facilitate small-bowel intubation and to aid in radiologic examinations –
Adults: 10 mg (2 ml) I.V. as a single dose over 1 to 2 minutes.
Children 6 to 14 years: 2.5 to 5 mg I.V. (0.5 to 1 ml).
Children under 6 years: 0.1 mg/kg I.V.
Delayed gastric emptying secondary to diabetic gastroparesis –
Adults: 10 mg P.O. 30 minutes before meals and h.s. for 2 to 8 weeks, depending on response.
Treatment of gastroesophageal reflux –
Adults: 10 to 15 mg P.O. q.i.d., p.r.n. Take 30 minutes before meals.

ADVERSE REACTIONS
Common reactions are in italics; life-threatening reactions are in bold italics.
CNS: *restlessness, anxiety, drowsiness,* fatigue, *lassitude,* insomnia, headache, dizziness, *extrapyramidal symptoms, tardive dyskinesia, dystonic reactions,* sedation.
CV: transient hypertension.
GI: nausea, bowel disturbances.
Skin: rash.
Other: fever, prolactin secretion, loss of libido.

INTERACTIONS
Alcohol, CNS depressants: additive CNS depression. Avoid concomitant use.

*Liquid form contains alcohol. **May contain tartrazine.

Anticholinergics, narcotic analgesics: antagonize GI motility effects of metoclopramide. Use together cautiously.
Phenothiazines, butyrophenones: increased risk of extrapyramidal effects. Monitor closely.

NURSING CONSIDERATIONS
- *Contraindicated* whenever stimulation of GI motility might be dangerous (hemorrhage, obstruction, or perforation), and in pheochromocytoma or seizure disorder.
- Elderly patients are more likely to experience extrapyramidal symptoms and tardive dyskinesia.
- Safety and effectiveness have not been established for therapy that continues longer than 12 weeks.
- Monitor blood pressure frequently in patients receiving I.V. dosage.
- **I.V. use:** I.V. infusions should be given slowly over at least 15 minutes. Protection from light is unnecessary if the infusion mixture is administered within 24 hours.
- Diphenhydramine 25 mg I.V. may be prescribed to counteract the extrapyramidal side effects associated with high metoclopramide doses.
- Warn patient to avoid activities requiring alertness for 2 hours after taking each dose.
- Oral form is being used investigationally to treat nausea and vomiting.

ondansetron hydrochloride
Zofran
Pregnancy Risk Category: B

HOW SUPPLIED
Tablets: 4 mg, 8 mg
Injection: 2 mg/ml

MECHANISM OF ACTION
A selective antagonist of a specific type of serotonin receptor (5-HT_3), which is located in the CNS at the area postrema (chemoreceptor trigger zone) and in the peripheral nervous system on nerve terminals of the vagus nerve. The blocking action of the drug may occur at both sites.

INDICATIONS & DOSAGE
Prevention of nausea and vomiting associated with emetogenic chemotherapy –
Adults and children over 12 years: 8 mg P.O. 30 minutes before the start of chemotherapy. Follow with 8 mg 4 hours and 8 hours after the first dose. Then follow with 8 mg q 8 hours for 1 to 2 days. Alternatively, administer a single dose of 32 mg I.V. infused over 15 minutes beginning 30 minutes before chemotherapy. Drug may also be administered in three doses of 0.15 mg/kg I.V. Give first dose 30 minutes before chemotherapy; administer subsequent doses 4 and 8 hours after the first dose. Infuse drug over 15 minutes.
Children age 4 to 11: 4 mg P.O. 30 minutes before the start of chemotherapy. Follow with 4 mg 4 hours and 8 hours after the first dose. Then follow with 4 mg q 8 hours for 1 to 2 days. Alternatively, administer a single dose of 32 mg I.V. infused over 15 minutes beginning 30 minutes before chemotherapy. Drug may also be administered in three doses of 0.15 mg/kg I.V. Give first dose 30 minutes before chemotherapy; administer subsequent doses 4 and 8 hours after the first dose. Infuse drug over 15 minutes.

ADVERSE REACTIONS
Common reactions are in italics; life-threatening reactions are in bold italics.
CNS: headache.
GI: *diarrhea, constipation.*
Metabolic: transient elevations in AST (SGOT) and ALT (SGPT) levels.
Skin: rash.
Other: ***bronchospasm (rare).***

INTERACTIONS

Drugs that alter hepatic drug metabolizing enzymes, such as phenobarbital or cimetidine: may alter pharmacokinetics of ondansetron. No dosage adjustment appears necessary.

NURSING CONSIDERATIONS

• *Contraindicated* in patients hypersensitive to the drug.
• *Use cautiously* in patients with hepatic failure. Limit daily dosage (oral or I.V.) to 8 mg.
• **I.V. use:** Dilute the drug in 50 ml of dextrose 5% in water injection or 0.9% sodium chloride injection before administration. The drug is also stable for up to 48 hours after dilution in 5% dextrose in 0.9% sodium chloride injection, 5% dextrose in 0.45% sodium chloride injection, and 3% sodium chloride injection.
• Decreased ondansetron clearance and prolonged half-life are reported in patients over 75 years. However, there are no recommendations for reducing dosage because these pharmacokinetic changes have not been associated with reduced safety or efficacy.

prochlorperazine
Compazine, Stemetil†‡

prochlorperazine edisylate
Compazine

prochlorperazine maleate
Anti-Naus‡, Chlorpazine, Compazine, Stemetil†‡

Pregnancy Risk Category: C

HOW SUPPLIED

prochlorperazine
Injection: 5 mg/ml
Suppositories: 2.5 mg, 5 mg, 25 mg
prochlorperazine edisylate
Syrup: 1 mg/ml
prochlorperazine maleate
Tablets: 5 mg, 10 mg, 25 mg
Capsules (sustained-release): 10 mg, 15 mg, 30 mg

MECHANISM OF ACTION

Acts on the chemoreceptor trigger zone to inhibit nausea and vomiting, and in larger doses, partially depresses the vomiting center as well.

INDICATIONS & DOSAGE

Preoperative nausea control –
Adults: 5 to 10 mg I.M. 1 to 2 hours before induction of anesthetic, repeat once in 30 minutes, if necessary; or 5 to 10 mg I.V. 15 to 30 minutes before induction of anesthetic (repeat once if necessary); or 20 mg/liter dextrose 5% in water and 0.9% sodium chloride solution by I.V. infusion, added to infusion 15 to 30 minutes before induction. Maximum parenteral dosage is 40 mg daily.
Severe nausea, vomiting –
Adults: 5 to 10 mg P.O. t.i.d. or q.i.d.; or 15 mg sustained-release form P.O. on arising; or 10 mg sustained-release form P.O. q 12 hours; or 25 mg rectally b.i.d.; or 5 to 10 mg I.M. injected deeply into upper outer quadrant of gluteal region. Repeat q 3 to 4 hours, p.r.n. Maximum I.M. dosage is 40 mg daily.
Children 18 to 39 kg: 2.5 mg P.O. or rectally t.i.d.; or 5 mg P.O. or rectally b.i.d. Maximum dosage is 15 mg daily; or 0.132 mg/kg deep I.M. injection. (Control usually obtained with 1 dose.)
Children 14 to 17 kg: 2.5 mg P.O. or rectally b.i.d. or t.i.d. Maximum dosage is 10 mg daily; or 0.132 mg/kg deep I.M. injection. (Control usually obtained with 1 dose.)
Children 9 to 13 kg: 2.5 mg P.O. or rectally daily or b.i.d. Maximum dosage is 7.5 mg daily; or 0.132 mg/kg deep I.M. injection. (Control usually obtained with 1 dose.)
Symptomatic management of psychotic disorders –

*Liquid form contains alcohol. **May contain tartrazine.

Adults: 5 to 10 mg, P.O. t.i.d. or q.i.d.
Children 2 to 12 years: 2.5 mg P.O. or P.R. b.i.d. or t.i.d. Do not exceed 10 mg on day 1. Increase dosage gradually to recommended maximum (if necessary).
Children 6 to 10 years: maximum 25 mg P.O. daily.
Children 2 to 5 years: maximum 20 mg P.O. daily.
Symptomatic management of severe psychoses –
Adults: 10 to 20 mg I.M. May be repeated in 1 to 4 hours. Rarely, patients may receive 10 to 20 mg q 4 to 6 hours. Oral therapy should be instituted after symptoms are controlled.
Children: 0.13 mg/kg I.M.
Management of excessive anxiety –
Adults: 5 to 10 mg by deep I.M. injection every 3 to 4 hours, not to exceed 40 mg daily; or 5 to 10 mg P.O. t.i.d. or q.i.d.; alternatively, give 15 mg (as the extended-release capsule) once daily, or 10 mg (extended-release capsule) q 12 hours.

ADVERSE REACTIONS

Common reactions are in italics; life-threatening reactions are in bold italics.
Blood: *transient leukopenia, **agranulocytosis.***
CNS: *extrapyramidal reactions,* sedation, pseudoparkinsonism, EEG changes, dizziness.
CV: *orthostatic hypotension,* tachycardia, ECG changes.
EENT: *ocular changes, blurred vision.*
GI: *dry mouth, constipation.*
GU: *urine retention,* dark urine, menstrual irregularities, gynecomastia, inhibited ejaculation.
Hepatic: *cholestatic jaundice.*
Metabolic: hyperprolactinemia.
Skin: *mild photosensitivity,* dermal allergic reactions, ***exfoliative dermatitis.***
Other: weight gain, increased appetite.

INTERACTIONS

Antacids: inhibited absorption of oral phenothiazines. Separate antacid and phenothiazine doses by at least 2 hours.
Anticholinergics, including antidepressants and antiparkinsonian agents: increased anticholinergic activity and aggravated parkinsonian symptoms. Use together cautiously.
Barbiturates: may decrease phenothiazine effect. Monitor patient for decreased antiemetic effect.

NURSING CONSIDERATIONS

- *Contraindicated* in phenothiazine hypersensitivity, CNS depression, bone marrow suppression, or subcortical damage; during pediatric surgery, use of spinal or epidural anesthetic or adrenergic blocking agents, alcohol usage, and those in a coma or depression.
- *Use cautiously* in combination with other CNS depressants; in hepatic disease, arteriosclerosis or cardiovascular disease (may cause sudden drop in blood pressure), exposure to extreme heat or cold (including antipyretic therapy), respiratory disorders, hypocalcemia, convulsive disorders or severe reactions to insulin or electroshock therapy, suspected brain tumor or intestinal obstruction, glaucoma, or prostatic hypertrophy; in acutely ill, dehydrated, or vomiting children; and in elderly or debilitated patients.
- Elderly patients should usually receive dosages in the lower range.
- Store in light-resistant container. Slight yellowing does not affect potency; discard very discolored solutions.
- Use only when vomiting can't be controlled by other measures, or when only a few doses are required. If more than 4 doses needed in 24-hour period, notify doctor.
- Not effective in motion sickness.
- To prevent contact dermatitis, avoid

getting concentrate or injection solution on hands or clothing.

- Dilute oral solution with tomato or fruit juice, milk, coffee, carbonated beverage, tea, water, soup, or pudding.
- Monitor CBC and liver function studies during prolonged therapy. Warn patients to wear protective clothing when exposed to sunlight.
- **I.V. use:** Infuse slowly, never as a bolus injection.
- Watch for orthostatic hypotension, especially when giving I.V.
- Do not give subcutaneously or mix in syringe with another drug. Give deep I.M.

thiethylperazine maleate

Norzine, Torecan**

Pregnancy Risk Category: C

HOW SUPPLIED

Tablets: 10 mg
Injection: 5 mg/ml
Suppositories: 10 mg

MECHANISM OF ACTION

Acts on the chemoreceptor trigger zone to inhibit nausea and vomiting.

INDICATIONS & DOSAGE

Nausea and vomiting –
Adults: 10 mg P.O., I.M., or rectally daily, b.i.d., or t.i.d.

ADVERSE REACTIONS

Common reactions are in italics; life-threatening reactions are in bold italics.

Blood: *transient leukopenia,* ***agranulocytosis.***
CNS: *extrapyramidal reactions (high incidence),* sedation (low incidence), pseudoparkinsonism, EEG changes, dizziness.
CV: *orthostatic hypotension,* tachycardia, EKG changes.
EENT: *ocular changes, blurred vision.*
GI: *dry mouth, constipation.*
GU: *urine retention,* dark urine, menstrual irregularities, gynecomastia, inhibited ejaculation.
Hepatic: *cholestatic jaundice.*
Metabolic: hyperprolactinemia.
Skin: *mild photosensitivity,* dermal allergic reactions.
Other: weight gain, increased appetite.

INTERACTIONS

Antacids: inhibited absorption of oral phenothiazines. Separate antacid and phenothiazine dosage by at least 2 hours.
Anticholinergics, including antidepressants and antiparkinsonian agents: increased anticholinergic activity, aggravated parkinson-like symptoms. Use together cautiously.
Barbiturates: may decrease phenothiazine effect. Monitor for decreased antiemetic effect.

NURSING CONSIDERATIONS

- *Contraindicated* in severe CNS depression, hepatic disease, coma, phenothiazine hypersensitivity.
- Don't give I.V. May cause severe hypotension.
- For nausea and vomiting associated with anesthesia and surgery, give deep I.M. injection on or shortly before terminating anesthesia.
- Possibly effective in dizziness; not effective in motion sickness.
- Use only when vomiting can't be controlled by other measures, or when only a few doses are required.
- Warn patient about hypotension. Advise him to stay in bed for 1 hour after receiving the drug.
- Store suppositories tightly covered and at temperatures below 77° F (25° C).
- If drug gets on skin, wash off at once to prevent contact dermatitis.

*Liquid form contains alcohol. **May contain tartrazine.

trimethobenzamide hydrochloride

Tebamide, Tegamide, Ticon, Tigan, Tiject-20

Pregnancy Risk Category: C

HOW SUPPLIED

Capsules: 100 mg, 250 mg
Injection: 100 mg/ml
Suppositories: 100 mg, 200 mg

MECHANISM OF ACTION

Acts on the chemoreceptor trigger zone to inhibit nausea and vomiting.

INDICATIONS & DOSAGE

Nausea and vomiting (treatment) –
Adults: 250 mg P.O. t.i.d. or q.i.d.; or 200 mg I.M. or rectally t.i.d. or q.i.d.
Postoperative nausea and vomiting (prevention) –
Adults: 200 mg I.M. or rectally (single dose) before or during surgery; may repeat 3 hours after termination of anesthesia, p.r.n.
Children 13 to 40 kg: 100 to 200 mg P.O. or rectally t.i.d. or q.i.d.
Children under 13 kg: 100 mg rectally t.i.d. or q.i.d. Limited to prolonged vomiting of known etiology.

ADVERSE REACTIONS

Common reactions are in italics; life-threatening reactions are in bold italics.
CNS: *drowsiness,* dizziness (in large doses).
CV: hypotension.
GI: diarrhea, exaggeration of preexisting nausea (in large doses).
Hepatic: *liver toxicity.*
Skin: skin hypersensitivity reactions.
Local: pain, stinging, burning, redness, swelling at I.M. injection site.
Other: antiemetic effect may mask signs of overdosage of toxic agents, or intestinal obstruction, brain tumor, or other conditions.

INTERACTIONS

Alcohol, CNS depressants: additive CNS depression. Avoid concomitant use.

NURSING CONSIDERATIONS

- *Contraindicated* in children with viral illness (a possible cause of vomiting in children); may contribute to the development of Reye's syndrome, a potentially fatal acute childhood encephalopathy, characterized by fatty degeneration of the liver.
- Suppositories contraindicated in hypersensitivity to benzocaine hydrochloride or similar local anesthetic.
- Stop drug if allergic skin reaction occurs.
- Give I.M. dose by deep injection into upper outer quadrant of gluteal region to reduce pain and local irritation.
- Warn patient of the possibility of drowsiness and dizziness, and caution him against driving or other activities requiring alertness until CNS effects of the drug are known.
- Store suppositories in refrigerator.
- Has little or no value in preventing motion sickness; limited value as antiemetic.

50

Antiulcer agents

cimetidine
famotidine
misoprostol
nizatidine
omeprazole
ranitidine hydrochloride
sucralfate

COMBINATION PRODUCTS
None.

cimetidine

Doractin‡, Tagamet

Pregnancy Risk Category: B

HOW SUPPLIED
Tablets: 200 mg, 300 mg, 400 mg, 800 mg
Oral liquid: 300 mg/5 ml
Injection: 150 mg/ml, 200 mg/2 ml‡

MECHANISM OF ACTION
Competitively inhibits the action of histamine (H_2) at receptor sites of the parietal cells, decreasing gastric acid secretion.

INDICATIONS & DOSAGE
Duodenal ulcer (short-term treatment) –
Adults and children over 16 years: 800 mg P.O. h.s. Alternatively, 400 mg P.O. b.i.d., or 300 mg P.O. q.i.d. (with meals and h.s.). Continue treatment for 4 to 6 weeks unless endoscopy shows healing. Maintenance therapy: 400 mg h.s. Parenteral: 300 mg diluted to 20 ml with 0.9% sodium chloride solution or other compatible I.V. solution by I.V. push over 1 to 2 minutes q 6 hours. Or 300 mg diluted in 50 ml dextrose 5% solution or other compatible I.V. solution by I.V. infusion over 15 to 20 minutes q 6 hours. Or 300 mg I.M. q 6 hours (no dilution necessary). To increase dose, give 300 mg doses more frequently to maximum daily dosage of 2,400 mg. Alternatively, give by continuous I.V. infusion. 900 mg/day (37.5 mg/hour) diluted in 100 to 1,000 ml of compatible solution.
Duodenal ulcer prophylaxis –
Adults and children over 16 years: 400 mg P.O. h.s.
Active benign gastric ulcer –
Adults: 300 mg P.O. q.i.d. with meals and h.s. for up to 8 weeks.
Pathologic hypersecretory conditions (such as Zollinger-Ellison syndrome, systemic mastocytosis, and multiple endocrine adenomas) –
Adults and children over 16 years: 300 mg P.O. q.i.d. with meals and h.s.; adjust to individual needs. Maximum daily dosage is 2,400 mg. Parenteral: 300 mg diluted to 20 ml with 0.9% sodium chloride solution or other compatible I.V. solutions by I.V. push over 1 to 2 minutes q 6 hours. Or 300 mg diluted in 50 ml dextrose 5% solution or other compatible I.V. solution by I.V. infusion over 15 to 20 minutes q 6 hours. To increase dosage, give 300-mg doses more frequently to maximum daily dosage of 2,400 mg.
Gastroesophageal reflux disease (GERD) –
Adults: 800 mg P.O. b.i.d. or 400 mg q.i.d. before meals and h.s.
Prevention of upper GI bleeding in critically ill patients –
Adults: 50 mg/hour by continuous I.V. infusion for up to 7 days. Patients with creatinine clearance below 30 ml/minute/1.73 m^2 should receive 25 mg/hour.

ADVERSE REACTIONS
Common reactions are in italics; life-threatening reactions are in bold italics.
Blood: ***agranulocytosis, neutropenia, thrombocytopenia, aplastic anemia*** (rare).
CNS: mental confusion, dizziness, headaches, peripheral neuropathy.
CV: bradycardia.
GI: *mild and transient diarrhea.*
GU: transient elevations in serum creatinine.
Hepatic: jaundice (rare).
Skin: acne-like rash, urticaria.
Other: hypersensitivity, muscle pain, mild gynecomastia after use longer than 1 month.

INTERACTIONS
Antacids: interfere with absorption of cimetidine. Separate cimetidine and antacids by at least 1 hour if possible.

Cimetidine may inhibit hepatic microsomal enzyme metabolism of some drugs, like warfarin, phenytoin, some benzodiazepines, lidocaine, theophylline, and propranolol. Monitor serum levels of these drugs closely during cimetidine therapy.

NURSING CONSIDERATIONS
- *Contraindicated* in patients with hypersensitivity to the drug.
- I.M. route of administration may be painful.
- Hemodialysis reduces blood levels of cimetidine. Schedule cimetidine dose at end of hemodialysis treatment. Dosage adjustments are necessary in patients with renal failure.
- Up to 10 g overdosage has been reported without adverse reactions.
- Taking tablets with meals will ensure a more consistent therapeutic effect.
- Remind patient that if he's taking cimetidine once daily, he should take it at bedtime for best results.
- Identify tablet strength when obtaining a drug history.
- Elderly or debilitated patients may be more susceptible to cimetidine-induced mental confusion.
- Urge patient to avoid cigarette smoking, as this may increase gastric acid secretion and worsen disease.
- **I.V. use:** Don't infuse I.V. too rapidly. May cause bradycardia. When administering cimetidine I.V. in 100 ml of diluent solution, do not infuse so rapidly that circulatory overload is produced. Some authorities recommend that the drug be infused over at least 30 minutes, to minimize the risk of adverse cardiac effects. Sometimes administered as continuous I.V. infusion. Use an infusion pump if given in a total volume of 250 ml per 24 hours or less.
- I.V. solutions compatible for dilution with cimetidine: 0.9% sodium chloride solution, dextrose 5% and 10% (and combinations of these) in water solutions, lactated Ringer's solution, and 5% sodium bicarbonate injection. Do not dilute with sterile water for injection.
- Has many investigational uses. Used before anesthesia for prophylaxis of aspiration pneumonitis; also used to treat hyperparathyroidism, herpes zoster, chronic hives, and as an adjunct in the treatment of acetaminophen overdose.
- Effectiveness in treatment of gastric ulcers not as great as in duodenal ulcer. Cimetidine may prove useful but is still unapproved in pancreatic insufficiency, short-bowel syndrome, psoriasis, prevention and treatment of GI bleeding, and prevention of gastric inactivation of oral enzyme preparations by gastric acid and pepsin.

famotidine
Pepcid, Pepcidine‡

Pregnancy Risk Category: B

HOW SUPPLIED

Tablets: 20 mg, 40 mg
Powder for oral suspension: 40 mg/5 ml after reconstituting
Injection: 10 mg/ml

MECHANISM OF ACTION

Competitively inhibits the action of histamine (H_2) at receptor sites of the parietal cells, decreasing gastric acid secretion.

INDICATIONS & DOSAGE

Duodenal ulcer–
Adults: For acute therapy, 40 mg P.O. once daily h.s. For maintenance therapy, 20 mg P.O. once daily h.s.
Pathologic hypersecretory conditions (such as Zollinger-Ellison syndrome)–
Adults: 20 mg P.O. q 6 hours. As much as 160 mg q 6 hours may be administered.
Hospitalized patients with intractable ulcers or hypersecretory conditions, or patients who cannot take oral medication–
Adults: 20 mg I.V. q 12 hours.
Gastroesophageal reflux disease (GERD)–
Adults: 20 mg P.O. b.i.d. for up to 6 weeks. For esophagitis caused by GERD, give 20 to 40 mg b.i.d. for up to 12 weeks.

ADVERSE REACTIONS

Common reactions are in italics; life-threatening reactions are in bold italics.
Blood: ***thrombocytopenia*** (rare).
CNS: *headache,* dizziness, hallucinations.
GI: diarrhea, constipation, nausea, flatulence.
GU: increased BUN and creatinine.
Skin: acne, pruritus, rash.
Local: transient irritation at I.V. site.

INTERACTIONS

None significant.

NURSING CONSIDERATIONS

- *Contraindicated* in patients with hypersensitivity to the drug.
- Gastric cancer must be ruled out before famotidine therapy.
- Advise patient not to take the drug for longer than 8 weeks unless doctor specifically orders it.
- Especially at the beginning of therapy when pain is severe and with doctor's knowledge, patient may take antacids concomitantly.
- Store reconstituted suspension below 86° F (30° C). Discard after 30 days.
- Urge patient to avoid cigarette smoking as this may increase gastric acid secretion and worsen disease.
- Patient may take famotidine with a snack if he desires. Remind patient that this drug is most effective if taken at bedtime.
- Some patients may have this drug prescribed to be taken 20 mg twice daily instead of 40 mg at bedtime. This alternate dosing schedule is also effective. However, at least one dose should be taken at bedtime.
- **I.V. use:** To prepare I.V. injection, dilute 2 ml (20 mg) famotidine with compatible I.V. solution to a total volume of either 5 or 10 ml, and inject slowly (over at least 2 minutes). Compatible solutions include sterile water for injection, 0.9% sodium chloride injection, 5% or 10% dextrose injection, 5% sodium bicarbonate injection, or lactated Ringer's injection.
- Alternatively, famotidine may be given by intermittent I.V. infusion. Dilute 20 mg (2 ml) famotidine in 100 ml of compatible solution, and infuse over 15 to 30 minutes. Solution is stable for 48 hours at room temperature after dilution.
- Store I.V. injection in refrigerator at 35.6° to 46.4° F (2° to 8° C).

misoprostol
Cytotec
Pregnancy Risk Category: X

HOW SUPPLIED
Tablets: 100 mcg, 200 mcg

MECHANISM OF ACTION
A synthetic prostaglandin E_1 analog, misoprostol replaces gastric prostaglandins that are depleted by NSAID therapy. It also decreases basal and stimulated gastric acid secretion, and may increase gastric mucus and bicarbonate production.

INDICATIONS & DOSAGE
Prevention of NSAID-induced gastric ulcers in elderly or debilitated patients at high risk of complications from gastric ulcer, and patients with a history of NSAID-induced ulcers –
Adults: 200 mcg P.O. q.i.d. with food. If this dosage isn't tolerated, it may be decreased to 100 mcg P.O. q.i.d.

ADVERSE REACTIONS
Common reactions are in italics; life-threatening reactions are in bold italics.
CNS: headache.
GI: diarrhea, abdominal pain, nausea, flatulence, dyspepsia, vomiting, constipation.
GU: hypermenorrhea, dysmenorrhea, spotting, cramps, menstrual disorders.

INTERACTIONS
Antacids: reduced plasma levels when administered concomitantly. Not considered significant.

NURSING CONSIDERATIONS
• *Contraindicated* for use in pregnant women and in patients who have a history of an allergic response to prostaglandins.
• Misoprostol should not be routinely administered to women of childbearing age unless they are at high risk of developing ulcers or complications from NSAID-induced ulcers.
• Special precautions must be taken to prevent the use of this drug during pregnancy. The patient must be fully aware of the dangers of misoprostol to a fetus, and must receive both oral and written warnings regarding these dangers. She must be capable of complying with effective contraceptive means, and must have a negative serum pregnancy test within 2 weeks of initiating therapy.
• Misoprostol therapy must not begin until the second or third day of the next normal menstrual period.
• Instruct *ALL* patients not to share misoprostol with anyone else. They should be aware that when taken by a pregnant patient this drug may cause miscarriage, often with potentially life-threatening bleeding. Concomitant ingestion of food or antacids seems to reduce maximal plasma concentrations of misoprostol, but this doesn't appear to impair the drug's effectiveness.
• Use investigationally for the prophylaxis and treatment of gastric ulcers, reflux esophagitis, alcohol-induced gastritis, hemorrhagic gastritis, and fat malabsorptions in patients with cystic fibrosis.

nizatidine
Axid
Pregnancy Risk Category: C

HOW SUPPLIED
Capsules: 150 mg, 300 mg

MECHANISM OF ACTION
Competitively inhibits the action of histamine at H_2 receptor sites of the parietal cells, decreasing gastric acid secretion.

INDICATIONS & DOSAGE
Active duodenal ulcer treatment –
Adults: 300 mg P.O. daily h.s. Alternatively, patient may receive 150 mg b.i.d.
Maintenance therapy of duodenal ulcer –
Adults: 150 mg daily h.s.
Gastroesophageal reflux disease (GERD) –
Adults: 150 mg P.O. b.i.d.

ADVERSE REACTIONS
Common reactions are in italics; life-threatening reactions are in bold italics.
Blood: ***thrombocytopenia.***
CNS: *somnolence.*
CV: arrhythmias.
Skin: *sweating,* rash, urticaria, ***exfoliative dermatitis.***
Other: hepatic damage, hyperuricemia, gynecomastia.

INTERACTIONS
Aspirin: nizatidine may elevate serum salicylate levels in patients taking high doses of aspirin.

NURSING CONSIDERATIONS
- *Contraindicated* in patients with hypersensitivity to H_2-receptor antagonists.
- Dosage should be reduced in patients with impaired renal function. Patients with a creatinine clearance of 20 to 50 ml/minute should receive 150 mg daily for treatment of active duodenal ulcer, or 150 mg every other day for maintenance therapy. Patients with a creatinine clearance below 20 ml/minute should receive 150 mg every other day for treatment or 150 mg every third day for maintenance.
- False-positive test results for urobilinogen may occur.
- Nizatidine has not been associated with antiandrogenic activity and does not appear to affect hepatic drug-metabolizing enzyme systems.
- Urge patient to avoid cigarette smoking, which will increase gastric acid secretion and worsen disease.
- Capsules may be opened and contents mixed with apple juice. However, drug has been shown to lose some potency when combined with tomato-based mixed-vegetable juices. Check with pharmacist for compatibility.

omeprazole
Prilosec, Losec†
Pregnancy Risk Category: C

HOW SUPPLIED
Capsules (delayed-release): 20 mg

MECHANISM OF ACTION
Inhibits the activity of the acid (proton) pump, H+/K+ ATPase, located at the secretory surface of the gastric parietal cell. This blocks the formation of gastric acid.

INDICATIONS & DOSAGE
Severe erosive esophagitis; symptomatic, poorly responsive gastroesophageal reflux disease (GERD) –
Adults: 20 mg P.O. daily for 4 to 8 weeks. Patients with GERD should have failed initial therapy with a histamine H_2 antagonist.
Pathologic hypersecretory conditions (such as Zollinger-Ellison syndrome) –
Adults: initially, 60 mg P.O. daily, with dosage titrated according to patient response. Daily dosage exceeding 80 mg should be administered in divided doses. Dosages up to 120 mg t.i.d. have been administered. Therapy should continue as long as clinically indicated.
Treatment of duodenal ulcers –
Adults: 20 mg P.O. daily for 4 to 8 weeks.

ADVERSE REACTIONS
Common reactions are in italics; life-threatening reactions are in bold italics.

CNS: headache, dizziness.
GI: diarrhea, abdominal pain, nausea, vomiting, constipation, flatulence.
Respiratory: cough.
Skin: rash.
Other: back pain.

INTERACTIONS

Diazepam, warfarin, and phenytoin: Decreased hepatic clearance possibly leading to increased serum levels. Monitor closely.
Ketoconazole, iron derivatives, and ampicillin esters: may exhibit poor bioavailability in patients taking omeprazole because optimal absorption of these drugs requires a low gastric pH.

NURSING CONSIDERATIONS

- *Contraindicated* in patients hypersensitive to the drug or any component of the enteric formulation.
- Prolonged (2-year) studies in rats revealed a dose-related increase in gastric carcinoid tumors; studies in humans have not detected a risk from short-term exposure to the drug. Further study is needed to assess the impact of sustained hypergastrinemia and hypochlorhydria. The manufacturer recommends that therapy with omeprazole not exceed the indicated duration.
- Capsules should be swallowed whole and not opened or crushed.
- Omeprazole increases its own bioavailability with repeated administration. The drug is labile in gastric acid, and less drug is lost to hydrolysis as the drug increases gastric pH.
- Dosage adjustments are not required for renal or hepatic impairment.
- Most patients with duodenal ulcers heal within 4 weeks. Omeprazole should not be used for maintenance therapy.

ranitidine hydrochloride

Zantac*

Pregnancy Risk Category: B

HOW SUPPLIED

Tablets: 150 mg, 300 mg
Dispersible tablets: 150 mg‡
Syrup: 15 mg/ml*
Injection: 25 mg/ml
Infusion: 0.5 mg/ml in 100-ml containers

MECHANISM OF ACTION

Competitively inhibits the action of histamine (H_2) at receptor sites of the parietal cells, decreasing gastric acid secretion.

INDICATIONS & DOSAGE

Duodenal and gastric ulcer (short-term treatment); pathological hypersecretory conditions, such as Zollinger-Ellison syndrome –
Adults: 150 mg P.O. b.i.d. or 300 mg daily h.s. Dosages up to 6 g daily may be prescribed in patients with Zollinger-Ellison syndrome. May also be administered parenterally: 50 mg I.V. or I.M. q 6 to 8 hours. When administering I.V. push, dilute to a total volume of 20 ml and inject over a period of 5 minutes. No dilution necessary when administering I.M. May also be administered by intermittent I.V. infusion. Dilute 50 mg ranitidine in 100 ml of dextrose 5% in water and infuse over 15 to 20 minutes. May also be given by continuous I.V. infusion, 150 mg in 250 mg compatible solution. Administer at 6.25 mg/hour using an infusion pump.
Maintenance therapy of duodenal ulcer –
Adults: 150 mg P.O. h.s.
Gastroesophageal reflux disease (GERD) –
Adults: 150 mg P.O. b.i.d.
Erosive esophagitis –
Adults: 150 mg P.O. q.i.d.

ADVERSE REACTIONS
Common reactions are in italics; life-threatening reactions are in bold italics.
Blood: ***neutropenia, thrombocytopenia.***
CNS: headache, malaise, dizziness, confusion.
CV: bradycardia.
GI: nausea, constipation.
Hepatic: elevated liver enzymes, jaundice.
Skin: rash.
Local: burning and itching at injection site.

INTERACTIONS
Antacids: may interfere with absorption of ranitidine (conflicting data). Stagger doses if possible.
Diazepam: decreased absorption when administered concomitantly with ranitidine.
Glipizide: possibly increased hypoglycemic effect. Dosage adjustment of glipizide may be necessary.
Procainamide: ranitidine may decrease renal clearance (conflicting data).
Warfarin: ranitidine may interfere with warfarin clearance (conflicting data).

NURSING CONSIDERATIONS
- *Contraindicated* in patients with hypersensitivity to the drug.
- *Use cautiously* in hepatic dysfunction. Dosage should be adjusted in patients with impaired renal function.
- Can be taken without regard to meals. Absorption not affected by food.
- Remind patient that if he's taking ranitidine once daily, he should take it at bedtime for best results.
- Urge patient to avoid smoking, as this may increase gastric acid secretion and worsen disease.
- **I.V. use:** When administering premixed I.V. infusion, give by slow I.V. drip (over 15 to 20 minutes). Do not add other drugs to the solution. If used with a primary I.V. fluid system, the primary solution should be discontinued during the infusion.
- To prepare I.V. injection, dilute 50 mg (2 ml) in 100 ml of compatible solution and infuse over 15 to 20 minutes. Compatible solutions include 0.9% sodium chloride injection, 5% or 10% dextrose injection, 5% sodium bicarbonate injection, or lactated Ringer's injection.
- Drug is incompatible with aluminum. Avoid using aluminum-based needles or other equipment when mixing or administering drug.

sucralfate
Carafate, Sulcrate†
Pregnancy Risk Category: B

HOW SUPPLIED
Tablets: 1 g

MECHANISM OF ACTION
Adheres to and protects the ulcer surface by forming a barrier.

INDICATIONS & DOSAGE
Short-term (up to 8 weeks) treatment of duodenal ulcer–
Adults: 1 g P.O. q.i.d. 1 hour before meals and h.s.
Maintenance therapy of duodenal ulcer–
Adults: 1 g P.O. b.i.d.

ADVERSE REACTIONS
Common reactions are in italics; life-threatening reactions are in bold italics.
CNS: dizziness, sleepiness.
GI: *constipation,* nausea, gastric discomfort, diarrhea, bezoar formation.

INTERACTIONS
Antacids: may decrease binding of drug to gastroduodenal mucosa, impairing effectiveness. Don't give within 30 minutes of each other.
Ciprofloxacin, norfloxacin, digoxin, cimetidine, ranitidine, phenytoin, tet-

racycline, theophylline: decreased absorption. Separate administration times by at least 2 hours.

NURSING CONSIDERATIONS

- No known contraindications.
- Drug is minimally absorbed. Incidence of adverse reactions is low.
- Tell patient for best results to take sucralfate on an empty stomach (1 hour before each meal and at bedtime).
- Pain and ulcer symptoms may subside within first few weeks of therapy. However, for complete healing, be sure patient continues on prescribed regimen.
- Monitor for severe, persistent constipation.
- Studies suggest that drug is as effective as cimetidine in healing duodenal ulcers.
- Drug has been used to treat gastric ulcers, but effectiveness of this use is still under investigation.
- Drug contains aluminum but isn't classified as an antacid.
- Urge patient to avoid smoking, as this may increase gastric acid secretion and worsen disease.

51
Corticosteroids

beclomethasone dipropionate
betamethasone
betamethasone acetate and betamethasone sodium phosphate
betamethasone sodium phosphate
cortisone acetate
dexamethasone
dexamethasone acetate
dexamethasone sodium phosphate
fludrocortisone acetate
flunisolide
hydrocortisone
hydrocortisone acetate
hydrocortisone cypionate
hydrocortisone sodium phosphate
hydrocortisone sodium succinate
methylprednisolone
methylprednisolone acetate
methylprednisolone sodium succinate
paramethasone acetate
prednisolone
prednisolone acetate
prednisolone sodium phosphate
prednisolone steaglate
prednisolone tebutate
prednisone
triamcinolone
triamcinolone acetonide
triamcinolone diacetate
triamcinolone hexacetonide

COMBINATION PRODUCTS

DECADRON WITH XYLOCAINE: dexamethasone phosphate 4 mg and lidocaine hydrochloride 10 mg/ml.

beclomethasone dipropionate

Aldecin Aqueous Nasal Spray‡, Aldecin Inhaler‡, Becloforte Inhaler‡, Beclovent, Beclovent Rotacaps†, Vanceril

Pregnancy Risk Category: C

HOW SUPPLIED

Oral inhalation aerosol: 42 mcg/metered spray, 50 mcg/metered spray‡, 250 mcg/metered spray‡

MECHANISM OF ACTION

Decreases inflammation, mainly by stabilizing leukocyte lysosomal membranes. Also suppresses the immune response, stimulates bone marrow, and influences protein, fat, and carbohydrate metabolism.

INDICATIONS & DOSAGE

Steroid-dependent asthma –
Adults: 2 to 4 inhalations t.i.d. or q.i.d. Maximum dosage is 20 inhalations daily.
Children 6 to 12 years: 1 to 2 inhalations t.i.d. or q.i.d. Maximum dosage is 10 inhalations daily.

ADVERSE REACTIONS

Common reactions are in italics; life-threatening reactions are in bold italics.
EENT: hoarseness, fungal infections of mouth and throat, throat irritation.
GI: dry mouth.

INTERACTIONS

None significant.

NURSING CONSIDERATIONS

- *Contraindicated* in status asthmaticus. Not for use in asthma controlled by bronchodilators or other noncorticosteroids alone, or for nonasth-

matic bronchial diseases. Also contraindicated in patients hypersensitive to any component of the formulation (fluorocarbons, oleic acid), and in patients with systemic fungal infections.
• Oral glucocorticoid therapy should be tapered slowly. Acute adrenal insufficiency and death have occurred in asthmatics who changed abruptly from oral corticosteroids to beclomethasone. Be sure patient reports symptoms associated with corticosteroid withdrawal, including fatigue, weakness, arthralgia, orthostatic hypotension, and dyspnea.
• Periodic measurement of growth and development may be necessary during high-dose or prolonged therapy in children.
• During times of stress (trauma, surgery, or infection) systemic corticosteroids may be needed to prevent adrenal insufficiency in previously steroid-dependent patients.
• Instruct patient to carry a card indicating his need for supplemental systemic glucocorticoids during stress.
• Patient requiring bronchodilator should use it several minutes before beclomethasone.
• Tell patient to allow 1 minute to elapse before taking subsequent puffs of medication, and to hold breath for a few seconds to enhance action of drug.
• Inform patient that beclomethasone doesn't provide relief for emergency asthma attacks. Patients using nasal form should understand that full therapeutic effect may take from a few days to a couple of weeks.
• Instruct patient to contact doctor if he notices a decreased response or if symptoms don't improve within 3 weeks of initiating therapy. Dose may have to be adjusted. Patient shouldn't exceed recommended dose on his own.
• Check mucous membranes frequently for signs of fungal infection.
• Patient can prevent oral fungal infections by gargling or rinsing mouth with water after each use of the inhaler. However, tell patient not to swallow the water.
• Tell patient to keep inhaler clean and unobstructed. Wash with warm water and dry thoroughly.
• A spacer device may help ensure delivery of the proper dose of medication. However, use of a spacer device with the Becloforte Inhaler is not recommended.
• Store medication between 36° and 86° F (2° and 30° C). Tell patient that before using medication or when carrying canister to gently warm the canister to room temperature by keeping it in his pocket. If the canister is cold, the proper dose of medication may not be delivered.

betamethasone
Betnelan†, Celestone*

betamethasone acetate and betamethasone sodium phosphate
Celestone Chronodose‡, Celestone Soluspan

betamethasone sodium phosphate
Betameth, Betnesol†, B.S.P., Celestone Phosphate, Cel-U-Jec, Prelestone, Selestoject

Pregnancy Risk Category: C

HOW SUPPLIED

betamethasone
Tablets: 600 mcg
Tablets (extended-release): 1 mg
Tablets (effervescent): 500 mcg†
Syrup: 600 mcg/5 ml
betamethasone acetate and betamethasone sodium phosphate
Injection: betamethasone acetate 3 mg and betamethasone sodium phosphate (equivalent to 3-mg base)/ml
betamethasone sodium phosphate
Effervescent tablets: 500 mcg*

Injection: 4 mg (3-mg base)/ml in 5-ml vials

MECHANISM OF ACTION
Decreases inflammation, mainly by stabilizing leukocyte lysosomal membranes. Also suppresses the immune response, stimulates bone marrow, and influences protein, fat, and carbohydrate metabolism.

INDICATIONS & DOSAGE
Severe inflammation or immunosuppression –
Adults: 0.6 to 7.2 mg P.O. daily; or 0.5 to 9 mg (sodium phosphate) I.M., I.V., or into joint or soft tissue daily; or 1.5 to 12 mg (sodium phosphate-acetate suspension) into joint or soft tissue q 1 to 2 weeks, p.r.n.
Prevention of neonatal respiratory distress syndrome –
Adults (pregnant women): 12 mg I.M. Celestone Soluspan 36 to 48 hours before premature delivery. Repeat in 24 hours.

ADVERSE REACTIONS
Common reactions are in italics; life-threatening reactions are in bold italics.

Most adverse reactions of corticosteroids are dose- or duration-dependent.
CNS: *euphoria, insomnia,* psychotic behavior, pseudotumor cerebri.
CV: ***CHF,*** hypertension, edema.
EENT: cataracts, glaucoma.
GI: *peptic ulcer,* GI irritation, increased appetite.
Metabolic: possible hypokalemia, hyperglycemia and carbohydrate intolerance, growth suppression in children.
Skin: delayed wound healing, acne, various skin eruptions.
Other: muscle weakness, osteoporosis, pancreatitis, hirsutism, susceptibility to infections. Acute adrenal insufficiency may follow increased stress (infection, surgery, or trauma) or abrupt withdrawal after long-term therapy.
Withdrawal symptoms: rebound inflammation, fatigue, weakness, arthralgia, fever, dizziness, lethargy, depression, fainting, orthostatic hypotension, dyspnea, anorexia, hypoglycemia. ***Sudden withdrawal may be fatal.***

INTERACTIONS
Barbiturates, phenytoin, rifampin: decreased corticosteroid effect. Corticosteroid dose may need to be increased.
Indomethacin, aspirin, NSAIDs: increased risk of GI distress and bleeding. Give together cautiously.
Oral anticoagulants: altered dosage requirements. Monitor prothrombin times closely.
Potassium-depleting drugs such as thiazide diuretics: enhanced potassium-wasting effects of betamethasone. Monitor serum potassium levels.
Skin-test antigens: decreased response. Defer skin testing until therapy is completed.
Vaccines and toxoids: decreased antibody response and increased risk of neurologic complications. Avoid concomitant use.

NURSING CONSIDERATIONS
- *Contraindicated* in systemic fungal infections. *Use cautiously* in patients with GI ulceration or renal disease, hypertension, osteoporosis, varicella, vaccinia, exanthema, diabetes mellitus, Cushing's syndrome, thromboembolic disorders, seizures, myasthenia gravis, CHF, tuberculosis, ocular herpes simplex, hypoalbuminemia, emotional instability, and psychotic tendencies.
- Elderly patients may be more susceptible to osteoporosis. Patients receiving long-term therapy should consider exercise or physical therapy.

*Liquid form contains alcohol. **May contain tartrazine.

Give vitamin D or calcium supplements as ordered.
- Don't use for alternate-day therapy.
- Adrenal suppression may last up to 1 year after drug is stopped. Gradually reduce drug dosage after long-term therapy. Tell patient not to stop drug abruptly or without doctor's consent. Be sure patient reports symptoms associated with corticosteroid withdrawal, including fatigue, weakness, arthralgia, orthostatic hypotension, and dyspnea.
- Always titrate to lowest effective dose.
- Be sure patient understands that he should contact doctor if his symptoms are worsening or the medication is no longer effective. However, patient should not increase dosage on his own.
- To prevent muscle atrophy, give I.M. injection deeply. Rotate injection sites.
- Monitor blood sugar and serum potassium regularly. Diabetic patients may require adjustments in insulin dosage.
- Teach patients about the effects of the drug. Warn those on long-term therapy about cushingoid symptoms.
- Observe for signs of infection, especially after steroid withdrawal. Tell patients to report slow healing.
- Instruct patient to carry a card indicating his need for supplemental glucocorticoids during stress.
- Give a daily dose in the morning for better results and less toxicity.
- Give with milk or food to reduce GI irritation.
- A glucocorticoid with little mineralocorticoid effect.
- Watch for additional potassium depletion from diuretics and amphotericin B. Potassium supplements may be necessary for patients receiving long-term therapy.
- A calorie- or sodium-restricted diet with protein supplementation may be necessary for patients receiving long-term therapy. Obtain baseline weight before starting therapy, and weigh patient daily; report any sudden weight gain to doctor.
- Betamethasone sometimes prescribed to treat respiratory distress syndrome in premature infants.
- Tell patient who is using the effervescent tablets to dissolve them in water immediately before ingestion.
- Patients receiving prolonged therapy should have periodic ophthalmic examinations. Periodic measurement of growth and development may be necessary during high-dose or prolonged therapy in children.
- Monitor for depression or mood changes, especially in patients receiving long-term therapy.

cortisone acetate

Cortate‡, Cortone Acetate

Pregnancy Risk Category: D

HOW SUPPLIED

Tablets: 5 mg, 10 mg, 25 mg
Injection (suspension): 25 mg/ml, 50 mg/ml

MECHANISM OF ACTION

Decreases inflammation, mainly by stabilizing leukocyte lysosomal membranes. Also suppresses the immune response, stimulates bone marrow, and influences protein, fat, and carbohydrate metabolism.

INDICATIONS & DOSAGE

Adrenal insufficiency, allergy, inflammation –
Adults: 25 to 300 mg P.O. or I.M. daily or on alternate days. Dosages highly individualized, depending on severity of disease.

ADVERSE REACTIONS

Common reactions are in italics; life-threatening reactions are in bold italics.

Most adverse reactions of cortico-

steroids are dose- or duration-dependent.
CNS: *euphoria, insomnia,* psychotic behavior, pseudotumor cerebri.
CV: ***CHF,*** hypertension, edema.
EENT: cataracts, glaucoma.
GI: *peptic ulcer,* GI irritation, increased appetite.
Metabolic: possible hypokalemia, hyperglycemia and carbohydrate intolerance, growth suppression in children.
Skin: delayed wound healing, acne, various skin eruptions.
Local: atrophy at I.M. injection sites.
Other: muscle weakness, osteoporosis, pancreatitis, hirsutism, susceptibility to infections. Acute adrenal insufficiency may follow increased stress (infection, surgery, or trauma) or abrupt withdrawal after long-term therapy.
Withdrawal symptoms: rebound inflammation, fatigue, weakness, arthralgia, fever, dizziness, lethargy, depression, fainting, orthostatic hypotension, dyspnea, anorexia, hypoglycemia. ***Sudden withdrawal may be fatal.***

INTERACTIONS
Barbiturates, phenytoin, rifampin: decreased corticosteroid effect. Corticosteroid dose may need to be increased.
Indomethacin, aspirin, NSAIDs: increased risk of GI distress and bleeding. Give together cautiously.
Live attenuated virus vaccines, other vaccines and toxoids: decreased antibody response and increased risk of neurologic complications. Avoid concomitant use.
Oral anticoagulants: altered dosage requirements. Monitor prothrombin times closely.
Potassium-depleting drugs such as thiazide diuretics: enhanced potassium-wasting effects of cortisone. Monitor serum potassium levels.
Skin-test antigens: decreased response. Defer skin testing until therapy is completed.

NURSING CONSIDERATIONS
- *Contraindicated* in systemic fungal infections. Injection is contraindicated in patients with sulfite sensitivity.
- *Use cautiously* in patients with GI ulceration or renal disease, hypertension, osteoporosis, varicella, vaccinia, exanthema, diabetes mellitus, Cushing's syndrome, thromboembolic disorders, seizures, myasthenia gravis, congestive heart failure, tuberculosis, ocular herpes simplex, hypoalbuminemia, emotional instability, and psychotic tendencies.
- Elderly patients may be more susceptible to osteoporosis. Patients receiving long-term therapy should consider exercise or physical therapy. Give vitamin D or calcium supplements as ordered.
- Gradually reduce drug dosage after long-term therapy. Tell patient not to discontinue drug abruptly or without doctor's consent.
- Always titrate to lowest effective dose.
- Patient may need low-sodium diet and potassium supplement.
- I.M. route causes slow onset of action. Don't use in acute conditions where rapid effect required. May use on a twice-daily schedule matching diurnal variation. Rotate injection sites to prevent muscle atrophy.
- A glucocorticoid with potent mineralocorticoid effect; report sudden weight gain or edema to doctor.
- Observe for signs of infection, especially after steroid withdrawal. Tell patient to report slow healing.
- Drug of choice for replacement therapy in adrenal insufficiency.
- Monitor serum electrolytes and blood sugar.
- Warn patients on long-term therapy about cushingoid symptoms.

*Liquid form contains alcohol. **May contain tartrazine.

• Give with milk or food to reduce GI irritation.
• Instruct patient to carry a card indicating his need for supplemental glucocorticoids during stress.
• Give a daily dose in the morning for better results and less toxicity.
• Not for I.V. use.
• Watch for additional potassium depletion from diuretics and amphotericin B.
• Immunizations may show decreased antibody response.

dexamethasone
Decadron, Deronil, Dexasone†, Dexone, Hexadrol, Mymethasone

dexamethasone acetate
Dalalone D.P., Dalalone L.A., Decadron L.A., Decaject-L.A., Decameth L.A., Dexacen LA, Dexasone-LA, Dexone LA, Dexon LA, Solurex-LA

dexamethasone sodium phosphate
Ak-Dex, Dalalone, Decadrol, Decadron Phosphate, Decaject, Decameth, Dex, Dexacen, Dexasone, Dexon, Dexone, Hexadrol Phosphate, Solurex

Pregnancy Risk Category: C

HOW SUPPLIED
dexamethasone
Tablets: 0.25 mg, 0.5 mg, 0.75 mg, 1 mg, 1.5 mg, 2 mg, 4 mg, 6 mg
Oral solution: 0.5 mg/5 ml, 0.5 mg/0.5 ml
Elixir: 0.5 mg/5 ml
dexamethasone acetate
Injection: 8 mg/ml, 16 mg/ml suspension
dexamethasone sodium phosphate
Injection: 4 mg/ml, 10 mg/ml, 20 mg/ml, 24 mg/ml

MECHANISM OF ACTION
Decreases inflammation, mainly by stabilizing leukocyte lysosomal membranes. Also suppresses the immune response, stimulates bone marrow, and influences protein, fat, and carbohydrate metabolism.

INDICATIONS & DOSAGE
Cerebral edema –
Adults: initially, 10 mg (phosphate) I.V., then 4 to 6 mg I.M. q 6 hours for 2 to 4 days, then tapered over 5 to 7 days.
Children: initially, 0.5 to 1.5 mg/kg I.V. daily; then 0.2 to 0.5 mg/kg I.V. daily in divided doses q 6 hours.
Inflammatory conditions, allergic reactions, neoplasias –
Adults: 0.25 to 4 mg P.O. b.i.d., t.i.d., or q.i.d.; or 4 to 16 mg (acetate) I.M. into joint or soft tissue q 1 to 3 weeks; or 0.8 to 1.6 mg (acetate) into lesions q 1 to 3 weeks.
Shock –
Adults: 1 to 6 mg/kg (phosphate) I.V. single dosage; or 40 mg I.V. q 2 to 6 hours, p.r.n.
Dexamethasone suppression test –
Adults: 0.5 mg P.O. q 6 hours for 48 hours.

ADVERSE REACTIONS
Common reactions are in italics; life-threatening reactions are in bold italics.

Most adverse reactions of corticosteroids are dose- or duration-dependent.

CNS: *euphoria, insomnia,* psychotic behavior, pseudotumor cerebri.
CV: ***CHF,*** hypertension, edema.
EENT: cataracts, glaucoma.
GI: *peptic ulcer,* GI irritation, increased appetite.
Metabolic: possible hypokalemia, hyperglycemia and carbohydrate intolerance, growth suppression in children.
Skin: delayed wound healing, acne, various skin eruptions.
Local: atrophy at I.M. injection sites.

Other: muscle weakness, osteoporosis, pancreatitis, hirsutism, susceptibility to infections. Acute adrenal insufficiency may follow increased stress (infection, surgery, or trauma) or abrupt withdrawal after long-term therapy.
Withdrawal symptoms: rebound inflammation, fatigue, weakness, arthralgia, fever, dizziness, lethargy, depression, fainting, orthostatic hypotension, dyspnea, anorexia, hypoglycemia. ***Sudden withdrawal may be fatal.***

INTERACTIONS

Barbiturates, phenytoin, rifampin: decreased corticosteroid effect. Corticosteroid dose may need to be increased.
Indomethacin, aspirin, NSAIDs: increased risk of GI distress and bleeding. Give together cautiously.
Oral anticoagulants: altered dosage requirements. Monitor prothrombin times closely.
Potassium-depleting drugs such as thiazide diuretics: enhanced potassium-wasting effects of dexamethasone. Monitor serum potassium levels.
Skin-test antigens: decreased response. Defer skin testing until therapy is completed.
Vaccines and toxoids: decreased antibody response and increased risk of neurologic complications. Avoid concomitant use.

NURSING CONSIDERATIONS

- *Contraindicated* in systemic fungal infections and for alternate-day therapy. Also contraindicated in patients hypersensitive to any component of the drug. Injectable forms may contain sulfites, which can cause an allergic reaction in sensitive patients.
- *Use cautiously* in GI ulceration or renal disease, hypertension, osteoporosis, varicella, vaccinia, exanthema, diabetes mellitus, Cushing's syndrome, thromboembolic disorders, seizures, myasthenia gravis, metastatic cancer, CHF, tuberculosis, ocular herpes simplex, hypoalbuminemia, emotional instability, and psychotic tendencies, and in children.
- Elderly patients may be more susceptible to osteoporosis. Patients receiving long-term therapy should consider exercise or physical therapy. Give vitamin D or calcium supplements as ordered.
- Gradually reduce drug dosage after long-term therapy. Tell patient not to discontinue drug abruptly or without doctor's consent.
- Always titrate to lowest effective dose.
- Monitor patient's weight, blood pressure, serum electrolytes.
- Instruct patient to carry a card indicating his need for supplemental systemic glucocorticoids during stress, especially as dosage is decreased.
- Give a daily dose in the morning for better results and less toxicity.
- Teach patient signs of early adrenal insufficiency: fatigue, muscular weakness, joint pain, fever, anorexia, nausea, dyspnea, dizziness, and fainting.
- May mask or exacerbate infections, including latent amebiasis.
- Watch for depression or psychotic episodes, especially in high-dose therapy.
- Inspect patient's skin for petechiae. Warn patient about easy bruising.
- Patients with diabetes may need increased insulin; monitor blood glucose.
- Monitor growth in infants and children on long-term therapy. Patients receiving long-term therapy should have periodic ophthalmic examinations.
- **I.V. use:** When administering as direct injection, inject undiluted over at least 1 minute. When administering as an intermittent or continuous infusion, dilute solution according to manufacturer's instructions and give over the prescribed duration. If used

*Liquid form contains alcohol. **May contain tartrazine.

for continuous infusion, change solution every 24 hours.
- Give I.M. injection deep into gluteal muscle. Rotate injection sites to prevent muscle atrophy. Avoid S.C. injection, as atrophy and sterile abscesses may occur.
- Give P.O. dose with food when possible.
- Warn patients on long-term therapy about cushingoid symptoms.
- Watch for additional potassium depletion from diuretics and amphotericin B. Potassium supplements may be necessary.
- Not used for alternate-day therapy.
- Dexamethasone most recently used in the diagnosis of depression. It is also an effective antiemetic.

fludrocortisone acetate
Florinef

Pregnancy Risk Category: C

HOW SUPPLIED
Tablets: 0.1 mg

MECHANISM OF ACTION
Increases sodium reabsorption, and potassium and hydrogen secretion at the nephron's distal convoluted tubule.

INDICATIONS & DOSAGE
Adrenal insufficiency (partial replacement), adrenogenital syndrome –
Adults: 0.1 to 0.2 mg P.O. daily.

ADVERSE REACTIONS
Common reactions are in italics; life-threatening reactions are in bold italics.
CV: *sodium and water retention,* hypertension, cardiac hypertrophy, edema.
Metabolic: hypokalemia.

INTERACTIONS
Potassium-depleting drugs such as thiazide diuretics: enhanced potassium-wasting effects of fludrocortisone. Monitor serum potassium levels.

NURSING CONSIDERATIONS
- *Contraindicated* in hypertension, CHF, or cardiac disease.
- *Use cautiously* in patients with Addison's disease.
- Monitor patient's blood pressure and serum electrolytes. Weigh patient daily; report sudden weight gain to doctor.
- Tell patient to report worsening symptoms, such as hypotension, weakness, cramping, and palpitations, to the doctor.
- Warn patient that mild peripheral edema is common.
- Unless contraindicated, give low-sodium diet high in potassium and protein. Potassium supplement may be needed.
- Has potent mineralocorticoid effects. Little glucocorticoid effect with usual doses.
- Used with cortisone or hydrocortisone in adrenal insufficiency.
- Watch for additional potassium depletion from diuretics and amphotericin B.
- Fludrocortisone is also prescribed to treat chronic severe orthostatic hypotension caused by levodopa therapy or diabetes mellitus.

flunisolide
AeroBid

Pregnancy Risk Category: C

HOW SUPPLIED
Oral inhalant: 250 mcg/metered spray, 50 doses/inhaler

MECHANISM OF ACTION
Decreases inflammation, mainly by stabilizing leukocyte lysosomal membranes. Also suppresses the immune response, stimulates bone marrow, and influences protein, fat, and carbohydrate metabolism.

INDICATIONS & DOSAGE

Steroid-dependent asthma –
Adults and children over 6 years: AeroBid Inhaler 2 inhalations (500 mcg) b.i.d. Don't exceed 4 inhalations b.i.d.

ADVERSE REACTIONS

Common reactions are in italics; life-threatening reactions are in bold italics.
CNS: headache.
EENT: watery eyes, throat irritation, hoarseness.
GI: nausea, vomiting, dry mouth.
Other: development of nasopharyngeal fungal infections.

INTERACTIONS

None significant.

NURSING CONSIDERATIONS

- *Contraindicated* in patients with hypersensitivity to the drug and in those with status asthmaticus or respiratory infections. Not recommended for use in asthma controlled by bronchodilators or other noncorticosteroids alone or for nonasthmatic bronchial diseases.
- Children receiving long-term therapy should have periodic growth measurements and should be checked for evidence of hypothalamic-pituitary-adrenal axis suppression.
- A spacer device may be useful to ensure proper dosage administration.
- Patients who have received long-term oral corticosteroid therapy should have their medication withdrawn slowly.
- Check mucous membranes frequently for signs of fungal infection. To prevent such infection, tell patient to gargle or rinse his mouth with water after using the inhaler. Caution him not to swallow the water.
- Tell patient to keep inhaler clean and unobstructed. Wash with warm water and dry thoroughly after use.
- Patient requiring bronchodilator should use it several minutes before flunisolide.
- Tell patient to allow 1 minute to elapse before repeating inhalations, and to hold breath for a few seconds to enhance action of drug.
- Warn patient that flunisolide doesn't relieve emergency asthma attacks.
- Store medication between 36° and 86° F (2° and 30° C). Tell patient that before using medication or when carrying canister to gently warm the canister to room temperature by keeping it in his pocket. If the canister is cold, the proper dose of medication may not be delivered.

---

hydrocortisone
Cortef, Cortenema, Hycort†, Hydrocortone

hydrocortisone acetate
Biosone, Cortifoam, Cortamed, Hydrocortone Acetate

hydrocortisone cypionate
Cortef

hydrocortisone sodium phosphate
Hydrocortone Phosphate

hydrocortisone sodium succinate
A-HydroCort, Solu-Cortef

Pregnancy Risk Category: C

HOW SUPPLIED

hydrocortisone
Tablets: 5 mg, 10 mg, 20 mg
Injection: 25 mg/ml, 50 mg/ml suspension
Enema: 100 mg/60 ml
hydrocortisone acetate
Injection: 25 mg/ml, 50 mg/ml suspension
Enema: 10% aerosol foam (provides 90 mg/application)
hydrocortisone cypionate

*Liquid form contains alcohol. **May contain tartrazine.

Oral suspension: 10 mg/5 ml
hydrocortisone sodium phosphate
Injection: 50 mg/ml solution
hydrocortisone sodium succinate
Injection: 100 mg, 250 mg, 500 mg, 1,000 mg/vial

MECHANISM OF ACTION

Decreases inflammation, mainly by stabilizing leukocyte lysosomal membranes. Also suppresses the immune response, stimulates bone marrow, and influences protein, fat, and carbohydrate metabolism.

INDICATIONS & DOSAGE

Severe inflammation, adrenal insufficiency–
Adults: 5 to 30 mg P.O. b.i.d., t.i.d., or q.i.d. (as much as 80 mg P.O. q.i.d. may be given in acute situations); or initially, 100 to 250 mg (succinate) I.M. or I.V., then 50 to 100 mg I.M., as indicated; or 15 to 240 mg (phosphate) I.M. or I.V. q 12 hours; or 5 to 75 mg (acetate) into joints and soft tissue. Dosage varies with size of joint. Often local anesthetics are injected with dose.
Shock–
Adults: 500 mg to 2 g (succinate) q 2 to 6 hours.
Children: 0.16 to 1 mg/kg (phosphate or succinate) I.M. or I.V., b.i.d. or t.i.d.
Adjunctive treatment of ulcerative colitis and proctitis–
Adults: 1 enema (100 mg) nightly for 21 days.

ADVERSE REACTIONS

Common reactions are in italics; life-threatening reactions are in bold italics.

Most adverse reactions of corticosteroids are dose- or duration-dependent.
CNS: *euphoria, insomnia,* psychotic behavior, pseudotumor cerebri.
CV: ***CHF,*** hypertension, edema.
EENT: cataracts, glaucoma.
GI: *peptic ulcer,* GI irritation, increased appetite.
Metabolic: possible hypokalemia, hyperglycemia and carbohydrate intolerance, growth suppression in children.
Skin: delayed wound healing, acne, various skin eruptions.
Other: muscle weakness, osteoporosis, pancreatitis, hirsutism, susceptibility to infections. Acute adrenal insufficiency may occur with increased stress (infection, surgery, or trauma) or abrupt withdrawal after long-term therapy.
Withdrawal symptoms: rebound inflammation, fatigue, weakness, arthralgia, fever, dizziness, lethargy, depression, fainting, orthostatic hypotension, dyspnea, anorexia, hypoglycemia. ***Sudden withdrawal may be fatal.***

INTERACTIONS

Barbiturates, phenytoin, rifampin: decreased corticosteroid effect. Corticosteroid dose may need to be increased.
Indomethacin, aspirin, NSAIDs: increased risk of GI distress and bleeding. Give together cautiously.
Live attenuated virus vaccines, other vaccines and toxoids: decreased antibody response and increased risk of neurologic complications. Avoid concomitant use.
Oral anticoagulants: altered dosage requirements. Monitor prothrombin times closely.
Potassium-depleting drugs such as thiazide diuretics: enhanced potassium-wasting effects of hydrocortisone. Monitor serum potassium levels.
Skin-test antigens: decreased response. Defer skin testing until therapy is completed.

NURSING CONSIDERATIONS

• *Contraindicated* in systemic fungal infections. Also contraindicated in patients allergic to any component of the formulation. Certain injectable forms contain sulfites, which can cause an allergic reaction in sensitive patients.

• *Use cautiously* in patients with GI ulceration or renal disease, hypertension, osteoporosis, varicella, vaccinia, exanthema, diabetes mellitus, Cushing's syndrome, thromboembolic disorders, seizures, myasthenia gravis, metastatic cancer, CHF, tuberculosis, ocular herpes simplex, hypoalbuminemia, emotional instability, and psychotic tendencies, and in children.

• Elderly patients may be more susceptible to osteoporosis. Patients receiving long-term therapy should consider exercise or physical therapy. Give vitamin D or calcium supplements as ordered.

• Gradually reduce drug dosage after long-term therapy. Tell patient not to discontinue drug abruptly or without doctor's consent.

• Always titrate to lowest effective dose.

• Has a glucocorticoid and mineralocorticoid effect.

• Monitor patient's weight, blood pressure, and serum electrolytes.

• May mask or exacerbate infections, including latent amebiasis.

• Stress (fever, trauma, surgery, and emotional problems) may increase adrenal insufficiency. Dose may have to be increased.

• Instruct patient to carry a card identifying his need for supplemental systemic glucocorticoids during stress.

• Give a daily dose in the morning for better results and less toxicity.

• Teach patient signs of early adrenal insufficiency: fatigue, muscular weakness, joint pain, fever, anorexia, nausea, dyspnea, dizziness, and fainting.

• Watch for depression or psychotic episodes, especially in high-dose therapy.

• Inspect patient's skin for petechiae. Warn patient about easy bruising.

• Patients with diabetes may need increased insulin; monitor blood glucose.

• Patients receiving prolonged therapy should have periodic ophthalmic examinations. Periodic measurement of growth and development may be necessary during high-dose or prolonged therapy in children.

• **I.V. use:** Do not use the acetate or suspension form for I.V. use. When administering as direct injection, inject directly into vein or into an I.V. line containing a free-flowing compatible solution over 30 seconds to several minutes. When administering as an intermittent or continuous infusion, dilute solution according to manufacturer's instructions and give over the prescribed duration. If used for continuous infusion, change solution every 24 hours.

• Hydrocortisone sodium phosphate may be added directly to dextrose or 0.9% sodium chloride injection for I.V. administration.

• Hydrocortisone sodium succinate must be reconstituted with bacteriostatic water or bacteriostatic sodium chloride solution before adding to I.V. solutions. When giving by direct I.V. injection, inject over at least 30 seconds. For infusion, dilute with 5% dextrose injection, 0.9% sodium chloride injection, or 5% dextrose in 0.9% sodium chloride injection to a concentration of 1 mg/ml or less.

• Give I.M. injection deep into gluteal muscle. Rotate injection sites to prevent muscle atrophy. Avoid S.C. injection, as atrophy and sterile abscesses may occur.

• Unless contraindicated, give low-sodium diet high in potassium and protein. Potassium supplement may be needed. Watch for additional potassium depletion from diuretics and amphotericin B.

• Give P.O. dose with food when possible.

• Warn patients on long-term therapy

*Liquid form contains alcohol. **May contain tartrazine.

about cushingoid symptoms, regardless of route of administration.

- Enema may produce same systemic effects as other forms of hydrocortisone. If enema therapy must exceed 21 days, discontinue gradually by reducing administration to every other night for 2 or 3 weeks.
- Do not confuse Solu-Cortef with Solu-Medrol.
- Injectable forms not used for alternate-day therapy.

methylprednisolone
Medrol**, Meprolone

methylprednisolone acetate
depMedalone, Depoject, Depo-Medrol, Depopred, Depo-Predate, D-Med, Duralone, Durameth, Medralone, Medrol Enpak, Medrone, Methylone, M-Prednisol, Rep-Pred

methylprednisolone sodium succinate
A-Metha-pred, Medrol†, Solu-Medrol

Pregnancy Risk Category: C

HOW SUPPLIED
methylprednisolone
Tablets: 2 mg, 4 mg, 8 mg, 16 mg, 24 mg, 32 mg
methylprednisolone acetate
Injection (suspension): 20 mg/ml, 40 mg/ml, 80 mg/ml
methylprednisolone sodium succinate
Injection: 40 mg, 125 mg, 500 mg, 1,000 mg, 2,000 mg/vial

MECHANISM OF ACTION
Decreases inflammation, mainly by stabilizing leukocyte lysosomal membranes. Also suppresses the immune response, stimulates bone marrow, and influences protein, fat, and carbohydrate metabolism.

INDICATIONS & DOSAGE
Severe inflammation or immunosuppression –
Adults: 2 to 60 mg P.O. in four divided doses; or 40 to 80 mg (acetate) I.M. daily, or 10 to 250 mg (succinate) I.M. or I.V. q 4 hours; or 4 to 30 mg (acetate) into joints and soft tissue, p.r.n.
Children: 117 mcg to 1.66 mg/kg (succinate) I.V. in three or four divided doses.
Shock –
Adults: 100 to 250 mg (succinate) I.V. at 2- to 6-hour intervals.
To decrease residual damage following spinal cord trauma –
Adults: 30 mg/kg (succinate) I.V. as a bolus injection within 8 hours of the injury, followed by a continuous infusion of 5.4 mg/kg/hour for the next 23 hours.

ADVERSE REACTIONS
Common reactions are in italics; life-threatening reactions are in bold italics.

Most adverse reactions of corticosteroids are dose- or duration-dependent.

CNS: *euphoria, insomnia,* psychotic behavior, pseudotumor cerebri.
CV: ***CHF,*** hypertension, edema.
EENT: cataracts, glaucoma.
GI: *peptic ulcer,* GI irritation, increased appetite.
Metabolic: possible hypokalemia, hyperglycemia and carbohydrate intolerance, growth suppression in children.
Skin: delayed wound healing, acne, various skin eruptions.
Other: muscle weakness, osteoporosis, pancreatitis, hirsutism, susceptibility to infections. Acute adrenal insufficiency may occur with increased stress (infection, surgery, or trauma) or abrupt withdrawal after long-term therapy.
Withdrawal symptoms: rebound inflammation, fatigue, weakness, arthralgia, fever, dizziness, lethargy,

depression, fainting, orthostatic hypotension, dyspnea, anorexia, hypoglycemia. ***Sudden withdrawal may be fatal.***

INTERACTIONS

Barbiturates, phenytoin, rifampin: decreased corticosteroid effect. Corticosteroid dose may need to be increased.
NSAIDs, indomethacin, aspirin: increased risk of GI distress and bleeding. Give together cautiously.
Oral anticoagulants: altered dosage requirements. Monitor prothrombin times closely.
Potassium-depleting drugs such as thiazide diuretics: enhanced potassium-wasting effects of methylprednisolone. Monitor serum potassium levels.
Skin-test antigens: decreased response. Defer skin testing until therapy is completed.
Vaccines and toxoids: decreased antibody response and increased risk of neurologic complications. Avoid concomitant use.

NURSING CONSIDERATIONS

- *Contraindicated* in systemic fungal infections. Also contraindicated in patients allergic to any component of the formulation. Certain injectable forms contain sulfites, which can cause an allergic reaction in sensitive patients.
- *Use cautiously* in patients with GI ulceration or renal disease, hypertension, osteoporosis, varicella, vaccinia, exanthema, diabetes mellitus, Cushing's syndrome, thromboembolic disorders, seizures, myasthenia gravis, metastatic cancer, CHF, tuberculosis, ocular herpes simplex, hypoalbuminemia, emotional instability, and psychotic tendencies.
- Elderly patients may be more susceptible to osteoporosis. Patients receiving long-term therapy should consider exercise or physical therapy. Give vitamin D or calcium supplements as ordered.
- Gradually reduce drug dosage after long-term therapy. Tell patient not to discontinue drug abruptly or without doctor's consent.
- Always titrate to lowest effective dose.
- A glucocorticoid with little mineralocorticoid effect.
- Discard reconstituted solutions after 48 hours.
- Don't use acetate salt when immediate onset of action is needed.
- Dermal atrophy may occur with large doses of acetate salt. Use multiple small injections rather than a single large dose and rotate injection sites.
- Monitor weight, blood pressure, serum electrolytes, and sleep patterns. Euphoria may initially interfere with sleep, but patient generally adjusts to the medication after 1 to 3 weeks.
- May mask or exacerbate infections, including latent amebiasis.
- Instruct patient to carry a card identifying his need for supplemental systemic glucocorticoids during stress.
- Give a daily dose in the morning for better results and less toxicity.
- Teach patient signs of early adrenal insufficiency: fatigue, muscular weakness, joint pain, fever, anorexia, nausea, dyspnea, dizziness, and fainting.
- Watch for depression or psychotic episodes, especially in high-dose therapy.
- Patients with diabetes may need increased insulin; monitor blood glucose.
- **I.V. use:** Use only methylprednisolone sodium succinate; never use acetate form for I.V. use. Reconstitute according to the manufacturer's directions using the supplied diluent, or use bacteriostatic water for injection with benzyl alcohol.
- When administering as direct injection, inject diluted drug into a vein or

free-flowing compatible I.V. solution over at least 1 minute. For treatment of shock, give massive doses over at least 10 minutes to prevent cardiac arrhythmias and circulatory collapse. When administering as an intermittent or continuous infusion, dilute solution according to manufacturer's instructions and give over the prescribed duration. If used for continuous infusion, change solution every 24 hours. Compatible solutions include dextrose 5% in water, 0.9% sodium chloride injection, and dextrose 5% in 0.9% sodium chloride injection.
- Give I.M. injection deep into gluteal muscle. Avoid S.C. injection, as atrophy and sterile abscesses may occur.
- Unless contraindicated, give low-sodium diet high in potassium and protein. Potassium supplement may be needed. Watch for additional potassium depletion from diuretics and amphotericin B.
- Give P.O. dose with food when possible. Critically ill patients may require concomitant antacid or H_2-receptor antagonist therapy.
- Warn patients on long-term therapy about cushingoid symptoms.
- Do not confuse Solu-Medrol with Solu-Cortef.
- Patients with hypothyroidism or cirrhosis may show an enhanced response to the drug.
- May be used for alternate-day therapy.

paramethasone acetate
Haldrone

Pregnancy Risk Category: C

HOW SUPPLIED
Tablets: 1 mg, 2 mg

MECHANISM OF ACTION
Decreases inflammation, mainly by stabilizing leukocyte lysosomal membranes. Also suppresses the immune response, stimulates bone marrow, and influences protein, fat, and carbohydrate metabolism.

INDICATIONS & DOSAGE
Inflammatory conditions –
Adults: 0.5 to 6 mg P.O. t.i.d. or q.i.d.
Children: 58 to 800 mcg/kg P.O. daily divided t.i.d. or q.i.d.

ADVERSE REACTIONS
Common reactions are in italics; life-threatening reactions are in bold italics.

Most adverse reactions of corticosteroids are dose- or duration-dependent.

CNS: *euphoria, insomnia,* psychotic behavior, pseudotumor cerebri.
CV: ***CHF,*** hypertension, edema.
EENT: cataracts, glaucoma.
GI: *peptic ulcer,* GI irritation, increased appetite.
Metabolic: possible hypokalemia, hyperglycemia and carbohydrate intolerance, growth suppression in children.
Skin: delayed wound healing, acne, various skin eruptions.
Other: muscle weakness, osteoporosis, pancreatitis, hirsutism, susceptibility to infections. Acute adrenal insufficiency may occur with increased stress (infection, surgery, or trauma) or abrupt withdrawal after long-term therapy.
Withdrawal symptoms: rebound inflammation, fatigue, weakness, arthralgia, fever, dizziness, lethargy, depression, fainting, orthostatic hypotension, dyspnea, anorexia, hypoglycemia. ***Sudden withdrawal may be fatal.***

INTERACTIONS
Barbiturates, phenytoin, rifampin: decreased corticosteroid effect. Corticosteroid dose may need to be increased.
NSAIDs, indomethacin, aspirin: in-

creased risk of GI distress and bleeding. Give together cautiously.
Oral anticoagulants: altered dosage requirements. Monitor prothrombin times closely.
Potassium-depleting drugs such as thiazide diuretics: enhanced potassium-wasting effects of paramethasone. Monitor serum potassium levels.
Skin-test antigens: decreased response. Defer skin testing until therapy is completed.
Vaccines and toxoids: decreased antibody response and increased risk of neurologic complications. Avoid concomitant use.

NURSING CONSIDERATIONS

- *Contraindicated* in systemic fungal infections and alternate-day therapy.
- *Use cautiously* in GI ulceration or renal disease, hypertension, osteoporosis, varicella, vaccinia, exanthema, diabetes mellitus, Cushing's syndrome, thromboembolic disorders, seizures, myasthenia gravis, metastatic cancer, CHF, tuberculosis, ocular herpes simplex, hypoalbuminemia, emotional instability, and psychotic tendencies.
- Elderly patients may be more susceptible to osteoporosis. Patients receiving long-term therapy should consider exercise or physical therapy. Give vitamin D or calcium supplements as ordered.
- Gradually reduce drug dosage after long-term therapy. Tell patient not to discontinue drug abruptly or without doctor's consent.
- Titrate to lowest effective dose.
- Has little mineralocorticoid effect.
- Monitor patient's weight, blood pressure, and serum electrolytes.
- May mask or exacerbate infections.
- Instruct patient to carry a card identifying his need for supplemental systemic glucocorticoids during stress.
- Give a daily dose in the morning for better results and less toxicity.
- Teach patient signs of early adrenal insufficiency: fatigue, muscular weakness, joint pain, fever, anorexia, nausea, dyspnea, dizziness, and fainting.
- Watch for depression or psychotic episodes with high-dose therapy.
- Patients with diabetes may need increased insulin; monitor blood glucose.
- Monitor growth in infants and children on long-term therapy.
- Periodic ophthalmic examinations are recommended in patients receiving long-term therapy.
- Unless contraindicated, give low-sodium diet high in potassium and protein. Potassium supplement may be needed.
- Watch for additional hypokalemia from diuretics and amphotericin B.
- Give P.O. dose with food when possible, especially if GI irritation occurs.
- Warn patients on long-term therapy about cushingoid symptoms.

prednisolone

Cortalone, Delta-Cortef, Deltasolone‡, Novo-prednisolone†, Panafcortelone‡, Prelone, Solone‡

prednisolone acetate

Articulose, Key-Pred, Niscort, Predaject, Predalone, Predate, Predcor, Predicort

prednisolone sodium phosphate

Codesol, Hydeltrasol, Key-Pred-SP, Pediapred, Predate-S, Predicort RP, Predsol Retention Enema‡, Predsol Suppositories‡

prednisolone steaglate

Sintisone‡

*Liquid form contains alcohol. **May contain tartrazine.

prednisolone tebutate

Hydeltra-TBA, Metalone-TBA, Nor-Pred TBA, Predalone TBA, Predate TBA, Predcor TBA, Prednisol TBA

Pregnancy Risk Category: B

HOW SUPPLIED

prednisolone
Tablets: 1 mg‡, 5 mg, 25 mg‡
Syrup: 15 mg/5 ml
prednisolone acetate
Injection (suspension): 25 mg/ml, 50 mg/ml, 100 mg/ml
prednisolone acetate and prednisolone sodium phosphate
Injection (suspension): 80 mg acetate and 20 mg sodium phosphate/ml
prednisolone sodium phosphate
Oral liquid: 6.7 mg (5-mg base)/5 ml
Injection: 20 mg/ml
Retention enema: 20 mg/100 ml‡
Suppositories: 5 mg‡
prednisolone steaglate
Tablets: 6.65 mg (equal to 3.5 mg prednisolone)‡
prednisolone tebutate
Injection (suspension): 20 mg/ml

MECHANISM OF ACTION

Decreases inflammation, mainly by stabilizing leukocyte lysosomal membranes. Also suppresses the immune response, stimulates bone marrow, and influences protein, fat, and carbohydrate metabolism.

INDICATIONS & DOSAGE

Severe inflammation or immunosuppression –
Adults: 2.5 to 15 mg P.O. b.i.d., t.i.d., or q.i.d.; 2 to 30 mg I.M. (acetate, phosphate), or I.V. (phosphate) q 12 hours; or 2 to 30 mg (phosphate) into joints, lesions, and soft tissue; or 4 to 40 mg (tebutate) into joints and lesions; or 0.25 to 1 ml (acetate-phosphate suspension) into joints weekly, p.r.n.

Treatment of proctitis‡ –
Adults: 1 suppository b.i.d., preferably in the morning and h.s.

Treatment of ulcerative colitis‡ –
Adults: 1 retention enema h.s. nightly for 2 to 4 weeks. The contents of the enema should be retained overnight.

ADVERSE REACTIONS

Common reactions are in italics; life-threatening reactions are in bold italics.

Most adverse reactions of corticosteroids are dose- or duration-dependent.

CNS: *euphoria, insomnia,* psychotic behavior, pseudotumor cerebri.
CV: ***CHF,*** hypertension, edema.
EENT: cataracts, glaucoma.
GI: *peptic ulcer,* GI irritation, increased appetite.
Metabolic: possible hypokalemia, hyperglycemia and carbohydrate intolerance, growth suppression in children.
Skin: delayed wound healing, acne, various skin eruptions.
Other: muscle weakness, osteoporosis, pancreatitis, hirsutism, susceptibility to infections. Acute adrenal insufficiency may occur with increased stress (infection, surgery, or trauma) or abrupt withdrawal after long-term therapy.
Withdrawal symptoms: rebound inflammation, fatigue, weakness, arthralgia, fever, dizziness, lethargy, depression, fainting, orthostatic hypotension, dyspnea, anorexia, hypoglycemia. ***Sudden withdrawal may be fatal.***

INTERACTIONS

Barbiturates, phenytoin, rifampin: decreased corticosteroid effect. Corticosteroid dose may need to be increased.
NSAIDs, indomethacin, aspirin: increased risk of GI distress and bleeding. Give together cautiously.
Oral anticoagulants: altered dosage

requirements. Monitor prothrombin times closely.
Potassium-depleting drugs such as thiazide diuretics: enhanced potassium-wasting effects of prednisolone. Monitor serum potassium levels.
Skin-test antigens: decreased response. Defer skin testing until therapy is completed.
Vaccines and toxoids: decreased antibody response and increased risk of neurologic complications. Avoid concomitant use.

NURSING CONSIDERATIONS

- *Contraindicated* in systemic fungal infections. *Use cautiously* in GI ulceration or renal disease, hypertension, osteoporosis, varicella, vaccinia, exanthema, diabetes mellitus, Cushing's syndrome, thromboembolic disorders, seizures, myasthenia gravis, metastatic cancer, CHF, tuberculosis, ocular herpes simplex, hypoalbuminemia, emotional instability, and psychotic tendencies.
- Don't confuse with prednisone.
- Elderly patients may be more susceptible to osteoporosis. Patients receiving long-term therapy should consider exercise or physical therapy. Give vitamin D or calcium supplements as ordered.
- Gradually reduce drug dosage after long-term therapy. Tell patient not to discontinue drug abruptly or without doctor's consent.
- Always titrate to lowest effective dose.
- A glucocorticoid with slight mineralocorticoid action.
- Prednisolone salts (acetate, sodium phosphate, and tebutate) are used parenterally less often than other corticosteroids that have more potent anti-inflammatory action.
- May be used for alternate-day therapy.
- Monitor patient's weight, blood pressure, and serum electrolytes.
- May mask or exacerbate infections. Tell patient to report slow healing.
- Instruct patient to carry a card identifying his need for supplemental systemic glucocorticoids during stress.
- Teach patient signs of early adrenal insufficiency: fatigue, muscular weakness, joint pain, fever, anorexia, nausea, dyspnea, dizziness, and fainting.
- Watch for depression or psychotic episodes, especially in high-dose therapy.
- Patients with diabetes may need increased insulin; monitor blood glucose.
- **I.V. use:** use only prednisolone sodium phosphate; never give acetate form I.V. When administering as direct injection, inject undiluted over at least 1 minute. When administering as an intermittent or continuous infusion, dilute solution according to manufacturer's instructions and give over the prescribed duration. Dextrose 5% in water or 0.9% sodium chloride injection are recommended as diluents for I.V. infusions.
- Give I.M. injection deep into gluteal muscle. Rotate injection sites to prevent muscle atrophy. Avoid S.C. injection, as atrophy and sterile abscesses may occur.
- Unless contraindicated, give low-sodium diet high in potassium and protein. Potassium supplement may be needed.
- Give P.O. dose with food when possible to reduce GI irritation.
- Warn patients on long-term therapy about cushingoid symptoms.
- Watch for additional potassium depletion from diuretics and amphotericin B.

prednisone

Apo-Prednisone†, Deltasone, Liquid Pred*, Meticorten, Novo-prednisone†, Orasone, Panafcort‡, Panasol, Prednicen-M, Prednisone

*Liquid form contains alcohol. **May contain tartrazine.

Intensol*, Sone‡, Sterapred, Winpred†

Pregnancy Risk Category: B

HOW SUPPLIED

Tablets: 1 mg, 2.5 mg, 5 mg, 10 mg, 20 mg, 25 mg, 50 mg
Oral solution: 5 mg/5 ml*, 5 mg/ml (concentrate)*
Syrup: 5 mg/5 ml*

MECHANISM OF ACTION

Decreases inflammation, mainly by stabilizing leukocyte lysosomal membranes. Also suppresses the immune response, stimulates bone marrow, and influences protein, fat, and carbohydrate metabolism.

INDICATIONS & DOSAGE

Severe inflammation or immunosuppression –
Adults: 2.5 to 15 mg P.O. b.i.d., t.i.d., or q.i.d. Maintenance dosage given once daily or every other day. Dosage must be individualized.
Children: 0.14 to 2 mg/kg P.O. daily divided q.i.d.
Acute exacerbations of multiple sclerosis –
Adults: 200 mg P.O. daily for 1 week, then 80 mg every other day for 1 month.

ADVERSE REACTIONS

Common reactions are in italics; life-threatening reactions are in bold italics.

Most adverse reactions of corticosteroids are dose- or duration-dependent.
CNS: *euphoria, insomnia,* psychotic behavior, pseudotumor cerebri.
CV: ***CHF,*** hypertension, edema.
EENT: cataracts, glaucoma.
GI: *peptic ulcer,* GI irritation, increased appetite.
Metabolic: possible hypokalemia, hyperglycemia and carbohydrate intolerance, growth suppression in children.
Skin: delayed wound healing, acne, various skin eruptions.
Other: muscle weakness, osteoporosis, pancreatitis, hirsutism, susceptibility to infections. Acute adrenal insufficiency may occur with increased stress (infection, surgery, or trauma) or abrupt withdrawal after long-term therapy.
Withdrawal symptoms: rebound inflammation, fatigue, weakness, arthralgia, fever, dizziness, lethargy, depression, fainting, orthostatic hypotension, dyspnea, anorexia, hypoglycemia. ***Sudden withdrawal may be fatal.***

INTERACTIONS

Barbiturates, phenytoin, rifampin: decreased corticosteroid effect. Corticosteroid dose may need to be increased.
NSAIDs, indomethacin, aspirin: increased risk of GI distress and bleeding. Give together cautiously.
Oral anticoagulants: altered dosage requirements. Monitor prothrombin times closely.
Potassium-depleting drugs such as thiazide diuretics: enhanced potassium-wasting effects of prednisone. Monitor serum potassium levels.
Skin-test antigens: decreased response. Defer skin testing until therapy is completed.
Vaccines and toxoids: decreased antibody response and increased risk of neurologic complications. Avoid concomitant use.

NURSING CONSIDERATIONS

- *Contraindicated* in systemic fungal infections.
- *Use cautiously* in GI ulceration or renal disease, hypertension, osteoporosis, varicella, vaccinia, exanthema, diabetes mellitus, Cushing's syndrome, thromboembolic disorders, seizures, myasthenia gravis, metastatic cancer, CHF, tuberculosis, ocular herpes simplex, hypoalbumin-

emia, emotional instability, and psychotic tendencies.
- Don't confuse with prednisolone.
- Elderly patients may be more susceptible to osteoporosis. Patients receiving long-term therapy should consider exercise or physical therapy. Give vitamin D or calcium supplements as ordered.
- Gradually reduce drug dosage after long-term therapy. Tell patient not to discontinue drug abruptly or without doctor's consent.
- Always titrate to lowest effective dose.
- Monitor patient's blood pressure, sleep patterns, and serum potassium.
- Weigh patient daily; report sudden weight gain to doctor.
- May mask or exacerbate infections, including latent amebiasis. Tell patient to report slow healing.
- Instruct patient to carry a card identifying his need for supplemental systemic glucocorticoids during stress.
- Give a daily dose in the morning for better results and less toxicity.
- Teach patient signs of early adrenal insufficiency: fatigue, muscular weakness, joint pain, fever, anorexia, nausea, dyspnea, dizziness, and fainting.
- Watch for depression or psychotic episodes, especially in high-dose therapy.
- Diabetic patients may need increased insulin; monitor blood glucose.
- Monitor growth in infants and children on long-term therapy.
- Periodic ophthalmic examinations are recommended in patients receiving long-term therapy.
- Unless contraindicated, give low-sodium diet high in potassium and protein. Potassium supplement may be needed.
- Unless contraindicated, give P.O. dose with food when possible to reduce GI irritation.
- May be used for alternate-day therapy.
- Watch for additional potassium depletion from diuretics and amphotericin B.
- Warn patients on long-term therapy about cushingoid symptoms.

triamcinolone

Aristocort, Atolone, Kenacort**, Tricilone

triamcinolone acetonide

Cenocort A, Cinonide, Kenaject, Kenalog, Kenalone, Tac-3, Tramacort, Triam-A, Triamonide, Tri-Kort, Trilog

triamcinolone diacetate

Amcort, Aristocort Forte, Aristocort Intralesional, Articulose-L.A., Cenocort Forte, Cinalone, Kenacort, Triam-Forte, Trilone, Tristoject

triamcinolone hexacetonide

Aristospan Intra-articular, Aristospan Intralesional

Pregnancy Risk Category: C

HOW SUPPLIED

triamcinolone
Tablets: 1 mg, 2 mg, 4 mg, 8 mg
Syrup: 2 mg/ml, 4 mg/ml
triamcinolone acetonide
Injection (suspension): 3 mg/ml, 10 mg/ml, 40 mg/ml
triamcinolone diacetate
Injection (suspension): 25 mg/ml, 40 mg/ml
triamcinolone hexacetonide
Injection (suspension): 5 mg/ml, 20 mg/ml
Oral inhalation aerosol: 100 mcg/metered spray, 240 doses/inhaler

MECHANISM OF ACTION

Decreases inflammation, mainly by stabilizing leukocyte lysosomal mem-

*Liquid form contains alcohol. **May contain tartrazine.

branes. Also suppresses the immune response, stimulates bone marrow, and influences protein, fat, and carbohydrate metabolism.

INDICATIONS & DOSAGE

Severe inflammation or immunosuppression –
Adults: 4 to 48 mg P.O. daily divided b.i.d., t.i.d., or q.i.d., or 40 mg I.M. (diacetate or acetonide) weekly; or 5 to 48 mg (diacetate or acetonide) into lesions; or 2 to 40 mg (diacetate or acetonide) into joints and soft tissue; or up to 0.5 mg (hexacetonide) per square inch of affected skin intralesional; or 2 to 20 mg (hexacetonide) intra-articular or intrasynovial into soft tissue or into joint or lesion. Often, a local anesthetic is injected into the joint with triamcinolone.
Steroid-dependent asthma –
Adults: 2 inhalations t.i.d. to q.i.d. Maximum 16 inhalations daily.
Children 6 to 12 years: 1 to 2 inhalations t.i.d. to q.i.d. Maximum 12 inhalations daily.

ADVERSE REACTIONS

Common reactions are in italics; life-threatening reactions are in bold italics.

Most adverse reactions of corticosteroids are dose- or duration-dependent.
CNS: *euphoria, insomnia,* psychotic behavior, pseudotumor cerebri.
CV: ***CHF,*** hypertension, edema.
EENT: cataracts, glaucoma.
GI: *peptic ulcer,* GI irritation, increased appetite.
Metabolic: possible hypokalemia, hyperglycemia and carbohydrate intolerance, growth suppression in children.
Skin: delayed wound healing, acne, various skin eruptions.
Other: muscle weakness, osteoporosis, pancreatitis, hirsutism, susceptibility to infections. Acute adrenal insufficiency may occur with increased stress (infection, surgery, or trauma) or abrupt withdrawal after long-term therapy.
Withdrawal symptoms: rebound inflammation, fatigue, weakness, arthralgia, fever, dizziness, lethargy, depression, fainting, orthostatic hypotension, dyspnea, anorexia, hypoglycemia. ***Sudden withdrawal may be fatal.***
Inhalation:
EENT: hoarseness, fungal infections of mouth and throat.
GI: dry mouth.

INTERACTIONS

Systemic:
Barbiturates, phenytoin, rifampin: decreased corticosteroid effect. Corticosteroid dose may need to be increased.
NSAIDs, indomethacin, aspirin: increased risk of GI distress and bleeding. Give together cautiously.
Oral anticoagulants: altered dosage requirements. Monitor prothrombin times closely.
Potassium-depleting drugs such as thiazide diuretics: enhanced potassium-wasting effects of triamcinolone. Monitor serum potassium levels.
Skin-test antigens: decreased response. Defer skin testing until therapy is completed.
Vaccines and toxoids: decreased antibody response and increased risk of neurologic complications. Avoid concomitant use.

NURSING CONSIDERATIONS

Systemic:
- *Contraindicated* in systemic fungal infections. Also contraindicated in patients with hypersensitivity to any component of the formulation. Injectable form may contain sulfites, which can cause an allergic response in sensitive patients.
- *Use cautiously* in GI ulceration or renal disease, hypertension, osteoporosis, varicella, vaccinia, exanthema, diabetes mellitus, Cushing's syn-

drome, thromboembolic disorders, seizures, myasthenia gravis, metastatic cancer, CHF, tuberculosis, ocular herpes simplex, hypoalbuminemia, emotional instability, and psychotic tendencies.

• Elderly patients may be more susceptible to osteoporosis. Patients receiving long-term therapy should consider exercise or physical therapy. Give vitamin D or calcium supplements as ordered.

• Gradually reduce drug dosage after long-term therapy. Tell patient not to discontinue drug abruptly or without doctor's consent.

• Always titrate to lowest effective dose.

• Monitor patient's weight, blood pressure, and serum electrolytes.

• May mask or exacerbate infections. Tell patient to report slow healing.

• Instruct patient to carry a card identifying his need for supplemental systemic glucocorticoids during stress.

• Give a daily dose in the morning for better results and less toxicity.

• Teach patient signs of early adrenal insufficiency: fatigue, muscular weakness, joint pain, fever, anorexia, nausea, dyspnea, dizziness, and fainting.

• Watch for depression or psychotic episodes, especially in high-dose therapy.

• Patients with diabetes may need increased insulin; monitor blood glucose.

• Give I.M. injection deep into gluteal muscle. Rotate injection sites to prevent muscle atrophy.

• Unless contraindicated, give low-sodium diet high in potassium and protein. Potassium supplement may be needed. Watch for additional potassium depletion from diuretics and amphotericin B.

• Give P.O. dose with food when possible to reduce GI irritation.

• Don't use diluents that contain preservatives. Flocculation may occur.

• Warn patients on long-term therapy about cushingoid symptoms.

• Not used for alternate-day therapy.

• Parenteral form is *not* for I.V. use.

Inhalation:

• Contraindicated in status asthmaticus. Not for use in asthma controlled by bronchodilators or other noncorticosteroids alone, or for nonasthmatic bronchial diseases.

• Oral therapy should be tapered slowly.

• Instruct patient to carry a card indicating his need for supplemental systemic glucocorticoids during stress.

• Patient requiring bronchodilator should use it several minutes before triamcinolone inhaler. Tell patient to allow 1 minute to elapse before repeat inhalations and to hold breath for a few seconds to enhance action of drug.

• Inform patient that inhaled corticosteroids don't provide relief for emergency asthma attacks.

• Instruct patient to contact doctor if he notices a decreased response. Dose may have to be adjusted. Patient shouldn't exceed recommended dose on his own.

• Teach patient using the inhaler to check mucous membranes frequently for signs of fungal infection. Tell patient to follow inhalations with glass of water to help prevent fungal infections.

• Tell patient to keep inhaler clean and unobstructed. Wash with warm water and dry thoroughly after use.

• Store medication between 36° and 86° F (2° and 30° C). Tell patient that before using medication or when carrying canister to gently warm the canister to room temperature by keeping it in his pocket. If the canister is cold, the proper dose of medication may not be delivered.

52

Androgens and anabolic steroids

danazol
fluoxymesterone
methyltestosterone
nandrolone decanoate
nandrolone phenpropionate
oxandrolone
oxymetholone
stanozolol
testosterone
testosterone cypionate
testosterone enanthate
testosterone propionate

COMBINATION PRODUCTS
DELADUMONE: testosterone enanthate 90 mg/ml, estradiol valerate 4 mg/ml, and chlorobutanol 0.5% in sesame oil.
DEPO-TESTADIOL (oil): testosterone cypionate 50 mg, estradiol cypionate 2 mg, and chlorobutanol 0.5%.
DITATE-DS: estradiol valerate 8 mg, and testosterone enanthate 180 mg.
ESTRATEST: esterified estrogens 1.25 mg, and methyltestosterone 2.5 mg.
ESTRATEST H.S.: esterified estrogens 0.625 mg, and methyltestosterone 1.25 mg.
HALODRIN: fluoxymesterone 1 mg with ethinyl estradiol 0.02 mg
PREMARIN WITH METHYLTESTOSTERONE: conjugated estrogens 0.625 mg and methyltestosterone 5 mg.

---

danazol
Cyclomen†, Danocrine
Pregnancy Risk Category: X

HOW SUPPLIED
Capsules: 50 mg, 100 mg, 200 mg

MECHANISM OF ACTION
Gonadotropin inhibitor that suppresses the pituitary-ovarian axis. Also acts on estrogen receptors to inhibit estrogenic effects.

INDICATIONS & DOSAGE
Mild endometriosis –
Women: initially, 100 to 200 mg P.O. b.i.d. Subsequent dosage based upon patient response.
Moderate to severe endometriosis –
Women: 400 mg P.O. b.i.d. uninterrupted for 3 to 6 months; may continue for 9 months.
Fibrocystic breast disease –
Women: 100 to 400 mg P.O. daily in 2 divided doses uninterrupted for 2 to 6 months.
Prevention of hereditary angioedema –
Adults: 200 mg P.O. 2 to 3 times a day, continued until favorable response is achieved. Then dosage should be decreased by half at 1- to 3-month intervals.

ADVERSE REACTIONS
Common reactions are in italics; life-threatening reactions are in bold italics.
Androgenic: in women – acne, edema, *weight gain, hirsutism,* hoarseness, clitoral enlargement, *decrease in breast size,* changes in libido, male pattern baldness, *oiliness of skin or hair.*
Blood: thrombocytopenia.
CNS: dizziness, headache, sleep disorders, fatigue, tremor, irritability, excitation, lethargy, mental depression, chills, paresthesia.
CV: elevated blood pressure.
EENT: visual disturbances.
GI: gastric irritation, nausea, vomiting, diarrhea, constipation, change in appetite.
GU: hematuria.
Hepatic: reversible jaundice.
Hypoestrogenic: flushing; sweating;

vaginitis, including itching, dryness, burning, and vaginal bleeding; nervousness, emotional lability, menstrual irregularities.
Other: muscle cramps or spasms.

INTERACTIONS
None significant.

NURSING CONSIDERATIONS
- *Contraindicated* in undiagnosed abnormal genital bleeding; impaired renal, cardiac, or hepatic function; during pregnancy; and in breast-feeding women.
- *Use cautiously* in epilepsy or migraine headache.
- Avoid use in women of childbearing age until pregnancy is ruled out. Be sure they understand the importance of effective nonhormonal contraception.
- Use with diet high in calories and protein unless contraindicated.
- Monitor closely for signs of virilization. Some androgenic effects, such as deepening of voice, may not be reversible upon discontinuation of drug.
- Periodically evaluate hepatic function.
- Periodic dosage decreases or gradual drug withdrawal should be considered.
- Advise patient who is taking danazol for fibrocystic disease to examine breasts regularly, and to call doctor immediately if breast nodule enlarges during treatment.
- Advise washing after intercourse to decrease the risk of vaginitis. Instruct patient to wear only cotton underwear.
- Has been used investigationally with impressive results in treating hemophilia and Christmas disease; also used to decrease symptoms of systemic lupus erythematosus in women and to treat gynecomastia in men.

fluoxymesterone
Android F, Halotestin**, Ora-Testryl
Controlled Substance Schedule III

Pregnancy Risk Category: X

HOW SUPPLIED
Tablets: 2 mg, 5 mg, 10 mg

MECHANISM OF ACTION
Stimulates target tissues to develop normally in androgen-deficient men.

INDICATIONS & DOSAGE
Hypogonadism and impotence caused by testicular deficiency–
Adults: 2 to 10 mg P.O. daily.
Palliation of breast cancer in women–
Adults: 15 to 30 mg P.O. daily in divided doses. All dosages should be individualized and reduced to minimum when effect is noted.
Postpartum breast engorgement–
Adults: 2.5 mg P.O. followed by 5 to 10 mg daily for 5 days.

ADVERSE REACTIONS
Common reactions are in italics; life-threatening reactions are in bold italics.
Androgenic: in women–*acne, edema, oily skin, weight gain, hirsutism, hoarseness,* clitoral enlargement, change in libido. In men–prepubertal: premature epiphyseal closure, *acne,* priapism, *growth of body and facial hair,* phallic enlargement; postpubertal: testicular atrophy, oligospermia, decreased ejaculatory volume, impotence, gynecomastia, epididymitis.
CV: edema.
GI: gastroenteritis, nausea, vomiting, constipation, change in appetite, diarrhea.
GU: bladder irritability.
Hepatic: reversible jaundice.
Hypoestrogenic: in women–flushing; sweating; vaginitis with itching, drying, burning, or bleeding; menstrual irregularities; emotional lability.

*Liquid form contains alcohol. **May contain tartrazine.

Other: hypercalcemia.

INTERACTIONS

Hepatotoxic medications: increased risk of hepatotoxicity. Monitor closely.
Hypoglycemic agents: altered dosage requirements. Monitor blood glucose levels in diabetics.
Oral anticoagulants: altered dosage requirements. Monitor prothrombin time.

NURSING CONSIDERATIONS

- *Contraindicated* in prostatic hypertrophy with obstruction; carcinoma of male breast; prostatic cancer; cardiac, hepatic, or renal decompensation; nephrosis; hypercalcemia; and in premature infants. Also contraindicated during pregnancy and in breast-feeding women.
- *Use cautiously* in prepubertal males; patients with diabetes or coronary disease; and patients taking ACTH, corticosteroids, or anticoagulants.
- Avoid use in women of childbearing age until pregnancy is ruled out. Be sure they understand the importance of using an effective, nonhormonal contraceptive during therapy.
- Advise washing after intercourse to decrease the risk of vaginitis. Instruct patient to wear only cotton underwear.
- Hypercalcemia symptoms may be difficult to distinguish from symptoms associated with condition being treated unless anticipated and thought of as a symptom cluster. Hypercalcemia is particularly likely to occur in patients with metastatic breast cancer and may indicate bone metastases.
- Explain to patient on drug for palliation of breast cancer that virilization usually occurs at dosage used. Give emotional support. Tell patient to report androgenic effects immediately. Stopping drug will prevent further androgenic changes but will probably not reverse those present.
- When used in breast cancer, subjective effects may not be seen for about 1 month; objective effects on clinical symptoms not for 3 months.
- Tell women to report menstrual irregularities; therapy should be discontinued pending etiologic determination.
- Edema is generally controllable with salt restriction or diuretics. Monitor weight routinely.
- Watch for symptoms of jaundice. Dosage adjustment may reverse condition. If liver function tests are abnormal, therapy should be stopped.
- Observe patient on concomitant anticoagulant therapy for ecchymotic areas, petechiae, or abnormal bleeding. Monitor prothrombin time.
- Watch for symptoms of hypoglycemia in patients with diabetes. Check blood glucose levels. Dosage of antidiabetic drug may need adjustment.
- Use with diet high in calories and protein unless contraindicated. Give small, frequent feedings.
- Patient should take drug with food or meals if GI upset occurs.

methyltestosterone

Android, Metandren**, Metandren Linguets, Oreton Methyl, Testomet‡, Testred, Virilon
Controlled Substance Schedule III
Pregnancy Risk Category: X

HOW SUPPLIED

Tablets: 5 mg‡, 10 mg, 25 mg, 50 mg‡
Tablets (buccal): 5 mg, 10 mg
Capsules: 10 mg

MECHANISM OF ACTION

Stimulates target tissues to develop normally in androgen-deficient males.

INDICATIONS & DOSAGE
Breast engorgement of nonnursing mothers –
Adults: 80 mg P.O. daily, or 40 mg buccal daily for 3 to 5 days.
Breast cancer in women 1 to 5 years postmenopausal –
Adults: 200 mg P.O. daily; or 100 mg buccal daily.
Eunuchoidism and eunuchism, male climacteric symptoms –
Adults: 10 to 40 mg P.O. daily; or 5 to 20 mg buccal daily.
Postpubertal cryptorchidism –
Adults: 30 mg P.O. daily; or 15 mg buccal daily.

ADVERSE REACTIONS
Common reactions are in italics; life-threatening reactions are in bold italics.
Androgenic: in women – *acne, edema, oily skin, weight gain, hirsutism, hoarseness,* clitoral enlargement, changes in libido. In men – prepubertal: premature epiphyseal closure, *acne,* priapism, *growth of body and facial hair,* phallic enlargement; postpubertal: testicular atrophy, oligospermia, decreased ejaculatory volume, impotence, gynecomastia, epididymitis.
CV: edema.
GI: gastroenteritis, constipation, nausea, vomiting, diarrhea, change in appetite.
GU: bladder irritability.
Hepatic: reversible jaundice.
Hypoestrogenic: in women – flushing; sweating; vaginitis with itching, drying, burning, or bleeding; menstrual irregularities.
Local: irritation of oral mucosa with buccal administration.
Other: hypercalcemia.

INTERACTIONS
Hepatotoxic medications: increased risk of hepatotoxicity. Monitor closely.
Hypoglycemic agents: altered dosage requirements. Monitor blood glucose levels in diabetics.
Oral anticoagulants: altered dosage requirements. Monitor prothrombin time.

NURSING CONSIDERATIONS
- *Contraindicated* in pregnancy and in breast-feeding women; in elderly, asthenic men who may react adversely to androgen overstimulation; in hypercalcemia; cardiac, hepatic, or renal decompensation; prostatic or breast cancer in men; benign prostatic hypertrophy with obstruction; conditions aggravated by fluid retention; hypertension; and in premature infants.
- *Use cautiously* in myocardial infarction or coronary artery disease.
- In children, X-ray of wrist bones should establish level of bone maturation before therapy. During treatment, bone maturation may proceed more rapidly than linear growth; therefore, dosage should be intermittent and X-rays should be taken periodically to monitor bone maturation.
- Avoid use in women of childbearing age until pregnancy is ruled out. Be sure they understand the importance of using an effective, nonhormonal contraceptive during therapy.
- Treatment of breast cancer usually restricted to patients 1 to 5 years postmenopausal.
- Edema is generally controllable with salt restriction or diuretics. Check weight regularly.
- Periodic serum cholesterol and calcium determinations, and cardiac and liver function tests recommended. Usually only used for intermittent therapy. Because of potential hepatotoxicity, watch closely for jaundice.
- In metastatic breast cancer, hypercalcemia may indicate progression of bone metastases. Report signs of hypercalcemia.
- Therapeutic response in breast cancer is usually apparent within 3

months. Therapy should be stopped if signs of disease progression appear.
- Enhances hypoglycemia; teach patient signs of hypoglycemia and method for checking blood glucose level. Instruct patient to report hypoglycemia immediately.
- Watch for ecchymoses, petechiae, and abnormal bleeding in patients receiving concomitant anticoagulants.
- Promptly report signs of virilization in women.
- Use with diet high in calories and protein unless contraindicated. Give small, frequent feedings.
- Advise washing after intercourse to decrease the risk of vaginitis. Instruct patient to wear only cotton underwear.
- Buccal tablets twice as potent as oral tablets. Tell patient to avoid eating, drinking, chewing, or smoking while buccal tablet is in place, and that tablet is not to be swallowed. Place in upper or lower buccal pouch between cheek and gum. Tablet requires 30 to 60 minutes to dissolve. Instruct patient to change tablet absorption site with each dose to minimize risk of buccal irritation.
- Abused to enhance athletic ability.

nandrolone decanoate

Anabolin LA, Androlone-D, Deca-Durabolin, Decolone, Hybolin Decanoate, Kabolin, Nandrobolic L.A., Neo-Durabolic

nandrolone phenpropionate

Anabolin IM, Androlone, Durabolin, Hybolin Improved, Nandrobolic

Controlled Substance Schedule III
Pregnancy Risk Category: X

HOW SUPPLIED

decanoate
Injection (in oil): 50 mg/ml, 100 mg/ml, 200 mg/ml

phenpropionate
Injection (in oil): 25 mg/ml, 50 mg/ml

MECHANISM OF ACTION

Anabolic steroid that promotes tissue-building processes and reverses catabolism. Also stimulates erythropoiesis.

INDICATIONS & DOSAGI

Severe debility or disease states, refractory anemias (decanoate) –
Adults: 100 to 200 mg I.M. weekly. Therapy should be intermittent.
Tissue-building (decanoate) –
Adults: 50 to 100 mg I.M. q 3 to 4 weeks.
Children 2 to 13 years: 25 to 50 mg I.M. q 3 to 4 weeks.
Control of metastatic breast cancer (phenpropionate) –
Adults: 25 to 50 mg I.M. weekly.
Children 2 to 13 years: 12.5 to 25 mg I.M. every 2 to 4 weeks.

ADVERSE REACTIONS

Common reactions are in italics; life-threatening reactions are in bold italics.
Androgenic: in women – *acne, edema, oily skin, weight gain, hirsutism, hoarseness,* clitoral enlargement, decreased or increased libido. In men – prepubertal: premature epiphyseal closure, *acne,* priapism, *growth of body and facial hair,* phallic enlargement; postpubertal: testicular atrophy, oligospermia, decreased ejaculatory volume, impotence, gynecomastia, epididymitis.
CV: edema.
GI: gastroenteritis, nausea, vomiting, diarrhea, change in appetite.
GU: bladder irritability.
Hepatic: reversible jaundice, hepatotoxicity.
Hypoestrogenic: in women – flushing; sweating; vaginitis with itching, drying, burning, or bleeding; menstrual irregularities with large doses.
Local: pain at injection site, induration.

Other: hypercalcemia, hypercalciuria.

INTERACTIONS

Hepatotoxic medications: increased risk of hepatotoxicity. Monitor closely.

Hypoglycemic agents: altered dosage requirements. Monitor blood glucose levels in diabetics.

Oral anticoagulants: altered dosage requirements. Monitor prothrombin time.

NURSING CONSIDERATIONS

- *Contraindicated* in prostatic hypertrophy with obstruction; male breast and prostatic cancer; cardiac, hepatic, or renal decompensation; nephrosis; in pregnancy; in breast-feeding women; and in premature infants.
- *Use cautiously* in prepubertal males; patients with diabetes or coronary disease; and patients taking ACTH, corticosteroids, or anticoagulants.
- Avoid use in women of childbearing age until pregnancy is ruled out. Be sure they understand the importance of using an effective, nonhormonal contraceptive during therapy.
- Advise washing after intercourse to decrease the risk of vaginitis. Instruct patient to wear only cotton underwear.
- When used to promote erythropoiesis, be sure patient has adequate daily iron intake.
- Inject drug deep I.M., preferably into upper outer quadrant of gluteal muscle in adults. Rotate injection sites to prevent muscle atrophy.
- Hypercalcemia is most likely to occur in patients with mammary carcinoma; these patients should have quantitative urine and serum calcium level determinations.
- Tell women to report menstrual irregularities; therapy should be discontinued pending etiologic determination.
- Watch for signs of virilization; they may be irreversible despite prompt discontinuation of therapy.
- Closely observe boys under 7 years for precocious development of male sexual characteristics.
- In children, therapy should be preceded by X-ray of wrist bones to establish level of bone maturation. During treatment, bone maturation may proceed more rapidly than linear growth; dosage should be intermittent and X-rays taken periodically.
- Edema is generally controllable with salt restrictions or diuretics. Check weight regularly.
- Watch for jaundice. Dosage adjustment may reverse condition. If liver function tests are abnormal, therapy should be stopped.
- Observe patients receiving concomitant anticoagulant therapy for ecchymotic areas, petechiae, or abnormal bleeding. Monitor prothrombin time.
- Watch for symptoms of hypoglycemia in patients with diabetes. Check blood glucose levels. Dosage of antidiabetic drug may need adjustment.
- Use with diet high in calories and protein unless contraindicated. Give small, frequent feedings.
- Abused to enhance athletic ability.
- Considered an adjunctive therapy.
- Anabolic steroids may alter many laboratory studies during therapy and for 2 to 3 weeks after therapy ends.

oxandrolone

Anavar, Lonavar‡

Controlled Substance Schedule III

Pregnancy Risk Category: X

HOW SUPPLIED

Tablets: 2.5 mg

MECHANISM OF ACTION

Anabolic steroid that promotes tissue-building processes and reverses catabolism. Also stimulates erythropoiesis.

*Liquid form contains alcohol. **May contain tartrazine.

INDICATIONS & DOSAGE

To combat catabolic effects of corticosteroid therapy, osteoporosis, prolonged immobilization and debilitated states–

Adults: 2.5 mg P.O. b.i.d., t.i.d., or q.i.d.; up to 20 mg daily for 2 to 4 weeks.

Children: 0.25 mg/kg daily P.O. for 2 to 4 weeks.

Continuous therapy should not exceed 3 months.

ADVERSE REACTIONS

Common reactions are in italics; life-threatening reactions are in bold italics.

Androgenic: in women – *acne, edema, oily skin, weight gain, hirsutism, hoarseness,* clitoral enlargement, decreased or increased libido. In men – prepubertal: premature epiphyseal closure, *acne,* priapism, *growth of body and facial hair,* phallic enlargement; postpubertal: testicular atrophy, oligospermia, decreased ejaculatory volume, impotence, gynecomastia, epididymitis.

CV: edema.

GI: gastroenteritis, nausea, vomiting, constipation or diarrhea, change in appetite.

GU: bladder irritability.

Hepatic: reversible jaundice, hepatotoxicity.

Hypoestrogenic: in women – flushing; sweating; vaginitis with itching, drying, burning, or bleeding; menstrual irregularities.

Other: hypercalcemia.

INTERACTIONS

Hepatotoxic medications: increased risk of hepatotoxicity. Monitor closely.

Hypoglycemic agents: altered dosage requirements. Monitor blood glucose levels in diabetics.

Oral anticoagulants: altered dosage requirements. Monitor prothrombin time.

NURSING CONSIDERATIONS

- *Contraindicated* in prostatic hypertrophy with obstruction; prostatic and male breast cancer; cardiac, hepatic, or renal decompensation; nephrosis; in pregnancy; in breast-feeding women; and in premature infants.
- *Use cautiously* in prepubertal males; patients with diabetes or coronary disease; and patients taking ACTH, corticosteroids, or anticoagulants.
- Avoid use in women of childbearing age until pregnancy is ruled out. Be sure they understand the importance of using an effective, nonhormonal contraceptive during therapy.
- When used to promote erythropoiesis, be sure patient has adequate daily iron intake.
- Advise washing after intercourse to decrease the risk of vaginitis. Instruct patient to wear only cotton underwear.
- Hypercalcemia symptoms may be difficult to distinguish from symptoms of condition being treated unless anticipated and thought of as a cluster. Hypercalcemia most likely to occur with metastatic breast cancer and may indicate bone metastases.
- Tell women to report menstrual irregularities; therapy should be discontinued pending etiologic determination.
- Watch for signs of virilization; may be irreversible despite prompt discontinuation of therapy. Doctor must decide if benefits outweigh effects.
- Boys under 7 years should be observed for precocious development of male sexual characteristics.
- In children, therapy should be preceded by X-ray of wrist bones to establish level of bone maturation. During treatment, bone maturation may proceed more rapidly than linear growth; dosage should be intermittent and X-rays taken periodically.
- Edema is generally controllable

with salt restriction or diuretics. Monitor weight routinely.
- Watch for jaundice. Dosage adjustment may reverse condition. Periodic liver function tests are recommended.
- Observe patient on concomitant anticoagulant therapy for ecchymotic areas, petechiae, or abnormal bleeding. Monitor prothrombin time.
- Watch for symptoms of hypoglycemia in patients with diabetes. Check blood glucose levels. Dosage of antidiabetic drug may need adjustment.
- Use with diet high in calories and protein unless contraindicated. Give small, frequent feedings.
- Patient should take drug with food or meals if GI upset occurs.
- Abused to enhance athletic ability.
- Anabolic steroids may alter many laboratory studies during therapy and for 2 to 3 weeks after therapy ends.

oxymetholone

Anadrol-50, Anapolon†, Anapolon 50†‡
Controlled Substance Schedule III
Pregnancy Risk Category: X

HOW SUPPLIED
Tablets: 50 mg

MECHANISM OF ACTION
Anabolic steroid that promotes tissue-building processes and reverses catabolism. Also stimulates erythropoiesis.

INDICATIONS & DOSAGE
Aplastic anemia –
Adults and children: 1 to 5 mg/kg P.O. daily. Dosage highly individualized; response not immediate. Trial of 3 to 6 months required.
Osteoporosis, catabolic conditions –
Adults: 5 to 15 mg P.O. daily, or up to 30 mg P.O. daily.
Children over 6 years: up to 10 mg P.O. daily.
Children under 6 years: 1.25 mg P.O. daily or up to q.i.d. Continuous therapy should not exceed 30 days in children; 90 days in any patient.

ADVERSE REACTIONS
Common reactions are in italics; life-threatening reactions are in bold italics.
Androgenic: in women – *acne, edema, oily skin, weight gain, hirsutism, hoarseness,* clitoral enlargement, decreased or increased libido, male pattern baldness. In men – prepubertal: premature epiphyseal closure, *acne,* priapism, *growth of body and facial hair,* phallic enlargement; postpubertal: testicular atrophy, oligospermia, decreased ejaculatory volume, impotence, gynecomastia, epididymitis.
CV: edema.
GI: gastroenteritis, nausea, vomiting, constipation, diarrhea, change in appetite.
GU: bladder irritability.
Hepatic: reversible jaundice, hepatotoxicity.
Hypoestrogenic: in women – flushing; sweating; vaginitis with itching, drying, burning, or bleeding; menstrual irregularities.
Other: hypercalcemia.

INTERACTIONS
Hepatotoxic medications: increased risk of hepatotoxicity. Monitor closely.
Hypoglycemic agents: altered dosage requirements. Monitor blood glucose levels in diabetics.
Oral anticoagulants: altered dosage requirements. Monitor prothrombin time.

NURSING CONSIDERATIONS
- *Contraindicated* in prostatic hypertrophy with obstruction; prostatic and male breast cancer; cardiac, hepatic, or renal decompensation; nephrosis; in pregnancy; in breast-feeding women; and in premature infants.
- *Use cautiously* in prepubertal males; patients with diabetes or coro-

nary diseases; and patients taking ACTH, corticosteroids, or anticoagulants.

• When used to promote erythropoiesis, be sure patient has adequate daily iron intake.

• Avoid use in women of childbearing age until pregnancy is ruled out. Be sure they understand the importance of using an effective, nonhormonal contraceptive during therapy.

• Advise washing after intercourse to decrease the risk of vaginitis. Instruct patient to wear only cotton underwear.

• Hypercalcemia symptoms may be difficult to distinguish from symptoms of condition being treated unless anticipated and thought of as a cluster. Hypercalcemia most likely to occur in metastatic breast cancer and may indicate bone metastases.

• Supportive treatment of anemias (transfusions, correction of iron, folic acid, vitamin B_{12}, or pyridoxine deficiency). Give 3 to 6 months for response.

• Effects in osteoporosis usually seen in 4 to 6 weeks.

• Tell women to report menstrual irregularities; therapy should be discontinued pending etiologic determination.

• Watch for signs of virilization; may be irreversible despite prompt discontinuation of therapy. Doctor must decide if benefits outweigh effects.

• Boys under 7 years should be observed for precocious development of male sexual characteristics.

• In children, therapy should be preceded by X-ray of wrist bones to establish level of bone maturation. During treatment, bone maturation may proceed more rapidly than linear growth; dosage should be intermittent and X-rays taken periodically. Epiphyseal development may continue 6 months after stopping therapy.

• Edema is generally controllable with salt restriction or diuretics. Monitor weight routinely.

• Watch for symptoms of jaundice. Dosage adjustment may reverse condition; if liver function tests are abnormal, therapy should be stopped.

• Observe patient on concomitant anticoagulant therapy for ecchymotic areas, petechiae, or abnormal bleeding. Monitor prothrombin time.

• Watch for symptoms of hypoglycemia in patients with diabetes. Check blood glucose levels. Dosage of antidiabetic drug may need adjustment.

• Use with diet high in calories and protein unless contraindicated. Give small, frequent feedings.

• Take with food or meals if GI upset occurs.

• Abused to enhance athletic ability.

• Anabolic steroids may alter many laboratory studies during therapy and for 2 to 3 weeks after therapy ends.

• Has also been used to prevent hereditary angioedema.

stanozolol

Winstrol

Controlled Substance Schedule III

Pregnancy Risk Category: X

HOW SUPPLIED

Tablets: 2 mg

MECHANISM OF ACTION

Anabolic steroid that promotes tissue-building processes and reverses catabolism. Also stimulates erythropoiesis.

INDICATIONS & DOSAGE

Prevention of hereditary angioedema –

Adults: 2 mg P.O. t.i.d. to 4 mg P.O. q.i.d for 5 days initially. Dosage is gradually reduced at intervals of 1 to 3 months to a dosage of 2 mg daily.

Children age 6 to 12: Administer up to 2 mg P.O. daily.

Children under age 6: 1 mg. P.O. daily

Note: Stanozolol should be used in children only during an acute attack.

ADVERSE REACTIONS

Common reactions are in italics; life-threatening reactions are in bold italics.

Androgenic: in women – *acne, edema, oily skin, weight gain, hirsutism, hoarseness,* clitoral enlargement, decreased or increased libido. In men – prepubertal: premature epiphyseal closure, *acne,* priapism, *growth of body and facial hair,* phallic enlargement; postpubertal: testicular atrophy, oligospermia, decreased ejaculatory volume, impotence, gynecomastia, epididymitis.

CV: edema.

GI: gastroenteritis, nausea, vomiting, constipation, diarrhea, change in appetite.

GU: bladder irritability.

Hepatic: reversible jaundice, hepatotoxicity.

Hypoestrogenic: in women – flushing; sweating; vaginitis with itching, drying, burning or bleeding; menstrual irregularities.

Other: hypercalcemia.

INTERACTIONS

Hepatotoxic medications: increased risk of hepatotoxicity. Monitor closely.

Hypoglycemic agents: altered dosage requirements. Monitor blood glucose levels in diabetics.

Oral anticoagulants: altered dosage requirements. Monitor prothrombin time.

NURSING CONSIDERATIONS

• *Contraindicated* in prostatic hypertrophy with obstruction; prostatic and male breast cancer; cardiac, hepatic, or renal decompensation; nephrosis; in pregnancy; in breast-feeding women; and in premature infants.

• *Use cautiously* in prepubertal males; patients with diabetes or coronary disease; and patients taking ACTH, corticosteroids, or anticoagulants.

• Avoid use in women of childbearing age until pregnancy is ruled out. Be sure they understand the importance of using an effective, nonhormonal contraceptive during therapy.

• A lower dosage in young women (2 mg b.i.d.) is recommended to avoid virilization. Watch for these adverse reactions; may be irreversible despite prompt discontinuation of therapy. Doctor must decide if benefits outweigh adverse effects.

• Tell women to report menstrual irregularities; therapy should be discontinued pending etiologic determination.

• Boys under 7 years should be observed for precocious development of male sexual characteristics.

• In children, therapy should be preceded by X-ray of wrist bones to establish level of bone maturation. During treatment, bone maturation may proceed more rapidly than linear growth; dosage should be intermittent and X-rays taken periodically.

• Edema is generally controllable with salt restriction or diuretics. Monitor weight routinely.

• Watch for symptoms of jaundice. Dosage adjustment may reverse condition; check liver function tests regularly. If abnormal, therapy should be discontinued.

• Observe patient on concomitant anticoagulant therapy for ecchymotic areas, petechiae, or abnormal bleeding. Monitor prothrombin time.

• Watch for symptoms of hypoglycemia in patients with diabetes. Check blood glucose levels. Dosage of antidiabetic drug may need adjustment.

• Use with diet high in calories and protein unless contraindicated. Give small, frequent feedings.

• Administer before or with meals to minimize GI distress.

• Advise washing after intercourse to decrease the risk of vaginitis. Instruct

patient to wear only cotton underwear.
- Monitor serum cholesterol.
- Abused to enhance athletic ability.
- Anabolic steroids may alter many laboratory studies during therapy and for 2 to 3 weeks after therapy ends.

testosterone
Andro, Andronaq, Histerone, Malogen, Testaqua, Testoject

testosterone cypionate
Andro-Cyp, Andronaq-LA, Andronate, dep Andro, Depotest, Depo-Testosterone, Duratest, T-Cypionate, Tesionate, Testa-C, Testoject-LA, Testred Cypionate, Virilon IM

testosterone enanthate
Android-T, Andro-LA, Andryl, Delatestryl, Durathate, Everone, Malogex†, Testone LA, Testrin PA

testosterone propionate
Malogen†, Testex

Controlled Substance Schedule III
Pregnancy Risk Category: X

HOW SUPPLIED
testosterone
Injection (aqueous suspension): 25 mg/ml, 50 mg/ml, 100 mg/ml
testosterone cypionate
Injection (in oil): 50 mg/ml, 100 mg/ml, 200 mg/ml
testosterone enanthate
Injection (in oil): 100 mg/ml, 200 mg/ml
testosterone propionate
Injection (in oil): 25 mg/ml, 50 mg/ml, 100 mg/ml

MECHANISM OF ACTION
Stimulates target tissues to develop normally in androgen-deficient men. Testosterone may have some antiestrogen properties, making it useful to treat certain estrogen-dependent breast cancers. Its action in postpartum breast engorgement is not known because testosterone does not suppress lactation.

INDICATIONS & DOSAGE
Eunuchism, eunuchoidism, deficiency after castration and male climacteric –
Men: 10 to 25 mg I.M. 2 to 5 times weekly, or 200 to 400 mg (cypionate or enanthate) I.M. q 4 weeks, or 10 to 25 mg (propionate) I.M. 2 to 4 times weekly.
Oligospermia –
Men: 100 to 200 mg (cypionate or enanthate) I.M. q 4 to 6 weeks for development and maintenance of testicular function.
Breast engorgement of nonnursing mothers –
Women: 25 to 50 mg I.M. daily for 3 to 4 days, starting at delivery.
Metastatic breast cancer –
Women: 50 to 100 mg (propionate) I.M. 3 times weekly. 200 to 400 mg (cypionate or enanthate) I.M. q 2 to 4 weeks.
Postmenopausal or primary osteoporosis –
Adults: 200 to 400 mg (enanthate) I.M. q 4 weeks.
Breast cancer in women 1 to 5 years postmenopausal –
Women: 100 mg I.M. 3 times weekly as long as improvement maintained.

ADVERSE REACTIONS
Common reactions are in italics; life-threatening reactions are in bold italics.
Androgenic: in women – *acne, edema, oily skin, weight gain, hirsutism, hoarseness,* clitoral enlargement, decreased or increased libido. In men – prepubertal: premature epiphyseal closure, *acne,* priapism, *growth of body and facial hair,* phallic enlargement; postpubertal: testicular atrophy, oligospermia, decreased ejaculatory volume, impotence, gynecomastia, epididymitis.

CV: edema.
GI: gastroenteritis, nausea, vomiting, constipation, diarrhea, change in appetite.
GU: bladder irritability.
Hepatic: reversible jaundice.
Hypoestrogenic: in women—flushing; sweating; vaginitis with itching, drying, burning, or bleeding; menstrual irregularities.
Local: pain at injection site, induration, irritation and sloughing with pellet implantation, edema.
Other: hypercalcemia.

INTERACTIONS

Hepatotoxic medications: increased risk of hepatotoxicity. Monitor closely.
Hypoglycemic agents: altered dosage requirements. Monitor blood glucose levels in diabetics.
Oral anticoagulants: altered dosage requirements. Monitor prothrombin time.

NURSING CONSIDERATIONS

- *Contraindicated* in women of childbearing potential (possible masculinization of female infant); in elderly, asthenic men who may react adversely to androgen overstimulation; in hypercalcemia; cardiac, hepatic, or renal decompensation; prostatic or breast cancer in males; benign prostatic hypertrophy with obstruction; conditions aggravated by fluid retention; hypertension; in pregnancy; in breast-feeding women; and in premature infants.
- *Use cautiously* in myocardial infarction or coronary artery disease, and in prepubertal males.
- Avoid use in women of childbearing age until pregnancy is ruled out. Be sure they understand the importance of using an effective, nonhormonal contraceptive during therapy.
- Periodic liver function tests should be performed.
- In metastatic breast cancer, hypercalcemia usually indicates progression of bone metastases. Report signs of hypercalcemia.
- Therapeutic response in breast cancer is usually apparent within 3 months. Stop therapy if signs of disease progression appear.
- Enhances hypoglycemia; teach patient how to recognize signs of hypoglycemia and tell him to report them immediately.
- Instruct men to report priapism, reduced ejaculatory volume, and gynecomastia. Withdraw drug if these occur.
- Inject deep into upper outer quadrant of gluteal muscle. Rotate injection sites to prevent muscle atrophy. Report soreness at site. Possibility of postinfection furunculosis.
- Watch for ecchymotic areas, petechiae, or abnormal bleeding in patients on concomitant anticoagulant therapy. Monitor prothrombin time.
- Report signs of virilization in females; reevaluate treatment.
- Monitor prepubertal males by X-ray for rate of bone maturation.
- Edema is generally controllable with salt restriction or diuretics. Monitor weight routinely.
- Use with diet high in calories and protein unless contraindicated. Give small, frequent feedings.
- Advise washing after intercourse to decrease the risk of vaginitis. Instruct patient to wear only cotton underwear.
- Daily dosage requirement best administered in divided doses.
- Store I.M. preparations at room temperature. If crystals appear, warming and shaking the bottle will usually disperse them.
- Many laboratory studies may be altered during therapy and for 2 to 3 weeks after therapy is stopped.

53

Estrogens and progestins

chlorotrianisene
dienestrol
diethylstilbestrol
diethylstilbestrol diphosphate
esterified estrogens
estradiol
estradiol cypionate
estradiol valerate
estrogens, conjugated
estrone
estropipate
ethinyl estradiol
ethinyl estradiol and desogestrel
ethinyl estradiol and ethynodiol diacetate
ethinyl estradiol and levonorgestrel
ethinyl estradiol and norethindrone
ethinyl estradiol and norethindrone acetate
ethinyl estradiol and norgestimate
ethinyl estradiol and norgestrel
ethinyl estradiol, norethindrone acetate, and ferrous fumarate
mestranol and norethindrone
hydroxyprogesterone caproate
levonorgestrel
medroxyprogesterone acetate
norethindrone
norethindrone acetate
norgestrel
progesterone
quinestrol

COMBINATION PRODUCTS

MENRIUM 5-2: chlordiazepoxide 5 mg and esterified estrogens 0.2 mg.
MENRIUM 5-4: chlordiazepoxide 5 mg and esterified estrogens 0.4 mg.
MENRIUM 10-4: chlordiazepoxide 10 mg and esterified estrogens 0.4 mg.
MILPREM-200: conjugated estrogens 0.45 mg and meprobamate 200 mg.
MILPREM-400: conjugated estrogens 0.45 mg and meprobamate 400 mg.
PMB 200: conjugated estrogens 0.45 mg and meprobamate 200 mg.
PMB 400: conjugated estrogens 0.45 mg and meprobamate 400 mg.

chlorotrianisene

TACE**

Pregnancy Risk Category: X

HOW SUPPLIED

Capsules: 12 mg, 25 mg

MECHANISM OF ACTION

Increases the synthesis of DNA, RNA, and protein in responsive tissues. Also reduces FSH and LH release from the pituitary.

INDICATIONS & DOSAGE

Prostatic cancer –
Men: 12 to 25 mg P.O. daily.
Atrophic vaginitis –
Women: 12 to 25 mg P.O. daily for 30 to 60 days.
Female hypogonadism –
Women: 12 to 25 mg P.O. for 21 days, followed by 1 dose of progesterone 100 mg I.M. or 5 days of oral progestogen given concurrently with last 5 days of chlorotrianisene (for example, medroxyprogesterone 5 to 10 mg).
Menopausal symptoms –
Women: 12 to 25 mg P.O. daily for 30 days or cyclic (3 weeks on, 1 week off).
Vulvar squamous hyperplasia –
Women: 12 to 25 mg P.O. daily.

ADVERSE REACTIONS

Common reactions are in italics; life-threatening reactions are in bold italics.

CNS: headache, dizziness, chorea, migraine, depression, libido changes.
CV: thrombophlebitis; ***thromboembolism;*** hypertension; edema; ***increased risk of stroke, pulmonary embolism, and myocardial infarction.***
EENT: worsening of myopia or astigmatism, intolerance to contact lenses.
GI: *nausea,* vomiting, abdominal cramps, bloating, diarrhea, constipation, anorexia, increased appetite, excessive thirst, weight changes, pancreatitis.
GU: in women – breakthrough bleeding, altered menstrual flow, dysmenorrhea, amenorrhea, cervical erosion or abnormal secretions, enlargement of uterine fibromas, vaginal candidiasis. In men – *gynecomastia, testicular atrophy, impotence.*
Hepatic: cholestatic jaundice.
Metabolic: hyperglycemia, hypercalcemia, folic acid deficiency.
Skin: melasma, urticaria, acne, seborrhea, oily skin, hirsutism or loss of hair.
Other: leg cramps, purpura, breast changes (tenderness, enlargement, secretion).

INTERACTIONS

Bromocriptine: may cause amenorrhea, interfering with the effects of bromocriptine. Avoid concomitant use.
Carbamazepine, phenobarbital, rifampin: decreased effectiveness of estrogen therapy. Monitor closely.
Corticosteroids: possible enhanced effects. Monitor closely.
Cyclosporine: increased risk of toxicity. Use together with caution and frequently monitor cyclosporine levels.
Dantrolene, other hepatotoxic medications: increased risk of hepatotoxicity. Monitor closely.
Oral anticoagulants: dosage adjustments may be necessary. Monitor prothrombin time.
Tamoxifen: estrogens may interfere with the effectiveness of tamoxifen. Avoid concomitant use.

NURSING CONSIDERATIONS

- *Contraindicated* in thrombophlebitis or thromboembolic disorders; cancer of breast, reproductive organs, or genitals; undiagnosed abnormal genital bleeding; and pregnancy.
- *Use cautiously* in hypertension, asthma, mental depression, bone diseases, blood dyscrasias, gallbladder disease, migraine, seizures, diabetes mellitus, amenorrhea, heart failure, hepatic or renal dysfunction, uterine fibroids, hypercalcemia from metastatic breast disease, and family history (mother, grandmother, sister) of breast or genital tract cancer. Development or worsening of these conditions may require discontinuation of the drug.
- Studies suggest that postmenopausal women who use estrogen replacement for more than 5 years to treat menopausal symptoms may be at increased risk for endometrial carcinoma. This risk is reduced by the use of cyclic rather than continuous therapy and use of the lowest possible dosages of estrogen. Adding progestins to the regimen decreases the incidence of endometrial hyperplasia; however, it isn't known if progestins affect the incidence of endometrial carcinoma. Most studies show no increased risk of breast cancer. Emphasize the importance of regular physical examinations.
- Patients should have a thorough physical examination before initiating estrogen therapy. Patients receiving long-term therapy should have repeat examinations yearly. Periodically monitor blood pressure, hepatic function, and serum lipid levels.
- Patient package insert that describes estrogen's adverse reactions is available. However, provide verbal explanation also.
- Warn patient to immediately report

*Liquid form contains alcohol. **May contain tartrazine.

suspected pregnancy; abdominal pain; pain, numbness, or stiffness in legs or buttocks; pressure or pain in chest; shortness of breath; severe headaches; visual disturbances, such as blind spots, flashing lights, or blurriness; vaginal bleeding or discharge; breast lumps; swelling of hands or feet; yellow skin and sclera; dark urine; and light-colored stools.
- Not used for menstrual disorders because duration of action is very long.
- Pathologist should be advised of estrogen therapy when specimen is sent.
- Patients with diabetes should report elevated blood glucose test results so antidiabetic medication dose can be adjusted.
- Teach women how to perform routine breast self-examination.
- Explain to patient on cyclic therapy for postmenopausal symptoms that, although withdrawal bleeding may occur during week off drug, fertility has not been restored. Pregnancy is not possible since she has not ovulated.
- May cause fluid retention and edema. Monitor weight regularly and recommend sodium restriction, as needed.

dienestrol (dienoestrol)

DV, Ortho Dienestrol

Pregnancy Risk Category: X

HOW SUPPLIED

Vaginal cream: 0.01%

MECHANISM OF ACTION

Increases the synthesis of DNA, RNA, and protein in responsive tissues. Also reduces FSH and LH release from the pituitary.

INDICATIONS & DOSAGE

Atrophic vaginitis and kraurosis vulvae –

Postmenopausal women: 1 to 2 intravaginal applications of vaginal cream daily for 1 to 2 weeks (as directed), then half that dose for the same period. A maintenance dosage of 1 applicatorful one to three times a week may be ordered.

ADVERSE REACTIONS

Common reactions are in italics; life-threatening reactions are in bold italics.

GU: vaginal discharge; with excessive use, uterine bleeding.

Local: increased discomfort, burning sensation. Systemic effects possible.

Other: breast tenderness.

INTERACTIONS

Bromocriptine: may cause amenorrhea, interfering with the effects of bromocriptine. Avoid concomitant use.

Carbamazepine, phenobarbital, rifampin: decreased effectiveness of estrogen therapy. Monitor closely.

Corticosteroids: possible enhanced effects. Monitor closely.

Cyclosporine: increased risk of toxicity. Use together with caution and frequently monitor cyclosporine levels.

Dantrolene, other hepatotoxic medications: increased risk of hepatotoxicity. Monitor closely.

Oral anticoagulants: dosage adjustments may be necessary. Monitor prothrombin time.

Tamoxifen: estrogens may interfere with the effectiveness of tamoxifen. Avoid concomitant use.

NURSING CONSIDERATIONS

- *Contraindicated* in thrombophlebitis or thromboembolic disorders; cancer of breast, reproductive organs, or genitals; undiagnosed abnormal genital bleeding; and pregnancy.
- *Use cautiously* in menstrual irregularities or endometriosis.
- Patients should have a thorough physical examination before initiating estrogen therapy. Patients receiving long-term therapy should have repeat examinations yearly. Periodically moni-

tor body weight, blood pressure, hepatic function, and serum lipid levels.
- Instruct patient to apply drug at bedtime to increase effectiveness.
- Patient package insert that describes estrogen's adverse reactions is available. However, provide verbal explanation also.
- Systemic reactions possible with normal intravaginal use. Monitor closely.
- Warn patient not to exceed the prescribed dose.
- Withdrawal bleeding may occur if estrogen is suddenly stopped.
- Patient shouldn't wear tampon while receiving vaginal therapy. She may need to wear sanitary pad to protect clothing.
- Teach patient how to insert suppositories or cream. Wash vaginal area with soap and water before application.
- Instruct patient to remain recumbent for 30 minutes after administration to prevent loss of drug.
- Instruct patient to report breast pain or tenderness, vaginal discharge or bleeding, or swelling of the hands or feet.
- Teach patient how to perform breast self-examination.

diethylstilbestrol (stilboestrol)
DES

diethylstilbestrol diphosphate
Honvol†

Pregnancy Risk Category: X

HOW SUPPLIED

diethylstilbestrol
Tablets: 1 mg, 2.5 mg, 5 mg
diethylstilbestrol diphosphate
Tablets: 50 mg†, 83 mg†
Injection: 50 mg/ml†

MECHANISM OF ACTION

Increases the synthesis of DNA, RNA, and protein in responsive tissues. Also reduces FSH and LH release from the pituitary.

INDICATIONS & DOSAGE

Postcoital contraception ("morning-after pill") –
Women: 25 mg P.O. b.i.d. for 5 days, starting within 72 hours after coitus.
Prostatic cancer –
Men: initially, 1 to 3 mg P.O. daily; may be reduced to 1 mg P.O. daily, or 5 mg I.M. twice weekly initially, followed by up to 4 mg I.M. twice weekly. Or 50 to 200 mg (diphosphate) P.O. t.i.d.; or 0.25 to 1 g I.V. daily for 5 days, then once or twice weekly.
Breast cancer –
Men and postmenopausal women: 15 mg P.O. daily.

ADVERSE REACTIONS

Common reactions are in italics; life-threatening reactions are in bold italics.
CNS: headache, dizziness, chorea, depression, lethargy.
CV: thrombophlebitis; ***thromboembolism;*** hypertension; edema; ***increased risk of stroke, pulmonary embolism, and myocardial infarction.***
EENT: worsening of myopia or astigmatism, intolerance to contact lenses.
GI: *nausea,* vomiting, abdominal cramps, bloating, diarrhea, constipation, anorexia, increased appetite, excessive thirst, weight changes, pancreatitis.
GU: in women – breakthrough bleeding, altered menstrual flow, dysmenorrhea, amenorrhea, cervical erosion, altered cervical secretions, enlargement of uterine fibromas, vaginal candidiasis, loss of libido. In men – gynecomastia, testicular atrophy, impotence.
Hepatic: cholestatic jaundice.
Metabolic: hyperglycemia, hypercalcemia, folic acid deficiency.

Skin: melasma, urticaria, acne, seborrhea, oily skin, hirsutism or loss of hair.
Other: leg cramps, breast tenderness or enlargement.

INTERACTIONS
Bromocriptine: may cause amenorrhea, interfering with the effects of bromocriptine. Avoid concomitant use.
Carbamazepine, phenobarbital, rifampin: decreased effectiveness of estrogen therapy. Monitor closely.
Corticosteroids: possible enhanced effects. Monitor closely.
Cyclosporine: increased risk of toxicity. Use together with caution and frequently monitor cyclosporine levels.
Dantrolene, other hepatotoxic medications: increased risk of hepatotoxicity. Monitor closely.
Oral anticoagulants: dosage adjustments may be necessary. Monitor prothrombin time.
Tamoxifen: estrogens may interfere with the effectiveness of tamoxifen. Avoid concomitant use.

NURSING CONSIDERATIONS
• *Contraindicated* in thrombophlebitis or thromboembolic disorders; undiagnosed abnormal genital bleeding; and pregnancy.
• *Use cautiously* in hypertension, asthma, mental depression, bone disease, migraine, seizures, blood dyscrasias, diabetes mellitus, gallbladder disease, amenorrhea, heart failure, hepatic or renal dysfunction, and family history (mother, grandmother, sister) of breast or genital tract cancer. Development or worsening of these conditions may require discontinuation of the drug.
• Patients should have a thorough physical examination before initiating estrogen therapy. Patients receiving long-term therapy should have repeat examinations yearly. Periodically monitor body weight, blood pressure, hepatic function, and serum lipid levels.
• Patient package insert that describes estrogen's adverse reactions is available. However, provide verbal explanation also.
• Warn patient to stop taking drug immediately if she becomes pregnant, since it can affect the fetus adversely.
• Warn patient to immediately report abdominal pain; pain, numbness, or stiffness in legs or buttocks; pressure or pain in chest; shortness of breath; severe headache; visual disturbances, such as blind spots, flashing lights, or blurriness; vaginal bleeding or discharge; breast lumps; sudden weight gain; swelling of hands or feet; yellow sclera or skin; dark urine; or light-colored stools.
• Pathologist should be advised of estrogen therapy when specimen is sent.
• Patients with diabetes should report elevated blood glucose test results so antidiabetic medication dose can be adjusted.
• High incidence of gross nonmalignant genital changes in offspring of women taking drug during pregnancy. Female offspring have higher than normal risk of developing cervical and vaginal adenocarcinoma. Male offspring may have higher than normal risk of developing testicular tumors, epididymal cysts, and impaired fertility.
• Increased number of cardiovascular deaths reported in men taking diethylstilbestrol tablet (5 mg daily) for prostatic cancer over long period of time. This effect not associated with 1-mg daily dose.
• Teach women how to perform routine breast self-examination.
• If patient experiences GI upset, give drug with or immediately after meals.
• Do not crush, break, or chew enteric-coated tablets.
• **I.V. use:** Mix ordered dose in 250 to 500 ml of dextrose 5% in water or 0.9% sodium chloride injection. In-

fuse slowly at 1 to 2 ml/minute for the first 15 minutes; if no adverse reactions occur, increase infusion rate to administer entire dose within 1 hour.
• To administer I.M., give by deep injection. Rotate injection sites to prevent muscle atrophy.

esterified estrogens

Estratab, Estromed†, Menest, Neo-Estrone†

Pregnancy Risk Category: X

HOW SUPPLIED

Tablets: 0.3 mg, 0.625 mg, 1.25 mg, 2.5 mg

MECHANISM OF ACTION

Increases the synthesis of DNA, RNA, and protein in responsive tissues. Also reduces FSH and LH release from the pituitary.

INDICATIONS & DOSAGE

Inoperable prostatic cancer –
Men: 1.25 to 2.5 mg P.O. t.i.d.
Breast cancer –
Men and postmenopausal women: 10 mg P.O. t.i.d. for 3 or more months.
Hypogonadism, castration, primary ovarian failure –
Women: 2.5 mg P.O. daily to t.i.d. in cycles of 3 weeks on, 1 week off.
Menopausal symptoms –
Women: average 0.3 to 3.75 mg P.O. daily in cycles of 3 weeks on, 1 week off.

ADVERSE REACTIONS

Common reactions are in italics; life-threatening reactions are in bold italics.
CNS: headache, dizziness, chorea, depression, libido changes, lethargy.
CV: thrombophlebitis; ***thromboembolism;*** hypertension; edema; ***increased risk of stroke, pulmonary embolism, and myocardial infarction.***
EENT: worsening of myopia or astigmatism, intolerance to contact lenses.
GI: *nausea,* vomiting, abdominal cramps, bloating, diarrhea, constipation, anorexia, increased appetite, weight changes, pancreatitis.
GU: in women – breakthrough bleeding, altered menstrual flow, dysmenorrhea, amenorrhea, cervical erosion, altered cervical secretions, enlargement of uterine fibromas, vaginal candidiasis. In men – gynecomastia, testicular atrophy, impotence.
Hepatic: cholestatic jaundice.
Metabolic: hyperglycemia, hypercalcemia, folic acid deficiency.
Skin: melasma, rash, acne, hirsutism or hair loss, seborrhea, oily skin.
Other: breast changes (tenderness, enlargement, secretion).

INTERACTIONS

Bromocriptine: may cause amenorrhea, interfering with the effects of bromocriptine. Avoid concomitant use.
Carbamazepine, phenobarbital, rifampin: decreased effectiveness of estrogen therapy. Monitor closely.
Corticosteroids: possible enhanced effects. Monitor closely.
Cyclosporine: increased risk of toxicity. Use together with caution and frequently monitor cyclosporine levels.
Dantrolene, other hepatotoxic medications: increased risk of hepatotoxicity. Monitor closely.
Oral anticoagulants: dosage adjustments may be necessary. Monitor prothrombin time.
Tamoxifen: estrogens may interfere with the effectiveness of tamoxifen. Avoid concomitant use.

NURSING CONSIDERATIONS

• *Contraindicated* in thrombophlebitis or thromboembolic disorders; undiagnosed abnormal genital bleeding; and pregnancy.
• *Use cautiously* in patients with history of hypertension, mental depression, gallbladder disease, migraine, seizures, diabetes mellitus, amenor-

rhea, or family history (mother, grandmother, sister) of breast or genital tract cancer. Development or worsening of these conditions may require discontinuation of the drug.

- Patient package insert that describes estrogen's adverse reactions is available. However, provide verbal explanation also.
- Studies suggest that postmenopausal women who use estrogen replacement for more than 5 years to treat menopausal symptoms may be at increased risk for endometrial carcinoma. This risk is reduced by the use of cyclic rather than continuous therapy and use of the lowest possible dosages of estrogen. Adding progestins to the regimen decreases the incidence of endometrial hyperplasia; however, it isn't known if progestins affect the incidence of endometrial carcinoma. Most studies show no increased risk of breast cancer. Emphasize the importance of regular physical examinations.
- Patients should have a thorough physical examination before initiating estrogen therapy. Patients receiving long-term therapy should have repeat examinations yearly. Periodically monitor body weight, blood pressure, serum lipid levels, and hepatic function.
- Warn patient to immediately report abdominal pain; pain, numbness, or stiffness in legs or buttocks; pressure or pain in chest; shortness of breath; severe headaches; visual disturbances, such as blind spots, flashing lights, or blurriness; vaginal bleeding or discharge; breast lumps; swelling of hands or feet; yellow skin or sclera; dark urine; or light-colored stools.
- Pathologist should be advised of estrogen therapy when specimen is sent.
- Patients with diabetes should report elevated blood glucose test results so antidiabetic medication dosage can be adjusted.
- Explain to patient on cyclic therapy for postmenopausal symptoms that, although she may experience withdrawal bleeding during week off drug, fertility has not been restored. Pregnancy cannot occur since she has not ovulated.
- Teach women how to perform routine breast self-examination.

---

estradiol (oestradiol)
Estrace**, Estrace Vaginal Cream, Estraderm

estradiol cypionate
depGynogen, Depo-Estradiol, Dura-Estrin, E-Cypionate, Estro-Cyp, Estrofem, Estroject-L.A., Estronol-LA

estradiol valerate (oestradiol valerate)
Delestrogen, Dioval, Duragen 10, Duragen 20, Duragen 40, Estradiol L.A., Estraval, Estraval P.A., Estra-L 20, Estra-L 40, Feminate, Femogex, Gynogen L.A., L.A.E., Menaval, Primogyn Depot‡, Ru-Est-Span 20, Ru-Est-Span 40, Valergen 10, Valergen 20, Valergen 40

Pregnancy Risk Category: X

HOW SUPPLIED
estradiol
Tablets (micronized): 1 mg, 2 mg
Transdermal: 4 mg/10 cm² (delivers 0.05 mg/24 hours); 8 mg/20 cm² (delivers 0.1 mg/24 hours)
Vaginal cream (in nonliquefying base): 0.1 mg/g
estradiol cypionate
Injection (in oil): 1 mg/ml, 5 mg/ml
estradiol valerate
Injection (in oil): 10 mg/ml, 20 mg/ml, 40 mg/ml

MECHANISM OF ACTION
Increases the synthesis of DNA, RNA, and protein in responsive tis-

sues. Also reduces FSH and LH release from the pituitary.

INDICATIONS & DOSAGE

Menopausal symptoms, hypogonadism, castration, primary ovarian failure –
Women: 1 to 2 mg P.O. daily, in cycles of 21 days on and 7 days off, or cycles of 5 days on and 2 days off; or 0.2 to 1 mg I.M. weekly.
Kraurosis vulvae –
Women: 1 to 1.5 mg I.M. once or more per week.
Atrophic vaginitis –
Women: 2 to 4 g intravaginal applications of cream daily for 1 to 2 weeks. When vaginal mucosa is restored, begin maintenance dosage of 1 g one to three times weekly.
Menopausal symptoms –
Women: 1 to 5 mg (cypionate) I.M. q 3 to 4 weeks. Or 5 to 20 mg (valerate) I.M., repeated once after 2 to 3 weeks.
Postpartum breast engorgement –
Women: 10 to 25 mg (valerate) I.M. at end of first stage of labor.
Inoperable breast cancer –
Women: 10 mg P.O. (oral estradiol) t.i.d. for 3 months.
Treatment of moderate to severe symptoms of menopause, female hypogonadism, female castration, primary ovarian failure, and atrophic conditions caused by deficient endogenous estrogen production –
Women: place one Estraderm transdermal patch on trunk of the body twice weekly. Administer on an intermittent cyclic schedule (3 weeks of therapy followed by discontinuation for 1 week).
Inoperable prostatic cancer –
Men: 30 mg (valerate) I.M. q 1 to 2 weeks. Or, 1 to 2 mg (oral estradiol) t.i.d.

ADVERSE REACTIONS

Common reactions are in italics; life-threatening reactions are in bold italics.
CNS: headache, dizziness, chorea, depression, libido changes, lethargy.
CV: thrombophlebitis, ***thromboembolism,*** hypertension, edema.
EENT: worsening of myopia or astigmatism, intolerance to contact lenses.
GI: *nausea,* vomiting, abdominal cramps, bloating, diarrhea, constipation, anorexia, increased appetite, weight changes, pancreatitis.
GU: in women – breakthrough bleeding, altered menstrual flow, dysmenorrhea, amenorrhea, cervical erosion, altered cervical secretions, enlargement of uterine fibromas, vaginal candidiasis. In men – gynecomastia, testicular atrophy, impotence.
Hepatic: cholestatic jaundice.
Metabolic: hyperglycemia, hypercalcemia, folic acid deficiency.
Skin: melasma, urticaria, acne, seborrhea, oily skin, hirsutism or hair loss.
Other: breast changes (tenderness, enlargement, secretion), leg cramps.

INTERACTIONS

Bromocriptine: may cause amenorrhea, interfering with the effects of bromocriptine. Avoid concomitant use.
Carbamazepine, phenobarbital, rifampin: decreased effectiveness of estrogen therapy. Monitor closely.
Corticosteroids: possible enhanced effects. Monitor closely.
Cyclosporine: increased risk of toxicity. Use together with caution and frequently monitor cyclosporine levels.
Dantrolene, other hepatotoxic medications: increased risk of hepatotoxicity. Monitor closely.
Oral anticoagulants: dosage adjustments may be necessary. Monitor prothrombin time.
Tamoxifen: estrogens may interfere with the effectiveness of tamoxifen. Avoid concomitant use.

*Liquid form contains alcohol. **May contain tartrazine.

NURSING CONSIDERATIONS

- *Contraindicated* in thrombophlebitis or thromboembolic disorders; cancer of breast, reproductive organs; undiagnosed abnormal genital bleeding; and pregnancy.
- *Use cautiously* in hypertension, mental depression, bone diseases, blood dyscrasias, migraine, seizures, diabetes mellitus, amenorrhea, heart failure, hepatic or renal dysfunction, or family history (mother, grandmother, sister) of breast or genital tract cancer. Development or worsening of these conditions may require discontinuation of the drug.
- Studies suggest that postmenopausal women who use estrogen replacement for more than 5 years to treat menopausal symptoms may be at increased risk for endometrial carcinoma. This risk is reduced by the use of cyclic rather than continuous therapy and use of the lowest possible dosages of estrogen. Adding progestins to the regimen decreases the incidence of endometrial hyperplasia; however, it isn't known if progestins affect the incidence of endometrial carcinoma. Most studies show no increased risk of breast cancer. Emphasize the importance of regular physical examinations.
- Patients should have a thorough physical examination before initiating estrogen therapy. Patients receiving long-term therapy should have repeat examinations yearly. Periodically monitor serum lipid levels, blood pressure, body weight, and hepatic function.
- Patient package insert that describes estrogen's adverse reactions is available. However, provide verbal explanation also.
- Warn patient to immediately report abdominal pain; pain, numbness, or stiffness in legs or buttocks; pressure or pain in chest; shortness of breath; severe headaches; visual disturbances, such as blind spots, flashing lights, or blurriness; vaginal bleeding or discharge; breast lumps; swelling of hands or feet; yellow skin or sclera; dark urine; or light-colored stools.
- Patients with diabetes should report elevated blood glucose test results so antidiabetic medication dosage can be adjusted.
- Pathologist should be advised of estrogen therapy when specimen is sent.
- Ask patient about allergies, especially to foods or plants. Estradiol is available as an aqueous solution or as a solution in peanut oil. Estradiol cypionate is available as a solution in cottonseed oil or vegetable oil. Estradiol valerate is available as a solution in castor oil, sesame oil, or vegetable oil.
- Teach patient how to use vaginal cream. Patient should wash vaginal area with soap and water before applying. Tell her to take drug at bedtime or to lie flat for 30 minutes after instillation to minimize drug loss.
- To administer as an injection, make sure drug is well dispersed in solution by rolling vial between palms. Inject deep I.M. into large muscle. Rotate injection sites to prevent muscle atrophy. Drug should never be given I.V.
- Transdermal patch should be applied to clean, dry, hairless, intact skin on abdomen or buttocks. Do not apply to breasts, waistline, or other areas where clothing can loosen the patch. When applying, ensure good contact with the skin, especially around the edges, and hold in place with the palm for about 10 seconds. Rotate application sites.
- In women who are currently taking oral estrogen, treatment with the Estraderm transdermal patch can begin 1 week after withdrawal of oral therapy or sooner if symptoms appear before the end of the week.
- Teach women how to perform routine breast self-examination.
- Explain to patient on cyclic therapy for postmenopausal symptoms that,

although withdrawal bleeding may occur during week off drug, fertility has not been restored. Pregnancy cannot occur since she has not ovulated.

estrogens, conjugated (estrogenic substances, conjugated; oestrogens, conjugated)

C.E.S.†, Conjugated Estrogens C.S.D.†, Premarin, Premarin Intravenous, Progens

Pregnancy Risk Category: X

HOW SUPPLIED

Tablets: 0.3 mg, 0.625 mg, 0.9 mg, 1.25 mg, 2.5 mg
Injection: 25 mg/5 ml
Vaginal cream: 0.625 mg/g

MECHANISM OF ACTION

Increases the synthesis of DNA, RNA, and protein in responsive tissues. Also reduces FSH and LH release from the pituitary.

INDICATIONS & DOSAGE

Abnormal uterine bleeding (hormonal imbalance) –
Women: 25 mg I.V. or I.M. Repeat in 6 to 12 hours.
Breast cancer (at least 5 years after menopause) –
Women: 10 mg P.O. t.i.d. for 3 months or more.
Castration, primary ovarian failure, and osteoporosis –
Women: 1.25 mg P.O. daily in cycles of 3 weeks on, 1 week off.
Hypogonadism –
Women: 2.5 mg P.O. b.i.d. or t.i.d. for 20 consecutive days each month.
Menopausal symptoms –
Women: 0.3 to 1.25 mg P.O. daily in cycles of 3 weeks on, 1 week off.
Postpartum breast engorgement –
Women: 3.75 mg P.O. q 4 hours for five doses or 1.25 mg q 4 hours for 5 days.
Treatment of atrophic vaginitis, kraurosis vulvae associated with menopause –
Women: 2 to 4 g intravaginally on a cyclical basis (3 weeks on, 1 week off).
Inoperable prostatic cancer –
Men: 1.25 to 2.5 mg P.O. t.i.d.

ADVERSE REACTIONS

Common reactions are in italics; life-threatening reactions are in bold italics.
CNS: headache, dizziness, chorea, depression, libido changes, lethargy.
CV: thrombophlebitis; ***thromboembolism;*** hypertension; edema; ***increased risk of stroke, pulmonary embolism, and myocardial infarction.***
EENT: worsening of myopia or astigmatism, intolerance to contact lenses.
GI: *nausea,* vomiting, abdominal cramps, bloating, diarrhea, constipation, anorexia, increased appetite, weight changes, pancreatitis.
GU: in women – breakthrough bleeding, altered menstrual flow, dysmenorrhea, amenorrhea, cervical erosion, altered cervical secretions, enlargement of uterine fibromas, vaginal candidiasis. In men – gynecomastia, testicular atrophy, impotence.
Hepatic: cholestatic jaundice.
Metabolic: hyperglycemia, hypercalcemia, folic acid deficiency.
Skin: melasma, urticaria, acne, seborrhea, oily skin, flushing (when given rapidly I.V.), hirsutism or loss of hair.
Other: breast changes (tenderness, enlargement, secretion), leg cramps.

INTERACTIONS

Bromocriptine: may cause amenorrhea, interfering with the effects of bromocriptine. Avoid concomitant use.
Carbamazepine, phenobarbital, rifampin: decreased effectiveness of estrogen therapy. Monitor closely.
Corticosteroids: possible enhanced effects. Monitor closely.
Cyclosporine: increased risk of toxic-

*Liquid form contains alcohol. **May contain tartrazine.

ity. Use together with caution and frequently monitor cyclosporine levels.
Dantrolene, other hepatotoxic medications: increased risk of hepatotoxicity. Monitor closely.
Oral anticoagulants: dosage adjustments may be necessary. Monitor prothrombin time.
Tamoxifen: estrogens may interfere with the effectiveness of tamoxifen. Avoid concomitant use.

NURSING CONSIDERATIONS

- *Contraindicated* in thrombophlebitis or thromboembolic disorders; undiagnosed abnormal genital bleeding; and pregnancy.
- *Use cautiously* in hypertension, gallbladder disease, bone diseases, blood dyscrasias, migraine, seizures, diabetes mellitus, amenorrhea, heart failure, hepatic or renal dysfunction, or family history (mother, grandmother, sister) of breast or genital tract cancer. Development or worsening of these conditions may require discontinuation of the drug.
- Studies suggest that postmenopausal women who use estrogen replacement for more than 5 years to treat menopausal symptoms may be at increased risk for endometrial carcinoma. This risk is reduced by the use of cyclic rather than continuous therapy and use of the lowest possible dosages of estrogen. Adding progestins to the regimen decreases the incidence of endometrial hyperplasia; however, it isn't known if progestins affect the incidence of endometrial carcinoma. Most studies show no increased risk of breast cancer. Emphasize the importance of regular physical examinations.
- Patients should have a thorough physical examination before initiating estrogen therapy. Patients receiving long-term therapy should have repeat examinations yearly. Periodically monitor serum lipid levels, blood pressure, body weight, and hepatic function.
- Patient package insert that describes estrogen's adverse reactions is available. However, provide verbal explanation also.
- Warn patient to immediately report abdominal pain; pain, numbness, or stiffness in legs or buttocks; pressure or pain in chest; shortness of breath; severe headaches; visual disturbances, such as blind spots, flashing lights, or blurriness; vaginal bleeding or discharge; breast lumps; swelling of hands or feet; yellow skin or sclera; dark urine; or light-colored stools.
- Teach patient how to use vaginal cream. Patient should wash the vaginal area with soap and water before applying. Tell her to take drug at bedtime or to lie flat for 30 minutes after instillation to minimize drug loss.
- I.M. or I.V. use preferred for rapid treatment of dysfunctional uterine bleeding or reduction of surgical bleeding.
- **I.V. use:** When giving by direct I.V. injection, administer slowly to avoid flushing reaction. If drug is to be infused, mix with dextrose, saline, or invert sugar solutions. Avoid mixing with solutions of acidic pH to prevent incompatibility.
- Refrigerate before reconstituting. Agitate gently after adding diluent.
- When administering by I.M. injection, inject deep into large muscle. Rotate injection sites to prevent muscle atrophy.
- Pathologist should be advised of estrogen therapy when specimen is sent.
- Patients with diabetes should report elevated blood glucose test results so antidiabetic medication dosage can be adjusted.
- Teach women how to perform routine breast self-examination.
- Explain to patient on cyclic therapy for postmenopausal symptoms that, although withdrawal bleeding may occur during week off drug, fertility has

not been restored. Pregnancy cannot occur since she has not ovulated.

estrone (oestrone)

Estrone "5", Estrone Aqueous, Estronol, Kestrone, Theelin Aqueous

Pregnancy Risk Category: X

HOW SUPPLIED

Injection (aqueous suspension): 2 mg/ml, 5 mg/ml

MECHANISM OF ACTION

Increases the synthesis of DNA, RNA, and protein in responsive tissues. Also reduces FSH and LH release from the pituitary.

INDICATIONS & DOSAGE

Atrophic vaginitis and menopausal symptoms –
Women: 0.1 to 0.5 mg I.M. two or three times weekly.
Female hypogonadism and primary ovarian failure –
Women: 0.1 to 1 mg I.M. weekly in single or divided doses.
Inoperable prostatic cancer –
Men: 2 to 4 mg I.M. 2 to 3 times weekly.

ADVERSE REACTIONS

Common reactions are in italics; life-threatening reactions are in bold italics.
CNS: headache, dizziness, chorea, depression, libido changes, lethargy.
CV: thrombophlebitis, ***thromboembolism,*** hypertension, edema.
EENT: worsening of myopia or astigmatism, intolerance to contact lenses.
GI: *nausea,* vomiting, abdominal cramps, bloating, diarrhea, constipation, anorexia, increased appetite, weight changes, pancreatitis.
GU: in women – breakthrough bleeding, altered menstrual flow, dysmenorrhea, amenorrhea, cervical erosion, altered cervical secretions, enlargement of uterine fibromas, vaginal candidiasis. In men – gynecomastia, testicular atrophy, impotence.
Hepatic: cholestatic jaundice.
Metabolic: hyperglycemia, hypercalcemia, folic acid deficiency.
Skin: melasma, urticaria, acne, seborrhea, oily skin, hirsutism or hair loss.
Other: breast changes (tenderness, enlargement, secretion), leg cramps.

INTERACTIONS

Bromocriptine: may cause amenorrhea, interfering with the effects of bromocriptine. Avoid concomitant use.
Carbamazepine, phenobarbital, rifampin: decreased effectiveness of estrogen therapy. Monitor closely.
Corticosteroids: possible enhanced effects. Monitor closely.
Cyclosporine: increased risk of toxicity. Use together with caution and frequently monitor cyclosporine levels.
Dantrolene, other hepatotoxic medications: increased risk of hepatotoxicity. Monitor closely.
Oral anticoagulants: dosage adjustments may be necessary. Monitor prothrombin time.
Tamoxifen: estrogens may interfere with the effectiveness of tamoxifen. Avoid concomitant use.

NURSING CONSIDERATIONS

- *Contraindicated* in thrombophlebitis or thromboembolic disorders; cancer of breast or reproductive organs; undiagnosed abnormal genital bleeding; and pregnancy.
- *Use cautiously* in hypertension, mental depression, migraine, seizures, diabetes mellitus, amenorrhea, hepatic or renal dysfunction, or family history (mother, grandmother, sister) of breast or genital tract cancer. Development or worsening of these conditions may require discontinuation of the drug.
- Estrone must be administered I.M.

Rotate injection sites to prevent muscle atrophy.
- Studies suggest that postmenopausal women who use estrogen replacement for more than 5 years to treat menopausal symptoms may be at increased risk for endometrial carcinoma. This risk is reduced by the use of cyclic rather than continuous therapy and use of the lowest possible dosages of estrogen. Adding progestins to the regimen decreases the incidence of endometrial hyperplasia; however, it isn't known if progestins affect the incidence of endometrial carcinoma. Most studies show no increased risk of breast cancer. Emphasize the importance of regular physical examinations.
- Patients should have a thorough physical examination before initiating estrogen therapy. Patients receiving long-term therapy should have repeat examinations yearly. Periodically monitor serum lipid levels, blood pressure, body weight, and hepatic function.
- Patient package insert that describes estrogen's adverse reactions is available. However, provide verbal explanation also.
- Warn patient to immediately report abdominal pain; pain, numbness, or stiffness in legs or buttocks; pressure or pain in chest; shortness of breath; severe headaches; visual disturbances, such as blind spots, flashing lights, or blurriness; vaginal bleeding or discharge; breast lumps; swelling of hands or feet; yellow skin and sclera; dark urine; or light-colored stools.
- Pathologist should be advised of estrogen therapy when specimen is sent.
- Patients with diabetes should report elevated blood glucose test results so antidiabetic medication dosage can be adjusted.
- Teach women how to perform routine breast self-examination.
- Explain to patient on cyclic therapy for postmenopausal symptoms that, although withdrawal bleeding may occur during week off drug, fertility has not been restored. Pregnancy cannot occur since she has not ovulated.

estropipate (piperazine estrone sulfate)

Ogen,† OrthoEST

Pregnancy Risk Category: X

HOW SUPPLIED

Tablets: 0.625 mg, 1.25 mg, 1.5 mg, 2.5 mg, 5 mg
Vaginal cream: 1.5 mg estropipate/g

MECHANISM OF ACTION

Increases the synthesis of DNA, RNA, and proteins in responsive tissues.

INDICATIONS & DOSAGE

Atrophic vaginitis, kraurosis vulvae, or moderate to severe vasomotor symptoms associated with menopause –
Women: 0.625 to 5 mg P.O. daily. Dosage is usually given on a cyclical, short-term basis.
Primary ovarian failure, female castration, or female hypogonadism –
Women: administer on a cyclical basis – 1.25 to 7.5 mg P.O. daily for the first 3 weeks, followed by a rest period of 8 to 10 days. If bleeding does not occur by the end of the rest period, repeat cycle.
Atrophic vaginitis or kraurosis vulvae –
Women: 2 to 4 g of vaginal cream daily. Administration should be cyclic and short term (3 weeks on and 1 week off)
Prevention of osteoporosis –
Women: 0.625 mg P.O. daily for 25 days of a 31-day cycle each month.

ADVERSE REACTIONS

Common reactions are in italics; life-threatening reactions are in bold italics.

CNS: depression, headache, dizziness, migraine, changes in libido.
CV: edema, thrombophlebitis; ***increased risk of stroke, pulmonary embolism, and myocardial infarction.***
GI: nausea, vomiting, abdominal cramps, bloating, cholestatic jaundice.
GU: increased size of uterine fibromyomata, vaginal candidiasis, cystitis-like syndrome, dysmenorrhea, amenorrhea, breakthrough bleeding, premenstrual-like syndrome.
Skin: hemorrhagic eruption, erythema nodosum, erythema multiforme, hirsutism, chloasma, hair loss.
Other: breast engorgement or enlargement, weight changes, aggravation of porphyria.

INTERACTIONS

Bromocriptine: may cause amenorrhea, interfering with the effects of bromocriptine. Avoid concomitant use.
Carbamazepine, phenobarbital, rifampin: decreased effectiveness of estrogen therapy. Monitor closely.
Corticosteroids: possible enhanced effects. Monitor closely.
Cyclosporine: increased risk of toxicity. Use together with caution and frequently monitor cyclosporine levels.
Dantrolene, other hepatotoxic medications: increased risk of hepatotoxicity. Monitor closely.
Oral anticoagulants: dosage adjustments may be necessary. Monitor prothrombin time.
Tamoxifen: estrogens may interfere with the effectiveness of tamoxifen. Avoid concomitant use.

NURSING CONSIDERATIONS

- *Contraindicated* in thrombophlebitis or thromboembolic disorders; cancer of the breast, reproductive organs, or genitals; undiagnosed genital bleeding; and pregnancy.
- *Use cautiously* in hypertension, asthma, mental depression, bone diseases, blood dyscrasias, gallbladder disease, migraine, seizures, diabetes mellitus, amenorrhea, heart failure, hepatic or renal dysfunction, and a family history of breast or genital cancer. Development or worsening of any of these conditions may require discontinuation of the drug.
- Studies suggest that postmenopausal women who use estrogen replacement for more than 5 years to treat menopausal symptoms may be at increased risk for endometrial carcinoma. This risk is reduced by the use of cyclic rather than continuous therapy and use of the lowest possible dosages of estrogen. Adding progestins to the regimen decreases the incidence of endometrial hyperplasia; however, it isn't known if progestins effect the incidence of endometrial carcinoma. Most studies show no increased risk of breast cancer. Stress the importance of regular physical examinations.
- Patients should have a thorough physical examination before initiating estrogen therapy. Patients receiving long-term therapy should have repeat examinations yearly. Periodically monitor serum lipid levels, blood pressure, body weight, and hepatic function.
- A patient package insert is available to describe the adverse reactions of estrogens, including the increased risk of endometrial carcinoma. However, provide a verbal explanation as well.
- Warn patient to immediately report abdominal pain; pain, stiffness, or numbness in the legs or buttocks; pressure or pain in the chest; shortness of breath; severe headaches; visual disturbances, such as blind spots or flashing lights; vaginal bleeding or discharge; breast lumps; swelling of the hands or feet; yellow skin or sclera; dark urine; or light-colored stools.

• Teach patient how to perform breast self-examination.
• When used to treat hypogonadism, the duration of therapy necessary to produce withdrawal bleeding depends upon the individual's endometrial response to the drug. If satisfactory withdrawal bleeding does not occur, an oral progestin may have to be added to the regimen. Explain to the patient that, despite the return of withdrawal bleeding, pregnancy is not possible since she is not ovulating.

ethinyl estradiol (ethinyloestradiol)

Estinyl**, Feminone

Pregnancy Risk Category: X

HOW SUPPLIED

Tablets: 0.02 mg, 0.05 mg, and 0.5 mg

MECHANISM OF ACTION

Increases the synthesis of DNA, RNA, and protein in responsive tissues. Also reduces FSH and LH release from the pituitary.

INDICATIONS & DOSAGE

Breast cancer (at least 5 years after menopause) –
Women: 1 mg P.O. t.i.d.
Hypogonadism –
Women: 0.05 mg P.O. daily to t.i.d. for 2 weeks a month, followed by 2 weeks progesterone therapy; continue for 3 to 6 monthly dosing cycles, followed by 2 months off.
Menopausal symptoms –
Women: 0.02 to 0.05 mg P.O. daily for cycles of 3 weeks on, 1 week off.
Inoperable prostatic cancer –
Men: 0.15 to 2 mg P.O. daily.

ADVERSE REACTIONS

Common reactions are in italics; life-threatening reactions are in bold italics.
CNS: headache, dizziness, chorea, depression, libido changes, lethargy.
CV: thrombophlebitis, ***thromboembolism***, hypertension, edema.
EENT: worsening of myopia or astigmatism, intolerance to contact lenses.
GI: *nausea,* vomiting, abdominal cramps, bloating, diarrhea, constipation, anorexia, increased appetite, weight changes.
GU: in women – breakthrough bleeding, altered menstrual flow, dysmenorrhea, amenorrhea, cervical erosion, altered cervical secretions, enlargement of uterine fibromas, vaginal candidiasis. In men – gynecomastia, testicular atrophy, impotence.
Hepatic: cholestatic jaundice.
Metabolic: hyperglycemia, hypercalcemia, folic acid deficiency.
Skin: melasma, urticaria, acne, seborrhea, oily skin, hirsutism or hair loss.
Other: breast changes (tenderness, enlargement, secretion), leg cramps.

INTERACTIONS

Bromocriptine: may cause amenorrhea, interfering with the effects of bromocriptine. Avoid concomitant use.
Carbamazepine, phenobarbital, rifampin: decreased effectiveness of estrogen therapy. Monitor closely.
Corticosteroids: possible enhanced effects. Monitor closely.
Cyclosporine: increased risk of toxicity. Use together with caution and frequently monitor cyclosporine levels.
Dantrolene, other hepatotoxic medications: increased risk of hepatotoxicity. Monitor closely.
Oral anticoagulants: dosage adjustments may be necessary. Monitor prothrombin time.
Tamoxifen: estrogens may interfere with the effectiveness of tamoxifen. Avoid concomitant use.

NURSING CONSIDERATIONS

• *Contraindicated* in thrombophlebitis or thromboembolic disorders; undiagnosed abnormal genital bleeding; and pregnancy.

• *Use cautiously* in hypertension, mental depression, bone diseases, migraine, seizures, blood dyscrasias, diabetes mellitus, amenorrhea, heart failure, hepatic or renal dysfunction, or family history (mother, grandmother, sister) of breast or genital tract cancer. Development or worsening of these conditions may require discontinuation of the drug.

• Studies suggest that postmenopausal women who use estrogen replacement for more than 5 years to treat menopausal symptoms may be at increased risk for endometrial carcinoma. This risk is reduced by the use of cyclic rather than continuous therapy and use of the lowest possible dosages of estrogen. Adding progestins to the regimen decreases the incidence of endometrial hyperplasia; however, it isn't known if progestins affect the incidence of endometrial carcinoma. Most studies show no increased risk of breast cancer. Emphasize the importance of regular physical examinations.

• Patients should have a thorough physical examination before initiating estrogen therapy. Patients receiving long-term therapy should have repeat examinations yearly. Periodically monitor serum lipid levels, blood pressure, body weight, and hepatic function.

• Patient package insert that describes estrogen's adverse reactions is available. However, provide verbal explanation also.

• Warn patient to immediately report abdominal pain; pain, numbness, or stiffness in legs or buttocks; pressure or pain in chest; shortness of breath; severe headaches; visual disturbances, such as blind spots, flashing lights, or blurriness; vaginal bleeding or discharge; breast lumps; swelling of hands or feet; yellow skin or sclera; dark urine; or light-colored stools.

• Pathologist should be advised of estrogen therapy when specimen is sent.

• Patients with diabetes should report elevated blood glucose test results so antidiabetic medication dosage can be adjusted.

• Teach women how to perform routine breast self-examination.

• Explain to patient on cyclic therapy for postmenopausal symptoms that, although withdrawal bleeding may occur during week off drug, fertility has not been restored. Pregnancy cannot occur because she has not ovulated.

ethinyl estradiol and desogestrel

monophasic: Desogen

ethinyl estradiol and ethynodiol diacetate

monophasic: Demulen 1/35, Demulen 1/50

ethinyl estradiol and levonorgestrel

monophasic: Levlen, Nordette
triphasic: Tri-Levlen, Triphasil

ethinyl estradiol and norethindrone

monophasic: Brevicon, Genora 0.5/35, Genora 1/35, Modicon, N.E.E. 1/35, Nelova 0.5/35 E, Nelova 1/35 E, Norcept-E 1/35, Norethin 1/35 E, Norinyl 1 + 35, Ortho-Novum 1/35, Ovcon-35, Ovcon-50
biphasic: Nelova 10/11, Ortho Novum 10/11
triphasic: Ortho Novum 7/7/7, Tri-Norinyl

ethinyl estradiol and norethindrone acetate

monophasic: Loestrin 21 1/20, Loestrin 21 1.5/30, Norlestrin 21 1/50, Norlestrin 21 2.5/50

*Liquid form contains alcohol. **May contain tartrazine.

ethinyl estradiol and norgestimate
monophasic: Ortho Cyclen

ethinyl estradiol and norgestrel
monophasic: Lo/Ovral, Ovral

ethinyl estradiol, norethindrone acetate, and ferrous fumarate
monophasic: Loestrin Fe 1/20, Loestrin Fe 1.5/30, Norlestrin Fe 1/50, Norlestrin Fe 2.5/50

mestranol and norethindrone
monophasic: Genora 1/50, Nelova 1/50 M, Norethin 1/50 M, Norinyl 1 + 50, Ortho-Novum 1/50

Pregnancy Risk Category: X

HOW SUPPLIED

Monophasic oral contraceptives

ethinyl estradiol and desogestrel
Tablets: ethinyl estradiol 30 mcg and desogestrel 0.15 mg (Desogen)

ethinyl estradiol and ethynodiol diacetate
Tablets: ethinyl estradiol 35 mcg and ethynodiol diacetate 1 mg (Demulen 1/35); ethinyl estradiol 50 mcg and ethynodiol diacetate 1 mg (Demulen 1/50)

ethinyl estradiol and levonorgestrel
Tablets: ethinyl estradiol 30 mcg and levonorgestrel 0.15 mg (Levlen, Nordette)

ethinyl estradiol and norethindrone
Tablets: ethinyl estradiol 35 mcg and norethindrone 0.4 mg (Ovcon-35); ethinyl estradiol 35 mcg and norethindrone 0.5 mg (Brevicon, Genora 0.5/35, Modicon, Nelova 0.5/35E); ethinyl estradiol 35 mcg and norethindrone 1 mg (Genora 1/35, N.E.E. 1/35, Nelova 1/35 E, Norcept-E 1/35, Norethin 1/35 E, Norinyl 1 + 35, Ortho-Novum 1/35), ethinyl estradiol 50 mcg and norethindrone 1 mg (Ovcon-50)

ethinyl estradiol and norethindrone acetate
Tablets: ethinyl estradiol 20 mcg and norethindrone acetate 1 mg (Loestrin 21 1/20); ethinyl estradiol 30 mcg and norethindrone acetate 1.5 mg (Loestrin 21 1.5/30); ethinyl estradiol 50 mcg and norethindrone acetate 1 mg (Norlestrin 21 1/50); ethinyl estradiol 50 mcg and norethindrone acetate 2.5 mg (Norlestrin 21 2.5/50)

ethinyl estradiol and norgestrel
Tablets: ethinyl estradiol 30 mcg and norgestrel 0.3 mg (Lo/Ovral); ethinyl estradiol 50 mcg and norgestrel 0.5 mg (Ovral)

ethinyl estradiol, norethindrone acetate, and ferrous fumarate
Tablets: ethinyl estradiol 20 mcg, norethindrone acetate 1 mg, and ferrous fumarate 75 mg (Loestrin Fe 1/20); ethinyl estradiol 30 mcg, norethindrone acetate 1.5 mg, and ferrous fumarate 75 mg (Loestrin Fe 1.5/30); ethinyl estradiol 50 mcg, norethindrone acetate 1 mg, and ferrous fumarate 75 mg (Norlestrin Fe 1/50); ethinyl estradiol 50 mcg, norethindrone acetate 2.5 mg, and ferrous fumarate 75 mg (Norlestrin Fe 2.5/50)

ethinyl estradiol and norgestimate
Tablets: ethinyl estradiol 35 mcg and norgestimate 0.250 mg (Ortho Cyclen)

mestranol and norethindrone
Tablets: mestranol 50 mcg and norethindrone 1 mg (Genora 1/50, Nelova 1/50 M, Norethin 1/50 M, Norinyl 1 + 50, Ortho-Novum 1/50)

Biphasic oral contraceptives

ethinyl estradiol and norethindrone
Tablets: ethinyl estradiol 35 mcg and norethindrone 0.5 mg during phase 1 [10 days]; ethinyl estradiol 35 mcg and norethindrone 1 mg during phase 2 [11 days] (Nelova 10/11, Ortho Novum 10/11)

Triphasic oral contraceptives

ethinyl estradiol and levonorgestrel
Tablets: (Tri-Levlen, Triphasil) ethinyl estradiol 35 mcg and levonorges-

trel 0.05 mg during phase 1 [6 days]; ethinyl estradiol 35 mcg and levonorgestrel 0.075 mg during phase 2 [5 days]; ethinyl estradiol 35 mcg and levonorgestrel 0.125 mg during phase 3 [10 days]

ethinyl estradiol and norethindrone
Tablets: (Tri-Norinyl) ethinyl estradiol 35 mcg and norethindrone 0.5 mg during phase 1 [7 days]; ethinyl estradiol 35 mcg and norethindrone 1 mg during phase 2 [9 days]; ethinyl estradiol 35 mcg and norethindrone 0.5 mg during phase 3 [5 days]; (Ortho Novum 7/7/7) ethinyl estradiol 35 mcg and norethindrone 0.5 mg during phase 1 [7 days]; ethinyl estradiol 35 mcg and norethindrone 0.75 mg during phase 2 [7 days]; ethinyl estradiol 35 mcg and norethindrone 1 mg during phase 3 [7 days]

MECHANISM OF ACTION

Oral contraceptives inhibit ovulation through a negative feedback mechanism directed at the hypothalamus. They may also prevent transport of the ovum through the fallopian tubes.

Estrogen suppresses secretion of follicle-stimulating hormone, blocking follicular development and ovulation.

Progestin suppresses luteinizing hormone secretion so ovulation can't occur even if the follicle develops. Progestin thickens cervical mucus, which interferes with sperm migration, and also causes endometrial changes that prevent implantation of the fertilized ovum.

INDICATIONS & DOSAGE

Contraception –
Women: 1 tablet P.O. daily, beginning on day 5 of menstrual cycle (first day of menstrual flow is day 1). With 20- and 21-tablet packages, new dosing cycle begins 7 days after last tablet taken. With 28-tablet packages, dosage is 1 tablet daily without interruption; extra tablets are placebos or contain iron. If only 1 or 2 doses are missed, dosage may continue on schedule. If 3 or more doses are missed, remaining tablets in monthly package must be discarded and another contraceptive method substituted. If next menstrual period doesn't begin on schedule, rule out pregnancy before starting new dosing cycle. If menstrual period begins, start new dosing cycle 7 days after last tablet was taken. If all doses have been taken on schedule and 1 menstrual period is missed, continue dosing cycle. If 2 consecutive menstrual periods are missed, pregnancy test is required before new dosing cycle is started.
Biphasic oral contraceptives –
1 color tablet P.O. daily for 10 days, then next color tablet for 11 days.
Triphasic oral contraceptives –
1 tablet P.O. daily in the sequence specified by the brand.
Endometriosis –
Women: Enovid 5 mg or 10 mg – 1 tablet P.O. daily for 2 weeks starting on day 5 of menstrual cycle. Continue without interruption for 6 to 9 months, increasing dose by 5 to 10 mg q 2 weeks, up to 20 mg daily. Up to 40 mg daily may be needed if breakthrough bleeding occurs.

ADVERSE REACTIONS

Common reactions are in italics; life-threatening reactions are in bold italics.
CNS: *headache, dizziness,* depression, libido changes, lethargy, migraine.
CV: ***thromboembolism,*** hypertension, edema.
EENT: worsening of myopia or astigmatism, intolerance to contact lenses.
GI: *nausea,* vomiting, abdominal cramps, bloating, diarrhea, constipation, anorexia, changes in appetite, weight gain, *bowel ischemia,* pancreatitis.
GU: *breakthrough bleeding,* granulomatous colitis, dysmenorrhea, amen-

*Liquid form contains alcohol. **May contain tartrazine.

orrhea, cervical erosion or abnormal secretions, enlargement of uterine fibromas, vaginal candidiasis.
Hepatic: gallbladder disease, cholestatic jaundice, liver tumors.
Metabolic: hyperglycemia, hypercalcemia, folic acid deficiency.
Skin: rash, acne, seborrhea, oily skin, ***erythema multiforme,*** hyperpigmentation.
Other: *breast tenderness,* enlargement, secretion.

Adverse reactions may be more serious, frequent, and rapid in onset with high-dose than with low-dose combinations.

INTERACTIONS

Bromocriptine: may cause amenorrhea, interfering with the effects of bromocriptine. Avoid concomitant use.
Carbamazepine, phenobarbital, rifampin: decreased effectiveness of estrogen therapy. Monitor closely.
Corticosteroids: possible enhanced effects. Monitor closely.
Cyclosporine: increased risk of toxicity. Use together with caution and frequently monitor cyclosporine levels.
Dantrolene, other hepatotoxic medications: increased risk of hepatotoxicity. Monitor closely.
Oral anticoagulants: dosage adjustments may be necessary. Monitor prothrombin time.
Tamoxifen: estrogens may interfere with the effectiveness of tamoxifen. Avoid concomitant use.

NURSING CONSIDERATIONS

- *Contraindicated* in thromboembolic disorders, cerebrovascular or coronary artery disease, myocardial infarction, known or suspected cancer of breasts or reproductive organs, benign or malignant liver tumors, undiagnosed abnormal vaginal bleeding, known or suspected pregnancy, lactation; and in adolescents with incomplete epiphyseal closure. Also contraindicated in women 35 years or older who smoke more than 15 cigarettes a day, and in all women over 40 years.
- *Use cautiously* in patients with systemic lupus erythematosus, hypertension, mental depression, migraine, epilepsy, asthma, diabetes mellitus, amenorrhea, scanty or irregular periods, fibrocystic breast disease, family history (mother, grandmother, sister) of breast or genital tract cancer, renal or gallbladder disease. Report development or worsening of these conditions to doctor. Prolonged therapy inadvisable in women who plan to become pregnant.
- Discontinue if patient develops granulomatous colitis while on oral contraceptives.
- Discontinue at least 1 week before surgery to decrease risk of thromboembolism. Use an alternative method of birth control.
- If one menstrual period is missed and tablets have been taken on schedule, tell patient to continue taking them. If two consecutive menstrual periods are missed, tell patient to stop drug and to have pregnancy test. Progestins may cause birth defects if taken early in pregnancy.
- Missed doses in midcycle greatly increase likelihood of pregnancy.
- If one tablet is missed, tell patient to take it as soon as remembered, or take two tablets the next day and continue regular schedule. If patient misses 2 consecutive days, she should take two tablets daily for 2 days, and resume normal schedule. Patient should use an additional method of birth control for 7 days after two missed doses.
- Warn patient that headache, nausea, dizziness, breast tenderness, spotting, and breakthrough bleeding are common at first. These should diminish after 3 to 6 dosing cycles (months). However, breakthrough bleeding in patients taking high-dose estrogen-progestin combinations for menstrual

disorders may necessitate dosage adjustment.

- Warn patient to immediately report abdominal pain; numbness, stiffness, or pain in legs or buttocks; pressure or pain in chest; shortness of breath; severe headache; visual disturbances, such as blind spots, blurriness, or flashing lights; undiagnosed vaginal bleeding or discharge; two consecutive missed menstrual periods; lumps in the breast; swelling of hands or feet; or severe pain in the abdomen (tumor rupture in the liver).
- Advise patient to use an additional method of birth control for the first week of administration in the initial cycle. Some doctors instruct patients to also use condoms or a diaphragm with spermicide.
- Tell patient to take tablets at same time each day; nighttime dosing may reduce nausea and headaches.
- Advise patient not to take same drug for longer than 12 months without consulting doctor. Stress importance of Pap smears and annual gynecologic examinations.
- Warn the patient of possible delay in achieving pregnancy when drug is discontinued.
- Many doctors recommend that women not become pregnant within 2 months after stopping drug. Advise patient to check with her doctor about how soon pregnancy may be attempted after hormonal therapy is stopped.
- Teach the patient how to perform a breast self-examination.
- Advise the patient of increased risks associated with simultaneous use of cigarettes and oral contraceptives.
- Periodically monitor serum lipid levels, blood pressure, body weight, and hepatic function.
- Many laboratory tests are affected by oral contraceptives; some include increase in serum bilirubin, alkaline phosphatase, AST (SGOT), ALT (SGPT), and protein-bound iodine; decrease in glucose tolerance and urinary excretion of 17-hydroxycorticosteroids (17-OHCS).
- Estrogens and progestins may alter glucose tolerance, thus changing requirements for antidiabetic drugs. Monitor blood glucose levels.
- Instruct patient to weigh herself at least twice a week and to report any sudden weight gain or edema to doctor.
- Warn patient to avoid exposure to ultraviolet light or prolonged exposure to sunlight.
- Many doctors advise women on prolonged therapy with oral contraceptives (5 years or longer) to stop drug and use other birth control methods in order to periodically reassess patient while off hormone therapy.
- The Centers for Disease Control and Prevention (CDC) reports that the use of oral contraceptives *may decrease* the incidence of ovarian and endometrial cancers. Also, oral contraceptives do not appear to increase a woman's risk of breast cancer. However, FDA reports that they may be linked to an increased risk of cervical cancer.
- Ovral has been prescribed as a postcoital contraceptive ("morning-after pill"). Patients are given 2 tablets at the initial visit and 2 tablets 12 hours later.
- Triphasic oral contraceptives may cause fewer adverse reactions such as breakthrough bleeding and spotting.

hydroxyprogesterone caproate

Delalutin†, Duralutin, Gesterol L.A., Hy-Gesterone, Hylutin, Hyprogest, Hyproval P.A., Hyroxon, Pro-Depo, Prodrox

Pregnancy Risk Category: X

HOW SUPPLIED

Injection: 125 mg/ml, 250 mg/ml

*Liquid form contains alcohol. **May contain tartrazine.

MECHANISM OF ACTION
Suppresses ovulation, possibly by inhibiting pituitary gonadotropin secretion. Forms a thick cervical mucus.

INDICATIONS & DOSAGE
Menstrual disorders –
Women: 125 to 375 mg I.M. q 4 weeks. Stop after 4 cycles.
Uterine cancer –
Women: 1 to 5 g I.M. weekly.

ADVERSE REACTIONS
Common reactions are in italics; life-threatening reactions are in bold italics.
CNS: dizziness, migraine headache, lethargy, depression.
CV: hypertension, thrombophlebitis, ***pulmonary embolism***, edema.
GI: nausea, vomiting, abdominal cramps.
GU: breakthrough bleeding, dysmenorrhea, amenorrhea, cervical erosion, or abnormal secretions, uterine fibromas, vaginal candidiasis.
Hepatic: cholestatic jaundice.
Metabolic: hyperglycemia.
Skin: melasma, rash.
Local: irritation and pain at injection site.
Other: breast tenderness, enlargement, or secretion; decreased libido.

INTERACTIONS
Barbiturates, carbamazepine, rifampin: decreased progestogen effects. Monitor for diminished therapeutic response.
Bromocriptine: may cause amenorrhea, interfering with the effects of bromocriptine. Avoid concomitant use.
Corticosteroids: possible enhanced effects. Monitor closely.
Dantrolene, other hepatotoxic medications: increased risk of hepatotoxicity. Monitor closely.
Oral anticoagulants: dosage adjustments may be necessary. Monitor prothrombin time.

NURSING CONSIDERATIONS
- *Contraindicated* in thromboembolic disorders, breast cancer, undiagnosed abnormal vaginal bleeding, severe hepatic disease, missed abortion, or in pregnant women.
- *Use cautiously* in diabetes mellitus, seizure disorder, migraine, cardiac or renal disease, asthma, and mental illness.
- FDA regulations require that, before receiving first dose, patients read package insert explaining possible progestin adverse reactions. Provide verbal explanation also. Patient should report any unusual symptoms immediately and should stop drug and call doctor if visual disturbances or migraine occurs.
- Hydroxyprogesterone should not be used to induce withdrawal bleeding or as a test for pregnancy; drug may cause birth defects and masculinization of female fetus.
- Warn patient that edema and weight gain are likely. Monitor weight routinely and recommend sodium-restricted diet as needed.
- Instruct patient to report breast pain or tenderness, vaginal discharge or bleeding, and swelling of the hands or feet.
- Give oil solutions (sesame oil and castor oil) deep I.M. in gluteal muscle. Rotate injection sites to prevent muscle atrophy.
- Effect lasts 7 to 14 days.
- Teach patient how to perform a monthly breast self-examination.
- Instruct patient that normal menstrual cycles may not resume for 2 to 3 months after drug is stopped.

levonorgestrel
Norplant System
Pregnancy Risk Category: X

HOW SUPPLIED
Implants: 36 mg per capsule; each kit contains six capsules

MECHANISM OF ACTION

Slowly releases the synthetic progestin levonorgestrel into the bloodstream. How progestins provide contraception is not fully understood, but they alter the mucus covering the cervix, prevent implantation of the egg, and in some patients prevent ovulation.

INDICATIONS & DOSAGE

Prevention of pregnancy—
Women: six capsules implanted subdermally in the midportion of the upper arm, about 8 cm above the elbow crease, during the first 7 days of the onset of menses. Capsules should be placed fanlike, 15 degrees apart (total of 75 degrees). Contraceptive efficacy lasts for 5 years.

ADVERSE REACTIONS

Common reactions are in italics; life-threatening reactions are in bold italics.
CNS: headache, nervousness, dizziness, change of appetite.
GI: nausea, *abdominal discomfort.*
GU: *amenorrhea, many bleeding days or prolonged bleeding, spotting, irregular onset of bleeding, frequent onset of bleeding, scanty bleeding, cervicitis, vaginitis, leukorrhea.*
Skin: dermatitis, acne, hirsutism, hypertrichosis, scalp hair loss.
Local: infection at implant site, transient pain or itching at implant site.
Other: adnexal enlargement, mastalgia, weight gain, *musculoskeletal pain, removal difficulty, breast discharge.*

INTERACTIONS

Carbamazepine, phenytoin, rifampin: may reduce the contraceptive efficacy of levonorgestrel implants.

NURSING CONSIDERATIONS

- *Contraindicated* in patients with thrombophlebitis or thromboembolic disorders, undiagnosed abnormal genital bleeding, acute liver disease, malignant or benign liver tumors, breast carcinoma, and known or suspected pregnancy.
- *Use cautiously* in patients with a history of depression because progestins can worsen depression; in diabetic and prediabetic patients because progestins may alter carbohydrate metabolism. (Patients using oral contraceptives containing progestins may show a decreased glucose tolerance; this has yet to be demonstrated with the implant system); and in patients with hyperlipidemias because progestins may alter lipid metabolism. (In clinical trials of the implant, patients experienced decreased cholesterol, low-density lipoprotein, and triglyceride levels, but both increased and decreased high-density lipoprotein levels. The long-term effects of these changes are not known.)
- Most patients develop variations in menstrual bleeding patterns, including irregular bleeding, prolonged bleeding, spotting, and amenorrhea. In most patients, these irregularities diminish over time.
- Be aware that irregular bleeding may mask symptoms of cervical or endometrial cancer.
- Warn patients that missed menstrual periods are not an accurate indicator of early pregnancy because the drug may induce amenorrhea. Advise patients that 6 weeks or more of amenorrhea (after a pattern of regular menstrual periods) could indicate pregnancy. If pregnancy is confirmed, the implants must be removed.
- The implants should be removed if the patient develops active thrombophlebitis or thromboembolic disease or will be immobilized for a significant length of time because of illness or some other factor.
- If jaundice develops, the capsules should be removed because steroid hormone metabolism is impaired in patients with liver failure.
- Closely monitor patients with con-

ditions that may be aggravated by fluid retention because steroid hormones may cause fluid retention.

- Encourage regular (at least annual) physical examinations.
- Tell patient to report to the doctor immediately if one of the implant capsules falls out (before the skin heals over the implant). Contraceptive efficacy may be impaired.
- Retinal thrombosis after use of oral contraceptives has been reported; however, there are no similar reports after use of the implant system.
- Patients with sudden unexplained vision problems, including users of contact lenses who develop vision changes or changes in lens tolerance, should be immediately evaluated by an ophthalmologist.
- Laboratory tests for sex hormone-binding globulin and thyroxine concentrations may show decreased values; for triiodothyronine uptake, increased values.
- Implants do not contain estrogen. Levonorgestrel is a totally synthetic progestin.

medroxyprogesterone acetate

Amen, Curretab, Cycrin, Depo-Provera, Provera

Pregnancy Risk Category: X

HOW SUPPLIED

Tablets: 2.5 mg, 5 mg, 10 mg
Injection (suspension): 100 mg/ml, 150 mg/ml, 400 mg/ml

MECHANISM OF ACTION

Suppresses ovulation, possibly by inhibiting pituitary gonadotropin secretion. Also forms a thick cervical mucus.

INDICATIONS & DOSAGE

Abnormal uterine bleeding due to hormonal imbalance –
Women: 5 to 10 mg P.O. daily for 5 to 10 days beginning on the 16th day of menstrual cycle. If patient has received estrogen – 10 mg P.O. daily for 10 days beginning on 16th day of cycle.
Secondary amenorrhea –
Women: 5 to 10 mg P.O. daily for 5 to 10 days.
Endometrial or renal carcinoma –
Adults: 400 to 1,000 mg/week I.M.
Contraception –
Women: 150 mg I.M. once q 3 months.

ADVERSE REACTIONS

Common reactions are in italics; life-threatening reactions are in bold italics.
CNS: dizziness, migraine headache, lethargy, depression.
CV: hypertension, thrombophlebitis, ***pulmonary embolism,*** edema.
GI: nausea, vomiting, abdominal cramps.
GU: breakthrough bleeding, dysmenorrhea, amenorrhea, cervical erosion, or abnormal secretions, uterine fibromas, vaginal candidiasis.
Hepatic: cholestatic jaundice.
Metabolic: hyperglycemia.
Skin: melasma, rash.
Local: pain, induration, sterile abscesses.
Other: breast tenderness, enlargement, or secretion; decreased libido.

INTERACTIONS

Aminoglutethimide, rifampin: decreased progestin effects. Monitor for diminished therapeutic response. If medroxyprogesterone is used as a contraceptive, patient should use a nonhormonal contraceptive during therapy with these drugs.
Bromocriptine: may cause amenorrhea, interfering with the effects of bromocriptine. Avoid concomitant use.

NURSING CONSIDERATIONS

- *Contraindicated* in thromboembolic disorders, breast cancer, undiagnosed

abnormal vaginal bleeding, missed abortion, hepatic dysfunction, or in pregnant women.
- *Use cautiously* in diabetes mellitus, seizure disorder, migraine, cardiac or renal disease, asthma, and mental illness.
- I.M. injection may be painful. Monitor sites for evidence of sterile abscess. Rotate injection sites to prevent muscle atrophy.
- FDA regulations require that, before receiving first dose, patients read package insert explaining possible progestin adverse reactions. Provide verbal explanation also. Patient should report any unusual symptoms immediately and should stop drug and call doctor if visual disturbances or migraine occurs.
- Don't use as test for pregnancy; drug may cause birth defects and masculinization of female fetus.
- Teach patient how to perform a monthly breast self-examination.
- Has been used effectively to treat obstructive sleep apnea.
- Drug has a prolonged but reversible contraceptive effect. Studies have shown that the median time to conception after discontinuation of drug is 10 months (range 4 to 31 months) in 93% of women; median time to conception is not related to duration of use of drug.

norethindrone

Micronor, Norlutin, Nor-Q.D.

Pregnancy Risk Category: X

HOW SUPPLIED

Tablets: 0.35 mg, 5 mg

MECHANISM OF ACTION

Suppresses ovulation, possibly by inhibiting pituitary gonadotropin secretion. Also forms a thick cervical mucus.

INDICATIONS & DOSAGE

Amenorrhea, abnormal uterine bleeding–

Women: 5 to 20 mg P.O. daily on days 5 to 25 of menstrual cycle.

Endometriosis–

Women: 10 mg P.O. daily for 14 days, then increase by 5 mg P.O. daily q 2 weeks up to 30 mg daily.

Contraception–

Women: initiate therapy with 0.35 mg P.O. on the first day of menstruation. Then, 0.35 mg P.O. daily.

ADVERSE REACTIONS

Common reactions are in italics; life-threatening reactions are in bold italics.

CNS: dizziness, migraine headache, lethargy, depression.

CV: hypertension, thrombophlebitis, ***pulmonary embolism,*** edema.

GI: nausea, vomiting, abdominal cramps.

GU: breakthrough bleeding, dysmenorrhea, amenorrhea, cervical erosion, or abnormal secretions, uterine fibromas, vaginal candidiasis.

Hepatic: cholestatic jaundice.

Metabolic: hyperglycemia.

Skin: melasma, rash.

Other: breast tenderness, enlargement, or secretion; decreased libido.

INTERACTIONS

Barbiturates, carbamazepine, rifampin: decreased progestogen effects. Monitor for diminished therapeutic response.

NURSING CONSIDERATIONS

- *Contraindicated* in thromboembolic disorders, breast cancer, undiagnosed abnormal vaginal bleeding, severe hepatic disease, missed abortion, or in pregnant women.
- *Use cautiously* in diabetes mellitus, seizure disorder, migraine, cardiac or renal disease, asthma, and mental illness.
- Don't use as test for pregnancy;

*Liquid form contains alcohol. **May contain tartrazine.

drug may cause birth defects and masculinization of female fetus.

- FDA regulations require that, before receiving first dose, patients read package insert explaining possible progestin adverse reactions. Provide verbal explanation also. Patient should report any unusual symptoms immediately and should stop drug and call doctor if visual disturbances or migraine occurs.
- Watch patient carefully for signs of edema.
- Preliminary estrogen treatment is usually needed in menstrual disorders.
- Teach the patient how to perform a monthly breast self-examination.

norethindrone acetate

Aygestin, Aygestin Cycle Pack, Norlutate

Pregnancy Risk Category: X

HOW SUPPLIED

Tablets: 5 mg

MECHANISM OF ACTION

Suppresses ovulation, possibly by inhibiting pituitary gonadotropin secretion. Also forms a thick cervical mucus.

INDICATIONS & DOSAGE

Amenorrhea, abnormal uterine bleeding –

Women: 2.5 to 10 mg P.O. daily on days 5 to 25 of menstrual cycle.

Endometriosis –

Women: 5 mg P.O. daily for 14 days, then increase by 2.5 mg daily q 2 weeks up to 15 mg daily.

ADVERSE REACTIONS

Common reactions are in italics; life-threatening reactions are in bold italics.

CNS: dizziness, migraine headache, lethargy, depression.

CV: hypertension, thrombophlebitis, ***pulmonary embolism,*** edema.

GI: nausea, vomiting, abdominal cramps.

GU: breakthrough bleeding, dysmenorrhea, amenorrhea, cervical erosion, or abnormal secretions, uterine fibromas, vaginal candidiasis.

Hepatic: cholestatic jaundice.

Metabolic: hyperglycemia.

Skin: melasma, rash.

Other: breast tenderness, enlargement, or secretion; decreased libido.

INTERACTIONS

Barbiturates, carbamazepine, rifampin: decreased progestogen effects. Monitor for diminished therapeutic response.

Bromocriptine: may cause amenorrhea, interfering with bromocriptine effects. Avoid concomitant use.

NURSING CONSIDERATIONS

- *Contraindicated* in thromboembolic disorders, breast cancer, undiagnosed abnormal vaginal bleeding, severe hepatic disease, missed abortion, or in pregnant women.
- *Use cautiously* in diabetes mellitus, seizure disorder, migraine, cardiac or renal disease, asthma, and mental illness.
- FDA regulations require that, before receiving first dose, patients read package insert explaining possible progestin adverse reactions. Provide verbal explanation also. Patient should report any unusual symptoms immediately and should stop drug and call doctor if visual disturbances or migraine occurs.
- Don't use as test for pregnancy; drug may cause birth defects and masculinization of female fetus.
- Preliminary estrogen treatment is usually needed in menstrual disorders.
- Twice as potent as norethindrone.
- Teach patient how to perform a monthly breast self-examination.

norgestrel

Ovrette**

Pregnancy Risk Category: X

HOW SUPPLIED

Tablets: 0.075 mg

MECHANISM OF ACTION

Suppresses ovulation, possibly by inhibiting pituitary gonadotropin secretion. Also forms a thick cervical mucus.

INDICATIONS & DOSAGE

Contraception –

Women: 0.075 mg P.O. daily.

ADVERSE REACTIONS

Common reactions are in italics; life-threatening reactions are in bold italics.

CNS: cerebral thrombosis or hemorrhage, migraine headache, lethargy, depression.

CV: hypertension, thrombophlebitis, ***pulmonary embolism,*** edema.

GI: nausea, vomiting, abdominal cramps, gallbladder disease.

GU: *breakthrough bleeding, change in menstrual flow,* dysmenorrhea, spotting, amenorrhea, cervical erosion, vaginal candidiasis.

Hepatic: cholestatic jaundice.

Skin: melasma, rash.

Other: breast tenderness, enlargement, or secretion.

INTERACTIONS

Barbiturates, carbamazepine, rifampin: decreased progestogen effects. Monitor for diminished therapeutic response.

Bromocriptine: may cause amenorrhea, interfering with bromocriptine effects. Avoid concomitant use.

NURSING CONSIDERATIONS

- *Contraindicated* in thromboembolic disorders, breast cancer, undiagnosed abnormal vaginal bleeding, severe hepatic disease, missed abortion, or in pregnant women.
- *Use cautiously* in diabetes mellitus, seizure disorder, migraine, cardiac or renal disease, asthma, and mental illness.
- FDA regulations require that, before receiving first dose, patients read package insert explaining possible progestin adverse reactions. Provide verbal explanation also. Patient should report any unusual symptoms immediately and should stop drug and call doctor if visual disturbances, migraine, or numbness or tingling in limbs occurs.
- Tell patient to take pill every day, even if menstruating. Pill should be taken at the same time every day.
- A progestogen-only oral contraceptive known as "minipill."
- Teach the patient how to perform a monthly breast self-examination.
- Women using oral contraceptives should be advised of the increased risk of serious cardiovascular adverse reactions associated with heavy cigarette smoking (15 or more cigarettes per day). These risks are quite marked in women over 35 years.
- Risk of pregnancy increases with each tablet missed. A patient who misses one tablet should take it as soon as she remembers; she should then take the next tablet at the regular time. A patient who misses two tablets should take one as soon as she remembers and then take the next regular dose at the usual time; she should use a nonhormonal method of contraception in addition to norgestrel until 14 tablets have been taken. A patient who misses three or more tablets should discontinue the drug and use a nonhormonal method of contraception until after her menses. If her menstrual period does not occur within 45 days, pregnancy testing is necessary.
- Instruct the patient to immediately report excessive bleeding or bleeding

*Liquid form contains alcohol. **May contain tartrazine.

between menstrual cycles, breast pain or tenderness, vaginal discharge, or swelling of the hands or feet.

progesterone

Gesterol 50, Progestaject, Progestilin†

Pregnancy Risk Category: X

HOW SUPPLIED

Injection (in oil): 50 mg/ml

MECHANISM OF ACTION

Suppresses ovulation, possibly by inhibiting pituitary gonadotropin secretion. Also forms a thick cervical mucus.

INDICATIONS & DOSAGE

Amenorrhea –
Women: 5 to 10 mg I.M. daily for 6 to 8 days.
Dysfunctional uterine bleeding –
Women: 5 to 10 mg I.M. daily for 6 doses.
Management of premenstrual syndrome (PMS) –
Women: 200 to 400 mg as a suppository administered either rectally or vaginally.

ADVERSE REACTIONS

Common reactions are in italics; life-threatening reactions are in bold italics.
CNS: dizziness, migraine headache, lethargy, depression.
CV: hypertension, thrombophlebitis, ***pulmonary embolism,*** edema.
GI: nausea, vomiting, abdominal cramps.
GU: breakthrough bleeding, dysmenorrhea, amenorrhea, cervical erosion, or abnormal secretions, uterine fibromas, vaginal candidiasis.
Hepatic: cholestatic jaundice.
Local: pain at injection site.
Metabolic: hyperglycemia.
Skin: melasma, rash.
Other: breast tenderness, enlargement, or secretion; decreased libido.

INTERACTIONS

Barbiturates, carbamazepine, rifampin: decreased progestogen effects. Monitor for diminished therapeutic response.
Bromocriptine: may cause amenorrhea, interfering with bromocriptine effects. Avoid concomitant use.

NURSING CONSIDERATIONS

- *Contraindicated* in thromboembolic disorders, breast cancer, undiagnosed abnormal vaginal bleeding, severe hepatic disease, or missed abortion.
- *Use cautiously* in diabetes mellitus, seizure disorder, migraine, cardiac or renal disease, asthma, and mental illness.
- FDA regulations require that, before receiving first dose, patients read package insert explaining possible progestin adverse reactions. Provide verbal explanation also. Patient should report any unusual symptoms immediately and should stop drug and call doctor if visual disturbances or migraine occurs.
- Give oil solutions (peanut oil or sesame oil) deep I.M. Check sites frequently for irritation. Rotate injection sites.
- Preliminary estrogen treatment is usually needed in menstrual disorders.
- Teach the patient how to perform a monthly breast self-examination.
- Progesterone suppositories are not commercially available and must be made by the pharmacist.
- Progesterone has been used during the first trimester of pregnancy to treat habitual abortion or pending spontaneous abortion.

quinestrol

Estrovis

Pregnancy Risk Category: X

HOW SUPPLIED

Tablets: 100 mcg

MECHANISM OF ACTION

Increases the synthesis of DNA, RNA, and protein in responsive tissues. Also reduces FSH and LH release from the pituitary.

INDICATIONS & DOSAGE

Moderate to severe vasomotor symptoms associated with menopause, and for atrophic vaginitis, kraurosis vulvae, female hypogonadism, female castration, and primary ovarian failure –

Women: 100 mcg P.O. once daily for 7 days, followed by 100 mcg weekly as maintenance dosage beginning 2 weeks after start of treatment. Dosage may be increased to 200 mcg weekly.

ADVERSE REACTIONS

Common reactions are in italics; life-threatening reactions are in bold italics.

CNS: headache, dizziness, chorea, migraine, depression, libido changes.

CV: thrombophlebitis; ***thromboembolism;*** hypertension; edema; ***increased risk of stroke, pulmonary embolism, and myocardial infarction.***

EENT: worsening of myopia or astigmatism, intolerance to contact lenses.

GI: *nausea,* vomiting, abdominal cramps, bloating, diarrhea, constipation, anorexia, increased appetite, excessive thirst, weight changes.

GU: breakthrough bleeding, altered menstrual flow, dysmenorrhea, amenorrhea, cervical erosion or abnormal secretions, enlargement of uterine fibromas, vaginal candidiasis.

Hepatic: cholestatic jaundice.

Metabolic: hyperglycemia, hypercalcemia, folic acid deficiency.

Skin: melasma, urticaria, acne, seborrhea, oily skin, hirsutism or loss of hair.

Other: leg cramps, purpura, breast changes (tenderness, enlargement, secretion).

INTERACTIONS

Bromocriptine: may cause amenorrhea, interfering with the effects of bromocriptine. Avoid concomitant use.

Carbamazepine, phenobarbital, rifampin: decreased effectiveness of estrogen therapy. Monitor closely.

Corticosteroids: possible enhanced effects. Monitor closely.

Cyclosporine: increased risk of toxicity. Use together with caution and frequently monitor cyclosporine levels.

Dantrolene, other hepatotoxic medications: increased risk of hepatotoxicity. Monitor closely.

Oral anticoagulants: dosage adjustments may be necessary. Monitor prothrombin time.

Tamoxifen: estrogens may interfere with the effectiveness of tamoxifen. Avoid concomitant use.

NURSING CONSIDERATIONS

- *Contraindicated* in thrombophlebitis or thromboembolic disorders; cancer of breast or reproductive organs; undiagnosed abnormal genital bleeding; and pregnancy.
- *Use cautiously* in hypertension, mental depression, migraine, seizures, diabetes mellitus, amenorrhea, hepatic or renal dysfunction, or family history (mother, grandmother, sister) of breast or genital tract cancer. Development or worsening of these may require discontinuation of the drug.
- Studies suggest that postmenopausal women who use estrogen replacement for more than 5 years to treat menopausal symptoms may be at increased risk for endometrial carcinoma. This risk is reduced by the use of cyclic rather than continuous therapy and use of the lowest possible dosages of estrogen. Adding progestins to the regimen decreases the incidence of endometrial hyperplasia; however, it isn't known if progestins affect the incidence of endometrial

carcinoma. Most studies show no increased risk of breast cancer. Emphasize the importance of regular physical examinations.

• Patients should have a thorough physical examination before initiating estrogen therapy. Patients receiving long-term therapy should have repeat examinations yearly. Periodically monitor body weight, blood pressure, hepatic function, and serum lipid levels.

• Patient package insert that describes estrogen's adverse reactions is available. However, provide verbal explanation also.

• Warn patient to immediately report abdominal pain; pain, numbness, or stiffness in legs or buttocks; pressure or pain in chest; shortness of breath; severe headaches; visual disturbances, such as blind spots, flashing lights, or blurriness; vaginal bleeding or discharge; breast lumps; swelling of hands or feet; yellow skin or sclera; dark urine; or light-colored stools.

• Pathologist should be advised of estrogen therapy when specimen is sent.

• Patients with diabetes should report elevated blood glucose test results so antidiabetic medication dosage can be adjusted.

• Attempts to discontinue medication should be made at 3- to 6-month intervals.

• Similar in effectiveness to conjugated estrogens in treating postmenopausal symptoms. Biggest advantage is that quinestrol can be taken once a week.

• Explain to patients on replacement therapy for postmenopausal symptoms that, although menstrual-like bleeding or spotting may occur, fertility has not been restored.

• Teach women how to perform breast self-examination.

54

Gonadotropins

gonadorelin acetate
gonadorelin hydrochloride
gonadotropin, chorionic
histrelin acetate
menotropins
nafarelin acetate

COMBINATION PRODUCTS
None.

gonadorelin acetate

Lutrepulse
Pregnancy Risk Category: B

HOW SUPPLIED
Injection: 0.8-mg/10-ml, 3.2-mg/10-ml vials; supplied as a kit with I.V. supplies and ambulatory infusion pump

MECHANISM OF ACTION
Mimics the action of gonadotropin releasing hormone, which results in the synthesis and release of luteinizing hormone (LH) from the anterior pituitary. LH subsequently acts upon the reproductive organs to regulate hormone synthesis.

INDICATIONS & DOSAGE
Induction of ovulation in women with primary hypothalamic amenorrhea – **Women:** 5 mcg I.V. q 90 minutes for 21 days. If no response follows three treatment intervals, dosage may be increased.

ADVERSE REACTIONS
Common reactions are in italics; life-threatening reactions are in bold italics.
GU: ovarian hyperstimulation.
Local: hematoma, infection, inflammation, mild phlebitis.
Other: multiple pregnancy.

INTERACTIONS
None reported.

NURSING CONSIDERATIONS
- *Contraindicated* in patients hypersensitive to the drug, in any women with conditions that could be complicated by pregnancy (such as pituitary prolactinoma), in patients who are anovulatory from any cause other than a hypothalamic disorder, and in patients with ovarian cysts.
- Anaphylaxis has been reported with similar drugs. Teach the patient how to recognize the signs and symptoms of hypersensitivity reactions (hives, wheezing, difficulty breathing) and encourage her to report these as soon as possible.
- Patients should understand that a multiple pregnancy is possible (incidence about 12%). Close monitoring of dosage as well as ultrasonography of the ovaries to monitor drug response is necessary.
- Patients usually require pelvic ultrasound on days 7 and 14 after establishment of a baseline scan. Some clinicians prefer shorter intervals between scans.
- Encourage patients to adhere to the close monitoring schedule required by the therapy. Regular pelvic examinations, midluteal phase serum progesterone determinations, and multiple ovarian ultrasound scans are necessary. Inspect the I.V. site at each visit.
- **I.V. use:** To mimic the naturally occurring hormone, gonadorelin acetate must be administered in a pulsatile fashion with the available ambulatory infusion pump. The pulse period is set at 1 minute (drug is infused over 1 minute) and pulse interval is set at 90 minutes.
- To administer 2.5 mcg/pulse, re-

constitute the 0.8-mg vial with 8 ml of supplied diluent, and set the pump to deliver 25 microliters/pulse. To administer 5 mcg/pulse, use the same dosage strength and dilution but set the pump to deliver 50 microliters/pulse.

- Some patients may require higher I.V. doses. To administer 10 mcg/pulse, reconstitute the 3.2-mg vial with 8 ml of supplied diluent, and set the pump to deliver 25 microliters/pulse. To administer 20 mcg/pulse, use the same dosage strength and dilution but set the pump to deliver 50 microliters/pulse.
- Instruct the patient about proper aseptic technique and care of the I.V. site. Cannula and I.V. site should be changed every 48 hours. Written instructions are available for the patient.
- Advise patient to report signs of infection, hematoma, inflammation, or phlebitis at the injection site. Patient should also immediately report severe abdominal pain, bloating, swelling of the hands or feet, nausea, vomiting, diarrhea, substantial weight gain, or shortness of breath.

gonadorelin hydrochloride (luteinizing hormone-releasing hormone, LHRH; gonadotropin releasing hormone, GnRH)

Factrel

Pregnancy Risk Category: B

HOW SUPPLIED
Injection: 100 mcg, 500 mcg

MECHANISM OF ACTION
A synthetic luteinizing hormone that releases LHRH.

INDICATIONS & DOSAGE
Evaluation of the functional capacity and response of gonadotropic hormones –

Adults: 100 mcg S.C. or I.V. In women for whom the phase of the menstrual cycle can be established, perform the test between day 1 and day 7.

ADVERSE REACTIONS
Common reactions are in italics; life-threatening reactions are in bold italics.

CNS: headache, flushing, light-headedness.

GI: nausea, abdominal discomfort.

Local: swelling, occasionally with pain and pruritus when administered S.C.; skin rash after chronic S.C. administration.

INTERACTIONS
Digoxin, oral contraceptives: may depress gonadotropin levels. Monitor results carefully.

Levodopa, spironolactone: may elevate gonadotropin levels. Monitor results carefully.

NURSING CONSIDERATIONS
- *Use cautiously* in patients who are allergic to other drugs, although hypersensitivity reactions have not yet been reported. Keep epinephrine readily available.
- The gonadorelin test can be performed concomitantly with other post-treatment evaluations.
- For specific test methodology and interpretation of test results, refer to the manufacturer's full product information. Ask pharmacist for a copy.
- **I.V. use:** Reconstitute vial with 1 to 2 ml of accompanying sterile diluent. Inject drug directly into vein over 3 to 5 minutes. Alternatively, inject into an I.V. line containing a free-flowing compatible solution. Prepare solution immediately before use. After reconstitution, store at room temperature and use within 1 day. Discard unused reconstituted solution and diluent.
- As a single injection, gonadorelin can evaluate the functional capacity and response of the gonadotropins of

the anterior pituitary. Prolonged or repeated administration may be necessary to measure pituitary gonadotropic reserve.

gonadotropin, chorionic (HCG)

Antuitrin, A.P.L., Chorex, Follutein, Pregnyl, Profasi HP

Pregnancy Risk Category: C

HOW SUPPLIED

Injection: 200 units/ml, 500 units/ml, 1,000 units/ml, 2,000 units/ml (after reconstitution)

MECHANISM OF ACTION

Serves as a substitute for luteinizing hormone to stimulate ovulation of an human menopausal gonadotropin-prepared follicle. Also promotes secretion of gonadal steroid hormones by stimulating production of androgen by the interstitial cells of the testes (Leydig's cells).

INDICATIONS & DOSAGE

Anovulation and infertility –
Women: 10,000 units I.M. 1 day after last dose of menotropins.
Hypogonadism –
Men: 500 to 1,000 units I.M. three times weekly for 3 weeks, then twice weekly for 3 weeks; or 4,000 units I.M. three times weekly for 6 to 9 months, then 2,000 units three times weekly for 3 more months.
Nonobstructive cryptorchidism –
Boys 4 to 9 years: 5,000 units I.M. every other day for four doses.

ADVERSE REACTIONS

Common reactions are in italics; life-threatening reactions are in bold italics.
CNS: headache, fatigue, irritability, restlessness, depression.
GU: early puberty (growth of testes, penis, pubic and axillary hair; voice change; down on upper lip; growth of body hair).
Local: *pain at injection site.*
Other: gynecomastia, edema.

INTERACTIONS

None significant.

NURSING CONSIDERATIONS

• *Contraindicated* in patients with pituitary hypertrophy or tumor, prostate cancer, and early puberty (usual onset between ages 10 and 13), undiagnosed vaginal bleeding, uterine fibroids, ovarian cyst, and a history of thrombophlebitis.
• *Use cautiously* in epilepsy, migraine, asthma, and cardiac or renal disease.
• When used with menotropins to induce ovulation, multiple births are possible.
• Usually used only after failure of clomiphene in anovulatory patients.
• In infertility, encourage daily intercourse from day before chorionic gonadotropin is given until ovulation occurs.
• Inspect genitalia of boys for signs of early puberty.
• Be alert to symptoms of ectopic pregnancy. Usually evident between week 8 to 12 of gestation.
• Reconstitute with 1 to 2 ml of supplied diluent just before use. Use reconstituted solutions within 24 hours.
• For I.M. use only. Don't inject I.V. Rotate injection sites to prevent muscle atrophy.
• Instruct the patient to immediately report severe abdominal pain, bloating, swelling of the hands or feet, nausea, vomiting, diarrhea, substantial weight gain, or shortness of breath.

histrelin acetate

Supprelin

Pregnancy Risk Category: X

HOW SUPPLIED
Injection: 120 mcg/0.6 ml, 300 mcg/0.6 ml, 600 mcg/0.6 ml

MECHANISM OF ACTION
An agonist that mimics the effects of gonadotropin releasing hormone (GnRH; also called luteinizing hormone-releasing hormone, or LHRH) but that is more potent than the naturally occurring hormone. Chronic administration desensitizes the responsiveness of the pituitary gonadotropin, resulting in a decrease in sex hormone production by the testes or ovaries.

INDICATIONS & DOSAGE
Centrally mediated (idiopathic or neurogenic) precocious puberty –
Children (girls 2 to 8 years; boys 2 to 9½ years): 10 mg/kg S.C. daily as a single injection.

ADVERSE REACTIONS
Common reactions are in italics; life-threatening reactions are in bold italics.
Blood: hyperlipidemia, anemia.
CNS: migraine headache, *headache, visual disturbances, mood changes, nervousness, dizziness, depression, libido changes, insomnia, anxiety,* paresthesia, cognitive changes, syncope, somnolence, lethargy, impaired consciousness, tremor, hyperkinesia, increased frequency of seizures, hot flashes, conduct disorder.
CV: *vasodilation,* edema, palpitations, tachycardia, hypertension, pallor.
EENT: epistaxis, ear congestion, abnormal pupillary function, otalgia, hearing loss, polyopia, pharyngitis, photophobia, rhinorrhea, sinusitis.
Endocrine: goiter.
GI: *abdominal pain, nausea, vomiting, diarrhea, flatulence, decreased appetite, dyspepsia,* cramps, constipation, thirst, gastritis.
GU: *menstrual changes, vaginal dryness, leukorrhea, menorrhagia, breast pain or edema,* breast discharge, decreased breast size, tenderness of female genitalia, glycosuria.
Respiratory: *upper respiratory infection, respiratory congestion, cough,* asthma, breathing disorder, bronchitis, hyperventilation.
Other: urticaria, *pyrexia, arthralgia, muscle stiffness, muscle cramps,* muscle pain, hypotonia, ***acute hypersensitivity reactions (anaphylaxis, angioedema).***

INTERACTIONS
None reported.

NURSING CONSIDERATIONS
- *Contraindicated* in patients with hypersensitivity to any component of the drug and in pregnant or breast-feeding women.
- Safety and efficacy have not been established in children under 2 years.
- Drug is indicated only for patients who will comply with the daily administration schedule. Noncompliance or inadequate dosing may result in inadequate control of the pubertal process, which can result in recurrence of symptoms, including onset of menses, breast development, or testicular growth; long-term consequences may involve decreased adult height.
- A complete physical and endocrinologic evaluation is necessary before drug therapy is initiated; several indices will be reexamined at 3 months, then every 6 to 12 months thereafter. Such evaluations should include determinations of height and weight, hand and wrist X-ray for bone age determination, sex steroid (estradiol or testosterone) levels, and GnRH stimulation test. These tests should be repeated periodically to determine effectiveness of therapy.
- Additional tests to rule out other causes of precocious puberty include beta human chorionic gonadotropin levels (to detect chorionic gonadotropin-secreting tumor), pelvic/adrenal/testicular ultrasound (to detect ste-

roid-secreting tumor); and computed tomography scan of the head (to detect any previously undiagnosed intracranial tumor). Workup also establishes baseline of gonad size for serial monitoring).

• Because drug is a peptide, it is destroyed in the GI tract and therefore must be administered parenterally. Administer S.C. and rotate injection site to minimize local reactions.

• Decreases in follicle-stimulating hormone, luteinizing hormone, and sex steroid levels are seen within 3 months.

• Drug should be stored in the refrigerator (36° to 46° F [2° to 8° C]) protected from light and in its original container. Vials should be used only once because drug does not contain preservatives. Allow medication to reach room temperature before giving.

• Drug is dispensed as a 7-day kit that contains a patient information leaflet. Caregivers should read and understand the leaflet.

• Before initiating therapy, both patient and parents should understand the importance of adhering to the daily administration schedules. To facilitate compliance and ensure adequate dosing, drug should be given at about the same time each day.

• Explain the importance of rotating injection sites daily. Sites should include upper arms, thighs, and abdomen.

• Warn patients of the potential risks of therapy and potential adverse effects. During the first month of treatment, girls commonly experience a slight menstrual flow, which is probably related to decreasing estrogen levels brought on by treatment. As estrogen levels drop, menses begins because estrogens support the endometrium.

• Advise patients to seek immediate medical attention if they have any signs of a hypersensitivity reaction: sudden development of skin rash, difficulty in breathing or swallowing, or rapid heartbeat. Notify doctor if severe or persistent swelling, redness, or irritation is present at the injection site.

• Patients should be reevaluated if prepubertal levels of sex steroids or GnRH test responses are not achieved within 3 months of therapy.

menotropins

Pergonal

Pregnancy Risk Category: C

HOW SUPPLIED

Injection: 75 IU of luteinizing hormone (LH) and 75 IU of follicle-stimulating hormone (FSH) activity/ampule; 150 IU of LH and 150 IU of FSH activity/ampule

MECHANISM OF ACTION

Menotropins, when administered to women who have not had primary ovarian failure, mimics follicle-stimulating hormone (FSH) in inducing follicular growth and luteinizing hormone (LH) in aiding follicular maturation.

INDICATIONS & DOSAGE

Anovulation –

Women: 75 IU each FSH and LH I.M. daily for 9 to 12 days, followed by 10,000 units chorionic gonadotropin I.M. 1 day after last dose of menotropins. Repeat for one to three menstrual cycles until ovulation occurs.

Infertility with ovulation –

Women: 75 IU each of FSH and LH I.M. daily for 9 to 12 days, followed by 10,000 units chorionic gonadotropin I.M. 1 day after last dose of menotropins. Repeat for two menstrual cycles and then increase to 150 IU each FSH and LH I.M. daily for 9 to 12 days, followed by 10,000 units chorionic gonadotropin I.M. 1 day after last dose of menotropins. Repeat for two menstrual cycles.

Infertility –

Men: 1 ampule I.M. three times weekly (given concomitantly with HCG 2,000 units twice weekly) for at least 4 months.

Menotropins are available in ampules containing 75 IU each FSH and LH.

ADVERSE REACTIONS

Common reactions are in italics; life-threatening reactions are in bold italics.

Blood: hemoconcentration with fluid loss into abdomen.

GI: nausea, vomiting, diarrhea.

GU: in women – *ovarian enlargement with pain and abdominal distention,* multiple births, ovarian hyperstimulation syndrome (sudden ovarian enlargement, ascites with or without pain, or pleural effusion); in men – *gynecomastia.*

Other: fever.

INTERACTIONS

None significant.

NURSING CONSIDERATIONS

- *Contraindicated* in patients with hypersensitivity to the drug; in those with ovarian failure, high urinary gonadotropin levels, thyroid or adrenal dysfunction, pituitary tumor, abnormal uterine bleeding, uterine fibroids, or ovarian cysts or enlargement; and in pregnant patients.
- *Use cautiously* in patients with cardiac, renal, or pulmonary disease; seizure disorder; migraine headache; history of thrombophlebitis; or polycystic ovary syndrome.
- Close monitoring of patient response is critical to ensure adequate ovarian stimulation without hyperstimulation.
- Tell patient that there is a possibility of multiple births.
- In infertility, encourage daily intercourse from day before chorionic gonadotropin is given until ovulation occurs.
- Pregnancy usually occurs 4 to 6 weeks after therapy.
- Reconstitute with 1 to 2 ml sterile saline injection. Use immediately.
- Rotate injection sites to prevent muscle atrophy.
- Instruct patient to immediately report severe abdominal pain, bloating, swelling of the hands or feet, nausea, vomiting, diarrhea, substantial weight gain, or shortness of breath.

nafarelin acetate

Synarel

Pregnancy Risk Category: X

HOW SUPPLIED

Nasal solution: 200 mcg/spray in metered-dose spray bottle (2 mg/ml)

MECHANISM OF ACTION

A gonadotropin-releasing hormone (GnRH) analog that acts on the pituitary to decrease the release of follicle-stimulating hormone (FSH) and luteinizing hormone (LH). The result is decreased ovarian stimulation, lowered circulating estrogens, and improvement of the symptoms associated with endometriosis.

INDICATIONS & DOSAGE

Management of endometriosis –

Women 18 years and older: 1 spray in one nostril b.i.d. Maximum duration of therapy is 6 months.

ADVERSE REACTIONS

Common reactions are in italics; life-threatening reactions are in bold italics.

CNS: *headaches, emotional lability, insomnia,* depression.

CV: edema.

EENT: *nasal irritation.*

GU: *vaginal dryness.*

Skin: *acne,* seborrhea, hirsutism.

Other: *hot flashes, decreased libido, myalgia,* reduced breast size, weight gain or loss, increased libido, decreased bone density.

INTERACTIONS
None reported.

NURSING CONSIDERATIONS
• *Contraindicated* in patients hypersensitive to GnRH analogs or any components of the formulation (benzalkonium chloride, sorbitol, purified water, glacial acetic acid, hydrochloric acid, or sodium hydroxide). Also contraindicated in the presence of undiagnosed vaginal bleeding, in breast-feeding women, and during pregnancy (because it may harm the fetus).
• Studies have confirmed a small loss in bone density after 6 months of therapy, probably caused by the hypoestrogenic state induced by the drug. Patients with major risk factors for osteoporosis (chronic alcohol or tobacco users, strong family history of osteoporosis, or patients who are using drugs that may reduce bone mass such as anticonvulsants or corticosteroids) should not receive additional courses of therapy and should strongly weigh the risks and benefits before an initial trial of the drug.
• Advise patient to contact her doctor if she develops a cold or rhinitis during therapy. If she requires a topical nasal decongestant, the manufacturer suggests that it be used at least 30 minutes after nafarelin treatment to reduce possible interference with nafarelin absorption.
• Advise patient to use nonhormonal form of contraception (such as barrier contraception). Although the drug will usually inhibit ovulation and stop menstruation, it is not a reliable contraceptive, particularly if the patient misses a few doses. She should stop the drug immediately and contact her doctor if she believes that she is pregnant.
• Teach patient that menstruation will stop with regular use of the drug. She should contact her doctor if menstruation persists or breakthrough bleeding occurs.
• Instruct patient to immediately report severe abdominal pain, bloating, swelling of the hands or feet, nausea, vomiting, diarrhea, substantial weight gain, or shortness of breath.

55

Antidiabetic agents and glucagon

acetohexamide
chlorpropamide
glipizide
glucagon
glyburide
insulins
tolazamide
tolbutamide

COMBINATION PRODUCTS
MIXTARD INJECTION◊: 100 mg/ml isophane purified pork insulin suspension and purified pork insulin injection.

acetohexamide
Dimelor†, Dymelor
Pregnancy Risk Category: D

HOW SUPPLIED
Tablets: 250 mg, 500 mg

MECHANISM OF ACTION
Stimulates insulin release from the pancreatic beta cells and reduces glucose output by the liver. An extrapancreatic effect increases peripheral sensitivity to insulin. A sulfonylurea.

INDICATIONS & DOSAGE
Adjunct to diet to lower the blood glucose in patients with non-insulin-dependent diabetes mellitus (type II) –
Adults: initially, 250 mg P.O. daily before breakfast; may increase dosage q 5 to 7 days (by 250 to 500 mg) as needed to maximum of 1.5 g daily, divided b.i.d. to t.i.d. before meals.
To replace insulin therapy –
Adults: if insulin dosage is less than 20 units daily, insulin may be stopped and oral therapy started with 250 mg P.O. daily, before breakfast, increased as above if needed. If insulin dosage is 20 to 40 units daily, start oral therapy with 250 mg P.O. daily, before breakfast, while reducing insulin dosage 25% to 30% daily or every other day, depending on response to oral therapy.

ADVERSE REACTIONS
Common reactions are in italics; life-threatening reactions are in bold italics.
GI: nausea, heartburn, vomiting.
Metabolic: sodium loss, ***hypoglycemia.***
Skin: rash, pruritus, facial flushing.
Other: ***hypersensitivity reactions.***

INTERACTIONS
Anabolic steroids, chloramphenicol, clofibrate, guanethidine, MAO inhibitors, phenylbutazone, salicylates, sulfonamides: increased hypoglycemic activity. Monitor blood glucose level.
Beta blockers, clonidine: prolonged hypoglycemic effect and masked symptoms of hypoglycemia. Use together cautiously.
Corticosteroids, glucagon, rifampin, thiazide diuretics: decreased hypoglycemic response. Monitor blood glucose level.
Hydantoins: increased blood levels of hydantoins. Monitor blood levels closely.
Oral anticoagulants: increased hypoglycemic activity or enhanced anticoagulant effect. Monitor blood glucose and prothrombin time.

NURSING CONSIDERATIONS
- *Contraindicated* for treating type I diabetes (insulin-dependent); diabetes adequately controlled by diet; and type II diabetes (non-insulin-dependent) complicated by ketosis, acidosis, diabetic coma, Raynaud's disease, gangrene, renal or hepatic impairment, or thyroid or other endo-

crine dysfunction. This drug also should not be used during pregnancy or breast-feeding.

- *Use cautiously* in patients with sulfonamide hypersensitivity.
- Instruct patient about nature of disease; importance of following therapeutic regimen, adhering to specific diet, weight reduction, exercise, and personal hygiene programs, and avoiding infection; how and when to perform self-monitoring of blood glucose level; and recognition of hypoglycemia and hyperglycemia.
- Make sure patient understands that therapy relieves symptoms but doesn't cure the disease.
- Patient transferring from another oral sulfonylurea antidiabetic drug usually needs no transition period.
- Patient transferring from insulin therapy to an oral antidiabetic requires blood glucose monitoring at least t.i.d. before meals. Patient may require hospitalization during transition.
- During periods of increased stress, such as infection, fever, surgery, or trauma, patient may require insulin therapy. Monitor patient closely for hyperglycemia in these situations.
- Advise patient to avoid moderate to large intake of alcohol; disulfiram-like reaction possible.
- Teach patient not to change drug dosage without doctor's approval. Report abnormal blood or urine glucose tests.
- Be sure patient understands that he should not take any other medication, including OTC drugs, without first checking with the doctor.
- Advise patient to carry a medical identification bracelet identifying him as a diabetic patient.

chlorpropamide

Apo-Chlorpropamide†, Diabinese, Glucamide, Novo-propamide†

Pregnancy Risk Category: D

HOW SUPPLIED

Tablets: 100 mg, 250 mg

MECHANISM OF ACTION

Stimulates insulin release from the pancreatic beta cells and reduces glucose output by the liver. An extrapancreatic effect increases peripheral sensitivity to insulin. Also exerts an antidiuretic effect in patients with pituitary-deficient diabetes insipidus. A sulfonylurea.

INDICATIONS & DOSAGE

Adjunct to diet to lower blood glucose in patients with non-insulin-dependent diabetes mellitus (type II) –

Adults: 250 mg P.O. daily with breakfast or in divided doses if GI disturbances occur. First dosage increase may be made after 5 to 7 days because of extended duration of action, then dosage may be increased q 3 to 5 days by 50 to 125 mg, if needed, to maximum of 750 mg daily.

Adults over 65 years: initial dose should be in the range of 100 to 125 mg P.O. daily.

To change from insulin to oral therapy –

Adults: if insulin dosage is less than 40 units daily, insulin may be stopped and oral therapy started as above. If insulin dosage is 40 units or more daily, start oral therapy as above with insulin reduced 50%. Further insulin reductions should be made according to patient response.

ADVERSE REACTIONS

Common reactions are in italics; life-threatening reactions are in bold italics.

GI: nausea, heartburn, vomiting.

GU: tea-colored urine.

Metabolic: ***prolonged hypoglycemia, dilutional hyponatremia.***
Skin: rash, pruritus, facial flushing.
Other: ***hypersensitivity reactions.***

INTERACTIONS

Anabolic steroids, chloramphenicol, clofibrate, guanethidine, MAO inhibitors, phenylbutazone, salicylates, sulfonamides: increased hypoglycemic activity. Monitor blood glucose level.
Beta blockers, clonidine: prolonged hypoglycemic effect and masked symptoms of hypoglycemia. Use together cautiously.
Corticosteroids, glucagon, rifampin, thiazide diuretics: decreased hypoglycemic response. Monitor blood glucose level.
Hydantoins: increased blood levels of hydantoins. Monitor blood levels closely.
Oral anticoagulants: increased hypoglycemic activity or enhanced anticoagulant effect. Monitor blood glucose and prothrombin time.

NURSING CONSIDERATIONS

- *Contraindicated* for treating type I diabetes (insulin-dependent); diabetes adequately controlled by diet; and type II diabetes (non-insulin-dependent) complicated by fever, ketosis, acidosis, diabetic coma, major surgery, severe trauma, Raynaud's disease, gangrene, renal or hepatic impairment, or thyroid or other endocrine dysfunction. This drug also should not be used during pregnancy or breast-feeding.
- *Use cautiously* in patients with sulfonamide hypersensitivity.
- Elderly patients may be more sensitive to this drug's adverse reactions.
- Instruct patient about nature of the disease; importance of following therapeutic regimen, adhering to specific diet, weight reduction, exercise, and personal hygiene programs, and avoiding infection; how and when to perform self-monitoring of blood glucose level; and recognition of and intervention for hypoglycemia and hyperglycemia.
- Make sure patient understands that therapy relieves symptoms but doesn't cure the disease.
- Adverse effects, especially hypoglycemia, may be more frequent or severe than with some other sulfonylurea drugs (acetohexamide, tolazamide, and tolbutamide) because of its long duration of effect (36 hours).
- If hypoglycemia occurs, patient should be monitored closely for a minimum of 3 to 5 days.
- Patient transferring from another oral sulfonylurea antidiabetic drug usually needs no transition period.
- Patient may require hospitalization during transition from insulin therapy to an oral antidiabetic. Monitor patient for blood glucose levels at least t.i.d., before meals. If performing both urine glucose and urine ketone testing, emphasize the need for a double-voided specimen.
- Drug may accumulate in patients with renal insufficiency.
- Advise patient to avoid intake of alcohol. Chlorpropamide-alcohol flush (CPAF) is characterized by facial flushing, light-headedness, headache, and occasional breathlessness. Even very small amounts of alcohol can produce this reaction.
- Watch for signs of impending renal insufficiency, such as dysuria, anuria, and hematuria, and report them to the doctor immediately.
- May potentiate antidiuretic hormone. Sometimes used to treat diabetes insipidus.
- Teach patient not to change drug dosage without doctor's approval. Report abnormal blood or urine glucose tests.
- Be sure patient understands that he should not take any other medication, including OTC drugs, without first checking with the doctor.
- Advise patient to carry a medical

identification bracelet identifying him as a diabetic patient.

glipizide

Glucotrol, Minidiab‡

Pregnancy Risk Category: C

HOW SUPPLIED

Tablets: 5 mg, 10 mg

MECHANISM OF ACTION

Stimulates insulin release from the pancreatic beta cells and reduces glucose output by the liver. An extrapancreatic effect increases peripheral sensitivity to insulin. A sulfonylurea.

INDICATIONS & DOSAGE

Adjunct to diet to lower the blood glucose in patients with non-insulin-dependent diabetes mellitus (type II) –
Adults: initially, 5 mg P.O. daily given before breakfast. Elderly patients or those with liver disease may be started on 2.5 mg. Usual maintenance dosage is 10 to 15 mg. Maximum recommended daily dosage is 40 mg.

To replace insulin therapy –
Adults: if insulin dosage is more than 20 units daily, patient may be started at usual dosage in addition to 50% of the insulin. If insulin dosage is less than 20 units, insulin may be discontinued.

ADVERSE REACTIONS

Common reactions are in italics; life-threatening reactions are in bold italics.
CNS: dizziness.
GI: nausea, vomiting, constipation.
Hepatic: cholestatic jaundice.
Metabolic: ***hypoglycemia.***
Skin: rash, pruritus, facial flushing.

INTERACTIONS

Anabolic steroids, chloramphenicol, clofibrate, guanethidine, MAO inhibitors, phenylbutazone, probenecid, salicylates, sulfonamides: increased hypoglycemic activity. Monitor blood glucose level.
Beta blockers, clonidine: prolonged hypoglycemic effect and masked symptoms of hypoglycemia. Use together cautiously.
Corticosteroids, glucagon, rifampin, thiazide diuretics: decreased hypoglycemic response. Monitor blood glucose level.
Hydantoins: increased blood levels of hydantoins. Monitor blood levels closely.
Oral anticoagulants: increased hypoglycemic activity or enhanced anticoagulant effect. Monitor blood glucose and prothrombin time.

NURSING CONSIDERATIONS

- *Contraindicated* in diabetic ketoacidosis, with or without coma. This drug also should not be used during pregnancy or breast-feeding.
- *Use cautiously* in renal and hepatic disease and sulfonamide hypersensitivity.
- Elderly patients may be more sensitive to this drug's adverse reactions.
- Patient transferring from insulin therapy to an oral antidiabetic requires blood glucose monitoring at least t.i.d. before meals. May require hospitalization during transition.
- During periods of increased stress, such as infection, fever, surgery, or trauma, patient may require insulin therapy. Monitor patient closely for hyperglycemia in these situations.
- Instruct patient about nature of disease; importance of following therapeutic regimen, adhering to specific diet, weight reduction, exercise, and personal hygiene programs, and avoiding infection; how and when to perform self-monitoring of blood glucose level; recognition of hypoglycemia and hyperglycemia.
- Some patients taking glipizide may be effectively controlled on a once-daily regimen, while others show better response with divided dosing.

- Give approximately 30 minutes before meals.
- Glipizide is a second-generation sulfonylurea oral hypoglycemic. The frequency of adverse reactions appears to be lower than with first-generation drugs such as chlorpropamide and tolbutamide.
- Glipizide has a mild diuretic effect. May be useful in patients who have CHF or cirrhosis.
- Teach patient not to change drug dosage without the doctor's orders. Report abnormal blood or urine glucose tests.
- Be sure patient understands that he should not take any other medication, including OTC drugs, without first checking with the doctor.
- Advise patient to carry a medical identification bracelet identifying him as a diabetic patient.

glucagon

Pregnancy Risk Category: B

HOW SUPPLIED

Powder for injection: 1 mg (1 unit)/vial, 10 mg (10 units)/vial

MECHANISM OF ACTION

Raises blood glucose level by promoting catalytic depolymerization of hepatic glycogen to glucose.

INDICATIONS & DOSAGE

Coma of insulin-shock therapy –
Adults: 0.5 to 1 mg S.C., I.M., or I.V. 1 hour after coma develops; may repeat within 25 minutes, if necessary. In very deep coma, also give glucose 10% to 50% I.V. for faster response. When patient responds, give additional carbohydrate immediately.

Severe insulin-induced hypoglycemia during diabetic therapy –
Adults and children: 0.5 to 1 mg S.C., I.M., or I.V.; may repeat q 20 minutes for 2 doses, if necessary. If coma persists, give glucose 10% to 50% I.V.

Diagnostic aid for radiologic examination –
Adults: 0.25 to 2 mg I.V. or I.M. before initiation of radiologic procedure.

ADVERSE REACTIONS

Common reactions are in italics; life-threatening reactions are in bold italics.
GI: nausea, vomiting.
Other: ***hypersensitivity***.

INTERACTIONS

Phenytoin: inhibited glucagon-induced insulin release. Use cautiously.

NURSING CONSIDERATIONS

- *Use cautiously* in patients with insulinoma pheochromocytoma.
- Unstable hypoglycemic diabetics may not respond to glucagon. Give dextrose I.V. instead.
- It is vital to arouse the patient from coma as quickly as possible and to give additional carbohydrates orally to prevent secondary hypoglycemic reactions.
- **I.V. use:** Reconstitute 1-unit vial with 1 ml of diluent; reconstitute 10-unit vial with 10 ml of diluent. Use only the diluent supplied by the manufacturer when preparing doses of 2 mg or less. For larger doses, dilute with sterile water for injection.
- For I.V. drip infusion, use dextrose solution, which is compatible with glucagon; drug forms a precipitate in chloride solutions. Give directly into vein or into I.V. tubing of a free-flowing compatible solution over 2 to 5 minutes. Interrupt primary infusion during glucagon injection if you're using the same I.V. line.
- Instruct patient and family in proper glucagon administration, recognition of hypoglycemia, and urgency of calling a doctor immediately in emergencies.
- May be used as diagnostic aid in ra-

diologic examination of the stomach, duodenum, small bowel, and colon when a hypotonic state is advantageous.

• Has a positive inotropic and chronotropic action on the heart. May be used to treat overdosage of beta-adrenergic blockers.

glyburide (glibenclamide)

DiaBeta**, Euglucon†, Glynase Prestab, Micronase

Pregnancy Risk Category: B

HOW SUPPLIED

Tablets: 1.25 mg, 2.5 mg, 5 mg
Tablets (micronized): 1.5 mg, 3 mg

MECHANISM OF ACTION

Stimulates insulin release from the pancreatic beta cells and reduces glucose output by the liver. An extrapancreatic effect increases peripheral sensitivity to insulin and causes a mild diuretic effect. A sulfonylurea.

INDICATIONS & DOSAGE

Adjunct to diet to lower the blood glucose in patients with non-insulin-dependent diabetes mellitus (type II) –
Adults: initially, 2.5 to 5 mg P.O. (regular tablets) daily administered with breakfast. Patients who are more sensitive to hypoglycemic drugs should be started at 1.25 mg daily. Usual maintenance dosage is 1.25 to 20 mg daily, given either as a single dose or in divided doses.

Alternatively, use micronized formulation. Initial dose is 1.5 to 3 mg daily. Patients who are more sensitive to hypoglycemic agents should be started at 0.75 mg daily.

To replace insulin therapy –
Adults: if insulin dosage is more than 40 units daily, patient may be started on 5 mg glyburide (regular tablets) or 3 mg glyburide (micronized formulation) daily in addition to 50% of the insulin dosage.

ADVERSE REACTIONS

Common reactions are in italics; life-threatening reactions are in bold italics.
GI: nausea, epigastric fullness, heartburn.
Hepatic: cholestatic jaundice.
Metabolic: ***hypoglycemia.***
Skin: rash, pruritus, facial flushing.

INTERACTIONS

Anabolic steroids, chloramphenicol, clofibrate, guanethidine, MAO inhibitors, phenylbutazone, salicylates, sulfonamides: increased hypoglycemic activity. Monitor blood glucose level.
Beta blockers, clonidine: prolonged hypoglycemic effect and masked symptoms of hypoglycemia. Use together cautiously.
Corticosteroids, glucagon, rifampin, thiazide diuretics: decreased hypoglycemic response. Monitor blood glucose level.
Hydantoins: increased blood levels of hydantoins. Monitor blood levels closely.
Oral anticoagulants: increased hypoglycemic activity or enhanced anticoagulant effect. Monitor blood glucose and prothrombin time.

NURSING CONSIDERATIONS

• *Contraindicated* in diabetic ketoacidosis, with or without coma. This drug also should not be used during pregnancy or breast-feeding.
• *Use cautiously* in sulfonamide hypersensitivity and severe renal impairment.
• Micronized glyburide contains the drug in a smaller particle size and is not bioequivalent to regular glyburide tablets. Patients who have been taking Micronase or DiaBeta should be retitrated.
• Elderly patients may be more sensitive to this drug's adverse reactions.
• Patient transferring from insulin therapy to an oral antidiabetic requires blood glucose monitoring at least t.i.d. before meals. Patient may

*Liquid form contains alcohol. **May contain tartrazine.

require hospitalization during transition.
• During periods of increased stress, such as infection, fever, surgery, or trauma, patient may require insulin therapy. Monitor patient closely for hyperglycemia in these situations.
• Instruct patient about nature of disease; importance of following therapeutic regimen, adhering to specific diet, weight reduction, exercise, and personal hygiene programs, and avoiding infection; how and when to perform self-monitoring of blood glucose level; recognition of hypoglycemia and hyperglycemia.
• A maintenance dosage of 5 mg glyburide (regular tablets) provides approximately the same degree of blood glucose control as 250 to 375 mg chlorpropamide, 250 to 375 mg tolazamide, 500 to 750 mg acetohexamide, or 1,000 to 1,500 mg tolbutamide.
• Although most patients may take glyburide once daily, patients taking more than 10 mg daily may achieve better results with twice-daily dosage.
• Glyburide is a second-generation sulfonylurea oral hypoglycemic. The frequency of adverse effects appears to be lower than with first-generation drugs such as chlorpropamide and tolbutamide.
• Glyburide exerts a mild diuretic effect. May be useful in patients who have CHF or cirrhosis.
• Teach patient not to change drug dosage without the doctor's orders. Report abnormal blood or urine glucose tests.
• Be sure patient understands that he should not take any other medication, including OTC drugs, without first checking with the doctor.
• Advise patient to carry a medical identification bracelet identifying him as a diabetic patient.

insulins

insulin injection (regular insulin, crystalline zinc insulin)

Actrapid HM‡, Actrapid HM Penfill‡, Actrapid MC‡, Actrapid MC Penfill‡, Humulin R◇, Hypurin Neutral‡, Insulin 2‡, Novolin R◇, Novolin R Penfill◇, Pork Regular Iletin II◇, Regular (Concentrated) Iletin II, Regular Iletin I◇, Regular Purified Pork Insulin◇, Velosulin◇, Velosulin Human‡, Velosulin Insuject◇

insulin zinc suspension, prompt (semilente)

Semilente Insulin◇, Semilente MC‡, Semilente Purified Pork◇

isophane insulin suspension (neutral protamine Hagedorn insulin, NPH)

Humulin N◇, Humulin NPH‡, Hypurin Isophane‡, Insulatard‡, Insulatard Human†, Insulatard NPH◇, Isotard MC‡, Novolin N◇, NPH Iletin I◇, NPH Insulin◇, NPH Purified Pork◇, Pork NPH Iletin II◇, Protaphane HM‡, Protaphane HM Penfill‡, Protaphane MC‡

isophane insulin suspension with insulin injection

Actraphane HM‡, Actraphane HM Penfill‡, Actraphane MC‡, Mixtard◇, Mixtard Human‡, Novolin 70/30

insulin zinc suspension (lente)

Humulin L◇, Lente Iletin I◇, Lente Insulin◇, Lente MC‡, Lente Purified Pork Insulin◇, Monotard HM‡, Monotard MC‡, Novolin L◇

†Available in Canada only. ‡Available in Australia only. ◇Available OTC.

protamine zinc suspension (PZI)

Protamine, Zinc & Iletin I◇; Protamine, Zinc & Iletin II (Beef)◇; Protamine, Zinc & Iletin II (Pork)◇; Protamine Zinc Insulin MC‡

insulin zinc suspension, extended (ultralente)

Ultralente Insulin◇, Ultralente Purified Beef◇, Ultratard HM‡, Ultratard MC‡

Pregnancy Risk Category: B

HOW SUPPLIED

insulin injection

Injection (from beef and pork): 40 units/ml◇, 100 units/ml◇ (Regular Iletin I◇)

Injection (human): 100 units/ml (Actrapid HM‡, Humulin R◇, Novolin R◇, Velosulin◇, Velosulin Human‡); 100 units/ml in 1.5-ml cartridge system◇ (Actrapid HM Penfill‡, Novolin R Penfill◇)

Injection (from pork): 100 units/ml◇

Injection (purified beef): 100 units/ml (Hypurin Neutral‡, Insulin 2‡)

Injection (purified pork): 100 units/ml (Actrapid MC‡, Pork Regular Iletin II◇, Regular Purified Pork Insulin◇, Velosulin◇); 100 units/ml in 1.5-ml cartridge system‡ (Actrapid MC Penfill‡); 100 units/ml in 2-ml cartridge system‡ (Velosulin Insuject‡); 500 units/ml (Regular [Concentrated] Iletin II)

insulin zinc suspension, prompt

Injection (from beef): 100 units/ml◇ (Semilente Insulin◇)

Injection (purified pork): 100 units/ml◇ (Semilente MC‡, Semilente Purified Pork◇)

isophane insulin suspension

Injection (from beef): 100 units/ml◇ (NPH Insulin◇)

Injection (from beef and pork): 40 units/ml◇, 100 units/ml◇ (NPH Iletin I◇)

Injection (human, recombinant): 100 units/ml (Humulin N◇, Humulin NPH‡, Insulatard Human†, Insulatard NPH◇, Novolin N◇, Protaphane HM‡); 100 units/ml in 1.5-ml cartridge system‡ (Protaphane HM Penfill‡)

Injection (purified beef): 100 units/ml (Hypurin Isophane‡, Isotard MC‡)

Injection (purified pork): 100 units/ml (Insulatard‡, Insulatard NPH◇, NPH Purified Pork◇, Pork NPH Iletin II, Protaphane MC‡)

isophane insulin suspension with insulin injection

Injection (human): 100 units/ml (Actraphane HM‡, Mixtard Human‡, Novolin 70/30◇); 100 units/ml in 1.5-ml cartridge system‡ (Actraphane HM Penfill‡)

Injection (purified pork): 100 units/ml (Actraphane MC‡, Mixtard◇)

insulin zinc suspension

Injection (from beef): 100 units/ml (Lente Insulin◇, Lente MC‡)

Injection (from beef and pork): 40 units/ml◇, 100 units/ml◇ (Lente Iletin I◇)

Injection (purified beef): 100 units/ml (Lente MC‡)

Injection (purified pork): 100 units/ml (Monotard MC‡, Lente Purified Pork Insulin◇)

Injection (human): 100 units/ml◇ (Humulin L◇, Monotard HM‡, Novolin I◇)

protamine zinc suspension

Injection (from beef and pork): 40 units/ml◇, 100 units/ml◇ (Protamine, Zinc & Iletin I◇)

Injection (purified beef): 100 units/ml◇ (Protamine, Zinc & Iletin II [Beef]◇)

Injection (purified pork): 100 units/ml (Protamine, Zinc & Iletin II [Pork]◇, Protamine Zinc Insulin MC‡)

insulin zinc suspension, extended

Injection (from beef): 100 units/ml◇ (Ultralente Purified Beef◇)

Injection (human): 100 units/ml‡ (Ultratard HM‡)

Injection (purified pork): 100 units/ml‡ (Ultratard MC‡)

*Liquid form contains alcohol. **May contain tartrazine.

MECHANISM OF ACTION

Increases glucose transport across muscle and fat cell membranes to reduce blood glucose level. Promotes conversion of glucose to its storage form, glycogen; triggers amino acid uptake and conversion to protein in muscle cells and inhibits protein degradation; stimulates triglyceride formation and inhibits release of free fatty acids from adipose tissue; and stimulates lipoprotein lipase activity, which converts circulating lipoproteins to fatty acids.

INDICATIONS & DOSAGE

Diabetic ketoacidosis (use regular insulin only) –

Adults: 25 to 150 units I.V. immediately, then additional doses may be given q 1 hour based on blood sugar level until patient is out of acidosis; then give S.C. q 6 hours thereafter. Alternative dosage schedule: 50 to 100 units I.V. and 50 to 100 units S.C. stat; additional doses may be given q 2 to 6 hours based on blood sugar levels; or 0.33 units/kg I.V. bolus, followed by 7 to 10 units/hour I.V. by continuous infusion. Continue infusion until blood sugar drops to 250 mg/dl, then start S.C. insulin q 6 hours.

Children: 0.5 to 1 unit/kg in two divided doses, 1 given I.V. and the other S.C., followed by 0.5 to 1 unit/kg I.V. q 1 to 2 hours; or 0.1 unit/kg I.V. bolus, then 0.1 unit/kg hourly continuous I.V. infusion until blood sugar drops to 250 mg/dl, then start S.C. insulin. Preparation of infusion: add 100 units regular insulin and 1 g albumin to 100 ml 0.9% sodium chloride solution. Insulin concentration will be 1 unit/ml. (The albumin will adsorb to plastic, preventing loss of the insulin to plastic.)

Type I (insulin-dependent) diabetes mellitus, ketosis-prone diabetics, diabetes mellitus inadequately controlled by diet and oral hypoglycemics –

Adults and children: therapeutic regimen prescribed by doctor and adjusted according to patient's blood and urine glucose concentrations.

ADVERSE REACTIONS

Common reactions are in italics; life-threatening reactions are in bold italics.

Metabolic: ***hypoglycemia,*** hyperglycemia (rebound, or Somogyi, effect).

Skin: urticaria.

Local: *lipoatrophy, lipohypertrophy,* itching, swelling, redness, stinging, warmth at site of injection.

Other: ***anaphylaxis.***

INTERACTIONS

Alcohol, beta blockers, clofibrate, fenfluramine, guanethidine, MAO inhibitors, salicylates, tetracycline: prolonged hypoglycemic effect. Monitor blood glucose level carefully.

Corticosteroids, epinephrine, dextrothyroxine, thiazide diuretics: diminished insulin response. Monitor for hyperglycemia.

NURSING CONSIDERATIONS

- Use only regular insulin in patients with circulatory collapse, diabetic ketoacidosis, or hyperkalemia. Do not use regular insulin concentrated (500 units/ml) I.V. Do not use intermediate or long-acting insulins for coma or other emergency requiring rapid drug action.
- *Use cautiously* in surgery and in patients with high fever, thyroid disease, severe infections, trauma, impaired hepatic or renal function, eating disorders, nausea, vomiting, or diarrhea.
- Accuracy of measurement is very important, especially with regular insulin concentrated. Aids, such as magnifying sleeve, dose magnifier, or cornwall syringe, may help improve accuracy.
- Dosage is always expressed in USP units.
- Don't interchange single-source

beef or pork insulins; a dosage adjustment may be required.

• Lente, semilente, and ultralente insulins may be mixed in any proportion.

• Regular insulin may be mixed with NPH or lente insulins in any proportion.

• Advise patient not to alter the order of mixing insulins or change the model or brand of syringe or needle.

• Note that switching from separate injections to a prepared mixture may alter patient's response. Whenever NPH or lente is mixed with regular insulin in the same syringe, be sure to administer immediately to avoid binding.

• Store insulin in cool area. Refrigeration desirable but not essential, except with regular insulin concentrated.

• Don't use insulin that has changed color or becomes clumped or granular in appearance.

• Check expiration date on vial before using contents.

• **I.V. use:** Only regular insulin should be administered I.V. Inject directly into vein, through an intermittent infusion device, or into a port close to I.V. access site at ordered rate. Intermittent infusion is not recommended. If given by continuous infusion, infuse drug diluted in 0.9% sodium chloride at a rate sufficient to reverse ketoacidosis.

• Usual administration route is S.C. because absorption rate and pain are less than with I.M. injections.

• Ketosis-prone type I diabetics, severely ill, and newly diagnosed diabetics with very high blood sugar level may require hospitalization and I.V. treatment with regular fast-acting insulin.

• Ketosis-resistant diabetics may be treated as outpatients with intermediate-acting insulin and instructions on how to alter dosage according to self-performed blood glucose determinations.

• Instruct patients on proper use of equipment for performing self-monitoring of blood glucose.

• Press but do not rub site after injection. Rotate injection sites and chart to avoid overuse of one area. However, unstable diabetics may achieve better control if injection site is rotated within same anatomic region.

• To mix insulin suspension, swirl vial gently or rotate between palms or between palm and thigh. Don't shake vigorously: this causes bubbling and air in syringe.

• Insulin requirements increase, sometimes drastically, in pregnant diabetics, then decline immediately postpartum.

• Be sure the patient knows that therapy relieves symptoms but doesn't cure the disease.

• Instruct patient about nature of disease; the importance of following the therapeutic regimen, adhering to specific diet, weight reduction, exercise, and personal hygiene programs, and avoiding infection; and timing of injection and eating. Emphasize that meals must not be omitted. Teach that self-monitoring of blood glucose tests and urine ketone tests are essential guides to dosage and success of therapy; important to recognize hypoglycemic symptoms because insulin-induced hypoglycemia is hazardous and may cause brain damage if prolonged; most adverse effects are self-limiting and temporary.

• Advise patient to wear medical identification alert at all times; to carry ample insulin supply and syringes on trips; to have carbohydrates (lump of sugar or candy) on hand for emergency; to take note of time zone changes for dose schedule when traveling.

• Marijuana use may increase insulin requirements.

• Cigarette smoking decreases the

*Liquid form contains alcohol. **May contain tartrazine.

amount of absorption of insulin administered subcutaneously. Advise patient not to smoke within 30 minutes after insulin injection.
• Some patients may develop insulin resistance and require large insulin doses to control symptoms of diabetes. U-500 insulin is available as Regular (Concentrated) Iletin I for such patients. Although every pharmacy may not normally stock it, it is readily available. Patient should notify pharmacist several days before refill of prescription is needed. Nurse should give hospital pharmacy sufficient notice before needing to refill in-house prescription. Never store U-500 insulin in same area with other insulin preparations because of danger of severe overdose if given accidentally to other patients. U-500 insulin must be administered with a U-100 syringe since no syringes are made for this drug.
• Humulin is synthesized by a strain of *Escherichia coli* that has been genetically altered. Novolin is derived from enzymatic alteration of pork insulin.

tolazamide

Ronase, Tolamide, Tolinase

Pregnancy Risk Category: C

HOW SUPPLIED

Tablets: 100 mg, 250 mg, 500 mg

MECHANISM OF ACTION

Stimulates insulin release from the pancreatic beta cells and reduces glucose output by the liver. An extrapancreatic effect increases peripheral sensitivity to insulin. A sulfonylurea.

INDICATIONS & DOSAGE

Adjunct to diet to lower the blood glucose in patients with non-insulin-dependent diabetes mellitus (type II) –
Adults: initially, 100 mg P.O. daily with breakfast if fasting blood sugar (FBS) is under 200 mg/dl; or 250 mg if FBS is over 200 mg/dl. May adjust dosage at weekly intervals by 100 to 250 mg. Maximum dosage is 500 mg b.i.d. before meals.
Adults over 65: 100 mg P.O. once daily.
To change from insulin to oral therapy –
Adults: if insulin dosage is under 20 units daily, insulin may be stopped and oral therapy started at 100 mg P.O. daily with breakfast. If insulin dosage is 20 to 40 units daily, insulin may be stopped and oral therapy started at 250 mg P.O. daily with breakfast. If insulin dosage is over 40 units daily, decrease insulin 50% and start oral therapy at 250 mg P.O. daily with breakfast. Increase dosages as above.

ADVERSE REACTIONS

Common reactions are in italics; life-threatening reactions are in bold italics.
GI: nausea, vomiting.
Metabolic: ***hypoglycemia.***
Skin: rash, urticaria, facial flushing.
Other: ***hypersensitivity reactions.***

INTERACTIONS

Anabolic steroids, chloramphenicol, clofibrate, guanethidine, MAO inhibitors, phenylbutazone, salicylates, sulfonamides: increased hypoglycemic activity. Monitor blood glucose level.
Beta blockers, clonidine: prolonged hypoglycemic effect and masked symptoms of hypoglycemia. Use together cautiously.
Corticosteroids, glucagon, rifampin, thiazide diuretics: decreased hypoglycemic response. Monitor blood glucose level.
Hydantoins: increased blood levels of hydantoins. Monitor blood levels closely.
Oral anticoagulants: increased hypoglycemic activity or enhanced anticoagulant effect. Monitor blood glucose and prothrombin time.

NURSING CONSIDERATIONS

• *Contraindicated* for treating type I diabetes (insulin-dependent); diabetes adequately controlled by diet; and type II diabetes (non-insulin-dependent) complicated by fever, ketosis, acidosis, coma, major surgery, severe trauma, Raynaud's disease, renal or hepatic impairment, or thyroid or other endocrine dysfunction. This drug also should not be used during pregnancy or breast-feeding.
• *Use cautiously* in sulfonamide hypersensitivity and in elderly, debilitated, or malnourished patients.
• Elderly patients may be more sensitive to this drug's adverse reactions.
• Instruct patient about nature of disease; importance of following therapeutic regimen, adhering to specific diet, weight reduction, exercise, and personal hygiene programs, and avoiding infection; how and when to perform self-monitoring of blood glucose level; and recognition of hypoglycemia and hyperglycemia.
• Be sure patient knows that therapy relieves symptoms but doesn't cure disease.
• Patient transferring from another oral sulfonylurea antidiabetic drug usually needs no transition period.
• Patient transferring from insulin therapy to an oral hypoglycemic should test for blood glucose at least t.i.d. before meals. Hospitalization may be required during the transition.
• Advise patient to avoid moderate to large intake of alcohol; disulfiram-like reaction possible.
• Teach patient not to change drug dosage without the doctor's orders. Report abnormal blood or urine glucose tests.
• Be sure patient understands that he should not take any other medication, including OTC drugs, without first checking with the doctor.
• Advise patient to carry a medical identification bracelet identifying him as a diabetic patient.

tolbutamide

Apo-Tolbutamide, Mobenol†, Novobutamide†, Oramide, Orinase

Pregnancy Risk Category: C

HOW SUPPLIED

Tablets: 250 mg, 500 mg

MECHANISM OF ACTION

Stimulates insulin release from the pancreatic beta cells and reduces glucose output by the liver. An extrapancreatic effect increases peripheral sensitivity to insulin. A sulfonylurea.

INDICATIONS & DOSAGE

Stable, maturity-onset (Type II) nonketotic diabetes mellitus uncontrolled by diet alone and previously untreated –
Adults: initially, 1 to 2 g P.O. daily as single dose or divided b.i.d. to t.i.d. May adjust dosage to maximum of 3 g daily.
To change from insulin to oral therapy –
Adults: if insulin dosage is under 20 units daily, insulin may be stopped and oral therapy started at 1 to 2 g P.O. daily. If insulin dosage is 20 to 40 units daily, insulin is reduced 30% to 50% and oral therapy started as above. If insulin dosage is over 40 units daily, insulin is decreased 20% and oral therapy started as above. Further reductions in insulin are based on patient's response to oral therapy.

ADVERSE REACTIONS

Common reactions are in italics; life-threatening reactions are in bold italics.
GI: nausea, heartburn.
Metabolic: ***hypoglycemia, dilutional hyponatremia.***
Skin: rash, pruritus, facial flushing.
Other: ***hypersensitivity reactions.***

INTERACTIONS

Anabolic steroids, chloramphenicol, clofibrate, guanethidine, MAO inhibi-

tors, phenylbutazone, salicylates, sulfonamides: increased hypoglycemic activity. Monitor blood glucose level.
Beta blockers, clonidine: prolonged hypoglycemic effect and masked symptoms of hypoglycemia. Use together cautiously.
Corticosteroids, glucagon, rifampin, thiazide diuretics: decreased hypoglycemic response. Monitor blood glucose level.
Hydantoins: increased blood levels of hydantoins. Monitor blood levels closely.
Oral anticoagulants: increased hypoglycemic activity or enhanced anticoagulant effect. Monitor blood glucose and prothrombin time.

NURSING CONSIDERATIONS

- *Contraindicated* for treating type I diabetes (insulin-dependent); diabetes adequately controlled by diet; and type II diabetes (non-insulin-dependent) complicated by fever, ketosis, acidosis, coma, major surgery, severe trauma, Raynaud's disease, renal or hepatic impairment, or thyroid or other endocrine dysfunction. This drug also should not be used during pregnancy or breast-feeding.
- *Use cautiously* in patients with sulfonamide hypersensitivity.
- Elderly patients may be more sensitive to this drug's adverse reactions.
- Instruct patient about nature of disease; importance of following therapeutic regimen, adhering to specific diet, weight reduction, exercise, and personal hygiene program, and avoiding infection; how and when to perform self-monitoring of blood glucose level; and recognition of hypoglycemia and hyperglycemia.
- Be sure patient knows that therapy relieves symptoms but doesn't cure disease.
- Patient transferring from another oral sulfonylurea antidiabetic drug usually needs no transition period.
- Patient transferring from insulin therapy to an oral hypoglycemic should test for blood glucose at least t.i.d. before meals. Hospitalization may be required during the transition.
- Advise patient to avoid moderate to large intake of alcohol: disulfiram-like reaction possible.
- Teach patient not to change drug dosage without the doctor's approval. Report abnormal blood or urine glucose tests.
- Be sure patient understands that he should not take any other medication, including OTC drugs, without first checking with the doctor.
- Advise patient to carry a medical identification bracelet identifying him as a diabetic patient.

56

Thyroid hormones

levothyroxine sodium
liothyronine sodium
liotrix
thyroglobulin
thyroid desiccated
thyrotropin

COMBINATION PRODUCTS

EUTHROID-½: levothyroxine sodium 30 mcg and liothyronine sodium 7.5 mcg.
EUTHROID-1: levothyroxine sodium 60 mcg and liothyronine sodium 15 mcg.
EUTHROID-2: levothyroxine sodium 120 mcg and liothyronine sodium 30 mcg.
EUTHROID-3: levothyroxine sodium 180 mcg and liothyronine sodium 45 mcg.
THYROLAR-¼: levothyroxine sodium 12.5 mcg and liothyronine sodium 3.1 mcg.
THYROLAR-½: levothyroxine sodium 25 mcg and liothyronine sodium 6.25 mcg.
THYROLAR-1: levothyroxine sodium 50 mcg and liothyronine sodium 12.5 mcg.
THYROLAR-2: levothyroxine sodium 100 mcg and liothyronine sodium 25 mcg.
THYROLAR-3: levothyroxine sodium 150 mcg and liothyronine sodium 37.5 mcg.

levothyroxine sodium (T₄ or L-thyroxine sodium)

Eltroxin†, Levoid, Levothroid, Levoxine, Oroxine‡, Synthroid**, Synthrox

Pregnancy Risk Category: A

HOW SUPPLIED
Tablets: 25 mcg, 50 mcg, 75 mcg, 100 mcg, 112 mcg, 125 mcg, 150 mcg, 175 mcg, 200 mcg, 300 mcg
Injection: 200 mcg/vial, 500 mcg/vial

MECHANISM OF ACTION
Stimulates the metabolism of all body tissues by accelerating the rate of cellular oxidation.

INDICATIONS & DOSAGE
Cretinism –
Children under 1 year: initially, 0.025 to 0.05 mg P.O. daily, increased by 0.05 mg P.O. q 2 to 3 weeks to total daily dosage of 0.1 to 0.4 mg P.O.
Myxedema coma –
Adults: 0.4 mg I.V., then 0.1 to 0.3 mg I.V. daily. After condition is stabilized, gradually decrease dosage to 0.05 to 0.1 mg daily. Switch to oral maintenance as soon as possible.
Thyroid hormone replacement –
Adults: initially, 0.025 to 0.1 mg P.O. daily, increased by 0.05 to 0.1 mg P.O. q 1 to 4 weeks until desired response. Maintenance dosage is 0.1 to 0.4 mg daily. May be administered I.V. or I.M. when P.O. ingestion is precluded for long periods.
Adults over 65 years: 0.025 mg P.O. daily. May be increased by 0.025 mg at 3- to 4-week intervals depending on response.
Children: initially, maximum 0.05 mg P.O. daily, gradually increased by 0.025 to 0.05 mg P.O. q 1 to 4 weeks until desired response.

ADVERSE REACTIONS
Common reactions are in italics; life-threatening reactions are in bold italics.

Adverse reactions of thyroid hormones are extensions of their pharma-

cologic properties and reflect patient sensitivity to them.
Signs of overdosage:
CNS: *nervousness, insomnia, tremor.*
CV: *tachycardia, palpitations, arrhythmias, angina pectoris,* hypertension.
GI: appetite change, nausea, diarrhea.
Other: headache, leg cramps, weight loss, sweating, heat intolerance, fever, menstrual irregularities.

INTERACTIONS
Cholestyramine and colestipol: levothyroxine absorption impaired. Separate doses by 4 to 5 hours.
Hypoglycemic agents: change in serum glucose levels. Monitor blood glucose levels. Dosage adjustments may be necessary.
I.V. phenytoin: free thyroid released. Monitor for tachycardia.
Oral anticoagulants: change in prothrombin time. Monitor prothrombin time. Dosage adjustments may be necessary.
Sympathomimetics such as epinephrine: increased risk of coronary insufficiency. Monitor closely.

NURSING CONSIDERATIONS
- *Contraindicated* in myocardial infarction, thyrotoxicosis (except with antithyroid drugs), or uncorrected adrenal insufficiency (thyroid hormones increase tissue demand for adrenocortical hormone and may cause acute adrenal crisis).
- *Use with extreme caution* in angina pectoris, hypertension, or other cardiovascular disorders; renal insufficiency; and ischemic states.
- Thyroid hormone replacement requirements are about 25% lower in patients over 60 years than in young adults.
- *Use cautiously* in myxedema; patients are unusually sensitive to thyroid hormone. Dose varies widely among patients; start at lowest and titrate in higher doses according to patient's symptoms and laboratory data until euthyroid state is reached.
- High initial I.V dosage is usually well tolerated by patients in myxedema coma; however, monitor blood pressure and heart rate closely. Normal serum levels of T_4 should be seen within 24 hours, followed in 3 days by a threefold increase in serum T_3.
- Rapid replacement in patients with arteriosclerosis may precipitate angina, coronary occlusion, or stroke. *Use cautiously* in these patients.
- In patients with coronary artery disease who must receive thyroid hormone, observe carefully for possible coronary insufficiency.
- Potentially dangerous; not indicated to relieve such vague symptoms as sluggishness, irritability, depression, and ill-defined pains; to treat obesity in euthyroid persons; to treat metabolic insufficiency not associated with thyroid insufficiency; or to treat menstrual disorders or male infertility, unless associated with hypothyroidism.
- When changing from levothyroxine to liothyronine, stop levothyroxine and begin liothyronine. Increase in small increments after residual effects of levothyroxine have disappeared. When changing from liothyronine to levothyroxine, start levothyroxine several days before withdrawing liothyronine to avoid relapse.
- To avoid problems with bioequivalence, patient who has achieved a stable response should not change product brands.
- Warn patient (especially elderly patients) to tell doctor at once if chest pain, palpitations, sweating, nervousness, shortness of breath, or other signs of overdosage or aggravated cardiovascular disease occur.
- Be sure patient understands the importance of compliance. Tell patient to take thyroid hormones at the same time each day, preferably before breakfast, to maintain constant hor-

mone levels. Suggest morning dosage to prevent insomnia.

- Monitor pulse and blood pressure.
- **I.V. use:** Prepare I.V. dosage immediately before injection. Do not mix with other solutions. Inject into vein over 1 to 2 minutes.
- Thyroid hormones alter thyroid function test results. Monitor prothrombin time; patients taking these hormones usually require less anticoagulant. Alert patients to report unusual bleeding and bruising.
- Patients taking levothyroxine who need to have radioactive iodine uptake studies must discontinue drug 4 weeks before test.

liothyronine sodium (T_3)

Cyronine, Cytomel, Tertroxin‡

Pregnancy Risk Category: A

HOW SUPPLIED

Tablets: 5 mcg, 25 mcg, 50 mcg

MECHANISM OF ACTION

Stimulates the metabolism of all body tissues by accelerating the rate of cellular oxidation.

INDICATIONS & DOSAGE

Cretinism –
Children 3 years and older: 50 to 100 mcg P.O. daily.
Children under 3 years: 5 mcg P.O. daily, increased by 5 mcg q 3 to 4 days until desired response occurs.
Myxedema –
Adults: initially, 5 mcg P.O. daily, increased by 5 to 10 mcg q 1 or 2 weeks. Maintenance dosage is 50 to 100 mcg daily.
Nontoxic goiter –
Adults: initially, 5 mcg P.O. daily; may be increased by 12.5 to 25 mcg daily q 1 to 2 weeks. Usual maintenance dosage is 75 mcg daily.
Adults over 65 years: initially, 5 mcg P.O. daily, increased by 5-mcg increments at weekly intervals until desired response.
Children: initially, 5 mcg P.O. daily, increased by 5-mcg increments at weekly intervals until desired response.
Thyroid hormone replacement –
Adults: initially, 25 mcg P.O. daily, increased by 12.5 to 25 mcg q 1 to 2 weeks until satisfactory response. Usual maintenance dosage is 25 to 75 mcg daily.
T_3 suppression test to differentiate hyperthyroidism from euthyroidism –
Adults: 75 to 100 mcg P.O. daily for 7 days.

ADVERSE REACTIONS

Common reactions are in italics; life-threatening reactions are in bold italics.

Adverse reactions to thyroid hormones are extensions of their pharmacologic properties and reflect patient sensitivity to them.

CNS: hyperirritability, *nervousness, insomnia,* twitching, *tremors,* headache.
CV: increased cardiac output, *tachycardia,* ***arrhythmias,*** angina pectoris, increased blood pressure, ***cardiac decompensation and collapse.***
GI: diarrhea, abdominal cramps, vomiting.
Other: weight loss, heat intolerance, hyperhidrosis, menstrual irregularities; in infants and children – accelerated rate of bone maturation.

INTERACTIONS

Cholestyramine and colestipol: liothyronine absorption impaired. Separate doses by 4 to 5 hours.
Hypoglycemic agents: change in serum glucose levels. Monitor blood glucose levels. Dosage adjustments may be necessary.
I.V. phenytoin: free thyroid released. Monitor for tachycardia.
Oral anticoagulants: change in prothrombin time. Monitor prothrombin

time. Dosage adjustments may be necessary.

Sympathomimetics such as epinephrine: increased risk of coronary insufficiency. Monitor closely.

NURSING CONSIDERATIONS

- *Contraindicated* in myocardial infarction, thyrotoxicosis (except with antithyroid drugs), or uncorrected adrenal insufficiency (thyroid hormones increase tissue demand for adrenocortical hormone and may cause acute adrenal crisis).
- *Use with extreme caution* in angina pectoris, hypertension, or other cardiovascular disorders; renal insufficiency; and ischemic states.
- Thyroid hormone replacement requirements are about 25% lower in patients over 60 years than in young adults.
- Rapid replacement in patients with arteriosclerosis may precipitate angina, coronary occlusion, or stroke. *Use cautiously* in these patients.
- In patients with coronary artery disease who must receive thyroid hormones, observe carefully for possible coronary insufficiency.
- *Use cautiously* in myxedema; these patients are unusually sensitive to thyroid hormone.
- Potentially dangerous; not indicated to relieve vague symptoms, such as sluggishness, irritability, depression, and ill-defined aches and pains; to treat obesity in euthyroid persons; to treat metabolic insufficiency; or to treat menstrual disorders or male infertility, unless associated with hypothyroidism.
- When changing from levothyroxine to liothyronine, stop levothyroxine and begin liothyronine. Increase in small increments after residual effects of levothyroxine have disappeared. When changing from liothyronine to levothyroxine, start levothyroxine several days before withdrawing liothyronine to avoid relapse.
- To avoid problems with bioequivalence, patient who has achieved a stable response should not change product brands.
- Warn patient (especially elderly patients) to tell doctor at once if chest pain, palpitations, sweating, nervousness, or other signs of overdosage occur. Also notify doctor immediately if any signs of aggravated cardiovascular disease develop (chest pain, dyspnea, and tachycardia).
- Be sure patient understands the importance of compliance. Tell patient to take thyroid hormones at the same time each day, preferably before breakfast, to maintain constant hormone levels. Suggest morning dosage to prevent insomnia.
- Monitor pulse and blood pressure.
- Thyroid hormones alter thyroid function tests. Monitor prothrombin time; patients taking these hormones usually require less anticoagulant. Alert patients to report unusual bleeding and bruising.
- Patients taking liothyronine who need to have radioactive iodine uptake studies must discontinue drug 7 to 10 days before test.

liotrix

Euthroid**, Thyrolar

Pregnancy Risk Category: A

HOW SUPPLIED

Tablets: levothyroxine sodium 30 mcg and liothyronine sodium 7.5 mcg (Euthroid-½); levothyroxine sodium 60 mcg and liothyronine sodium 15 mcg (Euthroid-1); levothyroxine sodium 120 mcg and liothyronine sodium 30 mcg (Euthroid-2); levothyroxine sodium 180 mcg and liothyronine sodium 45 mcg (Euthroid-3); levothyroxine sodium 12.5 mcg and liothyronine sodium 3.1 mcg (Thyrolar-¼); levothyroxine sodium 25 mcg and liothyronine sodium 6.25 mcg (Thyrolar-½); levothyroxine sodium 50 mcg and liothyronine sodium 12.5 mcg (Thyrolar-1); levothyroxine sodium 100 mcg and liothyronine sodium 25 mcg (Thyrolar-2); levothyroxine sodium 150 mcg and liothyronine sodium 37.5 mcg (Thyrolar-3)

MECHANISM OF ACTION

Stimulates the metabolism of all body tissues by accelerating the rate of cellular oxidation.

INDICATIONS & DOSAGE

Dosages are expressed in thyroid equivalents and must be individualized to approximate the deficit in the patient's thyroid secretion.

Hypothyroidism –

Adults and children: initially, 15 to 30 mg P.O. daily, increasing by 15 to 30 mg q 1 to 2 weeks to desired response; increments in children's dosage q 2 weeks.

Adults over 65 years: initially, 15 to 30 mg P.O. Usual adult dosage doubled q 6 to 8 weeks to desired response.

ADVERSE REACTIONS

Common reactions are in italics; life-threatening reactions are in bold italics.

Adverse reactions of thyroid hormones are extensions of their pharmacologic properties and reflect patient sensitivity to them.

CNS: hyperirritability, *nervousness, insomnia,* twitching, *tremors.*

CV: increased cardiac output, *tachycardia,* ***arrhythmias,*** angina pectoris, increased blood pressure, ***cardiac decompensation and collapse.***

GI: diarrhea, abdominal cramps, vomiting.

Other: weight loss, menstrual irregularities, heat intolerance, hyperhidrosis; infants and children – accelerated rate of bone maturation.

INTERACTIONS

Cholestyramine and colestipol: liotrix absorption impaired. Separate doses by 4 to 5 hours.

Hypoglycemic agents: change in serum glucose levels. Monitor blood glucose levels. Dosage adjustments may be necessary.

I.V. phenytoin: free thyroid released. Monitor for tachycardia.

Oral anticoagulants: change in prothrombin time. Monitor prothrombin time. Dosage adjustments may be necessary.

Sympathomimetics such as epinephrine: increased risk of coronary insufficiency. Monitor closely.

NURSING CONSIDERATIONS

- *Contraindicated* in myocardial infarction, thyrotoxicosis (except with antithyroid drugs), or uncorrected adrenal insufficiency (thyroid hormones increase tissue demand for adrenocortical hormone and may cause acute adrenal crisis).
- *Use with extreme caution* in angina pectoris, hypertension, or other cardiovascular disorders; renal insufficiency; and ischemic states.
- Thyroid hormone replacement requirements are about 25% lower in patients over 60 years than in young adults.
- Rapid replacement in arteriosclerosis may precipitate angina, coronary occlusion, or stroke. *Use cautiously* in these patients.
- *Use cautiously* in myxedema; these patients are unusually sensitive to thyroid hormone.
- In patients with coronary artery disease who must receive thyroid hormones, observe carefully for possible coronary insufficiency. Also observe carefully during surgery, since cardiac arrhythmias can be precipitated.
- Potentially dangerous; not indicated to relieve vague symptoms, such as sluggishness, irritability, depression, and ill-defined pains; to treat obesity in euthyroid persons; to treat metabolic insufficiency not associated with thyroid insufficiency; or to treat menstrual

*Liquid form contains alcohol. **May contain tartrazine.

disorders or male infertility, unless associated with hypothyroidism.

- Be sure patient understands the importance of compliance. Tell patient to take thyroid hormones at the same time each day, preferably before breakfast, to maintain constant hormone levels. Suggest morning dosage to prevent insomnia.
- To avoid problems with bioequivalence, patient who has achieved a stable response should not change product brands.
- Warn patient (especially elderly patients) to tell doctor at once if chest pain, palpitations, sweating, nervousness, or other signs of overdosage occur. Also notify doctor immediately if any signs of aggravated cardiovascular disease develop (chest pain, dyspnea, and tachycardia).
- The two commercially prepared liotrix drugs contain different amounts of each ingredient; do not change from one brand to the other without considering the differences in potency: Thyrolar-½ contains 25 mcg T_4 and 6.25 mcg T_3; Euthroid-½ contains 30 mcg T_4 and 7.5 mcg T_3.
- Monitor pulse and blood pressure.
- Thyroid hormones alter thyroid function test results. Monitor prothrombin time; patients taking these hormones usually require less anticoagulant. Alert patients to report unusual bleeding and bruising.

thyroglobulin

Proloid

Pregnancy Risk Category: A

HOW SUPPLIED

Tablets: 32 mg, 65 mg, 100 mg, 130 mg, 200 mg

MECHANISM OF ACTION

Stimulates the metabolism of all body tissues by accelerating the rate of cellular oxidation.

INDICATIONS & DOSAGE

Cretinism and juvenile hypothyroidism – **Children 1 year and older:** dosage may approach adult dosage (60 to 180 mg P.O. daily), depending on response.
Children 4 to 12 months: 60 to 80 mg P.O. daily.
Children 1 to 4 months: initially, 15 to 30 mg P.O. daily, increased at 2-week intervals. Usual maintenance dosage is 30 to 45 mg P.O. daily.
Hypothyroidism or myxedema –
Adults: initially, 15 to 30 mg P.O. daily, increased by 15 to 30 mg at 2-week intervals until desired response. Usual maintenance dosage is 60 to 180 mg P.O. daily, as a single dose.
Adults over 65 years: initially, 7.5 to 15 mg P.O. daily; dosage is doubled at 6- to 8-week intervals until desired response is obtained.

ADVERSE REACTIONS

Common reactions are in italics; life-threatening reactions are in bold italics.

Adverse reactions of thyroid hormones are extensions of their pharmacologic properties and reflect patient sensitivity to them.

CNS: hyperirritability, *nervousness, insomnia,* twitching, *tremors,* headache.
CV: increased cardiac output, *tachycardia,* ***arrhythmias,*** angina pectoris, increased blood pressure, ***cardiac decompensation and collapse.***
GI: diarrhea, abdominal cramps, vomiting.
Other: weight loss, heat intolerance, hyperhidrosis, menstrual irregularities; in infants and children – accelerated rate of bone maturation.

INTERACTIONS

Cholestyramine and colestipol: thyroglobulin absorption impaired. Separate doses by 4 to 5 hours.
Hypoglycemic agents: change in serum glucose levels. Monitor blood glucose levels. Dosage adjustments may be necessary.

I.V. phenytoin: free thyroid released. Monitor for tachycardia.
Oral anticoagulants: change in prothrombin time. Monitor prothrombin time. Dosage adjustments may be necessary.
Sympathomimetics such as epinephrine: increased risk of coronary insufficiency. Monitor closely.

NURSING CONSIDERATIONS

- *Contraindicated* in myocardial infarction, thyrotoxicosis (except with antithyroid drugs), or uncorrected adrenal insufficiency (thyroid hormones increase tissue demand for adrenocortical hormone and may cause acute adrenal crisis).
- *Use with extreme caution* in angina pectoris, hypertension, or other cardiovascular disorders; renal insufficiency; and ischemic states.
- Thyroid hormone replacement requirements are about 25% lower in patients over 60 years than in young adults.
- In patients with coronary artery disease who must receive thyroid hormones, observe carefully for possible coronary insufficiency.
- *Use cautiously* in myxedema; these patients are unusually sensitive to thyroid hormone.
- Potentially dangerous; not indicated to relieve vague symptoms, such as sluggishness, irritability, depression, and ill-defined pains; to treat obesity in euthyroid persons; to treat metabolic insufficiency not associated with thyroid insufficiency; or to treat menstrual disorders or male infertility, unless associated with hypothyroidism.
- Tell patient to take thyroid hormones at the same time each day, to maintain constant hormone levels.
- Warn patient (especially elderly patients) to tell doctor at once if chest pain, palpitations, sweating, nervousness, or other signs of overdosage occur. Also notify doctor immediately if chest pain, dyspnea, or tachycardia develop.
- To avoid problems with bioequivalence, patient who has achieved a stable response should not change product brands.
- Suggest morning dosage to prevent insomnia.
- Monitor pulse and blood pressure.
- Monitor prothrombin time; patients taking these hormones usually require less anticoagulant. Alert patients to report unusual bleeding and bruising.

thyroid dessicated

Armour Thyroid, S-P-T, Thyrar, Thyroid Strong, Thyroid USP Enseals, Thyro-Teric

Pregnancy Risk Category: A

HOW SUPPLIED

Tablets: 16 mg, 32 mg, 65 mg, 98 mg, 130 mg, 195 mg, 260 mg, 325 mg
Tablets (bovine origin): 32 mg, 65 mg, 130 mg
Tablets (enteric-coated): 32 mg, 65 mg, 130 mg
Strong tablets (50% stronger than thyroid USP, and containing 0.3% iodine): 32 mg, 65 mg, 130 mg, 195 mg
Capsules (porcine origin): 65 mg, 130 mg, 195 mg, 325 mg

MECHANISM OF ACTION

Stimulates the metabolism of all body tissues by accelerating the rate of cellular oxidation.

INDICATIONS & DOSAGE

Hypothyroidism –
Adults: initially, 60 mg P.O. daily, increased by 60 mg q 30 days until desired response. Usual maintenance dosage is 60 to 180 mg P.O. daily, as a single dose.
Adults over 65 years: 7.5 to 15 mg P.O. daily; dosage is doubled at 6- to 8-week intervals.

Myxedema –
Adults: 16 mg P.O. daily. May double dosage q 2 weeks to maximum 120 mg.
Cretinism and juvenile hypothyroidism –
Children 1 year and older: dosage may approach adult dosage (60 to 180 mg P.O.) daily, depending on response.
Children 4 to 12 months: 30 to 60 mg P.O. daily.
Children 1 to 4 months: initially, 15 to 30 mg P.O. daily, increased at 2-week intervals. Usual maintenance dosage is 30 to 45 mg P.O. daily.

ADVERSE REACTIONS

Common reactions are in italics; life-threatening reactions are in bold italics.

Adverse reactions of thyroid hormones are extensions of their pharmacologic properties and reflect patient sensitivity to them.
CNS: *hyperirritability, nervousness, insomnia,* twitching, tremors, headache.
CV: increased cardiac output, *tachycardia,* ***arrhythmias,*** angina pectoris, increased blood pressure, ***cardiac decompensation and collapse.***
GI: diarrhea, abdominal cramps, vomiting.
Other: weight loss, heat intolerance, hyperhidrosis, menstrual irregularities; in infants and children – accelerated rate of bone maturation.

INTERACTIONS

Cholestyramine: thyroid absorption impaired. Separate doses by 4 to 5 hours.
Hypoglycemic agents: change in serum glucose levels. Monitor blood glucose levels. Dosage adjustments may be necessary.
I.V. phenytoin: free thyroid released. Monitor for tachycardia.
Oral anticoagulants: change in prothrombin time. Monitor prothrombin time. Dosage adjustments may be necessary.
Sympathomimetics such as epinephrine: increased risk of coronary insufficiency. Monitor closely.

NURSING CONSIDERATIONS

- *Contraindicated* in myocardial infarction, thyrotoxicosis (except with antithyroid drugs), or uncorrected adrenal insufficiency (thyroid hormones increase tissue demand for adrenocortical hormone and may cause acute adrenal crisis).
- *Use with extreme caution* in angina pectoris, hypertension, or other cardiovascular disorders; renal insufficiency; and ischemic states.
- Thyroid hormone replacement requirements are about 25% lower in patients over 60 years than in young adults.
- *Use cautiously* in myxedema; these patients are unusually sensitive to thyroid hormone.
- In patients with coronary artery disease who must receive thyroid hormones, observe carefully for possible coronary insufficiency.
- Potentially dangerous; not indicated to relieve vague symptoms, such as sluggishness, irritability, depression, and ill-defined pains; to treat obesity in euthyroid persons; to treat metabolic insufficiency not associated with thyroid insufficiency; or to treat menstrual disorders or male infertility, unless caused by hypothyroidism.
- Tell patient to take thyroid hormones at the same time each day to maintain constant hormone levels.
- To avoid problems with bioequivalence, patient who has achieved a stable response should not change product brands.
- Warn patient (especially elderly patients) to tell doctor at once if chest pain, palpitations, sweating, nervousness, or other signs of overdosage occur. Also notify doctor immediately if any signs of aggravated cardiovascular disease develop (chest pain, dyspnea, and tachycardia).

• Suggest morning dosage to prevent insomnia.
• Monitor pulse and blood pressure.
• In children, sleeping pulse rate and basal morning temperature are guides to treatment.
• Thyroid hormones alter thyroid function test results. Monitor prothrombin time; patients taking these hormones usually require less anticoagulant. Alert patients to report unusual bleeding and bruising.

thyrotropin (thyroid-stimulating hormone, or TSH)

Thytropar

Pregnancy Risk Category: C

HOW SUPPLIED
Powder for injection: 10 IU/vial

MECHANISM OF ACTION
Stimulates the uptake of radioactive iodine in patients with thyroid carcinoma. Also promotes thyroid hormone production by the anterior pituitary.

INDICATIONS & DOSAGE
Diagnosis of thyroid cancer remnant with ^{131}I after surgery –
Adults: 10 IU I.M. or S.C. for 3 to 7 days.
Differential diagnosis of primary and secondary hypothyroidism –
Adults: 10 IU I.M. or S.C. for 1 to 3 days.
In PBI or ^{131}I uptake determinations for differential diagnosis of subclinical hypothyroidism or low thyroid reserve –
Adults: 10 IU I.M. or S.C.
Therapy for thyroid carcinoma (local or metastatic) with ^{131}I –
Adults: 10 IU I.M. or S.C. for 3 to 8 days.
To determine thyroid status of patient receiving thyroid hormone –
Adults: 10 units I.M. or S.C. for 1 to 3 days.

ADVERSE REACTIONS
Common reactions are in italics; life-threatening reactions are in bold italics.
CNS: headache.
CV: *tachycardia,* atrial fibrillation, angina pectoris, ***CHF,*** hypotension.
GI: nausea, vomiting.
Other: thyroid hyperplasia (large doses), fever, menstrual irregularities, allergic reactions (postinjection flare, urticaria, ***anaphylaxis***).

INTERACTIONS
Hypoglycemic agents: change in serum glucose levels. Monitor blood glucose levels. Dosage adjustments may be necessary.
Oral anticoagulants: change in prothrombin time. Monitor prothrombin time. Dosage adjustments may be necessary.
Sympathomimetics such as epinephrine: increased risk of coronary insufficiency. Monitor closely.

NURSING CONSIDERATIONS
• *Contraindicated* in patients hypersensitive to the drug, and in coronary thrombosis and untreated Addison's disease.
• *Use cautiously* in angina pectoris, CHF, hypopituitarism, and adrenocortical suppression.
• May cause thyroid hyperplasia.
• Diagnostic use: to identify subclinical hypothyroidism or low thyroid reserve, to evaluate need for thyroid hormone therapy, to distinguish between primary and secondary hypothyroidism, and to detect thyroid remnants and metastases of thyroid carcinoma.
• Three-day dosage schedule may be used in long-standing pituitary myxedema or with prolonged use of thyroid medication.

57

Thyroid hormone antagonists

methimazole
potassium iodide
potassium iodide, saturated solution
strong iodine solution
propylthiouracil
radioactive iodine (sodium iodide) ^{131}I

COMBINATION PRODUCTS
None.

methimazole

Tapazole
Pregnancy Risk Category: D

HOW SUPPLIED
Tablets: 5 mg, 10 mg

MECHANISM OF ACTION
Inhibits oxidation of iodine in the thyroid gland, blocking iodine's ability to combine with tyrosine to form thyroxine. May also prevent the coupling of monoiodotyrosine and diiodotyrosine to form thyroxine and triiodothyronine.

INDICATIONS & DOSAGE
Hyperthyroidism –
Adults: 5 mg P.O. t.i.d. if mild; 10 to 15 mg P.O. t.i.d. if moderately severe; and 20 mg P.O. t.i.d. if severe. Continue until patient is euthyroid, then start maintenance dosage of 5 mg daily to t.i.d. Maximum dosage 150 mg daily.
Children: 0.4 mg/kg P.O. daily divided q 8 hours. Continue until patient is euthyroid, then start maintenance dosage of 0.2 mg/kg daily divided q 8 hours.
Preparation for thyroidectomy –
Adults and children: same doses as for hyperthyroidism until patient is euthyroid; then iodine may be added for 10 days before surgery.
Thyrotoxic crisis –
Adults and children: same doses as for hyperthyroidism, with concomitant iodine therapy and propranolol.

ADVERSE REACTIONS
Common reactions are in italics; life-threatening reactions are in bold italics.
Blood: ***agranulocytosis,*** leukopenia, granulopenia, thrombocytopenia (appear to be dose-related).
CNS: headache, drowsiness, vertigo.
GI: diarrhea, nausea, vomiting (may be dose-related).
Hepatic: jaundice.
Skin: rash, urticaria, skin discoloration.
Other: arthralgia, myalgia, salivary gland enlargement, loss of taste, drug fever, lymphadenopathy.

INTERACTIONS
None significant.

NURSING CONSIDERATIONS
- *Use cautiously* in pregnancy. Pregnant women may require less drug as pregnancy progresses. Monitor thyroid function studies closely. Thyroid may be added to regimen. Drugs may be stopped during last few weeks of pregnancy.
- *Also use cautiously* in breast-feeding women. Although drug is excreted in breast milk, small doses given to the mother (15 mg/day or less) do not pose a major risk to the infant if infant's thyroid function is monitored frequently (at biweekly or weekly intervals).
- Watch for signs of hypothyroidism (mental depression; cold intolerance; hard, nonpitting edema). Dosage may need to be adjusted.

- Monitor CBC periodically to detect impending leukopenia, thrombocytopenia, and agranulocytosis. Also monitor hepatic function.
- Doses of over 30 mg/day increase the risk of agranulocytosis.
- Warn patient to report immediately: fever, sore throat, or mouth sores (possible signs of developing agranulocytosis). Agranulocytosis can develop too rapidly to be detected by periodic blood cell counts. Tell patient also to immediately report skin eruptions (sign of hypersensitivity).
- Drug should be stopped if severe rash or enlarged cervical lymph nodes develop.
- Tell patient to ask doctor about using iodized salt and eating shellfish during treatment.
- Warn patient against over-the-counter cough medicines; many contain iodine.
- Give with meals to reduce GI adverse reactions.
- Store in light-resistant container.

potassium iodide
Pima

potassium iodide, saturated solution (SSKI)

strong iodine solution (Lugol's solution)

Pregnancy Risk Category: D

HOW SUPPLIED
potassium iodide
Tablets (enteric-coated): 300 mg
Oral solution: 500 mg/15 ml
Syrup: 325 mg/5 ml
potassium iodide, saturated solution
Oral solution: 1 g/ml
strong iodine solution
Oral solution: iodine 50 mg/ml and potassium iodide 100 mg/ml

MECHANISM OF ACTION
Inhibits thyroid hormone formation by blocking iodotyrosine and iodothyronine synthesis. It also limits iodide transport into the thyroid gland and blocks thyroid hormone release.

INDICATIONS & DOSAGE
Preparation for thyroidectomy –
Adults and children: Strong Iodine Solution, USP, 0.1 to 0.3 ml P.O. t.i.d., or Potassium Iodide Solution, USP, 5 drops in water P.O. t.i.d. after meals for 2 to 3 weeks before surgery.
Thyrotoxic crisis –
Adults and children: Strong Iodine Solution, USP, 1 ml in water P.O. t.i.d. after meals.
Radiation protectant for thyroid gland –
Adults: 100 to 150 mg P.O. 24 hours before and for 3 to 10 days after radiation exposure
Expectorant –
Adults: 0.3 to 0.6 ml SSKI diluted in water three or four times a day.

ADVERSE REACTIONS
Common reactions are in italics; life-threatening reactions are in bold italics.
EENT: acute rhinitis, inflammation of salivary glands, periorbital edema, conjunctivitis, hyperemia.
GI: burning, irritation, *nausea,* vomiting, *metallic taste.*
Skin: acneiform rash, mucous membrane ulceration.
Other: fever, frontal headache, tooth discoloration, ***hypersensitivity, including symptoms resembling serum sickness.***

INTERACTIONS
Angiotensin-converting enzyme inhibitors, potassium-sparing diuretics: risk of hyperkalemia. Avoid concomitant use.
Antithyroid medications: potassium iodide may potentiate hypothyroid or goiterogenic effects. Monitor closely.

*Liquid form contains alcohol. **May contain tartrazine.

Lithium carbonate: hypothyroidism may occur. Use with caution.

NURSING CONSIDERATIONS
- *Contraindicated* in tuberculosis, iodide hypersensitivity, hyperkalemia; after meals that contain excessive starch; in laryngeal edema, swelling of salivary glands.
- Earliest signs of delayed hypersensitivity caused by iodides are irritation and swelling of the eyelids.
- Dilute oral doses in water, milk, or fruit juice, and give after meals to prevent gastric irritation, to hydrate the patient, and to mask the very salty taste.
- Tell patient to ask the doctor about using iodized salt and eating shellfish during treatment. Iodine-rich foods may not be permitted.
- Warn the patient that sudden withdrawal may precipitate thyroid storm.
- Avoid using enteric-coated tablets, which have been associated with small bowel lesions and can lead to serious complications, including perforation, hemorrhage, or obstruction.
- Store in light-resistant container.
- Give iodides through straw to avoid tooth discoloration.
- Usually given with other antithyroid drugs.

propylthiouracil (PTU)
Propyl-Thyracil†

Pregnancy Risk Category: D

HOW SUPPLIED
Tablets: 50 mg, 100 mg†

MECHANISM OF ACTION
Inhibits oxidation of iodine in the thyroid gland, blocking iodine's ability to combine with tyrosine to form thyroxine. May also prevent the coupling of monoiodotyrosine and diiodotyrosine to form thyroxine and triiodothyronine.

INDICATIONS & DOSAGE
Hyperthyroidism –
Adults: 100 mg P.O. t.i.d.; up to 300 mg q 8 hours have been used in severe cases. Continue until patient is euthyroid, then start maintenance dosage of 100 mg daily to t.i.d.
Children over 10 years: 100 mg P.O. t.i.d. Continue until patient is euthyroid, then start maintenance dosage of 25 mg t.i.d. to 100 mg b.i.d.
Children 6 to 10 years: 50 to 150 mg P.O. divided doses q 8 hours.
Preparation for thyroidectomy –
Adults and children: same doses as for hyperthyroidism, then iodine may be added 10 days before surgery.
Thyrotoxic crisis –
Adults and children: same doses as for hyperthyroidism, with concomitant iodine therapy and propranolol.

ADVERSE REACTIONS
Common reactions are in italics; life-threatening reactions are in bold italics.
Blood: ***agranulocytosis,*** leukopenia, thrombocytopenia (appear to be dose-related).
CNS: headache, drowsiness, vertigo.
EENT: visual disturbances.
GI: diarrhea, *nausea, vomiting* (may be dose-related).
Hepatic: jaundice, ***hepatotoxicity.***
Skin: rash, urticaria, skin discoloration, pruritus.
Other: arthralgia, myalgia, salivary gland enlargement, loss of taste, drug fever, lymphadenopathy, vasculitis.

INTERACTIONS
None significant.

NURSING CONSIDERATIONS
- *Use cautiously* in pregnancy. Pregnant women may require less drug as pregnancy progresses. Monitor thyroid function studies closely. Thyroid may be added to regimen. Drugs may be stopped during last few weeks of pregnancy.
- Also *use cautiously* in breast-feed-

ing women. Although small amounts of drug are excreted in breast milk, it appears safe for use by breast-feeding mothers if the infant's thyroid function is monitored at weekly or biweekly intervals.
- Watch for signs of hypothyroidism (mental depression; cold intolerance; hard, nonpitting edema). Dosage may need to be adjusted.
- Monitor CBC periodically to detect impending leukopenia, thrombocytopenia, and agranulocytosis.
- Warn patient to report immediately: fever, sore throat, or mouth sores (possible signs of developing agranulocytosis). Agranulocytosis can develop too rapidly to be detected by periodic blood cell counts. Tell patient to also report skin eruptions (sign of hypersensitivity) immediately.
- Drug should be stopped if severe rash or enlarged cervical lymph nodes develop.
- Tell patient to ask doctor about using iodized salt and eating shellfish during treatment.
- Warn patient against over-the-counter cough medicines; many contain iodine.
- Give with meals to reduce GI adverse reactions.
- Store in light-resistant container.

radioactive iodine (sodium iodide) ^{131}I

Iodotope Therapeutic, Sodium Iodide ^{131}I Therapeutic

Pregnancy Risk Category: X

HOW SUPPLIED

All radioactivity concentrations are determined at the time of calibration; ^{131}I has a physical half-life of about 8 days.

Iodotope Therapeutic

Capsules: radioactivity range is 1 to 50 millicuries (mCi)/capsule at time of calibration

Oral solution: radioactivity concentration is 7.05 mCi/ml at time of calibration; in vials containing approximately 7, 14, 28, 70, or 106 mCi at time of calibration

Sodium Iodide ^{131}I Therapeutic

Capsules: radioactivity range is 0.8 to 100 mCi/capsule

Oral solution: radioactivity range is 3.5 to 150 mCi/vial

MECHANISM OF ACTION

Limits thyroid hormone secretion by destroying thyroid tissue. The affinity of thyroid tissue for radioactive iodine facilitates uptake of the drug by cancerous thyroid tissue that has metastasized to other sites in the body.

INDICATIONS & DOSAGE

Hyperthyroidism –

Adults: usual dosage is 4 to 10 mCi P.O. Dosage based on estimated weight of thyroid gland and thyroid uptake. Treatment may be repeated after 6 weeks, according to serum thyroxine.

Thyroid cancer –

Adults: 50 to 150 mCi P.O. Dosage based on estimated malignant thyroid tissue and metastatic tissue as determined by total body scan. Treatment may be repeated according to clinical status.

ADVERSE REACTIONS

Common reactions are in italics; life-threatening reactions are in bold italics.

EENT: *feeling of fullness in neck,* metallic taste, "radiation mumps."

Endocrine: hypothyroidism, radiation thyroiditis.

Other: possible increased risk of developing ***leukemia*** later in life after sufficient ^{131}I dose for thyroid ablation following cancer surgery; possible increased risk of birth defects in offspring after sufficient ^{131}I dose for thyroid ablation following cancer surgery.

*Liquid form contains alcohol. **May contain tartrazine.

INTERACTIONS

Lithium carbonate: hypothyroidism may occur. Use with caution.

NURSING CONSIDERATIONS

- *Contraindicated* in pregnancy except to treat thyroid cancer. Also contraindicated during breast-feeding.
- Stop all antithyroid medications and thyroid preparations 1 week before ^{131}I dose. If medications are not stopped, patient may receive thyroid-stimulating hormone for 3 days before ^{131}I dose. When treating women of childbearing age, give dose during menstruation or within 7 days after menstruation.
- Many drugs can interfere with the action of ^{131}I. The following drugs should be withheld for the specified time before giving ^{131}I: adrenocorticoids, 1 week; benzodiazepines, 1 month; contrast media containing iodine, 1 to 2 months; cholecystographic agents, 6 to 9 months; iodine-containing products, including vitamins, expectorants, antitussives, and topical agents, 2 weeks; salicylates, 1 to 2 weeks.
- Food may delay absorption. Patient should fast overnight before administration.
- After therapy for hyperthyroidism, patient should not resume antithyroid drugs, but should continue propranolol or other drugs used to treat symptoms of hyperthyroidism until onset of full ^{131}I effect (usually 6 weeks).
- Monitor thyroid function with serum thyroxine.
- After dose for hyperthyroidism, patient's urine and saliva are slightly radioactive for 24 hours; vomitus is highly radioactive for 6 to 8 hours. Institute full radiation precautions during this time. Instruct patient to use appropriate disposal methods when coughing and expectorating.
- After dose for thyroid cancer, patient's urine, saliva, and perspiration remain radioactive for 3 days. Isolate patient and observe the following precautions: pregnant personnel should not take care of patient; disposable eating utensils and linens should be used; instruct patient to save all urine in lead containers for 24 to 48 hours so amount of radioactive material excreted can be determined. Patient should drink as much fluid as possible for 48 hours after drug administration to facilitate excretion. Limit contact with patient to 30 minutes per shift per person the first day. May increase time to 1 hour second day and longer on third day.
- If patient is discharged less than 7 days after ^{131}I dose for thyroid cancer, warn him to avoid close, prolonged contact with small children (for example, holding children on lap), and instruct him not to sleep in same room with spouse for 7 days after treatment because of increased risk of thyroid cancer in persons exposed to ^{131}I. Tell patient he may use same bathroom facilities as rest of family.

58

Pituitary hormones

corticotropin
cosyntropin
desmopressin acetate
leuprolide acetate
(See Chapter 71, ANTINEOPLASTICS ALTERING HORMONE BALANCE.)
lypressin
sermorelin acetate
somatrem
vasopressin
vasopressin tannate

COMBINATION PRODUCTS

None.

corticotropin (adrenocorticotropic hormone, ACTH)

ACTH, Acthar, Acthar Gel (H.P.)†, ACTH Gel, Cortigel-40, Cortigel-80, Cortrophin Gel, Cortropic-Gel-40, Cortropic-Gel-80, H.P. Acthar Gel

Pregnancy Risk Category: C

HOW SUPPLIED

Aqueous injection: 25 units/vial, 40 units/vial
Repository injection: 40 units/ml, 80 units/ml

MECHANISM OF ACTION

By replacing the body's own tropic hormone, stimulates the adrenal cortex to secrete its entire spectrum of hormones.

INDICATIONS & DOSAGE

Diagnostic test of adrenocortical function –
Adults: up to 80 units I.M. or S.C. in divided doses; or a single dose of repository form; or 10 to 25 units (aqueous form) in 500 ml dextrose 5% in water I.V. over 8 hours, between blood samplings.

Individual dosages generally vary with adrenal glands' sensitivity to stimulation as well as with specific disease. Infants and younger children require larger doses per kilogram than do older children and adults.

For therapeutic use –
Adults: 40 units S.C. or I.M. in 4 divided doses (aqueous); 40 units q 12 to 24 hours (gel or repository form).

ADVERSE REACTIONS

Common reactions are in italics; life-threatening reactions are in bold italics.
CNS: ***seizures,*** *dizziness,* papilledema, headache, *euphoria, insomnia,* mood swings, personality changes, depression, psychosis.
EENT: cataracts, glaucoma.
GI: peptic ulcer with perforation and hemorrhage, pancreatitis, abdominal distention, ulcerative esophagitis, nausea, vomiting.
GU: menstrual irregularities.
Metabolic: *sodium and fluid retention,* calcium and potassium loss, hypokalemic alkalosis, negative nitrogen balance.
Skin: impaired wound healing, thin fragile skin, petechiae, ecchymoses, facial erythema, increased sweating, acne, hyperpigmentation, allergic skin reactions, hirsutism.
Other: muscle weakness, steroid myopathy, loss of muscle mass, osteoporosis, vertebral compression fractures, cushingoid state, suppression of growth in children, activation of latent diabetes mellitus, progressive increase in antibodies, loss of ACTH stimulatory effect, and ***hypersensitivity.***

INTERACTIONS

Anticonvulsants, barbiturates, rifampin: increased metabolism of ACTH and decreased effectiveness. Monitor for lack of effect.
Estrogens: may potentiate the effects of cortisol. Dosage adjustments may be necessary.
NSAIDs, salicylates: increased risk of GI bleeding. Avoid concomitant use.
Oral anticoagulants: change in prothrombin time. Monitor prothrombin time. Dosage adjustments may be necessary.
Potassium-wasting diuretics: increased risk of hypokalemia. Monitor serum potassium levels.

NURSING CONSIDERATIONS

- *Contraindicated* in scleroderma, osteoporosis, systemic fungal infections, ocular herpes simplex, recent surgery, peptic ulcer, congestive heart failure, hypertension, sensitivity to pork and pork products, concomitant smallpox vaccination, adrenocortical hyperfunction or primary insufficiency, or Cushing's syndrome.
- *Use cautiously* in pregnant women or breast-feeding mothers and in women of childbearing age; patients being immunized; latent tuberculosis or tuberculin reactivity; hypothyroidism; cirrhosis; infection (use anti-infective therapy during and after ACTH treatment); acute gouty arthritis (limit ACTH treatment to a few days, and use conventional therapy during and for several days after ACTH treatment); emotional instability or psychotic tendencies; diabetes; abscess; pyogenic infections; renal insufficiency; myasthenia gravis.
- ACTH treatment should be preceded by verification of adrenal responsiveness and test for hypersensitivity and allergic reactions.
- ACTH should be adjunctive; not sole therapy. Oral agents are preferred for long-term therapy.
- Unusual stress may require additional use of rapidly acting corticosteroids. When possible, gradually reduce ACTH dosage to smallest effective dose to minimize induced adrenocortical insufficiency. Reinstitute therapy if stressful situation (trauma, surgery, severe illness) occurs shortly after stopping drug.
- Watch neonates of ACTH-treated mothers for signs of hypoadrenalism.
- Counteract edema by low-sodium, high-potassium intake; nitrogen loss by high-protein diet; and psychotic changes by reducing ACTH dosage or administering sedatives.
- ACTH may mask signs of chronic disease and decrease host resistance and ability to localize infection.
- Note and record weight changes, fluid exchange, and resting blood pressures until minimal effective dose is achieved.
- Refrigerate reconstituted solution and use within 24 hours.
- If administering gel, warm it to room temperature, draw into large needle, and give slowly deep I.M. with 21G or 22G needle. Warn patient that injection is painful.
- **I.V. use:** Use only the aqueous form for I.V. administration. Dilute in 500 ml dextrose 5% in water and infuse over 8 hours.

---

cosyntropin

Cortrosyn

Pregnancy Risk Category: C

HOW SUPPLIED

Injection: 0.25 mg/vial

MECHANISM OF ACTION

By replacing the body's own tropic hormone, stimulates the adrenal cortex to secrete its entire spectrum of hormones.

INDICATIONS & DOSAGE

Diagnostic test of adrenocortical function –

Adults and children: 0.25 to 1 mg I.M. or I.V. (unless label prohibits I.V. administration) between blood samplings.
Children under 2 years: 0.125 mg I.M. or I.V.

ADVERSE REACTIONS
Common reactions are in italics; life-threatening reactions are in bold italics.
Skin: pruritus.
Other: flushing, ***hypersensitivity***, ***anaphylaxis*** (rare).

INTERACTIONS
None significant.

NURSING CONSIDERATIONS
- *Use cautiously* in patients with hypersensitivity to natural corticotropin.
- Drug is synthetic duplication of the biologically active part of the ACTH molecule. It is less likely to produce sensitivity than natural ACTH from animal sources.
- **I.V. use:** Reconstitute with 1 ml of supplied diluent. For direct injection, administer over at least 2 minutes. May be further diluted with dextrose 5% in water or 0.9% sodium chloride injection and infused over 6 hours. Solution is stable for 12 hours at room temperature.
- Monitor patient for allergic reactions, rashes, dyspnea, wheezing, or evidence of anaphylaxis.

desmopressin acetate
DDAVP, Minirin‡, Stimate

Pregnancy Risk Category: B

HOW SUPPLIED
Nasal solution: 0.1 mg/ml
Injection: 4 mcg/ml

MECHANISM OF ACTION
Increases the permeability of the renal tubular epithelium to adenosine monophosphate and water; the epithelium promotes reabsorption of water and produces a concentrated urine (antidiuretic hormone effect). Desmopressin also increases Factor VIII activity by releasing endogenous Factor VIII from plasma storage sites.

INDICATIONS & DOSAGE
Nonnephrogenic diabetes insipidus, temporary polyuria and polydipsia associated with pituitary trauma –
Adults: 0.1 to 0.4 ml intranasally daily in 1 to 3 doses. Adjust morning and evening doses separately for adequate diurnal rhythm of water turnover. Alternatively, may administer injectable form in dosage of 0.5 to 1 ml I.V. or S.C. daily, usually in two divided doses.
Children 3 months to 12 years: 0.05 to 0.3 ml intranasally daily in 1 or 2 doses.
Treatment of hemophilia A and von Willebrand's disease –
Adults and children: 0.3 mcg/kg diluted in normal saline and infused I.V. slowly over 15 to 30 minutes. May repeat dose if necessary as indicated by laboratory response and the patient's clinical condition.
Primary nocturnal enuresis –
Children 5 years and over: initially, 20 mcg intranasally h.s. Adjust dose according to response. Maximum recommended dose is 40 mcg daily.

ADVERSE REACTIONS
Common reactions are in italics; life-threatening reactions are in bold italics.
CNS: headache.
CV: slight rise in blood pressure at high dosage.
EENT: nasal congestion, rhinitis.
GI: nausea, abdominal cramps.
GU: vulval pain.
Other: flushing.

INTERACTIONS
Demeclocycline, ethanol, epinephrine, heparin, lithium: increased risk of adverse effects. Monitor closely.

NURSING CONSIDERATIONS
• *Contraindicated* in patients with hypersensitivity to the drug, patients with type IIb von Willebrand's disease, and in children under age 3 months.
• *Use cautiously* in coronary artery insufficiency or hypertensive cardiovascular disease.
• Advise patient to wear medical alert identification.
• Adjust fluid intake to reduce risk of water intoxication and sodium depletion, especially in children or elderly patients. Warn these patients to drink only enough water to satisfy thirst.
• Overdose may cause oxytocic or vasopressor activity. Withhold drug until effects subside. Furosemide may be used if fluid retention is excessive.
• Some patients may have difficulty measuring and inhaling drug into nostrils. Teach patient and caregiver correct method of administration.
• Instruct patient to clear nasal passages before administering drug.
• Nasal congestion, allergic rhinitis, or upper respiratory infections may impair drug absorption. Advise patient to report such conditions to the doctor because they may require dosage adjustment.
• For treating nocturnal enuresis, the recommended method of administration is one-half of the calculated dose in each nostril.
• Intranasal use can cause changes in the nasal mucosa resulting in erratic, unreliable absorption. Report any patient's worsening condition to doctor, who may prescribe injectable DDAVP.
• Teach patients using S.C. desmopressin to rotate injection sites to prevent tissue damage.
• Desmopressin injection should not be used to treat hemophilia A with Factor VIII levels of 0% to 5%, or severe cases of von Willebrand's disease.
• In patients treated for hemophilia A and von Willebrand's disease, use of desmopressin may avoid the hazards of using blood products.
• Has been used successfully to reduce blood loss during cardiac surgery.

lypressin
Diapid

Pregnancy Risk Category: B

HOW SUPPLIED
Nasal spray: 0.185 mg/ml

MECHANISM OF ACTION
Increases the permeability of the renal tubular epithelium to adenosine monophosphate and water; the epithelium promotes reabsorption of water and produces a concentrated urine (antidiuretic hormone effect).

INDICATIONS & DOSAGE
Nonnephrogenic diabetes insipidus –
Adults and children: 1 or 2 sprays (approximately 2 USP posterior pituitary pressor units/spray) in either or both nostrils q.i.d. and an additional dose at bedtime, if needed, to prevent nocturia. If usual dosage is inadequate, increase frequency rather than number of sprays.

ADVERSE REACTIONS
Common reactions are in italics; life-threatening reactions are in bold italics.
CNS: headache, dizziness.
EENT: nasal congestion or ulceration, irritation, pruritus of nasal passages, rhinorrhea, conjunctivitis.
GI: heartburn due to drip of excess spray into pharynx, abdominal cramps, frequent bowel movements.
GU: possible transient fluid retention from overdose.
Skin: hypersensitivity reaction.

INTERACTIONS
None significant.

NURSING CONSIDERATIONS

- *Contraindicated* in patients with hypersensitivity to the drug.
- *Use cautiously* in patients with coronary artery disease, hypertension, allergic rhinitis, or upper airway infection.
- Patients should understand that the drug is for topical application to the nasal mucosa. It should not be inhaled.
- Instruct patient to clear nasal passage before administering drug.
- Inadvertent inhalation of spray may cause tightness in chest, coughing, and transient dyspnea.
- To administer a uniform, well-diffused spray, hold bottle upright with patient in vertical position holding head upright.
- Particularly useful if diabetes insipidus is unresponsive to other therapy, or if antidiuretic hormones of animal origin cause adverse effects.
- Nasal congestion, allergic rhinitis, or upper respiratory infections may diminish drug absorption and require larger dose or adjunctive therapy.
- Test patients sensitive to antidiuretic hormone for sensitivity to lypressin.
- Instruct the patient to carry the medication with him at all times because of its fairly short duration.
- Instruct patient to wear medical alert identification.

sermorelin acetate

Geref

Pregnancy Risk Category: C

HOW SUPPLIED

Powder for injection: 50 mcg/ampule

MECHANISM OF ACTION

A synthetic polypeptide that mimics the aminoterminal segment of the naturally occurring human growth hormone (GH).

INDICATIONS & DOSAGE

Diagnostic aid to determine the pituitary gland's ability to secrete GH– **Adults and children:** 1 mcg/kg as a single I.V. injection.

ADVERSE REACTIONS

Common reactions are in italics; life-threatening reactions are in bold italics.

CNS: headache.

GI: nausea.

Local: pain, redness, or swelling at injection site.

Other: transient warmth or flushing of face, unusual taste in mouth, antibody formation, paleness, tightness in chest.

INTERACTIONS

Antithyroid medications (such as propylthiouracil), anticholinergics: decreased response to sermorelin.

Clonidine, levodopa, or insulin-induced hypoglycemia: may elevate somatotropin levels.

Corticosteroids, insulin, cyclooxygenase inhibitors (for example, aspirin, acetaminophen, or NSAIDs): alter the pituitary secretion of somatotropin. Don't perform the test in patients receiving these drugs.

NURSING CONSIDERATIONS

- *Contraindicated* in patients with hypersensitivity to the drug or any components of the formulation.
- Response to drug may be blunted in hypothyroid patients.
- Although hypersensitivity reactions have been reported with the administration of other polypeptide hormones, none have been reported to date with sermorelin. About 25% of patients develop antibody formation with prolonged use; however, no symptomatic allergic reactions have been reported to date.
- In clinical trials, GH peak plasma levels of 28 ± 15 ng/ml occur at 30 ± 27 minutes after the injection.

• Discontinue GH therapy 1 week before the test.
• **I.V. use:** Reconstitute each ampule with a minimum of 0.5 ml of the supplied diluent. One ampule contains 50 mcg of drug, which is sufficient to test a 110-lb (50-kg) subject. Larger subjects will require the use of multiple ampules.
• Venous blood samples for GH determinations should be drawn 15 minutes before and immediately before injection. Administer bolus injection (1 mcg/kg I.V.) and follow with a 3-ml sodium chloride solution flush. Venous samples for GH determinations should be drawn at 15-minute intervals after injection (15 minutes, 30 minutes, 45 minutes, and 60 minutes).
• Baseline GH levels are generally low (< 4 ng/ml). Provocative tests such as sermorelin are useful in determining that the pituitary somatotroph can respond. However, a normal response doesn't rule out GH deficiency if the deficit is caused by hypothalamic dysfunction. This test is most easily interpreted if patient has had a subnormal response to conventional provocative testing (such as clonidine, levodopa, or arginine) and a normal response to sermorelin, suggesting that the cause of GH deficiency is hypothalamic dysfunction. Abnormal results from both conventional tests and sermorelin can't locate the dysfunction.
• Be sure patient understands that the test must be performed in the morning after an overnight fast. He should take nothing by mouth after midnight.

somatrem

Protropin

Pregnancy Risk Category: C

HOW SUPPLIED

Injectable lyophilized powder: 5 mg (10 IU)/vial

MECHANISM OF ACTION

Purified growth hormone of recombinant DNA origin that stimulates linear, skeletal muscle, and organ growth.

INDICATIONS & DOSAGE

Long-term treatment of children who have growth failure because of lack of adequate endogenous growth hormone secretion –
Children (prepuberty): 0.1 mg/kg I.M. or S.C. given three times weekly.

ADVERSE REACTIONS

Common reactions are in italics; life-threatening reactions are in bold italics.
Endocrine: hypothyroidism, hyperglycemia.
Other: antibodies to growth hormone.

INTERACTIONS

Glucocorticoids: may inhibit growth-promoting action of somatrem. Glucocorticoid dose may need to be adjusted.

NURSING CONSIDERATIONS

• *Contraindicated* in patients with closed epiphyses, an active underlying intracranial lesion, or known sensitivity to benzyl alcohol.
• *Use cautiously* in patients with hypothyroidism and in those whose growth hormone deficiency results from an intracranial lesion. Patient should be examined frequently for progression or recurrence of the underlying disease.
• Regular checkups with monitoring of height and of blood and radiologic studies are necessary.
• Observe patient for signs of glucose intolerance and hyperglycemia.
• Monitor periodic thyroid function tests for hypothyroidism, which may require treatment with a thyroid hormone.
• This drug replaces pituitary-derived

human growth hormone, which was removed from the market in 1985 because of an association with a rare but fatal virus infection (Jakob-Creutzfeldt disease). Reassure your patient and his family that somatrem is *pure* and that it is *safe*.

- To prepare the solution, inject the bacteriostatic water for injection (which is supplied) into the vial containing the drug. Then swirl the vial with a gentle rotary motion until the contents are completely dissolved. *Don't shake* the vial.
- After reconstitution, vial solution should be clear. Don't inject into the patient if the solution is cloudy or contains any particles.
- Store reconstituted vial in refrigerator. Must use within 7 days.
- Be sure to check this product's expiration date.

vasopressin (antidiuretic hormone)
Pitressin

vasopressin tannate
Pitressin Tannate

Pregnancy Risk Category: B

HOW SUPPLIED
vasopressin
Injection: 0.5-ml and 1-ml ampules, 20 units/ml
vasopressin tannate
Injection: 1-ml ampules, 5 units/ml

MECHANISM OF ACTION
Increases the permeability of the renal tubular epithelium to adenosine monophosphate and water; the epithelium promotes reabsorption of water and produces a concentrated urine (antidiuretic hormone effect).

INDICATIONS & DOSAGE
Nonnephrogenic, nonpsychogenic diabetes insipidus –
Adults: 5 to 10 units I.M. or S.C. b.i.d. to q.i.d., p.r.n.; or intranasally (aqueous solution used as spray or applied to cotton balls) in individualized doses, based on response. For chronic therapy, inject 2.5 to 5 units Pitressin Tannate in oil suspension I.M. or S.C. q 2 to 3 days.
Children: 2.5 to 10 units I.M. or S.C. b.i.d. to q.i.d., p.r.n.; or intranasally (aqueous solution used as spray or applied to cotton balls) in individualized doses. For chronic therapy, inject 1.25 to 2.5 units Pitressin Tannate in oil suspension I.M. or S.C. q 2 to 3 days.
Postoperative abdominal distention –
Adults: 5 units (aqueous) I.M. initially, then q 3 to 4 hours, increasing dose to 10 units, if needed. Reduce dose proportionately for children.
To expel gas before abdominal X-ray –
Adults: inject 10 units S.C. at 2 hours, then again at 30 minutes before X-ray. Enema before first dose may also help to eliminate gas.
Upper GI tract hemorrhage –
Adults: 0.2 to 0.4 units/minute by intraarterial injection. Do not use tannate in oil suspension.

ADVERSE REACTIONS
Common reactions are in italics; life-threatening reactions are in bold italics.
CNS: tremor, dizziness, headache.
CV: angina in patients with vascular disease, vasoconstriction. Large doses may cause hypertension, electrocardiographic changes. (With intraarterial infusion: ***bradycardia, cardiac arrhythmias, pulmonary edema.***)
GI: abdominal cramps, nausea, vomiting, diarrhea, intestinal hyperactivity.
GU: uterine cramps, anuria.
Skin: circumoral pallor.
Other: water intoxication (drowsiness, listlessness, headache, confusion, weight gain), hypersensitivity reactions (urticaria, angioneurotic

*Liquid form contains alcohol. **May contain tartrazine.

edema, bronchoconstriction, fever, rash, wheezing, dyspnea, ***anaphylaxis***), sweating.

INTERACTIONS

Carbamazepine, chlorpropamide, clofibrate: increased antidiuretic response. Use together cautiously.
Demeclocycline, lithium, norepinephrine: reduced antidiuretic activity. Use together cautiously.

NURSING CONSIDERATIONS

- *Contraindicated* in chronic nephritis with nitrogen retention. Use cautiously in children, elderly persons, pregnant women, and patients with epilepsy, migraine, asthma, cardiovascular disease, or fluid overload.
- Never inject vasopressin tannate in oil I.V.
- Never inject during first stage of labor; may cause ruptured uterus.
- Monitor specific gravity of urine and intake and output to aid evaluation of drug effectiveness.
- Place tannate in oil in warm water for 10 to 15 minutes. Then shake thoroughly to make suspension uniform before withdrawing I.M. injection dose. Small brown particles must be seen in suspension. Use absolutely dry syringe to avoid dilution.
- Instruct patient to rotate injection sites to prevent tissue damage.
- Give with 1 to 2 glasses of water to reduce adverse reactions and to improve therapeutic response.
- To prevent possible seizures, coma, and death, observe patient closely for early signs of water intoxication.
- Overhydration more likely with long-acting tannate oil suspension than with aqueous vasopressin solution.
- Use minimum effective dosage to reduce adverse reactions.
- May be used for transient polyuria resulting from antidiuretic hormone deficiency related to neurosurgery or head injury.
- Synthetic desmopressin is sometimes preferred because of longer duration and less frequent adverse reactions. Desmopressin is also commercially available as a nasal solution.
- Monitor blood pressure of patient on vasopressin twice daily. Watch for excessively elevated blood pressure or lack of response to drug, which may be indicated by hypotension. Also monitor fluid intake and output and daily weights.
- A rectal tube will facilitate gas expulsion following vasopressin injection.

59
Parathyroid-like agents

calcifediol
calcitonin (human)
calcitonin (salmon)
calcitriol
dihydrotachysterol
etidronate disodium

COMBINATION PRODUCTS
None.

calcifediol
Calderol

Pregnancy Risk Category: A

HOW SUPPLIED
Capsules: 20 mcg, 50 mcg

MECHANISM OF ACTION
Stimulates calcium absorption from the GI tract and promotes secretion of calcium from bone to blood.

INDICATIONS & DOSAGE
Treatment and management of metabolic bone disease associated with chronic renal failure –
Adults: initially, 300 to 350 mcg P.O. weekly, given on a daily or alternate-day schedule. Dosage may be increased at 4-week intervals. Optimal dosage must be carefully determined for each patient.

ADVERSE REACTIONS
Common reactions are in italics; life-threatening reactions are in bold italics.
Vitamin D intoxication associated with hypercalcemia:
CNS: headache, somnolence.
EENT: conjunctivitis, photosensitivity, rhinorrhea.
GI: nausea, vomiting, constipation, metallic taste, dry mouth, anorexia, diarrhea.
GU: polyuria.
Other: weakness, bone and muscle pain.

INTERACTIONS
Cholestyramine, colestipol: decreased absorption of orally administered vitamin D analogs. Avoid concomitant use.
Magnesium-containing antacids: possible hypermagnesemia, especially in patients with chronic renal failure. Avoid concomitant use.
Other vitamin D analogs: additive effects and increased toxicity. Avoid concomitant use.

NURSING CONSIDERATIONS
- *Contraindicated* in hypercalcemia or vitamin D toxicity. Withhold all preparations containing vitamin D in patients taking calcifediol.
- *Use cautiously* in patients with renal function impairment and in patients on digitalis because hypercalcemia may precipitate cardiac arrhythmias.
- Monitor serum calcium; serum calcium times serum phosphate should not exceed 70. During titration, serum calcium should be determined at least weekly. If hypercalcemia occurs, calcifediol should be discontinued but resumed after serum calcium returns to normal.
- Patient should receive adequate daily intake of calcium.
- Advise patient to adhere to diet and calcium supplementation and to avoid nonprescription drugs.
- Teach patient to report signs and symptoms of hypercalcemia.

calcitonin (human)
Cibacalcin

calcitonin (salmon)

Calcimar, Miacalcin

Pregnancy Risk Category: B

HOW SUPPLIED

human

Injection: 0.5 mg/vial

salmon

Injection: 100 IU/ml, 1-ml ampules; 200 IU/ml, 2-ml ampules

MECHANISM OF ACTION

Decreases osteoclastic activity by inhibiting osteocytic osteolysis. Also decreases mineral release and matrix or collagen breakdown in bone.

INDICATIONS & DOSAGE

Paget's disease of bone (osteitis deformans) –

Adults: initially, 100 IU of calcitonin (salmon) daily S.C. or I.M. Maintenance dosage is 50 to 100 IU daily or every other day. Alternatively, give calcitonin (human) 0.5 mg S.C. daily. If patient obtains sufficient improvement, dosage may be reduced to 0.25 mg. daily 2 or 3 times per week. Some patients may need as much as 1 mg daily.

Hypercalcemia –

Adults: 4 IU/kg of calcitonin (salmon) q 12 hours I.M.

Postmenopausal osteoporosis –

Women: 100 of calcitonin (salmon) daily I.M. or S.C.

ADVERSE REACTIONS

Common reactions are in italics; life-threatening reactions are in bold italics.

CNS: headaches.

GI: transient nausea with or without vomiting, diarrhea, anorexia.

GU: transient diuresis.

Metabolic: hyperglycemia.

Local: inflammation at injection site, skin rashes.

Other: *facial flushing;* hypocalcemia; swelling, tingling, and tenderness of hands; unusual taste sensation; ***anaphylaxis***.

INTERACTIONS

None significant.

NURSING CONSIDERATIONS

- *Contraindicated* in allergy to gelatin diluent used to prepare drug. Not recommended for breast-feeding mothers, or women who are or may become pregnant. Safe use in children not established.
- Periodic serum alkaline phosphatase and 24-hour urine hydroxyproline levels should be determined to evaluate drug effect.
- Skin test is usually done before beginning therapy.
- Systemic allergic reactions possible since hormone is protein. Keep epinephrine handy when administering.
- Patients with good initial clinical response to calcitonin who suffer relapse should be evaluated for antibody formation response to the hormone protein.
- Tell patient in whom calcitonin loses its hypocalcemic activity that further medication or increased dosages will be of no value.
- Facial flushing and warmth occur in 20% to 30% of all patients within minutes of injection; usually last about 1 hour. Reassure patient that this is a transient effect.
- Observe patient for signs of hypocalcemic tetany during therapy (muscle twitching, tetanic spasms, and seizures if hypocalcemia is severe).
- Monitor calcium closely. Watch for signs of hypercalcemic relapse: bone pain, renal calculi, polyuria, anorexia, nausea, vomiting, thirst, constipation, lethargy, bradycardia, muscle hypotonicity, pathologic fracture, psychosis, and coma.
- Periodic examinations of urine sediment are advisable.
- Calcitonin (human) is indicated especially in patients who have developed resistance to calcitonin (salmon). Calcitonin (human) is associated with risk of diminishing effi-

cacy caused by antibody formation or hypersensitivity reactions.
• Administer the drug at bedtime when possible to minimize nausea and vomiting.
• Treatment should continue for at least 6 months. Then, if symptoms have been relieved, it may be discontinued until symptoms or radiologic signs recur.
• Store calcitonin (human) at room temperature (77° F [25° C]); store calcitonin (salmon) in the refrigerator (36° to 46° F [2° to 8° C]).
• Be sure to use the freshly reconstituted solution within 2 hours.
• I.M. route is preferred if the volume of the dose to be administered exceeds 2 ml.
• When administered for postmenopausal osteoporosis, remind patient to take adequate calcium and vitamin D supplementation.

calcitriol (1,25-dihydroxycholecalciferol)

Rocaltrol

Pregnancy Risk Category: A (D if used in doses > RDA)

HOW SUPPLIED
Capsules: 0.25 mcg, 0.5 mcg

MECHANISM OF ACTION
Stimulates calcium absorption from the GI tract and promotes secretion of calcium from bone to blood.

INDICATIONS & DOSAGE
Management of hypocalcemia in patients undergoing chronic dialysis – **Adults:** initially, 0.25 mcg P.O. daily. Dosage may be increased by 0.25 mcg daily at 2- to 4-week intervals. Maintenance dosage is 0.25 mcg every other day up to 0.5 to 1.25 mcg daily.
Management of hypoparathyroidism and pseudohypoparathyroidism – **Adults and children over 1 year:** initially, 0.25 mcg P.O. daily. Dosage may be increased at 2- to 4-week intervals. Maintenance dosage is 0.25 to 2 mcg daily.

ADVERSE REACTIONS
Common reactions are in italics; life-threatening reactions are in bold italics.
Vitamin D intoxication associated with hypercalcemia:
CNS: headache, somnolence.
EENT: conjunctivitis, photophobia, rhinorrhea.
GI: nausea, vomiting, constipation, metallic taste, dry mouth, anorexia.
GU: polyuria.
Other: weakness, bone and muscle pain.

INTERACTIONS
Cholestyramine, colestipol: decreased absorption of orally administered vitamin D analogs. Avoid concomitant use.
Magnesium-containing antacids: possible hypermagnesemia, especially in patients with chronic renal failure. Avoid concomitant use.

NURSING CONSIDERATIONS
• *Contraindicated* in hypercalcemia or vitamin D toxicity. Withhold all preparations containing vitamin D in patients taking calcitriol. Not recommended in breast-feeding mothers.
• *Use cautiously* in patients on digitalis; hypercalcemia may precipitate cardiac arrhythmias.
• Monitor serum calcium; serum calcium times serum phosphate should not exceed 70. During titration, determine serum calcium twice weekly. If hypercalcemia occurs, discontinue, but resume after serum calcium returns to normal. Patient should receive adequate daily intake of calcium – 1,000 mg.
• Protect from heat and light.
• Instruct patient to adhere to diet and calcium supplementation and to avoid unapproved nonprescription drugs.
• Patients should not use magnesium-

*Liquid form contains alcohol. **May contain tartrazine.

containing antacids while taking this drug.

- Patients should report to doctor immediately any of the following symptoms: weakness, nausea, vomiting, dry mouth, constipation, muscle or bone pain, or metallic taste – early symptoms of vitamin D intoxication.
- Tell patient that although this drug is a vitamin, it must not be taken by anyone for whom it was not prescribed because of its potentially serious toxicities.
- Most potent form of vitamin D available.

dihydrotachysterol

AT-10‡, DHT Intensol*, Hytakerol

Pregnancy Risk Category: A (D if used in doses > RDA)

HOW SUPPLIED

Tablets: 0.125 mg, 0.2 mg, 0.4 mg
Capsules: 0.125 mg
Oral solution: 0.2 mg/5 ml, 0.2 mg/ml* (DHT Intensol*), 0.25 mg/ml (in sesame oil)

MECHANISM OF ACTION

Stimulates calcium absorption from the GI tract and promotes secretion of calcium from bone to blood.

INDICATIONS & DOSAGE

Familial hypophosphatemia –
Adults and children: 0.5 to 2 mg P.O. daily. Maintenance dosage is 0.3 to 1.5 mg daily.

Hypocalcemia associated with hypoparathyroidism and pseudohypoparathyroidism –
Adults: initially, 0.8 to 2.4 mg P.O. daily for several days. Maintenance dosage is 0.2 to 2 mg daily, as required for normal serum calcium. Average dose is 0.6 mg daily.
Children: initially, 1 to 5 mg P.O. for several days. Maintenance dosage is 0.2 to 1 mg daily, as required for normal serum calcium.

Renal osteodystrophy in chronic uremia –
Adults: 0.1 to 0.6 mg P.O. daily.

Prophylaxis of hypocalcemic tetany following thyroid surgery –
Adults: 0.25 mg P.O. daily (with calcium supplements).

ADVERSE REACTIONS

Common reactions are in italics; life-threatening reactions are in bold italics.

Vitamin D intoxication associated with hypercalcemia:
CNS: headache, somnolence.
EENT: conjunctivitis, photophobia, rhinorrhea.
GI: nausea, vomiting, constipation, metallic taste, dry mouth, anorexia, diarrhea.
GU: polyuria.
Other: weakness, bone and muscle pain.

INTERACTIONS

Cholestyramine, colestipol: decreased absorption of orally administered vitamin D analogs. Avoid concomitant use.
Thiazide diuretics: possible hypercalcemia in hypoparathyroid patients. Avoid concomitant use.

NURSING CONSIDERATIONS

- *Contraindicated* in hypercalcemia, hypocalcemia associated with renal insufficiency and hyperphosphatemia, renal stones, hypersensitivity to vitamin D, and in breast-feeding mothers.
- Monitor serum and urine calcium. Watch for signs of hypercalcemia.
- Adequate dietary calcium intake is necessary; usually supplemented with 10 to 15 g oral calcium lactate or gluconate daily.
- Report hypercalcemia reactions to doctor. Early signs of hypercalcemia include thirst, headache, vertigo, tinnitus, anorexia.
- 1 mg equal to 120,000 units ergocalciferol (vitamin D_2).

• Store in tightly closed, light-resistant container. Don't refrigerate.

etidronate disodium

Didronel

Pregnancy Risk Category: B

HOW SUPPLIED

Tablets: 200 mg, 400 mg

MECHANISM OF ACTION

Decreases osteoclastic activity by inhibiting osteocytic osteolysis. Also decreases mineral release and matrix or collagen breakdown in bone.

INDICATIONS & DOSAGE

Symptomatic Paget's disease –
Adults: 5 mg/kg P.O. daily as a single dose 2 hours before a meal with water or juice. Patient should not eat for 2 hours after dose. May give up to 10 mg/kg daily in severe cases. Maximum dosage is 20 mg/kg daily.
Heterotopic ossification in spinal cord injuries –
Adults: 20 mg/kg P.O. daily for 2 weeks, then 10 mg/kg daily for 10 weeks. Total treatment period is 12 weeks.
Heterotopic ossification after total hip replacement –
Adults: 20 mg/kg daily P.O.for 1 month before total hip replacement and for 3 months afterward.

ADVERSE REACTIONS

Common reactions are in italics; life-threatening reactions are in bold italics.
GI: (seen most frequently at 20 mg/kg daily) diarrhea, increased frequency of bowel movements, nausea.
Other: increased or recurrent bone pain at pagetic sites, pain at previously asymptomatic sites, increased risk of fracture, *elevated serum phosphate.*

INTERACTIONS

None significant.

NURSING CONSIDERATIONS

• *Use cautiously* in enterocolitis, impaired renal function.
• Therapy should not last more than 6 months. After 3 months, resume if needed. Don't give longer than 3 months at doses above 10 mg/kg daily.
• Don't give drug with food, milk, or antacids; may reduce absorption.
• Monitor renal function before and during therapy.
• Elevated serum phosphate may occur, especially in patients receiving higher doses. However, serum phosphate usually returns to normal 2 to 4 weeks after drug's discontinued.
• Monitor drug effect by serum alkaline phosphatase and urinary hydroxyproline excretion (both lowered if therapy effective).
• Tell patient that improvement may not occur for up to 3 months but may continue for months after drug is stopped. Stress importance of good nutrition, especially diet high in calcium and vitamin D.
• Has been used investigationally to prevent or treat osteoporosis.

60

Diuretics

acetazolamide
acetazolamide sodium
amiloride hydrochloride
bendroflumethiazide
benzthiazide
bumetanide
chlorothiazide
chlorothiazide sodium
chlorthalidone
dichlorphenamide
ethacrynate sodium
ethacrynic acid
furosemide
hydrochlorothiazide
hydroflumethiazide
indapamide
mannitol
methazolamide
methyclothiazide
metolazone
polythiazide
quinethazone
spironolactone
triamterene
trichlormethiazide
urea

COMBINATION PRODUCTS

ALAZIDE: spironolactone 25 mg and hydrochlorothiazide 25 mg.
ALDACTAZIDE: spironolactone 25 mg and hydrochlorothiazide 25 mg.
ALDACTAZIDE 50/50: spironolactone 50 mg and hydrochlorothiazide 50 mg.
ALTEXIDE: spironolactone 25 mg and hydrochlorothiazide 25 mg.
DYAZIDE: triamterene 50 mg and hydrochlorothiazide 25 mg.
MAXZIDE: triamterene 75 mg and hydrochlorothiazide 50 mg.
MODURETIC: amiloride hydrochloride 5 mg and hydrochlorothiazide 50 mg.
SPIRONAZIDE: spironolactone 25 mg and hydrochlorothiazide 25 mg.
SPIROZIDE: spironolactone 25 mg and hydrochlorothiazide 25 mg.

acetazolamide

Acetazolam†, Ak-Zol, Apo-Acetazolamide†, Dazamide, Diamox, Diamox Sequels, Storzolamide

acetazolamide sodium

Diamox Parenteral, Diamox Sodium†

Pregnancy Risk Category: C

HOW SUPPLIED

Tablets: 125 mg, 250 mg
Capsules (extended-release): 500 mg
Injection: 500 mg/vial

MECHANISM OF ACTION

Blocks the action of carbonic anhydrase, thereby promoting the renal excretion of sodium, potassium, bicarbonate, and water. Bicarbonate ion excretion makes the urine alkaline. Also decreases secretion of aqueous humor in the eye, thereby lowering intraocular pressure. As an anticonvulsant, may inhibit carbonic anhydrase in the CNS and decrease abnormal paroxysmal or excessive neuronal discharge. In acute mountain sickness, carbonic anhydrase inhibitors produce a respiratory and metabolic acidosis that may stimulate ventilation, increase cerebral blood flow, promote the release of oxygen from hemoglobin, and increase ventilation.

INDICATIONS & DOSAGE

Narrow-angle glaucoma –
Adults: 250 mg q 4 hours; or 250 mg P.O., I.M., or I.V. b.i.d. for short-term therapy.
Edema in congestive heart failure –

Adults: 250 to 375 mg P.O., I.M., or I.V. daily in a.m.
Children: 5 mg/kg daily in a.m.
Open-angle glaucoma –
Adults: 250 mg daily to 1 g P.O., I.M., or I.V. divided q.i.d.
Prevention or amelioration of acute mountain sickness –
Adults: 250 mg P.O. q 8 to 12 hours.
Adjunctive treatment of myoclonic, refractory generalized tonic-clonic, absence, or mixed seizures –
Adults: 375 mg P.O., I.M., or I.V. daily up to 250 mg q.i.d. Alternatively, use sustained-release form 250 to 500 mg P.O. daily or b.i.d. Initial dosage when used with other anticonvulsants usually is 250 mg daily.
Children: 8 to 30 mg/kg P.O. daily, divided t.i.d. or q.i.d. Maximum dosage is 1.5 g daily, or 300 to 900 mg/m^2 daily.

ADVERSE REACTIONS
Common reactions are in italics; life-threatening reactions are in bold italics.
Blood: ***aplastic anemia,*** hemolytic anemia, leukopenia.
CNS: drowsiness, paresthesias, confusion.
EENT: transient myopia.
GI: nausea, vomiting, anorexia.
GU: crystalluria, renal calculi, hematuria.
Metabolic: hyperchloremic acidosis, hypokalemia, asymptomatic hyperuricemia.
Skin: rash.
Local: *pain at injection site,* sterile abscesses.

INTERACTIONS
None significant.

NURSING CONSIDERATIONS
- *Contraindicated* in long-term therapy for chronic noncongestive narrow-angle glaucoma; also in hyponatremia or hypokalemia, renal or hepatic disease or dysfunction, adrenal gland failure, or hyperchloremic acidosis.
- *Use cautiously* in patients with respiratory acidosis, emphysema, chronic pulmonary disease, and in those patients receiving other diuretics.
- Monitor intake and output and electrolytes, especially serum potassium. When used in diuretic therapy, consult with doctor and dietitian to provide high-potassium diet.
- Weigh patient daily. Rapid or excessive fluid loss causes weight loss and hypotension.
- Diuretic effect is decreased when acidosis occurs but can be reestablished by withdrawing drug for several days and then restarting, or by intermittent administration schedules.
- Reconstitute 500-mg vial with at least 5 ml sterile water for injection. Use within 24 hours of reconstitution.
- I.M. injection is painful because of alkalinity of solution.
- **I.V. use:** Administer direct I.V. using a 21G or 23G needle. Inject 100 to 500 mg/minute into a large vein. Intermittent or continuous infusion is not recommended.
- Elderly patients are especially susceptible to excessive diuresis.
- May cause false-positive urine protein tests by alkalinizing the urine.
- To make an oral liquid: soften 1 tablet in 2 teaspoonfuls of very warm water and add to 2 teaspoonfuls honey or syrup (chocolate or cherry). Don't use fruit juice.

amiloride hydrochloride
Kaluril‡, Midamor

Pregnancy Risk Category: B

HOW SUPPLIED
Tablets: 5 mg

MECHANISM OF ACTION
A potassium-sparing diuretic that inhibits sodium reabsorption and potas-

*Liquid form contains alcohol. **May contain tartrazine.

sium excretion by direct action on the distal tubule.

INDICATIONS & DOSAGE

Hypertension; edema associated with congestive heart failure, usually in patients who are also taking thiazide or other potassium-wasting diuretics –

Adults: usual dosage is 5 mg P.O. daily. Dosage may be increased to 10 mg daily, if necessary. As much as 20 mg daily can be given.

ADVERSE REACTIONS

Common reactions are in italics; life-threatening reactions are in bold italics.

CNS: *headache,* weakness, dizziness.

CV: orthostatic hypotension.

GI: *nausea, anorexia, diarrhea, vomiting,* abdominal pain, constipation.

GU: impotence.

Metabolic: hyperkalemia.

INTERACTIONS

ACE inhibitors, potassium-sparing diuretics, potassium supplements: possible hyperkalemia. Avoid concomitant use.

NSAIDs: decreased diuretic effectiveness. Avoid concomitant use.

NURSING CONSIDERATIONS

- *Contraindicated* in patients with elevated serum potassium level (greater than 5.5 mEq/liter). Don't administer to patients receiving other potassium-sparing diuretics, such as spironolactone and triamterene. Also contraindicated in anuria and acute or chronic renal insufficiency because potassium retention is increased.
- Risk of hyperkalemia is greater when a potassium-wasting drug is not taken concurrently. When amiloride is taken this way, be sure to monitor daily potassium.
- Discontinue immediately if potassium level exceeds 6.5 mEq/liter.
- Advise patient to avoid sudden posture changes and rise slowly to avoid orthostatic hypotension.
- Warn patient to avoid excessive ingestion of potassium-rich foods or potassium-containing salt substitutes. Concomitant potassium supplement can lead to serious hyperkalemia.
- Administer amiloride with meals to prevent nausea.

bendroflumethiazide (bendrofluazide)

Aprinox‡, Aprinox-M‡, Benzide‡, Naturetin

Pregnancy Risk Category: B

HOW SUPPLIED

Tablets: 2.5 mg, 5 mg, 10 mg

MECHANISM OF ACTION

A thiazide diuretic that increases urine excretion of sodium and water by inhibiting sodium reabsorption in the cortical diluting site of the ascending loop of Henle.

INDICATIONS & DOSAGE

Edema, hypertension –

Adults: 5 to 20 mg P.O. daily or divided b.i.d.

Children: initially, 0.1 to 0.4 mg/kg (3 to 12 mg/m^2) P.O. daily or divided b.i.d.

Maintenance: 0.05 to 0.1 mg/kg (1.5 to 3 mg/m^2) P.O. daily or divided b.i.d.

ADVERSE REACTIONS

Common reactions are in italics; life-threatening reactions are in bold italics.

Blood: ***aplastic anemia, agranulocytosis,*** leukopenia, thrombocytopenia.

CV: volume depletion and dehydration, orthostatic hypotension.

GI: anorexia, nausea, pancreatitis.

Hepatic: hepatic encephalopathy.

Metabolic: hypokalemia, asymptomatic hyperuricemia, hyperglycemia and impairment of glucose tolerance, fluid and electrolyte imbalances including dilutional hyponatremia and

hypochloremia, metabolic alkalosis, hypercalcemia, gout.
Skin: dermatitis, photosensitivity, rash.
Other: hypersensitivity reactions, such as pneumonitis and vasculitis.

INTERACTIONS
Cholestyramine, colestipol: intestinal absorption of thiazides decreased. Keep doses as separate as possible.
Diazoxide: increased antihypertensive, hyperglycemic, and hyperuricemic effects. Use together cautiously.
NSAIDs: may decrease diuretic effectiveness. Avoid concomitant use.

NURSING CONSIDERATIONS
- *Contraindicated* in anuria or hypersensitivity to other thiazides or other sulfonamide-derived drugs.
- *Use cautiously* in severe renal disease and impaired hepatic function.
- Monitor intake and output, weight, and serum electrolytes regularly. Monitor serum creatinine and BUN regularly. Not as effective if these are more than twice normal.
- Consult with doctor and dietitian to provide high-potassium diet. Watch for signs of hypokalemia (for example, muscle weakness and cramps). Patients on digitalis have an increased risk of digitalis toxicity from potassium-depleting adverse effect of this diuretic. May be used with potassium-sparing diuretic to prevent potassium loss.
- Foods rich in potassium include citrus fruits, bananas, tomatoes, dates, and apricots.
- Monitor blood glucose levels. Check insulin requirements in patients with diabetes. May treat severe hyperglycemia with oral antidiabetic agents.
- Monitor blood uric acid, especially in patients with a history of gout.
- Elderly patients are especially susceptible to excessive diuresis.
- Give in a.m. to prevent nocturia.
- In hypertension, therapeutic response may be delayed several days.
- Thiazides and thiazide-like diuretics should be discontinued before tests for parathyroid function are performed.
- Advise patient to avoid sudden posture changes and rise slowly to avoid orthostatic hypotension.
- Advise patient to use a sunscreen.

benzthiazide
Aquatag**, Exna**, Hydrex, Proaqua**

Pregnancy Risk Category: D

HOW SUPPLIED
Tablets: 50 mg

MECHANISM OF ACTION
A thiazide diuretic that increases urine excretion of sodium and water by inhibiting sodium reabsorption in the cortical diluting site of the nephron.

INDICATIONS & DOSAGE
Edema, hypertension –
Adults: 50 to 200 mg P.O. daily or in divided doses.
Children: 1 to 4 mg/kg P.O. daily in three divided doses.

ADVERSE REACTIONS
Common reactions are in italics; life-threatening reactions are in bold italics.
Blood: ***aplastic anemia, agranulocytosis,*** leukopenia, thrombocytopenia.
CV: volume depletion and dehydration, orthostatic hypotension.
GI: anorexia, nausea, pancreatitis.
Hepatic: hepatic encephalopathy.
Metabolic: hypokalemia, asymptomatic hyperuricemia, hyperglycemia and impairment of glucose tolerance, fluid and electrolyte imbalances including dilutional hyponatremia and hypochloremia, metabolic alkalosis, hypercalcemia, gout.

Skin: dermatitis, photosensitivity, rash.
Other: hypersensitivity reactions, such as pneumonitis and vasculitis.

INTERACTIONS
Cholestyramine, colestipol: intestinal absorption of thiazides decreased. Keep doses as separate as possible.
Diazoxide: increased antihypertensive, hyperglycemic, and hyperuricemic effects. Use together cautiously.
NSAIDs: may decrease diuretic effectiveness. Avoid concomitant use.

NURSING CONSIDERATIONS
- *Contraindicated* in anuria or hypersensitivity to other thiazides or other sulfonamide-derived drugs.
- *Use cautiously* in severe renal disease and impaired hepatic function.
- Monitor intake and output, weight, and serum electrolytes regularly. Consult with doctor and dietitian to provide high-potassium diet. Watch for signs of hypokalemia (for example, muscle weakness and cramps). Patients on digitalis have an increased risk of digitalis toxicity from the potassium-depleting adverse effect of this diuretic. May use with potassium-sparing diuretic to prevent potassium loss.
- Foods rich in potassium include citrus fruits, bananas, tomatoes, dates, and apricots.
- Monitor blood pressure routinely. If possible, teach patient or family how to check blood pressure.
- Monitor serum creatinine and BUN regularly. Not as effective if these levels are more than twice normal.
- Monitor blood glucose levels. Check insulin requirements in patients with diabetes. May treat severe hyperglycemia with oral antidiabetic agents.
- Monitor blood uric acid level, especially in patients with a history of gout.
- Give in a.m. to prevent nocturia.
- Elderly patients are especially susceptible to excessive diuresis.
- In hypertension, therapeutic response may be delayed several days.
- Thiazides and thiazide-like diuretics should be discontinued before tests for parathyroid function are performed.
- Advise patient to avoid sudden posture changes and rise slowly to avoid orthostatic hypotension.
- Advise patient to use a sunscreen.

bumetanide
Bumex, Burinex‡

Pregnancy Risk Category: C

HOW SUPPLIED
Tablets: 0.5 mg, 1 mg, 2 mg
Injection: 0.25 mg/ml

MECHANISM OF ACTION
A loop diuretic that inhibits reabsorption of sodium and chloride at the proximal portion of the ascending loop of Henle.

INDICATIONS & DOSAGE
Edema in congestive heart failure, or hepatic or renal disease –
Adults: 0.5 to 2 mg P.O. once daily. If diuretic response not adequate, a second or third dose may be given at 4- to 5-hour intervals. Maximum dosage is 10 mg/day. May be administered parenterally when P.O. not feasible. Usual initial dose is 0.5 to 1 mg I.V. or I.M. If response is not adequate, a second or third dose may be given at 2- to 3-hour intervals. Maximum dosage is 10 mg/day.
Children: 0.02 to 0.1 mg/kg P.O., I.M., or I.V. q 12 hours.

ADVERSE REACTIONS
Common reactions are in italics; life-threatening reactions are in bold italics.
CNS: dizziness, headache.
CV: volume depletion and dehydra-

tion, orthostatic hypotension, ECG changes.
EENT: transient deafness.
GI: nausea.
Metabolic: hypokalemia; hypochloremic alkalosis; asymptomatic hyperuricemia; fluid and electrolyte imbalances, including dilutional hyponatremia, hypocalcemia, hypomagnesemia; hyperglycemia and impairment of glucose tolerance.
Skin: rash.
Other: muscle pain and tenderness.

INTERACTIONS

Aminoglycoside antibiotics: potentiated ototoxicity. Use together cautiously.
Antihypertensive agents: increased risk of hypotension. Use together cautiously.
Probenecid, indomethacin, NSAIDs: inhibited diuretic response. Use cautiously.

NURSING CONSIDERATIONS

- *Contraindicated* in anuria, hepatic coma, or in states of severe electrolyte depletion.
- *Use cautiously* in patients with hepatic cirrhosis and ascites. Supplemental potassium or potassium-sparing diuretics may be used to prevent hypokalemia and metabolic alkalosis in these patients. Use cautiously in patients with depressed renal function. Also use cautiously in patients allergic to sulfonamides, who may show hypersensitivity to bumetanide.
- Use in children is not FDA-approved. Do not use in neonates because it contains benzyl alcohol.
- Potent loop diuretic; can lead to profound water and electrolyte depletion. Monitor blood pressure and pulse rate during rapid diuresis. Use cautiously with other potassium-wasting drugs.
- If oliguria or azotemia develops or increases, may require stopping drug.
- Monitor serum electrolytes, BUN, and CO_2 frequently.
- Watch for signs of hypokalemia (for example, muscle weakness and cramps). Patients also receiving digitalis have an increased risk of digitalis toxicity from the potassium-depleting effect of this diuretic.
- Consult with doctor and dietitian to provide high-potassium diet.
- Foods rich in potassium include citrus fruits, tomatoes, bananas, dates, and apricots.
- Monitor blood glucose levels in patients with diabetes. May treat severe hyperglycemia with oral antidiabetic agents.
- Monitor blood uric acid, especially in patients with a history of gout.
- **I.V. use:** Give I.V. doses by direct I.V. using a 21G or 23G needle over 1 to 2 minutes. For intermittent infusion, give diluted drug through an intermittent infusion device or piggyback into an I.V. line containing a free-flowing compatible solution. Infuse at ordered rate. Continuous infusion not needed.
- Advise patients taking bumetanide to stand up slowly to prevent dizziness and to limit alcohol intake and strenuous exercise in hot weather since these exacerbate orthostatic hypotension.
- Bumetanide can be safely prescribed in patients allergic to furosemide; 1 mg of bumetanide is equal to 40 mg of furosemide.
- May be less ototoxic than furosemide, but the clinical relevance of this has not been determined.
- Give in a.m. to prevent nocturia. If second dose is necessary, give in the early afternoon.
- Intermittent dosage given on alternate days, or for 3 to 4 days with 1 or 2 days intervening, is recommended as the safest and most effective dosage schedule for control of edema.

chlorothiazide

Azide‡, Chlotride‡, Diachlor, Diuret‡, Diurigen, Diuril

chlorothiazide sodium

Diuril Sodium

Pregnancy Risk Category: D

HOW SUPPLIED

Tablets: 250 mg, 500 mg
Oral suspension: 250 mg/5 ml
Injection: 500-mg vial

MECHANISM OF ACTION

A thiazide diuretic that increases urine excretion of sodium and water by inhibiting sodium reabsorption in the cortical diluting site of the nephron.

INDICATIONS & DOSAGE

Edema, hypertension –
Adults: 500 mg to 2 g P.O. or I.V. daily or in two divided doses.
Diuresis –
Children over 6 months: 20 mg/kg P.O. or I.V. daily in divided doses.
Children under 6 months: may require 30 mg/kg P.O. or I.V. daily in two divided doses.

ADVERSE REACTIONS

Common reactions are in italics; life-threatening reactions are in bold italics.
Blood: ***aplastic anemia, agranulocytosis,*** leukopenia, thrombocytopenia.
CV: volume depletion and dehydration, orthostatic hypotension.
GI: anorexia, nausea, pancreatitis.
Hepatic: hepatic encephalopathy.
Metabolic: hypokalemia, asymptomatic hyperuricemia, hyperglycemia and impairment of glucose tolerance, fluid and electrolyte imbalances including dilutional hyponatremia and hypochloremia, metabolic alkalosis, hypercalcemia, gout.
Skin: dermatitis, photosensitivity, rash.
Other: hypersensitivity reactions, such as pneumonitis and vasculitis.

INTERACTIONS

Cholestyramine, colestipol: intestinal absorption of thiazides decreased. Keep doses as separate as possible.
Diazoxide: increased antihypertensive, hyperglycemic, and hyperuricemic effects. Use together cautiously.
NSAIDs: decreased diuretic effectiveness. Avoid concomitant use.

NURSING CONSIDERATIONS

- *Contraindicated* in anuria, hypersensitivity to other thiazides or other sulfonamide-derived drugs, impaired hepatic function, or progressive hepatic disease.
- *Use cautiously* in severe renal disease.
- Monitor intake and output, weight, blood pressure, and serum electrolytes.
- Consult with doctor and dietitian to provide high-potassium diet. Watch for signs of hypokalemia (for example, muscle weakness, and cramps). Patients on digitalis have an increased risk of digitalis toxicity from the potassium-depleting effect of the diuretic. May use with potassium-sparing diuretic to prevent potassium loss.
- Foods rich in potassium include citrus fruits, tomatoes, bananas, dates, and apricots.
- Monitor blood glucose levels. Check insulin requirements in patients with diabetes. May treat severe hyperglycemia with oral antidiabetic agents.
- Monitor serum creatinine and BUN regularly. Not as effective if these levels are more than twice normal.
- Monitor blood uric acid, especially in patients with a history of gout.
- Monitor serum calcium and watch for progressive renal impairment.
- **I.V. use:** Only injectable thiazide. For I.V. use only – not I.M. or S.C.

†Available in Canada only. ‡Available in Australia only. ◇Available OTC.

Reconstitute 500 mg with 18 ml of sterile water for injection. May store reconstituted solutions at room temperature up to 24 hours. Compatible with I.V. dextrose or sodium chloride solutions. Inject reconstituted drug directly into vein, through an I.V. line containing a free-flowing compatible solution, or through an intermittent infusion device.

- Avoid I.V. infiltration; can be very painful.
- Give in a.m. to prevent nocturia. Administering oral form with food may enhance absorption.
- In hypertension, therapeutic response may be delayed several days.
- Elderly patients are especially susceptible to excessive diuresis.
- Thiazides and thiazide-like diuretics should be stopped before tests for parathyroid function are performed.
- Advise patient to avoid sudden posture changes and rise slowly to avoid orthostatic hypotension.
- Advise patient to use a sunscreen.

chlorthalidone

Apo-Chlorthalidone†, Hygroton, Novothalidone†, Thalitone, Uridon†

Pregnancy Risk Category: D

HOW SUPPLIED

Tablets: 25 mg, 50 mg, 100 mg

MECHANISM OF ACTION

Although not a thiazide, chlorthalidone acts in a similar fashion. It increases urine excretion of sodium and water by inhibiting sodium reabsorption in the cortical diluting site of the nephron.

INDICATIONS & DOSAGE

Edema, hypertension –

Adults: 25 to 100 mg P.O. daily, or 100 mg 3 times weekly or on alternate days.

Children: 2 mg/kg P.O. 3 times weekly.

ADVERSE REACTIONS

Common reactions are in italics; life-threatening reactions are in bold italics.

Blood: ***aplastic anemia, agranulocytosis,*** leukopenia, thrombocytopenia.

CV: volume depletion and dehydration, orthostatic hypotension.

GI: anorexia, nausea, pancreatitis.

GU: impotence.

Hepatic: hepatic encephalopathy.

Metabolic: hypokalemia, asymptomatic hyperuricemia, hyperglycemia and impairment of glucose tolerance, fluid and electrolyte imbalances including dilutional hyponatremia and hypochloremia, metabolic alkalosis, hypercalcemia, gout.

Skin: dermatitis, photosensitivity, rash.

Other: hypersensitivity reactions, such as pneumonitis and vasculitis.

INTERACTIONS

Cholestyramine, colestipol: intestinal absorption of thiazides decreased. Keep doses as separate as possible.

Diazoxide: increased antihypertensive, hyperglycemic, and hyperuricemic effects. Use together cautiously.

NSAIDs: decreased diuretic effectiveness. Avoid concomitant use.

NURSING CONSIDERATIONS

- *Contraindicated* in anuria or in hypersensitivity to thiazides or other sulfonamide-derived drugs.
- *Use cautiously* in severe renal disease, progressive hepatic disease, and impaired hepatic function.
- Monitor intake and output, weight, blood pressure, and serum electrolytes.
- Consult with doctor and dietitian to provide high-potassium diet. Watch for signs of hypokalemia (for example, muscle weakness, and cramps). Patients on digitalis have an increased

*Liquid form contains alcohol. **May contain tartrazine.

risk of digitalis toxicity from the potassium-depleting effect of this diuretic. May use with potassium-sparing diuretic to prevent potassium loss.
- Foods rich in potassium include citrus fruits, tomatoes, bananas, dates, and apricots.
- Monitor serum creatinine and BUN regularly. Not as effective if these levels are more than twice normal.
- Monitor blood uric acid, especially in patients with a history of gout.
- Monitor blood glucose levels. Check insulin requirements in patients with diabetes. May treat severe hyperglycemia with oral antidiabetic agents.
- In hypertension, therapeutic response may be delayed several days.
- Give in a.m. to prevent nocturia.
- Elderly patients are especially susceptible to excessive diuresis.
- Thiazides and thiazide-like diuretics should be stopped before tests for parathyroid function are performed.
- Advise patient to avoid sudden posture changes and rise slowly to avoid orthostatic hypotension.
- Advise patient to use a sunscreen.
- Notice that Uridon tablets (available in Canada only) should not be confused with the urinary anti-infective Uridon Modified (available in the United States).

dichlorphenamide
Daranide
Pregnancy Risk Category: C

HOW SUPPLIED
Tablets: 50 mg

MECHANISM OF ACTION
A carbonic anhydrase inhibitor that decreases secretion of aqueous humor in the eye, thereby lowering intraocular pressure.

INDICATIONS & DOSAGE
Adjunct in glaucoma –
Adults: initially, 100 to 200 mg P.O., followed by 100 mg q 12 hours until desired response obtained. Maintenance dosage is 25 to 50 mg P.O. daily b.i.d. or t.i.d. Give miotics concomitantly.

ADVERSE REACTIONS
Common reactions are in italics; life-threatening reactions are in bold italics.
Blood: ***aplastic anemia,*** hemolytic anemia, leukopenia.
CNS: drowsiness, paresthesia.
EENT: transient myopia.
GI: nausea, vomiting, anorexia.
GU: crystalluria, renal calculi.
Metabolic: hyperchloremic acidosis, hypokalemia, asymptomatic hyperuricemia.
Skin: rash.

INTERACTIONS
None significant.

NURSING CONSIDERATIONS
- *Contraindicated* in hepatic insufficiency, renal failure, adrenocortical insufficiency, hyperchloremic acidosis, depressed sodium or potassium levels, severe pulmonary obstruction with inability to increase alveolar ventilation, or Addison's disease. Long-term use contraindicated in severe, absolute, or chronic noncongestive narrow-angle glaucoma.
- *Use cautiously* in respiratory acidosis, monitoring blood pH and blood gases.
- Monitor electrolytes, especially serum potassium in initial treatment. Usually no problem in long-term glaucoma therapy unless risk of hypokalemia from other causes; potassium supplements may be necessary.
- May cause false-positive results in urine protein tests.
- Anticipate that drug will be given every day for glaucoma but intermittently for edema.

• Evaluate patient with glaucoma for eye pain to make sure drug is effective in decreasing intraocular pressure.

ethacrynate sodium

Edecrin Sodium

ethacrynic acid

Edecril‡, Edecrin

Pregnancy Risk Category: D

HOW SUPPLIED

Tablets: 25 mg, 50 mg
Injection: 50 mg (with 62.5 mg of mannitol and 0.1 mg of thimerosal)

MECHANISM OF ACTION

A loop diuretic that inhibits reabsorption of sodium and chloride at the proximal portion of the ascending loop of Henle.

INDICATIONS & DOSAGE

Acute pulmonary edema –
Adults: 50 to 100 mg of ethacrynate sodium I.V. slowly over several minutes.
Edema –
Adults: 50 to 200 mg P.O. daily. Refractory cases may require up to 200 mg b.i.d.
Children: initial dose is 25 mg P.O., cautiously, increased in 25-mg increments daily until desired effect is achieved.

ADVERSE REACTIONS

Common reactions are in italics; life-threatening reactions are in bold italics.
Blood: ***agranulocytosis,*** neutropenia, thrombocytopenia.
CV: volume depletion and dehydration, orthostatic hypotension.
EENT: transient deafness with too-rapid I.V. injection.
GI: abdominal discomfort and pain, diarrhea.
Metabolic: hypokalemia; hypochloremic alkalosis; asymptomatic hyperuricemia; fluid and electrolyte imbalances including dilutional hyponatremia, hypocalcemia, hypomagnesemia; hyperglycemia and impairment of glucose tolerance.
Skin: dermatitis.

INTERACTIONS

Aminoglycoside antibiotics: potentiated ototoxic adverse reactions of both ethacrynic acid and aminoglycosides. Use together cautiously.
Antihypertensive agents: increased risk of hypotension. Use together cautiously.
NSAIDs: decreased diuretic effectiveness. Use together cautiously.
Warfarin: potentiated anticoagulant effect. Use together cautiously.

NURSING CONSIDERATIONS

• *Contraindicated* in patients with anuria and in infants.
• *Use cautiously* in patients with electrolyte abnormalities. If electrolyte imbalance, azotemia, or oliguria develops, may require discontinuing drug.
• This drug is a very potent diuretic.
• Monitor intake and output, weight, blood pressure, and serum electrolytes.
• Consult with doctor and dietitian to provide high-potassium diet. Watch for signs of hypokalemia (for example, muscle weakness and cramps).
• Foods rich in potassium include citrus fruits, tomatoes, bananas, dates, and apricots.
• Patients also on digitalis have an increased risk of digitalis toxicity from the potassium-depleting effect.
• Don't give subcutaneously or I.M.
• **I.V. use:** Reconstitute vacuum vial with 50 ml of dextrose 5% injection or sodium chloride injection. Discard unused solution after 24 hours. Don't use cloudy or opalescent solutions. Give slowly through tubing of running infusion over several minutes.
• Sodium and potassium chloride supplement may be needed.

• Reconstitute vacuum vial with 50 ml of dextrose 5% injection or sodium chloride injection. Discard unused solution after 24 hours. Don't use cloudy or opalescent solutions.
• Elderly patients are especially susceptible to excessive diuresis.
• Give P.O. doses in a.m. to prevent nocturia.
• Severe diarrhea may necessitate discontinuing drug.
• Monitor blood uric acid, especially in patients with a history of gout.
• Advise patient to avoid sudden posture changes and rise slowly to avoid orthostatic hypotension.

furosemide (frusemide)

Apo-Furosemide†, Furomide M.D., Furoside†, Lasix*, Lasix Special†, Myrosemide*, Novosemide†, Urex‡, Urex-M‡, Uritol†
Pregnancy Risk Category: C

HOW SUPPLIED

Tablets: 20 mg, 40 mg, 80 mg, 500 mg†
Oral solution: 8 mg/ml, 10 mg/ml, 50 mg/ml
Injection: 10 mg/ml

MECHANISM OF ACTION

A loop diuretic that inhibits reabsorption of sodium and chloride at the proximal portion of the ascending loop of Henle.

INDICATIONS & DOSAGE

Acute pulmonary edema –
Adults: 40 mg I.V. injected slowly; then 40 mg I.V. in 1 to 1½ hours if needed.
Edema –
Adults: 20 to 80 mg P.O. daily in a.m., second dose can be given in 6 to 8 hours; carefully titrated up to 600 mg daily if needed; or 20 to 40 mg I.M. or I.V. Increase by 20 mg q 2 hours until desired response is achieved. I.V. dose should be given slowly over 1 to 2 minutes.
Hypertension –
Adults: 40 mg P.O. b.i.d. Adjust dose according to response.
Infants and children: 2 mg/kg P.O. daily; dose increased by 1 to 2 mg/kg in 6 to 8 hours if needed; carefully titrated up to 6 mg/kg daily if needed.
Hypertensive crisis, acute renal failure –
Adults: 100 to 200 mg I.V. over 1 to 2 minutes.
Chronic renal failure –
Adults: initially, 80 mg P.O. daily. Increase by 80 to 120 mg daily until desired response is achieved.
Hypercalcemia –
Adults: 80 to 100 mg I.V. every 1 to 2 hours as needed and tolerated.

ADVERSE REACTIONS

Common reactions are in italics; life-threatening reactions are in bold italics.
Blood: ***agranulocytosis,*** leukopenia, thrombocytopenia.
CV: volume depletion and dehydration, orthostatic hypotension.
EENT: transient deafness with too rapid I.V. injection.
GI: abdominal discomfort and pain, diarrhea (with oral solution).
Metabolic: hypokalemia; hypochloremic alkalosis; asymptomatic hyperuricemia, fluid and electrolyte imbalances including dilutional hyponatremia, hypocalcemia, hypomagnesemia; hyperglycemia and impairment of glucose tolerance.
Skin: dermatitis.

INTERACTIONS

Aminoglycoside antibiotics: potentiated ototoxicity. Use together cautiously.
Antihypertensive agents: increased risk of hypotension. Use together cautiously.
Chloral hydrate: sweating, flushing with I.V. furosemide.

Clofibrate: enhanced furosemide effects. Use cautiously.
NSAIDs: inhibited diuretic response. Use cautiously.

NURSING CONSIDERATIONS

- *Contraindicated* in patients with a history of hypersensitivity to the drug, and in patients with anuria.
- *Use cautiously* in cardiogenic shock complicated by pulmonary edema, anuria, hepatic coma, or electrolyte imbalances. Drug is not routinely administered to women of childbearing age because its safety in pregnancy hasn't been established.
- Potent loop diuretic; can lead to profound water and electrolyte depletion. Monitor blood pressure and pulse rate during rapid diuresis and routinely with chronic use.
- Sulfonamide-sensitive patients may have allergic reactions to furosemide.
- If oliguria or azotemia develops or increases, may require stopping drug.
- Monitor serum electrolyte, BUN, and CO_2 frequently.
- Monitor serum potassium level. Watch for signs of hypokalemia (for example, muscle weakness and cramps). Patients also on digitalis have an increased risk of digitalis toxicity from the potassium-depleting effect.
- Consult with doctor and dietitian to provide high-potassium diet.
- Foods rich in potassium include citrus fruits, tomatoes, bananas, dates, and apricots.
- Monitor blood glucose levels in patients with diabetes. May treat severe hyperglycemia with oral antidiabetic agents.
- Monitor blood uric acid, especially in patients with a history of gout.
- **I.V. use:** Promotes calcium excretion. I.V. furosemide often used to treat hypercalcemia.
- To prepare parenteral furosemide for I.V. infusion, mix drug with dextrose 5% in water, 0.9% sodium chloride solution, or lactated Ringer's solution. Use prepared infusion solution within 24 hours.
- Don't use parenteral route in infants and children unless oral dosage form is not practical.
- Give P.O. and I.M. preparations in a.m. to prevent nocturia. Give second doses in early afternoon.
- Elderly patients are especially susceptible to excessive diuresis, with potential for circulatory collapse and thromboembolic complications.
- Store tablets in light-resistant container to prevent discoloration (doesn't affect potency). Don't use discolored (yellow) injectable preparation. Oral furosemide solution should be stored in the refrigerator to ensure stability of the drug.
- Advise patients taking furosemide to stand slowly to prevent dizziness, and to limit alcohol intake and strenuous exercise in hot weather because these exacerbate orthostatic hypotension.
- Advise patients to report immediately ringing in ears, severe abdominal pain, or sore throat and fever; may indicate furosemide toxicity.
- Discourage patients receiving furosemide therapy at home from storing different types of medication in the same container. This increases the risk of drug errors, especially for patients taking both furosemide and digoxin, since the most popular strengths of these drugs' pills are white tablets approximately equal in size.

hydrochlorothiazide

Apo-Hydro†, Dichlotride‡, Diuchlor H†, Esidrix, HydroDIURIL, Mictrin, Natrimax†, Novohydrazide†, Oretic, Thiuretic, Urozide†

Pregnancy Risk Category: D

HOW SUPPLIED

Tablets: 25 mg, 50 mg, 100 mg
Oral solution: 10 mg/ml, 100 mg/ml

MECHANISM OF ACTION

A thiazide diuretic that increases urine excretion of sodium and water by inhibiting sodium reabsorption in the cortical diluting site of the nephron.

INDICATIONS & DOSAGE

Edema –
Adults: initially, 25 to 100 mg P.O. daily or intermittently for maintenance dosage.
Children over 6 months: 2.2 mg/kg P.O. daily divided b.i.d.
Children under 6 months: up to 3.3 mg/kg P.O. daily divided b.i.d.
Hypertension –
Adults: 25 to 100 mg P.O. daily or divided dosage. Daily dosage increased or decreased according to blood pressure.

ADVERSE REACTIONS

Common reactions are in italics; life-threatening reactions are in bold italics.
Blood: ***aplastic anemia, agranulocytosis,*** leukopenia, thrombocytopenia.
CV: volume depletion and dehydration, orthostatic hypotension.
GI: anorexia, nausea, pancreatitis.
Hepatic: hepatic encephalopathy.
Metabolic: hypokalemia, asymptomatic hyperuricemia, hyperglycemia and impairment of glucose tolerance, fluid and electrolyte imbalances including dilutional hyponatremia and hypochloremia, metabolic alkalosis, hypercalcemia, gout.
Skin: dermatitis, photosensitivity, rash.
Other: hypersensitivity reactions, such as pneumonitis and vasculitis.

INTERACTIONS

Cholestyramine, colestipol: intestinal absorption of thiazides decreased. Keep doses as separate as possible.
Diazoxide: increased antihypertensive, hyperglycemic, and hyperuricemic effects. Use together cautiously.
Hypoglycemic agents: dosage adjustments may be necessary. Monitor blood glucose levels.
NSAIDs: decreased diuretic effectiveness. Avoid concomitant use.

NURSING CONSIDERATIONS

- *Contraindicated* in anuria or hypersensitivity to other thiazides or other sulfonamide derivatives.
- *Use cautiously* in severe renal disease, impaired hepatic function, and progressive hepatic disease.
- Monitor intake and output, weight, blood pressure, and serum electrolytes.
- Consult with doctor and dietitian to provide high-potassium diet. Watch for hypokalemia (for example, muscle weakness and cramps). Patients also on digitalis have an increased risk of digitalis toxicity from the potassium-depleting effect of this diuretic. May use with potassium-sparing diuretic to prevent potassium loss.
- Foods rich in potassium include citrus fruits, tomatoes, bananas, dates, and apricots.
- Monitor serum creatinine and BUN regularly. Not as effective if these levels are more than twice normal.
- Monitor blood uric acid, especially in patients with a history of gout.
- Check insulin requirements in patients with diabetes. May treat severe hyperglycemia with oral antidiabetic agents.
- In hypertension, therapeutic response may be delayed several days.
- Give in a.m. to prevent nocturia. Studies have shown that the drug is as effective when administered once daily as it is when given more frequently.
- Elderly patients are especially susceptible to excessive diuresis.
- Thiazides and thiazide-like diuret-

ics should be stopped before tests for parathyroid function are performed.
- Advise patient to avoid sudden posture changes and rise slowly to avoid orthostatic hypotension.
- Advise patient to use a sunscreen.

hydroflumethiazide

Diucardin, Saluron

Pregnancy Risk Category: B

HOW SUPPLIED

Tablets: 50 mg

MECHANISM OF ACTION

A thiazide diuretic that increases urine excretion of sodium and water by inhibiting sodium reabsorption in the cortical diluting site of the ascending loop of Henle.

INDICATIONS & DOSAGE

Edema—

Adults: 25 to 200 mg P.O. daily in divided doses. Maintenance dosages may be on intermittent or alternate-day schedule.

Children: 1 mg/kg P.O. daily.

Hypertension—

Adults: 50 to 100 mg P.O. daily or b.i.d.

ADVERSE REACTIONS

Common reactions are in italics; life-threatening reactions are in bold italics.

Blood: ***aplastic anemia, agranulocytosis,*** leukopenia, thrombocytopenia.

CV: volume depletion and dehydration, orthostatic hypotension.

GI: anorexia, nausea, pancreatitis.

Hepatic: hepatic encephalopathy.

Metabolic: hypokalemia, asymptomatic hyperuricemia, hyperglycemia and impairment of glucose tolerance, fluid and electrolyte imbalances including dilutional hyponatremia and hypochloremia, metabolic alkalosis, hypercalcemia, gout.

Skin: dermatitis, photosensitivity, rash.

Other: hypersensitivity reactions, such as pneumonitis and vasculitis.

INTERACTIONS

Cholestyramine, colestipol: intestinal absorption of thiazides decreased. Keep doses as separate as possible.

Diazoxide: increased antihypertensive, hyperglycemic, and hyperuricemic effects. Use together cautiously.

NSAIDs: decreased diuretic effectiveness.

NURSING CONSIDERATIONS

- *Contraindicated* in anuria or hypersensitivity to other thiazides or other sulfonamide-derived drugs.
- *Use cautiously* in severe renal disease, impaired hepatic function, and progressive hepatic disease.
- Monitor intake and output, weight, blood pressure, and serum electrolytes.
- Consult with doctor and dietitian to provide high-potassium diet. Foods rich in potassium include citrus fruits, tomatoes, bananas, dates, and apricots. Watch for hypokalemia (for example, muscle weakness and cramps). May use with potassium-sparing diuretic to prevent potassium loss. Patients also on digitalis have an increased risk of digitalis toxicity from the potassium-depleting effects of this diuretic.
- Monitor serum creatinine and BUN regularly. Not as effective if these levels are more than twice normal.
- Monitor blood uric acid, especially in patients with a history of gout.
- Check insulin requirements in patients with diabetes. May treat severe hyperglycemia with oral antidiabetic agents.
- Give in a.m. to prevent nocturia.
- In hypertension, therapeutic response may be delayed several days.
- Elderly patients are especially susceptible to excessive diuresis.
- Thiazides and thiazide-like diuret-

ics should be stopped before tests for parathyroid function are performed.
- Advise patient to avoid sudden posture changes and rise slowly to avoid orthostatic hypotension.
- Advise patient to use a sunscreen.

indapamide

Lozide†, Lozol, Natrilix‡

Pregnancy Risk Category: B

HOW SUPPLIED

Tablets: 2.5 mg

MECHANISM OF ACTION

A thiazide-like diuretic that inhibits sodium reabsorption in the cortical diluting site of the nephron. Also has a direct vasodilating effect that may be a result of calcium channel-blocking action.

INDICATIONS & DOSAGE

Edema, hypertension –

Adults: 2.5 mg P.O. as a single daily dose taken in the morning. Dosage may be increased to 5 mg daily.

ADVERSE REACTIONS

Common reactions are in italics; life-threatening reactions are in bold italics.

CNS: headache, irritability, nervousness.

CV: volume depletion and dehydration, orthostatic hypotension.

GI: anorexia, nausea, pancreatitis.

Metabolic: hypokalemia; asymptomatic hyperuricemia; fluid and electrolyte imbalances, including dilutional hyponatremia and hypochloremia; metabolic alkalosis; gout.

Skin: dermatitis, photosensitivity, rash.

Other: muscle cramps and spasms.

INTERACTIONS

Diazoxide: increased antihypertensive, hyperglycemic, and hyperuricemic effects. Use together cautiously.

NSAIDs: decreased diuretic effectiveness. Avoid concomitant use.

NURSING CONSIDERATIONS

- *Contraindicated* in anuria or hypersensitivity to other sulfonamide-derived drugs.
- *Use cautiously* in severe renal disease, impaired hepatic function, and progressive hepatic disease.
- Monitor intake and output, weight, blood pressure, and serum electrolytes.
- Consult with doctor and dietitian to provide high-potassium diet. Foods rich in potassium include citrus fruits, tomatoes, bananas, dates, and apricots. Watch for symptoms of hypokalemia (for example, muscle weakness and cramps). May use with potassium-sparing diuretic to prevent potassium loss. Patients also receiving digitalis have an increased risk of digitalis toxicity from the potassium-depleting effects of this diuretic.
- Monitor serum creatinine and BUN regularly. Not as effective if these levels are more than twice normal.
- Monitor blood uric acid level, especially in patients with a history of gout.
- Check insulin requirements in patients with diabetes. May treat severe hyperglycemia with oral antidiabetic agents.
- Give in a.m. to prevent nocturia.
- In hypertension, therapeutic response may be delayed several days.
- Elderly patients are especially susceptible to excessive diuresis.
- Thiazides and thiazide-like diuretics should be stopped before tests for parathyroid function are performed.
- Advise patient to avoid sudden posture changes and rise slowly to avoid orthostatic hypotension.
- Advise patient to use a sunscreen.

†Available in Canada only. ‡Available in Australia only. ◇Available OTC.

mannitol
Osmitrol†

Pregnancy Risk Category: C

HOW SUPPLIED
Injection: 5%, 10%, 15%, 20%, 25%

MECHANISM OF ACTION
An osmotic diuretic that increases the osmotic pressure of glomerular filtrate, inhibiting tubular reabsorption of water and electrolytes. Also elevates blood plasma osmolality, resulting in enhanced flow of water into extracellular fluid.

INDICATIONS & DOSAGE
Test dose for marked oliguria or suspected inadequate renal function –
Adults and children over 12 years: 200 mg/kg or 12.5 g as a 15% or 20% solution I.V. over 3 to 5 minutes. Response adequate if 30 to 50 ml urine/hour is excreted over 2 to 3 hours.
Treatment of oliguria –
Adults and children over 12 years: 50 to 100 g I.V. as a 15% to 20% solution over 90 minutes to several hours.
Prevention of oliguria or acute renal failure –
Adults and children over 12 years: 50 to 100 g I.V. of a concentrated (5% to 25%) solution. Exact concentration is determined by fluid requirements.
Edema –
Adults and children over 12 years: 100 g I.V. as a 10% to 20% solution over 2- to 6-hour period.
To reduce intraocular pressure or intracranial pressure –
Adults and children over 12 years: 1.5 to 2 g/kg as a 15% to 25% solution I.V. over 30 to 60 minutes.
To promote diuresis in drug intoxication –
Adults and children over 12 years: 5% to 10% solution continuously up to 200 g I.V., while maintaining 100 to 500 ml urine output/hour and a positive fluid balance.
Irrigating solution during transurethral resection of the prostate –
Men: 2.5% to 5% solution as needed.

ADVERSE REACTIONS
Common reactions are in italics; life-threatening reactions are in bold italics.
CNS: rebound increase in intracranial pressure 8 to 12 hours after diuresis, headache, confusion.
CV: transient expansion of plasma volume during infusion causing circulatory overload and ***pulmonary edema,*** tachycardia, angina-like chest pain.
EENT: blurred vision, rhinitis.
GI: thirst, nausea, vomiting.
GU: urine retention.
Metabolic: fluid and electrolyte imbalance, water intoxication, cellular dehydration.

INTERACTIONS
None significant.

NURSING CONSIDERATIONS
- *Contraindicated* in anuria, severe pulmonary congestion, frank pulmonary edema, severe congestive heart disease, severe dehydration, metabolic edema, progressive renal disease or dysfunction, progressive heart failure during administration, or active intracranial bleeding except during craniotomy.
- Monitor vital signs (including central venous pressure) at least hourly; intake and output hourly (report increasing oliguria). Monitor weight, renal function, fluid balance, and serum and urine sodium and potassium levels daily.
- Solution often crystallizes, especially at low temperatures. To redissolve, warm bottle in hot water bath, shake vigorously. Cool to body temperature before giving. Concentrations greater than 15% have greater tendency to crystallize. Do not use solution with undissolved crystals.
- **I.V. use:** Always use an in-line filter

and an infusion pump. Direct injection is not recommended. Administer as intermittent or continuous infusion at prescribed rate. Check I.V. line patency at infusion site before and during administration.

- Avoid infiltration; if it occurs, observe for inflammation, edema, and necrosis.
- For maximum intraocular pressure reduction before surgery, give 1 to 1½ hours preoperatively.
- Can be used to measure glomerular filtration rate.
- Give frequent mouth care or fluids as permitted to relieve thirst.
- Urethral catheter is inserted in comatose or incontinent patients because therapy is based on strict evaluation of intake and output. In patients with urethral catheters, use an hourly urometer collection bag to facilitate accurate evaluation of output.
- When used as an irrigating solution, limited evidence suggests that concentrations of at least 3.5% are necessary to avoid hemolysis.

methazolamide

Neptazane

Pregnancy Risk Category: C

HOW SUPPLIED

Tablets: 25 mg, 50 mg

MECHANISM OF ACTION

A carbonic anhydrase inhibitor that decreases secretion of aqueous humor in the eye, thereby lowering intraocular pressure.

INDICATIONS & DOSAGE

Glaucoma (open-angle, or preoperatively in obstructive or narrow-angle) –

Adults: 50 to 100 mg b.i.d. or t.i.d.

ADVERSE REACTIONS

Common reactions are in italics; life-threatening reactions are in bold italics.

Blood: ***aplastic anemia,*** hemolytic anemia, leukopenia.
CNS: drowsiness, paresthesias.
EENT: transient myopia.
GI: nausea, vomiting, anorexia.
GU: crystalluria, renal calculi.
Metabolic: hyperchloremic acidosis, hypokalemia, asymptomatic hyperuricemia.
Skin: rash.

INTERACTIONS

NSAIDs: decreased diuretic effectiveness. Avoid concomitant use.

NURSING CONSIDERATIONS

- *Contraindicated* in severe or absolute glaucoma; for long-term use in chronic noncongestive narrow-angle glaucoma; in patients with depressed serum sodium or potassium levels, renal or hepatic disease or dysfunction, adrenal gland dysfunction, or hyperchloremic acidosis.
- *Use cautiously* in respiratory acidosis, emphysema, and chronic pulmonary disease.
- Monitor intake and output, weight, and serum electrolytes.
- May cause false-positive urine protein tests by alkalinizing urine.
- Elderly patients are especially susceptible to excessive diuresis.
- Diuretic effect decreases in acidosis.
- Anticipate that drug will be given every day for glaucoma but intermittently for edema. Caution patient to comply with prescribed dosage to lessen risk of metabolic acidosis.
- Evaluate the patient with glaucoma for eye pain to make sure drug is effective in decreasing intraocular pressure.

methyclothiazide

Aquatensen, Duretic†, Enduron, Enduron M‡

Pregnancy Risk Category: D

HOW SUPPLIED
Tablets: 2.5 mg, 5 mg

MECHANISM OF ACTION
A thiazide diuretic that increases urine excretion of sodium and water by inhibiting sodium reabsorption in the cortical diluting site of the nephron.

INDICATIONS & DOSAGE
Edema, hypertension –
Adults: 2.5 to 10 mg P.O daily.
Children: 0.05 to 2 mg/kg or 1.5 to 6 mg/m² P.O. as a single daily dose.

ADVERSE REACTIONS
Common reactions are in italics; life-threatening reactions are in bold italics.
Blood: ***aplastic anemia, agranulocytosis,*** leukopenia, thrombocytopenia.
CV: volume depletion and dehydration, orthostatic hypotension.
GI: anorexia, nausea, pancreatitis.
Hepatic: hepatic encephalopathy.
Metabolic: hypokalemia, asymptomatic hyperuricemia, hyperglycemia and impairment of glucose tolerance, fluid and electrolyte imbalances including dilutional hyponatremia and hypochloremia, metabolic alkalosis, hypercalcemia, gout.
Skin: dermatitis, photosensitivity, rash.
Other: hypersensitivity reactions, such as pneumonitis and vasculitis.

INTERACTIONS
Cholestyramine, colestipol: intestinal absorption of thiazides decreased. Keep doses as separate as possible.
Diazoxide: increased antihypertensive, hyperglycemic, and hyperuricemic effects. Use together cautiously.

NURSING CONSIDERATIONS
- *Contraindicated* in renal decompensation, anuria, or hypersensitivity to other thiazides or other sulfonamide-derived drugs.
- *Use cautiously* in potassium depletion, renal disease or dysfunction, impaired hepatic function, and progressive hepatic disease.
- Monitor intake and output, weight, blood pressure, and serum electrolytes.
- Consult with doctor and dietitian to provide high-potassium diet. Foods rich in potassium include citrus fruits, tomatoes, bananas, dates, and apricots. Watch for hypokalemia (for example, muscle weakness and cramps). Patients also on digitalis have an increased risk of digitalis toxicity from the potassium-depleting effect of this diuretic. May use with potassium-sparing diuretic to prevent potassium loss.
- Check insulin requirements in patients with diabetes. May treat severe hyperglycemia with oral antidiabetic agents.
- Monitor serum creatinine and BUN regularly. Not as effective if these level are more than twice normal.
- Monitor blood uric acid, especially in patients with a history of gout.
- In hypertension, therapeutic response may be delayed several days.
- Give in a.m. to prevent nocturia.
- Elderly patients are especially susceptible to excessive diuresis.
- Thiazides and thiazide-like diuretics should be stopped before tests for parathyroid function are performed.
- Advise patient to avoid sudden posture changes and rise slowly to avoid orthostatic hypotension.
- Advise patient to use a sunscreen.

metolazone
Diulo, Mykrox, Zaroxolyn**
Pregnancy Risk Category: D

HOW SUPPLIED
Tablets: 0.5 mg, 2.5 mg, 5 mg, 10 mg

*Liquid form contains alcohol. **May contain tartrazine.

MECHANISM OF ACTION
Although not a thiazide diuretic, metolazone acts in a similar fashion. It increases urine excretion of sodium and water by inhibiting sodium reabsorption in the cortical diluting site of the ascending loop of Henle.

INDICATIONS & DOSAGE
Edema in congestive heart failure –
Adults: 5 to 10 mg P.O. daily.
Edema in renal disease –
Adults: 5 to 20 mg P.O. daily.
Hypertension –
Adults: 2.5 to 5 mg (Diulo or Zaroxolyn) P.O. daily. Maintenance dosage determined by patient's blood pressure. Or 0.5 mg (Mykrox) once daily in the morning. Increase to 1 mg P.O. daily as needed. If response is inadequate, add another antihypertensive agent.

ADVERSE REACTIONS
Common reactions are in italics; life-threatening reactions are in bold italics.
Blood: ***aplastic anemia, agranulocytosis,*** leukopenia, thrombocytopenia.
CV: volume depletion and dehydration, orthostatic hypotension.
GI: anorexia, nausea, pancreatitis.
Hepatic: hepatic encephalopathy.
Metabolic: hypokalemia, asymptomatic hyperuricemia, hyperglycemia and impairment of glucose tolerance, fluid and electrolyte imbalances including dilutional hyponatremia and hypochloremia, metabolic alkalosis, hypercalcemia, gout.
Skin: dermatitis, photosensitivity, rash.
Other: hypersensitivity reactions, such as pneumonitis and vasculitis.

INTERACTIONS
Cholestyramine, colestipol: intestinal absorption of thiazides decreased. Keep doses as separate as possible.
Diazoxide: increased antihypertensive, hyperglycemic, and hyperuricemic effects. Use together cautiously.
NSAIDs: decreased diuretic effect. Avoid concomitant use.

NURSING CONSIDERATIONS
- *Contraindicated* in anuria, hepatic coma or precoma, or hypersensitivity to thiazides or other sulfonamide-derived drugs.
- *Use cautiously* in hyperuricemia or gout and impaired renal or hepatic function.
- Mykrox tablets are more rapidly and completely absorbed than other brands; their absorption characteristics mimic those of an oral solution. Dosage is different; do not interchange Mykrox with Diulo or Zaroxolyn.
- Monitor intake and output, weight, blood pressure, and serum electrolytes.
- Consult with doctor and dietitian to provide high-potassium diet. Foods rich in potassium include citrus fruits, tomatoes, bananas, dates, and apricots. Watch for hypokalemia (for example, muscle weakness and cramps). Patients also on digitalis may have an increased risk of digitalis toxicity from the potassium-depleting effect of this diuretic. May use with potassium-sparing diuretic to prevent potassium loss.
- Check insulin requirements in patients with diabetes. May treat severe hyperglycemia with oral antidiabetic agents.
- Monitor blood uric acid, especially in patients with a history of gout.
- In hypertension, therapeutic response may be delayed several days.
- Give in a.m. to prevent nocturia.
- Elderly patients are especially susceptible to excessive diuresis.
- A thiazide-related diuretic. However, unlike thiazide diuretics, metolazone is effective in patients with decreased renal function.

- Used as an adjunct in furosemide-resistant edema.
- Thiazides and thiazide-like diuretics should be stopped before tests for parathyroid function are performed.
- Advise patient to avoid sudden posture changes and rise slowly to avoid orthostatic hypotension.
- Advise patient to use a sunscreen.

polythiazide

Renese

Pregnancy Risk Category: D

HOW SUPPLIED

Tablets: 1 mg, 2 mg, 4 mg

MECHANISM OF ACTION

A thiazide diuretic that increases urine excretion of sodium and water by inhibiting sodium reabsorption in the cortical diluting site of the nephron.

INDICATIONS & DOSAGE

Hypertension –
Adults: 2 to 4 mg P.O. daily.
Edema in heart failure or renal failure –
Adults: 1 to 4 mg P.O. daily.
Children: 0.02 to 0.08 mg/kg P.O. daily.

ADVERSE REACTIONS

Common reactions are in italics; life-threatening reactions are in bold italics.
Blood: ***aplastic anemia, agranulocytosis,*** leukopenia, thrombocytopenia.
CV: volume depletion and dehydration, orthostatic hypotension.
GI: anorexia, nausea, pancreatitis.
Hepatic: hepatic encephalopathy.
Metabolic: hypokalemia, asymptomatic hyperuricemia, hyperglycemia and impairment of glucose tolerance, fluid and electrolyte imbalances including dilutional hyponatremia and hypochloremia, metabolic alkalosis, hypercalcemia, gout.
Skin: dermatitis, photosensitivity, rash.
Other: hypersensitivity reactions, such as pneumonitis and vasculitis.

INTERACTIONS

Cholestyramine, colestipol: intestinal absorption of thiazides decreased. Keep doses as separate as possible.
Diazoxide: increased antihypertensive, hyperglycemic, and hyperuricemic effects. Use together cautiously.

NURSING CONSIDERATIONS

- *Contraindicated* in anuria or hypersensitivity to other thiazides or other sulfonamide-derived drugs.
- *Use cautiously* in severe renal disease, impaired hepatic function, and allergies.
- Monitor intake and output, weight, blood pressure, and serum electrolytes.
- Consult with doctor and dietitian to provide high-potassium diet. Foods rich in potassium include citrus fruits, tomatoes, bananas, dates, and apricots. Watch for hypokalemia (for example, muscle weakness and cramps). Patients also on digitalis may have an increased risk of digitalis toxicity from the potassium-depleting effect of this diuretic. May use with potassium-sparing diuretic to prevent potassium loss.
- Monitor blood uric acid, especially in patients with a history of gout.
- Check insulin requirements in patients with diabetes. May treat severe hyperglycemia with oral antidiabetic agents.
- In hypertension, therapeutic response may be delayed several days.
- Give in a.m. to prevent nocturia.
- Elderly patients are especially susceptible to excessive diuresis.
- Thiazides and thiazide-like diuretics should be stopped before tests for parathyroid function are performed.
- Advise patient to avoid sudden pos-

ture changes and rise slowly to avoid orthostatic hypotension.
- Advise patient to use a sunscreen.

quinethazone

Aquamox‡, Hydromox

Pregnancy Risk Category: D

HOW SUPPLIED

Tablets: 50 mg

MECHANISM OF ACTION

Although not a thiazide diuretic, quinethazone acts in a similar fashion. It increases urine excretion of sodium and water by inhibiting sodium reabsorption in the cortical diluting site of the nephron.

INDICATIONS & DOSAGE

Management of edema or hypertension –

Adults: 50 to 100 mg P.O. daily or 50 mg P.O. b.i.d. Occasionally, up to 150 to 200 mg P.O. daily may be needed.

ADVERSE REACTIONS

Common reactions are in italics; life-threatening reactions are in bold italics.

Blood: ***aplastic anemia, agranulocytosis,*** leukopenia, thrombocytopenia.
CV: volume depletion and dehydration, orthostatic hypotension.
GI: anorexia, nausea, pancreatitis.
Hepatic: hepatic encephalopathy.
Metabolic: hypokalemia, asymptomatic hyperuricemia, hyperglycemia and impairment of glucose tolerance, fluid and electrolyte imbalances including dilutional hyponatremia and hypochloremia, metabolic alkalosis, hypercalcemia, gout.
Skin: dermatitis, photosensitivity, rash.
Other: hypersensitivity reactions, such as pneumonitis and vasculitis.

INTERACTIONS

Cholestyramine, colestipol: intestinal absorption of thiazides decreased. Keep doses as separate as possible.
Diazoxide: increased antihypertensive, hyperglycemic, and hyperuricemic effects. Use together cautiously.

NURSING CONSIDERATIONS

- *Contraindicated* in anuria or hypersensitivity to quinethazones, thiazides, or other sulfonamide-derived drugs.
- *Use cautiously* in severe renal disease, impaired hepatic function, and allergies.
- Monitor intake and output, weight, blood pressure, and serum electrolytes.
- Consult with doctor and dietitian to provide high-potassium diet. Foods rich in potassium include citrus fruits, tomatoes, bananas, dates, and apricots. Watch for hypokalemia (for example, muscle weakness and cramps). Patients also on digitalis have an increased risk of digitalis toxicity from the potassium-depleting effect of this diuretic. May use with potassium-sparing diuretic to prevent potassium loss.
- Monitor serum creatinine and BUN regularly.
- Check insulin requirements in patients with diabetes. May treat severe hyperglycemia with oral hypoglycemics.
- Monitor blood uric acid, especially in patients with a history of gout.
- In hypertension, therapeutic response may be delayed several days.
- Give in a.m. to prevent nocturia.
- Elderly patients are especially susceptible to excessive diuresis.
- Thiazides and thiazide-like diuretics should be stopped before tests for parathyroid function are performed.
- Advise patient to avoid sudden posture changes and rise slowly to avoid orthostatic hypotension.

• Advise patient to use a sunscreen.

spironolactone

Aldactone, Novospiroton†, Sincomen†, Spirotone‡

Pregnancy Risk Category: D

HOW SUPPLIED

Tablets: 25 mg, 50 mg, 100 mg

MECHANISM OF ACTION

A potassium-sparing diuretic that antagonizes aldosterone in the distal tubule, increasing excretion of sodium and water but sparing potassium.

INDICATIONS & DOSAGE

Edema –

Adults: 25 to 200 mg P.O. daily in divided doses.

Children: initially, 3.3 mg/kg P.O. daily in divided doses.

Hypertension –

Adults: 50 to 100 mg P.O. daily in divided doses.

Treatment of diuretic-induced hypokalemia –

Adults: 25 to 100 mg P.O. daily when oral potassium supplements are considered inappropriate.

Detection of primary hyperaldosteronism –

Adults: 400 mg P.O. daily for 4 days (short test) or 3 to 4 weeks (long test). If hypokalemia and hypertension are corrected, a presumptive diagnosis of primary hyperaldosteronism is made.

ADVERSE REACTIONS

Common reactions are in italics; life-threatening reactions are in bold italics.

CNS: headache.

GI: anorexia, nausea, diarrhea.

Metabolic: ***hyperkalemia,*** dehydration, hyponatremia, transient elevation in BUN, acidosis.

Skin: urticaria.

Other: gynecomastia in men, breast soreness and menstrual disturbances in women.

INTERACTIONS

ACE inhibitors, potassium supplements: concomitant use may result in hyperkalemia. Don't use together.

Aspirin: possible blocked spironolactone effect. Watch for diminished spironolactone response.

Digoxin: may alter digoxin clearance and increase risk of toxicity. Monitor digoxin levels.

NURSING CONSIDERATIONS

• *Contraindicated* in anuria, acute or progressive renal insufficiency, or hyperkalemia.

• *Use cautiously* in fluid or electrolyte imbalances, impaired renal function, and hepatic disease.

• A mild acidosis may occur during therapy. This may be dangerous in patients with hepatic cirrhosis.

• Monitor serum electrolytes, intake and output, weight, and blood pressure.

• Potassium-sparing diuretic; useful as an adjunct to other diuretic therapy. Less potent diuretic than thiazide and loop types. Diuretic effect delayed 2 to 3 days when used alone.

• Maximum antihypertensive response may be delayed up to 2 weeks.

• Warn patient to avoid excessive ingestion of potassium-rich foods or potassium-containing salt substitutes. Concomitant potassium supplement can lead to serious hyperkalemia.

• Elderly patients are more susceptible to excessive diuresis.

• Protect drug from light.

• Breast cancer reported in some patients taking spironolactone, but cause-and-effect relationship not confirmed. Warn against taking drug indiscriminately.

• Give with meals to enhance absorption.

• Because of its antiandrogenic properties, spironolactone has been prescribed to treat hirsutism. The dose for this indication is 200 mg daily.

• Spironolactone may interfere with

*Liquid form contains alcohol. **May contain tartrazine.

some laboratory tests that measure digoxin levels. Inform laboratory that patient is taking spironolactone.

triamterene

Dyrenium, Dytac‡

Pregnancy Risk Category: D

HOW SUPPLIED

Tablets: 50 mg, 100 mg

MECHANISM OF ACTION

A potassium-sparing diuretic that inhibits sodium reabsorption and potassium excretion by direct action on the distal tubule.

INDICATIONS & DOSAGE

Edema –

Adults: initially, 100 mg P.O. b.i.d. after meals. Total daily dosage should not exceed 300 mg.

ADVERSE REACTIONS

Common reactions are in italics; life-threatening reactions are in bold italics.

Blood: megaloblastic anemia related to low folic acid levels.

CNS: dizziness.

CV: hypotension.

EENT: sore throat.

GI: dry mouth, nausea, vomiting.

Metabolic: ***hyperkalemia,*** dehydration, hyponatremia, transient elevation in BUN, acidosis.

Skin: photosensitivity, rash.

Other: ***anaphylaxis,*** muscle cramps.

INTERACTIONS

ACE inhibitors, potassium supplements: increased risk of hyperkalemia. Don't use together.

Indomethacin, NSAIDs: may enhance the risk of nephrotoxicity. Avoid concomitant use.

Quinidine: may interfere with some laboratory tests that measure quinidine levels. Inform laboratory that patient is taking triamterene.

NURSING CONSIDERATIONS

- *Contraindicated* in anuria, severe or progressive renal disease or dysfunction, severe hepatic disease, or hyperkalemia.
- *Use cautiously* in impaired hepatic function, diabetes mellitus, pregnancy, or lactation.
- Watch for blood dyscrasias.
- Monitor blood pressure, BUN, and serum electrolytes.
- A potassium-sparing diuretic, useful as an adjunct to other diuretic therapy. Less potent than thiazides and loop diuretics. Usually used with potassium-wasting diuretics. Full effect delayed 2 to 3 days when used alone.
- Warn patients to avoid excessive ingestion of potassium-rich foods or potassium-containing salt substitutes. Concomitant potassium supplement can lead to serious hyperkalemia.
- Give medication after meals to prevent nausea.
- Withdraw gradually to prevent excessive rebound potassium excretion.

trichlormethiazide

Aquazide, Diurese, Metahydrin**, Naqua

Pregnancy Risk Category: D

HOW SUPPLIED

Tablets: 2 mg, 4 mg

MECHANISM OF ACTION

A thiazide diuretic that increases urine excretion of sodium and water by inhibiting sodium reabsorption in the cortical diluting site of the nephron.

INDICATIONS & DOSAGE

Edema –

Adults: 1 to 4 mg P.O. daily or in two divided doses.

Children over 6 months: 0.07 mg/kg (2 mg/m^2) P.O. daily or in two divided doses.

Hypertension –
Adults: 2 to 4 mg P.O. daily.
Children over 6 months: 0.07 mg/kg (2 mg/m²) P.O. daily or in two divided doses.

ADVERSE REACTIONS
Common reactions are in italics; life-threatening reactions are in bold italics.
Blood: ***aplastic anemia, agranulocytosis,*** leukopenia, thrombocytopenia.
CV: volume depletion and dehydration, orthostatic hypotension.
GI: anorexia, nausea, pancreatitis.
Hepatic: hepatic encephalopathy.
Metabolic: hypokalemia, asymptomatic hyperuricemia, hyperglycemia and impairment of glucose tolerance, fluid and electrolyte imbalances including dilutional hyponatremia and hypochloremia, metabolic alkalosis, hypercalcemia, gout.
Skin: dermatitis, photosensitivity, rash.
Other: hypersensitivity reactions, such as pneumonitis and vasculitis.

INTERACTIONS
Cholestyramine, colestipol: intestinal absorption of thiazides decreased. Keep doses as separate as possible.
Diazoxide: increased antihypertensive, hyperglycemic, and hyperuricemic effects. Use together cautiously.

NURSING CONSIDERATIONS
- *Contraindicated* in anuria or hypersensitivity to other thiazides or other sulfonamide-derived drugs.
- *Use cautiously* in severe renal disease and impaired hepatic function.
- Monitor intake and output, weight, blood pressure, and serum electrolytes.
- Consult with doctor and dietitian to provide high-potassium diet. Foods rich in potassium include citrus fruits, tomatoes, bananas, dates, and apricots. Watch for hypokalemia (muscle weakness and cramps). Patients also on digitalis have an increased risk of digitalis toxicity from the potassium-depleting effect of this diuretic. May use with potassium-sparing diuretic to prevent hypokalemia.
- Monitor serum creatinine and BUN regularly. Not as effective if these levels are more than twice normal.
- Check insulin requirements in patients with diabetes. May treat severe hyperglycemia with oral antidiabetic agents. Monitor blood glucose levels.
- Monitor blood uric acid, especially in patients with a history of gout.
- In hypertension, therapeutic response may be delayed several days.
- Give in a.m. to prevent nocturia.
- Elderly patients are especially susceptible to excessive diuresis.
- Thiazides and thiazide-like diuretics should be stopped before tests for parathyroid function are performed.
- Advise patient to avoid sudden posture changes and rise slowly to avoid orthostatic hypotension.
- Advise patient to use a sunscreen.

urea (carbamide)
Ureaphil

Pregnancy Risk Category: C

HOW SUPPLIED
Injection: 40 g/150 ml

MECHANISM OF ACTION
An osmotic diuretic that increases the osmotic pressure of glomerular filtrate, inhibiting tubular reabsorption of water and electrolytes. Also elevates blood plasma osmolality, resulting in enhanced flow of water into extracellular fluid.

INDICATIONS & DOSAGE
Intracranial or intraocular pressure –
Adults: 1 to 1.5 g/kg as a 30% solution by slow I.V. infusion over 1 to 2.5 hours.
Children over 2 years: 0.5 to 1.5 g/kg slow I.V. infusion.

Children under 2 years: as little as 0.1 g/kg slow I.V. infusion. Maximum rate is 4 ml/minute.

Maximum adult daily dosage is 120 g. To prepare 135 ml 30% solution, mix contents of 40-g vial of urea with 105 ml dextrose 5% or 10% in water or 10% invert sugar in water. Each ml of 30% solution provides 300 mg urea.

ADVERSE REACTIONS
Common reactions are in italics; life-threatening reactions are in bold italics.
CNS: *headache.*
CV: tachycardia, CHF, *pulmonary edema.*
GI: *nausea, vomiting.*
Metabolic: sodium and potassium depletion.
Local: irritation or necrotic sloughing may occur with extravasation.

INTERACTIONS
None significant.

NURSING CONSIDERATIONS
- *Contraindicated* in severely impaired renal function, marked dehydration, frank hepatic failure, or active intracranial bleeding.
- *Use cautiously* in pregnancy, lactation, cardiac disease, hepatic impairment, and sickle cell disease with CNS involvement.
- **I.V. use:** Avoid rapid I.V. infusion; may cause hemolysis or increased capillary bleeding. Avoid extravasation; may cause reactions ranging from mild irritation to necrosis.
- Use freshly reconstituted urea only for I.V. infusion; solution becomes ammonia upon standing.
- Don't infuse into leg veins; may cause phlebitis or thrombosis, especially in elderly patients.
- Watch for hyponatremia or hypokalemia (muscle weakness, lethargy); may indicate electrolyte depletion before serum levels are reduced.
- Maintain adequate hydration; monitor blood pressure, intake and output, and serum electrolytes.
- In renal disease, monitor BUN.
- Indwelling urethral catheter should be used in comatose patients to ensure bladder emptying. Use an hourly urometer collection bag for accurate evaluation of diuresis.
- If satisfactory diuresis does not occur in 6 to 12 hours, urea should be discontinued and renal function reevaluated.
- Use within minutes of reconstitution.
- Assess breath sounds for crackles, indicating pulmonary edema.

61

Electrolytes and replacement solutions

calcium acetate
calcium carbonate
calcium chloride
calcium citrate
calcium glubionate
calcium gluceptate
calcium gluconate
calcium lactate
calcium phosphate, dibasic
calcium phosphate, tribasic
dextran, low molecular weight
dextran, high molecular weight
hetastarch
magnesium chloride
magnesium sulfate
potassium acetate
potassium bicarbonate
potassium chloride
potassium gluconate
Ringer's injection
Ringer's injection, lactated
sodium chloride

COMBINATION PRODUCTS
KAOCHLOR-EFF: 20 mEq potassium, 20 mEq chloride (from potassium chloride, potassium citrate, potassium bicarbonate, and betaine hydrochloride).
KLORVESS*: 20 mEq each potassium and chloride (from potassium chloride, potassium bicarbonate, and l-lysine monohydrochloride).
KOLYUM: 20 mEq potassium, 3.4 mEq chloride (from potassium gluconate and potassium chloride).
NEUTRA-PHOS: phosphorus 250 mg, sodium 164 mg, potassium 278 mg (from dibasic and monobasic sodium and potassium phosphate).
TWIN-K-CL: 15 ml supplies 15 mEq of potassium ions as a combination of potassium gluconate, potassium citrate, and ammonium chloride.

calcium acetate
Phos-Ex◊, Phos-Lo

calcium carbonate
Alka-Mints◊, Amitone◊, Cal Carb-HD◊, Cal-Plus◊, Chooz◊, Dicarbosil◊, Equilet◊, Mallamint◊, Rolaids Calcium Rich◊, Tums◊, Tums E-X Extra Strength◊, Tums Extra Strength◊

calcium chloride◊

calcium citrate◊

calcium glubionate◊

calcium gluceptate◊

calcium gluconate
Kalcinate◊

calcium lactate◊

calcium phosphate, dibasic◊

calcium phosphate, tribasic
Posture◊

Pregnancy Risk Category: C

HOW SUPPLIED

acetate
Tablets: 250 mg◊, 500 mg◊, 667 mg, 668 mg◊, 1,000 mg◊ (contains 253 mg/calcium/g)
Injection: 0.5 mEq Ca^{++} per ml

carbonate
Tablets◊*:* 650 mg, 667 mg, 750 mg, 1.25 g, 1.5 g (contains 400 mg calcium/g)
Tablets (chewable)◊*:* 350 mg, 420 mg, 500 mg, 625 mg, 750 mg, 850 mg, 1.25 g

*Liquid form contains alcohol. **May contain tartrazine.

Capsules: 1.512 g◊
Oral suspension: 1.25 g/5 ml (contains 400 mg of elemental calcium/g)◊
Chewy squares: 1.5 g◊
Powder packets: 6.5 g (2,400 mg calcium) per packet◊
chloride
Injection: 10% solution in 10-ml ampules, vials, and syringes
citrate
Tablets: 950 mg (contains 211 mg of elemental calcium/g)◊
glubionate
Syrup: 1.8 g/5 ml (contains 64 mg of elemental calcium/g)
gluceptate
Injection: 1.1 g/5 ml in 5-ml ampules or 50-ml vials
gluconate
Tablets: 500 mg◊, 650 mg◊, 975 mg◊, 1 g◊ (contains 90 mg of elemental calcium/g)
Injection: 10% solution in 10-ml ampules and vials, 10-ml or 20-ml vials
lactate
Tablets: 325 mg, 650 mg (contains 130 mg of elemental calcium/g)
phosphate, dibasic
Tablets: 468 mg (contains 230 mg of elemental calcium/g)◊
phosphate, tribasic
Tablets: 300 mg◊, 600 mg◊ (contains 400 mg of elemental calcium/g)

MECHANISM OF ACTION

Replaces and maintains calcium.

INDICATIONS & DOSAGE

Hypocalcemia, hypocalcemic tetany, hypocalcemia during exchange transfusions, cardiac resuscitation for inotropic effect when epinephrine has failed; magnesium intoxication; hypoparathyroidism –
Adults and children: initially, 500 mg to 1 g calcium salt I.V., with further dosage based on serum calcium determinations and specific calcium salt. See below for dosages with specific calcium salts.

Dosage with calcium acetate (1g yields 12.6 mEq Ca^{++}):
Hypophosphatemia –
Adults: 1,334 to 2,000 mg P.O. t.i.d. with meals. Most dialysis patients will require 3 to 4 tablets with each meal.

Dosage with calcium chloride (1 g [10 ml] yields 13.5 mEq Ca^{++}):
Magnesium intoxication –
Adults and children: initially, 500 mg I.V., with further doses based on calcium and magnesium determinations.
Cardiac arrest –
Adults: 0.5 to 1 g I.V., not to exceed 1 ml/minute; or 200 to 800 mg into the ventricular cavity.
Hypocalcemia –
Adults: 500 mg to 1 g I.V. at intervals of 1 to 3 days, determined by serum calcium levels.
Calcium supplementation during total parenteral nutrition –
Adults: 10 to 15 mEq I.V. daily.
Children: 5 to 20 mEq I.V. daily.
Neonates: 0.5 to 3 mEq/kg I.V. daily.

Dosage with calcium gluconate (1 g [10 ml] yields 4.5 mEq Ca^{++}):
Hypocalcemia –
Adults: 500 mg to 1 g I.V., repeated q 1 to 3 days p.r.n. as determined by serum calcium levels. Further doses depend on serum calcium determinations.
Children: 100 to 150 mg/kg I.V. three to four times daily. Rate of infusion should not exceed 0.5 ml/minute.

Dosage with calcium gluceptate (1.1 g [5 ml] yields 4.5 mEq Ca^{++}) and calcium salts (18 mg [1 ml] yields 0.898 mEq Ca^{++}):
Hypocalcemia –
Adults: initially, 5 to 20 ml I.V., with further doses based on serum calcium determinations. If I.V. injection is impossible, 2 to 5 ml I.M. Average adult oral dose is 1 to 2 g elemental calcium P.O. daily, divided t.i.d. or q.i.d. Average oral dose for children is 45 to 65

mg/kg P.O. daily, divided t.i.d. or q.i.d.
During exchange transfusions – **Adults and children:** 0.5 ml I.V. after each 100 ml blood exchanged.

ADVERSE REACTIONS
Common reactions are in italics; life-threatening reactions are in bold italics.
CNS: from I.V. use, tingling sensations, sense of oppression or heat waves; with rapid I.V. injection, syncope.
CV: mild fall in blood pressure; with rapid I.V. injection, vasodilation, bradycardia, ***cardiac arrhythmias, cardiac arrest.***
GI: with oral ingestion, irritation, hemorrhage, *constipation;* with I.V. administration, chalky taste; with oral calcium chloride, GI hemorrhage, nausea, vomiting, thirst, abdominal pain.
GU: hypercalcemia, polyuria, renal calculi.
Skin: local reaction if calcium salts given I.M., burning, necrosis, tissue sloughing, cellulitis, soft tissue calcification.
Local: with S.C. injection, pain and irritation; *with I.V., vein irritation.*

INTERACTIONS
Digitalis glycosides: increased digitalis toxicity; administer calcium very cautiously (if at all) to digitalized patients.

NURSING CONSIDERATIONS
• *Contraindicated* in ventricular fibrillation, hypercalcemia, or renal calculi.
• *Use cautiously* in patients with sarcoidosis and renal or cardiac disease, and in digitalized patients. Use calcium chloride cautiously in cor pulmonale, respiratory acidosis, and respiratory failure.
• **I.V. use (direct injection):** Administer slowly through a small needle into a large vein or through an I.V. line containing a free-flowing, compatible solution at a rate not exceeding 1 ml/minute (1.5 mEq/minute) for calcium chloride, 1.5 to 5 ml/minute for calcium gluconate, and 2 ml/minute for calcium gluceptate. Do not use scalp veins in children.
• **I.V. use (intermittent infusion):** Infuse diluted solution through an I.V. line containing a compatible solution. Maximum rate of 200 mg/minute suggested for calcium gluceptate and calcium gluconate.
• Calcium chloride should be given I.V. only. When adding to parenteral solutions that contain other additives (especially phosphorus or phosphate), observe closely for precipitate. Use an inline filter.
• Monitor ECG when giving calcium I.V. Stop if patient complains of discomfort. Following I.V. injection, patient should remain recumbent for 15 minutes.
• I.M. injection should be given in the gluteal region in adults; lateral thigh in infants. I.M. route used only in emergencies when no I.V. route available.
• Monitor blood calcium frequently. Report abnormalities.
• Hypercalcemia may result after large doses in chronic renal failure.
• Solutions should be warmed to body temperature before administration.
• Severe necrosis and tissue sloughing follow extravasation. Calcium gluconate is less irritating to veins and tissues than calcium chloride.
• If GI upset occurs, give oral calcium products 1 to 1½ hours after meals.
• Oxalic acid (found in rhubarb and spinach), phytic acid (in bran and whole cereals), and phosphorus (in milk and dairy products) may interfere with absorption of calcium.
• Crash carts usually contain both calcium gluconate and calcium chlo-

*Liquid form contains alcohol. **May contain tartrazine.

ride. Make sure doctor specifies form he wants administered.

dextran, low molecular weight (dextran 40)

Gentran 40, Rheomacrodex LMD

Pregnancy Risk Category: C

HOW SUPPLIED

Injection: 10% dextran in dextrose 5% or 0.9% sodium chloride

MECHANISM OF ACTION

Expands plasma volume and provides fluid replacement.

INDICATIONS & DOSAGE

Plasma volume expansion –
Adults: Dosage of 10% solution by I.V. infusion depends on amount of fluid loss.

First 500 ml of dextran may be infused rapidly with central venous pressure monitoring. Infuse remaining dose slowly. Total daily dosage not to exceed 2 g/kg body weight. If therapy continued past 24 hours, do not exceed 1 g/kg daily. Continue for no longer than 5 days.

Reduction of blood sludging –
Adults: 500 ml of 10% solution by I.V. infusion.

Prophylaxis of venous thrombosis –
Adults: 10 ml/kg (500 to 1,000 ml) of a 10% solution I.V. on the day of the procedure; 500 ml on days 2 and 3.

ADVERSE REACTIONS

Common reactions are in italics; life-threatening reactions are in bold italics.
Blood: *decreased level of hemoglobin and hematocrit;* with higher doses, increased bleeding time.
GI: nausea, vomiting.
GU: tubular stasis and blocking, increased viscosity of urine.
Hepatic: increased AST (SGOT) and ALT (SGPT) levels.
Skin: hypersensitivity reaction, urticaria.
Other: ***anaphylaxis.***

INTERACTIONS

None significant.

NURSING CONSIDERATIONS

- *Contraindicated* in marked hemostatic defects; marked cardiac decompensation or pulmonary edema; renal disease with severe oliguria or anuria; or extreme dehydration.
- *Use cautiously* in active hemorrhage; may cause additional blood loss. Evaluate patient's hydration status before administration.
- Doctor may order dextran 1 (Promit) to protect against dextran-induced anaphylaxis. Administer Promit, 20 ml I.V. over 60 seconds, 1 to 2 minutes before the I.V. infusion of dextran.
- **I.V. use:** Observe patient closely during early phase of infusion; most anaphylactoid reactions occur during this time.
- Hazardous for patients with heart failure, especially if in sodium chloride solution. Use dextrose in water solution instead.
- Works as plasma expander via colloidal osmotic effect, thereby drawing fluid from interstitial to intravascular space. Provides plasma expansion slightly greater than volume infused. Watch for circulatory overload and a rise in central venous pressure.
- Monitor urine flow rate during administration. If oliguria or anuria occurs or is not relieved by infusion, stop dextran and give loop diuretic.
- Assess hydration before starting therapy; otherwise, use urine or serum osmolarity because urine specific gravity is affected by urine dextran concentration.
- Check hemoglobin and hematocrit; don't allow to fall below 30% by volume.
- May interfere with analyses of blood grouping, cross matching, bilirubin, blood glucose, and protein.

• Store at constant 77° F (25° C). May precipitate in storage, but can be heated to dissolve if necessary.

dextran, high molecular weight (dextran 70, dextran 75)

Gentran 75, Macrodex

Pregnancy Risk Category: C

HOW SUPPLIED

Injection: 6% dextran 70 in 0.9% sodium chloride or dextrose 5%; 6% dextran 75 in 0.9% sodium chloride or dextrose 5%

MECHANISM OF ACTION

Expands plasma volume and provides fluid replacement.

INDICATIONS & DOSAGE

Plasma expander –

Adults: usual dose 30 g (500 ml of 6% solution) I.V. In emergency situations, may be administered at rate of 1.2 to 2.4 g (20 to 40 ml) per minute. In normovolemic or nearly normovolemic patients, rate of infusion should not exceed 240 mg (4 ml)/minute.

Total dosage during first 24 hours not to exceed 1.2 g/kg; actual dosage depends on amount of fluid loss and resultant hemoconcentration, and must be determined for each patient.

ADVERSE REACTIONS

Common reactions are in italics; life-threatening reactions are in bold italics.

Blood: *decreased level of hemoglobin and hematocrit;* with doses of 15 ml/kg body weight, prolonged bleeding time and significant suppression of platelet function.

GI: nausea, vomiting.

GU: increased specific gravity and viscosity of urine, tubular stasis and blocking.

Hepatic: increased AST (SGOT) and ALT (SGPT) levels.

Skin: hypersensitivity reaction, urticaria.

Other: fever, arthralgia, nasal congestion, ***anaphylaxis.***

INTERACTIONS

None significant.

NURSING CONSIDERATIONS

• *Contraindicated* in marked hemostatic defects; marked cardiac decompensation or pulmonary edema; renal disease with severe oliguria or anuria; or extreme dehydration.

• *Use cautiously* in active hemorrhage; may cause additional blood loss.

• Doctor may order dextran 1 (Promit) to protect against dextran-induced anaphylaxis. Administer Promit, 20 ml I.V. over 60 seconds, 1 to 2 minutes before the I.V. infusion of dextran 70.

• **I.V. use:** Observe patient closely during early phase of infusion; most anaphylactoid reactions occur during this time.

• Hazardous for patients with heart failure, especially if in sodium chloride solution. Use dextrose in water solution instead.

• Works as plasma expander via colloidal osmotic effect, thereby drawing fluid from interstitial to intravascular space. Provides plasma expansion slightly greater than volume infused. Watch for circulatory overload.

• Monitor urine flow rate during administration. If oliguria or anuria occurs or is not relieved by infusion, stop dextran and give loop diuretic.

• Assess hydration before starting therapy; otherwise, use urine or serum osmolarity because urine specific gravity is affected by the urine dextran concentration.

• Check hemoglobin and hematocrit; don't allow to fall below 30% by volume.

• Draw blood samples *before* starting infusion.

• May interfere with analyses of blood grouping, cross matching, bilirubin, blood glucose, and protein.
• May precipitate in storage, but can be heated to dissolve if necessary.

hetastarch

Hespan

Pregnancy Risk Category: C

HOW SUPPLIED

Injection: 500 ml (6 g/100 ml in 0.9% sodium chloride solution)

MECHANISM OF ACTION

Expands plasma volume and provides fluid replacement.

INDICATIONS & DOSAGE

Plasma expander –

Adults: 500 to 1,000 ml I.V. depending on amount of blood lost and resultant hemoconcentration. Total dosage usually not to exceed 1,500 ml/day. Up to 20 ml/kg hourly may be used in hemorrhagic shock.

ADVERSE REACTIONS

Common reactions are in italics; life-threatening reactions are in bold italics.
CNS: headaches.
CV: peripheral edema of lower extremities.
EENT: periorbital edema.
GI: nausea, vomiting.
Skin: urticaria.
Other: wheezing, mild fever.

INTERACTIONS

None significant.

NURSING CONSIDERATIONS

• *Contraindicated* in severe bleeding disorders, with severe congestive heart failure, or renal failure with oliguria and anuria.
• To avoid circulatory overload, monitor patients with impaired renal function carefully.
• Discontinue if allergic or sensitivity reactions occur. If necessary, administer an antihistamine.
• When used in continuous-flow centrifugation, leukapheresis ratio is usually 1 part hetastarch to 8 parts venous whole blood.
• Hetastarch is *not* a substitute for blood or plasma.
• Available in 500-ml I.V. infusion bottles.
• Discard partially used bottles.

magnesium chloride

Slow-Mag◊

magnesium sulfate

Pregnancy Risk Category: B

HOW SUPPLIED

chloride

Tablets (delayed-release): 64 mg

sulfate

Injectable solutions: 10%, 12.5%, 25%, 50% in 2-ml, 5-ml, 10-ml, 20-ml, and 30-ml ampules, vials, and prefilled syringes

MECHANISM OF ACTION

Replaces and maintains magnesium levels. As an anticonvulsant, reduces muscle contractions by interfering with the release of acetylcholine at the myoneural junction.

INDICATIONS & DOSAGE

Hypomagnesemia –

Adults: 1 g, or 8.12 mEq, of 50% solution (2 ml) I.M. q 6 hours for 4 doses, depending on serum magnesium level.

Severe hypomagnesemia (serum magnesium 0.8 mEq/liter or less, with symptoms) –

Adults: 6 g, or 50 mEq, of 50% solution I.V. in 1 liter of solution over 4 hours.

Subsequent doses depend on serum magnesium levels.

Magnesium supplementation –

Adults: 64 mg (1 tablet) P.O. t.i.d.

Magnesium supplementation in total parenteral nutrition (TPN) –
Adults: 8 to 24 mEq I.V. daily added to TPN solution.
Children over 6 years: 2 to 10 mEq I.V. daily added to TPN solution.

Each 2 ml of 50% solution contains 1 g, or 8.12 mEq, magnesium sulfate.

Acute treatment of preeclampsia and eclampsia –
Women: loading dose: 2 to 4 g (4 to 8 ml of 50% solution) given by slow I.V. bolus (over 5 minutes).
Maintenance dosage: 1 to 2 g hourly as a constant infusion. Prepare by adding 8 ml of 50% solution to 250 ml dextrose 5% in water.

Hypomagnesemic seizures –
Adults: 1 to 2 g (as 10% solution) I.V. over 15 minutes, then 1 g I.M. q 4 to 6 hours, based on patient response and magnesium blood level.

Seizures secondary to hypomagnesemia in acute nephritis –
Adults: 0.2 ml/kg of 50% solution I.M. q 4 to 6 hours, p.r.n. or 100 mg/kg of 10% solution I.V. very slowly. Titrate dosage according to magnesium blood level and seizure response.

Paroxysmal atrial tachycardia unresponsive to other treatments –
Adults: 3 to 4 g I.V. (as a 10% solution) over 30 seconds, with close monitoring of ECG.

ADVERSE REACTIONS

Common reactions are in italics; life-threatening reactions are in bold italics.

CNS: toxicity: *weak or absent deep tendon reflexes,* flaccid paralysis, hypothermia, drowsiness, hypocalcemia (perioral paresthesias, twitching carpopedal spasm, tetany, and seizures).

CV: slow, weak pulse; cardiac arrhythmias (hypocalcemia); *hypotension.*

Skin: flushing, sweating.

Other: *respiratory paralysis,* hypocalcemia.

INTERACTIONS

Neuromuscular blocking agents: may cause increased neuromuscular blockage. Use cautiously.

NURSING CONSIDERATIONS

- *Contraindicated* in impaired renal function, myocardial damage, or heart block, and in actively progressing labor.
- *Use parenteral magnesium with extreme caution* in patients receiving digitalis preparations. Treating magnesium toxicity with calcium in such patients could cause serious alterations in cardiac conduction; heart block may result.
- **I.V. use:** Inject I.V. bolus dose slowly to avoid respiratory or cardiac arrest. If available, use infusion pump for continuous infusion. Maximum infusion rate is 150 mg/minute. Rapid drip causes feeling of heat.
- Keep I.V. calcium available to reverse magnesium intoxication.
- Monitor vital signs every 15 minutes when giving I.V. for severe hypomagnesemia. Watch for respiratory depression and signs of heart block. Respirations should be more than 16/minute before dose is given.
- Monitor intake and output. Output should be 100 ml or more during 4-hour period before dose.
- Test knee-jerk and patellar reflexes before each additional dose. If absent, give no more magnesium until reflexes return; otherwise, patient may develop temporary respiratory failure and need cardiopulmonary resuscitation or I.V. administration of calcium.
- Check magnesium level after repeated doses.
- After giving to toxemic mothers within 24 hours before delivery, watch neonate for signs of magnesium toxicity, including neuromuscular and respiratory depression.

potassium acetate

Pregnancy Risk Category: C

HOW SUPPLIED

Injection: 2 mEq/ml in 20-ml, 30-ml vials.

MECHANISM OF ACTION

Replaces and maintains potassium level.

INDICATIONS & DOSAGE

Treatment of hypokalemia –
Adults: I.V. should be used for life-threatening hypokalemia or when oral replacement not feasible. Give no more than 20 mEq hourly in concentration of 40 mEq/liter or less. Total 24-hour dosage should not exceed 150 mEq (3 mEq/kg in children). Potassium replacement should be done with ECG monitoring and frequent serum potassium determinations.
Prevention of hypokalemia –
Adults: dosage is individualized according to patient's needs. In most cases, dosage should not exceed 150 mEq/day. Administer as an additive to I.V. infusions. Usual dose is 40 mEq/liter, and solutions are usually infused at a rate not to exceed 20 mEq/hour.
Children: individualize dose. Usual dose should not exceed 3 mEq/kg/day. Administer as an additive to I.V. infusions.

ADVERSE REACTIONS

Common reactions are in italics; life-threatening reactions are in bold italics.
Signs of hyperkalemia:
CNS: paresthesias of the extremities, listlessness, mental confusion, weakness or heaviness of legs, flaccid paralysis.
CV: ***peripheral vascular collapse with fall in blood pressure, cardiac arrhythmias,*** heart block, possible cardiac arrest, ECG changes (prolonged P-R intervals; wide QRS complex; ST segment depression; tall, tented T waves).
GI: nausea, vomiting, abdominal pain, diarrhea, bowel ulceration.
GU: oliguria.
Skin: cold skin, gray pallor.

INTERACTIONS

None significant.

NURSING CONSIDERATIONS

- *Contraindicated* in severe renal impairment with oliguria, anuria, azotemia; untreated Addison's disease; or in acute dehydration, hyperkalemia, hyperkalemic form of familial periodic paralysis, and conditions associated with extensive tissue breakdown.
- *Use cautiously* in patients with cardiac disease, patients receiving potassium-sparing diuretics, and those with renal impairment.
- During therapy, monitor ECG, renal function, intake and output, and serum potassium, serum creatinine, and BUN levels. Never give potassium postoperatively until urine flow is established.
- Give slowly as diluted solution; potentially fatal hyperkalemia may result from too-rapid infusion.
- **I.V. use:** Parenteral potassium given by I.V. infusion only; never I.V. push or I.M.Observe for pain and redness at infusion site. Large-bore needle reduces local irritation.
- Watch for signs of GI ulceration: obstruction, hemorrhage, pain, distention, severe vomiting, and bleeding.
- Reconstitute potassium acetate powder with liquids; give after meals with a full glass of water or fruit juice to minimize GI irritation.
- To prevent serious hyperkalemia, potassium deficits must be replaced gradually.

potassium bicarbonate

K + Care ET, K-Gen ET, K-Ide, Klor-Con/EF, K-Lyte ET

Pregnancy Risk Category: A

HOW SUPPLIED

Effervescent tablets: 25 mEq

MECHANISM OF ACTION

Replaces and maintains potassium.

INDICATIONS & DOSAGE

Hypokalemia –

Adults: 25 to 50 mEq dissolved in ½ to a full glass of water (120 to 240 ml) once daily to q.i.d.

ADVERSE REACTIONS

Common reactions are in italics; life-threatening reactions are in bold italics.

CNS: paresthesias of the extremities, listlessness, mental confusion, weakness or heaviness of legs, flaccid paralysis.

CV: ***cardiac arrhythmias,*** ECG changes (prolonged P-R interval; wide QRS complex; ST segment depression; tall, tented T waves).

GI: *nausea, vomiting, abdominal pain,* diarrhea, ulcerations, hemorrhage, obstruction, perforation.

INTERACTIONS

None significant.

NURSING CONSIDERATIONS

- *Contraindicated* in severe renal impairment with oliguria, anuria, azotemia, and untreated Addison's disease; also in acute dehydration, hyperkalemia, hyperkalemic form of familial periodic paralysis, and conditions associated with extensive tissue breakdown.
- *Use cautiously* in patients with cardiac disease and in those receiving potassium-sparing diuretics.
- Monitor BUN, serum potassium and creatinine, and intake and output.
- Never switch potassium products without a doctor's order.
- Dissolve potassium bicarbonate tablets in 6 to 8 ounces of cold water. Dissolve completely to minimize GI irritation.
- Don't administer potassium supplements postoperatively until urine flow has been established.
- Have patient take with meals and sip slowly over 5 to 10 minutes.
- Potassium bicarbonate cannot be given instead of potassium chloride.
- Potassium bicarbonate does not correct hypochloremic alkalosis.
- Available in lime and orange flavors. Ask patient's flavor preference.

potassium chloride

Cena-K, K + 10, K + Care, Kaochlor 10%*, Kaochlor S-F 10%*, Kaon-Cl, Kaon-Cl 20%*, Kato Powder, Kay Ciel*, K-Dur, K-Lease, K-Lor, Klor-10%*, Klor-Con, Klorvess, Klotrix, K-Lyte/Cl, K-Norm, K-Tab, Micro-K Extencaps, Rum-K, Slow-K, Ten-K

Pregnancy Risk Category: A

HOW SUPPLIED

Tablets: 1.22 mEq (99 mg), 8 mEq (600 mg), 10 mEq (750 mg), 20 mEq (1,500 mg), 25 mEq (1,875 mg)
Tablets (controlled-release): 6.7 mEq (500 mg), 8 mEq (600 mg), 10 mEq (750 mg), 20 mEq (1,500 mg)
Tablets (enteric-coated): 4 mEq (300 mg), 13.4 mEq (1,000 mg)
Capsules (controlled-release): 8 mEq (600 mg), 10 mEq (750 mg)
Oral liquid: 5% (10 mEq/15 ml), 7.5% (15 mEq/15 ml), 10% (20 mEq/15 ml), 15% (30 mEq/15 ml), 20% (40 mEq/15 ml)
Powder for oral use: 15 mEq/packet, 20 mEq/packet, 25 mEq/packet, 25 mEq/dose
Injection: 20 mEq, 40 mEq ampules; additive syringes containing 30 mEq or 40 mEq; 10 mEq, 20 mEq, 30

*Liquid form contains alcohol. **May contain tartrazine.

mEq, 40 mEq, 45 mEq, 60 mEq, 100 mEq, 200 mEq, 400 mEq, or 1,000 mEq vials

MECHANISM OF ACTION
Replaces and maintains potassium level.

INDICATIONS & DOSAGE
Hypokalemia –
Adults: 40 to 100 mEq P.O. daily in three or four divided doses for treatment; 20 mEq for prevention. Further dosage based on serum potassium.

Use I.V. route when oral replacement not feasible or when hypokalemia is life-threatening. Usual dose 20 mEq hourly in concentration of 40 mEq/liter or less. Total daily dosage not to exceed 150 mEq (3 mEq/kg in children). Potassium replacement should be done only with ECG monitoring and frequent serum potassium determinations.

ADVERSE REACTIONS
Common reactions are in italics; life-threatening reactions are in bold italics.
Signs of hyperkalemia –
CNS: paresthesias of the extremities, listlessness, mental confusion, weakness or heaviness of limbs, flaccid paralysis.
CV: ***peripheral vascular collapse with fall in blood pressure, cardiac arrhythmias, heart block, possible cardiac arrest,*** ECG changes (prolonged P-R interval; wide QRS; ST segment depression; tall, tented T waves).
GI: *nausea, vomiting, abdominal pain,* diarrhea, GI ulcerations (possible stenosis, hemorrhage, obstruction, perforation).
GU: oliguria.
Skin: cold skin, gray pallor.
Local: *postinfusion phlebitis.*

INTERACTIONS
None significant.

NURSING CONSIDERATIONS
- *Contraindicated* in severe renal impairment with oliguria, anuria, azotemia, and untreated Addison's disease; also in acute dehydration, hyperkalemia, hyperkalemic form of familial periodic paralysis, and conditions associated with extensive tissue breakdown.
- *Use cautiously* in patients with cardiac disease and in those receiving potassium-sparing diuretics.
- Potassium should not be given during immediate postoperative period until urine flow is established.
- **I.V. use:** Parenteral potassium given by infusion only; never I.V. push or I.M. Give slowly as dilute solution; potentially fatal hyperkalemia may result from too-rapid infusion.
- Small amounts of lidocaine injection (1 to 3 ml of the 1% strength) may be added directly to the potassium chloride solution. This will help reverse postinfusion phlebitis.
- Give oral potassium supplements with extreme caution because its many forms deliver varying amounts of potassium. Never switch products without a doctor's order.
- Sugar-free liquid available (Kaochlor S-F 10%).
- Use a liquid preparation if tablet or capsule passage is likely to be delayed, such as in GI obstruction.
- Have patient sip liquid potassium slowly to minimize GI irritation.
- Give with or after meals with full glass of water or fruit juice to lessen GI distress.
- Patient should make sure powders are completely dissolved before ingesting.
- Enteric-coated tablets not recommended due to potential for GI bleeding and small-bowel ulcerations.
- Tablets in wax matrix sometimes lodge in esophagus and cause ulceration in cardiac patients who have esophageal compression from enlarged left atrium. In such patients

and in those with esophageal stasis or obstruction, use liquid form.

- Microencapsulated form (Micro-K) has been shown in one study to cause less GI bleeding than the wax matrix tablets. However, this hasn't been completely confirmed.
- Often used orally with diuretics that cause potassium excretion. Potassium chloride most useful since diuretics waste chloride ion. Hypokalemic alkalosis treated best with potassium chloride.
- Monitor ECG and serum electrolytes during therapy.
- Don't crush sustained-release potassium products.

potassium gluconate

Glu-K, Kaon Liquid*, Kaon Tablets, Kaylixer*, K-G Elixir*, Potassium Rougier†

Pregnancy Risk Category: A

HOW SUPPLIED

Tablets: 500 mg (2 mEq K^+), 1,170 mg (5 mEq K^+)†
Elixir: 4.68 g (20 mEq K^+)/15 ml*

MECHANISM OF ACTION

Replaces and maintains potassium.

INDICATIONS & DOSAGE

Hypokalemia –
Adults: 40 to 100 mEq P.O. daily in three or four divided doses for treatment; 20 mEq daily for prevention. Further dosage based on serum potassium determinations.

ADVERSE REACTIONS

Common reactions are in italics; life-threatening reactions are in bold italics.
CNS: paresthesias of the extremities, listlessness, mental confusion, weakness or heaviness of legs, flaccid paralysis.
CV: ***cardiac arrhythmias,*** ECG changes (prolonged P-R interval; wide QRS complex; ST segment depression; tall, tented T waves).
GI: *nausea, vomiting, abdominal pain,* diarrhea, GI ulcerations with oral products (especially enteric-coated tablets); ulcerations may be accompanied by stenosis, hemorrhage, obstruction, perforation.

INTERACTIONS

None significant.

NURSING CONSIDERATIONS

- *Contraindicated* in severe renal impairment with oliguria, anuria, azotemia, and untreated Addison's disease; also in acute dehydration, hyperkalemia, hyperkalemic form of familial periodic paralysis, and conditions associated with extensive tissue breakdown.
- *Use cautiously* in patients with cardiac disease and in those receiving potassium-sparing diuretics.
- Monitor ECG, serum potassium and creatinine levels, BUN, and intake and output.
- Give oral potassium supplements with extreme caution because their many forms deliver varying amounts of potassium. Never switch products without a doctor's order.
- Don't administer potassium supplements postoperatively until urine flow has been established.
- Have patient sip liquid potassium slowly to minimize GI irritation.
- Give with or after meals with full glass of water or fruit juice to lessen GI distress.
- Potassium gluconate does not correct hypokalemic hypochloremic alkalosis.
- Enteric-coated tablets not recommended because of potential for GI bleeding and small-bowel ulcerations.

Ringer's injection

Pregnancy Risk Category: C

HOW SUPPLIED
Injection: 250 ml, 500 ml, 1,000 ml

MECHANISM OF ACTION
Replaces fluids and electrolytes.

INDICATIONS & DOSAGE
Fluid and electrolyte replacement –
Adults and children: dose highly individualized, but usually 1.5 to 3 liters (2% to 6% body weight) infused I.V. over 18 to 24 hours.

ADVERSE REACTIONS
Common reactions are in italics; life-threatening reactions are in bold italics.
CV: fluid overload.

INTERACTIONS
None significant.

NURSING CONSIDERATIONS
- *Contraindicated* in renal failure, except as emergency volume expander.
- *Use cautiously* in congestive heart failure, circulatory insufficiency, renal dysfunction, hypoproteinemia, and pulmonary edema.
- Ringer's injection contains sodium, 147 mEq/liter; potassium, 4 mEq/liter; calcium, 4.5 mEq/liter; and chloride, 155.5 mEq/liter. This electrolyte content is insufficient for treating severe electrolyte deficiencies, although it does provide electrolytes in levels approximately equal to those of the blood.

Ringer's injection, lactated
(Hartmann's solution, Ringer's lactate solution)

Pregnancy Risk Category: C

HOW SUPPLIED
Injection: 250 ml, 500 ml, 1,000 ml

MECHANISM OF ACTION
Replaces fluids and electrolytes.

INDICATIONS & DOSAGE
Fluid and electrolyte replacement –
Adults and children: dosage highly individualized, but usually 1.5 to 3 liters (2% to 6% body weight) infused I.V. over 18 to 24 hours.

ADVERSE REACTIONS
Common reactions are in italics; life-threatening reactions are in bold italics.
CV: fluid overload.

INTERACTIONS
None significant.

NURSING CONSIDERATIONS
- *Contraindicated* in renal failure, except as emergency volume expander.
- *Use cautiously* in congestive heart failure, circulatory insufficiency, renal dysfunction, hypoproteinemia, and pulmonary edema.
- Lactated Ringer's injection contains sodium, 130 mEq/liter; potassium, 4 mEq/liter; calcium, 3 mEq/liter; chloride, 109.7 mEq/liter; and lactate, 28 mEq/liter.
- Approximates more closely the electrolyte concentration in blood plasma than Ringer's injection.

sodium chloride
Pregnancy Risk Category: C

HOW SUPPLIED
Tablets (enteric-coated): 1 g
Tablets (slow-release): 600 mg
Injection: 0.45% sodium chloride 500 ml, 1,000 ml; 0.9% sodium chloride 50 ml, 100 ml, 150 ml, 250 ml, 500 ml, 1,000 ml; 3% sodium chloride 500 ml; 5% sodium chloride 500 ml

MECHANISM OF ACTION
Replaces and maintains sodium and chloride levels.

INDICATIONS & DOSAGE
Highly individualized fluid and electrolyte replacement in hyponatremia

caused by electrolyte loss or in severe salt depletion –
Adults: 400 ml of 3% or 5% solution only with frequent electrolyte determination and only if given slow I.V.; with 0.45% solution: 3% to 8% of body weight, according to deficiencies, over 18 to 24 hours; with 0.9% solution: 2% to 6% of body weight, according to deficiencies, over 18 to 24 hours.
Management of "heat cramp" caused by excessive perspiration –
Adults: 1 g P.O. with every glass of water.

ADVERSE REACTIONS
Common reactions are in italics; life-threatening reactions are in bold italics.
CV: aggravation of congestive heart failure; edema and ***pulmonary edema*** if too much given or given too rapidly.
Metabolic: hypernatremia and aggravation of existing acidosis with excessive infusion; serious electrolyte disturbance, loss of potassium.

INTERACTIONS
None significant.

NURSING CONSIDERATIONS
- *Use cautiously* in congestive heart failure, circulatory insufficiency, renal dysfunction, and hypoproteinemia.
- **I.V. use:** Infuse 3% and 5% solutions very slowly and with caution to avoid pulmonary edema. Use only for critical situations. Observe patient continually.
- Concentrates available for addition to parenteral nutrient solutions. Don't confuse these small volumes of parenterals with normal saline injection. *Read label carefully.*
- Monitor serum electrolytes.

62

Acidifier and alkalinizers

ammonium chloride
sodium bicarbonate
sodium lactate
tromethamine

COMBINATION PRODUCTS
None.

ammonium chloride◊

Pregnancy Risk Category: B

HOW SUPPLIED
Tablets: 500 mg◊
Tablets (enteric-coated): 500 mg◊, 1,000 mg◊
Injection: 2.14% (0.4 mEq/ml), 26.75% (5 mEq/ml)

MECHANISM OF ACTION
Increases free hydrogen ion (H^+) concentration. Also acts as an expectorant by causing reflex stimulation of bronchial mucous glands.

INDICATIONS & DOSAGE
Metabolic alkalosis; chloride replacement –
Adults and children: I.V. dose (in mEq) is equal to the serum chloride deficit (in mEq/ml) multiplied by the extracellular fluid volume (estimated as 20% of the body weight in kilograms). One-half the calculated volume should be given, then patient should be reassessed.
As an acidifying agent –
Adults: 4 to 12 g P.O. daily in divided doses.
Children: 75 mg/kg P.O. daily in four divided doses.
As expectorant –
Adults: 250 to 500 mg P.O. q 2 to 4 hours.

ADVERSE REACTIONS
Common reactions are in italics; life-threatening reactions are in bold italics.

Adverse reactions usually result from ammonia toxicity or too-rapid I.V. administration.
CNS: headache, confusion, progressive drowsiness, excitement alternating with ***coma,*** hyperventilation, ***calcium-deficient tetany, twitching,*** hyperreflexia, EEG abnormalities.
CV: bradycardia.
GI: (with oral dose) *gastric irritation, nausea, vomiting,* thirst, anorexia, retching.
GU: glycosuria.
Metabolic: ***acidosis, hyperchloremia, hypokalemia,*** hyperglycemia.
Skin: rash, pallor.
Local: pain at injection site.
Other: irregular respirations with periods of apnea.

INTERACTIONS
Spironolactone: systemic acidosis. Use together cautiously.

NURSING CONSIDERATIONS
- *Contraindicated* in severe hepatic or renal dysfunction.
- *Use cautiously* in pulmonary insufficiency or cardiac edema and in infants.
- **I.V. use:** Dilute concentrated form (26.75%) before administration. Add 100 to 200 mEq (20 to 40 ml of the 26.75% solution) to 500 or 1,000 ml of normal saline injection. Administer via infusion pump not exceeding 5 ml/min in adults.
- Give oral form after meals to decrease GI adverse reactions. Enteric-coated tablets may also minimize GI symptoms but are absorbed erratically.
- Do not administer drug with milk or

other alkaline solutions because they are not compatible.
- Pain of I.V. injection may be lessened by decreasing infusion rate.
- Determine CO_2 combining power and serum electrolytes before and during therapy to prevent acidosis.
- Monitor urine pH and output. Diuresis is normal for first 2 days.
- Monitor rate and depth of respirations frequently.
- When using as an expectorant, give with full glass of water.

sodium bicarbonate◇

Pregnancy Risk Category: C

HOW SUPPLIED

Tablets: 300 mg◇, 325 mg◇, 600 mg◇, 650 mg◇
Injection: 4% (2.4 mEq/5 ml), 4.2% (5 mEq/10 ml), 5% (297.5 mEq/500 ml), 7.5% (8.92 mEq/10 ml and 44.6 mEq/50 ml), 8.4% (10 mEq/10 ml and 50 mEq/50 ml)

MECHANISM OF ACTION

Restores buffering capacity of the body and neutralizes excess acid.

INDICATIONS & DOSAGE

Cardiac arrest –
Adults and children: as a 7.5% or 8.4% solution, 1 mEq/kg I.V. followed by 0.5 mEq/kg I.V. every 10 minutes depending on blood gases. Further dosages based on blood gases. If blood gases unavailable, use 0.5 mEq/kg I.V. q 10 minutes until spontaneous circulation returns.
Infants up to 2 years: 4.2% solution, I.V. infusion. Rate not to exceed 8 mEq/kg daily.
Metabolic acidosis –
Adults and children: dosage depends on blood CO_2 content, pH, and patient's clinical condition. Generally, 2 to 5 mEq/kg I.V. infused over 4- to 8-hour period.
Systemic or urinary alkalinization –
Adults: 325 mg to 2 g P.O. q.i.d.
Children: 12 to 120 mg/kg P.O. daily.
Antacid –
Adults: 300 mg to 2 g P.O. chewed and taken with glass of water.

ADVERSE REACTIONS

Common reactions are in italics; life-threatening reactions are in bold italics.
GI: gastric distention, belching, flatulence.
GU: renal calculi or crystals.
Metabolic: (with overdose) ***alkalosis,*** hypernatremia, ***hyperkalemia,*** hyperosmolarity.

INTERACTIONS

I.V. solutions containing calcium: precipitate may form. Don't mix together. Take care to flush I.V. lines adequately.

NURSING CONSIDERATIONS

- No contraindications for use in life-threatening emergencies. *Contraindicated* in hypertension, in patients with tendency toward edema, in patients who are losing chlorides by vomiting or from continuous GI suction, in patients receiving diuretics known to produce hypochloremic alkalosis, and in patients on sodium-restricted diets or with renal disease.
- **I.V. use:** May be added to other I.V. fluids. Because sodium bicarbonate inactivates such catecholamines as norepinephrine and dopamine, do not mix with I.V. solutions of these agents.
- To avoid risk of alkalosis, determine blood pH, PaO_2, $PaCO_2$, and serum electrolytes. Keep doctor informed of serum laboratory results.
- Tell patient not to take with milk. May cause hypercalcemia, alkalosis, and possibly renal calculi.
- Discourage use as an antacid. Offer a nonabsorbable alternative antacid if it is to be used repeatedly.

- May cause enteric-coated drugs to be prematurely released in the stomach.
- Sodium bicarbonate is not routinely recommended for use in cardiac arrest because it may produce a paradoxical acidosis from CO_2 production. It should not be routinely administered during the early stages of resuscitation unless preexisting acidosis is clearly present. May be used at team leader's discretion after such interventions as defibrillation, cardiac compression, and administration of first-line drugs.
- If sodium bicarbonate is being used to produce an alkaline urine, monitor urine pH q 4 to 6 hours (should be >7.0).

sodium lactate

Pregnancy Risk Category: C

HOW SUPPLIED

Injection: ⅙ molar solution
Injection (for preparations of I.V. admixtures): 2.5 mEq/ml

MECHANISM OF ACTION

Metabolized to sodium bicarbonate. Then produces buffering effect.

INDICATIONS & DOSAGE

Alkalinize urine –
Adults: 30 ml of ⅙ molar solution/kg of body weight I.V. given in divided doses over 24 hours.
Metabolic acidosis –
Adults: usually given as $^1/_6$ molar injection (167 mEq lactate/liter I.V.). Dosage depends on degree of bicarbonate deficit.

ADVERSE REACTIONS

Common reactions are in italics; life-threatening reactions are in bold italics.
Metabolic: (with overdose) ***alkalosis,*** hypernatremia, hyperosmolarity.

INTERACTIONS

None significant.

NURSING CONSIDERATIONS

- *Contraindicated* in severe hepatic and renal disease, respiratory alkalosis, or acidosis associated with congenital heart disease with persistent cyanosis.
- Sodium lactate should not be used in patients with severe acidosis because rapid replacement of serum bicarbonate is required. Sodium lactate is slowly metabolized to bicarbonate by the liver; serum bicarbonate levels may not rise for 1 to 2 hours after administration.
- Monitor serum electrolytes to avoid alkalosis.

tromethamine

Tham

Pregnancy Risk Category: C

HOW SUPPLIED

Injection: 18 g/500 ml

MECHANISM OF ACTION

Combines with hydrogen ions and associated acid anions; the resulting salts are excreted.

INDICATIONS & DOSAGE

Metabolic acidosis (associated with cardiac bypass surgery or with cardiac arrest) –
Adults: dosage depends on bicarbonate deficit. Calculate as follows: ml of 0.3 M tromethamine solution required = weight in kg × bicarbonate deficit (mEq/liter). Additional therapy based on serial determinations of existing bicarbonate deficit.
Children: calculate dosage as above. Give slowly over 3 to 6 hours. Additional therapy based on degree of acidosis. Total 24-hour dosage should not exceed 33 to 40 ml/kg.

ADVERSE REACTIONS

Common reactions are in italics; life-threatening reactions are in bold italics.
CNS: ***respiratory depression.***

Metabolic: hypoglycemia, ***hyperkalemia*** (with decreased urine output).
Local: venospasm; I.V. thrombosis; inflammation, necrosis, and sloughing if extravasation occurs.

INTERACTIONS
None significant.

NURSING CONSIDERATIONS
- *Contraindicated* in anuria, uremia, chronic respiratory acidosis, or pregnancy (except in acute, life-threatening situations).
- *Use cautiously* in renal disease and poor urine output. Monitor ECG and serum potassium in these patients.
- To prevent blood pH from rising above normal, adjust dosage carefully.
- **I.V. use:** Give slowly through large needle (18G to 20G) into largest antecubital vein or by indwelling I.V. catheter.
- Before, during, and after therapy make the following determinations: blood pH; carbon dioxide tension; bicarbonate, glucose, and electrolyte levels.
- When giving drug to patient with associated respiratory acidosis, mechanical ventilation should be readily available.
- Except in life-threatening situations, do not use longer than 1 day.
- If extravasation occurs, infiltrate area with 1% procaine and hyaluronidase 150 units; may reduce vasospasm and dilute remaining drug in local area.

63

Hematinics

ferrous fumarate
ferrous gluconate
ferrous sulfate
iron dextran

COMBINATION PRODUCTS

FERMALOX◊: ferrous sulfate 200 mg, and magnesium hydroxide and dried aluminum hydroxide gel 200 mg.
FEROCYL◊: iron (as fumarate) 50 mg and docusate sodium 100 mg.
FERRO-SEQUELS◊: iron (as fumarate) 50 mg and docusate sodium 100 mg.
SIMRON◊: iron (as gluconate) 10 mg and polysorbate 20, 400 mg.

ferrous fumarate

Eldofe◊, Feostat◊, Ferranol◊, Fersamal†, Fumasorb◊, Fumerin◊, Hemocyte◊, Ircon◊, Maniron◊, Novofumar†, Palafer†, Span-FF◊
Pregnancy Risk Category: A

HOW SUPPLIED

Tablets◊: 63 mg, 195 mg, 200 mg, 324 mg, 325 mg
Tablets (chewable): 100 mg◊
Capsules (controlled-release): 325 mg◊
Oral suspension: 100 mg/5 ml◊
Drops: 45 mg/0.6 ml◊

MECHANISM OF ACTION

Provides elemental iron, an essential component in the formation of hemoglobin. Each 100 mg of ferrous fumarate provides 33 mg of elemental iron.

INDICATIONS & DOSAGE

Iron deficiency–
Adults: 200 mg P.O. t.i.d. or q.i.d.
Children: 3 mg/kg P.O. t.i.d., increased to 6 mg/kg P.O. t.i.d. as needed and tolerated.

ADVERSE REACTIONS

Common reactions are in italics; life-threatening reactions are in bold italics.
GI: *nausea,* vomiting, *constipation, black stools.*
Other: elixir may stain teeth.

INTERACTIONS

Antacids, levodopa, penicillamine, quinolones, tetracycline, vitamin E: decreased iron absorption. Separate doses by 2 to 4 hours.
Chloramphenicol: watch for delayed response to iron therapy.
Vitamin C: concurrent administration may increase iron absorption. Beneficial drug interaction.

NURSING CONSIDERATIONS

- *Contraindicated* in hemosiderosis; also contraindicated in patients with hemochromatosis and hemolytic anemia unless an iron deficiency anemia is also present.
- *Use cautiously* in peptic ulcer, regional enteritis, and ulcerative colitis. Also use cautiously on long-term basis.
- GI upset related to dose. Between-meal dosing preferable, but can be given with some foods although absorption may be decreased. Enteric-coated products reduce GI upset but also reduce amount of iron absorbed.
- Iron is toxic; parents should be aware of iron poisoning in children. As few as 3 or 4 tablets can cause serious poisoning in children.
- Tablets may be given with juice or water, but not in milk or antacids. Give with orange juice to promote iron absorption.
- To avoid staining teeth, give elixir iron preparations with straw.
- Check for constipation; record color

and amount of stool. Teach dietary measures for preventing constipation.

- Oral iron may turn stools black. This unabsorbed iron is harmless; however, it could mask the presence of melena.
- Monitor hemoglobin and reticulocyte counts during therapy.
- Do not crush or chew sustained-release iron preparations.
- If the patient misses a dose, tell him to take it as soon as he remembers, unless it's time for the next dose. Do not double-dose.
- Combination products – Simron, Ferro-Sequels, Ferocyl, Fer-Regules – contain stool softeners to help prevent constipation. Fermalox contains antacids to help relieve GI upset, if present; don't use this product unless absolutely necessary because of decreased iron absorption. Usually, combination iron products should be avoided.
- Certain foods may impair oral iron absorption, including yogurt, cheese, eggs, milk, whole-grain breads and cereals, tea, and coffee.

ferrous gluconate

Fergon*◊, Ferralet◊, Fertinic†, Novoferrogluc†

Pregnancy Risk Category: A

HOW SUPPLIED

Tablets: 300 mg◊, 320 mg◊, 325 mg◊ (320-mg tablet contains 37 mg Fe^{+})
Capsules: 86 mg◊, 325 mg◊, 435 mg◊
Elixir: 300 mg/5 ml (contains 35 mg Fe^{+})*◊

MECHANISM OF ACTION

Provides elemental iron, an essential component in the formation of hemoglobin. Each 100 mg of ferrous gluconate provides 11.6 mg of elemental iron.

INDICATIONS & DOSAGE

Iron deficiency –
Adults: 300 to 325 mg P.O. q.i.d., increased to 650 mg q.i.d. as needed and tolerated.
Children 2 years or older: 8 mg/kg P.O. t.i.d., increased to 16 mg P.O. t.i.d. as needed and tolerated.

ADVERSE REACTIONS

Common reactions are in italics; life-threatening reactions are in bold italics.
GI: *nausea,* vomiting, *constipation, black stools.*
Other: elixir may stain teeth.

INTERACTIONS

Antacids, levodopa, penicillamine, quinolones, tetracycline, vitamin E: decreased iron absorption. Separate doses if possible.
Chloramphenicol: watch for delayed response to iron therapy.
Vitamin C: may increase iron absorption. Beneficial drug interaction.

NURSING CONSIDERATIONS

- *Contraindicated* in peptic ulcer, regional enteritis, ulcerative colitis, hemosiderosis, and hemochromatosis. Also contraindicated in patients with a hemolytic anemia unless an iron deficiency anemia is also present.
- *Use cautiously* on long-term basis.
- GI upset related to dose. Between-meal dosing preferable, but can be given with some foods although absorption may be decreased. Enteric-coated products reduce GI upset but also reduce amount of iron absorbed.
- Tell patient to continue regular dosing schedule if he misses a dose. Patient shouldn't double the dose.
- Iron is toxic; parents should be aware of iron poisoning in children. As few as 3 or 4 tablets can cause serious poisoning in children.
- Dilute liquid preparations in juice (preferably orange juice) or water, but not in milk or antacids. Give tablets

*Liquid form contains alcohol. **May contain tartrazine.

with orange juice to promote absorption.
• To avoid staining teeth, give elixir iron preparations with straw; patient may take with water or fruit juice.
• Check for constipation; record color and amount of stool. Teach dietary measures for preventing constipation.
• Oral iron may turn stools black. This unabsorbed iron is harmless; however, it could mask melena.
• Monitor hemoglobin and reticulocyte counts during therapy.
• If the patient misses a dose, tell him to take it as soon as he remembers, unless it is time for the next dose. Do not double-dose.
• Certain foods may impair oral iron absorption, including yogurt, cheese, eggs, milk, whole-grain breads and cereals, tea, and coffee.

ferrous sulfate

Feosol*◇, Fer-In-Sol*◇, Feritard‡, Fero-Grad†, Fero-Gradumet◇, Ferolix*◇, Ferospace◇, Ferralyn◇, Fespan‡, Irospan◇, Mol-Iron*◇, Novoferrosulfa†, Slow-Fe, Telefon◇

Pregnancy Risk Category: A

HOW SUPPLIED

Ferrous sulfate is 20% elemental iron; dried and powdered (exsiccated), it is about 32% elemental iron.
Tablets: 195 mg◇, 250 mg◇, 300 mg◇, 325 mg◇; 200 mg (exsiccated)◇
Tablets (extended-release): 160 mg (exsiccated)◇, 525 mg
Capsules: 150 mg◇, 159 mg (exsiccated), 190 mg (exsiccated)◇, 225 mg◇, 250 mg◇, 250 mg (exsiccated), 390 mg◇
Capsules (extended-release): 150 mg◇, 167 mg (exsiccated)◇, 525 mg◇
Elixir: 220 mg/5 ml*◇
Liquid: 75 mg/0.6 ml◇, 125 mg/ml
Syrup: 90 mg/5 ml◇

MECHANISM OF ACTION

Provides elemental iron, an essential component in the formation of hemoglobin.

INDICATIONS & DOSAGE

Iron deficiency –
Adults: 325 mg P.O. t.i.d. or q.i.d. Alternatively, give 1 delayed release capsule (160 or 525 mg) P.O. twice daily.
Children: 4 to 6 mg/kg daily in 3 divided doses.
Prophylaxis for iron deficiency anemia –
Pregnant women: 150 mg P.O. daily during the last 2 trimesters.
Premature or undernourished infants: 1 to 2 mg/kg P.O. daily (as elemental iron) in divided doses.

ADVERSE REACTIONS

Common reactions are in italics; life-threatening reactions are in bold italics.
GI: *nausea,* vomiting, *constipation, black stools.*
Other: elixir may stain teeth.

INTERACTIONS

Antacids, levodopa, penicillamine, quinolones, tetracycline, vitamin E: decreased iron absorption. Separate doses if possible.
Chloramphenicol: watch for delayed response to iron therapy.
Vitamin C: may increase iron absorption. Beneficial drug interaction.

NURSING CONSIDERATIONS

• *Contraindicated* in hemosiderosis and hemochromatosis. Also contraindicated in patients with hemolytic anemia unless iron deficiency anemia is also present.
• *Use cautiously* in peptic ulcer, ulcerative colitis, and regional enteritis. Also use cautiously on long-term basis.
• GI upset related to dose. Between-meal dosing preferable, but can be given with some foods although ab-

sorption may be decreased. Enteric-coated products reduce GI upset but also reduce amount of iron absorbed.

- Tell patient to continue regular dosing schedule if he misses a dose. Patient shouldn't double the dose.
- Iron is toxic; parents should be aware of potential for iron poisoning in children. As few as 3 or 4 tablets can cause serious poisoning in children.
- Dilute liquid preparations in juice or water, but not in milk or antacids. Dilute liquids in orange juice; give tablets with orange juice to promote iron absorption.
- To avoid staining teeth, give elixir iron preparations with straw.
- Check for constipation; record color and amount of stool. Teach dietary measures for preventing constipation.
- Oral iron may turn stools black. This unabsorbed iron is harmless; however, it could mask melena.
- Monitor hemoglobin and reticulocyte counts during therapy.
- Do not crush or chew sustained-release preparations.
- If the patient misses a dose, tell him to take it as soon as he remembers, unless it is almost time for the next dose. Do not double-dose.
- Certain foods may impair oral iron absorption, including yogurt, cheese, eggs, milk, whole grain breads and cereals, coffee, and tea.

iron dextran

Hydextran, Imferon, K-FeRON

Pregnancy Risk Category: C

HOW SUPPLIED

Injection: 50 mg elemental iron/ml

MECHANISM OF ACTION

Provides elemental iron, an essential component in the formation of hemoglobin; 1 ml iron dextran provides 50 mg elemental iron.

INDICATIONS & DOSAGE

Iron deficiency anemia –

Adults: I.M. or I.V. injections of iron are advisable only for patients for whom oral administration is impossible or ineffective. Test dose (0.5 ml) required before administration.

I.M. (by Z-track): inject 0.5 ml test dose. If no reactions next daily dose should ordinarily not exceed 0.5 ml (25 mg) for infants under 5 kg; 1 ml (50 mg) for children under 9 kg; 2 ml (100 mg) for patients under 50 kg; 5 ml (250 mg) for patients over 50 kg.

I.V. push: inject 0.5 ml test dose. If no reaction, within 2 to 3 days the dosage may be raised to 2 ml daily I.V., 1 ml/minute undiluted and infused slowly until total dose is achieved. No single dose should exceed 100 mg.

I.V. infusion: dosages are expressed in terms of elemental iron. Dilute in 250 to 1,000 ml of normal saline solution; dextrose increases local vein irritation. Infuse test dose of 25 mg slowly over 5 minutes. If no reaction occurs in 5 minutes, infusion may be started. Infuse total dose slowly over approximately 6 to 12 hours.

ADVERSE REACTIONS

Common reactions are in italics; life-threatening reactions are in bold italics.

CNS: headache, transitory paresthesias, arthralgia, myalgia, dizziness, malaise, syncope.

CV: *hypotensive reaction, peripheral vascular flushing with overly rapid I.V. administration, tachycardia.*

GI: nausea, vomiting, metallic taste, transient loss of taste perception.

Local: *soreness and inflammation at injection site (I.M.); brown skin discoloration at injection site (I.M.); local phlebitis at injection site (I.V.),* sterile abscess, necrosis, atrophy, fibrosis.

Skin: rash, urticaria.

Other: ***anaphylaxis, bronchospasm,*** delayed sensitivity reactions.

INTERACTIONS
None significant.

NURSING CONSIDERATIONS

- *Contraindicated* in all anemias except iron deficiency anemia.
- *Use with extreme caution* in patients with impaired hepatic function or rheumatoid arthritis and in infants.
- Patients with certain inflammatory diseases (such as rheumatoid arthritis or ankylosing spondylitis) may be at higher risk for certain delayed reactions.
- Monitor vital signs for drug reaction. Reactions are varied, ranging from pain, inflammation, and myalgia to hypotension, shock, and death.
- Inject deeply into upper outer quadrant of buttock – never into arm or other exposed area – with a 2- to 3-inch, 19G or 20G needle. Use Z-track technique to avoid leakage into subcutaneous tissue and staining of skin.
- Skin staining may be minimized by using a separate needle to withdraw the drug from its container.
- Monitor hemoglobin concentration, hematocrit, and reticulocyte count.
- **I.V. use:** Check hospital policy before administering I.V. Some do not permit infusion method because its safety is controversial.
- Use I.V. in these situations: insufficient muscle mass for deep intramuscular injection; impaired absorption from muscle due to stasis or edema; possibility of uncontrolled intramuscular bleeding from trauma (as may occur in hemophilia); and with massive and prolonged parenteral therapy (as may be necessary in cases of chronic substantial blood loss).
- Upon completion of I.V. iron dextran infusion, flush the vein with 10 ml of 0.9% sodium chloride solution. Patient should rest 15 to 30 minutes after I.V. administration.
- Not removed by hemodialysis.

Anticoagulants

dicumarol
heparin calcium
heparin sodium
warfarin sodium

COMBINATION PRODUCTS
None.

dicumarol (bishydroxycoumarin)

Pregnancy Risk Category: D

HOW SUPPLIED
Tablets: 25 mg, 50 mg

MECHANISM OF ACTION
Inhibits vitamin K-dependent activation of clotting factors II, VII, IX, and X, which are formed in the liver.

INDICATIONS & DOSAGE
Prophylaxis and treatment of pulmonary emboli; prevention and treatment of emboli associated with deep vein thrombosis, myocardial infarction, rheumatic heart disease with heart valve damage, prosthetic heart valves, atrial arrhythmias –
Adults: 200 to 300 mg P.O. on first day, 25 to 200 mg P.O. daily thereafter, based on prothrombin times.

ADVERSE REACTIONS
Common reactions are in italics; life-threatening reactions are in bold italics.
Blood: ***hemorrhage with excessive dosage,*** eosinophilia, leukopenia, ***agranulocytosis.***
GI: anorexia, nausea, vomiting, cramps, *diarrhea,* mouth ulcers.
GU: hematuria.
Skin: dermatitis, urticaria, necrosis, gangrene, alopecia, *rash.*
Other: *fever,* hepatitis, jaundice.

INTERACTIONS
Acetaminophen: increased bleeding possible with chronic (greater than 2 weeks) therapy with acetaminophen. Monitor very carefully.
Allopurinol, amiodarone, cephalosporins, chloramphenicol, ciprofloxacin, clofibrate, diflunisal, thyroid drugs, heparin, anabolic steroids, cimetidine, disulfiram, glucagon, methimazole, metronidazole, propylthiouracil, sulindac, sulfinpyrazone, sulfonamides, tricyclic antidepressants, vitamin E: increased prothrombin time. Monitor patient carefully for bleeding. Consider anticoagulant dosage reduction.
Barbiturates: inhibition of hypoprothrombinemic effect of anticoagulants. If barbiturates are withdrawn, reduce anticoagulant dosage; inhibition may last weeks after barbiturate is withdrawn, but fatal hemorrhage can occur when inhibiting effect disappears.
Cholestyramine: decreased response when administered too close together. Administer 6 hours after oral anticoagulants.
Glutethimide, chloral hydrate, sulfinpyrazone, triclofos sodium: increased or decreased prothrombin time. Avoid use if possible, or monitor patient carefully.
Griseofulvin, ethchlorvynol, carbamazepine, rifampin: decreased prothrombin time with reduced anticoagulant effect. Monitor patient carefully.
Hydantoins: increased serum levels of hydantoin. Monitor closely.
Indomethacin, mefenamic acid, oxyphenbutazone, phenylbutazone, salicylates: increased prothrombin time; ulcerogenic effects. Don't use together.

Sulfonylureas (oral hypoglycemic agents): increased hypoglycemic response. Monitor blood glucose levels.

NURSING CONSIDERATIONS

- *Contraindicated* in hemophilia, thrombocytopenic purpura, polycythemia vera, leukemia with pronounced bleeding tendency, open wounds or ulcers, GI, GU, or respiratory tract ulcers, cerebrovascular hemorrhage, aneurysms, pericarditis, pericardial effusions, vasculitis, diverticulitis, pregnancy, impaired hepatic or renal function, severe hypertension, acute nephritis, subacute bacterial endocarditis. Also contraindicated in patients with recent eye, CNS, or spinal cord surgery.
- *Use with extreme caution* (if at all) in psychiatric patients, debilitated patients, or cachectic patients. Also use cautiously in breast-feeding women. Monitor infants for evidence of easy bruising or bleeding.
- *Use cautiously* during menses, during use of any drainage tube, and in any patient in whom slight bleeding is dangerous.
- Use caution when adding or stopping any drug for patient receiving anticoagulants. May change the clotting status and result in hemorrhage.
- Fever and skin rash signal severe adverse reactions. Withhold drug and call doctor.
- Give drug at same time daily. Stress importance of complying with recommended dosage and keeping follow-up appointments. Patient should carry a card that identifies him as a potential bleeder.
- Regularly inspect patient for bleeding gums, bruises on arms or legs, petechiae, nosebleeds, melena, tarry stools, hematuria, hematemesis. Tell patient and family to watch for these signs and notify doctor immediately.
- Warn patient to avoid OTC products containing aspirin, other salicylates, or drugs that may interact with dicumarol.
- **I.V. use:** Because onset of action is delayed, heparin sodium is often given during first few days of treatment. When heparin is being given simultaneously, don't draw blood for prothrombin time within 5 hours of intermittent I.V. heparin administration. However, prothrombin time may be drawn at any time during continuous heparin infusion.
- Dose given depends on prothrombin time (PT). Doctors usually try to maintain PT at 1.5 to 2 times normal. PT values depend on procedure and reagents used in individual laboratory.
- Tell patient to notify doctor if menses is heavier than usual.
- Tell patient to use electric razor when shaving to avoid scratching skin and to brush teeth with a soft toothbrush.
- May turn alkaline urine red-orange.
- Duration of action 2 to 6 days.
- Light to moderate alcohol intake does not significantly affect prothrombin times.
- Tell patient to eat a consistent amount of leafy green vegetables every day. These contain vitamin K, and eating different amounts daily may alter anticoagulant effect.

heparin calcium

Calcilean†, Calciparine, Caprin‡, Uniparin-Ca‡

heparin sodium

Hepalean†, Heparin Lock Flush Solution (Tubex), Hep Lock, Liquaemin Sodium, Uniparin‡

Pregnancy Risk Category: C

HOW SUPPLIED

Products are derived from beef lung or porcine intestinal mucosa.

calcium
Ampule: 12,500 units/0.5 ml; 20,000 units/0.8 ml
Syringe: 5,000 units/0.2 ml
sodium
Carpuject: 5,000 units/ml
Disposable syringes: 1,000 units/ml, 2,500 units/ml, 5,000 units/ml, 7,500 units/ml, 10,000 units/ml, 15,000 units/ml, 20,000 units/ml, 40,000 units/ml
Premixed I.V. solutions: 1,000 units in 500 ml normal saline solution; 2,000 units in 1,000 ml normal saline solution; 12,500 units in 250 ml 0.45% saline solution; 25,000 units in 250 ml 0.45% saline solution; 25,000 units in 500 ml 0.45% saline solution; 10,000 units in 100 ml dextrose 5% in water (D_5W); 12,500 units in 250 ml D_5W; 25,000 units in 250 ml D_5W; 25,000 units in 500 ml D_5W; 20,000 units in 500 ml D_5W
Unit-dose ampules: 1,000 units/ml, 5,000 units/ml, 10,000 units/ml
Vials: 1,000 units/ml, 2,500 units/ml, 5,000 units/ml, 7,500 units/ml, 10,000 units/ml, 15,000 units/ml, 20,000 units/ml, 40,000 units/ml
heparin sodium flush
Disposable syringes: 10 units/ml, 100 units/ml
Vials: 10 units/ml, 100 units/ml

MECHANISM OF ACTION

Accelerates formation of an antithrombin III-thrombin complex. It inactivates thrombin and prevents conversion of fibrinogen to fibrin.

INDICATIONS & DOSAGE

Treatment of deep vein thrombosis, myocardial infarction –
Adults: initially, 5,000 to 7,500 units I.V. push, then adjusted according to PTT and given I.V. q 4 hours (usually 4,000 to 5,000 units); or 5,000 to 7,500 units I.V. bolus, then 1,000 units/hour by I.V. infusion pump. Wait 8 hours following bolus dose, and adjust hourly rate according to PTT.
Treatment of pulmonary embolism; diagnosis and treatment of consumptive coagulopathy (such as disseminated intravascular coagulation) –
Adults: initially, 7,500 to 10,000 units I.V. push, then adjusted according to PTT and given I.V. q 4 hours (usually 4,000 to 5,000 units); or 7,500 to 10,000 units I.V. bolus, then 1,000 units hourly by I.V. infusion pump. Wait 8 hours following bolus dose, and adjust hourly rate according to PTT.
Prophylaxis of embolism, venous thrombosis, pulmonary embolism, atrial fibrillation with embolism; prophylaxis of postoperative deep vein thrombosis –
Adults: 5,000 units S.C. q 12 hours. In surgical patients, give first dose 2 hours before procedure; follow with 5,000 units S.C. q 8 to 12 hours for 5 to 7 days or until patient is fully ambulatory.
Open heart surgery –
Adults: (total body perfusion) 150 to 300 units/kg continuous I.V infusion.
Treatment of pulmonary emboli; prevention and treatment of deep vein thrombosis –
Children: initially, 50 units/kg I.V. drip. Maintenance dose is 100 units/kg I.V. drip q 4 hours. Constant infusion: 20,000 units/m² daily. Dosages adjusted according to PTT.
As an I.V. flush to maintain patency of I.V. indwelling catheters –
Adults: 10 to 100 units as an I.V. flush. Use a sufficient volume of solution to fill the device. Not intended for therapeutic use.

Heparin dosing is highly individualized, depending upon disease state, age, renal and hepatic status.

ADVERSE REACTIONS

Common reactions are in italics; life-threatening reactions are in bold italics.
Blood: ***hemorrhage with excessive***

*Liquid form contains alcohol. **May contain tartrazine.

dosage, *overly prolonged clotting time,* ***thrombocytopenia.***
Local: irritation, mild pain, hematoma, ulceration, cutaneous or subcutaneous necrosis.
Other: ***"white clot" syndrome,*** hypersensitivity reactions including chills, fever, pruritus, rhinitis, burning of feet, conjunctivitis, lacrimation, arthralgia, urticaria.

INTERACTIONS

Anticoagulants, oral: additive anticoagulation. Monitor prothrombin time and partial thromboplastin time.
Salicylates: increased anticoagulant effect. Don't use together.
Thrombolytics: increased risk of hemorrhage. Monitor closely.

NURSING CONSIDERATIONS

- *Contraindicated* in patients hypersensitive to the drug. Conditionally contraindicated in active bleeding; blood dyscrasias; or bleeding tendencies such as hemophilia, thrombocytopenia, or hepatic disease with hypoprothrombinemia; suspected intracranial hemorrhage; suppurative thrombophlebitis; inaccessible ulcerative lesions (especially of GI tract); open ulcerative wounds; extensive denudation of skin; ascorbic acid deficiency and other conditions causing increased capillary permeability; during or after brain, eye, or spinal cord surgery; during spinal tap or spinal anesthesia; during continuous tube drainage of stomach or small intestine; in subacute bacterial endocarditis; shock; advanced renal disease; threatened abortion; severe hypertension. Although the use of heparin is clearly hazardous in these conditions, a decision to use it depends on the comparative risk in failure to treat the coexisting thromboembolic disorder.
- *Use cautiously* during menses; in mild hepatic or renal disease; alcoholism; in patients in occupations with the risk of physical injury; immediately postpartum; and in patients with history of allergies, asthma, or GI ulcers.
- When patient requires anticoagulation during pregnancy, most clinicians use heparin.
- Monitor platelet counts regularly. Thrombocytopenia caused by heparin may be associated with a type of arterial thrombosis known as "white clot" syndrome.
- Measure partial thromboplastin time (PTT) carefully and regularly. Anticoagulation present when PTT values are 1.5 to 2 times control values.
- Drug requirements are higher in early phases of thrombogenic diseases and febrile states; lower when patient becomes stabilized.
- Regularly inspect patient for bleeding gums, bruises on arms or legs, petechiae, nosebleeds, melena, tarry stools, hematuria, hematemesis. Tell patient and family to watch for these signs and notify doctor immediately.
- Tell patient to avoid OTC medications containing aspirin, other salicylates, or drugs that may interact with heparin.
- Heparin comes in various concentrations. Check order and vial carefully.
- Low-dose injections given sequentially between iliac crests in lower abdomen deep into subcutaneous fat. Inject drug slowly subcutaneously into fat pad. Leave needle in place for 10 seconds after injection; then withdraw needle. Alternate site every 12 hours – right for a.m., left for p.m.
- Don't massage after subcutaneous injection. Watch for signs of bleeding at injection site. Rotate sites and keep accurate record.
- **I.V. use:** I.V. administration preferred because of long-term effect and irregular absorption when given subcutaneously. Whenever possible, administer I.V. heparin using infusion pump to provide maximum safety.

Check constant I.V. infusions regularly, even when pumps are in good working order, to prevent overdosage or underdosage. Place notice above patient's bed to inform I.V. team or lab personnel to apply pressure dressings after taking blood.
• During intermittent I.V. therapy, always draw blood ½ hour before next scheduled dose to avoid falsely elevated PTT.
• Give on time; do not skip a dose or "catch up" with an I.V. containing heparin. If I.V. is out, restart it as soon as possible, and reschedule bolus dose immediately.
• Concentrated heparin solutions (greater than 100 units/ml) can irritate blood vessels.
• I.M. administration not recommended.
• Avoid excessive I.M. injections of other drugs to prevent or minimize hematomas. If possible, don't give I.M. injections at all.
• Elderly patients should usually start at lower doses.
• Blood for PTT can be drawn any time after 8 hours of initiation of continuous I.V. heparin therapy. Never draw blood for PTT from the I.V. tubing of the heparin infusion, or from vein of infusion. Falsely elevated PTT will result. Always draw blood from opposite arm.
• Never piggyback other drugs into an infusion line while heparin infusion is running. Many antibiotics and other drugs inactivate heparin. Never mix any drug with heparin in syringe when bolus therapy is used.
• Abrupt withdrawal may cause increased coagulability. Usually, heparin therapy is followed by oral anticoagulants for prophylaxis.
• Protamine sulfate, a heparin antagonist, may be used to treat severe heparin calcium or heparin sodium overdose. Dosage is based on the dose of heparin, its route of administration, and the time elapsed since it was given. As a general rule, give 1 to 1.5 units of protamine/100 units of heparin administered if only a few minutes have elapsed. If 30 to 60 minutes have elapsed, give 0.5 to 0.75 mg protamine/100 units heparin; if 2 hours or more have elapsed, give 0.25 to 0.375 mg protamine/100 units heparin.

warfarin sodium

Coumadin, Panwarfin**, Warfilone Sodium†

Pregnancy Risk Category: D

HOW SUPPLIED

Tablets: 1 mg, 2 mg, 2.5 mg, 5 mg, 7.5 mg, 10 mg
Injection: 50 mg/vial

MECHANISM OF ACTION

Inhibits vitamin K-dependent activation of clotting factors II, VII, IX, and X, which are formed in the liver.

INDICATIONS & DOSAGE

Prophylaxis and treatment of pulmonary emboli; prevention and treatment of emboli associated with deep vein thrombosis, myocardial infarction, rheumatic heart disease with heart valve damage, prosthetic heart valves, atrial arrhythmias –
Adults: 10 to 15 mg P.O. for 3 days, then dosage based on daily prothrombin (PT) times. Usual maintenance dosage is 2 to 10 mg P.O. daily. Alternative regimen: initially, 40 to 60 mg P.O. as a single dose, or 20 to 30 mg for elderly patients; then 2 to 10 mg daily based on PT determinations.

Warfarin sodium also available for I.V. use (50 mg/vial). Reconstitute with sterile water for injection. I.V. form rarely used and may be in periodic short supply.

ADVERSE REACTIONS

Common reactions are in italics; life-threatening reactions are in bold italics.

*Liquid form contains alcohol. **May contain tartrazine.

Blood: ***hemorrhage with excessive dosage,*** eosinophilia, leukopenia.
GI: paralytic ileus, intestinal obstruction (both resulting from hemorrhage), diarrhea, vomiting, cramps, nausea.
GU: excessive uterine bleeding.
Skin: dermatitis, urticaria, *rash,* necrosis, gangrene, alopecia.
Other: *fever,* hepatitis, jaundice.

INTERACTIONS

Acetaminophen: increased bleeding possible with chronic (greater than 2 weeks) therapy with acetaminophen. Monitor very carefully.
Amiodarone, cephalosporins, chloramphenicol, ciprofloxacin, clofibrate, diflunisal, thyroid drugs, heparin, anabolic steroids, cimetidine, disulfiram, glucagon, methimazole, metronidazole, propylthiouracil, sulindac, sulfinpyrazone, sulfonamides, vitamin E: increased prothrombin time. Monitor patient carefully for bleeding. Consider anticoagulant dosage reduction.
Barbiturates: inhibition of hypoprothrombinemic effect of anticoagulants. If barbiturates are withdrawn, reduce anticoagulant dose; inhibition may last weeks after barbiturate is withdrawn, but fatal hemorrhage can occur when inhibition disappears.
Cholestyramine: decreased response when used too close together. Administer 6 hours after oral anticoagulants.
Glutethimide, chloral hydrate, triclofos sodium: increased or decreased prothrombin time. Avoid use if possible, or monitor patient carefully.
Griseofulvin, ethchlorvynol, carbamazepine, paraldehyde, rifampin: decreased prothrombin time with reduced anticoagulant effect. Monitor patient carefully.
Hydantoins: increased serum levels of hydantoins. Monitor closely.
Indomethacin, mefenamic acid, oxyphenbutazone, phenylbutazone, salicylates: increased prothrombin time; ulcerogenic effects. Don't use together.
Sulfonylureas (oral hypoglycemic agents): increased hypoglycemic response. Monitor blood glucose levels.

NURSING CONSIDERATIONS

- *Contraindicated* in bleeding or hemorrhagic tendencies resulting from open wounds, visceral cancer, GI ulcers, severe hepatic or renal disease, severe uncontrolled hypertension, subacute bacterial endocarditis, polycythemia vera, vitamin K deficiency; after recent operations in eye, brain, or spinal cord.
- *Use cautiously* in diverticulitis, colitis, mild or moderate hypertension, mild or moderate hepatic or renal disease, lactation; with drainage tubes in any orifice; with regional or lumbar block anesthesia; or in any condition increasing risk of hemorrhage.
- Observe breast-feeding infants of mothers on drug for unexpected bleeding.
- PT determinations essential for proper control. High incidence of bleeding when PT exceeds 2.5 times control values. Doctors usually try to maintain PT at 1.5 to 2 times normal.
- Give at same time daily. Stress importance of complying with prescribed dosage and follow-up appointments. Patient should carry a card that identifies him as a potential bleeder.
- Elderly patients and patients with renal or hepatic failure are especially sensitive to warfarin effect.
- Half-life of warfarin's anticoagulant effect is 36 to 44 hours. Effect can be neutralized by vitamin K injections.
- Regularly inspect patient for bleeding gums, bruises on arms or legs, petechiae, nosebleeds, melena, tarry stools, hematuria, hematemesis. Tell patient and family to watch for these signs and notify doctor immediately.
- Warn patient to avoid OTC products containing aspirin, other salicylates, or drugs that interact with warfarin.

- Food and enteral feedings that contain vitamin K may impair anticoagulation. Warn patient to read labels.
- Because onset of action is delayed, heparin sodium is often given during first few days of treatment. When heparin is being given simultaneously, don't draw blood for prothrombin time within 5 hours of intermittent I.V. heparin administration. However, blood for prothrombin time may be drawn at any time during continuous heparin infusion.
- Fever and skin rash signal severe adverse reactions. Withhold drug and call doctor immediately.
- Tell patient to notify doctor if menses is heavier than usual. May require dosage adjustment.
- Tell patient to use electric razor when shaving to avoid scratching skin and to use a soft toothbrush.
- Best oral anticoagulant for patient taking antacids or phenytoin.
- Light to moderate alcohol intake does not significantly affect prothrombin time.
- Possibly effective in treatment of transient cerebral ischemic attacks.
- Tell patient to eat a daily, consistent amount of leafy green vegetables, which contain vitamin K. Eating different amounts daily may alter anticoagulant effects.

*Liquid form contains alcohol. **May contain tartrazine.

65
Hemostatics

absorbable gelatin sponge
microfibrillar collagen hemostat
oxidized cellulose
thrombin

COMBINATION PRODUCTS
None.

absorbable gelatin sponge
Gelfoam

HOW SUPPLIED
Sponges: 20 mm × 60 mm × 3 mm, 20 mm × 60 mm × 7 mm, 80 mm × 62.5 mm × 10 mm, 80 mm × 125 mm × 10 mm, 80 mm × 250 mm × 10 mm, 80 mm × 125 mm (compressed)
Packs: 40 cm × 2 cm, 40 cm × 6 cm
Dental packs: 10 mm × 20 mm × 7 mm, 20 mm × 20 mm × 7 mm
Prostatectomy cones: 13 cm (5″) diameter, 18 cm (7″) diameter

MECHANISM OF ACTION
Absorbs and holds many times its weight in blood. Also provides a framework for growth of granulation tissue.

INDICATIONS & DOSAGE
Decubitus ulcers –
Adults: place aseptically deep into ulcer. Don't disturb or remove; may add extra p.r.n.
To provide hemostasis in surgery (adjunct) –
Adults: apply saturated with isotonic sodium chloride injection or thrombin solution. Hold in place for 10 to 15 seconds. When oozing is controlled, allow material to remain in place.

ADVERSE REACTIONS
Common reactions are in italics; life-threatening reactions are in bold italics.
CNS: ***compression of brain or spinal cord,*** neurologic symptoms, headache, hearing loss.
Local: infection, giant cell granuloma.
Other: fever, ***toxic shock syndrome.***

INTERACTIONS
None significant.

NURSING CONSIDERATIONS
- *Contraindicated* in frank infection, or postpartum bleeding or hemorrhage; also for use as a sole hemostatic agent in abnormal bleeding.
- Should not be used in closure of skin incisions.
- Avoid overpacking when placed into body cavities or closed tissue spaces.
- Systemically absorbed within 4 to 6 weeks; no need to remove except when used in laminectomy procedures or when used to pack foramen in bone.

microfibrillar collagen hemostat
Avitene

Pregnancy Risk Category: C

HOW SUPPLIED
Nonwoven web: 70 mm × 70 mm × 1 mm, 70 mm × 35 mm × 1 mm
Fibrous form: 1-g, 5-g jars

MECHANISM OF ACTION
Attracts and aggregates platelets.

INDICATIONS & DOSAGE
To provide hemostasis in surgery (adjunct) –
Adults and children: amount de-

pends on severity of bleeding. Compress area with dry sponges. Apply drug directly to bleeding site for 1 to 5 minutes. Gently remove excess. Reapply if needed.

ADVERSE REACTIONS
Common reactions are in italics; life-threatening reactions are in bold italics.
Blood: hematoma.
Local: exacerbation of wound dehiscence, abscess formation, foreign body reaction, adhesion formation.
Other: enhanced infection in contaminated wounds, mediastinitis, hypersensitivity, allergic reactions.

INTERACTIONS
None significant.

NURSING CONSIDERATIONS
- *Contraindicated* in closure of skin incisions; hemostat may interfere with healing. Should not be used on bone surfaces where cement needed to attach prostheses.
- Not for injection.
- Don't spill on nonbleeding surfaces.
- Don't dilute. Always apply dry.
- Adheres to wet gloves, instruments, or tissue surfaces. Handle and apply with smooth, dry forceps. Apply directly to source of bleeding.
- Autoclaving inactivates product. Ethylene oxide sterilization should be avoided.

oxidized cellulose
Oxycel, Surgicel

HOW SUPPLIED
Pads: 3″ × 3″, 8 ply
Pledgets: 2″ × 1″ × 1″
Strips: ½ × 2″, ½ × 5″, ½ × 36″; 2″ × 3″, 2″ × 14″, 2″ × 18″; 4″ × 8″

MECHANISM OF ACTION
Absorbs and holds many times its weight in blood.

INDICATIONS & DOSAGE
To provide hemostasis in surgery (adjunct); external bleeding at tumor sites –
Adults and children: apply with sterile technique, p.r.n. Remove after hemostasis, if possible, with dry sterile forceps. Leave in place if necessary.

ADVERSE REACTIONS
Common reactions are in italics; life-threatening reactions are in bold italics.
CNS: headache when used as packing for epistaxis, or after rhinologic procedures or application to surface wounds.
EENT: sneezing, epistaxis, stinging, or burning when used as packing for rhinologic procedures; nasal membrane necrosis or septal perforation.
GU: difficult urination (when used in GU procedures).
Local: encapsulation of fluid, foreign body reaction, burning or stinging after application to surface wounds.
Other: possible prolongation of drainage, ***intestinal obstruction*** following cholecystectomy.

INTERACTIONS
Thrombin: may decrease blood clotting effectiveness.

NURSING CONSIDERATIONS
- *Contraindicated* in controlling hemorrhage from large arteries; for use on nonhemorrhagic, serous, oozing surfaces; in implantation in bone defects.
- Don't pack or wad unless it will be removed after hemostasis. Don't apply too tightly when used as wrap sheet in vascular surgery. Apply loosely against bleeding surface.
- Always remove after hemostasis when used in laminectomies or near optic nerve chiasm.
- Don't autoclave this product.
- Use only amount needed to produce hemostasis. Remove excess before surgical closure.

- Use minimal amounts in urologic procedures.
- In large wounds, don't overlap skin edges.
- Use sterile technique to remove from open wounds after hemostasis. Don't remove without irrigating material first; otherwise, fresh bleeding may occur.
- Don't moisten. Hemostatic effect is greater when applied dry.
- Should not be used for permanent packing in fractures because it may result in cyst formation.

thrombin

Thrombinar, Thrombostat‡

Pregnancy Risk Category: C

HOW SUPPLIED

Powder: 1,000-, 5,000-, 10,000-, and 20,000-unit vials
Kit: 10,000-unit or 20,000-unit with sprayer assembly

MECHANISM OF ACTION

Converts fibrinogen to fibrin.

INDICATIONS & DOSAGE

Bleeding from parenchymatous tissue, cancellous bone, dental sockets, nasal and laryngeal surgery, and in plastic surgery and skin-grafting procedures –

Adults: apply 100 units per ml of sterile isotonic sodium chloride solution or sterile distilled water to area where clotting needed (or may apply dry powder in bone surgery); in major bleeding, apply 1,000 to 2,000 units/ml sterile isotonic sodium chloride solution. Sponge blood from area before application, but avoid sponging area after application.

ADVERSE REACTIONS

Common reactions are in italics; life-threatening reactions are in bold italics.
Systemic: hypersensitivity and fever.

INTERACTIONS

None significant.

NURSING CONSIDERATIONS

- *Contraindicated* in patients with hypersensitivity to thrombin or bovine products.
- Obtain patient history of reactions to thrombin or bovine products.
- Observe patient for allergic reactions, and monitor vital signs regularly.
- Have blood typed and cross matched to treat possible hemorrhage.
- Don't inject topical thrombin or allow it to enter large blood vessels. I.V. injection may cause death because of severe intravascular clotting.
- May be used with absorbable gelatin sponge but not with oxidized cellulose. Check sponge labeling before use.
- Neutralize stomach acids before oral use in GI hemorrhage.
- Keep refrigerated, preferably frozen, until ready to use. Unstable in solution. Store away from heat. Solutions should be used within 3 hours. Excess solution may be refrigerated at 2° to 8° C or frozen for up to 48 hours.
- Broken down by diluted acid, alkali, and salts of heavy metals.

66

Blood derivatives

antihemophilic factor
antithrombin III, human
Factor IX complex
intravascular perfluorochemical emulsion
normal serum albumin 5%
normal serum albumin 25%
plasma protein fraction

COMBINATION PRODUCTS
None.

antihemophilic factor (AHF)
Hemofil M, Koate-HS, Koate-HT, Monoclate

Pregnancy Risk Category: C

HOW SUPPLIED
Injection: vials, with diluent. Number of units on label.

A new porcine product is now available for patients with congenital hemophilia A who have antibodies to human Factor VIII:C.

MECHANISM OF ACTION
Directly replaces deficient clotting factor.

INDICATIONS & DOSAGE
Prophylaxis of spontaneous hemorrhage in patients with hemophilia A (Factor VIII deficiency) –
Adults and children: dosage must be calculated using the formula:

$$\text{AHF required (IU)} = \text{body weight (kg)} \times \text{desired Factor VIII increase (\% of normal)} \times 0.5$$

To prevent spontaneous hemorrhage, the desired level of Factor VIII is 5% of normal; for mild hemorrhage, 30% of normal; for moderate hemorrhage and minor surgery, 30% to 50% of normal; for severe hemorrhage, 80% to 100% of normal.
Treatment of bleeding in patients with hemophilia A (Factor VIII deficiency) –
Adults and children: For minor hemorrhage into muscle and joints, 8 to 10 IU/kg I.V every 8 to 12 hours for 1 or more days. For overt bleeding, 15 to 25 IU/kg I.V. every 8 to 12 hours for 3 to 4 days. To treat massive bleeding or hemorrhage involving major organs, an initial dose of 40 to 50 IU/kg I.V. is followed by 20 to 25 IU/kg I.V. every 8 to 12 hours.

ADVERSE REACTIONS
Common reactions are in italics; life-threatening reactions are in bold italics.
CNS: headache, paresthesias, clouding or loss of consciousness, somnolence, lethargy.
CV: tachycardia, hypotension, possible ***intravascular hemolysis*** in patients with blood type A, B, or AB.
EENT: visual disturbances.
GI: nausea, vomiting.
Skin: erythema, *urticaria.*
Other: *chills, fever, backache, flushing,* chest constriction; ***hypersensitivity,*** rigor, stinging at injection site.

INTERACTIONS
None significant.

NURSING CONSIDERATIONS
- *Use cautiously* in neonates, infants, and patients with hepatic disease because of susceptibility to hepatitis, which may be transmitted in antihemophilic factor.
- Monitor vital signs regularly.
- **I.V. use:** For I.V. use only. Use plastic syringe; drug may interact with glass syringe and bind to its surface. Take baseline pulse rate before I.V.

administration. If pulse rate increases significantly, flow rate should be reduced or administration stopped.

- Monitor patient for allergic reactions.
- Refrigerate concentrate until ready to use, but not after reconstituted. Refrigeration after reconstitution may cause the active ingredient to precipitate. Before reconstituting, concentrate and diluent bottles should be warmed to room temperature. To mix drug, gently roll vial between hands. Reconstituted solution unstable; use within 3 hours. Store away from heat. Don't shake or mix with other I.V. solutions.
- As ordered, administer hepatitis B vaccine before administering antihemophilic factor.
- Risk of hepatitis, including non-A, non-B hepatitis, must be weighed against risk of the patient not receiving the drug.
- Because of the manufacturing process, the risk of HIV transmission is extremely low.
- Monitor coagulation studies before and during therapy.

antithrombin III, human (AT-III, heparin cofactor I)

ATnativ

Pregnancy Risk Category: C

HOW SUPPLIED

Injection: 500 IU

MECHANISM OF ACTION

Replaces deficient AT-III in patients with hereditary AT-III deficiency, normalizing coagulation-inhibiting capability and inhibiting formation of thromboemboli. Also inactivates plasmin but to a lesser extent than the clotting factor.

INDICATIONS & DOSAGE

Prophylaxis and adjunctive treatment of thromboembolism associated with hereditary AT-III deficiency –
Adults and children: initial dose is individualized to the quantity required to increase AT-III activity to 120% of normal activity as determined 30 minutes after administration. Usual dose is 50 to 100 IU/minute I.V., not to exceed 100 IU/minute. Dose is calculated based on anticipated 1% increase in plasma AT-III activity produced by 1 IU/kg of body weight using the formula:

$$\text{Dose (Units)} = \frac{(\text{desired activity } [\%] - \text{baseline activity } [\%]) \times \text{weight (kg)}}{1\% \text{ (IU/kg)}}$$

Maintenance dose is individualized to quantity required to increase AT-III activity to 80% of normal activity and is administered at 24-hour intervals.

To calculate the dose, multiply the desired AT-III activity (as % of normal) minus the baseline AT-III activity (as % of normal) by the body weight (in kg). Divide by actual increase in AT-III activity (in %) produced by 1 IU/kg as determined 30 minutes after administration of initial dose.

Treatment is usually continued for 2 to 8 days but may be prolonged in pregnancy or when used with surgery or immobilization.

ADVERSE REACTIONS

Common reactions are in italics; life-threatening reactions are in bold italics.
CV: vasodilation, lowered blood pressure.
GU: diuresis.

INTERACTIONS

Heparin: Concurrent administration with heparin increases the anticoagulant effect of both. Heparin dosage reduction may be necessary.

NURSING CONSIDERATIONS

- *Use with extreme caution* in children and neonates because safety and efficacy have not been established.
- *Use cautiously.* Because drug is prepared from pooled plasma from human donors, it carries with it a minimal risk of transmission of viruses, including hepatitis and human immunodeficiency virus. Plasma used in the manufacturing process is screened for these viruses, and the product is heat-treated for 10 hours at 140° F (60° C) to further reduce the risk of viral transmission.
- Not recommended for long-term prophylaxis of thrombotic episodes.
- Because of the risk of neonatal thromboembolism in children of parents with hereditary AT-III deficiency, measure AT-III levels immediately after birth. Fatal neonatal thromboembolism has been reported.
- Determinations of AT-III activity should be performed twice daily until the dosage requirement has stabilized, then daily immediately before dose. Functional assays are preferred because quantitative immunologic test results may be normal despite decreased AT-III activity.
- One IU is equivalent to the quantity of endogenous AT-III present in 1 ml of normal human plasma.
- Dyspnea and increased blood pressure may occur if administration rate is too rapid (1,500 IU in 5 minutes).
- Heparin binds to AT-III lysine binding sites in a 1:1 M ratio, which results in increased efficacy of heparin.
- **I.V. use:** Reconstitute using 10 ml sterile water (provided), normal saline solution, or dextrose 5% in water. *Do not shake vial. Further dilution in same diluent solution may occur if desired.*
- Store at 36° to 46° F (2° to 8° C).

Factor IX complex

Alpha-Nine, Konyne-HT, Profilnine Heat-Treated, Proplex T

Pregnancy Risk Category: C

HOW SUPPLIED

Injection: vials, with diluents. Units specified on label.

MECHANISM OF ACTION

Directly replaces deficient clotting factor.

INDICATIONS & DOSAGE

Factor IX deficiency (hemophilia B or Christmas disease), anticoagulant overdosage –

Adults and children: units required equal 0.8 to 1 × body weight in kg × percentage of desired increase of Factor IX level, by slow I.V. infusion or I.V. push. Dosage is highly individualized, depending on degree of deficiency, level of Factor IX desired, weight of patient, and severity of bleeding.

ADVERSE REACTIONS

Common reactions are in italics; life-threatening reactions are in bold italics.

CNS: somnolence, lethargy, headache.

CV: ***thromboembolic reactions; myocardial infarction; disseminated intravascular coagulation; pulmonary embolism;*** possible ***intravascular hemolysis*** in patients with blood types A, B, or AB; changes in blood pressure or heart rate.

GI: nausea, vomiting.

Skin: urticaria.

Other: *transient fever, chills, flushing, tingling,* ***hypersensitivity.***

INTERACTIONS

Aminocaproic acid: increased risk of thrombosis. Avoid concomitant use.

NURSING CONSIDERATIONS

- *Contraindicated* in hepatic disease, intravascular coagulation, or fibrinolysis.
- *Use cautiously* in neonates and infants because of susceptibility to hepatitis, which may be transmitted with Factor IX complex.
- Observe for allergic reactions, and monitor vital signs regularly.
- Risk of hepatitis, including non-A, non-B hepatitis, must be weighed against risk of not receiving the drug.
- Because of the manufacturing process, the risk of HIV transmission is extremely low.
- As ordered, administer hepatitis B vaccine before administering Factor IX complex.
- **I.V. use:** Avoid rapid infusion. If tingling sensation, fever, chills, or headache develops during I.V. infusion, decrease flow rate and notify the doctor.
- Reconstitute with 20 ml sterile water for injection for each vial of lyophilized drug. Keep refrigerated until ready to use; warm to room temperature before reconstituting. Use within 3 hours of reconstitution. Unstable in solution. Don't shake, refrigerate, or mix solution with other I.V. solutions. Store away from heat.

intravascular perfluorochemical emulsion

Fluosol

Pregnancy Risk Category: B

HOW SUPPLIED

Emulsion for injection: 20%; supplied in kit form with additive solutions (1 and 2) and materials to provide continuous oxygenation

MECHANISM OF ACTION

An emulsion of synthetic perfluorochemicals that acts as a carrier of oxygen.

INDICATIONS & DOSAGE

To prevent or decrease myocardial ischemia during percutaneous transluminal coronary angioplasty (PTCA) in patients at high risk for ischemic complications of angioplasty (including patients with a low baseline ejection fraction, patients with large areas of the myocardium at risk, patients with recent myocardial infarction, patients with unstable angina or refractory angina requiring hospitalization) –

Adults: first, a test dose of 0.5 ml should be withdrawn from the prepared solution and injected into a peripheral vein. If no adverse reactions occur within 10 minutes, warmed, oxygenated emulsion may be administered by intracoronary injection at a rate of 60 to 90 ml/minute. Administer through the central lumen of an angioplasty balloon catheter without removing the guide wire. Use an angiographic power injector with a warming jacket.

ADVERSE REACTIONS

Common reactions are in italics; life-threatening reactions are in bold italics.

CV: ***ventricular tachycardia or fibrillation,*** bradycardia, chest discomfort, hypotension.

Respiratory: dyspnea, increased respiratory rate, coughing.

Skin: mild pruritus.

INTERACTIONS

Anesthetics: may prolong the action of lipid-soluble anesthetics.

Hepatotoxic agents: animal studies revealed that perfluorochemicals enhanced the hepatotoxic effects of carbon tetrachloride.

NURSING CONSIDERATIONS

- *Contraindicated* in patients with hypersensitivity to any components of the compound and in patients with functionally critical secondary stenosis in areas distal to the site of the lesion being treated.

- Reportedly, this drug will accumulate in the body after repeated dosage. Intravascular perfluorochemical emulsion should not be given more than once every 6 months.
- Drug should be administered only by physicians familiar with PTCA. Follow institutional policy regarding emergency surgical procedures for coronary artery bypass graft surgery.
- When used with an angiographic power injector reservoir of 260 ml and a flow rate of 60 ml/minute, more than 4 minutes of perfusion time will be allowed. Perfusion time should be limited by patient tolerance and physician judgment.
- In the unlikely event that the patient reacts adversely to the test dose (1.2% of the patients in clinical trials reacted), the drug should not be given. Severe reactions can be managed with methylprednisolone or diphenhydramine.
- The emulsion must be oxygenated and warmed to approximately 98.6° F (37° C) before administration. Infusion of solutions at room temperature has been associated with ventricular fibrillation.
- The container of intravascular perfluorochemical emulsion must be stored in the freezer (between 23° and −22° F [−5° and −30° C]). Emulsions that appear to have thawed partially during storage should not be used. Use a warming cabinet or water bath set at 98.6° F to thaw the solution (do not use a microwave oven because this may cause uneven heating of the solution). Do not refreeze thawed solutions. Allow at least 30 minutes for thawing of the solution.
- The additive solutions (solutions 1 and 2) should not be frozen; they may be stored at room temperature not exceeding 86° F (30° C).
- Do not add anything other than solutions 1 and 2 or carbogen gas (95% oxygen, 5% carbon dioxide) to the emulsion. Do not oxygenate with 100% oxygen, because this will adversely affect the solution's final pH.
- **I.V. use:** When administering, do not use an in-line filter because it may damage the emulsion. Never administer any solution that has evidence of emulsion separation.
- Studies have shown that perfluorochemicals are excreted in breast milk. Breast-feeding after administration of intravascular perfluorochemical emulsion is not recommended.

normal serum albumin 5%
Albuminar 5%, Albutein 5%, Buminate 5%, Plasbumin 5%

normal serum albumin 25%
Albuminar 25%, Albumisol 25%, Buminate 25%, Plasbumin 25%

Pregnancy Risk Category: C

HOW SUPPLIED
albumin 5%
Injection: 5%, in 50-ml, 250-ml, 500-ml, 1,000-ml bottles
albumin 25%
Injection: 25%, in 10-ml, 20-ml, 50-ml, 100-ml vials

MECHANISM OF ACTION
Normal serum albumin 25% provides intravascular oncotic pressure in a 5:1 ratio, which causes a shift of fluid from interstitial spaces to the circulation and slightly increases plasma protein concentration. Normal serum albumin 5% supplies colloid to the blood and expands plasma volume.

INDICATIONS & DOSAGE
Shock –
Adults: initially, 500 ml (5% solution) by I.V. infusion, repeat q 30 minutes, p.r.n. Dosage varies with patient's condition and response.
Children: 25% to 50% adult dose in nonemergency.

*Liquid form contains alcohol. **May contain tartrazine.

Hypoproteinemia –
Adults: 1,000 to 1,500 ml 5% solution by I.V. infusion daily, maximum rate 5 to 10 ml/minute; or 25 to 100 g 25% solution by I.V. infusion daily, maximum rate 3 ml/minute. Dosage varies with patient's condition and response.
Burns –
Adults: dosage varies according to extent of burn and patient's condition. Usually maintain plasma albumin at 2 to 3 g/100 ml.
Hyperbilirubinemia –
Infants: 1 g albumin (4 ml 25%)/kg before transfusion.

ADVERSE REACTIONS
Common reactions are in italics; life-threatening reactions are in bold italics.
CV: ***vascular overload after rapid infusion,*** hypotension, altered pulse rate.
GI: increased salivation, nausea, vomiting.
Skin: urticaria.
Other: chills, fever, altered respiration.

INTERACTIONS
None significant.

NURSING CONSIDERATIONS
- *Contraindicated* in severe anemia or heart failure.
- *Use cautiously* in low cardiac reserve, absence of albumin deficiency, and sodium restriction.
- Do not give more than 250 g in 48 hours.
- Watch for hemorrhage or shock after surgery or injury. Rapid rise in blood pressure may cause bleeding from sites that are not apparent at lower pressures.
- Monitor vital signs carefully.
- Watch for signs of vascular overload (heart failure or pulmonary edema).
- Patient should be properly hydrated before infusion of solution.
- **I.V. use:** Avoid rapid I.V. infusion. Specific rate is individualized according to patient's age, condition, and diagnosis. Dilute with sterile water for injection, 0.9% sodium chloride solution, or dextrose 5% in water injection. Use solution promptly; contains no preservatives. Discard unused solution. Don't use cloudy solutions or those containing sediment. Solution should be clear amber color.
- Freezing may cause bottle to break. Follow storage instructions on bottle.
- One volume of 25% albumin is equivalent to five volumes of 5% albumin in producing hemodilution and relative anemia.
- This product is very expensive, and random supply shortages occur often.
- Monitor intake and output, hemoglobin, hematocrit, and serum protein and electrolytes during therapy.

plasma protein fraction
Plasmanate, Plasma-Plex, Plasmatein, Protenate

Pregnancy Risk Category: C

HOW SUPPLIED
Injection: 5% solution in 50-ml, 250-ml, 500-ml vials

MECHANISM OF ACTION
Supplies colloid to the blood and expands plasma volume.

INDICATIONS & DOSAGE
Shock –
Adults: varies with patient's condition and response, but usual dose is 250 to 500 ml I.V. (12.5 to 25 g protein), usually no faster than 10 ml/minute.
Children: 22 to 33 ml/kg I.V. infused at rate of 5 to 10 ml/minute.
Hypoproteinemia –
Adults: 1,000 to 1,500 ml I.V. daily. Maximum infusion rate 8 ml/minute.

ADVERSE REACTIONS
Common reactions are in italics; life-threatening reactions are in bold italics.
CNS: headache.
CV: variable effects on blood pressure after rapid infusion or intraarterial administration; ***vascular overload after rapid infusion.***
GI: nausea, vomiting, hypersalivation.
Skin: erythema, urticaria.
Other: flushing, chills, fever, back pain, dyspnea.

INTERACTIONS
None significant.

NURSING CONSIDERATIONS
- *Contraindicated* in patients with severe anemia or heart failure, and those patients undergoing cardiac bypass.
- *Use cautiously* in hepatic or renal failure, low cardiac reserve, and restricted sodium intake.
- Monitor blood pressure. Infusion should be slowed or stopped if hypotension suddenly occurs.
- Vital signs should return to normal gradually; monitor hourly.
- Watch for signs of vascular overload (heart failure or pulmonary edema).
- Monitor intake and output. Watch for and report decreased urine output.
- Check expiration date before using. Discard solutions in containers opened for more than 4 hours. Solution contains no preservatives.
- Don't use solutions that are cloudy, contain sediment, or have been frozen.
- If patient is dehydrated, give additional fluids either P.O. or I.V.
- Do not give more than 250 g (5,000 ml 5%) in 48 hours.
- Contains 130 to 160 mEq sodium/liter.

67

Thrombolytic enzymes

alteplase
anistreplase
streptokinase
urokinase

COMBINATION PRODUCTS
None.

alteplase (tissue plasminogen activator, recombinant; t-PA)

Actilyse‡, Activase

Pregnancy Risk Category: C

HOW SUPPLIED
Injection: 20-mg (11.6 million-IU), 50-mg (29 million-IU) vials

MECHANISM OF ACTION
Binds to fibrin in a thrombus, and locally converts plasminogen to plasmin, which initiates local fibrinolysis.

INDICATIONS & DOSAGE
Lysis of thrombi obstructing coronary arteries in acute MI –
Adults: 100 mg I.V. infusion over 3 hours as follows: 60 mg in the first hour, of which 6 to 10 mg is given as a bolus over the first 1 to 2 minutes. Then 20 mg/hr infusion for 2 hours. Smaller adults (< 65 kg) should receive a dose of 1.25 mg/kg in a similar fashion (60% in the first hour, with 10% as a bolus; then 20% of the total dose per hour for 2 hours).
Management of acute massive pulmonary embolism –
Adults: 100 mg I.V. infusion over 2 hours. Begin heparin at the end of the infusion when the partial thromboplastin time or thrombin time returns to twice normal or less.

ADVERSE REACTIONS
Common reactions are in italics; life-threatening reactions are in bold italics.
Blood: ***severe, spontaneous bleeding (cerebral, retroperitoneal, GU, GI).***
CNS: ***cerebral hemorrhage,*** fever.
CV: hypotension, arrhythmias.
GI: nausea, vomiting.
Local: bleeding at puncture sites.
Other: hypersensitivity, urticaria.

INTERACTIONS
Aspirin, dipyridamole, heparin, coumarin anticoagulants: increased risk of bleeding. Monitor patient carefully.

NURSING CONSIDERATIONS
- *Contraindicated* in active internal bleeding, intracranial neoplasm, arteriovenous malformation, aneurysm, and severe uncontrolled hypertension. Also *contraindicated* in patients with a history of CVA, recent (within 2 months) intraspinal or intracranial trauma or surgery, or known bleeding diathesis.
- Consider risk versus benefit in patients with recent (within 10 days) major surgery; in pregnancy and first 10 days postpartum; organ biopsy; trauma (including cardiopulmonary resuscitation); GI or GU bleeding; cerebrovascular disease; hypertension (systolic ≥ 180 mm Hg or diastolic ≥ 110 mm Hg); mitral stenosis, atrial fibrillation, or other condition that may lead to left heart thrombus; acute pericarditis or subacute bacterial endocarditis; septic thrombophlebitis; diabetic hemorrhagic retinopathy; in patients receiving anticoagulants; and in patients age 75 and older.
- Do not exceed dose of 100 mg. Higher doses may increase risk of intracranial bleeding.
- Coronary thrombolysis is associated

with arrhythmias induced by reperfusion of ischemic myocardium. Such arrhythmias do not differ from those commonly associated with MI. Have antiarrhythmic agents readily available, and carefully monitor ECG.

- Recanalization of occluded coronary arteries and improvement of heart function are time-dependent phenomena and require initiation of treatment with alteplase as soon as possible after the onset of symptoms.
- Bleeding is the most common adverse effect and may occur internally and at external puncture sites. Avoid invasive procedures during thrombolytic therapy. Carefully monitor patient for signs of internal bleeding and frequently check all puncture sites.
- Heparin therapy is frequently initiated after treatment with alteplase to decrease the risk of rethrombosis.
- Reconstitute drug with sterile water for injection (without preservatives) only. Do not use vial if the vacuum is not present. Reconstitute with a large-bore (18G) needle, directing the stream of sterile water at the lyophilized cake. Do not shake. Slight foaming is common, and solution should be clear or pale yellow.
- Drug may be administered as reconstituted (1 mg/ml) or diluted with an equal volume of 0.9% sodium chloride solution or dextrose 5% in water to make a 0.5 mg/ml solution. Adding other drugs to the infusion is not recommended.
- Reconstitute alteplase solution immediately before use, and administer it within 8 hours. The drug may be temporarily stored at 35° to 86° F (2° to 30° C), but it is stable for 8 hours at room temperature. Discard any solution unused after that time because it contains no preservatives.

anistreplase (anisoylated plasminogen-streptokinase activator complex; APSAC)

Eminase

Pregnancy Risk Category: C

HOW SUPPLIED

Injection: 30 units/vial

MECHANISM OF ACTION

Anistreplase is derived from Lys-plasminogen and streptokinase. It is formulated into a fibrinolytic enzyme plus activator complex with the activator temporarily blocked by an anisoyl group. The drug is activated in vivo by a nonenzymatic process that removes the anisoyl group. The active Lys-plasminogen-streptokinase activator complex is progressively formed in the bloodstream or within the thrombus.

INDICATIONS & DOSAGE

Lysis of cornary artery thrombi following acute MI –

Adults: 30 units I.V. over 2 to 5 minutes. Administer by direct injection.

ADVERSE REACTIONS

Common reactions are in italics; life-threatening reactions are in bold italics.

Blood: ***bleeding,*** eosinophilia.

CNS: ***intracranial hemorrhage.***

CV: arrhythmias, conduction disorders, hypotension.

EENT: hemoptysis, gum or mouth hemorrhage.

GI: ***bleeding.***

GU: hematuria.

Skin: hematomas, urticaria, itching, flushing, delayed (2 weeks after therapy) purpuric rash.

Local: bleeding at puncture sites.

Other: ***anaphylactoid reactions*** *(rare).*

INTERACTIONS

Heparin, oral anticoagulants, drugs that alter platelet function (including aspirin and dipyridamole): may increase the risk of bleeding. Use together cautiously.

NURSING CONSIDERATIONS

- *Contraindicated* in patients with a history of severe allergic reaction to anistreplase or streptokinase; active internal bleeding, history of CVA, recent (within the past 2 months) intraspinal or intracranial surgery or trauma, aneurysm, arteriovenous malformation, intracranial neoplasm, uncontrolled hypertension, or known bleeding diathesis.
- Consider risk versus benefit in patients with recent (within 10 days) major surgery; trauma (including cardiopulmonary resuscitation); GI or GU bleeding; cerebrovascular disease; hypertension (systolic ≥ 180 mm Hg or diastolic ≥ 110 mm Hg); mitral stenosis, atrial fibrillation, or other condition that may lead to left heart thrombus; acute pericarditis or subacute bacterial endocarditis; septic thrombophlebitis; diabetic hemorrhagic retinopathy; in pregnancy and first 10 days postpartum; in patients receiving anticoagulants, and in patients 75 years and older.
- Unlike other thrombolytics that must be infused, anistreplase is given by direct injection over 2 to 5 minutes.
- Thrombolytic therapy is associated with the occurrence of reperfusion arrhythmias that may signify successful thrombolysis. These arrhythmias are similar to those seen in the course of an acute MI and may include sinus bradycardia, accelerated idioventricular rhythm, ventricular tachycardia, or premature ventricular depolarizations. Be prepared to treat bradycardia or ventricular irritability during anistreplase therapy. Carefully monitor ECG during treatment with anistreplase.
- Anistreplase is derived from human plasma. No cases of hepatitis or HIV infection have been reported to date. The manufacturing process is designed to purify the plasma used in the preparation of the drug.
- Reconstitute the drug by slowly adding 5 ml of sterile water for injection. Direct the stream against the side of the vial, not at the drug itself. Gently roll the vial to mix the dry powder and water. To avoid excessive foaming, don't shake the vial. The reconstituted solution should be colorless to pale yellow. Inspect for particulate matter.
- Do not mix the drug with other medications; do not dilute the solution after reconstitution.
- If the drug is not administered within 30 minutes of reconstituting, discard the vial.
- In vitro coagulation tests will be affected by the presence of anistreplase. This can be attenuated if blood samples are collected in the presence of aprotinin (150 to 200 units/ml).
- Bleeding is the most common adverse reaction and may occur internally and at external puncture sites. Carefully monitor patient.
- Heparin therapy is frequently initiated after treatment with thrombolytics to decrease the risk of rethrombosis.
- Teach the patient signs of internal bleeding. Tell him to report these immediately. Advise the patient about proper dental care to avoid excessive gum trauma.

streptokinase

Kabikinase, Streptase

Pregnancy Risk Category: C

HOW SUPPLIED

Injection: 100,000 IU, 250,000 IU, 600,000 IU, 750,000 IU, 1,500,000 IU in vials for reconstitution

MECHANISM OF ACTION

Activates plasminogen in two steps. Plasminogen and streptokinase form a complex that exposes the plasminogen-activating site. Plasminogen is converted to plasmin by cleavage of the peptide bond.

INDICATIONS & DOSAGE

Arteriovenous cannula occlusion –
Adults: 250,000 IU in 2 ml I.V. solution by I.V. pump infusion into each occluded limb of the cannula over 25 to 35 minutes. Clamp off cannula for 2 hours. Then aspirate contents of cannula; flush with saline solution and reconnect.
Venous thrombosis, pulmonary embolism, and arterial thrombosis and embolism –
Adults: loading dose is 250,000 IU I.V. infusion over 30 minutes. Sustaining dose is 100,000 IU/hour I.V. infusion for 72 hours for deep vein thrombosis and 100,000 IU/hour over 24 to 72 hours by I.V. infusion pump for pulmonary embolism.
Lysis of coronary artery thrombi following acute MI –
Adults: 140,000 units administered as a loading dose followed by maintenance infusion. Loading dose is 20,000 IU via coronary catheter, followed by a maintenance dose of 2,000 IU/minute for 60 minutes as an infusion. Alternatively, may be administered as an I.V. infusion. Usual adult dose is 1.5 million units infused over 60 minutes.

ADVERSE REACTIONS

Common reactions are in italics; life-threatening reactions are in bold italics.
Blood: ***bleeding,*** low hematocrit.
CV: transient lowering or elevation of blood pressure.
EENT: periorbital edema.
Skin: urticaria.
Local: phlebitis at injection site.
Other: ***hypersensitivity to drug,*** fever, ***anaphylaxis,*** musculoskeletal pain, minor breathing difficulty, bronchospasms, angioneurotic edema.

INTERACTIONS

Anticoagulants: increased risk of bleeding. Monitor closely.
Aspirin, dipyridamole, indomethacin, phenylbutazone, drugs affecting platelet activity: increased risk of bleeding. Combined therapy with low-dose aspirin (162.5 mg) or dipyridamole has improved acute and long-term results.

NURSING CONSIDERATIONS

- *Contraindicated* in ulcerative wounds, active internal bleeding, and recent CVA; recent trauma with possible internal injuries; visceral or intracranial malignant neoplasms; ulcerative colitis; diverticulitis; severe hypertension; acute or chronic hepatic or renal insufficiency; uncontrolled hypocoagulation; chronic pulmonary disease with cavitation; subacute bacterial endocarditis or rheumatic valvular disease; recent cerebral embolism, thrombosis, or hemorrhage. Also contraindicated within 10 days after intra-arterial diagnostic procedure or any surgery, including liver or kidney biopsy, lumbar puncture, thoracentesis, paracentesis, or extensive or multiple cutdowns.
- *Use cautiously* when treating arterial emboli that originate from left side of heart because of danger of cerebral infarction.
- I.M. injections and other invasive procedures are contraindicated during streptokinase therapy.
- Before initiating therapy, draw blood to determine PTT and PT. Rate of I.V. infusion depends on thrombin time and streptokinase resistance.
- If the patient has had either a recent streptococcal infection or recent treatment with streptokinase, a higher loading dose may be necessary.
- **I.V. use:** Reconstitute each vial with 5 ml sodium chloride solution for injection. Further dilute to 45 ml.

Don't shake; roll gently to mix. Use within 24 hours. Store powder at room temperature and refrigerate after reconstitution.

- Monitor patient for excessive bleeding every 15 minutes for the first hour, every 30 minutes for the second through eighth hours, then once every shift. If bleeding is evident, stop therapy. Pretreatment with heparin or drugs affecting platelets causes high risk of bleeding, but may improve long-term results. Monitor closely.
- Monitor pulses, color, and sensation of extremities every hour.
- Have typed and crossmatched packed red cells and whole blood ready to treat possible hemorrhage.
- Keep aminocaproic acid available to treat bleeding. Corticosteroids are used to treat allergic reactions.
- Before using streptokinase to clear an occluded arteriovenous cannula, try flushing with heparinized sodium chloride solution.
- Bruising more likely during therapy; avoid unnecessary handling of patient. Side rails should be padded.
- Maintain the involved extremity in straight alignment to prevent bleeding from the infusion site.
- Keep venipuncture sites to a minimum; use pressure dressing on puncture sites for at least 15 minutes.
- Keep a laboratory flow sheet on patient's chart to monitor partial thromboplastin time, prothrombin time, hemoglobin, and hematocrit.
- To check for hypersensitivity, give 100 IU intradermally; a wheal and flare response within 20 minutes means patient is probably allergic. Monitor vital signs frequently.
- Watch for signs of hypersensitivity. Notify doctor immediately. Antihistamines or corticosteroids may be used to treat mild allergic reactions. If a severe reaction occurs, the infusion should be stopped immediately.
- Heparin by continuous infusion is usually started within an hour after stopping streptokinase. Use infusion pump to administer heparin.
- Should be used only by doctors with wide experience in thrombotic disease management where clinical and laboratory monitoring can be performed.
- Thrombolytic therapy in patients with acute MI may decrease infarct size, improve ventricular function, and decrease incidence of CHF. Streptokinase must be administered within 6 hours of the onset of symptoms for optimal effect.

urokinase

Abbokinase, Ukidan‡, Win-Kinase

Pregnancy Risk Category: B

HOW SUPPLIED

Injection: 5,000 IU/ml unit-dose vial; 250,000-IU vial

MECHANISM OF ACTION

Activates plasminogen by directly cleaving peptide bonds at two different sites.

INDICATIONS & DOSAGE

Lysis of acute massive pulmonary emboli and lysis of pulmonary emboli accompanied by unstable hemodynamics –

Adults: for I.V. infusion only by constant infusion pump that will deliver a total volume of 195 ml.

Priming dose: 4,400 IU/kg of urokinase-0.9% sodium chloride solution admixture given over 10 minutes. Follow with 4,400 IU/kg hourly for 12 to 24 hours. Total volume should not exceed 200 ml. Follow therapy with continuous I.V. infusion of heparin, then oral anticoagulants.

Coronary artery thrombosis –

Adults: following a bolus dose of heparin ranging from 2,500 to 10,000 units, infuse 6,000 IU/minute of urokinase into the occluded artery for up to 2 hours. Average total dosage is 500,000 IU.

Venous catheter occlusion—
Adults: Instill 5,000 IU into occluded line, wait 5 minutes, then aspirate. Repeat aspiration attempts q 5 minutes for 30 minutes. If not patent after 30 minutes, cap line and let urokinase work for 30 to 60 minutes before aspirating. May require second instillation.

ADVERSE REACTIONS

Common reactions are in italics; life-threatening reactions are in bold italics.
Blood: ***bleeding,*** low hematocrit.
Local: phlebitis at injection site.
Other: hypersensitivity (not as frequent as streptokinase), musculoskeletal pain, bronchospasm, ***anaphylaxis.***

INTERACTIONS

Anticoagulants: increased risk of bleeding. Monitor closely.
Aspirin, dipyridamole, indomethacin, phenylbutazone, other drugs affecting platelet activity: increased risk of bleeding.

NURSING CONSIDERATIONS

• *Contraindicated* in ulcerative wounds, active internal bleeding, and cerebrovascular accident; aneurysm; arteriovenous malformation; known bleeding diathesis, recent trauma with possible internal injuries; visceral or intracranial malignancy; pregnancy and first 10 days postpartum; ulcerative colitis; diverticulitis; severe hypertension; acute or chronic hepatic or renal insufficiency; uncontrolled hypocoagulation; chronic pulmonary disease with cavitation; subacute bacterial endocarditis or rheumatic valvular disease; and recent cerebral embolism, thrombosis, or hemorrhage. Also contraindicated within 10 days after intraarterial diagnostic procedure or any surgery (liver or kidney biopsy, lumbar puncture, thoracentesis, paracentesis, or extensive or multiple cutdowns); intracranial or intraspinal surgery in the past 2 months.
• I.M. injections and other invasive procedures are contraindicated during urokinase therapy.
• Maintain the involved extremity in straight alignment to prevent bleeding from the infusion site.
• **I.V. use:** Add 5 ml sterile water for injection to vial. Dilute further with 0.9% sodium chloride or 5% dextrose in water solution before infusion. The total volume of fluid administered should not exceed 200 ml. Don't use bacteriostatic water for injection to reconstitute; it contains preservatives.
• Monitor patient for bleeding every 15 minutes for the first hour; every 30 minutes for the second through eighth hours; then once every shift. Pretreatment with drugs affecting platelets places patient at high risk of bleeding.
• Monitor pulses, color, and sensation of extremities every hour.
• Have typed and crossmatched red cells, whole blood, and aminocaproic acid available to treat bleeding. Corticosteroids are used to treat allergic reactions.
• Keep a laboratory flow sheet on patient's chart to monitor partial thromboplastin time, prothrombin time, hemoglobin, and hematocrit.
• Although the incidence of hypersensitivity is low, watch for signs of this reaction.
• Monitor vital signs.
• Keep venipuncture sites to a minimum; use pressure dressing on puncture sites for at least 15 minutes.
• Heparin by continuous infusion is usually started within an hour after urokinase has been stopped to prevent recurrent thrombosis.
• Bruising is more likely during therapy; avoid unnecessary handling of patient. Side rails should be padded.
• Instruct the patient to report symptoms of bleeding.

68

Alkylating agents

busulfan
carboplatin
carmustine
chlorambucil
cisplatin
cyclophosphamide
dacarbazine
ifosfamide
lomustine
mechlorethamine hydrochloride
melphalan
streptozocin
thiotepa
uracil mustard

COMBINATION PRODUCTS
None.

busulfan

Myleran

Pregnancy Risk Category: D

HOW SUPPLIED
Tablets: 2 mg

MECHANISM OF ACTION
Cross-links strands of cellular DNA and interferes with RNA transcription, causing an imbalance of growth that leads to cell death. Cell cycle-nonspecific.

INDICATIONS & DOSAGE
Chronic myelocytic (granulocytic) leukemia –
Adults: 4 to 8 mg P.O. daily up to 12 mg P.O. daily until WBC falls to 15,000/mm³; stop drug until WBC rises to 50,000/mm³, then resume treatment as before; or 4 to 8 mg P.O. daily until WBC falls to 10,000 to 20,000/mm³, then reduce daily dosage as needed to maintain WBC at this level (usually 2 mg daily).
Children: 0.06 to 0.12 mg/kg or 1.8 to 4.6 mg/m²/day P.O.; adjust dosage to maintain WBC at 20,000/mm³, but never less than 10,000/mm³.

ADVERSE REACTIONS
Common reactions are in italics; life-threatening reactions are in bold italics.
Blood: WBC falling after about 10 days and continuing to fall for 2 weeks after stopping drug; ***thrombocytopenia, leukopenia, anemia.***
CNS: *seizures.*
GI: nausea, vomiting, diarrhea, cheilosis, glossitis.
GU: amenorrhea, testicular atrophy, impotence.
Metabolic: Addison-like wasting syndrome, profound hyperuricemia due to increased cell lysis.
Skin: transient hyperpigmentation, rash, urticaria, anhidrosis.
Other: gynecomastia; alopecia; ***irreversible pulmonary fibrosis, commonly termed "busulfan lung."***

INTERACTIONS
None significant.

NURSING CONSIDERATIONS
• *Contraindicated* in patients with chronic myelogenous leukemia, which is known to be resistant to the drug.
• *Use cautiously* in patients recently given other myelosuppressive drugs or radiation treatment and in those with depressed neutrophil or platelet count. Because high-dose therapy has been associated with seizures, use such therapy cautiously in patients with a history of head trauma or seizures or in patients receiving other drugs that lower the seizure threshold.
• Warn patient to watch for signs of infection (fever, sore throat, fatigue) and bleeding (easy bruising, nose-

bleeds, bleeding gums, melena). Take temperature daily.

- Pulmonary fibrosis may occur as late as 4 to 6 months after treatment with busulfan.
- Persistent cough and progressive dyspnea with alveolar exudate may result from drug toxicity, not pneumonia. Instruct patient to report symptoms so dosage adjustments can be made.
- To prevent hyperuricemia with resulting uric acid nephropathy, allopurinol may be used with adequate hydration. Monitor serum uric acid.
- Patient response usually begins within 1 to 2 weeks (increased appetite, sense of well-being, decreased total leukocyte count, reduction in size of spleen).
- Anticoagulants and aspirin products should be used cautiously. Watch closely for signs of bleeding. Instruct patient to avoid any OTC product containing aspirin.
- Avoid all I.M. injections when platelets are below 100,000/mm³.
- Therapeutic effects are often accompanied by toxicity.

carboplatin

Paraplatin

Pregnancy Risk Category: D

HOW SUPPLIED

Injection: 50-mg, 150-mg, 450-mg vials

MECHANISM OF ACTION

A non-cell-cycle-specific alkylating agent that produces cross-linking of strands of DNA.

INDICATIONS & DOSAGE

Palliative treatment of ovarian carcinoma –

Adults: 360 mg/m² I.V. on day 1 q 4 weeks; doses should not be repeated until platelet count exceeds 100,000/mm³ and neutrophil count exceeds 2,000/mm³. Subsequent doses are based on blood counts. Clinical trials have suggested the following dosage adjustments: if platelet count is above 100,000/mm³ and neutrophil count is above 2,000/mm³, dose administered should be 125% of the recommended starting dose. Dose should be reduced to 75% if platelet count falls below 50,000/mm³ or neutrophil count is below 500/mm³.

ADVERSE REACTIONS

Common reactions are in italics; life-threatening reactions are in bold italics.

Blood: ***thrombocytopenia, leukopenia, neutropenia, anemia.***

CNS: dizziness, confusion, peripheral neuropathy, ototoxicity, central neurotoxicity.

GI: constipation, diarrhea, *nausea, vomiting.*

Other: alopecia, hypersensitivity, hepatotoxicity, *increased BUN, creatinine, AST, or alkaline phosphatase.*

INTERACTIONS

Bone marrow depressants (including radiotherapy): increased hematologic toxicity.

Nephrotoxic agents: added nephrotoxicity of carboplatin.

NURSING CONSIDERATIONS

- *Contraindicated* in patients with a history of hypersensitivity to cisplatin, platinum-containing compounds, or mannitol. Carboplatin should be avoided in patients with severe bone marrow depression or bleeding.
- Administer this drug under the supervision of a doctor who is experienced in the use of chemotherapeutic agents.
- Determine serum electrolytes, creatinine, BUN, CBC, and creatinine clearance levels before the first infusion and before each course.
- Hydration or diuresis before or after treatment is not necessary.
- Transfusions may be necessary dur-

ing treatment because of cumulative anemia.
• Bone marrow depression may be more severe in patients with creatinine clearance below 60 ml/minute, and dosage adjustments are recommended for such patients. Patients with a creatinine clearance of 41 to 59 ml/minute should receive a starting dose of 250 mg/m²; patients with a creatinine clearance of 16 to 40 ml/minute should receive a starting dose of 200 mg/m². Recommended dosage adjustments are not available for patients with a creatinine clearance of 15 ml/minute or less.
• Patients over 65 years are at greater risk for neurotoxicity.
• Exercise extreme caution when preparing or administering carboplatin to avoid mutagenic, teratogenic, and carcinogenic risks. Use a biological containment cabinet, wear gloves and mask, and use syringes with Luer-Lok fittings to prevent leakage of drug solution. Also correctly dispose of needles, vials, and unused drug, and avoid contaminating work surfaces. Avoid inhalation of dust or vapors and contact with skin or mucous membranes.
• **I.V. use:** Reconstitute with dextrose 5% in water (D_5W), 0.9% sodium chloride solution, or sterile water for injection to make a concentration of 10 mg/ml. Add 5 ml diluent to the 50-mg vial, 15 ml diluent to the 150-mg vial, or 45 ml diluent to the 450-mg vial. It can then be further diluted for infusion with 0.9% sodium chloride solution or D_5W. A concentration as low as 0.5 mg/ml can be prepared. Drug may be given by continuous or intermittent infusion over at least 15 minutes.
• Do not use needles or I.V. administration sets containing aluminum because carboplatin may precipitate and lose potency.
• Carboplatin can produce severe vomiting. Administer antiemetic therapy as ordered.
• Monitor vital signs during infusion.
• Monitor CBC and platelet count frequently during therapy and, when indicated, until recovery. Leukocyte and platelet nadirs usually occur by day 21. Levels usually return to baseline by day 28. Don't repeat dose unless platelet count exceeds 100,000/mm³.
• Unopened vials should be stored at room temperature. Once reconstituted and diluted as directed, drug is stable at room temperature for 8 hours. Because the drug does not contain antibacterial preservatives, unused drug should be discarded after 8 hours.
• Check ordered dose against laboratory test results carefully. Only one increase in dosage is recommended. Subsequent doses should not exceed 125% of starting dose.
• Because of the possibility of infant toxicity, nursing mothers taking carboplatin should discontinue breast-feeding.
• Have epinephrine, corticosteroids, and antihistamines available when administering carboplatin because anaphylaxis-like reactions may occur within minutes of administration.
• Advise women of childbearing age to avoid becoming pregnant during therapy. Also recommend consulting with doctor before becoming pregnant.

carmustine (BCNU)
BiCNU

Pregnancy Risk Category: D

HOW SUPPLIED
Injection: 100-mg vial (lyophilized), with a 3-ml vial of absolute alcohol supplied as a diluent

MECHANISM OF ACTION
Cross-links strands of cellular DNA and interferes with RNA transcrip-

tion, causing an imbalance of growth that leads to cell death. Cell cycle-nonspecific.

INDICATIONS & DOSAGE

Brain, colon, and stomach cancer; Hodgkin's disease; non-Hodgkin's lymphomas; melanomas; multiple myeloma; and hepatoma –

Adults: 75 to 100 mg/m² I.V. by slow infusion daily for 2 days; repeat q 6 weeks if platelets are above 100,000/mm³ and WBC is above 4,000/mm³. Dosage is reduced by 30% when WBC is 2,000 to 3,000/mm³ and platelets are 25,000 to 75,000/mm³. Dosage is reduced by 50% when WBC is less than 2,000/mm³ and platelets are less than 25,000/mm³.

Alternative therapy: 200 mg/m² I.V. by slow infusion as a single dose, repeated q 6 to 8 weeks; or 40 mg/m² I.V. by slow infusion for 5 consecutive days, repeated q 6 weeks.

ADVERSE REACTIONS

Common reactions are in italics; life-threatening reactions are in bold italics.

Blood: ***cumulative bone marrow depression,*** *delayed 4 to 6 weeks, lasting 1 to 2 weeks;* ***leukopenia; thrombocytopenia.***

CNS: ataxia, drowsiness.

GI: *nausea, which begins in 2 to 6 hours (can be severe); vomiting.*

GU: nephrotoxicity.

Hepatic: hepatotoxicity.

Metabolic: possible hyperuricemia in lymphoma patients when rapid cell lysis occurs.

Skin: facial flushing.

Local: *intense pain at infusion site from venous spasm.*

Other: ***pulmonary fibrosis.***

INTERACTIONS

Cimetidine: may increase carmustine's bone marrow toxicity. Avoid combination if possible.

NURSING CONSIDERATIONS

- *Contraindicated* in patients with hypersensitivity to the drug. Drug should not be used or dosage reduced in hepatic or renal impairment, compromised hematologic status, or after recent exposure to cytotoxic or radiation therapy.
- Pulmonary toxicity appears to be dose-related. Baseline pulmonary function tests should be performed before therapy and periodically thereafter. Hepatic and renal function tests should also be performed periodically.
- Warn patient to watch for signs of infection (fever, sore throat, fatigue) and bleeding (easy bruising, nosebleeds, bleeding gums, melena). Take temperature daily.
- Monitor CBC.
- To reduce nausea, give antiemetic before administering.
- Don't mix with other drugs during administration.
- **I.V. use:** To reconstitute, dissolve 100 mg carmustine in 3 ml absolute alcohol provided by manufacturer. Dilute solution with 27 ml sterile water for injection. Resultant solution contains 3.3 mg carmustine/ml in 10% alcohol. Dilute in normal saline solution or dextrose 5% in water for I.V. infusion. Give at least 250 ml over 1 to 2 hours. To reduce pain on infusion, dilute further or slow infusion rate.
- Solution is unstable in plastic I.V. bags. Administer only in glass containers.
- May store reconstituted solution in refrigerator for 48 hours. May decompose at temperatures above 80° F (26.6° C).
- If powder liquefies or appears oily, it is a sign of decomposition. Discard.
- To prevent hyperuricemia with resulting uric acid nephropathy, allopurinol may be used with adequate hydration. Monitor serum uric acid.
- Avoid contact with skin, as carmus-

*Liquid form contains alcohol. **May contain tartrazine.

tine will cause a brown stain. If drug comes into contact with skin, wash off thoroughly.
• Anticoagulants and aspirin products should be used cautiously. Watch closely for signs of bleeding. Instruct patient to avoid any OTC product containing aspirin.
• Avoid all I.M. injections when platelets are below $100{,}000/mm^3$.
• Since carmustine crosses the blood-brain barrier, it may be used to treat primary brain tumors.
• Preparation of parenteral form is associated with carcinogenic, mutagenic, and teratogenic risks for personnel. Follow institutional policy to reduce risks.
• Therapeutic effects are often accompanied by toxicity.

chlorambucil

Leukeran

Pregnancy Risk Category: D

HOW SUPPLIED
Tablets: 2 mg

MECHANISM OF ACTION
Cross-links strands of cellular DNA and interferes with RNA transcription, causing an imbalance of growth that leads to cell death. Cell cycle-nonspecific.

INDICATIONS & DOSAGE
Chronic lymphocytic leukemia, diffuse lymphocytic lymphoma, nodular lymphocytic lymphoma, Hodgkin's disease, ovarian carcinoma, mycosis fungoides, polycythemia vera, nephrotic syndrome, testicular carcinoma –
Adults: 0.1 to 0.2 mg/kg P.O. daily for 3 to 6 weeks, then adjust for maintenance (usually 4 to 10 mg daily).
Children: 0.1 to 0.2 mg/kg P.O. daily or $4.5 mg/m^2$ daily as a single dose or in divided doses.

ADVERSE REACTIONS
Common reactions are in italics; life-threatening reactions are in bold italics.
Blood: ***leukopenia,*** delayed up to 3 weeks, lasting up to 10 days after last dose; ***thrombocytopenia; anemia;*** myelosuppression (usually moderate, gradual, and rapidly reversible).
CNS: seizures (with overdose).
GI: *nausea, vomiting, stomatitis*
GU: *azoospermia, infertility.*
Metabolic: hyperuricemia, hepatotoxicity (rare).
Respiratory: interstitial pneumonitis or ***pulmonary fibrosis*** (rare).
Skin: ***exfoliative dermatitis,*** rash.
Other: allergic febrile reaction.

INTERACTIONS
None significant.

NURSING CONSIDERATIONS
• *Contraindicated* in patients with hypersensitivity or resistance to previous therapy. Know that patients with hypersensitivity to melphalan may also have hypersensitivity to chlorambucil. Dosage adjustment is recommended in hematologic impairment.
• *Use cautiously* in patients with a history of seizures, head trauma, or use of epileptogenic drugs.
• Place patient on neutropenia precautions if WBC falls below $2{,}000/mm^3$ or granulocytes fall below $1{,}000/mm^3$.
• Severe neutropenia reversible up to cumulative dosage of 6.5 mg/kg in a single course.
• Warn patient to watch for signs of infection (fever, sore throat, fatigue) and bleeding (easy bruising, nosebleeds, bleeding gums, melena). Take temperature daily.
• Monitor CBC.
• To prevent hyperuricemia with resulting uric acid nephropathy, allopurinol may be used with adequate hydration. Monitor serum uric acid.

• Avoid all I.M. injections when platelets are below 100,000/mm³.
• Anticoagulants and aspirin products should be used cautiously. Watch closely for signs of bleeding. Instruct patient to avoid OTC products containing aspirin.
• Therapeutic effects are often accompanied by toxicity.

cisplatin (cis-platinum)

Platamine‡, Platinol AQ

Pregnancy Risk Category: D

HOW SUPPLIED

Injection: 10-mg, 50-mg vials

MECHANISM OF ACTION

Cross-links strands of cellular DNA and interferes with RNA transcription, causing an imbalance of growth that leads to cell death. Cell cycle-nonspecific.

INDICATIONS & DOSAGE

Adjunctive therapy in metastatic testicular cancer–

Adults: 20 mg/m² I.V. daily for 5 days. Repeat every 3 weeks for 3 cycles or longer.

Adjunctive therapy in metastatic ovarian cancer–

Adults: 100 mg/m² I.V. Repeat every 4 weeks; or 50 mg/m² I.V. every 3 weeks with concurrent doxorubicin therapy.

Treatment of advanced bladder cancer–

Adults: 50 to 70 mg/m² I.V. once every 3 to 4 weeks. Patients who have received other antineoplastics or radiation therapy should receive 50 mg/m² every 4 weeks.

Note: Prehydration and mannitol diuresis may reduce renal toxicity and ototoxicity significantly.

ADVERSE REACTIONS

Common reactions are in italics; life-threatening reactions are in bold italics.

Blood: *mild myelosuppression in 25% to 30% of patients,* ***leukopenia, thrombocytopenia, hypomagnesemia, hypocalcemia, anemia;*** nadirs in circulating platelets and leukocytes on days 18 to 23, with recovery by day 39.

CNS: peripheral neuritis, loss of taste, ***seizures.***

EENT: *tinnitus, hearing loss.*

GI: *nausea, vomiting, beginning 1 to 4 hours after dose and lasting 24 hours;* diarrhea; metallic taste.

GU: *more prolonged and severe renal toxicity with repeated courses of therapy.*

Other: ***anaphylactoid reaction.***

INTERACTIONS

Aminoglycoside antibiotics: additive nephrotoxicity. Monitor renal function studies very carefully.

Bumetanide, ethacrynic acid, furosemide: additive ototoxicity. Avoid concomitant use.

Phenytoin: decreased serum phenytoin levels. Monitor serum levels.

NURSING CONSIDERATIONS

• *Contraindicated* in patients with hypersensitivity to the drug or to carboplatin and in those with severe renal disease, hearing impairment, or myelosuppression.
• *Use cautiously* and with dosage modification as needed in preexisting renal impairment, myelosuppression, or hearing impairment.
• Hydrate patient with normal saline solution before giving drug. Maintain urine output of 100 ml/hour for 4 consecutive hours before therapy and for 24 hours after therapy.
• **I.V. use:** The manufacturer recommends that the drug be administered as an I.V. infusion in 2 liters normal saline solution with 37.5 g mannitol over 6 to 8 hours.
• Do not use needles or I.V. administration sets that contain aluminum because it will displace the platinum,

causing a loss of potency and formation of a black precipitate.
• Investigational protocols may include intense hydration of the patient with 0.9% sodium chloride. The cisplatin dose is then administered in 3% sodium chloride.
• Mannitol may be given as 12.5 g I.V. bolus before starting cisplatin infusion. Follow, if ordered, by infusion of mannitol at rate of up to 10 g/hour p.r.n. to maintain urine output during and 6 to 24 hours after cisplatin infusion.
• Some clinicians use I.V. sodium thiosulfate to minimize toxicity. Check current protocol.
• Do not repeat dosage unless platelets are over 100,000/mm³, WBC is over 4,000/mm³, creatinine is under 1.5 mg/dl, or BUN is under 25 mg/dl.
• Warn patient to watch for signs of infection (fever, sore throat, fatigue) and bleeding (easy bruising, nosebleeds, bleeding gums, melena). Take temperature daily.
• Monitor CBC, electrolytes (especially potassium and magnesium), platelets, and renal function studies before initial and subsequent dosages.
• To prevent deficiencies (10 to 20 mEq/L), potassium chloride is frequently added to I.V. fluids before and after cisplatin therapy.
• Tell patient to report tinnitus immediately to prevent permanent hearing loss. Do audiometry prior to initial dosage and subsequent courses.
• Nausea and vomiting may be severe and protracted (up to 24 hours). Administer antiemetics as ordered. Monitor intake and output. Continue I.V. hydration until patient can tolerate adequate oral intake.
• Ondansetron or high-dose metoclopramide has been used very effectively to treat and prevent nausea and vomiting. Some clinicians combine metoclopramide with dexamethasone and antihistamines.
• Delayed-onset vomiting (3 to 5 days after treatment) has been reported. Patients may need prolonged antiemetic treatment.
• Reconstitute with sterile water for injection. Stable for 24 hours in 0.9% sodium chloride solution at room temperature. Don't refrigerate.
• Infusions are most stable in chloride-containing solutions (such as 0.9% sodium chloride, 0.45% sodium chloride, and 0.22% sodium chloride).
• Given with bleomycin and vinblastine for testicular cancer and with doxorubicin for ovarian cancer.
• Renal toxicity is cumulative. Renal function must return to normal before next dose can be given.
• Avoid all I.M. injections when platelets are below 100,000/mm³.
• Anaphylactoid reaction usually responds to immediate treatment with epinephrine, corticosteroids, or antihistamines.
• Preparation of parenteral form is associated with carcinogenic, mutagenic, and teratogenic risks for personnel. Follow institutional policy to reduce risks.
• Therapeutic effects are often accompanied by toxicity.

cyclophosphamide

Cycoblastin‡, Cytoxan**, Cytoxan Lyophilized, Endoxan-Asta‡, Neosar, Procytox†

Pregnancy Risk Category: D

HOW SUPPLIED
Tablets: 25 mg, 50 mg
Injection: 100-mg, 200-mg, 500-mg, 1-g, 2-g vials

MECHANISM OF ACTION
Cross-links strands of cellular DNA and interferes with RNA transcription, causing an imbalance of growth that leads to cell death. Cell cycle-nonspecific.

INDICATIONS & DOSAGE

Breast, head, neck, lung, and ovarian cancer; Hodgkin's disease; chronic lymphocytic leukemia; chronic myelocytic leukemia; acute lymphoblastic leukemia; acute myelocytic leukemia; neuroblastoma; retinoblastoma; non-Hodgkin's lymphomas; multiple myeloma; mycosis fungoides; sarcomas; nephrotic syndrome –

Adults: initially, 40 to 50 mg/kg I.V. in divided doses over 2 to 5 days; then adjust for maintenance. Or 1 to 5 mg/kg P.O. daily, depending upon patient tolerance. Maintenance dosage is 1 to 5 mg/kg P.O. daily; or 10 to 15 mg/kg q 7 to 10 days I.V.; or 3 to 5 mg/kg I.V. twice weekly.

Children: 2 to 8 mg/kg daily or 60 to 250 mg/m² daily P.O. or I.V. for 6 days (dosage depends on susceptibility of neoplasm). Maintenance dosage is 2 to 5 mg/kg or 50 to 150 mg/m² P.O. twice weekly.

ADVERSE REACTIONS

Common reactions are in italics; life-threatening reactions are in bold italics.

Blood: ***leukopenia,*** nadir between days 8 to 15, recovery in 17 to 28 days; ***thrombocytopenia; anemia.***

CV: *cardiotoxicity* (with very high doses and in combination with doxorubicin).

GI: anorexia; *nausea and vomiting beginning within 6 hours, lasting 4 hours;* stomatitis; mucositis.

GU: gonadal suppression (may be irreversible), ***hemorrhagic cystitis,*** bladder fibrosis, nephrotoxicity.

Metabolic: hyperuricemia; syndrome of inappropriate antidiuretic hormone secretion (with high doses).

Other: *reversible alopecia in 50% of patients, especially with high doses;* secondary malignancies, ***pulmonary fibrosis*** (high doses), ***anaphylaxis.***

INTERACTIONS

Barbiturates: increased pharmacologic effect and enhanced cyclophosphamide toxicity due to induction of hepatic enzymes.

Cardiotoxic drugs: additive adverse cardiac effects.

Corticosteroids, chloramphenicol: reduced activity of cyclophosphamide. Use cautiously.

Digoxin: may decrease serum digoxin levels. Monitor levels closely.

Succinylcholine: prolonged neuromuscular blockade. Don't use together.

NURSING CONSIDERATIONS

- *Contraindicated* in patients with hypersensitivity to the drug. Repeat courses of the drug are contraindicated in patients in whom it causes hemorrhagic cystitis.
- *Use cautiously.* Dosage modification may be required in severe leukopenia, thrombocytopenia, malignant cell infiltration of bone marrow, recent radiation therapy or chemotherapy, or hepatic or renal disease.
- Advise both male and female patients to practice contraception while taking this drug and for 4 months after; drug is potentially teratogenic.
- Monitor CBC and renal and hepatic functions.
- Encourage fluid intake (3 liters daily) to prevent hemorrhagic cystitis. Don't give drug at bedtime, because voiding is too infrequent to avoid cystitis. If hemorrhagic cystitis occurs, discontinue drug. Cystitis can occur months after therapy has been stopped.
- Encourage patients to void every 1 to 2 hours while awake to minimize risk of hemorrhagic cystitis.
- Reconstituted solution is stable 6 days refrigerated or 24 hours at room temperature.
- Check reconstituted solution for small particles. Filter solution if necessary.
- Avoid all I.M. injections when platelets are below 100,000/mm³.
- **I.V. use:** Can be given by direct I.V.

*Liquid form contains alcohol. **May contain tartrazine.

push into a running I.V. line or by infusion in normal saline solution or dextrose 5% in water. Lyophilized preparation is much easier to reconstitute. Request this form from the pharmacy when preparing I.V.
• To prevent hyperuricemia with resulting uric acid nephropathy, allopurinol may be used with adequate hydration. Monitor serum uric acid.
• Warn patient that alopecia is likely to occur, but that it is reversible.
• Monitor for cyclophosphamide toxicity if patient's corticosteroid therapy is discontinued.
• Preparation of parenteral form is associated with carcinogenic, mutagenic, and teratogenic risks for personnel. Follow institutional policy to reduce risks.
• Therapeutic effects are often accompanied by toxicity.

dacarbazine (DTIC)

DTIC-Dome

Pregnancy Risk Category: C

HOW SUPPLIED

Injection: 100-mg, 200-mg vials

MECHANISM OF ACTION

Cross-links strands of cellular DNA and interferes with RNA transcription, causing an imbalance of growth that leads to cell death. Cell cycle-nonspecific.

INDICATIONS & DOSAGE

Metastatic malignant melanoma –
Adults: 2 to 4.5 mg/kg or 70 to 160 mg/m^2 I.V. daily for 10 days, then repeat q 4 weeks as tolerated; or 250 mg/m^2 I.V. daily for 5 days, repeated at 3-week intervals.
Hodgkin's disease –
Adults: 150 mg/m^2 I.V. daily (in combination with other agents) for 5 days, repeated q 4 weeks; or 375 mg/m^2 on the first day of a combination regimen, repeated q 15 days.

ADVERSE REACTIONS

Common reactions are in italics; life-threatening reactions are in bold italics.
Blood: ***leukopenia and thrombocytopenia,*** nadir between 3 and 4 weeks.
GI: *severe nausea and vomiting begin within 1 to 3 hours in 90% of patients, last 1 to 12 hours; anorexia.*
Metabolic: increased liver enzymes, hepatotoxicity (rare).
Skin: phototoxicity.
Local: severe pain if I.V. infiltrates or if solution is too concentrated; tissue damage.
Other: *flu-like syndrome* (fever, malaise, myalgia beginning 7 days after treatment stopped and possibly lasting 7 to 21 days), alopecia, ***anaphylaxis.***

INTERACTIONS

None significant.

NURSING CONSIDERATIONS

• *Contraindicated* in patients with hypersensitivity to the drug.
• *Use cautiously* at lower dosage if renal or bone marrow function is impaired. Stop drug if WBC falls to 3,000/mm^3 or platelets drop to 100,000/mm^3. Monitor CBC.
• Warn patient to watch for signs of infection (fever, sore throat, fatigue) and bleeding (easy bruising, nosebleeds, bleeding gums, melena). Take temperature daily.
• Discard refrigerated solution after 72 hours and room temperature solution after 8 hours.
• Avoid all I.M. injections when platelets are below 100,000/mm^3.
• **I.V. use:** Give I.V. infusion in 50 to 100 ml dextrose 5% in water over 30 minutes. During infusion, protect bag from direct sunlight to avoid possible drug breakdown. May dilute further or slow infusion to decrease pain at infusion site.
• Take care not to allow extravasation during infusion. If I.V. infiltrates, discontinue immediately and apply ice to area for 24 to 48 hours.

- For Hodgkin's disease, usually given with bleomycin, vinblastine, and doxorubicin.
- Advise patient to avoid sunlight and sunlamps for first 2 days after treatment.
- Anticoagulants and aspirin products should be used cautiously. Watch closely for signs of bleeding. Instruct patient to avoid OTC products containing aspirin.
- Administering antiemetics before giving dacarbazine may help decrease nausea. Nausea and vomiting may sometimes subside after several doses.
- Reassure patient that flulike syndrome may be treated with mild antipyretics, such as acetaminophen.
- Preparation of parenteral form is associated with carcinogenic, mutagenic, and teratogenic risks for personnel. Follow institutional policy to reduce risks.
- Therapeutic effects are often accompanied by toxicity.

ifosfamide

Ifex

Pregnancy Risk Category: D

HOW SUPPLIED

Injection: 1 g (supplied with 200-mg ampule of mesna), 2 g†, 3 g†

MECHANISM OF ACTION

Cross-links strands of cellular DNA, and interferes with RNA transcription causing an imbalance of growth that leads to cell death. Cell cycle-nonspecific.

INDICATIONS & DOSAGE

Testicular cancer–

Adults: 1.2 g/m²/day I.V. for 5 consecutive days. Treatment is repeated every 3 weeks or after the patient recovers from hematologic toxicity.

ADVERSE REACTIONS

Common reactions are in italics; life-threatening reactions are in bold italics.

Blood: ***leukopenia, thrombocytopenia, myelosuppression.***

CNS: *lethargy, somnolence, confusion, depressive psychosis,* ***coma.***

CV: supraventricular arrhythmias.

GI: *nausea, vomiting.*

GU: *hemorrhagic cystitis (dose-limiting adverse reaction occurring in up to 50% of patients), hematuria,* nephrotoxicity.

Hepatic: elevated liver enzymes.

Other: *alopecia.*

INTERACTIONS

Allopurinol: may produce excessive ifosfamide effect by prolonging half-life. Monitor for enhanced toxicity.

Barbiturates, phenytoin: induce hepatic enzymes, hastening the formation of toxic metabolites. Ifosfamide toxicity may be increased.

Corticosteroids: may inhibit hepatic enzymes, reducing ifosfamide's effect. Monitor for enhanced ifosfamide toxicity if concurrent steroid dosage is suddenly reduced or discontinued.

Myelosuppressants: enhanced hematologic toxicity. Dosage adjustment may be necessary.

NURSING CONSIDERATIONS

- *Contraindicated* in patients with hypersensitivity to the drug and in patients with severely depressed bone marrow function.
- *Use cautiously* in renal or hepatic impairment.
- Ifosfamide should be administered with a protecting agent (mesna) to prevent hemorrhagic cystitis. Adequate fluid intake (2 liters/day, either P.O. or I.V.) is essential.
- Obtain a urinalysis before each dose. If microscopic hematuria is present, the patient should be evaluated for hemorrhagic cystitis. Dosage adjustments of mesna may be necessary.
- Bladder irrigation with normal sa-

line solution may decrease the possibility of cystitis.
• Avoid giving the drug at bedtime, because infrequent voiding during the night may increase the possibility of cystitis. Stop the drug if patient develops cystitis.
• Warn patient to watch for signs of infection (fever, sore throat, fatigue) and bleeding (easy bruising, nosebleeds, bleeding gums, melena). Take temperature daily.
• Avoid all I.M. injections when platelets are below 100,000/mm^3.
• Anticoagulants and aspirin products should be used cautiously. Watch closely for signs of bleeding. Instruct patient to avoid OTC products containing aspirin.
• Administering antiemetics before giving ifosfamide may help decrease nausea.
• Assess patient for changes in mental status and cerebellar dysfunction. Dosage may have to be decreased.
• **I.V. use:** Prepare I.V. solution by reconstituting 1-g vial with 20 ml sterile water for injection or bacteriostatic water for injection to yield a solution of 50 mg/ml. It may then be further diluted with sterile water, dextrose 2.5% or 5% in water, 0.45% or 0.9% sodium chloride injection, 5% dextrose and 0.9% sodium chloride injection, or lactated Ringer's injection.
• Infusing each dose slowly (over at least 30 minutes) will decrease possibility of cystitis.
• Reconstituted solution is stable 1 week at room temperature or 3 weeks refrigerated. However, use solution within 6 hours if drug was reconstituted with sterile water without a preservative (such as benzyl alcohol or parabens).
• Monitor CBC and renal and liver function tests.
• Monitor patient for CNS changes.
• Preparation of parenteral form is associated with carcinogenic, mutagenic, and teratogenic risks for personnel. Follow institutional policy to reduce risks.

lomustine (CCNU)
CeeNU

Pregnancy Risk Category: D

HOW SUPPLIED
Capsules: 10 mg, 40 mg, 100 mg, dose pack (2 100-mg, 2 40-mg, 2 10-mg capsules)

MECHANISM OF ACTION
Cross-links strands of cellular DNA and interferes with RNA transcription, causing an imbalance of growth that leads to cell death. Cell cycle-nonspecific.

INDICATIONS & DOSAGE
Brain tumors, Hodgkin's disease –
Adults and children: 130 mg/m^2 P.O. as a single dose q 6 weeks. Reduce dosage according to degree of bone marrow suppression. Repeat doses should not be given until WBC is more than 4,000/mm^3 and platelet count is more than 100,000/mm^3.

ADVERSE REACTIONS
Common reactions are in italics; life-threatening reactions are in bold italics.
Blood: ***anemia, leukopenia,*** *delayed up to 6 weeks, lasting 1 to 2 weeks;* ***thrombocytopenia,*** *delayed up to 4 weeks, lasting 1 to 2 weeks.*
GI: *nausea and vomiting beginning within 4 to 5 hours, lasting 24 hours;* stomatitis.
GU: nephrotoxicity, progressive azotemia.

INTERACTIONS
None significant.

NURSING CONSIDERATIONS
• *Contraindicated* in patients with hypersensitivity to the drug.
• *Use cautiously.* Dosage modification may be required in patients with

decreased platelets, leukocytes, or erythrocytes, and in patients receiving other myelosuppressive drugs.

- Give 2 to 4 hours after meals. Lomustine will be more completely absorbed if taken when the stomach is empty. To avoid nausea, give antiemetic before administering.
- May be useful in cancer involving CNS, since cerebrospinal fluid level equals 30% to 50% of plasma level 1 hour after administration.
- Monitor CBC weekly. Usually not administered more often than every 6 weeks; bone marrow toxicity is cumulative and delayed.
- Warn patient to watch for signs of infection (fever, sore throat, fatigue) and bleeding (easy bruising, nosebleeds, bleeding gums, melena). Take temperature daily.
- Periodically monitor liver function.
- Avoid all I.M. injections when platelets are below 100,000/mm³.
- Anticoagulants and aspirin products should be used cautiously. Watch closely for signs of bleeding. Instruct patient to avoid OTC products containing aspirin.
- Therapeutic effects are often accompanied by toxicity.

mechlorethamine hydrochloride (nitrogen mustard)

Mustargen

Pregnancy Risk Category: D

HOW SUPPLIED

Injection: 10-mg vials

MECHANISM OF ACTION

Cross-links strands of cellular DNA and interferes with RNA transcription, causing an imbalance of growth that leads to cell death. Cell cycle-nonspecific.

INDICATIONS & DOSAGE

Polycythemia vera, chronic lymphocytic leukemia, chronic myelocytic leukemia, malignant effusions (pericardial, peritoneal, pleural), mycosis fungoides, Hodgkin's disease, non-Hodgkin's lymphomas, diffuse lymphocytic lymphoma –

Adults: 0.4 mg/kg or 10 mg/m² I.V. as a single dose or in divided doses q 3 to 6 weeks. Give through running I.V. infusion. Dosage reduced in prior radiation or chemotherapy to 0.2 to 0.4 mg/kg. Dosage based on ideal or actual body weight, whichever is less.

Neoplastic effusions –

Adults: 0.2 to 0.4 mg/kg intracavitarily.

Mycosis fungoides –

Adults: topical solution or ointment applied to lesion. Topical preparations must be compounded by pharmacist; drug concentration, frequency of application, and duration of therapy will vary according to patient tolerance and response. Mechlorethamine ointments of 0.01% to 0.02% and topical solutions containing 10 mg/50 to 60 ml have been used.

ADVERSE REACTIONS

Common reactions are in italics; life-threatening reactions are in bold italics.

Blood: ***thrombocytopenia, granulocytopenia, lymphocytopenia,*** *nadir of* ***myelosuppression*** *occurring by days 4 to 10, lasting 10 to 21 days;* mild anemia begins in 2 to 3 weeks, possibly lasting 7 weeks.

CNS: headache, weakness, drowsiness, vertigo, light-headedness, ***seizures,*** progressive paralysis, paresthesia, ***cerebral degeneration, coma.***

EENT: tinnitus; *metallic taste* (immediately after dose); deafness with high doses.

GI: *nausea, vomiting, and anorexia* begin within minutes, last 8 to 24 hours.

Metabolic: hyperuricemia.

Skin: rash.

*Liquid form contains alcohol. **May contain tartrazine.

Local: *thrombophlebitis, sloughing, severe irritation if drug extravasates or touches skin.*
Other: *alopecia,* may precipitate herpes zoster, ***anaphylaxis.***

INTERACTIONS
Procarbazine, cyclophosphamide: possible increased risk of hepatotoxicity.

NURSING CONSIDERATIONS
- *Contraindicated* in patients with hypersensitivity to the drug. Drug should not be used in patients with acute or chronic suppurative inflammation because it may promote the rapid development of amyloidosis. The manufacturer states that the drug is contraindicated in patients with known infectious diseases.
- *Use cautiously.* Dosage modification may be required in severe anemia, depressed neutrophil or platelet count, or in patients recently treated with radiation or chemotherapy. Monitor CBC.
- Neurotoxicity increases with dose and patient age.
- Avoid contact with skin or mucous membranes. Wear gloves when preparing solution to prevent accidental skin contact. If contact occurs, wash with copious amounts of water.
- **I.V. use:** Mechlorethamine is a potent vesicant. Be sure I.V. doesn't infiltrate. If drug extravasates, apply cold compresses and infiltrate the area with isotonic sodium thiosulfate.
- Very unstable solution. Prepare immediately before infusion. Visually inspect before using. Use within 15 minutes. Discard unused solution.
- Do not use solutions that are discolored or contain particulate matter. Do not use vials that appear to contain droplets of water.
- When given intracavitarily for sclerosing effect, turn patient from side to side every 15 minutes to 1 hour to distribute drug.
- To prevent hyperuricemia with resulting uric acid nephropathy, mechlorethamine may be used with adequate hydration. Monitor serum uric acid.
- Avoid all I.M. injections when platelets are below 100,000/mm^3.
- Warn patient to watch for signs of infection (fever, sore throat, fatigue) and bleeding (easy bruising, nosebleeds, bleeding gums, melena). Take temperature daily.
- Anticoagulants and aspirin products should be used cautiously. Watch closely for signs of bleeding. Instruct patient to avoid OTC products containing aspirin.
- Any equipment used in the preparation and administration of mechlorethamine should be disposed of properly and according to institutional policy. Unused solution should be neutralized with an equal volume of 5% sodium bicarbonate and 5% sodium thiosulfate.
- Preparation of parenteral form is associated with carcinogenic, mutagenic, and teratogenic risks for personnel. Follow institutional policy to reduce risks.
- Therapeutic effects are often accompanied by toxicity.

melphalan (L-phenylalanine mustard)
Alkeran

Pregnancy Risk Category: D

HOW SUPPLIED
Tablets (scored): 2 mg
Injection: 50 mg

MECHANISM OF ACTION
Cross-links strands of cellular DNA and interferes with RNA transcription, causing an imbalance of growth that leads to cell death. Cell cycle-nonspecific.

INDICATIONS & DOSAGE

Multiple myeloma –

Adults: initially, 6 mg P.O. daily for 2 to 3 weeks, then stop drug for up to 4 weeks or until WBC and platelets stop dropping and begin to rise again; resume with maintenance dosage of 2 mg daily. Stop drug if WBC is below 3,000/mm^3 or platelets are below 100,000/mm^3. Alternative therapy: 0.15 mg/kg P.O. daily for 7 days, or 0.25 mg/kg for 4 days; repeat q 4 to 6 weeks.

Alternatively, administer I.V. to patients who can't tolerate oral therapy. Give 16 mg/m^2 by infusion over 15 to 20 minutes. Give at 2-week intervals for four doses. After patient has recovered from toxicity, drug is given at 4-week intervals.

Nonresectable advanced ovarian cancer –

Adults: 0.2 mg/kg P.O. daily for 5 days. Repeat q 4 to 5 weeks, depending on bone marrow recovery.

ADVERSE REACTIONS

Common reactions are in italics; life-threatening reactions are in bold italics.

Blood: ***thrombocytopenia, leukopenia, agranulocytosis.***

Skin: dermatitis, pruritus, rash, alopecia.

Other: ***pneumonitis and pulmonary fibrosis, anaphylaxis.***

INTERACTIONS

Carmustine: I.V. melphalan may lower the threshold for carmustine lung toxicity. Monitor closely.

Cisplatin: may alter renal clearance of melphalan by causing nephrotoxicity. Monitor renal function; adjust dosage as ordered.

Cyclosporine: severe renal failure has been reported in patients who followed a single I.V. dose of melphalan with standard doses of cyclosporine. Avoid use.

Nalidixic acid: increased incidence of severe hemorrhagic necrotic enterocolitis in pediatric patients. Avoid use.

NURSING CONSIDERATIONS

- *Contraindicated* in patients with hypersensitivity to the drug and in patients whose disease is known to be resistant to the drug. Know that patients with hypersensitivity to chlorambucil may exhibit cross-sensitivity to melphalan.
- Not recommended in severe leukopenia, thrombocytopenia, or anemia; or in chronic lymphocytic leukemia.
- Monitor serum uric acid and CBC.
- Avoid all I.M. injections when platelets are below 100,000/mm^3.
- May need dosage reduction in renal impairment.
- Therapeutic effects are often accompanied by toxicity.
- Drug of choice in multiple myeloma in combination with prednisone.
- Anticoagulants and aspirin products should be used cautiously. Watch closely for signs of bleeding. Instruct patient to avoid OTC products containing aspirin.
- Administer on empty stomach, because absorption is decreased by food.
- Warn patient to watch for signs of infection (fever, sore throat, fatigue) and bleeding (easy bruising, nosebleeds, bleeding gums, melena). Take temperature daily.
- **I.V. use:** Because drug isn't stable in solution, reconstitute immediately before administering. Reconstitute drug with the 10 ml of sterile diluent supplied by the manufacturer. Shake vigorously until a clear solution is obtained. The resultant solution will contain 5 mg melphalan/ml. Immediately dilute the required dose in 0.9% sodium chloride injection. Final concentration shouldn't exceed 0.45 mg/ml. Give I.V. infusion over 15 to 20 minutes.
- Understand the importance of prompt dilution and administration.

Within 30 minutes, the reconstituted product begins to degrade. After final dilution, nearly 1% of the drug degrades every 10 minutes. Don't refrigerate the reconstituted product because a precipitate will form.
• Follow institutional guidelines for the safe handling, preparation, administration, and disposal of chemotherapeutic drugs.

streptozocin
Zanosar
Pregnancy Risk Category: C

HOW SUPPLIED
Injection: 1-g vials

MECHANISM OF ACTION
Cross-links strands of cellular DNA and interferes with RNA transcription, causing an imbalance of growth that leads to cell death. Cell cycle-nonspecific.

INDICATIONS & DOSAGE
Treatment of Hodgkin's disease, metastatic islet cell carcinoma of the pancreas; colon cancer; exocrine pancreatic tumors; and carcinoid tumors –
Adults and children: 500 mg/m² I.V. for 5 consecutive days q 6 weeks until maximum benefit or until toxicity is observed. Alternatively, 1,000 mg/m² at weekly intervals for the first 2 weeks. Don't exceed a single dose of 1,500 mg/m².

ADVERSE REACTIONS
Common reactions are in italics; life-threatening reactions are in bold italics.
Blood: ***anemia, leukopenia, thrombocytopenia.***
GI: *nausea, vomiting,* diarrhea.
Hepatic: elevated liver enzymes.
Metabolic: hyperglycemia and hypoglycemia.
Renal: *renal toxicity (evidenced by azotemia, glycosuria, and renal tubular acidosis),* mild proteinuria.
Local: *sloughing, severe irritation if extravasation occurs.*

INTERACTIONS
Doxorubicin: prolonged elimination half-life of doxorubicin if administered with streptozocin. Dose of doxorubicin should be reduced.
Other potentially nephrotoxic drugs such as aminoglycosides: increased risk of renal toxicity. Use cautiously.
Phenytoin: may decrease the effectiveness of streptozocin in pancreatic cancer. Monitor carefully.

NURSING CONSIDERATIONS
• *Contraindicated* in patients with hypersensitivity to the drug.
• *Use cautiously.* Dosage modification may be required in patients with preexisting renal or hepatic disease.
• Renal toxicity resulting from streptozocin therapy is dose-related and cumulative. Monitor renal function before and after each course of therapy. Urinalysis, BUN, creatinine, serum electrolytes, and creatinine clearance should be obtained before, and at least weekly during, drug administration. Weekly monitoring should continue for 4 weeks after each course.
• Mild proteinuria is one of the first signs of renal toxicity. Make sure doctor is aware if and when this occurs. The dosage of the drug may have to be reduced.
• Test urine for protein and glucose each nursing shift.
• Monitor CBC and liver function studies at least weekly.
• Warn patient to watch for signs of infection (fever, sore throat, fatigue) and bleeding (easy bruising, nosebleeds, bleeding gums, melena). Take temperature daily.
• Nausea and vomiting occurs in almost *all* patients. Make sure patient is being treated with an antiemetic.

• **I.V. use:** Reconstitute the streptozocin powder with 0.9% sodium chloride injection. This will produce a pale gold solution. Best to use within 12 hours of reconstitution.
• The product contains no preservatives and is not intended as a multiple-dose vial.
• When preparing the solution, wear gloves to protect the skin from contact. If contact occurs, wash with copious amounts of water.
• If extravasation occurs, stop infusion immediately.
• Unopened and unreconstituted vials of streptozocin should be stored in the refrigerator.
• Preparation of parenteral form is associated with carcinogenic, mutagenic, and teratogenic risks for personnel. Follow institutional policy to reduce risks.
• Therapeutic effects are often accompanied by toxicity.

thiotepa

Thiotepa

Pregnancy Risk Category: D

HOW SUPPLIED

Injection: 15-mg vials

MECHANISM OF ACTION

Cross-links strands of cellular DNA and interferes with RNA transcription, causing an imbalance of growth that leads to cell death. Cell cycle-nonspecific.

INDICATIONS & DOSAGE

Breast and ovarian cancer; lymphomas and bronchogenic carcinomas –
Adults and children over 12 years: 0.2 mg/kg I.V. daily for 4 to 5 days at intervals of 2 to 4 weeks.
Bladder tumor –
Adults and children over 12 years: 60 mg in 60 ml water instilled in bladder for 2 hours once weekly for 4 weeks.
Neoplastic effusions –
Adults and children over 12 years: 0.6 to 0.8 mg/kg intracavitarily, p.r.n. Stop drug or decrease dosage if WBC is below 4,000/mm^3 or if platelets are below 150,000/mm^3.
Malignant meningeal neoplasms –
Adults: 1 to 10 mg/m^2 intrathecally once or twice weekly.

ADVERSE REACTIONS

Common reactions are in italics; life-threatening reactions are in bold italics.
Blood: ***leukopenia** **begins within 5 to 30 days; thrombocytopenia; neutropenia, anemia.***
GI: *nausea, vomiting.*
GU: amenorrhea, decreased spermatogenesis.
Metabolic: hyperuricemia.
Skin: hives, rash.
Local: intense pain at administration site.
Other: headache, fever, tightness of throat, dizziness, alopecia.

INTERACTIONS

Succinylcholine: prolonged neuromuscular blockade. Monitor carefully.

NURSING CONSIDERATIONS

• *Contraindicated* in patients with hypersensitivity to the drug and in patients with severe bone marrow, hepatic, or renal dysfunction.
• *Use cautiously* in bone marrow suppression and renal or hepatic dysfunction.
• Monitor CBC weekly for at least 3 weeks after last dosage. Warn patient to report even mild infections.
• GU adverse reactions reversible in 6 to 8 months.
• May require use of local anesthetic at injection site if intense pain occurs.
• For bladder instillation: Dehydrate patient 8 to 10 hours before therapy. Instill drug into bladder by catheter; ask patient to retain solution for 2 hours. Volume may be reduced to 30

*Liquid form contains alcohol. **May contain tartrazine.

ml if discomfort is too great with 60 ml. Reposition patient every 15 minutes for maximum area contact.

• Toxicity delayed and prolonged because drug binds to tissues and stays in body several hours.
• To prevent hyperuricemia with resulting uric acid nephropathy, allopurinol may be used with adequate hydration. Monitor serum uric acid.
• Avoid all I.M. injections when platelets are below 100,000/mm^3.
• Warn patient to watch for signs of infection (fever, sore throat, fatigue) and bleeding (easy bruising, nosebleeds, bleeding gums, melena). Take temperature daily.
• Can be given by all parenteral routes, including direct injection into the tumor.
• **I.V. use:** Refrigerate and protect dry powder from direct sunlight to avoid possible drug breakdown. Exercise caution when preparing and administering this drug to avoid mutagenic, teratogenic, and carcinogenic risks. Use a biological containment cabinet, gloves, and mask, and avoid contaminating work surfaces. Reconstitute with sterile water for injection only. Discard refrigerated solution after 5 days. When administering the drug, if pain occurs at the insertion site, dilute the drug further or use a local anesthetic to reduce pain at infusion site. Make sure drug does not infiltrate.
• Anticoagulants and aspirin products should be used cautiously. Watch closely for signs of bleeding. Instruct patient to avoid OTC products containing aspirin.
• Therapeutic effects are often accompanied by toxicity.

uracil mustard

Uracil Mustard Capsules**

Pregnancy Risk Category: X

HOW SUPPLIED

Capsules: 1 mg

MECHANISM OF ACTION

Cross-links strands of cellular DNA and interferes with RNA transcription, causing an imbalance of growth that leads to cell death. Cell cycle-nonspecific.

INDICATIONS & DOSAGE

Chronic lymphocytic and myelocytic leukemia; Hodgkin's disease; non-Hodgkin's lymphomas of the histiocytic and lymphocytic types; reticulum cell sarcoma; lymphomas; mycosis fungoides; polycythemia vera; cancer of ovaries, cervix, and lungs – **Adults:** 1 to 2 mg P.O. daily for 3 months or until desired response or toxicity; maintenance dosage is 1 mg daily for 3 out of 4 weeks until optimum response or relapse; or 3 to 5 mg P.O. for 7 days not to exceed total dosage of 0.5 mg/kg, then 1 mg daily until response, then 1 mg daily 3 out of 4 weeks.

ADVERSE REACTIONS

Common reactions are in italics; life-threatening reactions are in bold italics.

Blood: bone marrow suppression, delayed 2 to 4 weeks; ***thrombocytopenia; leukopenia; anemia.***

CNS: irritability, nervousness, mental cloudiness, and depression.

GI: *nausea, vomiting, diarrhea, epigastric distress,* abdominal pain, anorexia.

Metabolic: hyperuricemia.

Skin: pruritus, dermatitis, hyperpigmentation, alopecia.

INTERACTIONS

None significant.

NURSING CONSIDERATIONS

• *Contraindicated* in patients with hypersensitivity to the drug and in patients with aplastic anemia, thrombocytopenia, or leukopenia.
• *Use cautiously.* Dosage modification may be required in patients with bone marrow suppression.

- Some commercially available capsules contain tartrazine dye, which may provoke allergic reactions in certain individuals. This reaction is rare but is more likely to occur in aspirin-sensitive persons.
- Give at bedtime to reduce nausea.
- Warn patient to watch for signs of infection (fever, sore throat, fatigue) and bleeding (easy bruising, nosebleeds, bleeding gums, melena). Take temperature daily.
- Monitor platelet count. Check CBC once or twice weekly for 4 weeks; then 4 weeks after stopping drug.
- To prevent hyperuricemia and resulting uric acid nephropathy, allopurinol may be used with adequate hydration. Monitor serum uric acid.
- Avoid all I.M. injections when platelets are below 100,000/mm^3.
- Warn patient to watch for signs of infection (fever, sore throat, fatigue) and bleeding (easy bruising, nosebleeds, bleeding gums, melena). Take temperature daily.
- Anticoagulants and aspirin products should be used cautiously. Watch closely for signs of bleeding. Instruct patient to avoid OTC products containing aspirin.
- Therapeutic effects are often accompanied by toxicity.

*Liquid form contains alcohol. **May contain tartrazine.

69

Antimetabolites

cladribine
cytarabine
floxuridine
fludarabine phosphate
fluorouracil
hydroxyurea
mercaptopurine
methotrexate
methotrexate sodium
thioguanine

COMBINATION PRODUCTS
None.

cladribine (2-chlorodeoxyadenosine)
Leustatin

Pregnancy Risk Category: D

HOW SUPPLIED
Injection: 1 mg/ml

MECHANISM OF ACTION
A purine nucleoside analog that enters tumor cells, is phosphorylated by deoxycytidine kinase, and is subsequently converted into an active triphosphate deoxynucleotide. This metabolite impairs synthesis of new DNA, inhibits repair of existing DNA, and disrupts cellular metabolism.

INDICATIONS & DOSAGE
Active hairy cell leukemia –
Adults: 0.09 mg/kg daily by continuous I.V. infusion for 7 days.

ADVERSE REACTIONS
Common reactions are in italics; life-threatening reactions are in bold italics.
Blood: ***severe neutropenia, anemia; thrombocytopenia,*** purpura, petechiae.
CNS: *headache, fatigue, dizziness, insomnia.*
CV: *tachycardia, edema.*
EENT: epistaxis.
GI: *nausea, decreased appetite, vomiting, diarrhea, constipation, abdominal pain.*
Respiratory: *abnormal breath or chest sounds, cough, shortness of breath.*
Skin: *rash, pruritus, pain, erythema.*
Other: *fever,* ***infection,*** *local reactions at the injection site, chills, asthenia, diaphoresis, malaise, trunk pain, myalgia, arthralgia.*

INTERACTIONS
None reported.

NURSING CONSIDERATIONS
- *Contraindicated in* patients with hypersensitivity to the drug.
- *Use cautiously* in patients with preexisting bone marrow suppression or renal or hepatic impairment. If possible, avoid using drug in patients with active infections.
- Cladribine is a toxic drug, and some toxicity is expected during treatment. Close monitoring of hematologic function, especially during the first 4 to 8 weeks of therapy, is recommended. Severe bone marrow suppression, including neutropenia, anemia, and thrombocytopenia, have been commonly observed in patients treated with this drug; many patients also have preexisting hematologic impairment from their disease.
- Fever is commonly observed during the first month of therapy. In clinical trials, virtually all patients received parenteral antibiotics.
- Because of the risk of fetal malformations, advise women of childbearing age to avoid becoming pregnant.

• **I.V. use:** For a 24-hour infusion, add the calculated dose to a 500-ml infusion bag of 0.9% sodium chloride injection and infuse over 24 hours. Once diluted, administer promptly or begin administration within 8 hours. Don't use solutions that contain dextrose because studies have shown increased degradation of the drug. Because the drug product doesn't contain any bacteriostatic agents, use strict aseptic technique to prepare the admixture. Repeat daily for 7 consecutive days.
• Alternatively, prepare a 7-day infusion using bacteriostatic sodium chloride injection, which contains 0.9% benzyl alcohol. Studies have shown acceptable physical and chemical stability using Pharmacia Deltec medication cassettes. First, pass the calculated amount of drug through a disposable 0.22-micron hydrophilic syringe filter into a sterile infusion reservoir. Next, add sufficient bacteriostatic sodium chloride injection to bring the total volume to 100 ml. Clamp off the line, then disconnect and discard the filter. If necessary, aseptically aspirate air bubbles from the reservoir using a new filter or a sterile vent filter assembly.
• Because the calculated dose dilutes the benzyl alcohol preservative, 7-day infusion solutions prepared for patients weighing more than 187 lb (85 kg) may have reduced preservative effectiveness.
• Refrigerate unopened vials at 36° to 46° F (2° to 8° C) and protect from light. Although freezing doesn't adversely affect the drug, a precipitate may form; this will disappear if the drug is allowed to warm to room temperature gradually and the vial is vigorously shaken. Don't heat or microwave; don't refreeze.
• Cladribine has also been used to treat advanced cutaneous T-cell lymphomas, chronic lymphocytic leukemia, malignant lymphomas, acute myeloid leukemias, mycosis fungoides, and Sézary syndrome.

cytarabine (ara-C, cytosine arabinoside)

Alexan‡, Cytosar-U, Tarabine PFS

Pregnancy Risk Category: D

HOW SUPPLIED

Injection: 40-mg‡, 100-mg, 500-mg, 1-g, 2-g vials

MECHANISM OF ACTION

Inhibits DNA synthesis.

INDICATIONS & DOSAGE

Acute myelocytic and other acute leukemias, non-Hodgkin's lymphoma –
Adults and children: 200 mg/m² daily by continuous I.V. infusion for 5 days. Repeat every 2 weeks.
Meningeal leukemias and meningeal neoplasms –
Adults and children: 10 to 30 mg/m² intrathecally once every 4 days.

ADVERSE REACTIONS

Common reactions are in italics; life-threatening reactions are in bold italics.
Blood: ***leukopenia,*** *WBC nadir 7 to 9 days after drug stopped;* anemia, reticulocytopenia; ***thrombocytopenia,*** platelet nadir occurring on day 10; *megaloblastosis.*
CNS: neurotoxicity with high doses.
EENT: *keratitis.*
GI: *nausea, vomiting,* diarrhea, dysphagia; reddened area at juncture of lips, followed by sore mouth, oral ulcers in 5 to 10 days; high dose given via rapid I.V. may cause projectile vomiting.
Hepatic: hepatotoxicity (usually mild and reversible).
Metabolic: hyperuricemia.
Skin: rash.
Other: flulike syndrome.

INTERACTIONS

Digoxin: serum digoxin levels may decrease. Monitor closely.

NURSING CONSIDERATIONS

- *Contraindicated* in patients with hypersensitivity to the drug.
- *Use cautiously.* Dosage modification may be required in thrombocytopenia, leukopenia, renal or hepatic disease, and after other chemotherapy or radiation therapy.
- Watch for signs of infection (cough, fever, sore throat) and bleeding (easy bruising, nosebleeds, bleeding gums). Monitor CBC.
- Excellent mouth care can help prevent stomatitis.
- **I.V. use:** Nausea and vomiting more frequent when large doses are administered rapidly by I.V. push. These reactions are less frequent with infusion. To reduce nausea, give antiemetic before administering.
- Steroid eye drops are prescribed to prevent drug-induced keratitis.
- Monitor intake and output carefully. Maintain high fluid intake and give allopurinol, if ordered, to avoid urate nephropathy in leukemia induction therapy. Monitor serum uric acid.
- Monitor hepatic and renal function.
- Use preservative-free 0.9% sodium chloride or Elliot's B solution for intrathecal use.
- Reconstituted solution is stable for 48 hours. Discard cloudy reconstituted solution.
- Avoid I.M. injections of any drugs in patients with thrombocytopenia to prevent bleeding.
- Warn patient to watch for signs of infection (fever, sore throat, fatigue) and bleeding (easy bruising, nosebleeds, bleeding gums, melena). Take temperature daily.
- Modify or discontinue therapy if polymorphonuclear granulocyte count is below 1,000/mm³ or if platelet count is below 50,000/mm³.
- Assess patients receiving high doses for neurotoxicity. May first appear as nystagmus, but can progress to ataxia and cerebellar dysfunction.
- Preparation of parenteral form is associated with carcinogenic, mutagenic, and teratogenic risks for personnel. Follow institutional policy to reduce risks.

floxuridine

FUDR

Pregnancy Risk Category: D

HOW SUPPLIED

Injection: 500-mg vials (50 mg/ml in 10-ml vials or 100 mg/ml in 5-ml vials)

MECHANISM OF ACTION

Inhibits DNA synthesis.

INDICATIONS & DOSAGE

Brain, breast, head, neck, liver, gallbladder, and bile duct cancer –
Adults: 0.1 to 0.6 mg/kg daily by intra-arterial infusion (use pump for continuous, uniform rate); or 0.4 to 0.6 mg/kg daily into hepatic artery.

ADVERSE REACTIONS

Common reactions are in italics; life-threatening reactions are in bold italics.
Blood: ***leukopenia, anemia,*** thrombocytopenia.
CNS: cerebellar ataxia, vertigo, nystagmus, seizures, depression, hemiplegia, hiccups, lethargy.
EENT: blurred vision.
GI: *anorexia, stomatitis, cramps, nausea, vomiting, diarrhea, bleeding, enteritis.*
Hepatic: cholangitis, jaundice, elevated liver enzymes.
Skin: *erythema,* dermatitis, pruritus, rash.

INTERACTIONS

None significant.

NURSING CONSIDERATIONS

• *Contraindicated* in patients with poor nutritional state, bone marrow suppression, or serious infection.
• *Use cautiously* following high-dose pelvic irradiation or use of alkylating agent, and in impaired hepatic or renal function.
• Severe skin and GI adverse reactions require stopping drug. Use of antacid eases but probably won't prevent GI distress.
• Excellent mouth care can help prevent stomatitis.
• Monitor intake and output, CBC, and renal and hepatic function.
• Discontinue if WBC falls below 3,500/mm³ or if platelet count falls below 100,000/mm³.
• Therapeutic effect may be delayed 1 to 6 weeks. Make sure patient is aware of time it may take for improvement to be noted.
• Reconstitute with sterile water for injection. Dilute further in dextrose 5% in water or 0.9% sodium chloride solution for actual infusion.
• Avoid I.M. injections of any drugs in patients with thrombocytopenia to prevent bleeding.
• Use an infusion pump with intra-arterial infusions.
• Refrigerated solution is stable for no more than 2 weeks.
• Check line for bleeding, blockage, displacement, or leakage.
• Preparation of parenteral form is associated with carcinogenic, mutagenic, and teratogenic risks for personnel. Follow institutional policy to reduce risks.

fludarabine phosphate

Fludara

Pregnancy Risk Category: D

HOW SUPPLIED

Powder for injection: 50 mg

MECHANISM OF ACTION

An antineoplastic antimetabolite whose exact mechanism of action is not fully established and may be multifaceted. After conversion to its active metabolite, fludarabine interferes with DNA synthesis by inhibiting DNA polymerase alpha, ribonucleotide reductase, and DNA primase.

INDICATIONS & DOSAGE

B-cell chronic lymphocytic leukemia (CLL) in patients who have either not responded or responded inadequately to at least one standard alkylating agent regimen –

Adults: 25 mg/m² I.V. over 30 minutes for 5 consecutive days. Repeat cycle q 28 days.

ADVERSE REACTIONS

Common reactions are in italics; life-threatening reactions are in bold italics.

Blood: ***myelosuppression.***

CNS: *fatigue, malaise, weakness,* paresthesia, headache, sleep disorder, depression, cerebellar syndrome, transient ischemic attack, agitation, *confusion;* ***coma, death*** (with high doses).

CV: *edema,* angina, phlebitis, ***arrhythmias, CHF,*** supraventricular tachycardia, deep venous thrombosis, ***aneurysm, CVA,*** hemorrhage.

EENT: *visual disturbances,* hearing loss; delayed blindness (with high doses); sinusitis, pharyngitis, epistaxis.

GI: *nausea, vomiting,* diarrhea, constipation, *anorexia,* stomatitis, GI bleeding, esophagitis, mucositis.

GU: dysuria, urinary infection, urinary hesitancy, proteinuria, hematuria, ***renal failure.***

Respiratory: cough, *pneumonia,* dyspnea, upper respiratory infection, allergic pneumonitis, hemoptysis, hypoxia, bronchitis.

Skin: rash, pruritus, seborrhea.

Other: *fever, chills, infection,* pain, myalgia, tumor lysis syndrome, alo-

*Liquid form contains alcohol. **May contain tartrazine.

pecia, ***anaphylaxis,*** diaphoresis, hyperglycemia, dehydration, liver failure, cholelithiasis.

INTERACTIONS
Other myelosuppressive agents: increased toxicity. Avoid concomitant use.

NURSING CONSIDERATIONS
- *Contraindicated* in patients sensitive to drug or components.
- *Use cautiously* in patients with renal insufficiency, hematologic impairment, and myelosuppression. Advanced age, renal insufficiency, and bone marrow impairment may predispose patient to increased or excessive toxicity. Monitor patient closely and modify dosage based on toxicity. Most toxic effects are dose-dependent.
- Bone marrow suppression can be severe. Careful hematologic monitoring is required, especially of neutrophil and platelet counts.
- Severe neurologic effects are seen when high doses are used to treat acute leukemia. Irreversible CNS toxicity characterized by delayed blindness, coma, and death is associated with high doses. No specific antidote exists.
- Optimal duration of therapy is not yet determined. Current recommendations suggest three additional cycles after achieving maximal response before discontinuing therapy.
- **I.V. use:** To prepare solution, add 2 ml of sterile water for injection to the solid cake of fludarabine. Dissolution should occur within 15 seconds; each ml will contain 25 mg of drug. Use within 8 hours of reconstitution. Fludarabine also can be diluted in 100 ml or 125 ml of 5% dextrose or normal saline solution.
- Follow institutional protocol regarding guidelines for proper handling and disposal of chemotherapeutic agents.
- Store drug in refrigerator at 36° to 36° F (2° to 8° C).
- Used investigationally to treat non-Hodgkin's lymphoma, macroglobulinemic lymphoma, prolymphocytic leukemia or prolymphocytoid variant of CLL, mycosis fungoides, hairy-cell leukemia, and Hodgkin's disease.

fluorouracil
(5-fluorouracil, 5-FU)

Adrucil, Efudex, Fluoroplex

Pregnancy Risk Category: D

HOW SUPPLIED
Injection: 50 mg/ml
Cream: 1%, 5%
Topical solution: 1%, 2%, 5%

MECHANISM OF ACTION
Inhibits DNA synthesis.

INDICATIONS & DOSAGE
Colon, rectal, breast, ovarian, cervical, bladder, liver, and pancreatic cancer –
Adults: 12.5 mg/kg I.V. daily for 3 to 5 days q 4 weeks; or 15 mg/kg weekly for 6 weeks. (Dosages recommended based on lean body weight.) Maximum single recommended dose is 800 mg, although higher single doses (up to 1.5 g) have been used. The injectable form has been given orally but is not recommended.
Multiple actinic (solar) keratoses; superficial basal cell carcinoma –
Adults: apply cream or topical solution b.i.d.

ADVERSE REACTIONS
Common reactions are in italics; life-threatening reactions are in bold italics.
Blood: ***leukopenia,*** thrombocytopenia, anemia; WBC nadir 9 to 14 days after first dose; platelet nadir in 7 to 14 days.
CNS: acute cerebellar syndrome, ataxia, confusion, disorientation, euphoria, headache, nystagmus.

GI: *stomatitis, GI ulcer (may precede leukopenia), nausea, vomiting in 30% to 50% of patients; diarrhea, anorexia.*
Skin: (I.V. use) *dermatitis,* hyperpigmentation (especially in blacks), nail changes, pigmented palmar creases.
Local: *erythema, pain, burning, scaling, pruritus;* (topical use) contact dermatitis, *hyperpigmentation,* soreness, suppuration, swelling.
Other: *reversible alopecia in 5% to 20% of patients, weakness, malaise.*

INTERACTIONS

Leucovorin calcium, prior treatment with alkylating agents: increased toxicity of fluorouracil. Use with extreme caution.

NURSING CONSIDERATIONS

• *Contraindicated* in patients with hypersensitivity to the drug; patients who are in a poor nutritional state; patients with bone marrow suppression (leukocyte counts less than or equal to 5,000/mm³ or platelet counts less than or equal to 100,000/mm³); and in those who have had major surgery within the previous month.
• *Use cautiously* after high-dose pelvic irradiation or use of alkylating agents or in patients with impaired hepatic or renal function or widespread neoplastic infiltration of bone marrow.
• Watch for stomatitis or diarrhea (signs of toxicity). May use topical oral anesthetic to soothe lesions. Discontinue if diarrhea occurs.
• Encourage good and frequent oral hygiene to prevent superinfection of denuded mucosa.
• Give antiemetic before administering drug to reduce nausea.
• Monitor WBC and platelet counts daily. Watch for ecchymoses, petechiae, easy bruising, and anemia.
• Consider protective isolation if WBC is less than 2,000/mm³.
• Dermatologic side effects reversible when drug is stopped. Patient should use highly protective sunscreens to avoid inflammatory erythematous dermatitis. Long-term use of the drug is associated with erythematous, desquamative rash of the hands and feet. May be treated with pyridoxine (50 to 150 mg P.O. daily) for 5 to 7 days.
• Therapeutic concentrations are not reached in cerebrospinal fluid.
• **I.V. use:** Slowing infusion rate so it takes from 2 to 8 hours lessens toxicity.
• Don't use cloudy solution. If crystals form, redissolve by warming.
• Solution is more stable in plastic I.V. bags than in glass bottles. Use plastic I.V. containers for administering continuous infusions.
• Monitor intake and output, CBC, and renal and hepatic functions.
• Don't refrigerate fluorouracil.
• Sometimes ordered as 5-fluorouracil or 5-FU. The numeral 5 is part of the drug name and should not be confused with dosage units.
• Sometimes administered via hepatic arterial infusion in treatment of hepatic metastases.
• Warn patient that alopecia may occur but is reversible.
• To prevent bleeding, avoid I.M. injections in patients with thrombocytopenia.
• Fluorouracil toxicity may be delayed for 1 to 3 weeks.
• Preparation of parenteral form is associated with carcinogenic, mutagenic, and teratogenic risks for personnel. Follow institutional policy to reduce risks.

For topical application:
• Avoid occlusive dressings as they increase the risk of inflammatory reactions in adjacent normal skin.
• Patient should avoid prolonged exposure to sunlight or ultraviolet light.
• Apply with caution near eyes, nose, and mouth.
• Warn patient that treated area may be unsightly during therapy and for

several weeks after therapy. Complete healing may take 1 or 2 months.
- Ingestion and systemic absorption may cause leukopenia, thrombocytopenia, stomatitis, diarrhea, or GI ulceration, bleeding, and hemorrhage.
- Application to large ulcerated areas may cause systemic toxicity.
- Expect to use 1% concentration on the face. Higher concentrations are used for thicker-skinned areas or resistant lesions.
- Expect to use 5% strength for superficial basal cell carcinoma confirmed by biopsy.
- Wash hands immediately after handling medication.

hydroxyurea
Hydrea**

Pregnancy Risk Category: D

HOW SUPPLIED
Capsules: 500 mg

MECHANISM OF ACTION
Inhibits DNA synthesis.

INDICATIONS & DOSAGE
Melanoma; resistant chronic myelocytic leukemia; recurrent, metastatic, or inoperable ovarian cancer; head and neck cancers –
Adults: 80 mg/kg P.O. as single dose q 3 days; or 20 to 30 mg/kg P.O. as a single daily dose.

ADVERSE REACTIONS
Common reactions are in italics; life-threatening reactions are in bold italics.
Blood: *leukopenia,* thrombocytopenia, anemia, *megaloblastosis; dose-limiting and dose-related **bone marrow suppression,** with rapid recovery.*
CNS: drowsiness, hallucinations.
GI: *anorexia, nausea, vomiting, diarrhea,* stomatitis.
GU: increased BUN and serum creatinine levels.
Metabolic: hyperuricemia.
Skin: rash, pruritus.

INTERACTIONS
Cytotoxic drugs, radiation therapy: enhanced toxicity of hydroxyurea. Use together cautiously.

NURSING CONSIDERATIONS
- *Contraindicated* in patients with hypersensitivity to the drug.
- *Use cautiously* in renal dysfunction. Discontinue if WBC is less than 2,500/mm³ or if platelet count is less than 100,000/mm³.
- Dosage modification may be required after chemotherapy or radiation therapy.
- Warn patient to watch for signs of infection (fever, sore throat, fatigue) and bleeding (easy bruising, nosebleeds, bleeding gums, melena). Take temperature daily.
- If patient can't swallow capsule, he may empty contents into water and take immediately.
- Monitor intake and output; keep patient hydrated.
- Routinely measure BUN, uric acid, and serum creatinine.
- Drug crosses blood-brain barrier.
- Auditory and visual hallucinations and blood toxicity increase when decreased renal function exists.
- When patients receive concomitant irradiation, they may experience an increased incidence or severity of GI distress or stomatitis.
- Avoid all I.M. injections when platelets are below 100,000/mm³.
- Has been used investigationally to relieve symptoms of sickle cell anemia. Dosage is highly variable; in early trials, the median dose was 20 mg/kg daily.

mercaptopurine (6-MP, 6-mercaptopurine)
Purinethol

Pregnancy Risk Category: D

HOW SUPPLIED
Tablets (scored): 50 mg

MECHANISM OF ACTION
Inhibits RNA and DNA synthesis.

INDICATIONS & DOSAGE
Acute lymphoblastic leukemia (in children), acute myeloblastic leukemia, chronic myelocytic leukemia –
Adults: 80 to 100 mg/m² (rounded to the nearest 25 mg) P.O. daily as a single dose up to 5 mg/kg daily.
Children: 75 mg/m² (rounded to the nearest 25 mg) P.O. daily.
Usual maintenance for adults and children: 1.5 to 2.5 mg/kg daily.

ADVERSE REACTIONS
Common reactions are in italics; life-threatening reactions are in bold italics.
Blood: ***leukopenia,*** *thrombocytopenia, and anemia; all may persist several days after drug is stopped.*
GI: *nausea, vomiting, and anorexia in 25% of patients;* painful oral ulcers.
Hepatic: biliary stasis, *jaundice,* ***hepatic necrosis.***
Metabolic: hyperuricemia.
Skin: rash, hyperpigmentation.

INTERACTIONS
Allopurinol: slowed inactivation of mercaptopurine. Decrease mercaptopurine to ¼ or ⅓ normal dose.
Hepatotoxic drugs: may enhance liver toxicity of mercaptopurine.
Nondepolarizing neuromuscular blockers: antagonized muscle relaxant effect. Notify anesthesiologist that patient is receiving mercaptopurine.
Warfarin: enhanced anticoagulant effect.

NURSING CONSIDERATIONS
- *Contraindicated* in patients whose disease has exhibited resistance to the drug.
- *Use cautiously.* Dosage modifications may be required following chemotherapy or radiation therapy, in depressed neutrophil or platelet count, and in impaired hepatic or renal function.
- Observe for signs of bleeding and infection.
- Hepatic dysfunction is reversible when drug is stopped. Watch for jaundice, clay-colored stools, and frothy dark urine. Drug should be stopped if hepatic tenderness occurs.
- Monitor blood counts, serum transaminase, alkaline phosphatase, and bilirubin weekly during induction and monthly during maintenance.
- Warn patient to watch for signs of infection (fever, sore throat, fatigue) and bleeding (easy bruising, nosebleeds, bleeding gums, melena). Take temperature daily.
- Monitor intake and output. Encourage fluid intake (3 liters daily).
- Sometimes ordered as 6-mercaptopurine or 6-MP. The numeral 6 is part of drug name and does not signify number of dosage units.
- Warn patient that improvement may take 2 to 4 weeks or longer.
- GI adverse reactions less common in children than in adults.
- Avoid all I.M. injections when platelets are below 100,000/mm³.
- Monitor serum uric acid. If allopurinol is necessary, use cautiously.

methotrexate

methotrexate sodium
Folex, Mexate, Rheumatrex
Pregnancy Risk Category: D

HOW SUPPLIED
Tablets (scored): 2.5 mg
Injection: 20-mg, 25-mg, 50-mg, 100-mg, 250-mg vials, lyophilized powder, preservative-free; 25-mg/ml vials, preservative-free solution; 2.5-mg/ml, 25-mg/ml vials, lyophilized powder, preserved

*Liquid form contains alcohol. **May contain tartrazine.

MECHANISM OF ACTION

Prevents reduction of folic acid to tetrahydrofolate by binding to dihydrofolate reductase.

INDICATIONS & DOSAGE

Trophoblastic tumors (choriocarcinoma, hydatidiform mole) –
Adults: 15 to 30 mg P.O. or I.M. daily for 5 days. Repeat after 1 or more weeks, according to response or toxicity.
Acute lymphoblastic and lymphatic leukemia –
Adults and children: 3.3 mg/m² P.O., I.M., or I.V. daily for 4 to 6 weeks or until remission occurs; then 20 to 30 mg/m² P.O. or I.M. twice weekly.
Meningeal leukemia –
Adults and children: 10 to 15 mg/m² intrathecally q 2 to 5 days until cerebrospinal fluid is normal. Use only 20-, 50-, or 100-mg vials of powder with no preservatives; dilute using 0.9% sodium chloride injection *without* preservatives or Elliot's B solution. Use only new vials of drug and diluent. Use immediately.
Burkitt's lymphoma (Stage I or Stage II) –
Adults: 10 to 25 mg P.O. daily for 4 to 8 days with 1-week rest intervals.
Lymphosarcoma (Stage III) –
Adults: 0.625 to 2.5 mg/kg daily P.O., I.M., or I.V.
Mycosis fungoides –
Adults: 2.5 to 10 mg P.O. daily or 50 mg I.M. weekly; or 25 mg I.M. twice weekly.
Psoriasis –
Adults: 10 to 25 mg P.O., I.M., or I.V. as single weekly dose.
Rheumatoid arthritis –
Adults: Initially 7.5 mg P.O. weekly, either in a single dose or divided as 2.5 mg P.O. q 12 hours for three doses once a week. Dosage may be gradually increased to a maximum of 20 mg weekly.

ADVERSE REACTIONS

Common reactions are in italics; life-threatening reactions are in bold italics.
Blood: WBC and platelet nadir occurring on day 7; ***anemia, leukopenia, thrombocytopenia*** (all dose-related).
CNS: ***arachnoiditis*** *within hours of intrathecal use;* subacute neurotoxicity which may begin a few weeks later; ***necrotizing demyelinating leukoencephalopathy*** a few years later.
EENT: pharyngitis.
GI: gingivitis, *stomatitis; diarrhea leading to* ***hemorrhagic enteritis and intestinal perforation;*** *nausea; vomiting.*
GU: nephropathy, *tubular necrosis.*
Hepatic: acute toxicity (elevated transaminases), *chronic toxicity* (cirrhosis, ***hepatic fibrosis***).
Metabolic: hyperuricemia.
Respiratory: ***pulmonary fibrosis,*** pneumonitis.
Skin: *urticaria;* pruritus; hyperpigmentation; exposure to sun may aggravate psoriatic lesions, rash, photosensitivity.
Other: alopecia; ***pulmonary interstitial infiltrates;*** long-term use in children may cause osteoporosis.

INTERACTIONS

Digoxin: serum digoxin levels may be decreased. Monitor closely.
Folic acid derivatives: antagonized methotrexate effect.
Phenytoin: serum phenytoin levels may be decreased. Monitor closely.
Probenecid, phenylbutazone, NSAIDs, salicylates, sulfonamides: increased methotrexate toxicity; don't use together if possible.
Vaccines: immunizations may be ineffective; risk of disseminated infection with live virus vaccines.

NURSING CONSIDERATIONS

- *Contraindicated* in patients with hypersensitivity to the drug.
- *Use cautiously* and with dosage modification in patients with im-

paired hepatic or renal function, bone marrow suppression, aplasia, leukopenia, thrombocytopenia, or anemia. Also *use cautiously* in infection, peptic ulcer, and ulcerative colitis and in very young, elderly, or debilitated patients.

- Therapy may be discontinued if ulcerative stomatitis or other severe GI adverse reaction occurs, or if pulmonary toxicity is detected.
- Warn patient to avoid conception during and immediately after therapy because of possible abortion or congenital anomalies.
- Rash, redness, or ulcerations in mouth or pulmonary adverse reactions may signal serious complications.
- Perform baseline pulmonary function tests and monitor periodically.
- Monitor serum uric acid.
- Monitor intake and output daily. Encourage fluid intake (2 to 3 liters daily).
- Alkalinize urine by giving sodium bicarbonate tablets to prevent precipitation of drug, especially with high doses. Maintain urine pH at more than 6.5. Reduce dosage if BUN 20 to 30 mg/dl or creatinine 1.2 to 2 mg/dl. Stop drug if BUN more than 30 mg/dl or creatinine more than 2 mg/dl.
- Watch for increases in AST (SGOT), ALT (SGPT), alkaline phosphatase; may signal hepatic dysfunction.
- Watch for bleeding (especially GI) and infection.
- Warn patient to use highly protective sunscreen when exposed to sunlight.
- Take temperature daily, and watch for cough, dyspnea, and cyanosis.
- Leucovorin rescue is necessary with high-dose (greater than 100 mg) protocols. Don't confuse with folic acid. This rescue technique is effective against systemic toxicity but does not interfere with the tumor cells' absorption of the methotrexate.
- **I.V. use:** May be administered undiluted by I.V. push injection.
- Avoid all I.M. injections in patients with thrombocytopenia.
- Advise patient not to discontinue leucovorin rescue if he experiences severe nausea and vomiting. Parenteral therapy may be necessary.
- Teach patient good oral care to prevent superinfection of oral cavity.
- Preparation of parenteral form is associated with carcinogenic, mutagenic, and teratogenic risks for personnel. Follow institutional policy to reduce risks.

thioguanine (6-thioguanine, 6-TG)

Lanvis†

Pregnancy Risk Category: D

HOW SUPPLIED

Tablets (scored): 40 mg

MECHANISM OF ACTION

Inhibits purine synthesis.

INDICATIONS & DOSAGE

Acute leukemia, chronic myelogenous leukemia –

Adults and children: initially, 2 mg/kg daily P.O. (usually calculated to nearest 20 mg). If necessary, dose is then increased gradually to 3 mg/kg daily as tolerated.

ADVERSE REACTIONS

Common reactions are in italics; life-threatening reactions are in bold italics.

Blood: ***leukopenia, anemia, thrombocytopenia*** (occurs slowly over 2 to 4 weeks).

GI: nausea, vomiting, stomatitis, diarrhea, anorexia.

Hepatic: ***hepatotoxicity,*** jaundice.

Metabolic: hyperuricemia.

INTERACTIONS

Myelosuppressive drugs: increased risk of toxicity, especially myelosuppression and bleeding. Use together cautiously.

NURSING CONSIDERATIONS

- *Contraindicated* in patients whose disease has shown resistance to the drug.
- *Use cautiously* and with dosage modification in patients with renal or hepatic dysfunction.
- Stop drug if hepatotoxicity or hepatic tenderness occurs. Watch for jaundice; may be reversible if drug is stopped promptly.
- Monitor CBC daily during induction, then weekly during maintenance therapy.
- Monitor serum uric acid.
- Sometimes ordered as 6-thioguanine. The numeral 6 is part of drug name and does not signify dosage units.
- Avoid all I.M. injections when platelets are below 100,000/mm^3.

70

Antibiotic antineoplastic agents

bleomycin sulfate
dactinomycin
daunorubicin hydrochloride
doxorubicin hydrochloride
idarubicin hydrochloride
interferon gamma-1b
mitomycin
plicamycin
procarbazine hydrochloride

COMBINATION PRODUCTS
None.

bleomycin sulfate
Blenoxane

Pregnancy Risk Category: D

HOW SUPPLIED
Injection: 15-unit vials (1 unit = 1 mg)

MECHANISM OF ACTION
Inhibits DNA synthesis and causes scission of single- and double-stranded DNA.

INDICATIONS & DOSAGE
Dosage and indications may vary. Check patient's protocol with doctor.
Cervical, esophageal, head, neck, and testicular cancer –
Adults: 10 to 20 units/m² I.V., I.M., or S.C. 1 or 2 times weekly to total 300 to 400 units.
Hodgkin's disease –
Adults: 10 to 20 units/m² I.V., I.M., or S.C. 1 or 2 times weekly. After 50% response, maintenance 1 unit I.M. or I.V. daily or 5 units I.M. or I.V. weekly.
Lymphomas –
Adults: first two doses should be 2 units or less, and patient should be monitored for any allergic reaction. If no reaction occurs, then follow above dosing schedule.

ADVERSE REACTIONS
Common reactions are in italics; life-threatening reactions are in bold italics.
CNS: hyperesthesia of scalp and fingers, headache.
GI: *stomatitis, prolonged anorexia in 13% of patients, nausea, vomiting,* diarrhea.
Skin: *erythema, vesiculation, and hardening and discoloration of palmar and plantar skin in 8% of patients;* desquamation of hands, feet, and pressure areas; *hyperpigmentation; acne.*
Other: *reversible alopecia,* swelling of interphalangeal joints, ***pulmonary fibrosis*** *in 10% of patients, pulmonary adverse reactions (fine crackles, fever, dyspnea), leukocytosis and nonproductive cough, allergic reaction (fever up to 106° F [41.1° C] with chills up to 5 hours after injection;* ***anaphylaxis*** *in 1% to 6% of patients).*

INTERACTIONS
Digitalis glycosides: decreased serum digoxin levels. Monitor closely.
Phenytoin: decreased serum phenytoin levels. Monitor closely.

NURSING CONSIDERATIONS
- *Contraindicated* in patients with hypersensitivity to the drug and during pregnancy.
- *Use cautiously* in renal or pulmonary impairment.
- Because of an increased risk of anaphylactoid reactions, the first two doses in patients with lymphoma should be limited to 2 units or less.
- Pulmonary adverse reactions common in patients over 70 years. Fatal pulmonary fibrosis occurs in 1% of

patients, especially when cumulative dose exceeds 400 units.
- Pulmonary function tests should be performed to establish pre-treatment baseline. Drug should be stopped if pulmonary function test shows a marked decline.
- Monitor chest X-ray and listen to lungs.
- Monitor injection site for signs of irritation.
- Drug concentrates in keratin of squamous epithelium. To prevent linear streaking, don't use adhesive dressings on skin.
- Allergic reactions may be delayed for several hours, especially in lymphoma.
- Advise patient that alopecia may occur, but is usually reversible.
- **I.V. use:** Refrigerated, reconstituted solution is stable for 4 weeks; at room temperature, it's stable for 2 weeks. Bleomycin may adsorb to plastic (PVC) I.V. bags. For prolonged stability, use glass containers.
- Bleomycin-induced fever is common and may be treated with antipyretics. This reaction usually occurs within 3 to 6 hours of administration.
- Refrigerate unopened vials containing dry powder.
- Preparation of parenteral form is associated with carcinogenic, mutagenic, and teratogenic risks for personnel. Follow institutional policy to reduce risks.

dactinomycin (actinomycin D)

Cosmegen

Pregnancy Risk Category: C

HOW SUPPLIED
Injection: 500 mcg/vial

MECHANISM OF ACTION
Interferes with DNA-dependent RNA synthesis by intercalation.

INDICATIONS & DOSAGE
Dosage and indications may vary. Check patient's protocol with doctor.

Sarcomas, trophoblastic tumors in women, testicular cancer –

Adults: 500 mcg I.V. daily for 5 days not to exceed 15 mg/kg or 400 to 600 mg/m^2 daily; wait 2 to 4 weeks and repeat. Or 2 mg I.V. single weekly dose for 3 weeks; wait for bone marrow recovery, then repeat in 3 to 4 weeks.

Wilms' tumor, rhabdomyosarcoma, Ewing's sarcoma –

Children: 15 mcg/kg I.V. daily for 5 days. Maximum dosage 500 mcg daily. Wait for bone marrow recovery.

ADVERSE REACTIONS
Common reactions are in italics; life-threatening reactions are in bold italics.

Blood: ***anemia, leukopenia, thrombocytopenia, pancytopenia.***

GI: *anorexia, nausea, vomiting,* abdominal pain, diarrhea, *stomatitis,* ulceration, proctitis.

Skin: *erythema;* desquamation; *hyperpigmentation of skin, especially in previously irradiated areas; acne-like eruptions (reversible).*

Local: phlebitis, severe damage to soft tissue.

Other: reversible alopecia, ***hepatotoxicity.***

INTERACTIONS
None significant.

NURSING CONSIDERATIONS
- *Contraindicated* in renal, hepatic, or bone marrow impairment and in patients with chickenpox or herpes zoster.
- Stomatitis, diarrhea, leukopenia, thrombocytopenia may require modifying dosage and schedule.
- Give antiemetic before administering to reduce nausea.
- Monitor renal and hepatic functions.
- Monitor CBC daily and platelet counts frequently.

• Warn patient to watch for signs of infection (fever, sore throat, fatigue) and bleeding (easy bruising, nosebleeds, bleeding gums, melena). Take temperature daily.
• Warn patient that alopecia may occur but is usually reversible.
• **I.V. use:** Use only sterile water (without preservatives) as diluent for injection. Discard unused solutions since they do not contain a preservative.
• Dactinomycin is a vesicant. Administer through a running I.V. with good blood return. If infiltration occurs, apply cold compresses to area.
• Preparation of parenteral form is associated with carcinogenic, mutagenic, and teratogenic risks for personnel. Follow institutional policy to reduce risks.

daunorubicin hydrochloride (DNR)

Cerubidin‡, Cerubidine

Pregnancy Risk Category: D

HOW SUPPLIED

Injection: 20 mg/vial

MECHANISM OF ACTION

Interferes with DNA-dependent RNA synthesis by intercalation.

INDICATIONS & DOSAGE

Dosage and indications may vary. Check patient's protocol with doctor.

Remission induction in acute nonlymphocytic leukemia (myelogenous, monocytic, erythroid), acute lymphocytic leukemias –

Adults: as a single agent, 60 mg/m² daily I.V. on days 1, 2, and 3 q 3 to 4 weeks; in combination, 45 mg/m² daily I.V. on days 1, 2, and 3 of the first course and on days 1 and 2 of subsequent courses with cytosine arabinoside infusions.

Note: Dose should be reduced if hepatic or renal function is impaired.

ADVERSE REACTIONS

Common reactions are in italics; life-threatening reactions are in bold italics.

Blood: ***bone marrow suppression*** (lowest blood counts 10 to 14 days after administration).

CV: ***irreversible cardiomyopathy*** (dose-related), ECG changes, arrhythmias, pericarditis, myocarditis.

GI: *nausea, vomiting, stomatitis, esophagitis,* anorexia, diarrhea.

GU: nephrotoxicity, transient red urine.

Hepatic: ***hepatotoxicity.***

Skin: rash, pigmentation of fingernails and toenails.

Local: *severe cellulitis or tissue sloughing if drug extravasates.*

Other: *generalized alopecia,* fever, chills, hyperuricemia.

INTERACTIONS

Dexamethasone, heparin: don't mix. May form a precipitate.

NURSING CONSIDERATIONS

• *Contraindicated* in patients who have received the lifetime dosage limitations of the drug: limit cumulative dose to 500 to 600 mg/m²; 450 mg/m² when patient has been receiving radiation therapy that encompasses the heart or any other cardiotoxic agent, such as cyclophosphamide.
• *Use cautiously* in myelosuppression and impaired cardiac, renal, and liver function.
• Stop drug immediately in signs of CHF or cardiomyopathy.
• Monitor ECG before treatment, monthly during therapy.
• Note if resting pulse rate is high (a sign of cardiac adverse reactions).
• *Never* give I.M. or S.C.
• **I.V. use:** *Avoid extravasation;* inject into tubing of freely flowing I.V. If extravasation occurs, discontinue I.V. immediately and apply ice to area for 24 to 48 hours. Local infiltration with hydrocortisone sodium succinate injection (50 to 100 mg) or sodium bi-

carbonate (5 ml of 8.4% injection) may be ordered.

- Monitor CBC and hepatic function.
- Warn patient that urine may be red for 1 to 2 days and that it's a normal adverse reaction, not hematuria.
- Advise patient that alopecia may occur but is usually reversible.
- Nausea and vomiting may be very severe and last 24 to 48 hours.
- Reconstituted solution is stable for 24 hours at room temperature or 48 hours refrigerated. Optimally, use within 8 hours of preparation.
- Reddish color looks very similar to doxorubicin (Adriamycin). *Do not confuse the two drugs.*
- Preparation of parenteral form is associated with carcinogenic, mutagenic, and teratogenic risks for personnel. Follow institutional policy to reduce risks.

doxorubicin hydrochloride

Adriamycin‡, Adriamycin PFS, Adriamycin RDF, Rubex

Pregnancy Risk Category: D

HOW SUPPLIED

Injection (preservative-free): 2 mg/ml
Powder for injection: 10-mg, 20-mg, 50-mg, 100-mg, 150-mg vials

MECHANISM OF ACTION

Interferes with DNA-dependent RNA synthesis by intercalation.

INDICATIONS & DOSAGE

Dosage and indications may vary. Check patient's protocol with doctor.
Bladder, breast, cervical, head, neck, liver, lung, ovarian, prostatic, stomach, testicular, and thyroid cancer; Hodgkin's disease; acute lymphoblastic and myeloblastic leukemia; Wilms' tumor; neuroblastomas; lymphomas; sarcomas –
Adults: 60 to 75 mg/m² I.V. as single dose q 3 weeks; or 30 mg/m² I.V. in single daily dose, days 1 to 3 of 4-week cycle. Alternatively, 20 mg/m² I.V. once weekly or 30 mg/m² I.V. on 3 successive days, repeated every 4 weeks. Maximum cumulative dose 550 mg/m².

ADVERSE REACTIONS

Common reactions are in italics; life-threatening reactions are in bold italics.
Blood: ***leukopenia, especially agranulocytosis, during days 10 to 15, with recovery by day 21; thrombocytopenia.***
CV: *cardiac depression, seen in such ECG changes as sinus tachycardia, T wave flattening, ST segment depression, voltage reduction; arrhythmias in 11% of patients;* ***irreversible cardiomyopathy (sometimes with pulmonary edema) with mortality of 30% to 75%.***
GI: *nausea, vomiting,* diarrhea, *stomatitis,* esophagitis.
GU: enhancement of cyclophosphamide-induced bladder injury, transient red urine.
Skin: *hyperpigmentation of nails, dermal creases, or skin, especially in previously irradiated areas.*
Local: *severe cellulitis or tissue sloughing if drug extravasates.*
Other: hyperuricemia, *complete alopecia within 3 to 4 weeks;* hair may regrow 2 to 5 months after drug is stopped.

INTERACTIONS

Aminophylline, dexamethasone, fluorouracil, heparin, hydrocortisone, or cephalothin: don't mix together. May form a precipitate.
Digoxin: serum digoxin levels may be decreased. Monitor closely.
Streptozocin: increased and prolonged blood levels. Dosage may have to be adjusted.

NURSING CONSIDERATIONS

- *Contraindicated* in patients who have received lifetime cumulative dose of 550 mg/m².

• Dosage modification may be required in myelosuppression and in impaired cardiac or hepatic function.
• Stop drug or slow rate of infusion if tachycardia develops.
• Stop drug immediately in signs of CHF. Prevent by limiting cumulative dose to 550 mg/m²; 400 mg/m² when patient is also receiving or has received cyclophosphamide or irradiation to cardiac area.
• Monitor ECG before treatment, monthly during therapy.
• *Never* give I.M. or S.C.
• **I.V. use:** *Avoid extravasation;* inject slowly by I.V. push into tubing of freely flowing I.V. Don't place I.V. line over joints or in extremities with poor venous or lymphatic drainage. If extravasation occurs, discontinue I.V. immediately and apply ice to area for 24 to 48 hours. Some clinicians will infiltrate the area with a parenteral corticosteroid. The area should be monitored closely. Because the extravasation reaction may be progressive, early consultation with a plastic surgeon may be advisable.
• If vein streaking occurs, slow administration rate. However, if welts occur, stop administration and report to doctor.
• Monitor CBC and hepatic function.
• Warn patient to watch for signs of infection (fever, sore throat, fatigue) and bleeding (easy bruising, nosebleeds, bleeding gums, melena). Take temperature daily.
• Warn patient urine will be orange to red for 1 to 2 days. Explain that this is not blood; it is caused by the appearance of the drug in the urine.
• Dosage should be reduced in hepatic dysfunction.
• Warn patient that alopecia will occur but is usually reversible.
• Refrigerated, reconstituted solution is stable for 48 hours; at room temperature, it's stable for 24 hours.
• If cumulative dose exceeds 550 mg/m² body surface area, 30% of patients develop cardiac adverse reactions, which begin 2 weeks to 6 months after stopping drug.
• The alternative dosage schedule (once-weekly dosing) has been found to cause a lower incidence of cardiomyopathy.
• Decrease dosage if serum bilirubin is increased: 50% dosage when bilirubin is 1.2 to 3 mg/100 ml; 25% dosage when bilirubin is greater than 3 mg/100 ml.
• Esophagitis is very common in patients who have also received radiation therapy.
• Premedicate with antiemetic to reduce nausea.
• Reddish color looks very similar to daunorubicin (Cerubidine). *Do not confuse the two drugs.*
• Preparation of parenteral form is associated with carcinogenic, mutagenic, and teratogenic risks for personnel. Follow institutional policy to reduce risks.

idarubicin hydrochloride

Idamycin

Pregnancy Risk Category: D

HOW SUPPLIED

Powder for injection: 5 mg, 10 mg

MECHANISM OF ACTION

An antineoplastic antibiotic that inhibits nucleic acid synthesis by intercalation and that interacts with the enzyme topoisomerase II. It is highly lipophilic, which results in an increased rate of cellular uptake.

INDICATIONS & DOSAGE

Dosage and indications may vary. Check current literature for recommended protocol.

Acute myeloid leukemia, including FAB (French-American-British) classifications M1 through M7, in combination with other approved antileukemic agents –

*Liquid form contains alcohol. **May contain tartrazine.

Adults: 12 mg/m² daily for 3 days by slow I.V. injection (over 10 to 15 minutes) in combination with 100 mg/m² of cytarabine daily for 7 days by continuous I.V. infusion or as a 25 mg/m² bolus followed by 200 mg/m² daily for 5 days by continuous infusion.
A second course may be administered if needed. If patient experiences severe mucositis, delay administration until recovery is complete and reduce dose by 25%. Dosage should also be reduced in patients with hepatic or renal impairment. Idarubicin should not be given if bilirubin level is above 5 mg/dl.

ADVERSE REACTIONS

Common reactions are in italics; life-threatening reactions are in bold italics.
Blood: *myelosuppression.*
CNS: headache, changed mental status, ***seizures.***
CV: ***CHF,*** atrial fibrillation, chest pain, ***MI,*** asymptomatic decline in left ventricular ejection fraction, ***myocardial insufficiency, arrhythmias,*** *hemorrhage,* myocardial toxicity.
GI: *nausea, vomiting,* cramps, diarrhea, *mucositis,* ***severe enterocolitis with perforation*** (rare).
GU: decreased renal function, hyperuricemia.
Skin: alopecia, rash, urticaria, bullous erythrodermatous rash on palms and soles, hives at injection site.
Other: *infection,* fever, changes in hepatic function, local tissue necrosis (if extravasation occurs), allergic reactions.

INTERACTIONS

Heparin, alkaline solutions: incompatible. Idarubicin should not be mixed with other drugs unless specific compatibility data is available.

NURSING CONSIDERATIONS

- *Contraindicated* in patients with severe myelosuppression, preexisting cardiac disease, and severe hemorrhagic conditions and in those with overwhelming infection.
- *Use with extreme caution* in hepatic or renal function impairment; dosage reduction is necessary.
- Monitor hepatic and renal function frequently. Frequent determination of CBC is also recommended.
- Hyperuricemia may result from rapid lysis of leukemic cells; take appropriate preventive measures (including adequate hydration) before starting treatment. Allopurinol may be ordered.
- Control systemic infections before therapy.
- Antiemetics may be used to prevent or treat nausea and vomiting.
- **I.V. use:** Reconstitute to a final concentration of 1 mg/ml using 0.9% sodium chloride injection without preservatives. Add 5 ml to the 5-mg vial or 10 ml to the 10-ml vial. *Do not use bacteriostatic saline.* Vial is under negative pressure.
- Administer over 10 to 15 minutes into a free-flowing I.V. infusion of 0.9% sodium chloride or 5% dextrose solution that is running into a large vein.
- Reconstituted solutions are stable for 3 days (72 hours) at room temperature (59° to 86° F [15° to 30° C]); 7 days if refrigerated. Discard unused solutions appropriately.
- If extravasation or signs of extravasation occur, discontinue infusion immediately and notify doctor. Treat with intermittent ice packs – ½ hour immediately, then ½ hour four times daily for 4 days.
- Follow institutional guidelines regarding storage, mixing, administration, and disposal of chemotherapeutic agents.
- Instruct patient to recognize signs and symptoms of extravasation and to call doctor or nurse if these occur.

interferon gamma-1b

Actimmune

Pregnancy Risk Category: C

HOW SUPPLIED

Injection: 100 mcg (3 million units)/vial

MECHANISM OF ACTION

Acts as an interleukin-type lymphokine. It has potent phagocyte-activating properties and enhances the oxidative metabolism of tissue macrophages.

INDICATIONS & DOSAGE

Chronic granulomatous disease – **Adults with a body surface area > 0.5 m²:** 50 mcg/m² (1.5 million units/m²) I.M. three times weekly, preferably h.s. The preferred injection site is the deltoid or anterior thigh.
Adults with a body surface area ≤ 0.5 m²: 1.5 mcg/kg/dose three times weekly.

ADVERSE REACTIONS

Common reactions are in italics; life-threatening reactions are in bold italics.
Blood: *myelosuppression* (at high doses).
CNS: *headache, chills (flulike syndrome),* fatigue, decreased mental status, gait disturbance.
GI: nausea, vomiting, diarrhea.
Metabolic: elevated hepatic enzymes (at high doses).
Skin: rash.
Local: erythema or tenderness at the injection site.
Other: fever, myalgia, arthralgia.

INTERACTIONS

Myelosuppressive agents: possible additive myelosuppression. Use together with caution.
Zidovudine: increased plasma levels of zidovudine. Dosage adjustments are necessary.

NURSING CONSIDERATIONS

- *Contraindicated* in patients hypersensitive to the drug, or to genetically engineered products derived from *Escherichia coli.*
- *Use cautiously* in patients with cardiac disease, including arrhythmias, ischemia, or CHF. The flulike syndrome commonly seen at high doses of the drug can exacerbate these conditions. Also *use cautiously* in patients with compromised CNS function or seizure disorders. CNS adverse reactions that may occur at high doses of the drug can exacerbate these conditions.
- Ensure that patient who will self-administer the drug has a copy of the patient information leaflet, which will aid the safe and effective use of the medication. Be sure patient understands the correct methods of drug administration and of disposal of medical waste.
- Note that discomfort from the flulike syndrome commonly associated with this drug may be minimized by taking the drug at bedtime. Acetaminophen may be useful in treating these symptoms.
- Refrigerate drug immediately. Vials must be stored in a refrigerator (36° to 46° F [2° to 8° C]); do not freeze. Do not shake the vial; avoid excessive agitation. Discard vials that have been left at room temperature for a total period of more than 12 hours.
- Each vial is for single dose only. Because the drug does not contain a preservative, discard the unused contents.

mitomycin (mitomycin-C)

Mutamycin

Pregnancy Risk Category: D

HOW SUPPLIED

Injection: 5-mg, 20-mg, 40-mg vials

MECHANISM OF ACTION
Acts like an alkylating agent, cross-linking strands of DNA. This causes an imbalance of cell growth, leading to cell death.

INDICATIONS & DOSAGE
Dosage and indications may vary. Check patient's protocol with doctor.
Breast, colon, head, neck, lung, pancreatic, and stomach cancer; malignant melanoma –
Adults: 2 mg/m² I.V. daily for 5 days. Stop drug for 2 days, then repeat dosage for 5 more days; or 20 mg/m² as a single dose. Repeat cycle after 6 to 8 weeks, when WBC has returned to 3,000/mm³ and platelets are 75,000/mm³.

ADVERSE REACTIONS
Common reactions are in italics; life-threatening reactions are in bold italics.
Blood: ***thrombocytopenia, leukopenia*** *(may be delayed up to 8 weeks and may be cumulative with successive doses).*
CNS: paresthesias.
GI: *nausea, vomiting,* anorexia, stomatitis.
Local: desquamation, induration, pruritus, *pain at injection site.* Extravasation causes cellulitis, ulceration, sloughing.
Other: *reversible alopecia; purple coloration of nail beds;* fever; ***microangiopathic hemolytic anemia,*** *syndrome characterized by* ***thrombocytopenia, renal failure, and hypertension; interstitial pneumonitis.***

INTERACTIONS
None significant.

NURSING CONSIDERATIONS
• *Contraindicated* in patients with a platelet count less than or equal to 75,000/mm³ or a WBC count less than or equal to 3,000 cells/mm³ and in patients with bleeding disorders, coagulopathy, serious infections, or impaired renal function. Because of the risk of generalized disease, do not give to patients who have recently had chicken pox or herpes zoster.
• Dosage modification is required when platelet count is below 75,000/mm³, WBC is less than 4,000/mm³; in coagulation or bleeding disorders, serious infections, and impaired renal function.
• *Use cautiously* and avoid extravasation. Stop infusion immediately if extravasation occurs because of the potential for severe ulceration and necrosis.
• **I.V. use:** Using sterile water for injection, constitute the 5-mg vials with 10 ml, the 20-mg vials with 40 ml, and the 40-mg vials with 80 ml.
• Follow institutional policy when preparing and administering this drug to avoid mutagenic, teratogenic, and carcinogenic risks.
• Be aware that reconstituted solution is stable for 1 week at room temperature and 2 weeks if refrigerated. Protect from light.
• Continue CBC and blood studies at least 7 weeks after therapy is stopped.
• Warn patient to watch for signs of infection (fever, sore throat, fatigue) and bleeding (easy bruising, nosebleeds, bleeding gums, melena). Take temperature daily.
• Advise patient that alopecia may occur, but that it's usually reversible.
• Has been administered topically by bladder instillation and intra-arterially through the hepatic artery.
• Monitor renal function.
• Never administer I.M. or S.C.

plicamycin (mithramycin)
Mithracin

Pregnancy Risk Category: X

HOW SUPPLIED
Injection: 2.5-mg vials

MECHANISM OF ACTION
Forms a complex with DNA, thus inhibiting RNA synthesis. Also inhibits osteocytic activity, blocking calcium and phosphorus resorption from bone.

INDICATIONS & DOSAGE
Dosage and indications may vary. Check patient's protocol with doctor.
Hypercalcemia associated with advanced malignancy–
Adults: 15 to 25 mcg/kg I.V. daily for 1 to 4 days.
Testicular cancer–
Adults: 25 to 30 mcg/kg I.V. daily for up to 10 days (based on ideal body weight or actual weight, whichever is less).

ADVERSE REACTIONS
Common reactions are in italics; life-threatening reactions are in bold italics.
Blood: ***leukopenia, thrombocytopenia; bleeding syndrome, from epistaxis to generalized hemorrhage;*** *facial flushing.*
GI: *nausea, vomiting,* anorexia, diarrhea, stomatitis, metallic taste.
GU: proteinuria; increased BUN, serum creatinine.
Metabolic: ***decreased serum calcium,*** potassium, and phosphorus; elevated liver enzymes.
Skin: periorbital pallor, usually the day before toxic symptoms occur.
Local: extravasation causes irritation, cellulitis.

INTERACTIONS
None significant.

NURSING CONSIDERATIONS
- *Contraindicated* in thrombocytopenia and in coagulation and bleeding disorders. Dosage modification may be required in renal, hepatic, or bone marrow impairment.
- Monitor LDH, AST (SGOT), ALT (SGPT), alkaline phosphatase, BUN, creatinine, potassium, calcium, and phosphorus levels.
- Monitor platelet count and prothrombin time before and during therapy.
- Warn patient to watch for signs of infection (fever, sore throat, fatigue) and bleeding (easy bruising, nosebleeds, bleeding gums, melena). Take temperature daily.
- Facial flushing is an early indicator of bleeding.
- Give antiemetic before administering to reduce nausea.
- **I.V. use:** To prepare solution, add 4.9 ml sterile water for injection to vial and shake to dissolve. Then dilute for I.V infusion in 1,000 ml D_5W or normal saline.
- Store lyophilized powder in refrigerator. Remains stable after reconstitution for 24 hours; 48 hours in refrigerator. Dilute solutions are stable for 4 to 6 hours. Discard unused drug properly.
- Preparation of parenteral form is associated with carcinogenic, mutagenic, and teratogenic risks for personnel. Follow institutional policy to reduce risks.
- Slow infusion reduces nausea that develops with I.V. push.
- Avoid extravasation. Plicamycin is a vesicant. If I.V. infiltrates, stop immediately; use ice packs. Restart I.V.
- Avoid contact with skin or mucous membranes.
- Therapeutic effect in hypercalcemia may not be seen for 24 to 48 hours; may last 3 to 15 days.
- Precipitous drop in calcium possible. Monitor patient for tetany, carpopedal spasm, Chvostek's sign, muscle cramps; check serum calcium.

procarbazine hydrochloride
Matulane, Natulan†‡

Pregnancy Risk Category: D

HOW SUPPLIED
Capsules: 50 mg

MECHANISM OF ACTION
Inhibits DNA, RNA, and protein synthesis.

INDICATIONS & DOSAGE
Dosage and indications may vary. Check patient's protocol with doctor.
Hodgkin's disease, lymphomas, brain and lung cancer–
Adults: 2 to 4 mg/kg P.O. daily in a single dose or divided doses for the first week. Then, 4 to 6 mg/kg daily until WBC falls below 4,000/mm^3 or platelets fall below 100,000/mm^3. After bone marrow recovers, resume maintenance dosage of 1 to 2 mg/kg/day.
Children: 50 mg/m^2 P.O. daily for first week, then 100 mg/m^2 until response or toxicity occurs. Maintenance dosage is 50 mg/m^2 P.O. daily after bone marrow recovery.

ADVERSE REACTIONS
Common reactions are in italics; life-threatening reactions are in bold italics.
Blood: ***bleeding tendency, thrombocytopenia, leukopenia, anemia.***
CNS: nervousness, depression, insomnia, nightmares, *hallucinations*, confusion, ***seizures.***
EENT: retinal hemorrhage, nystagmus, photophobia.
GI: *nausea, vomiting, anorexia,* stomatitis, dry mouth, dysphagia, diarrhea, constipation.
Skin: dermatitis.
Other: reversible alopecia, ***pleural effusion.***

INTERACTIONS
Alcohol: mild disulfiram-like reaction. Warn patient not to drink alcohol.
CNS depressants: additive depressant effects.
Digoxin: serum digoxin levels may be decreased. Monitor closely.
Meperidine: may cause severe hypotension and possible death. Don't give together.
Sympathomimetics, local anesthetics, antidepressants, foods high in tyramine content (Chianti wine, cheese): possible tremors, palpitations, increased blood pressure.

NURSING CONSIDERATIONS
- *Contraindicated* in patients with hypersensitivity to the drug and in patients with inadequate bone marrow reserve as documented by bone marrow aspiration.
- *Use cautiously* in leukopenia, thrombocytopenia, anemia, and impaired hepatic or renal function.
- Warn patient to watch for signs of infection (fever, sore throat, fatigue) and bleeding (easy bruising, nosebleeds, bleeding gums, melena). Take temperature daily.
- Nausea and vomiting may be decreased if taken at bedtime and in divided doses.
- Warn patient not to drink alcoholic beverages while taking this drug.
- Procarbazine inhibits MAO and can cause disulfiram-like reaction if taken with other MAO inhibitors, tricyclic antidepressants, or foods with a high tyramine content. Inhibition of MAO may persist for 2 weeks after discontinuing the drug.
- Instruct patient to stop medication and check with doctor immediately if disulfiram-like reaction occurs (chest pains, rapid or irregular heartbeat, severe headache, stiff neck).
- Monitor CBC and platelet counts.
- Avoid all I.M. injections in patients with thrombocytopenia.
- Warn patient to avoid hazardous tasks such as driving or operating heavy machinery until the adverse CNS reactions of the drug are known.

71

Antineoplastics altering hormone balance

aminoglutethimide
estramustine phosphate sodium
flutamide
goserelin acetate
leuprolide acetate
megestrol acetate
mitotane
tamoxifen citrate
testolactone
trilostane

COMBINATION PRODUCTS
None.

---

aminoglutethimide
Cytadren

Pregnancy Risk Category: D

HOW SUPPLIED
Tablets: 250 mg

MECHANISM OF ACTION
Blocks conversion of cholesterol to delta-5-pregnenolone in the adrenal cortex, inhibiting the synthesis of glucocorticoids, mineralocorticoids, and other steroids.

INDICATIONS & DOSAGE
Suppression of adrenal function in Cushing's syndrome and adrenal cancer; metastatic breast cancer; prostate cancer–
Adults: initially, 250 mg P.O. b.i.d. or t.i.d. for 14 days. Maintenance dosage is 250 mg q.i.d. at 6-hour intervals. Dosage may be increased in increments of 250 mg daily q 1 to 2 weeks to a maximum daily dosage of 2 g.

ADVERSE REACTIONS
Common reactions are in italics; life-threatening reactions are in bold italics.
Blood: transient leukopenia, ***agranulocytosis.***
CNS: *drowsiness,* headache, dizziness.
CV: hypotension, tachycardia.
Endocrine: adrenal insufficiency, masculinization, hirsutism.
GI: nausea, anorexia.
Skin: *morbilliform skin rash,* pruritus, urticaria.
Other: fever, myalgia.

INTERACTIONS
Alcohol: may potentiate the effects of aminoglutethimide.
Dexamethasone, medroxyprogesterone: aminoglutethimide increases hepatic metabolism of these agents.
Oral anticoagulants: decreased anticoagulant effect.

NURSING CONSIDERATIONS
- *Contraindicated* in patients with hypersensitivity to the drug.
- May cause adrenal hypofunction, especially under stressful conditions, such as surgery, trauma, or acute illness. Patients may need mineralocorticoid supplements to treat hyponatremia and orthostatic hypotension. Glucocorticoid replacement may also be necessary, especially in patients with breast cancer. Monitor such patients carefully.
- Monitor blood pressure frequently. Advise patient to stand up slowly to minimize orthostatic hypotension.
- May cause a decrease in thyroid hormone production. Monitor thyroid function studies.
- Perform baseline hematologic studies and monitor CBC periodically.
- Warn patient to watch for signs of infection (fever, sore throat, fatigue) and bleeding (easy bruising, nose-

bleeds, bleeding gums, melena). Take temperature daily.

- Warn patient that drug can cause drowsiness and dizziness. Advise him to avoid activities that require alertness and good psychomotor coordination until CNS effects of the drug are known.
- Tell patient to report if skin rash persists for more than 8 days. Reassure patient that drowsiness, nausea, and loss of appetite will diminish within 2 weeks after start of aminoglutethimide therapy. However, if these symptoms persist, tell patient to notify doctor.

estramustine phosphate sodium

Emcyt, Estracyst‡

Pregnancy Risk Category: D

HOW SUPPLIED

Capsules: 140 mg

MECHANISM OF ACTION

A combination of estrogen and an alkylating agent; acts by its ability to bind selectively to a protein present in the human prostate.

INDICATIONS & DOSAGE

Palliative treatment of metastatic or progressive cancer of the prostate –
Adults: 10 to 16 mg/kg P.O. in three to four divided doses. Usual dosage is 14 mg/kg daily. Therapy should continue for up to 3 months and, if successful, be maintained as long as the patient responds.

ADVERSE REACTIONS

Common reactions are in italics; life-threatening reactions are in bold italics.
Blood: ***leukopenia, thrombocytopenia.***
CNS: loss of libido.
CV: ***myocardial infarction, CVA,*** sodium and fluid retention, ***edema, pulmonary emboli,*** thrombophlebitis, ***CHF,*** hypertension.
GI: *nausea, vomiting,* diarrhea.
Skin: rash, pruritus.
Other: *painful gynecomastia and breast tenderness,* thinning of hair, hyperglycemia, fluid retention.

INTERACTIONS

Calcium-rich foods (milk and dairy products): impaired absorption of estramustine.

NURSING CONSIDERATIONS

- *Contraindicated* in patients hypersensitive to estradiol and nitrogen mustard. Also contraindicated in active thrombophlebitis or thromboembolic disorders, except in those cases where the actual tumor mass is the cause of the thromboembolic phenomenon.
- *Use cautiously* in patients with history of thrombophlebitis or thromboembolic disorders and cerebrovascular or coronary artery disease.
- Tell the patient to take this drug on an empty stomach (2 hours before or 1 hour after meals) and to avoid taking the drug with milk or dairy products.
- Estramustine may exaggerate preexisting peripheral edema or CHF. Weight gain should be monitored regularly in these patients.
- Monitor blood pressure and glucose tolerance periodically throughout therapy.
- Each 140-mg capsule contains 12.5 mg sodium.
- Because of the possibility of mutagenic effects, advise patient and spouse to use contraceptive measures if woman is of childbearing age.
- Estramustine is a combination of the estrogen estradiol and a nitrogen mustard. Shown to be effective in patients refractory to estrogen therapy alone.
- Patient may continue estramustine as long as he's responding favorably.

Some patients have taken the drug for more than 3 years.

- Store capsules in refrigerator.

flutamide

Eulexin

Pregnancy Risk Category: D

HOW SUPPLIED

Capsules: 125 mg

MECHANISM OF ACTION

Inhibits androgen uptake or prevents binding of androgens in nucleus of cells within target tissues.

INDICATIONS & DOSAGE

Treatment of metastatic prostatic carcinoma (stage D_2) in combination with luteinizing hormone-releasing hormone analogs such as leuprolide acetate –

Adults: 250 mg P.O. q. 8 hours.

ADVERSE REACTIONS

Common reactions are in italics; life-threatening reactions are in bold italics.

CNS: *loss of libido.*

CV: edema, hypertension.

GI: *diarrhea, nausea, vomiting.*

GU: *impotence.*

Metabolic: gynecomastia, elevated of hepatic enzymes, hepatitis.

Skin: rash, photosensitivity.

Other: *hot flashes.*

INTERACTIONS

None reported.

NURSING CONSIDERATIONS

- *Contraindicated* in patients with hypersensitivity to flutamide.
- Periodic liver tests should be performed in patients receiving chronic therapy with flutamide.
- Patients should understand that flutamide must be taken continuously with the agent used for medical castration (such as leuprolide acetate) to allow the full benefit of therapy. Leuprolide suppresses testosterone production, while flutamide inhibits testosterone action at the cellular level. Together they can impair the growth of androgen-responsive tumors. Patients should not discontinue either drug without consulting the doctor.

goserelin acetate

Zoladex

Pregnancy Risk Category: X

HOW SUPPLIED

Implants: 3.6 mg

MECHANISM OF ACTION

A luteinizing hormone-releasing hormone (LHRH) analog that acts on the pituitary to decrease the release of follicle-stimulating hormone (FSH) and luteinizing hormone (LH). In males, the result is dramatically lowered serum levels of testosterone.

INDICATIONS & DOSAGE

Palliative treatment of advanced carcinoma of the prostate –

Adults: 1 implant S.C. q 28 days into the upper abdominal wall.

ADVERSE REACTIONS

Common reactions are in italics; life-threatening reactions are in bold italics.

Blood: anemia.

CNS: lethargy, pain (worsened in the first 30 days), dizziness, insomnia, anxiety, depression, headache, chills, fever.

CV: edema, ***CHF, arrhythmias, CVA,*** hypertension, ***myocardial infarction,*** peripheral vascular disorder, chest pain.

EENT: upper respiratory infection.

GI: nausea, vomiting, diarrhea, constipation, ulcer.

GU: *decreased erections, lower urinary tract symptoms,* renal insufficiency, urinary obstruction, urinary tract infection.

Respiratory: COPD.
Skin: rash, sweating.
Other: *hot flashes, sexual dysfunction,* gout, hyperglycemia, weight increase, breast swelling and tenderness.

INTERACTIONS
None reported.

NURSING CONSIDERATIONS
- *Contraindicated* during pregnancy.
- At the beginning of therapy, LHRH analogs such as goserelin may cause a worsening of the symptoms of prostatic cancer because the drug initially causes an increase in testosterone serum levels. A few patients may experience increased bone pain. Rarely, disease exacerbation (either spinal cord compression or ureteral obstruction) has occurred.
- Advise the patient to report every 28 days for a new implant. A delay of a couple of days is permissible, however.
- The implant comes in a preloaded syringe. If the package is damaged, do not use the syringe. Make sure that the drug is visible in the translucent chamber of the syringe.
- The drug is administered into the upper abdominal wall using aspetic technique. After cleaning the area with an alcohol swab (and injecting a local anesthetic), stretch the patient's skin with one hand while grasping the barrel of the syringe with the other. Insert the needle into the S.C. fat, then change direction of the needle so that it parallels the abdominal wall. The needle should then be pushed in until the hub touches the patient's skin, then withdrawn about 1 cm (this creates a gap for the drug to be injected) before depressing the plunger completely.
- To avoid the need for a new syringe and injection site, do not aspirate after inserting the needle.

leuprolide acetate
Lucrin‡, Lupron, Lupron Depot
Pregnancy Risk Category: X

HOW SUPPLIED
Injection: 1 mg/0.2 ml (5 mg/ml) in 2.8-ml multiple-dose vials
Depot injection: 7.5 mg/ml

MECHANISM OF ACTION
Initially stimulates but then inhibits the release of follicle-stimulating and luteinizing hormone. This results in testosterone suppression.

INDICATIONS & DOSAGE
Management of advanced prostate cancer–
Men: 1 mg S.C. daily. Alternatively, give 7.5 mg I.M. (depot injection) monthly.
Endometriosis–
Women: 3.75 mg I.M (depot injection only) as a single injection once a month for up to 6 months.

ADVERSE REACTIONS
Common reactions are in italics; life-threatening reactions are in bold italics.
CNS: dizziness, depression, headache.
CV: arrhythmias, angina, MI.
Endocrine: *hot flashes.*
GI: nausea, vomiting.
Local: skin reactions at injection site.
Other: pulmonary embolus, peripheral edema, decreased libido, elevated liver enzymes, transient bone pain during first week of treatment.

INTERACTIONS
None significant.

NURSING CONSIDERATIONS
- *Contraindicated* in patients with hypersensitivity to the drug or other gonadotropin-releasing hormone analogues, during pregnancy, and in women with undiagnosed vaginal bleeding.

• *Use cautiously* in patients hypersensitive to benzyl alcohol.
• Never administer by I.V. injection.
• Leuprolide is a nonsurgical alternative to orchiectomy for prostate cancer.
• Studies show leuprolide is therapeutically equivalent to diethylstilbestrol in "medical castration" palliation treatment but has significantly milder and fewer adverse reactions.
• Reassure patient who has had undesirable effects from other endocrine therapies that leuprolide is much easier to tolerate.
• When treating prostate cancer, symptoms (bone pain, difficult urination, neurologic symptoms) may worsen when therapy is initiated. Reassure patient that these effects are transient and will disappear after about 1 week.
• If patient is going to self-administer S.C. injection, he should be carefully instructed about proper administration techniques, and he should be advised to use only the syringes provided by the manufacturer.
• If another syringe must be substituted, a low dose insulin syringe (U-100, 0.5 ml) may be an appropriate choice.
• Advise patients to store the drug at room temperature, protected from light and sources of heat.
• Once monthly depot injection should be administered under medical supervision. Use supplied diluent to reconstitute drug. Draw 1 ml into a syringe with a 22G needle (extra diluent is provided and should be discarded). Inject into vial, then shake well. Suspension will appear milky. Although the suspension is stable for 24 hours after reconstitution, it contains no bacteriostat. Use immediately.

megestrol acetate

Megace, Megostat‡

Pregnancy Risk Category: X

HOW SUPPLIED

Tablets: 20 mg, 40 mg

MECHANISM OF ACTION

Changes the tumor's hormonal environment and alters the neoplastic process.

INDICATIONS & DOSAGE

Breast cancer–
Women: 40 mg P.O. q.i.d.
Endometrial cancer–
Women: 40 to 320 mg P.O. daily in divided doses.

ADVERSE REACTIONS

Common reactions are in italics; life-threatening reactions are in bold italics.
GU: dysfunctional uterine bleeding when drug is discontinued.
Other: weight gain, increased appetite, carpal tunnel syndrome, thrombophlebitis, alopecia, hirsutism, breast tenderness.

INTERACTIONS

None significant.

NURSING CONSIDERATIONS

• *Contraindicated* in patients with hypersensitivity to the drug.
• *Use cautiously* in patients with history of thrombophlebitis.
• Megestrol is a relatively nontoxic drug with a low incidence of adverse effects.
• Adequate trial is 2 months. Reassure patient that therapeutic response isn't immediate.

mitotane

Lysodren

Pregnancy Risk Category: C

HOW SUPPLIED
Tablets (scored): 500 mg

MECHANISM OF ACTION
Selectively destroys adrenocortical tissue and hinders extraadrenal metabolism of cortisol.

INDICATIONS & DOSAGE
Inoperable adrenocortical cancer–
Adults: initially, 1 to 6 g P.O. daily divided t.i.d. or q.i.d.; increased to 9 to 10 g P.O. daily, divided t.i.d. or q.i.d. Dosage is adjusted until maximum tolerated dosage is achieved (varies from 2 to 16 g daily but is usually 8 to 10 g daily).
Children: initially, 0.1 to 0.5 mg/kg P.O. (1 to 2 g daily) in divided doses. Increase dosage based upon patient tolerance and response. Usual dose is 5 to 7 g daily in divided doses.

ADVERSE REACTIONS
Common reactions are in italics; life-threatening reactions are in bold italics.
CNS: *depression, somnolence, lethargy, vertigo;* brain damage and dysfunction in long-term, high-dose therapy.
GI: *severe nausea, vomiting,* diarrhea, anorexia.
Metabolic: adrenal insufficiency.
Skin: dermatitis, maculopapular rash.

INTERACTIONS
None significant.

NURSING CONSIDERATIONS
- *Contraindicated* in patients with hypersensitivity to the drug.
- *Use cautiously* in patients with hepatic disease; however, dosage need not be routinely reduced in such patients.
- Drug should not be used in a patient with shock or trauma. Use of corticosteroids may avoid acute adrenocorticoid insufficiency and is usually required. Glucocorticoid dosage should be increased in periods of physiologic stress such as infection or trauma.
- Assess and record behavioral and neurologic signs for baseline data daily throughout therapy. Prolonged therapy has been associated with significant neurologic impairment.
- Give antiemetic before administering to reduce nausea.
- Dosage may be reduced if GI or skin adverse reactions are severe.
- Obese patients may need higher dosage and may have longer-lasting adverse reactions, since drug distributes mostly to body fat.
- Warn ambulatory patient of CNS adverse reactions; advise him to avoid hazardous tasks requiring mental alertness or physical coordination.
- Monitor effectiveness by reduction in pain, weakness, anorexia.
- Adequate trial is at least 3 months, but therapy can continue if clinical benefits are observed.

tamoxifen citrate
Nolvadex, Nolvadex D†‡, Tamofen†

Pregnancy Risk Category: D

HOW SUPPLIED
Tablets: 10 mg, 15.2 mg†
Tablets (film-coated): 30.4 mg†

MECHANISM OF ACTION
Acts as an estrogen antagonist.

INDICATIONS & DOSAGE
Advanced premenopausal and postmenopausal breast cancer–
Women: 10 mg P.O. b.i.d. to t.i.d.

ADVERSE REACTIONS
Common reactions are in italics; life-threatening reactions are in bold italics.
Blood: transient fall in WBC or platelets.
GI: nausea in 10% of patients, vomiting, anorexia.
GU: vaginal discharge and bleeding.

Metabolic: hypercalcemia.
Skin: rash.
Other: temporary bone or tumor pain, hot flashes in 7% of patients. Brief exacerbation of pain from osseous metastases.

INTERACTIONS
None significant.

NURSING CONSIDERATIONS
- *Contraindicated* in patients with hypersensitivity to the drug.
- Monitor CBC closely in patients with preexisting leukopenia or thrombocytopenia.
- Acts as an "antiestrogen." Best results have been reported in patients with positive estrogen receptors.
- Adverse reactions are usually minor and well tolerated.
- Reassure patient that acute exacerbation of bone pain during tamoxifen therapy usually indicates drug will produce good response. Use analgesic to relieve pain.
- Short-term therapy induces ovulation in premenopausal women. Barrier form of contraception is recommended.
- Monitor serum calcium. Drug may compound hypercalcemia related to bone metastases during initiation of therapy.
- Also used to treat breast cancer in men and advanced ovarian cancer in women. Has been used to stimulate ovulation in women with oligomenorrhea or amenorrhea who previously used oral contraceptives.

testolactone
Teslac
Controlled Substance Schedule III
Pregnancy Risk Category: C

HOW SUPPLIED
Tablets: 50 mg

MECHANISM OF ACTION
Changes the tumor's hormonal environment and alters the neoplastic process.

INDICATIONS & DOSAGE
Advanced postmenopausal breast cancer–
Women: 250 mg P.O. q.i.d.

ADVERSE REACTIONS
Common reactions are in italics; life-threatening reactions are in bold italics.
CNS: paresthesias, peripheral neuropathy.
CV: increased blood pressure, edema.
GI: nausea, vomiting, diarrhea.
Metabolic: hypercalcemia.
Other: alopecia.

INTERACTIONS
Oral anticoagulants: increased pharmacologic effects. Monitor carefully.

NURSING CONSIDERATIONS
- *Contraindicated* in male breast cancer and not recommended for premenopausal women.
- Adequate trial is 3 months. Reassure patient that therapeutic response isn't immediate.
- Monitor fluids and electrolytes, especially calcium.
- Immobilized patients are prone to hypercalcemia. Exercise may prevent it. Force fluids to aid calcium excretion.
- Drug causes less virilization than testosterone.
- Higher-than-recommended doses do not increase incidence of remission.
- Testolactone is an androgen.

trilostane
Modrastane
Pregnancy Risk Category: X

HOW SUPPLIED
Capsules: 30 mg, 60 mg

MECHANISM OF ACTION
Reversibly lowers elevated circulating levels of glucocorticoids by inhibiting the enzyme system essential for their production in the adrenal gland.

INDICATIONS & DOSAGE
Adrenal cortical hyperfunction in Cushing's syndrome –
Adults: 30 mg P.O. q.i.d. initially. May be increased at intervals of 3 to 4 days to maximum of 480 mg daily.

ADVERSE REACTIONS
Common reactions are in italics; life-threatening reactions are in bold italics.
CNS: headache.
CV: *orthostatic hypotension.*
EENT: burning of oral and nasal membranes.
GI: *diarrhea, upset stomach,* nausea, flatulence, bloating.
Metabolic: hyperkalemia.
Skin: flushing, rash.
Other: fever, fatigue, hot flashes.

INTERACTIONS
Aminoglutethimide, mitotane: may cause severe adrenocortical hypofunction.
Thiazides, loop diuretics: decreased potassium loss because trilostane inhibits aldosterone production.

NURSING CONSIDERATIONS
- *Contraindicated* in patients with severe renal or hepatic disease.
- *Use cautiously* in patients who are receiving other drugs that suppress adrenal function.
- Trilostane may prevent normal response to physiologic stressful situation. Therefore, patients who develop a severe illness or need surgery may need to have this drug temporarily discontinued.
- Because the drug may cause orthostatic hypotension by suppressing aldosterone production, monitor blood pressure regularly in all patients.
- Patient should show therapeutic response within 2 weeks. If no response has occurred, the doctor may discontinue the drug.
- Most patients show a therapeutic response at doses below 360 mg/day.
- Trilostane is prescribed when surgery or pituitary radiation is inappropriate or must be delayed. Explain to patient that the drug does not cure the underlying disease.

72
Miscellaneous antineoplastic agents

altretamine
asparaginase
***Erwinia* asparaginase**
bacillus Calmette-Guérin (BCG), live intravesical
etoposide
mitoxantrone hydrochloride
paclitaxel
pentostatin
teniposide
vinblastine sulfate
vincristine sulfate

COMBINATION PRODUCTS
None.

altretamine (hexamethylmelamine; HMM)
Hexalen

Pregnancy Risk Category: D

HOW SUPPLIED
Capsules: 50 mg

MECHANISM OF ACTION
Unknown. Structurally similar to the alkylating agent triethylenemelamine but not an alkylating agent. However, metabolism is known to be important for antitumor activity; metabolites of the drug are known alkylating agents.

INDICATIONS & DOSAGE
Palliative treatment of patients with persistent or recurrent ovarian cancer after first-line therapy with cisplatin or alkylating agent-based combination therapy –
Adults: 260 mg/m² P.O. daily in four divided doses with meals and h.s. for 14 or 21 consecutive days in a 28-day cycle.

ADVERSE REACTIONS
Common reactions are in italics; life-threatening reactions are in bold italics.
Blood: *leukopenia, thrombocytopenia, anemia.*
CNS: *sensory neuropathy*, anorexia, ataxia, paresthesias, hyporeflexia, fatigue, ***seizures***.
GI: *nausea and vomiting.*
Skin: alopecia; erythematous macropapular eczema.
Other: increased serum creatinine and elevated BUN levels.

INTERACTIONS
Cimetidine: may increase the half-life and toxicity of altretamine. Monitor closely for toxicity.
MAO inhibitors: severe orthostatic hypotension. Avoid concomitant use.

NURSING CONSIDERATIONS
- *Contraindicated* in patients hypersensitive to the drug and in patients with preexisting bone marrow depression or severe neurologic toxicity. However, patients with preexisting cisplatin neuropathies caused by high-dose cisplatin therapy have been successfully treated with altretamine. Carefully monitor these patients for worsening neurologic function.
- Continuous high-dose daily treatment with altretamine is associated with a higher incidence of mild to moderate neurotoxicity. It appears to be reversible when therapy is discontinued.
- Discontinue the drug temporarily for at least 14 days if laboratory tests show a platelet count below 75,000/mm³, WBC count below 2,000/mm³, or granulocyte count below 1,000/mm³. Also discontinue temporarily if the patient experiences severe GI distress that is unresponsive to symptom-

atic treatment or develops signs of progressive neuropathy. Drug should be discontinued if neurologic symptoms fail to stabilize.
• Unconfirmed reports suggest that the severity and incidence of neurotoxicity may be decreased by concomitant administration of pyridoxine.
• A careful neurologic assessment should be performed before each course of therapy.
• Monitor CBC and platelet count before each course of therapy and monthly thereafter. Altretamine causes a mild to moderate dose-related myelosuppression. Nadirs of leukocyte and platelet counts are reached by 3 to 4 weeks. Normal counts are regained by 6 weeks. Be sure that the patient understands that the drug may cause fetal harm and advise patient to avoid pregnancy.
• Continuous daily administration of this drug is associated with nausea and vomiting, which is usually treatable with antiemetics. If nausea and vomiting is severe, dosage reduction or temporary discontinuation of the drug may be necessary.

asparaginase (L-asparaginase)
Elspar, Kidrolase†

Erwinia asparaginase (porton asparaginase)

Pregnancy Risk Category: C

HOW SUPPLIED
asparaginase
Injection: 10,000-IU vials
***Erwinia* asparaginase**
Available through National Cancer Institute
Injection: 10,000 IU/vial

MECHANISM OF ACTION
Destroys the amino acid asparagine, which is needed for protein synthesis in acute lymphocytic leukemia. This leads to death of the leukemic cell.

Asparaginase is derived from cultures of *Escherichia coli.* Some patients may develop hypersensitivity to this drug. *Erwinia* asparaginase is derived from cultures of *Erwinia carotovora* and has been used in these patients without cross-sensitivity reactions.

INDICATIONS & DOSAGE
Acute lymphocytic leukemia (when used along with other drugs) –
Adults and children: asparaginase – 1,000 IU/kg I.V. daily for 10 days, injected over 30 minutes or by slow I.V. push; or 6,000 IU/m² I.M. at intervals specified in protocol.
Sole induction agent for acute lymphocytic leukemia –
Adults: asparaginase – 200 IU/kg I.V. daily for 28 days.
Acute lymphocytic leukemia (in combination with other drugs) –
Adults: *Erwinia* asparaginase – 5,000 to 10,000 IU/m² daily for 7 days q 3 weeks or 10,000 to 40,000 IU/m² q 2 to 3 weeks. Doses may be given I.V. over 15 to 30 minutes or by I.M. injection.
Children: *Erwinia* asparaginase – 6,000 to 10,000 IU/m² I.V. or I.M. daily for 14 days; or 60,000 IU/m² every other day for a total of 12 doses; or 1,000 IU/kg for 10 days.

ADVERSE REACTIONS
Common reactions are in italics; life-threatening reactions are in bold italics.
Blood: ***anemia, hypofibrinogenemia*** and depression of other clotting factors, ***thrombocytopenia, leukopenia,*** depression of serum albumin.
CNS: confusion, drowsiness, depression, hallucinations, nervousness, lethargy, somnolence.
GI: *vomiting (may last up to 24 hours), anorexia, nausea,* cramps, weight loss.
GU: *azotemia,* ***renal failure,*** uric

acid nephropathy, glycosuria, polyuria.
Hepatic: elevated AST (SGOT), ALT (SGPT), ***hepatotoxicity***.
Metabolic: elevated alkaline phosphatase and bilirubin (direct and indirect); increase or decrease in total lipids; *hyperuricemia, hyperglycemia; increased blood ammonia.*
Skin: *rash, urticaria.*
Other: ***hemorrhagic pancreatitis and anaphylaxis*** *(relatively common)*, chills, fever.

INTERACTIONS

Methotrexate: decreased methotrexate effectiveness.
Vincristine, prednisone: concurrent use is associated with increased toxicity.

NURSING CONSIDERATIONS

- *Contraindicated* in pancreatitis and previous hypersensitivity unless desensitized. *Use cautiously* in preexisting hepatic dysfunction.
- *Use cautiously.* Because of the unpredictability of adverse reactions, drug should be administered in hospital setting with close supervision.
- Keep epinephrine, diphenhydramine, and I.V. corticosteroids available for treatment of anaphylaxis.
- Don't use as sole agent to induce remission unless combination therapy is inappropriate. Not recommended for maintenance therapy.
- Risk of hypersensitivity increases with repeated dosages. Patient may be desensitized, but this doesn't rule out risk of allergic reactions. Routine administration of 2 IU I.V. test dose may identify high-risk patients.
- **I.V. use:** Give I.V. injection over 30 minutes through a running infusion of sodium chloride injection or 5% dextrose injection.
- For I.M. injection, limit dose at single injection site to 2 ml.
- Because of vomiting, patient may need parenteral fluids for 24 hours or until oral fluids are tolerated.
- Monitor CBC and bone marrow function. Bone marrow regeneration may take 5 to 6 weeks.
- Obtain frequent serum amylase determinations to check pancreatic status. If elevated, asparaginase should be discontinued.
- Tumor lysis can result in uric acid nephropathy. Prevent occurrence by increasing fluid intake. Allopurinol should be started before therapy begins.
- Warn patient to watch for signs of infection (fever, sore throat, fatigue) and bleeding (easy bruising, nosebleeds, bleeding gums, melena). Take temperature daily.
- Monitor blood and urine glucose before and during therapy. Watch for signs of hyperglycemia, such as glycosuria and polyuria.
- Reconstitute with either 2 to 5 ml sterile water for injection or sodium chloride injection.
- Don't shake vial; may cause loss of potency. Don't use cloudy solutions.
- Refrigerate unopened dry powder. Reconstituted solution is stable for 6 hours at room temperature, 24 hours refrigerated.
- Preparation of parenteral form is associated with carcinogenic, mutagenic, and teratogenic risks for personnel. Follow institutional policy to reduce risks.

bacillus Calmette-Guérin (BCG), live intravesical

ImmuCyst†, TheraCys, TICE BCG

Pregnancy Risk Category: C

HOW SUPPLIED

TheraCys
Suspension (freeze-dried) for bladder instillation: 27 mg/vial
TICE BCG
Suspension (freeze-dried) for bladder

*Liquid form contains alcohol. **May contain tartrazine.

instillation: approximately 50 mg/ampule

MECHANISM OF ACTION

Exact mechanism unknown. Instillation of the live bacterial suspension causes a local inflammatory response. Local infiltration of histiocytes and leukocytes is followed by a decrease in the superficial tumors within the bladder.

INDICATIONS & DOSAGE

Treatment of in situ carcinoma of the urinary bladder (primary and relapsed) –

Adults: administer 3 reconstituted and diluted vials intravesically once weekly for 6 weeks (induction) followed by additional treatments at 3, 6, 12, 18, and 24 months (TheraCys); 1 bladder instillation (1 ampule suspended in 50 ml sterile, preservative-free saline solution) once weekly for 6 weeks, then once monthly for 6 to 12 months (TICE BCG).

ADVERSE REACTIONS

Common reactions are in italics; life-threatening reactions are in bold italics.

Blood: anemia, leukopenia, thrombocytopenia.

GI: nausea, vomiting, anorexia, diarrhea, mild abdominal pain.

GU: *dysuria, urinary frequency, hematuria,* cystitis, urinary urgency, urinary incontinence, urinary tract infection, cramps, pain, decreased bladder capacity, tissue in urine, local infection, renal toxicity, genital pain.

Other: malaise, *fever above 101° F (38.3° C),* chills, myalgia, arthralgia, elevated liver enzymes, ***disseminated mycobacterial infection.***

INTERACTIONS

Antibiotics: antimicrobial therapy for other infections may attenuate the response to BCG intravesical. Avoid concomitant use.

Immunosuppressants, bone marrow depressants, and radiation therapy: may impair the response to BCG intravesical because these treatments can decrease the patient's immune response and may also increase the risk of osteomyelitis or disseminated BCG infection. Avoid concomitant use.

NURSING CONSIDERATIONS

- *Contraindicated* in patients with compromised immune systems, in patients who are receiving immunosuppressive therapy because of the risk of bacterial infection, and in those with urinary tract infection because of the risk of increased bladder irritation or disseminated BCG infection. Also contraindicated in patients with fever of unknown origin. If the fever is caused by an infection, the drug should be withheld until the patient has recovered.
- Do not use as an immunizing agent for the prevention of cancer. Do not use to prevent tuberculosis because the drug should not be confused with BCG vaccine.
- This drug should not be handled or administered by caregiver with a known immunologic deficiency.
- BCG intravesical should not be administered within 7 to 14 days of transurethral resection or biopsy. Fatal disseminated BCG infection has occurred after traumatic catheterization.
- Carefully monitor patient's urinary status because the drug causes an inflammatory response in the bladder. It has been associated with bacterial urinary tract infection, hematuria, dysuria, and urinary frequency.
- Closely monitor patients for evidence of systemic BCG infection. BCG infections are rarely detected by positive cultures. Withhold therapy if systemic infection is suspected (short-term high fever above 103° F [39.4°]; persistent fever above 101° F over 2 days or with severe malaise). Contact infectious disease specialist for initia-

tion of fast-acting antituberculosis therapy.

• Patients with a small bladder capacity may experience increased local irritation with the usual dose of BCG intravesical.

• The drug has the potential to cause hypersensitivity reactions. Manage symptomatically.

• Tuberculin sensitivity may be rendered positive by BCG intravesical treatment. Determine patient's reactivity to tuberculin before therapy.

• Administration of this drug should be avoided by anyone with immune deficiency, and requires wearing of masks and gloves.

• To administer TheraCys, reconstitute the drug only with 1 ml of the provided diluent per vial, just before use. Do not remove the rubber stopper to prepare the solution. Use immediately. The contents of the three reconstituted vials are to be added to 50 ml of sterile, preservative-free saline solution (final volume 53 ml). A urethral catheter is instilled into the bladder under aseptic conditions, the bladder is drained, and then 53 ml of the prepared solution is infused by gravity feed. The catheter is then removed. Properly dispose of any unused drug.

• To administer TICE BCG, use thermosetting plastic or sterile glass containers and syringes. Draw 1 ml of sterile, preservative-free saline solution into a 3-ml syringe. Add to one ampule of the drug; gently expel back into the ampule three times to ensure thorough mixing. Use immediately. Dispense the cloudy suspension into the top end of a catheter-tipped syringe that contains 49 ml saline. Gently rotate the syringe. Properly dispose of any unsed drug.

• Handle the drug and all material used for the instillation of the drug as infectious material because it contains live attenuated mycobacteria. Dispose of all associated materials (syringes, catheters, and containers) as biohazardous waste.

• Use strict aseptic technique to administer the drug to minimize trauma to the GU tract and to prevent introducing other contaminants to the area.

• If there is evidence of traumatic catheterization, do not administer the drug. Subsequent treatment may resume after 1 week as if no interruption of the schedule has occurred.

• Bladder irritation can be treated symptomatically with phenazopyridine, acetaminophen, and propantheline. Systemic hypersensitivity reactions can be treated with diphenhydramine (Benadryl).

• Tell the patient to retain the drug in his bladder for 2 hours after instillation (if possible). For the first hour, he should lie 15 minutes prone, 15 minutes supine, and 15 minutes on each side. He may be sit up for the second hour.

• Instruct patient to sit when voiding.

• Patient should be instructed to disinfect any urine for 6 hours after instillation of the drug. To disinfect urine, add undiluted household bleach (5% sodium hypochlorite solution) in equal volume to voided urine to the toilet; allow to stand for 15 minutes before flushing.

• Tell the patient to call if symptoms worsen or if he develops any of the following symptoms: blood in the urine, fever and chills, frequent urge to urinate, painful urination, nausea, vomiting, joint pain, or rash.

• Tell the patient that a cough that develops after therapy could indicate a life-threatening BCG infection and should be reported to the doctor immediately.

etoposide (VP-16)

VePesid

Pregnancy Risk Category: D

*Liquid form contains alcohol. **May contain tartrazine.

HOW SUPPLIED
Capsules: 50 mg
Injection: 100-mg/5-ml multiple-dose vials

MECHANISM OF ACTION
A semisynthetic derivative of podophyllotoxin that arrests cell mitosis.

INDICATIONS & DOSAGE
Testicular cancer –
Adults: 50 to 100 mg/m² P.O. or I.V. on 5 consecutive days q 3 to 4 weeks; or 100 mg/m² on days 1, 3, and 5 q 3 to 4 weeks.
Small-cell carcinoma of the lung, acute nonlymphocytic leukemia, Hodgkin's disease, non-Hodgkin's lymphoma, Ewing's sarcoma –
Adults: 35 mg/m² I.V. or P.O. daily for 4 consecutive days or 50 mg/m² I.V. or P.O. daily for 5 consecutive days q 3 or 4 weeks.
Kaposi's sarcoma –
Adults: 150 mg/m² P.O. or I.V. daily for 3 consecutive days q 4 weeks.

ADVERSE REACTIONS
Common reactions are in italics; life-threatening reactions are in bold italics.
Blood: *anemia, **myelosuppression** (dose-limiting), **leukopenia, thrombocytopenia.***
CV: hypotension from rapid infusion.
GI: nausea and vomiting, anorexia, abdominal pain, *stomatitis.*
Local: infrequent phlebitis.
Other: occasional headache and fever, *reversible alopecia, **anaphylaxis*** (rare), peripheral neuropathy.

INTERACTIONS
Warfarin: etoposide may further increase prothrombin time.

NURSING CONSIDERATIONS
- *Contraindicated* for intrapleural and intrathecal administration.
- Oral dosage is calculated according to body surface area; dose is rounded to the nearest 50 mg.
- Store capsules in refrigerator.
- **I.V. use:** Give drug by slow I.V. infusion (over at least 30 minutes) to prevent severe hypotension.
- The drug may be diluted for infusion in either dextrose 5% in water or normal saline solution to a concentration of 0.2 or 0.4 mg/ml. Higher concentrations may crystallize.
- Solutions diluted to 0.2 mg/ml are stable for 96 hours at room temperature in plastic or glass unprotected from light; solutions diluted to 0.4 mg/ml are stable for 48 hours under the same conditions.
- Do not administer through membrane-type in-line filters because the diluent may dissolve the filter.
- Blood pressure should be monitored before infusion and at 30-minute intervals during infusion. If systolic blood pressure falls below 90 mm Hg, infusion should be stopped and doctor notified.
- Have diphenhydramine, hydrocortisone, epinephrine, and airway available in case of an anaphylactic reaction.
- Monitor CBC. Observe patient for signs of bone marrow suppression.
- Observe oral cavity for signs of ulceration.
- Etoposide has produced complete remissions in small-cell lung cancer and testicular cancer.
- Preparation of parenteral form is associated with carcinogenic, mutagenic, and teratogenic risks for personnel. Follow institutional policy to reduce risks.

mitoxantrone hydrochloride
Novantrone

Pregnancy Risk Category: D

HOW SUPPLIED
Injection: 2 mg/ml in 10-ml, 12.5-ml, 15-ml vials

MECHANISM OF ACTION
Not fully understood; probably non-cell-cycle specific. Reacts with DNA, producing cytotoxic effect.

INDICATIONS & DOSAGE
Combination initial therapy for acute nonlymphocytic leukemia (ANL) – **Adults:** induction begins with 12 mg/m² I.V. daily on days 1 through 3, in combination with cytosine arabinoside 100 mg/m² daily on days 1 through 7. A second induction may be given if response is not adequate. Maintenance therapy: 12 mg/m² on days 1 and 2 with cytosine arabinoside administered on days 1 through 5.

ADVERSE REACTIONS
Common reactions are in italics; life-threatening reactions are in bold italics.
Blood: ***myelosuppression.***
CNS: *seizures,* headache.
CV: ***CHF, arrhythmias,*** tachycardia.
EENT: conjunctivitis.
GI: *bleeding, abdominal pain, diarrhea, nausea, mucositis, stomatitis, vomiting.*
Respiratory: dyspnea, cough.
Skin: petechiae, ecchymoses.
Other: alopecia, jaundice, fever, hyperuricemia, renal failure.

INTERACTIONS
Heparin: incompatible when mixed together.

NURSING CONSIDERATIONS
- *Contraindicated* in patients with hypersensitivity to mitoxantrone.
- *Use cautiously* in patients with prior exposure to anthracyclines or other cardiotoxic drugs.
- Uric acid nephropathy can be avoided by adequately hydrating the patient before and during therapy. Be prepared to administer allopurinol as ordered.
- Patients with significant myelosuppression should not receive mitoxantrone unless the benefits outweigh the risks. Mitoxantrone should be prescribed only by doctors experienced with chemotherapy.
- Hematologic and chemistry laboratory parameters should be monitored closely.
- **I.V. use:** Available as an aqueous solution of 2 mg/ml in volumes of 10, 12.5, and 15 ml. The dose should be diluted in at least 50 ml of 0.9% sodium chloride injection or dextrose 5% in water (D_5W) injection. Administer by direct injection into a free-flowing I.V. of 0.9% sodium chloride or D_5W injection over at least 3 minutes. Mixing with other drugs is not recommended.
- Mitoxantrone is not a vesicant; however, if drug extravasates, discontinue infusion immediately.
- The undiluted solution should be stored at room temperature. Once diluted, the mixture is stable for 48 hours at room temperature.
- Exercise extreme caution when preparing or administering mitoxantrone to avoid mutagenic, teratogenic, and carcinogenic risks. Use a biological containment cabinet, wear gloves and mask, and use syringes with Luer-Lok fittings to prevent leakage of drug solution. Spills should be cleaned with a calcium hypochlorite solution (6 parts calcium hypochlorite to 13 parts of water for each 1 part of mitoxantrone). Also correctly dispose of needles, vials, and unused drug, and avoid contaminating work surfaces. Avoid inhalation of dust or vapors and contact with skin or mucous membranes. If contact with the eye occurs, irrigate with water or saline and consult an ophthalmologist. If the drug comes in contact with the skin, irrigate the area with water.
- Infections should be treated with antibiotics, as ordered. If severe nonhematologic toxicity occurs during the first course of therapy, the second course should be delayed until patient recovers.

- Patients should be informed that the urine may appear blue-green within 24 hours after administration and some bluish discoloration of the sclera may occur, but that these effects are not harmful.
- Monitor left ventricular ejection fraction during administration.

paclitaxel

Taxol

Pregnancy Risk Category: D

HOW SUPPLIED

Injection: 30 mg/5 ml

MECHANISM OF ACTION

Prevents depolymerization of cellular microtubules, thus inhibiting the normal reorganization of the microtubule network necessary for mitosis and other vital cellular functions.

INDICATIONS & DOSAGE

Metastatic ovarian carcinoma after failure of first-line or subsequent chemotherapy –

Women: 135 mg/m² I.V. over 24 hours q 3 weeks. Subsequent courses shouldn't be repeated until neutrophil count is ≥ 1,500 cells/mm³ and platelet count is ≥ 100,000 cells/mm³.

ADVERSE REACTIONS

Common reactions are in italics; life-threatening reactions are in bold italics.

Blood: ***neutropenia, leukopenia, thrombocytopenia,*** *anemia, infections, bleeding.*

CV: *bradycardia, hypotension, abnormal ECG.*

GI: *nausea, vomiting, diarrhea, mucositis.*

Skin: alopecia.

Other: ***hypersensitivity reactions,*** *peripheral neuropathy, myalgia, arthralgia.*

INTERACTIONS

Cisplatin: possible additive myelosuppressive effects. Use together cautiously.

Ketoconazole: inhibits paclitaxel metabolism. Use together cautiously.

NURSING CONSIDERATIONS

- *Contraindicated* in patients with hypersensitivity to the drug or polyoxyethylated castor oil, a vehicle used to solubilize the drug, and in patients with baseline neutrophil count below 1,500 cells/mm³.
- *Use cautiously* in patients who have received prior radiation therapy because these patients may display more frequent or more severe myelosuppression. Also use cautiously in patients with hepatic impairment.
- Severe hypersensitivity reactions have occurred in as many as 2% of patients treated in early clinical trials. To reduce the incidence or severity of these reactions, patients should be pretreated with corticosteroids, such as dexamethasone and antihistamines. Both H_1-receptor antagonists, such as diphenhydramine, and H_2-receptor antagonists, such as cimetidine or ranitidine, may be used.
- Bone marrow toxicity is the most frequent and dose-limiting toxicity. Frequent monitoring of blood counts is necessary during therapy. Packed RBC or platelet transfusions may be necessary in severe cases.
- If patient develops significant cardiac conduction abnormalities during treatment, appropriate therapy should be administered and continuous cardiac monitoring should be performed during subsequent infusions.
- **I.V. use:** Concentrate must be diluted before infusion. Compatible solutions include 0.9% sodium chloride injection, dextrose 5% in water, 5% dextrose in 0.9% sodium chloride injection, and 5% dextrose in Ringer's lactate injection. Dilute to a final concentration of 0.3 to 1.2 mg/ml. Infu-

sion solutions should be prepared and stored in glass containers. Drug should be administered using an in-line 0.22-micron filter.

- The undiluted concentrate shouldn't come in contact with polyvinylchloride plastic I.V. bags or tubing. Store diluted solution in glass or polypropylene plastic bottles, or use polypropylene or polyolefin bags. Administer through polyethylene-lined administration sets.
- Follow institutional protocol for the safe handling, preparation, and administration of chemotherapeutic drugs. Dispose of all waste materials properly.
- Warn patient that alopecia is common (up to 82% of patients).
- Teach patient the signs and symptoms of peripheral neuropathy, such as tingling or burning sensation or numbness in the extremities. Tell her to report these symptoms immediately. Although common, severe symptoms occur infrequently. Dosage reduction may be necessary.

pentostatin (2′-deoxycoformycin; DCF)

Nipent

Pregnancy Risk Category: D

HOW SUPPLIED

Powder for injection: 10 mg/vial

MECHANISM OF ACTION

Inhibits the enzyme adenosine deaminase (ADA), causing an increase in intracellular levels of deoxyadenosine triphosphate. This leads to cell damage and death. Because the greatest activity of ADA is in cells of the lymphoid system (especially malignant T cells), pentostatin is useful in treating leukemias.

INDICATIONS & DOSAGE

Alpha-interferon-refractory hairy-cell leukemia – **Adults:** 4 mg/m^2 every other week.

ADVERSE REACTIONS

Common reactions are in italics; life-threatening reactions are in bold italics.

Blood: ***myelosuppression, leukopenia, anemia, thrombocytopenia, lymphadenopathy.***

CNS: headache, neurologic symptoms, anxiety, confusion, depression, dizziness, insomnia, nervousness, paresthesia, somnolence, abnormal thinking.

CV: ***arrhythmias,*** *abnormal ECG, thrombophlebitis,* ***hemorrhage.***

EENT: *abnormal vision, conjunctivitis, ear pain, eye pain, epistaxis, pharyngitis, rhinitis, sinusitis.*

GI: *nausea, vomiting, anorexia, diarrhea, constipation, flatulence, stomatitis.*

GU: *GU disorder, hematuria, dysuria, increased BUN level, increased creatinine level.*

Hepatic: *elevated liver function tests.*

Metabolic: *weight loss, peripheral edema, increased lactate dehydrogenase.*

Respiratory: *cough, upper respiratory disorder, lung disorder, bronchitis, dyspnea, lung edema, pneumonia.*

Skin: *ecchymosis, petechiae, rash, skin disorder, eczema, dry skin, herpes simplex or zoster, maculopapular rash, vesiculobullous rash, pruritus, seborrhea, discoloration, sweating.*

Other: *fever, infection, fatigue, pain,* ***allergic reactions,*** *chills, sepsis, chest pain, abdominal pain, back pain, flu-like syndrome, asthenia, malaise, myalgia, arthralgia.*

INTERACTIONS

Fludarabine: risk of severe or fatal pulmonary toxicity. Don't use together.

Vidarabine: increased incidence or severity of adverse effects associated with either drug. Avoid concomitant use.

NURSING CONSIDERATIONS

- *Contraindicated* in patients with hypersensitivity to the drug.
- *Use cautiously* and only under the supervision of a doctor qualified and experienced in the use of chemotherapeutic agents. Adverse reactions after pentostatin therapy are common.
- Withhold drug or discontinue in patients with evidence of CNS toxicity, a severe rash, or an active infection. Drug may be resumed when the infection clears. Also avoid use in patients with renal damage (creatinine clearance of 60 ml/minute or less).
- Temporarily withhold drug if the absolute neutrophil count falls below 200 cells/mm^3 and the pretreatment level was over 500 cells/mm^3. No recommendations exist regarding dosage adjustments in patients with anemia, neutropenia, or thrombocytopenia.
- Drug should be used only in patients who have hairy-cell leukemia refractory to alpha interferon. This is defined as disease that progresses after a minimum of 3 months of treatment with alpha interferon or disease that does not exhibit a response after 6 months of therapy.
- The optimal duration of therapy is unknown. Current recommendations suggest two additional courses of therapy after a complete response. If the patient has not had a partial response after 6 months of therapy, discontinue drug. If the patient has had only a partial response, continue drug for another 6 months or for two courses of therapy after a complete response.
- **I.V. use:** Follow institutional guidelines for proper handling, administration, and disposal of chemotherapeutic agents. Treat all spills and waste products with 5% sodium hypochlorite. Wear protective clothing and polyethylene gloves. Add 5 ml sterile water for injection to the vial containing pentostatin powder for injection. Mix thoroughly to make a solution of 5 mg/ml. Drug may be administered by I.V. bolus injection or diluted further in 25 or 50 ml of dextrose 5% in water (D_5W) or 0.9% sodium chloride injection and infused over 20 to 30 minutes.
- Be sure patient is adequately hydrated before therapy. Administer 500 to 1,000 ml of D_5W in 0.45% sodium chloride injection. Give 500 ml of D_5W after drug is given.

teniposide (VM-26)

Vumon

Pregnancy Risk Category: C

HOW SUPPLIED

Injection: 10 mg/ml

MECHANISM OF ACTION

A semisynthetic derivative of podophyllotoxin that arrests cell mitosis and causes breaks in DNA.

INDICATIONS & DOSAGE

Refractory childhood acute lymphoblastic leukemia –

Children: optimum dosage hasn't been established. In clinical trials, dosages ranged from 165 to 250 mg/m^2 I.V. once or twice weekly for 4 to 6 weeks. Usually used in combination with other agents.

ADVERSE REACTIONS

Common reactions are in italics; life-threatening reactions are in bold italics.

Blood: ***myelosuppression*** *(dose-limiting), leukopenia, neutropenia, thrombocytopenia, anemia*.

CV: hypotension from rapid infusion.

GI: nausea and vomiting.

Local: *phlebitis,* extravasation.

Other: alopecia (rare), ***anaphylaxis*** (rare), sensitivity reactions (chills, fever, urticaria, tachycardia, ***bronchospasm,*** dyspnea, hypotension, flushing), mucositis.

INTERACTIONS

None significant.

NURSING CONSIDERATIONS

- *Contraindicated* in patients with hypersensitivity to the drug or to polyoxyethylated castor oil, an injection vehicle.
- *Use cautiously* in patients with a history of mild-to-moderate sensitivity reactions to the drug. Also use cautiously and in lower doses in patients with Down's syndrome because these patients may be particularly sensitive to myelosuppressive chemotherapy.
- Some clinicians may decide to use this drug despite the patient's history of hypersensitivity reactions because the drug's benefits may outweigh its risks. Such a patient should be pretreated with antihistamines and corticosteroids before the infusion begins and closely watched during drug administration.
- Baseline and periodic determinations of blood counts and renal and hepatic function studies should be performed.
- **I.V. use:** Dilute drug in either dextrose 5% in water or 0.9% sodium chloride injection to a final concentration of 0.1, 0.2, 0.4, or 1 mg/ml. Cloudy solutions should be discarded. Prepare and store the drug in glass containers. Infuse over 45 to 90 minutes to prevent hypotension.
- Solutions containing 0.5 to 1 mg/ml are stable for 4 hours; those containing 0.1 to 0.2 mg/ml are stable for 6 hours.
- Avoid extravasation. Because extravasation of drug can result in local tissue necrosis or sloughing, it's extremely important to ensure careful placement of the I.V. catheter.
- Monitor blood pressure before infusion and at 30-minute intervals during infusion. If systolic blood pressure falls below 90 mm Hg, stop infusion and notify doctor.
- Don't administer through a membrane-type in-line filter because the diluent may dissolve the filter.
- Have on hand diphenhydramine, hydrocortisone, epinephrine, and appropriate emergency equipment to establish an airway in case of anaphylaxis.
- Drug may be given by local bladder instillation for bladder cancer.
- Preparation of parenteral form is associated with carcinogenic, mutagenic, and teratogenic risks for personnel. Follow institutional policy to reduce risks.

vinblastine sulfate (VLB)

Alkaban-AQ, Velban, Velbe†‡, Velsar

Pregnancy Risk Category: D

HOW SUPPLIED

Injection: 10-mg vials (lyophilized powder), 10-mg/10-ml vials

MECHANISM OF ACTION

Arrests mitosis in metaphase, blocking cell division.

INDICATIONS & DOSAGE

Breast or testicular cancer, Hodgkin's and non-Hodgkin's lymphomas, choriocarcinoma, lymphosarcoma, neuroblastoma, mycosis fungoides, Kaposi's sarcoma, histiocytosis –

Adults: 0.1 mg/kg or 3.7 mg/m^2 I.V. weekly or q 2 weeks. May be increased to maximum dosage of 0.5 mg/kg or 18.5 mg/m^2 I.V. weekly according to response. Dosage should not be repeated if WBC less than 4,000/mm^3.

Children: initial dose 2.5 mg/m^2 I.V. Increase dose by 1.25 mg/m^2 until leukocytes are below 3,000/mm^3 or a tumor response is seen. Maximum dose is 7.5 mg/m^2.

ADVERSE REACTIONS

Common reactions are in italics; life-threatening reactions are in bold italics.

Blood: ***anemia, leukopenia*** (nadir

*Liquid form contains alcohol. **May contain tartrazine.

days 4 to 10 and lasts another 7 to 14 days), ***thrombocytopenia.***
CNS: depression, *paresthesias, peripheral neuropathy and neuritis, numbness, loss of deep tendon reflexes, muscle pain and weakness,* ***seizures,*** headache.
CV: hypertension.
EENT: pharyngitis.
GI: *nausea, vomiting, stomatitis,* ulcer and bleeding, *constipation, ileus, anorexia, weight loss,* abdominal pain.
GU: oligospermia, aspermia, urine retention.
Skin: dermatitis, vesiculation.
Local: *irritation, phlebitis,* cellulitis, necrosis if I.V. extravasates.
Other: ***acute bronchospasm,*** reversible alopecia in 5% to 10% of patients, *pain in tumor site,* low fever.

INTERACTIONS
Mitomycin: increased risk of bronchospasm and shortness of breath.
Phenytoin: decreased plasma phenytoin levels.

NURSING CONSIDERATIONS
- *Contraindicated* in severe leukopenia or bacterial infection.
- *Use cautiously* in jaundice or hepatic dysfunction.
- Do not administer into a limb with compromised circulation.
- Decrease dose by 50% if bilirubin levels are greater than 3 mg/100 ml.
- After administering, monitor for life-threatening acute bronchospasm reaction. If this occurs, notify doctor immediately. Reaction most likely to occur in patient who is also receiving mitomycin.
- Give antiemetic before administering to reduce nausea.
- Drug should be stopped if stomatitis occurs.
- Assess bowel activity. Give laxatives as needed. May use stool softeners prophylactically.
- Don't repeat dosage more frequently than every 7 days or severe leukopenia will develop.
- Less neurotoxic than vincristine.
- Assess for numbness and tingling in hands and feet. Assess gait for early evidence of footdrop.
- **I.V. use:** Should be injected directly into vein or tubing of running I.V. over 1 minute. May also be given in a 50-ml dextrose 5% in water or 0.9% sodium chloride solution and infused over 15 minutes. If extravasation occurs, stop infusion immediately. The manufacturer recommends that moderate heat be applied to the area of leakage. Local injection of hyaluronidase may help disperse the drug. Some clinicians prefer to apply ice packs on and off every 2 hours for 24 hours, with local injection of hydrocortisone or 0.9% sodium chloride.
- Warn patient that loss of all body hair may occur but is usually reversible.
- Adequate trial 12 weeks; reassure patient that therapeutic response isn't immediate.
- Reconstitute 10-mg vial with 10 ml of sodium chloride injection or sterile water. This yields 1 mg/ml. Refrigerate reconstituted solution. Discard after 30 days.
- Don't confuse vinblastine with vincristine or the investigational agent vindesine.
- Preparation of parenteral form is associated with carcinogenic, mutagenic, and teratogenic risks for personnel. Follow institutional policy to reduce risks.

vincristine sulfate
Oncovin, Vincasar PFS

Pregnancy Risk Category: D

HOW SUPPLIED
Injection: 1-mg/ml, 2-mg/2-ml, 5-mg/5-ml multiple-dose vials; 1-mg/1-ml, 2-mg/2-ml preservative-free vials

MECHANISM OF ACTION

Arrests mitosis in metaphase, blocking cell division.

INDICATIONS & DOSAGE

Acute lymphoblastic and other leukemias, Hodgkin's disease, non-Hodgkin's lymphoma, lymphosarcoma, reticulum cell sarcoma, neuroblastoma, rhabdomyosarcoma, Wilms' tumor, Ewing's sarcoma, osteogenic and other sarcomas, lung and breast cancer—

Adults: 0.4 to 1.4 mg/m² I.V. weekly.
Children over 10 kg: 1.5 to 2 mg/m² I.V. weekly.
Children 10 kg and under: initially, 0.05 mg/kg I.V. weekly.
Maximum single dosage (adults and children) is 2 mg.

ADVERSE REACTIONS

Common reactions are in italics; life-threatening reactions are in bold italics.
Blood: rapidly reversible mild anemia and leukopenia.
CNS: *peripheral neuropathy,* sensory loss, *loss of deep tendon reflexes, paresthesias, wristdrop and footdrop,* ataxia, cranial nerve palsies (headache, *jaw pain,* hoarseness, vocal cord paralysis, visual disturbances), *muscle weakness and cramps,* depression, agitation, insomnia; some neurotoxicities may be permanent.
CV: hypotension.
EENT: diplopia, optic and extraocular neuropathy, ptosis.
GI: diarrhea, *constipation, cramps,* ileus that mimics surgical abdomen, *nausea, vomiting,* anorexia, *stomatitis,* weight loss, dysphagia, ***intestinal necrosis.***
GU: urine retention, syndrome of inappropriate antidiuretic hormone (SIADH).
Local: severe local reaction when extravasated, *phlebitis,* cellulitis.
Other: ***acute bronchospasm,*** *reversible alopecia (up to 71% of patients),* fever.

INTERACTIONS

Asparaginase: decreased hepatic clearance of vincristine.
Calcium channel blockers: enhanced vincristine accumulation in cells.
Digoxin: decreased digoxin effects. Monitor serum digoxin.
Mitomycin: possibly increased frequency of bronchospasm and acute pulmonary reactions.

NURSING CONSIDERATIONS

- *Contraindicated* in patients with hypersensitivity to the drug. Do not administer the drug to patients who are concurrently receiving radiation therapy through ports that include the liver.
- *Use cautiously* in jaundice or hepatic dysfunction, neuromuscular disease, infection, and with other neurotoxic drugs. Dose may be reduced by 50% if bilirubin is above 3 mg/dl.
- After administering, monitor for life-threatening acute bronchospasm reaction. If this occurs, notify doctor immediately. Reaction most likely to occur in patient who is also receiving mitomycin.
- Monitor for hyperuricemia, especially in patients with leukemia or lymphoma. Maintain good hydration and administer allopurinol as ordered to prevent uric acid nephropathy.
- Because of neurotoxicity, don't give drug more than once a week. Children more resistant to neurotoxicity than adults. Neurotoxicity is dose-related and usually reversible.
- **I.V. use:** Should be given directly into vein or tubing of running I.V. slowly over 1 minute. May also be given in a 50-ml dextrose 5% in water or normal saline solution and infused over 15 minutes. If drug infiltrates, stop infusion immediately. Apply ice packs on and off every 2 hours for 24 hours.
- Check for depression of Achilles tendon reflex, numbness, tingling, footdrop or wristdrop, difficulty in

walking, ataxia, and slapping gait. Also check ability to walk on heels. Support patient when walking.

- Monitor bowel function. Give stool softener, laxative, or water before dosing. Constipation may be an early sign of neurotoxicity.
- Warn patient that alopecia may occur but is usually reversible.
- Be extremely careful about doses. Don't confuse vincristine with vinblastine or the investigational agent vindesine.
- 5-mg vials are for multiple-dose use only. Don't administer entire vial to one patient as a single dose.
- All vials (1-mg, 2-mg, 5-mg) contain 1 mg/ml solution and should be refrigerated.
- Preparation of parenteral form is associated with carcinogenic, mutagenic, and teratogenic risks for personnel. Follow institutional policy to reduce risks.

73

Immunosuppressants

azathioprine
cyclosporine
levamisole hydrochloride
lymphocyte immune globulin
muromonab-CD3

COMBINATION PRODUCTS
None.

azathioprine

Imuran, Thioprine‡

Pregnancy Risk Category: D

HOW SUPPLIED
Tablets: 50 mg
Injection: 100 mg

MECHANISM OF ACTION
Inhibits purine synthesis.

INDICATIONS & DOSAGE
Immunosuppression in renal transplants –
Adults and children: initially, 3 to 5 mg/kg P.O. or I.V. daily usually beginning on the day of transplantation. Maintain at 1 to 3 mg/kg daily (dosage varies considerably according to patient response).
Treatment of severe, refractory rheumatoid arthritis –
Adults: initially, 1 mg/kg P.O. taken as a single dose or as two doses. If patient response is not satisfactory after 6 to 8 weeks, dosage may be increased by 0.5 mg/kg daily (up to a maximum of 2.5 mg/kg daily) at 4-week intervals.

ADVERSE REACTIONS
Common reactions are in italics; life-threatening reactions are in bold italics.
Blood: ***leukopenia, bone marrow suppression,*** anemia, ***pancytopenia, thrombocytopenia.***
GI: nausea, vomiting, anorexia, ***pancreatitis,*** steatorrhea, mouth ulceration, esophagitis.
Hepatic: ***hepatotoxicity,*** jaundice.
Skin: rash.
Other: ***immunosuppression*** *(possibly profound),* arthralgia, muscle wasting, alopecia.

INTERACTIONS
Allopurinol: impaired inactivation of azathioprine. Decrease azathioprine dose to ¼ or ⅓ normal dose.
Nondepolarizing neuromuscular blocking agents: azathioprine may reverse the neuromuscular blockade.

NURSING CONSIDERATIONS
- *Contraindicated* in patients with hypersensitivity to the drug.
- *Use cautiously* in hepatic or renal dysfunction.
- Watch for clay-colored stools, dark urine, pruritus, and yellow skin and sclera; and for increased alkaline phosphatase, bilirubin, AST (SGOT), and ALT (SGPT).
- In renal homotransplants, start drug 1 to 5 days before surgery.
- Hemoglobin, WBC, and platelet count should be done at least once monthly; more often at beginning of treatment. Drug should be stopped immediately when WBC is less than 3,000/mm^3 to prevent irreversible bone marrow suppression.
- This is a potent immunosuppressive. Warn patient to report even mild infections (colds, fever, sore throat, and malaise).
- **I.V. use:** Only for patients unable to tolerate oral medications. Reconstitute 100-mg vial with 10 ml of sterile water for injection. Visually inspect for particles before giving. Drug may be administered by direct I.V. injec-

tion or further diluted in 0.9% sodium chloride injection or dextrose 5% in water and infused over 30 to 60 minutes.

- Instruct patient to avoid conception during therapy and for 4 months after stopping therapy.
- Warn patient that some thinning of hair is possible.
- Avoid I.M. injections of any drugs in patients with severely depressed platelet counts (thrombocytopenia) to prevent bleeding.
- Therapeutic response usually occurs within 8 weeks. When used for refractory rheumatoid arthritis, inform patient that it may take up to 12 weeks to be effective.

cyclosporine (cyclosporin)

Sandimmun‡, Sandimmune

Pregnancy Risk Category: C

HOW SUPPLIED

Oral solution: 100 mg/ml
Injection: 50 mg/ml

MECHANISM OF ACTION

Inhibits the proliferation of T lymphocytes.

INDICATIONS & DOSAGE

Prophylaxis of organ rejection in kidney, liver, bone marrow, and heart transplants –

Adults and children: 15 mg/kg P.O. (oral solution) 4 to 12 hours before transplantation. Continue this daily dosage postoperatively for 1 to 2 weeks. Then, gradually reduce dosage by 5%/week to maintenance level of 5 to 10 mg/kg/day. Alternatively, administer I.V. concentrate 4 to 5 mg/kg 4 to 12 hours before transplantation. Postoperatively, repeat this dosage daily until patient can tolerate oral solution.

ADVERSE REACTIONS

Common reactions are in italics; life-threatening reactions are in bold italics.

Blood: anemia, ***leukopenia, thrombocytopenia.***
CNS: *tremor,* headache.
CV: hypertension.
GI: *gum hyperplasia,* nausea, vomiting, diarrhea, oral thrush.
GU: ***nephrotoxicity.***
Hepatic: ***hepatotoxicity.***
Skin: *hirsutism,* acne.
Other: sinusitis, flushing, increased LDL cholesterol levels, ***infections.***

INTERACTIONS

Aminoglycosides, amphotericin B, co-trimoxazole, NSAIDs: increased risk of nephrotoxicity.
Azathioprine, corticosteroids, cyclophosphamide, verapamil: increased immunosuppression.
Carbamazepine, isoniazid, phenobarbital, phenytoin, rifampin: possible decreased immunosuppressant effect. May need to increase cyclosporine dosage.
Ketoconazole, amphotericin B, cimetidine, diltiazem, erythromycin, imipenem-cilastatin, metoclopramide, prednisolone: may increase blood levels of cyclosporine. Monitor for increased toxicity.

NURSING CONSIDERATIONS

- *Contraindicated* in patients with hypersensitivity to the drug. The injectable form contains polyoxylethylated castor oil (Cremophor EL), which may provoke hypersensitivity reactions in certain persons. Closely monitor patients receiving I.V. infusion of the drug for hypersensitivity reactions.
- Cyclosporine may cause nephrotoxicity. Monitor BUN and serum creatinine levels. Nephrotoxicity may develop 2 to 3 months after transplant surgery. Report these findings to doctor. He may reduce the dosage.
- Differentiation between trans-

planted kidney rejection and cyclosporine-induced nephrotoxicity must be made.
- Monitor liver function tests for hepatotoxicity, which usually occurs during first month post-organ transplant.
- Cyclosporine should always be given concomitantly with adrenal corticosteroids.
- Absorption of cyclosporine oral solution can be erratic. Monitor cyclosporine blood levels at regular intervals. In a recent study, absorption in children following liver transplant was enhanced by administering with water-soluble vitamin E.
- Measure oral doses carefully in an oral syringe. To increase palatability, mix with whole milk, chocolate milk, or fruit juice. Use a glass container to minimize adherence to container walls.
- Dosage should be given once daily in the morning. Encourage patient to take drug at the same time each day.
- Patient may take with meals if drug causes nausea. Anorexia, nausea, and vomiting are usually transient and occur during initiation of therapy.
- Stress to patient that therapy should not be stopped without doctor's approval.
- To prevent thrush, patient should swish and swallow nystatin four times daily.
- **I.V. use:** Usually reserved for patients who cannot tolerate oral medications. Cyclosporine I.V. concentrate is administered at one-third the oral dose and must be diluted before use. Each ml of the concentrate should be diluted in 20 to 100 ml of dextrose 5% in water or 0.9% sodium chloride injection. Dilute immediately before administration; infuse over 2 to 6 hours.
- If hirsutism occurs, tell patient she may use a depilatory.
- Cyclosporine has been used for various conditions, such as psoriatic arthritis or ulcerative colitis.

levamisole hydrochloride
Ergamisol

Pregnancy Risk Category: C

HOW SUPPLIED
Tablets: 50 mg (base)

MECHANISM OF ACTION
Unknown. The effects of the drug on the immune system are complex. It appears to restore depressed immune function and may potentiate the actions of monocytes and macrophages and enhance T cell responses.

INDICATIONS & DOSAGE
Adjuvant treatment of Dukes' stage C colon cancer (with fluorouracil) after surgical resection –
Adults: 50 mg P.O. q 8 hours for 3 days. Therapy should begin no sooner than 7 days and no later than 30 days after surgery, providing that the patient is out of the hospital, ambulating, maintaining normal oral nutrition, has well-healed wounds, and has recovered from any postoperative complications. Fluorouracil (450 mg/m^2/day I.V.) is given daily for 5 days starting 21 to 34 days after surgery.

Maintenance dosage is 50 mg P.O. q 8 hours for 3 days q 2 weeks for 1 year. Given in conjunction with fluorouracil maintenance therapy (450 mg/m^2/day by rapid I.V. push, once a week beginning 28 days after the initial 5-day course) for 1 year.

ADVERSE REACTIONS
Common reactions are in italics; life-threatening reactions are in bold italics.
Blood: ***agranulocytosis, leukopenia, thrombocytopenia, granulocytopenia.***
CNS: *dizziness, headache, paresthesia, somnolence, depression, nervousness, insomnia, anxiety, fatigue, fever.*
CV: chest pain, edema.
EENT: blurred vision, conjunctivitis.
GI: *nausea, diarrhea, stomatitis,*

*Liquid form contains alcohol. **May contain tartrazine.

vomiting, anorexia, abdominal pain, constipation, flatulence, dyspepsia.
Metabolic: hyperbilirubinemia.
Skin: *dermatitis, alopecia,* ***exfoliative dermatitis,*** *pruritus, urticaria.*
Other: rigors, *infection, dysgeusia, altered sense of smell, arthralgia, myalgia.*

INTERACTIONS
Alcohol: may precipitate a disulfiram-like (Antabuse) reaction. Avoid concomitant use.
Phenytoin: plasma levels may be elevated when administered with levamisole and fluorouracil. Monitor phenytoin plasma levels.

NURSING CONSIDERATIONS
• *Contraindicated* in patients with a known hypersensitivity to the drug. Use with close hematologic monitoring because there is an association with agranulocytosis, which is sometimes fatal. Neutropenia is usually reversible when therapy is discontinued.
• If levamisole therapy begins 7 to 20 days after surgery, fluorouracil should be started with the second course of levamisole therapy. It should begin no sooner than 21 days and no later than 35 days after surgery. If levamisole is deferred until 21 to 30 days after surgery, fluorouracil therapy should begin with the first course of levamisole.
• If stomatitis or diarrhea develops during the initial course of fluorouracil therapy, discontinue drug, then begin weekly fluorouracil therapy 28 days after the start of the initial course. If stomatitis or diarrhea develops during the weekly doses of fluorouracil, defer fluorouracil therapy until these symptoms subside. Then, restart fluorouracil therapy at reduced dosages (decrease dose by 20%).
• Do not exceed recommended doses. Higher doses are associated with greater incidence of agranulocytosis.
• Dosage modifications are based on hematologic parameters. If WBC count is 2,500/mm^3 to 3,500/mm^3, don't administer fluorouracil until WBC count is above 3,500/mm^3. When fluorouracil is restarted, reduce dosage by 20%. If WBC count stays below 2,500/mm^3 for over 10 days after flurouracil is withdrawn, discontinue levamisole.
• If platelet count is below 100,000/mm^3, discontinue therapy with both fluorouracil and levamisole.
• Baseline CBC with differential and platelets and electrolyte and liver function studies are necessary immediately before starting therapy. Then, a CBC with differential and platelets should be performed at weekly intervals before treatment with fluorouracil. Electrolyte and liver function studies should be repeated every 3 months for 1 year.
• Advise patients to immediately report any flulike symptoms, such as fever and chills.
• Tell patients to promptly report stomatitis or diarrhea during fluorouracil therapy.

lymphocyte immune globulin (antithymocyte globulin [equine], ATG)
Atgam
Pregnancy Risk Category: C

HOW SUPPLIED
Injection: 50 mg of equine IgG/ml, 5-ml ampules

MECHANISM OF ACTION
Inhibits cell-mediated immune responses by either altering T cell function or eliminating antigen-reactive T cells.

INDICATIONS & DOSAGE
Prevention of acute renal allograft rejection –
Adults and children: 15 mg/kg I.V. daily for 14 days followed by alternate-day dosing for 14 days; the first

dose should be given within 24 hours of transplantation.
Treatment of acute renal allograft rejection –
Adults and children: 10 to 15 mg/kg I.V. daily for 14 days followed by alternate-day dosing for 14 days. Therapy should be initiated when rejection is diagnosed.

ADVERSE REACTIONS

Common reactions are in italics; life-threatening reactions are in bold italics.
Blood: ***leukopenia, thrombocytopenia, hemolysis,*** hyperglycemia, elevated serum hepatic enzymes.
CNS: malaise, ***seizures,*** headache.
CV: ***hypotension,*** *chest pain,* thrombophlebitis, tachycardia, edema, ***pulmonary edema,*** iliac vein obstruction, renal artery stenosis.
EENT: *dyspnea,* ***laryngospasm.***
GI: *nausea, vomiting,* diarrhea, stomatitis, hiccups, epigastric pain, abdominal distension.
Other: febrile reactions, serum sickness, ***anaphylaxis,*** rash, infections, arthralgia, night sweats, lymphadenopathy.

INTERACTIONS

None reported.

NURSING CONSIDERATIONS

- *Contraindicated* in patients with hypersensitivity to the drug. An intradermal skin test is recommended at least 1 hour before the first dose. Marked local swelling or erythema larger than 10 mm indicates an increased potential for severe systemic reaction (such as anaphylaxis). Severe reactions to the skin test, such as hypotension, tachycardia, dyspnea, generalized rash, or anaphylaxis, usually preclude further administration of the drug.
- *Use cautiously* in patients receiving additional immunosuppressive therapy (such as corticosteroids, azathioprine) because of the increased potential for infection. ATG concentrate should not be diluted with dextrose solutions or solutions with a low salt concentration since a precipitate may form. The proteins in ATG can be denatured by air. ATG is unstable in acidic solutions.
- Monitor patient for signs of infection.
- ATG solutions must be filtered during administration; filters with pore sizes of 0.2 to 5 microns have been used.
- **I.V. use:** Concentrated drug for injection must be diluted before administration. Dilute the required dose in 250 to 1,000 ml of 0.45% or 0.9% sodium chloride injection. The final concentration of drug should not exceed 1 mg/ml. When adding ATG to the infusion solution, the container should be inverted so that the drug does not contact air inside the container. Gently rotate or swirl the container to mix contents; do not shake because this may cause excessive foaming or denature the drug protein. Infuse with an in-line filter with a pore size of 0.2 to 1 micron, over no less than 4 hours (most institutions infuse over 4 to 8 hours).
- ATG concentrate is very heat-sensitive; refrigerate at 2° to 8° C (do not freeze).
- Do not use solutions that are more than 12 hours old, including actual infusion time.

muromonab-CD3

Orthoclone OKT3

Pregnancy Risk Category: C

HOW SUPPLIED

Injection: 5 mg/5 ml in 5-ml ampules

MECHANISM OF ACTION

Muromonab-CD3 is an IgG antibody that reacts in the T-lymphocyte membrane with a molecule (CD3) needed for antigen recognition. This drug depletes the blood of CD3-positive T cells, which leads to restoration of allograft function and reversal of rejection.

INDICATIONS & DOSAGE

Treatment of acute allograft rejection in renal transplant patients –
Adults: 5 mg I.V. bolus once daily for 10 to 14 days.
Children: 2.5 mg I.V. bolus once daily for 10 to 14 days.

ADVERSE REACTIONS

Common reactions are in italics; life-threatening reactions are in bold italics.
CV: *chest pain.*
GI: *nausea, vomiting,* diarrhea.
Other: ***severe pulmonary edema,*** *fever, chills, tremors, dyspnea,* ***infection.***

INTERACTIONS

None reported.

NURSING CONSIDERATIONS

- *Contraindicated* in patients with fluid overload, as evidenced by chest X-ray or a weight gain greater than 3% within the week before treatment.
- Muromonab-CD3 is a monoclonal antibody preparation. Patients develop antibodies to this preparation that can lead to loss of effectiveness and more severe adverse reactions if a second course of therapy is attempted. Therefore, experts believe that this drug should be used for only a single course of treatment.
- Most adverse reactions develop within ½ hour to 6 hours after the first dose.
- Treatment should begin in a facility where the patient can be monitored closely and that is equipped and staffed for cardiopulmonary resuscitation.
- Assess patient for signs of fluid overload before treatment.
- Chest X-ray must be taken within 24 hours before starting drug treatment.
- Inform patient of expected adverse reactions. Reassure him that they will be less severe as treatment progresses.
- Administering an antipyretic before giving the drug may help lower incidence of expected pyrexia and chills. Corticosteroids may also be administered before first injection to help decrease incidence of adverse reactions. Methylprednisolone sodium succinate (1 mg/kg) preinjection, followed by hydrocortisone sodium succinate (100 mg) 30 minutes postinjection, have been recommended to alleviate the severity of the first dose reaction.

74

Vaccines and toxoids

BCG vaccine
cholera vaccine
diphtheria and tetanus toxoids, adsorbed
diphtheria and tetanus toxoids and pertussis vaccine
diphtheria and tetanus toxoids and acellular pertussis vaccine
Haemophilus b conjugate vaccines
hepatitis B vaccine, recombinant
influenza virus vaccine, 1993-1994 trivalent types A & B (purified surface antigen)
influenza virus vaccine, 1993-1994 trivalent types A & B (subvirion or split virion)
influenza virus vaccine, 1993-1994 trivalent types A & B (whole virion)
Japanese encephalitis virus vaccine, inactivated
measles, mumps, and rubella virus vaccine, live
measles (rubeola) and rubella virus vaccine, live attenuated
measles (rubeola) virus vaccine, live attenuated
meningitis vaccine
mumps virus vaccine, live
plague vaccine
pneumococcal vaccine, polyvalent
poliovirus vaccine, live, oral, trivalent
poliovirus vaccine, inactivated
rabies vaccine, human diploid cell
rubella and mumps virus vaccine, live
rubella virus vaccine, live attenuated
tetanus toxoid, adsorbed
tetanus toxoid, fluid
typhoid vaccine
typhoid vaccine, oral
yellow fever vaccine

COMBINATION PRODUCTS
TETRAMUNE: 10 mcg purified Haemophilus b saccharide and approximately 25 mcg CRM_{197} protein, 12.5 Lf units inactivated diphtheria, 5 Lf units inactivated tetanus, and 4 protective units pertussis/0.5 ml.

BCG vaccine

Pregnancy Risk Category: C

HOW SUPPLIED
Intradermal vaccine: 3 to 26 million colony-forming units (CFU)/ml (Glaxo strain)
Percutaneous vaccine: 1 to 8 × 10^8 CFU/vial (Tice strain)

MECHANISM OF ACTION
Promotes active immunity to tuberculosis.

INDICATIONS & DOSAGE
Tuberculosis exposure, cancer immunotherapy–
Adults and children 3 months and over: 0.1 ml (intradermal vaccine) or 0.2 to 0.3 ml (percutaneous vaccine) applied to cleansed area of skin followed by application of multiple puncture disk.
Children under 3 months: 0.05 ml (intradermal vaccine).

ADVERSE REACTIONS
Common reactions are in italics; life-threatening reactions are in bold italics.
Local: lymphangitis, lymph node and skin abscess, ulceration at site of injection (2 to 3 weeks after injection), lupus reaction.
Other: urticaria of trunk and limbs,

*Liquid form contains alcohol. **May contain tartrazine.

lymphadenitis, osteomyelitis, ***anaphylaxis.***

INTERACTIONS

Immunosuppressive therapy: may reduce response to BCG vaccine. Avoid if possible.
Isoniazid, rifampin, streptomycin: inhibited multiplication of BCG. Avoid using together.
Theophylline: BCG vaccine may impair theophylline elimination.

NURSING CONSIDERATIONS

- *Contraindicated* in hypogammaglobulinemia, positive tuberculin reaction (when meant for use as immunoprophylactic after exposure to tuberculosis), immunosuppression, fresh smallpox vaccination, burns, and in patients receiving corticosteroid therapy. Women should avoid this vaccine during pregnancy.
- *Use cautiously* in chronic skin disease. Inject in area of healthy skin only.
- Obtain history of allergies and reaction to immunization.
- Vaccine is of no value as immunoprophylactic in patients with positive tuberculin test.
- Keep epinephrine 1:1,000 available to treat anaphylaxis.
- Recommended injection site is over insertion of deltoid muscle.
- Do not shake vial following reconstitution. Use within 8 hours of reconsitution.
- Expected lesion forms in 7 to 10 days.
- Allow an interval of at least 3 weeks between BCG and rubella vaccination.
- Don't administer to children with febrile illness.
- Live vaccine; destroy by autoclaving or formaldehyde solution before disposal.
- Patient should have tuberculin skin test 2 to 3 months after BCG vaccination to determine success of vaccine.
- Use of BCG has shown some value in treatment of various cancers, such as leukemia, some lung cancers, malignant melanoma, multiple myeloma, and some breast tumors. Currently, researchers are trying to find ways of augmenting the immune system's response to cancer. They hope to stimulate the body to destroy tumor cells.

cholera vaccine

Pregnancy Risk Category: C

HOW SUPPLIED

Injection: suspension of killed *Vibrio cholerae* (each milliliter contains 8 units of Inaba and Ogawa serotypes) in 1-ml, 1.5-ml, and 20-ml vials

MECHANISM OF ACTION

Promotes active immunity to cholera.

INDICATIONS & DOSAGE

Primary immunization –
Adults and children over 10 years: two doses of 0.5 ml I.M. or 1 ml S.C., 1 week to 1 month apart, before traveling in cholera area. Booster is 0.5 ml q 6 months as long as protection is needed.
Children 5 to 10 years: 0.3 ml I.M. or S.C.
Children 6 months to 4 years: 0.2 ml I.M. or S.C. Boosters of same dose should be given q 6 months as long as protection is needed.

ADVERSE REACTIONS

Common reactions are in italics; life-threatening reactions are in bold italics.
Systemic: malaise, fever, flushing, urticaria, tachycardia, hypotension, diarrhea, headache, ***anaphylaxis.***
Local: *erythema, swelling, pain, induration.*

INTERACTIONS

Yellow fever vaccine: simultaneous administration may interfere with immune response to cholera vaccine and yellow fever vaccine. Administer 3 weeks apart.

NURSING CONSIDERATIONS

- *Contraindicated* in corticosteroid therapy or in immunosuppression. Not recommended for children under 6 months. Defer in acute illness.
- Vaccine is about 50% effective in reducing the incidence of clinical illness for 3 to 6 months.
- Obtain history of allergies and reaction to immunization.
- Keep epinephrine 1:1,000 available.
- May be given intradermally to adults and children over age 5, but the volume of injection is limited to 0.2 ml. I.M. and S.C. routes give higher levels of protection.
- Administer I.M. in deltoid muscle in adults and children over 3 years.
- Pain, induration, and swelling are common at the injection site for 24 to 48 hours.

diphtheria and tetanus toxoids, adsorbed

Pregnancy Risk Category: C

HOW SUPPLIED

Available in pediatric (DT) and adult (Td) strengths

Injection (for pediatric use): diphtheria toxoid 6.6 Lf units and tetanus toxoid 5 Lf units per 0.5 ml; diphtheria toxoid 10 Lf units and tetanus toxoid 5 Lf units per 0.5 ml; diphtheria toxoid 12.5 Lf units and tetanus toxoid 5 Lf units per 0.5 ml; diphtheria toxoid 15 Lf units and tetanus toxoid 10 Lf units per 0.5 ml

Injection (for adult use): diphtheria toxoid 1.5 Lf units and tetanus toxoid 5 Lf units per 0.5 ml; diphtheria toxoid 2 Lf units and tetanus toxoid 5 Lf units per 0.5 ml; diphtheria toxoid 2 Lf units and tetanus toxoid 10 Lf units per 0.5 ml

MECHANISM OF ACTION

Promotes immunity to diphtheria and tetanus by inducing production of antitoxins.

INDICATIONS & DOSAGE

Primary immunization –

Adults and children over 7 years: use adult strength; 0.5 ml I.M. 4 to 6 weeks apart for two doses and a third dose 1 year later. Booster is 0.5 ml I.M. q 10 years.

Children 1 to 6 years: use pediatric strength; 0.5 ml I.M. at least 4 weeks apart for two doses. Give booster dosage 6 to 12 months after the second injection. If the final immunizing dose is given after the 7th birthday, use the adult strength.

Infants 6 weeks to 1 year: use pediatric strength; 0.5 ml I.M. at least 4 weeks apart for three doses. Give booster dose 6 to 12 months after third injection.

ADVERSE REACTIONS

Common reactions are in italics; life-threatening reactions are in bold italics.

Systemic: chills, fever, malaise, ***anaphylaxis.***

Local: stinging, edema, erythema, pain, induration.

INTERACTIONS

None significant.

NURSING CONSIDERATIONS

- *Contraindicated* in immunosuppression, radiation, or corticosteroid therapy. Defer in respiratory illness or polio outbreaks, or acute illness except in emergency. Use single antigen during polio risks. In children under 6 years, use only when diphtheria, tetanus, and pertussis combination is contraindicated because of pertussis component.
- Verify strength (pediatric or adult) of toxoid used.
- Obtain history of allergies and reaction to immunization.

- Keep epinephrine 1:1,000 available.
- Give in site not recently used for vaccines or toxoids.

diphtheria and tetanus toxoids and pertussis vaccine (DTP, DPT)
Tri-Immunol

diphtheria and tetanus toxoids and acellular pertussis vaccine
Acel-Imune

HOW SUPPLIED
whole-cell vaccine
Injection: 6.7 Lf units inactivated diphtheria, 5 Lf units inactivated tetanus, and 4 protective units pertussis per 0.5 ml, in 7.5-ml vials; 12.5 Lf units inactivated diphtheria, 5 Lf units inactivated tetanus, and 4 protective units pertussis per 0.5 ml, in 7.5-ml vials (Tri-Immunol)
acellular vaccine
Injection: 7.5 Lf units inactivated diphtheria, 5 Lf units inactivated tetanus, and 300 hemagglutinating units of acellular pertussis vaccine per 0.5 ml

MECHANISM OF ACTION
Promotes active immunity to diphtheria, tetanus, and pertussis by inducing production of antitoxins and antibodies.

INDICATIONS & DOSAGE
Primary immunization –
Children 6 weeks to 6 years: 0.5 ml I.M. 2 months apart for three doses and a fourth dose 1 year later. Booster is 0.5 ml I.M. when starting school.

Not advised for adults or children over 6 years.

The acellular vaccine may be used only for the fourth or fifth dose in children 17 months to 7 years who have previously been immunized with three or four doses of the whole-cell vaccine.

ADVERSE REACTIONS
Common reactions are in italics; life-threatening reactions are in bold italics.
Systemic: slight fever, chills, malaise, ***seizures, encephalopathy, anaphylaxis,*** anorexia, vomiting.
Local: *soreness, redness,* expected nodule remaining several weeks.
Other: ***sudden infant death syndrome.***

INTERACTIONS
Immunosuppressive therapy: may reduce response to DPT vaccine. Avoid if possible.

NURSING CONSIDERATIONS
- *Contraindicated* in corticosteroid therapy, immunosuppression, and history of seizures. Defer in acute febrile illness.
- Children with preexisting neurologic disorders should not receive pertussis component. Also, children who react to any DPT injection by exhibiting neurologic signs shouldn't receive pertussis component in any succeeding injections. Diphtheria and tetanus toxoids (DT) should be given instead.
- Acellular vaccine may have a lower incidence of local pain and fever.
- DPT injection may be given at same time as trivalent oral polio vaccine.
- Obtain history of allergies and reaction to immunization.
- Keep epinephrine 1:1,000 available.
- Not to be used for active infection.
- Don't give subcutaneously.
- Shake before using. Refrigerate.
- Administer only by deep I.M. injection, preferably in thigh or deltoid muscle.
- An information booklet is available that describes the risks and benefits of this vaccine. Be sure parents read and understand the information before vaccine is administered.

Haemophilus b conjugate vaccines

Haemophilus b conjugate vaccine, diphtheria CRM_{197} protein conjugate (HbOC)
HibTITER

Haemophilus b conjugate vaccine, diphtheria toxoid conjugate (PRP-D)
ProHIBiT

Haemophilus b conjugate vaccine, meningococcal protein conjugate (PRP-OMP)
PedvaxHIB

HOW SUPPLIED

conjugate vaccine, diphtheria CRM_{197} protein conjugate

Injection: 10 mcg purified Haemophilus b saccharide and approximately 25 mcg CRM_{197} protein per 0.5 ml

conjugate vaccine, diphtheria toxoid conjugate

Injection: 25 mcg of *Haemophilus influenzae* type B (Hib) capsular polysaccharide and 18 mcg of diphtheria toxoid protein per 0.5 ml

conjugate vaccine, meningococcal protein conjugate

Powder for injection: 15 mcg Haemophilus b PRP, 250 mcg *Neisseria meningitidis* OMPC per dose

MECHANISM OF ACTION

Promotes active immunity to Hib.

The vaccine is a polymer of ribose, ribitol, and phosphate (PRP) and is covalently linked to highly antigenic substances, enabling the vaccine to promote an immune response in infants.

INDICATIONS & DOSAGE

Immunization against Hib infection –
conjugate vaccine, diphtheria CRM_{197} protein conjugate

Infants: 0.5 ml I.M. at age 2 months. Repeat at ages 4 months and 6 months. A booster dose is required at age 15 months.

Previously unvaccinated infants 2 to 6 months: 0.5 ml I.M. Repeat in 2 months and again in 4 months for a total of three doses. Give a booster dose at age 15 months.

Previously unvaccinated infants 7 to 11 months: 0.5 ml I.M. Repeat in 2 months, for a total of two doses. Give a booster dose at age 15 months (but no sooner than 2 months after the last vaccination).

Previously unvaccinated infants 12 to 14 months: 0.5 ml I.M. Give a booster dose at age 15 months (but no sooner than 2 months after the first vaccination).

Previously unvaccinated children 15 months to 5 years: 0.5 ml I.M. A booster dose is not required.

conjugate vaccine, diphtheria toxoid conjugate

Previously unvaccinated children 15 months to 5 years: 0.5 ml I.M. A booster dose is not required. Not recommended for use in children under age 15 months.

conjugate vaccine, meningococcal protein conjugate

Infants: 0.5 ml I.M. at age 2 months. Repeat at age 4 months. A booster dose is required at age 12 months.

Previously unvaccinated infants 2 to 6 months: 0.5 ml I.M. Repeat in 2 months. Give a booster dose at age 12 months.

Previously unvaccinated infants 7 to 11 months: 0.5 ml I.M. Repeat in 2 months. Give a booster dose at age 15 months (but no sooner than 2 months after the last vaccination).

Previously unvaccinated infants 12 to 14 months: 0.5 ml I.M. Give a booster dose at age 15 months (but no sooner than 2 months after the first vaccination).

Previously unvaccinated children 15 months to 5 years: 0.5 ml I.M. A booster dose is not required.

ADVERSE REACTIONS
Common reactions are in italics; life-threatening reactions are in bold italics.
Systemic: fever, ***anaphylaxis***.
Local: *erythema and pain at injection site.*

INTERACTIONS
Immunosuppressive agents: may suppress antibody response to Hib vaccine.

NURSING CONSIDERATIONS
- *Contraindicated* in immunosuppression. Defer immunization in acute illness.
- Hib is an important cause of meningitis in infants and preschool children.
- The conjugate vaccine is formed when Hib is chemically bound to other protein antigens. It produces a stronger immune response in most patients.
- Don't administer intradermally or I.V. Must administer I.M.
- Know that the diphtheria toxoid conjugate vaccine (ProHIBiT) is not recommended in children under age 15 months.
- Administer into the anterolateral aspect of the upper thigh in small children. Injections may be made into the deltoid of larger children if sufficient muscle mass is present.
- This vaccine will *not* protect children against any other microorganisms that cause meningitis. Will protect against Hib only.
- This vaccine and DPT can be given simultaneously. A combination product is commercially available.
- Don't administer to children with febrile illness.
- Not routinely given to adults or children over 5 years unless they are at high risk for infection (including patients with chronic conditions such as functional asplenia, splenectomy, Hodgkin's disease, or sickle cell anemia).
- Keep epinephrine 1:1,000 available in case of a severe allergic reaction.
- Children vaccinated with nonconjugated vaccine (no longer available in the United States) need not be routinely revaccinated if the primary immunization occurred at 24 months. However, if the first vaccination occurred at 18 to 23 months, the child should be revaccinated with conjugate vaccine, provided at least 2 months has elapsed.

hepatitis B vaccine, recombinant
Engerix-B, Recombivax HB

Pregnancy Risk Category: C

HOW SUPPLIED
Injection: 5 mcg HB_sAg/0.5 ml (Recombivax HB, pediatric injection); 10 mcg HB_sAg/0.5 ml (Engerix-B, pediatric injection); 10 mcg HB_sAg/ml (Recombivax HB); 20 mcg HB_sAg/ml (Engerix-B); 40 mcg HB_sAg/ml (Recombivax HB Dialysis Formulation)

MECHANISM OF ACTION
Promotes active immunity to hepatitis B.

INDICATIONS & DOSAGE
Immunization against infection from all known subtypes of hepatitis B; primary preexposure prophylaxis against hepatitis B; or postexposure prophylaxis (when given with hepatitis B immune globulin) –
Engerix-B
Adults and children over 10 years: initially, give 20 mcg (1-ml adult formulation) I.M., followed by a second dose of 20 mcg I.M. 30 days later. Give a third dose of 20 mcg I.M. 6 months after the initial dose.
Neonates and children up to 10 years: initially, give 10 mcg (0.5-ml pediatric formulation) I.M., followed by a second dose of 10 mcg I.M. 30 days later. Give a third dose of 10

mcg I.M. 6 months after the initial dose.

Adults undergoing dialysis or receiving immunosuppressant therapy: initially, give 40 mcg I.M. (divided into two 20-mcg doses and administered at different sites). Follow with a second dose of 40 mcg I.M. in 30 days, and a final dose of 40 mcg I.M. 6 months after the initial dose.

Note: Certain populations (neonates born to infected mothers, persons recently exposed to the virus, and travelers to high-risk areas) may receive the vaccine on an abbreviated schedule, with the initial dose followed by a second dose in 1 month, and the third dose after 2 months. For prolonged maintenance of protective antibody titers, a booster dose is recommended 12 months after the initial dose.

Recombivax HB

Adults: initially, give 10 mcg (1-ml adult formulation) I.M., followed by a second dose of 10 mcg I.M. 30 days later. Give a third dose of 10 mcg I.M. 6 months after the initial dose.

Children 11 to 19 years: initially, give 5 mcg (0.5-ml pediatric formulation) I.M., followed by a second dose of 5 mcg I.M. 30 days later. Give a third dose of 5 mcg I.M. 6 months after the initial dose.

Neonates and children to 11 years: initially, give 2.5 mcg (0.25-ml pediatric formulation) I.M., followed by a second dose of 2.5 mcg I.M. 30 days later. Give a third dose of 2.5 mcg I.M. 6 months after the initial dose.

Adults undergoing dialysis or receiving immunosuppressant therapy: initially, give 40 mcg I.M. (use dialysis formulation, which contains 40 mcg/ml). Follow with a second dose of 40 mcg I.M. in 30 days, and give a final dose of 40 mcg I.M. 6 months after the initial dose.

ADVERSE REACTIONS

Common reactions are in italics; life-threatening reactions are in bold italics.

Systemic: slight fever, transient malaise, headache, dizziness, nausea, vomiting, flulike symptoms, myalgia.

Local: discomfort at injection site, local inflammation.

INTERACTIONS

None reported.

NURSING CONSIDERATIONS

- *Contraindicated* in patients with a history of severe hypersensitivity reaction to yeast. Recombinant vaccines are derived from yeast cultures.
- *Use cautiously* in any serious, active infections; compromised cardiac or pulmonary status; and in those for whom a febrile or systemic reaction could pose a serious risk.
- Recombinant hepatitis B vaccine is not made with any human plasma products.
- The Centers for Disease Control and Prevention reports that response to hepatitis B vaccine is significantly better when administered in the arm rather than the buttock. Adults should receive the vaccine in the deltoid muscle; infants and young children should receive the vaccine in the anterolateral aspect of the thigh. Never administer I.V.
- May be administered S.C., but this route may lead to an increased incidence or severity of local reactions. Use only in persons at risk for hemorrhage, such as hemophiliacs.
- Although anaphylaxis has not been reported, epinephrine should always be available when administering this drug to counteract any possible reaction.
- The recommended dosage regimen provides immunity for at least 5 years.
- The following persons are at increased risk of infection and should be considered for the vaccine: certain

health care personnel (especially those working with dialysis patients, in blood banks, and in emergency medicine); selected patients and patient contacts; certain endemic populations (Alaskan Eskimos, Indo-Chinese and Haitian refugees); certain military personnel; morticians and embalmers; sexually active homosexuals; prostitutes; prisoners; and users of illicit injectable drugs.
- The American Academy of Pediatrics recommends hepatitis B vaccination for all neonates and encourages immunization for adolescents when resources allow.
- Thoroughly agitate vial just before administration to restore suspension.
- Store both opened and unopened vials in the refrigerator. Don't freeze.

---

influenza virus vaccine, 1993-1994 trivalent types A & B (purified surface antigen)
Flu-Imune

influenza virus vaccine, 1993-1994 trivalent types A & B (subvirion or split virion)
Fluogen Split, Fluzone Split, Flu-Shield

influenza virus vaccine, 1993-1994 trivalent types A & B (whole virion)
Fluzone (Whole)

Pregnancy Risk Category: C

HOW SUPPLIED
Injection: 15 mcg A/Texas/36/91-like (H1N1), 15 mcg A/Beijing/32/92-like (H3N2), and 15 mcg B/Panama/45/90-like hemagglutinin antigens per 0.5 ml

MECHANISM OF ACTION
Promotes immunity to influenza by inducing production of antibodies.

INDICATIONS & DOSAGE
Influenza prophylaxis –
Adults and children over 12 years: 0.5 ml whole or split virus I.M. Only one dose is required.
Children 9 to 12 years: 0.5 ml split virus I.M. Only one dose is required.
Children 3 to 8 years: 0.5 ml split virus I.M. Repeat dose in 4 weeks unless child has been previously vaccinated.
Children 6 to 35 months: 0.25 ml split virus I.M. Repeat dose in 4 weeks unless child has been previously vaccinated.

ADVERSE REACTIONS
Common reactions are in italics; life-threatening reactions are in bold italics.
Systemic: fever, malaise, myalgia, *anaphylaxis.*
Local: erythema, induration, soreness at the injection site.

Fever and malaise reactions occur most often in children and in others not exposed to influenza viruses. Severe reactions in adults are rare.

INTERACTIONS
Theophylline, warfarin: clearance may be impaired.

NURSING CONSIDERATIONS
- *Contraindicated* in egg allergy. Defer in acute respiratory or other active infection.
- *Use cautiously* in patients with a history of sulfite allergy. Obtain history of allergies, especially to eggs, and reaction to immunization.
- Pregnancy isn't a contraindication for influenza vaccination. According to the Centers for Disease Control and Prevention, this vaccine is considered safe in pregnant women. Vaccination shouldn't be postponed, regardless of the stage of pregnancy, in women who have high-risk conditions and who will be in the first trimester of pregnancy when the flu season begins.
- Patients with immunodeficiency

may receive two doses 1 month apart; however, there is little evidence to suggest that booster doses improve the immunogenic response to the vaccine. Chemoprophylaxis with amantadine may be helpful.

- Ideally, vaccinations should be performed in November, since outbreaks of influenza generally don't occur until December. Try to avoid administering the vaccine too early in the season because antibody titers may begin to decline prior to the flu season.
- Patients should understand that annual vaccination using the current vaccine is necessary because immunity to influenza decreases in the year following the injection.
- Note that the combination of antigens used to create influenza vaccine changes annually even though some antigens may be the same as previous years. It is important that leftover supplies of 1992-1993 vaccine not be used to immunize patients for the 1993-1994 flu season.
- Children 12 years and under should receive their second dose in December, if possible.
- Vaccines could be given to both children and adults throughout the flu season, even as late as April.
- Thoroughly agitate vial just before administration to restore suspension.
- Give injections for adults and older children in deltoid muscle; in anterolateral aspect of thigh for infants and children under 3 years.
- Keep epinephrine 1:1,000 available.
- Strongly recommended for anyone over 6 months; for patients with chronic disease, metabolic disorders, or medical conditions that put them at risk for complications from influenza; for health care workers, especially doctors, nurses, employees of nursing homes, volunteer workers, and other personnel in both hospital and outpatient settings; and for household members who may contact persons at high risk for medical complications of influenza. Vaccination is also recommended for anyone who wishes to reduce the chance of infection.
- Influenza vaccine available as whole virus, split virus, and purified surface antigen preparations. Split virus and purified surface antigen vaccines cause somewhat fewer adverse reactions than whole virus in children.
- Fever, malaise, and myalgia may begin 6 to 12 hours after vaccination and persist 1 to 2 days. These systemic reactions are not common. Patients should understand that the vaccine cannot cause influenza.
- Allergic reactions, which usually occur immediately, are extremely rare.
- Paralysis associated with Guillain-Barré syndrome is rare, and has only been associated with the 1976 vaccine.
- Patient should be made aware of risk as compared with risk of influenza and its complications.
- Children should not be given pertussis vaccine within 3 days of influenza virus vaccine. However, they may receive Haemophilus b vaccine, oral polio vaccine, measles-mumps-rubella vaccine, or pneumococcal vaccine at the same time. Injections should be made at different sites.
- Although there is little information regarding influenza in persons with human immunodeficiency virus, it is considered prudent for these persons to receive the vaccine. Persons with advanced disease may exhibit a low response; there is no evidence that a booster dose will improve the immune response.

Japanese encephalitis virus vaccine, inactivated

Je-Vax

Pregnancy Risk Category: C

*Liquid form contains alcohol. **May contain tartrazine.

HOW SUPPLIED

Injection: 1-ml, 10-ml vials

MECHANISM OF ACTION

Provides active immunity against Japanese encephalitis (JE), a mosquito-borne arboviral Flavivirus infection that's the leading cause of viral encephalitis in Asia.

INDICATIONS & DOSAGE

Active immunization against JE –
Primary immunization schedule
Adults and children 3 years and over: 1 ml S.C. on days 0, 7, and 30.
Children 1 to 3 years: 0.5 ml S.C. on days 0, 7, and 30.
Booster doses
Adults and children 3 years and over: 1 ml S.C. q 2 years.
Children 1 to 3 years: 0.5 ml S.C. q 2 years.

ADVERSE REACTIONS

Common reactions are in italics; life-threatening reactions are in bold italics.
CNS: *headache, dizziness.*
CV: hypotension.
GI: *nausea, vomiting, abdominal pain.*
Respiratory: ***respiratory distress.***
Skin: *rash,* generalized urticaria.
Local: *local tenderness and swelling.*
Other: *fever; malaise; chills; myalgia;* angioedema of the face, oropharynx, extremities, or lips; ***anaphylaxis.***

INTERACTIONS

None reported.

NURSING CONSIDERATIONS

- *Contraindicated* in persons with hypersensitivity to the drug or thimerosal, a preservative, and in persons who exhibited severe adverse reactions, such as generalized urticaria or angioedema, to a prior dose of the vaccine. Because the vaccine is derived from mouse brain, its use is *contraindicated* in persons with hypersensitivity to substances originating from murine or neural origin.
- *Use cautiously* in pregnant or breast-feeding patients, elderly patients, and patients with a history of urticaria after vaccines, drugs, or insect stings. Weigh known risk factors against benefits of the vaccine. Advanced age may be a risk factor for developing symptomatic illness after JE infection. JE acquired during pregnancy can cause intrauterine infection and fetal death.
- Before using the vaccine, the clinician must weigh the risks of adverse effects against the risks of exposure and illness as well as the availability, acceptability, and efficacy of repellents and other alternative protective measures.
- The vaccine has been associated with a moderate incidence of local and mild systemic adverse effects. Local tenderness and swelling have been reported in up to 20% of those receiving the vaccine; systemic effects, such as fever, headache, malaise, or rash, in up to 10%. Serious reactions, such as generalized urticaria or angioedema, are uncommon (1% or less of those vaccinated).
- Generalized urticaria or angioedema may occur within minutes of receiving the vaccine. However, adverse reactions that may be related to the vaccine have occurred as late as 17 days after the injection. Most reactions occur within the first 10 days, with the majority occurring within 48 hours. Monitor patient closely for 30 minutes after the injection. Warn him about the possibility of delayed generalized urticaria or delayed angioedema of the extremities, face, oropharynx or, especially, lips.
- Attempts have been made to characterize the time course of adverse reactions. Reactions to the first dose have occurred a median of 12 hours after injection (88% happened within 3 days). The delay between the second

dose and adverse effects was usually longer, with a median of 3 days and some effects not seen for 2 weeks. Some patients exhibited adverse reactions to the second or third dose, even when the first or second dose was well tolerated.
• Because of the possibility of delayed reactions, warn patient to remain in areas where he can obtain medical care for 10 days after injection. International travel shouldn't occur during this time. He should seek medical assistance as soon as any reaction appears.
• Encourage patients and parents to report adverse effects after vaccination. Health care providers should report these adverse effects to the U.S. Department of Health and Human Services (DHHS) Vaccine Adverse Event Reporting System (VAERS). Contact VAERS at (800) 822-7967 for information about the system and reporting forms.
• Vaccine should be used to provide protection against JE in persons planning to travel or reside in areas where the virus is endemic. It's not indicated for all persons traveling to or residing in Asia. The risk for acquiring JE among most travelers to Asia is extremely low. Contact the Centers for Disease Control and Prevention at (404) 332-4555 for current travel advisories.
• Teach patient personal precautions that may avoid exposure to mosquito bites, such as using insect repellents and wearing protective clothing. Avoiding outdoor activities, especially during twilight periods and in the evening, will further reduce risk.
• Be sure that resuscitative equipment and drugs, such as epinephrine 1:1,000, diphenhydramine, and corticosteroids, are readily available to treat adverse reactions.
• Patients should follow the recommended three-dose schedule for best results. When time constraints prohibit the use of this schedule, an abbreviated schedule with injections on days 0, 7, and 14 may be used.
• When it isn't possible to follow these schedules, a two-dose regimen with injections on days 0 and 7 may be used. Antibodies will be induced in about 80% of patients with this schedule. Don't use a two-dose regimen unless circumstances are unusual.
• Regardless of schedule used, remember to allow at least 10 days after the last dose before international travel begins.
• To prepare vaccine for injection, use supplied diluent (sterile water for injection). Add 1.3 ml diluent to the single-dose vial; 11 ml diluent to the 10-dose vial. Shake vial thoroughly to ensure dissolution of vaccine. After reconstitution, the vaccine may be stored in the refrigerator (36° to 46° F [2° to 8° C]) for 8 hours.

measles, mumps, and rubella virus vaccine, live

M-M-RII

Pregnancy Risk Category: X

HOW SUPPLIED

Injection: single-dose vial containing not less than 1,000 $TCID_{50}$ (tissue culture infective doses) of attenuated measles virus derived from Enders' attenuated Edmonston strain (grown in chick embryo culture), 5,000 $TCID_{50}$ of the Jeryl Lynn (B level) mumps strain (grown in chick embryo culture), and the Wistar RA 27/3 strain of rubella virus (propagated in human diploid cell culture)

MECHANISM OF ACTION

Promotes immunity to measles, mumps, and rubella virus by inducing production of antibodies.

*Liquid form contains alcohol. **May contain tartrazine.

INDICATIONS & DOSAGE

Routine vaccination –
Children: administer 1 vial S.C. A two-dose schedule is recommended, with the first dose given at 15 months (12 months in high-risk areas) and the second dose given at the entry of school (kindergarten or first grade).
Measles outbreak control –
Children: if cases are occurring in children under 1 year, vaccinate children as young as 6 months. All students and their siblings should be revaccinated if they are without documentation of measles immunity.
Adults: school personnel born in or after 1957 should be revaccinated if they are without proof of measles immunity. If the outbreak is in a medical facility, all workers born in or after 1957 should be revaccinated if they are without proof of immunity. Revaccination should be considered for persons born before 1957 as well.

ADVERSE REACTIONS

Common reactions are in italics; life-threatening reactions are in bold italics.
Systemic: fever, rash, regional lymphadenopathy, urticaria, ***anaphylaxis.***
Local: erythema.

INTERACTIONS

Immune serum globulin, whole blood, plasma: antibodies in serum may interfere with immune response. Don't use vaccine within 3 months of transfusion.

NURSING CONSIDERATIONS

- *Contraindicated* in immunosuppression; cancer; blood dyscrasias; corticosteroid or radiation therapy; gamma globulin disorders; fever; or active, untreated tuberculosis.
- *Use cautiously* in patients with hypersensitivity to neomycin, chickens, ducks, eggs, or feathers. Defer immunization in acute illness.
- Incidence of adverse effects is low (0.5 to 4%).
- Presence of maternal antibodies may prevent response in children under 12 months.
- Treat fever with antipyretics, such as acetaminophen.
- Store in refrigerator; protect from light. Solution may be used if red, pink, or yellow, but must be clear.
- Use only diluent supplied. Discard 8 hours after reconstituting.
- Obtain history of allergies, especially to ducks, rabbits, antibiotics, and reaction to immunization.
- Inject in outer aspect of upper arm. Don't give I.V.
- Keep epinephrine 1:1,000 available.
- Because of a recent rise in the incidence of measles, the Immunization Practices Advisory Committee (ACIP) recommends that colleges and other post-high school educational institutions, as well as medical institutions employing health care providers, obtain documentation of the receipt of two doses of vaccine after age 1 (or other proof of immunity, such as infection, documented by a physician). Combined measles, mumps, and rubella (MMR) vaccine is preferred.
- The Centers for Disease Control and Prevention (CDC) recommends that, during a measles outbreak in a health care facility, susceptible personnel exposed to the measles virus (whether or not they received measles vaccine or immunoglobulin) avoid patient contact for days 5 through 21 after such exposure. If they become ill, they should avoid patient contact for at least 7 days after developing rash.
- Clinical trials have shown that vitamin A supplementation reduces morbidity and mortality in children with measles. Studies have used 100,000 to 400,000 IU daily.

measles (rubeola) and rubella virus vaccine, live attenuated

M-R-Vax II

Pregnancy Risk Category: X

HOW SUPPLIED

Injection: single-dose vial containing not less than 1,000 $TCID_{50}$ (tissue culture infective doses) per 0.5 ml of attenuated measles virus derived from Enders' attenuated Edmonston strain (grown in chick embryo culture); 1,000 $TCID_{50}$ of the Wistar RA 27/3 strain of rubella virus

MECHANISM OF ACTION

Promotes immunity to measles and rubella virus by inducing production of antibodies.

INDICATIONS & DOSAGE

Immunization –

Children 15 months to puberty: 1 vial (1,000 units) S.C.

ADVERSE REACTIONS

Common reactions are in italics; life-threatening reactions are in bold italics.

Systemic: fever, rash, lymphadenopathy, ***anaphylaxis***.

INTERACTIONS

Immune serum globulin, whole blood, plasma: antibodies in serum may interfere with immune response. Don't use vaccine within 3 months of transfusion.

Tuberculin skin test: may temporarily decrease response to test. Defer skin testing.

NURSING CONSIDERATIONS

- *Contraindicated* in immunosuppression; cancer; blood dyscrasias; corticosteroid or radiation therapy; gamma globulin disorders; fever; or active, untreated tuberculosis.
- *Use cautiously* in patients with hypersensitivity to neomycin, chickens, ducks, eggs, or feathers; when there is a history of febrile seizures; or in cerebral injury. Defer immunization in acute illness.
- Do not give within 1 month of other live virus vaccines, except oral poliovirus vaccine.
- Allow an interval of at least 3 weeks between BCG and rubella vaccines.
- Store in refrigerator and protect from light. Solution may be used if red, pink, or yellow, but must be clear (with no precipitation).
- Use only diluent supplied. Discard 8 hours after reconstituting.
- Inject in outer aspect of upper arm. Don't inject I.V.
- Keep epinephrine 1:1,000 available.

measles (rubeola) virus vaccine, live attenuated

Attenuvax

Pregnancy Risk Category: X

HOW SUPPLIED

Injection: single-dose vial containing not less than 1,000 $TCID_{50}$ (tissue culture infective doses) of attenuated measles virus derived from Enders' attenuated Edmonston strain (grown in chick embryo culture)

MECHANISM OF ACTION

Promotes immunity to measles virus by inducing production of antibodies.

INDICATIONS & DOSAGE

Immunization –

Adults and children 15 months or over: 0.5 ml (1,000 units) S.C. A two-dose schedule is recommended, with the first dose given at 15 months (12 months in high-risk areas) and the second dose given at the entry of school (kindergarten or first grade).

Measles outbreak control –

Children: if cases are occurring in children under 1 year, vaccinate children as young as 6 months. All stu-

*Liquid form contains alcohol. **May contain tartrazine.

dents and their siblings should be revaccinated if they are without documentation of measles immunity.
Adults: school personnel born in or after 1957 should be revaccinated if they are without proof of measles immunity. If the outbreak is in a medical facility, all workers born in or after 1957 should be revaccinated if they are without proof of immunity. Revaccination should be considered for persons born before 1957 as well.

ADVERSE REACTIONS
Common reactions are in italics; life-threatening reactions are in bold italics.
Systemic: fever, rash, lymphadenopathy, ***anaphylaxis,*** febrile seizures in susceptible children, anorexia, leukopenia.
Local: erythema, swelling, tenderness.

INTERACTIONS
Immune serum globulin, whole blood, plasma: antibodies in serum may interfere with immune response. Don't use vaccine within 3 months of transfusion.
Tuberculin skin test: may temporarily decrease response to test. Defer skin testing.

NURSING CONSIDERATIONS
• *Contraindicated* in immunosuppression; cancer; blood dyscrasias; corticosteroid or radiation therapy; gamma globulin disorders; or active, untreated tuberculosis; fever.
• *Use cautiously* in patients with hypersensitivity to neomycin, chickens, eggs, or feathers. Defer in acute illness or after administration of blood or plasma.
• Warn patient to avoid pregnancy for 3 months after vaccination.
• Do not give I.V.
• Obtain history of allergies, especially to eggs, and reaction to immunization.
• Keep epinephrine 1:1,000 available.
• Store in refrigerator and protect from light. Solution may be used if red, pink, or yellow, but must be clear (with no precipitation).
• Use only diluent supplied. Discard 8 hours after reconstituting.
• May be given with oral poliovirus vaccine.
• Because of a recent rise in the incidence of measles, the Immunization Practices Advisory Committee (ACIP) recommends that colleges and other post-high school educational institutions, as well as medical institutions employing health care providers, obtain documentation of the receipt of two doses of vaccine after age 1 (or other proof of immunity, such as infection, documented by a physician). Combined measles, mumps, and rubella (MMR) vaccine is preferred.
• The Centers for Disease Control and Prevention (CDC) recommends that, during a measles outbreak in a health care facility, susceptible personnel exposed to the measles virus (whether or not they received measles vaccine or immunoglobulin) avoid patient contact for days 5 through 21 after such exposure. If they become ill, they should avoid patient contact for at least 7 days after developing rash.

meningitis vaccine
Menomune-A/C, Menomune-A/C/Y/W-135

Pregnancy Risk Category: C

HOW SUPPLIED
Injection: a killed bacterial vaccine in 10-dose and 50-dose vials with vial of diluent

MECHANISM OF ACTION
Promotes active immunity to meningitis.

INDICATIONS & DOSAGE
Meningococcal meningitis prophylaxis –
Adults and children over 2 years: 0.5 ml S.C.

ADVERSE REACTIONS
Common reactions are in italics; life-threatening reactions are in bold italics.
Systemic: headache, malaise, chills, fever, cramps, ***anaphylaxis.***
Local: *pain, erythema, induration.*

INTERACTIONS
None significant.

NURSING CONSIDERATIONS
- *Contraindicated* in immunosuppression. Defer in acute illness.
- Vaccine may be given with other immunizations.
- Tell patient to avoid pregnancy for 3 months after vaccination.
- Some clinicians will revaccinate children if they are at high risk and previously received vaccine before 4 years.
- Obtain history of allergies and reaction to immunization.
- Do not give I.V.
- Keep epinephrine 1:1,000 available.

mumps virus vaccine, live
Mumpsvax

Pregnancy Risk Category: X

HOW SUPPLIED
Injection: single-dose vial containing not less than 5,000 $TCID_{50}$ (tissue culture infective doses) of attenuated mumps virus derived from Jeryl Lynn mumps strain (grown in chick embryo culture), and vial of diluent

MECHANISM OF ACTION
Promotes active immunity to mumps.

INDICATIONS & DOSAGE
Immunization –
Adults and children over 1 year: 1 vial (5,000 units) S.C.

ADVERSE REACTIONS
Common reactions are in italics; life-threatening reactions are in bold italics.
Systemic: *slight fever,* rash, malaise, mild allergic reactions, febrile seizures (rare).

INTERACTIONS
Immune serum globulin, whole blood, plasma: antibodies in serum may interfere with immune response. Don't use vaccine within 3 months of transfusion.
Tuberculin skin test: may temporarily decrease response to test. Defer skin testing.

NURSING CONSIDERATIONS
- *Contraindicated* in immunosuppression; cancer; blood dyscrasias; corticosteroid or radiation therapy; gamma globulin disorders; active, untreated tuberculosis; or pregnancy.
- *Use cautiously* in patients with hypersensitivity to neomycin, chickens, ducks, eggs, or feathers. Defer in acute or febrile illness and for 3 months following transfusions or treatment with immune serum globulin.
- Keep epinephrine 1:1,000 available.
- Mumpsvax should not be given less than 1 month before or after immunization with other live virus vaccines, with the exception of Attenuvax, Meruvax, or monovalent or trivalent live, oral poliovirus vaccine, which may be administered simultaneously.
- Not recommended for infants under 12 months because retained maternal mumps antibodies may interfere with the immune response.
- Stress importance of avoiding pregnancy for 3 months after immuniza-

tion. If necessary, provide contraceptive information.
- Treat fever with antipyretics.
- Do not give I.V.
- Store in refrigerator and protect from light. Solution may be used if red, pink, or yellow (but must be clear).
- Use only diluent supplied. Discard 8 hours after reconstituting.
- Obtain history of allergies, especially to antibiotics, and reaction to immunization.

plague vaccine

Pregnancy Risk Category: C

HOW SUPPLIED
Injection: 2 billion killed plague bacilli (*Yersinia pestis*)/ml in 20-ml vials

MECHANISM OF ACTION
Promotes active immunity to plague.

INDICATIONS & DOSAGE
Primary immunization and booster–
Adults and children over 10 years: 1 ml I.M. followed by 0.2 ml in 4 weeks, then 0.2 ml 6 months after the first dose. Booster is 0.1 to 0.2 ml q 6 months while in plague area.
Children 5 to 10 years: 3/5 adult primary or booster dose.
Children 1 to 4 years: 2/5 adult primary or booster dose.
Children under 1 year: 1/5 adult primary or booster dose.

ADVERSE REACTIONS
Common reactions are in italics; life-threatening reactions are in bold italics.
Systemic: malaise, headache, slight fever, lymphadenopathy, ***anaphylaxis.***
Local: swelling, *induration, erythema.*

INTERACTIONS
None significant.

NURSING CONSIDERATIONS
- *Contraindicated* in patients with hypersensitivity to beef, soy, casein, or phenol, and in immunosuppression. Defer in respiratory infection.
- Deltoid area is the preferred injection site.
- Recommended for all laboratory and field personnel working with *Yersinia pestis.*
- Obtain history of allergies and reaction to immunization.
- Keep epinephrine 1:1,000 available.

pneumococcal vaccine, polyvalent

Pneumovax 23, Pnu-Imune 23

Pregnancy Risk Category: C

HOW SUPPLIED
Injection: 25 mcg each of 23 polysaccharide isolates/0.5 ml

MECHANISM OF ACTION
Promotes active immunity to infections caused by *Streptococcus pneumoniae.*

INDICATIONS & DOSAGE
Pneumococcal immunization–
Adults and children over 2 years: 0.5 ml I.M. or S.C.

Not recommended for children under 2 years.

ADVERSE REACTIONS
Common reactions are in italics; life-threatening reactions are in bold italics.
Systemic: *slight fever,* ***anaphylaxis.***
Local: soreness, severe, local reaction can occur when revaccination takes place within 3 years.

INTERACTIONS
None significant.

NURSING CONSIDERATIONS

- Check immunization history carefully to avoid revaccination within 3 years.
- Recomended for all adults over 65 years.
- Simultaneous administration with influenza vaccine is safe and effective.
- Inject in deltoid or midlateral thigh. Don't inject I.V.
- Keep refrigerated. Reconstitution or dilution not necessary.
- Treat fever with mild antipyretics.
- Protects against 23 pneumococcal types, which account for 90% of pneumococcal disease.
- Also may be administered to children to prevent pneumococcal otitis media.
- Obtain history of allergies and reaction to immunization. Eggs and egg protein are not used during the manufacture of the vaccine; contains phenol as a preservative.
- When splenectomy is being considered, vaccine should be given at least 2 weeks before procedure to ensure adequate antibody response. This vaccine may be less effective in splenectomized patients.
- Keep epinephrine 1:1,000 available.

poliovirus vaccine, live, oral, trivalent (TOPV)

Orimune

polovirus vaccine, inactivated (IPV)

IPOL, Polivax

Pregnancy Risk Category: C

HOW SUPPLIED

Oral vaccine: mixture of three viruses (types 1, 2, and 3), grown in monkey kidney tissue culture, in 0.5-ml single-dose Dispettes
Inactivated vaccine injection: mixture of three types of poliovirus (Types 1, 2, and 3) grown in tissue culture. IPOL employs monkey kidney cultures; Polivax employs human diploid cell cultures.

MECHANISM OF ACTION

Promotes immunity to poliomyelitis by inducing humoral antibodies and antibodies in the lymphatic tissue.

INDICATIONS & DOSAGE

Poliovirus immunization –
Children and nonimmunized adults: 0.5 ml P.O. (TOPV), followed by a second dose of 0.5 ml in 6 to 8 weeks. Give third 0.5-ml dose 6 to 12 months after second dose. A reinforcing dose of 0.5 ml should be given before entry to school.
Infants: administer 0.5 ml P.O. at 2 months, 4 months, and 18 months. Optional dose may be given at 6 months.
Poliovirus immunization in persons who cannot receive TOPV –
Adults: 0.5 ml S.C., followed by a second dose in 4 to 8 weeks. Administer a third dose in 6 to 12 months.
Children: 0.5 ml S.C. at 2 months and 4 months. Administer a third dose at 15 to 18 months. A reinforcing dose of 0.5 ml S.C. should be given before entry into school.

ADVERSE REACTIONS

Common reactions are in italics; life-threatening reactions are in bold italics.
Systemic: ***paralytic poliomyelitis.***

INTERACTIONS

Immune serum globulin, whole blood, plasma: antibodies in serum may interfere with immune response. Don't use vaccine within 3 months of transfusion.
Tuberculin skin test: skin test may be suppressed. Don't test for 6 weeks.

NURSING CONSIDERATIONS

- Oral vaccine is *contraindicated* in immunosuppression, cancer, and immunoglobulin abnormalities and in radiation, antimetabolite, alkylating agent, or corticosteroid therapy. These patients should receive IPV. Injectable vaccine is *contraindicated* in patients with hypersensitivity to neomycin or streptomycin.

- Defer oral vaccines in patients with vomiting or diarrhea. Defer both forms of vaccine in acute illness.
- Patients with immunodeficiency or altered immune status may be at risk for developing the disease if live vaccine is administered. These patients should receive parenteral form.
- The highest risk of poliovirus infection occurs after the first dose of the oral vaccine.
- Adults at high risk for exposure who have completed a primary course may receive another dose.
- Should not be administered to neonates under 6 weeks.
- *Use with caution* in siblings of child with known immunodeficiency syndrome. IPV is preferred.
- This vaccine is not effective in modifying or preventing existing or incubating poliomyelitis.
- Check the parents' immunization history when they bring in child for vaccine; this is an excellent time for parents to receive booster immunizations.
- Keep frozen until used. Once thawed, if unopened, may store refrigerated up to 30 days. Opened vials may be refrigerated up to 7 days. Thaw before administration.
- Color change from pink to yellow has no effect on efficacy of the vaccine. Yellow color results from vaccine being stored at low temperatures.
- Obtain history of allergies and reaction to immunization.
- Oral vaccine is not for parenteral use.
- An information booklet is available that describes the risks and benefits of this vaccine. Be sure parents read and understand this information before vaccine is administered.

rabies vaccine, human diploid cell (HDCV)

Imovax

Pregnancy Risk Category: C

HOW SUPPLIED

Intradermal injection: 0.25 IU rabies antigen/dose

I.M. injection: 2.5 IU of rabies antigen/ml, in single-dose vial with diluent

MECHANISM OF ACTION

Promotes active immunity to rabies.

INDICATIONS & DOSAGE

Postexposure antirabies immunization –

Adults and children: five 1-ml doses of HDCV I.M. (for example, in the deltoid region). Give first dose as soon as possible after exposure; give an additional dose on each of days 3, 7, 14, and 28 after first dose. If there is a lack of antibody response after this primary series, a booster dose is recommended.

Preexposure prophylaxis immunization for persons in high-risk groups –

Adults and children: three 1-ml injections administered I.M. Give first dose on day 0 (the first day of therapy), second dose on day 7, and third dose on either day 21 or 28. Alternatively, give 0.1 ml intradermally on the same dosage schedule.

ADVERSE REACTIONS

Common reactions are in italics; life-threatening reactions are in bold italics.

Systemic: headache, nausea, abdominal pain, muscle aches, dizziness, fever, diarrhea, ***anaphylaxis***, ***serum sickness.***

Local: *pain, erythema, swelling or itching at injection site.*

INTERACTIONS
Corticosteroids, immunosuppressive agents, antimalarial drugs: decreased response to rabies vaccine. Avoid concomitant use.

NURSING CONSIDERATIONS
• *Use cautiously* in persons with a history of hypersensitivity.
• Stop corticosteroids during immunizing period.
• When postexposure immunization is indicated, pregnancy is not a contraindication.
• Check serum levels for antibody titer 2 to 3 weeks after the last injection of the primary series.
• Some patients who receive booster doses experience serum sickness-like allergic reactions. These reactions usually respond to antihistamines.
• Keep epinephrine 1:1,000 available.
• The intradermal route is associated with suboptimal antibody response and high incidence of adverse effects. Do not use.
• The Centers for Disease Control and Prevention recommends a booster dose with Imovax for all persons who have been potentially exposed to rabies since October 15, 1984, and who have received postexposure prophylaxis with Wyvac unless acceptable titers were proven.
• The alternative regimen of 0.1-ml doses is only for *preexposure* prophylaxis. For postexposure prophylaxis, only the 1-ml doses should be used.

rubella and mumps virus vaccine, live
Biavax II
Pregnancy Risk Category: X

HOW SUPPLIED
Injection: single-dose vial containing not less than 1,000 $TCID_{50}$ (tissue culture infective doses) of the Wistar RA 27/3 rubella virus (propagated in human diploid cell culture) and not less than 5,000 $TCID_{50}$ of the Jeryl Lynn mumps strain (grown in chick embryo cell culture)

MECHANISM OF ACTION
Promotes immunity to rubella and mumps by inducing production of antibodies.

INDICATIONS & DOSAGE
Measles and mumps immunization –
Adults and children over 1 year: 1 vial (1,000 units) S.C.

ADVERSE REACTIONS
Common reactions are in italics; life-threatening reactions are in bold italics.
Systemic: fever, rash, thrombocytopenic purpura, urticaria, arthritis, arthralgia, polyneuritis, ***anaphylaxis.***
Local: pain, erythema, induration, lymphadenopathy.

INTERACTIONS
Immune serum globulin, whole blood, plasma: antibodies in serum may interfere with immune response. Don't give vaccine within 3 months of transfusion.
Tuberculin skin test: may temporarily decrease response to test. Defer skin testing.

NURSING CONSIDERATIONS
• *Contraindicated* in immunosuppression; cancer; blood dyscrasias; corticosteroid or radiation therapy; gamma globulin disorders; active, untreated tuberculosis; fever; or pregnancy.
• *Use cautiously* in patients with hypersensitivity to neomycin, chickens, ducks, eggs, or feathers. Defer in acute illness and after administration of immune serum globulin, blood, or plasma.
• Stress importance of avoiding pregnancy for 3 months after immunization. If necessary, provide contraceptive information.
• Store in refrigerator and protect

*Liquid form contains alcohol. **May contain tartrazine.

from light. Solution may be used if red, pink, or yellow (but must be clear).

- Use only diluent supplied. Discard 8 hours after reconstituting.
- Obtain history of allergies, especially to ducks, rabbits, and antibiotics, and reaction to immunization.
- Inject into outer aspect of upper arm. Don't inject I.V.
- Keep epinephrine 1:1,000 available.
- Allow an interval of at least 3 weeks between BCG and rubella vaccines.

rubella virus vaccine, live attenuated (RA 27/3)

Meruvax II

Pregnancy Risk Category: X

HOW SUPPLIED

Injection: single-dose vial containing not less than 1,000 $TCID_{50}$ (tissue culture infective doses) of the Wistar RA 27/3 strain of rubella (virus propagated in human diploid cell culture)

MECHANISM OF ACTION

Promotes immunity to rubella by inducing production of antibodies.

INDICATIONS & DOSAGE

Measles immunization–

Adults and children over 1 year: 1 vial (1,000 units) S.C.

ADVERSE REACTIONS

Common reactions are in italics; life-threatening reactions are in bold italics.

Systemic: *joint pain,* fever, rash, thrombocytopenic purpura, urticaria, arthritis, arthralgia, polyneuritis, ***anaphylaxis.***

Local: pain, erythema, induration, lymphadenopathy.

INTERACTIONS

Immune serum globulin, whole blood, plasma: antibodies in serum may interfere with immune response. Don't use vaccine within 3 months of transfusion. Immune serum globulin may be given 2 weeks before vaccine.

Tuberculin skin test: may temporarily decrease response to test. Defer skin testing.

NURSING CONSIDERATIONS

- *Contraindicated* in immunosuppression; cancer; blood dyscrasias; corticosteroid or radiation therapy; gamma globulin disorders; active, untreated tuberculosis; or fever.
- *Use cautiously* in patients with hypersensitivity to neomycin, chickens, ducks, eggs, or feathers. Defer in acute illness and after administration of human immune serum globulin, blood, or plasma.
- Stress importance of avoiding pregnancy for 3 months after immunization. If necessary, provide contraceptive information.
- Store in refrigerator and protect from light. Solution may be used if red, pink, or yellow (but must be clear).
- Use only diluent supplied. Discard 8 hours after reconstituting.
- Obtain history of allergies, especially to ducks and rabbits, and reaction to immunization.
- Inject into outer aspect of upper arm. Don't inject I.V.
- Keep epinephrine 1:1,000 available.
- Allow an interval of at least 3 weeks between BCG and rubella vaccines.

tetanus toxoid, adsorbed

tetanus toxoid, fluid

Pregnancy Risk Category: C

HOW SUPPLIED

adsorbed

Injection: 5 to 10 Lf units of inactivated tetanus/0.5-ml dose, in 0.5-ml syringes and 5-ml vials

fluid
Injection: 4 to 5 Lf units of inactivated tetanus/0.5-ml dose, in 0.5-ml syringes and 7.5-ml vials

MECHANISM OF ACTION
Promotes immunity to tetanus by inducing production of antitoxin.

INDICATIONS & DOSAGE
Primary immunization –
Adults and children: 0.5 ml (adsorbed) I.M. 4 to 6 weeks apart for two doses, then third dose 1 year after the second; 0.5 ml (fluid) I.M. or S.C. 4 to 8 weeks apart for three doses, then fourth dose of 0.5 ml 6 to 12 months after third dose. Booster is 0.5 ml I.M. at 10-year intervals.

ADVERSE REACTIONS
Common reactions are in italics; life-threatening reactions are in bold italics.
Systemic: slight fever, chills, malaise, aches and pains, flushing, urticaria, pruritus, tachycardia, hypotension, ***anaphylaxis***.
Local: erythema, induration, nodule.

INTERACTIONS
Chloramphenicol: may interfere with response to tetanus toxoid.

NURSING CONSIDERATIONS
- *Contraindicated* in immunosuppression and immunoglobulin abnormalities. Defer in acute illness and polio outbreaks, except in emergencies.
- For prevention, not treatment, of tetanus infections.
- Determine date of last tetanus immunization.
- Don't use hot or cold compresses; may increase severity of local reaction.
- Obtain history of allergies and reaction to immunization.
- Keep epinephrine 1:1,000 available.
- Adsorbed form produces longer duration of immunity. Fluid form provides quicker booster effect in patients actively immunized previously.
- Do not confuse this drug with tetanus immune globulin, human.

typhoid vaccine

typhoid vaccine, oral
Vivotif Berna Vaccine

Pregnancy Risk Category: C

HOW SUPPLIED
Injection: suspension of killed Ty-2 strain of Salmonella typhi; provides 8 units/ml in 5-ml, 10-ml, and 20-ml vials
Capsules (enteric-coated): 2 to 6 × 10^9 colony-forming units of viable *Salmonella typhi* $Ty^{21}a$ and 5 to 50 × 10^9 bacterial cells of nonviable $Ty^{21}a^2$

MECHANISM OF ACTION
Provides active immunity to typhoid fever.

INDICATIONS & DOSAGE
Primary immunization –
Adults and children over 10 years: 0.5 ml S.C.; repeat in 4 weeks. Booster is the same dose as primary immunization q 3 years.
Children 6 months to 10 years: 0.25 ml S.C.; repeat in 4 weeks. Booster is the same dose as primary immunization q 3 years.
Oral vaccine –
Adults: 1 capsule on alternate days taken 1 hour before meals. Booster dose is the same as the primary vaccine every 5 years.

ADVERSE REACTIONS
Common reactions are in italics; life-threatening reactions are in bold italics.
Systemic: *fever,* malaise, headache, nausea, ***anaphylaxis***.
Local: swelling, pain, inflammation.

*Liquid form contains alcohol. **May contain tartrazine.

INTERACTIONS
Sulfonamides, other antibiotics: may impair antibody response. Don't use together.

NURSING CONSIDERATIONS
- *Contraindicated* in immunosupression. Defer in acute illness.
- Treat fever with antipyretics.
- Do not give intradermally.
- Obtain history of allergies and reaction to immunization.
- Keep epinephrine 1:1,000 available.
- Store at 35.6° to 50° F (2° to 10° C).
- Shake thoroughly before withdrawing from vial.
- When administering oral vaccine, patient must understand the importance of taking all four doses. It is imperative that the alternate-day regimen be followed.
- Oral vaccine may be taken with cold or lukewarm water. Enteric-coated capsules should not be chewed or crushed.
- Store oral vaccine in refrigerator.

yellow fever vaccine
YF-Vax

Pregnancy Risk Category: D

HOW SUPPLIED
Injection: live, attenuated 17D yellow fever virus in 1- and 5-dose vials, with diluent; supplied only to designated yellow fever vaccination centers authorized to issue yellow fever vaccination certificates

MECHANISM OF ACTION
Provides active immunity to yellow fever.

INDICATIONS & DOSAGE
Primary vaccination –
Adults and children over 6 months: 0.5 ml deep S.C. booster is 0.5 ml S.C. q 10 years.

ADVERSE REACTIONS
Common reactions are in italics; life-threatening reactions are in bold italics.
Systemic: fever, malaise, ***anaphylaxis.***
Local: mild swelling, pain.

INTERACTIONS
Cholera vaccine: concurrent administration may interfere with immune response to both yellow fever vaccine and cholera vaccine. Administer 3 weeks apart.

NURSING CONSIDERATIONS
- *Contraindicated* in gamma globulin deficiency, immunosuppression, cancer, corticosteroid or radiation therapy, or allergies to chickens or eggs. Also *contraindicated* in pregnancy and in infants under 9 months except in high-risk areas. Information regarding these areas can be obtained from the Centers for Disease Control and Prevention, Division of Vector-Borne Infectious Diseases, at (303) 221-6400.
- Reconstitute with sodium chloride injection that contains no preservatives (preservatives decrease potency).
- Must be kept frozen. Don't use unless shipping case contains some dry ice upon arrival. Avoid vigorous shaking; carefully swirl mixture until suspension is uniform. Use within 1 hour after reconstitution. Discard remainder.
- Obtain history of allergies, especially to eggs, and reaction to immunization.
- Don't give within 1 month of other live virus vaccines; may be given concurrently with hepatitis B vaccine.
- Keep epinephrine 1:1,000 available.

75

Antitoxins and antivenins

black widow spider antivenin
botulism antitoxin, bivalent equine
crotaline antivenin, polyvalent
diphtheria antitoxin, equine
***Micrurus fulvius* antivenin**
tetanus antitoxin (TAT), equine

COMBINATION PRODUCTS
None.

black widow spider antivenin

Antivenin *(Latrodectus mactans)*
Pregnancy Risk Category: C

HOW SUPPLIED
Injection: combination package – 1 vial of antivenin (6,000 units/vial), one 2.5-ml vial of diluent (sterile water for injection), and one 1-ml vial of normal equine (horse) serum (1:10 dilution) for sensitivity testing

MECHANISM OF ACTION
Neutralizes and binds venom.

INDICATIONS & DOSAGE
Black widow spider bite –
Adults and children: 2.5 ml I.M. in deltoid. Second dose may be needed.

ADVERSE REACTIONS
Common reactions are in italics; life-threatening reactions are in bold italics.
Systemic: hypersensitivity, ***anaphylaxis, neurotoxicity.***

INTERACTIONS
None significant.

NURSING CONSIDERATIONS
• *Contraindicated* in patients with hypersensitivity to the drug.
• Immobilize patient; splint the bitten limb to prevent spread of venom.
• Test for sensitivity before giving. Use 0.2 ml of a 1:10 dilution in normal saline solution.
• Epinephrine 1:1,000 should be available in case of adverse reaction.
• Venom is neurotoxic and may cause respiratory paralysis and seizures. Watch patient carefully for 2 to 3 days.
• Obtain accurate patient history of allergies, especially to horses, and reaction to immunization.
• Earliest possible use of antivenin recommended for best results.
• Antivenin may be given I.V. in severe cases (when patient is in shock), in 10 to 50 ml of saline solution over 15 minutes.

botulism antitoxin, bivalent equine

Pregnancy Risk Category: D

HOW SUPPLIED
Available through your state health department or the office of the state epidemiologist.

MECHANISM OF ACTION
Neutralizes and binds toxin.

INDICATIONS & DOSAGE
Botulism –
Adults and children: 1 vial I.V. stat and q 4 hours, p.r.n., until patient's condition improves. Dilute antitoxin 1:10 in dextrose 5% or 10% in water or normal saline solution before giving. Give first 10 ml of dilution over 5 minutes; after 15 minutes, rate may be increased.

ADVERSE REACTIONS
Common reactions are in italics; life-threatening reactions are in bold italics.
Systemic: hypersensitivity, ***anaphylaxis,*** serum sickness (urticaria, pruritus, fever, malaise, arthralgia) may occur in 5 to 13 days.

INTERACTIONS
None significant.

NURSING CONSIDERATIONS
- *Contraindicated* in patients with hypersensitivity to the drug.
- Test for sensitivity before giving.
- Epinephrine 1:1,000 should be available in case of adverse reaction. Bivalent antitoxin contains antibodies against types A and B *Clostridium botulinum.* Antitoxins against all other types available only from Centers for Disease Control and Prevention in Atlanta: Monday to Friday, 8 a.m. to 4:30 p.m. (E.S.T.), (404) 329-3670; nights, weekends, and holidays (emergencies only), (404) 329-2888.
- Obtain accurate patient history of allergies, especially to horses, and reaction to immunization.
- Earliest possible use of antitoxin is recommended for best results.

crotaline antivenin, polyvalent

Pregnancy Risk Category: D

HOW SUPPLIED
Injection: combination package – one vial of lyophilized serum, one vial of diluent (10 ml bacteriostatic water for injection), and one 1-ml vial of normal horse serum (diluted 1:10) for sensitivity testing

MECHANISM OF ACTION
Neutralizes and binds venom of snakes of the species crotalids (pit vipers), including rattle snakes, water moccasins, and copperheads.

INDICATIONS & DOSAGE
Crotalid (rattlesnake) bites –
Adults and children: initially, 10 to 50 ml I.V., depending on severity of bite and patient response. If large amount of venom, 70 to 100 ml I.V. directly into superficial vein. Subsequent doses based on patient's response; may give 10 ml q ½ to 2 hours, p.r.n. If bite is in extremity, inject part of initial dose at various sites around limb above swelling; don't inject in finger or toe. The smaller the patient, the larger the initial dose.

ADVERSE REACTIONS
Common reactions are in italics; life-threatening reactions are in bold italics.
Systemic: *hypersensitivity,* ***anaphylaxis, neurotoxicity,*** *serum sickness.*

INTERACTIONS
Antihistamines: enhanced toxicity of crotaline venoms. Don't use together.

NURSING CONSIDERATIONS
- *Contraindicated* in patients with hypersensitivity to the drug.
- *Use cautiously.* In a recent study, 60% of patients treated with antivenin developed hypersensitivity.
- Test for sensitivity before giving. Give 0.02 to 0.03 ml of a 1:10 dilution in 0.9% sodium chloride solution intradermally. Read results after 5 to 10 minutes.
- Watch patient carefully for delayed allergic reaction or relapse.
- Immobilize patient immediately. Splint the bitten extremity.
- Epinephrine 1:1,000 should be available in case of adverse reaction.
- Type and cross match blood as soon as possible since hemolysis from venom prevents accurate cross matching.
- Early use of antivenin is recommended for best results.
- Children, who have less resistance and less body fluid to dilute venom, may need twice the adult dose.

- Obtain accurate patient history of allergies, especially to horses, and reaction to immunization.
- Discard unused reconstituted drug.
- If a large number of vials are administered, serum sickness is a likely complication. Corticosteroids should be administered.

diphtheria antitoxin, equine

Pregnancy Risk Category: D

HOW SUPPLIED

Injection: not less than 500 units/ml in 10,000-unit and 20,000-unit vials

MECHANISM OF ACTION

Neutralizes and binds toxin.

INDICATIONS & DOSAGE

Diphtheria prevention –

Adults and children: 1,000 to 5,000 units I.M.

Diphtheria treatment –

Adults and children: 20,000 to 80,000 units or more slow I.V. Additional doses may be given in 24 hours. I.M. route may be used in mild cases.

ADVERSE REACTIONS

Common reactions are in italics; life-threatening reactions are in bold italics.

Systemic: hypersensitivity, ***anaphylaxis,*** serum sickness (urticaria, pruritus, fever, malaise, arthralgia) may occur in 7 to 12 days.

INTERACTIONS

None significant.

NURSING CONSIDERATIONS

- *Contraindicated* in patients with hypersensitivity to the drug.
- Test for sensitivity before giving.
- Epinephrine 1:1,000 should be available in case of adverse reaction.
- Obtain accurate patient history of allergies, especially to horses, and reaction to immunization.
- Therapy should begin immediately, without delay for culture reports, if patient has symptoms of diphtheria (sore throat, fever, tonsillar membrane).
- For storage, refrigerate antitoxin at 35.6° to 50° F (2° to 10° C). Before administering, warm to 90° to 95° F (32.2° to 35° C), never higher.

Micrurus fulvius antivenin

Pregnancy Risk Category: D

HOW SUPPLIED

Injection: combination package with 10 ml diluent

MECHANISM OF ACTION

Neutralizes and binds coral snake venom.

INDICATIONS & DOSAGE

Eastern and Texas coral snake bite –

Adults and children: 3 to 5 vials slow I.V. through running I.V. of 0.9% normal saline solution. Give first 1 to 2 ml over 3 to 5 minutes, and watch for signs of allergic reaction. If no signs develop, continue injection. Up to 10 vials may be needed. Not effective for Sonoran or Arizona coral snake bites.

ADVERSE REACTIONS

Common reactions are in italics; life-threatening reactions are in bold italics.

Systemic: hypersensitivity, ***anaphylaxis.***

INTERACTIONS

None significant.

NURSING CONSIDERATIONS

- *Contraindicated* in patients with hypersensitivity to the drug.
- Test for sensitivity before giving.
- Immobilize patient or splint bitten limb to prevent spread of venom.
- Early use of antivenin (before onset of neurotoxic signs) recommended for best results. Because systemic signs

usually develop late, asymptomatic patients should be treated.

- Venom is neurotoxic and may cause respiratory paralysis. Watch patient carefully for 24 hours. Have epinephrine 1:1,000 available in case of adverse reaction.
- Obtain accurate patient history of allergies, especially to horses, and reaction to immunization.

tetanus antitoxin (TAT), equine

Pregnancy Risk Category: D

HOW SUPPLIED

Injection: not less than 400 units/ml in 1,500-unit and 20,000-unit vials

MECHANISM OF ACTION

Neutralizes and binds toxin.

INDICATIONS & DOSAGE

Tetanus prophylaxis –

Patients over 30 kg: 3,000 to 5,000 units I.M. or S.C.

Patients under 30 kg: 1,500 to 3,000 units I.M. or S.C.

Tetanus treatment –

All patients: 10,000 to 20,000 units injected into wound. Give additional 40,000 to 100,000 units I.V. Start tetanus toxoid at same time but at different site and with a different syringe.

ADVERSE REACTIONS

Common reactions are in italics; life-threatening reactions are in bold italics.

Systemic: joint pain, hypersensitivity,

Local: pain, numbness, skin rash, ***anaphylaxis,*** serum sickness.

INTERACTIONS

None significant.

NURSING CONSIDERATIONS

- *Contraindicated* in patients with hypersensitivity to the drug.
- Test for sensitivity before giving. Give 0.1 ml as a 1:1,000 dilution in normal saline solution intradermally.
- Use only when tetanus immune globulin (human) not available.
- Obtain accurate patient history of allergies, especially to horses, and reaction to immunization. If respiratory difficulty develops, give 0.4 ml of 1:1,000 solution epinephrine.
- Give preventive dose to those who have had two or fewer injections of tetanus toxoid and who have tetanus-prone injuries more than 24 hours old.

76

Immune serums

antirabies serum, equine
cytomegalovirus immune globulin, intravenous
hepatitis B immune globulin, human
immune globulin intramuscular
immune globulin intravenous
rabies immune globulin, human
Rh_o(D) immune globulin, human
tetanus immune globulin, human
varicella-zoster immune globulin

COMBINATION PRODUCTS
None.

antirabies serum, equine

Pregnancy Risk Category: C

HOW SUPPLIED
Injection: 125 IU/ml (1,000 IU/vial)

MECHANISM OF ACTION
Provides passive immunity to rabies.

INDICATIONS & DOSAGE
Rabies exposure –
Adults and children: 40 to 55 IU/kg at time of first dose of rabies vaccine. Use half of dose to infiltrate wound area. Give remainder I.M. Don't give rabies vaccine and antirabies serum in same syringe or at same site.

For wounds, including mucous membranes, the entire dose should be administered I.M.

ADVERSE REACTIONS
Common reactions are in italics; life-threatening reactions are in bold italics.
Systemic: within 6 to 12 days *serum sickness* occurs in 15% of children, up to 40% of adult patients. Symptoms are skin eruptions, arthralgia, pruritus, lymphadenopathy, fever, headache, malaise, abdominal pain; ***anaphylaxis.***
Local: pain at injection site.

INTERACTIONS
Corticosteroids and immunosuppressive agents: interferes with response. Avoid during postexposure immunization period.

NURSING CONSIDERATIONS
- *Contraindicated* in patients with hypersensitivity to the drug.
- Because of a significantly lower incidence of adverse reactions, rabies immune globulin (human) is preferred. This drug should be used only when the immune globulin is unavailable.
- Do sensitivity test on all patients before giving. Dilute serum 1:100 or 1:1,000 with normal saline solution for injection. Inject intradermally on inner forearm. Inject other arm with 0.1 ml of normal saline solution for injection intradermally as a control. Read within 20 minutes. Positive reaction: wheal 10 mm or more and erythematous flare 20 mm × 20 mm.
- Obtain history of animal bite, allergies (especially to equine serum and to eggs), and reaction to immunizations.
- Epinephrine solution 1:1,000 should always be available when administering this drug.
- This immune serum provides immediate passive immunity (short-term).
- Do not confuse this drug with rabies vaccine, which is a suspension of attenuated or killed microorganisms used to confer long-term active immunity. These two drugs are often administered together prophylactically

after exposure to known or suspected rabid animals.

- Ask patient when he received last tetanus immunization, since many doctors order a booster at this time.

cytomegalovirus immune globulin, intravenous (CMV-IGIV)

CytoGam

Pregnancy Risk Category: C

HOW SUPPLIED

Powder for injection: 2.5 g with 50 ml sterile water diluent supplied

MECHANISM OF ACTION

Provides passive immunity by supplying a relatively high concentration of immunoglobulin G (IgG) antibodies against CMV. Increasing these antibody levels in CMV-exposed patients may attenuate or reduce the incidence of serious CMV disease.

INDICATIONS & DOSAGE

To attenuate primary CMV disease in seronegative kidney transplant recipients who receive a kidney from a CMV seropositive donor–

Adults: administer according to the following schedule.

– within 72 hours of transplant: 150 mg/kg
– 2 weeks after transplant: 100 mg/kg
– 4 weeks after transplant: 100 mg/kg
– 6 weeks after transplant: 100 mg/kg
– 8 weeks after transplant: 100 mg/kg
– 12 weeks after transplant: 50 mg/kg
– 16 weeks after transplant: 50 mg/kg.

Administer initial dose at 15 mg/kg/hour. Increase to 30 mg/kg/hour after 30 minutes if no untoward reactions occur, then increase to 60 mg/kg/hour after another 30 minutes if no untoward reactions occur. Volume should not exceed 75 ml/hour. Subsequent doses may be administered at 15 mg/kg/hour for 15 minutes, increasing at 15-minute intervals in a stepwise fashion to 60 mg/kg/hour.

ADVERSE REACTIONS

Common reactions are in italics; life-threatening reactions are in bold italics.

CV: hypotension.

GI: nausea, vomiting.

Other: flushing, chills, muscle cramps, back pain, fever, wheezing, ***anaphylaxis***.

INTERACTIONS

Live virus vaccines: CMV immune serum may interfere with the immune response to live virus vaccines. Vaccination should be deferred for at least 3 months.

NURSING CONSIDERATIONS

- *Contraindicated* in patients with history of sensitivity to other human Ig preparations and in patients with selective IgA deficiency.
- **I.V. use:** Reconstitute as follows: Remove tab portion of vial cap and clean rubber stopper with 70% alcohol or equivalent. Add 50 ml sterile water for injection. *Do not shake vial; avoid foaming.* After adding water, release residual vacuum in vial to hasten dissolution. Rotate vial gently to wet all undissolved powder. Allow powder to dissolve for 30 minutes before administration. Inspect vial for clarity and particles.
- Infusion should begin within 6 hours of reconstitution and finish within 12 hours.
- Monitor patient closely during each change of infusion rate. Monitor vital signs preinfusion, midinfusion, postinfusion, and before any increase in infusion rate.
- If anaphylaxis or drop in blood pressure occurs, discontinue infusion and administer supportive therapy, including drugs such as diphenhydramine and epinephrine.
- Administer through a separate I.V.

line using a constant infusion pump. Filters are unnecessary.

- If unable to administer through separate line, piggyback into preexisting line of sodium chloride injection or one of the following dextrose solutions with or without sodium chloride: dextrose 2.5% in water, dextrose 5% in water, dextrose 10% in water, or dextrose 20% in water. Do not dilute more than 1:2 with any of the above solutions.
- Store powder for injection in refrigerator at 36° to 46° F (2° to 8° C). Do not store reconstituted drug.
- Drug has also been used for liver transplants and allogenic bone marrow transplants.

hepatitis B immune globulin, human

H-BIG, Hep-B-Gammagee, HyperHep

Pregnancy Risk Category: C

HOW SUPPLIED

Injection: 1-ml, 4-ml, 5-ml vials

MECHANISM OF ACTION

Provides passive immunity to hepatitis B.

INDICATIONS & DOSAGE

Hepatitis B exposure in high-risk patients –

Adults and children: 0.06 ml/kg I.M. within 7 days after exposure. Repeat 28 days after exposure.

Neonates born to women who test positive for hepatitis B surface antigen (HB_sAg): 0.5 ml within 12 hours of birth. Repeat dose at ages 3 months and 6 months.

ADVERSE REACTIONS

Common reactions are in italics; life-threatening reactions are in bold italics.

Systemic: ***anaphylaxis.***

INTERACTIONS

Other vaccines: Hepatitis B immune globulin may interfere with response to live virus vaccines. Defer administration for 3 months.

NURSING CONSIDERATIONS

- *Contraindicated* in patients with a history of anaphylactic reactions to immune serum.
- Anterolateral aspect of thigh or deltoid areas are the preferred injection sites in adults; anterolateral aspect of thigh is preferred for neonates and children under 3 years.
- Health-care personnel should receive immunization if exposed to hepatitis B (for example, needle-stick, direct contact).
- Obtain history of allergies and reaction to immunizations.

immune globulin intramuscular (IGIM, IG, gamma globulin)

Gamastan, Gammar

immune globulin intravenous (IGIV)

Gamimune N, Gammagard, Gammar-IV, Iveegam, Sandoglobulin, Venoglobulin-I

Pregnancy Risk Category: C

HOW SUPPLIED

intramuscular

Injection: 2-ml, 10-ml vials

intravenous

Injection: 5% in 10-ml, 50-ml, 100-ml vials (Gamimune N)

Powder for injection: 50 mg protein/ml in 0.5-g, 2.5-g, 5-g, 10-g vials (Gammagard); 2.5-g vials (Gammar-IV); 500-mg and 1-g vials, and 2.5-g and 5-g infusion bottles (Iveegam), 1-g, 3-g, 6-g vials (Sandoglobulin); 2.5-g, 5-g vials (Venoglobulin-I)

MECHANISM OF ACTION

Provides passive immunity by increasing antibody titer. The primary component is IgG.

INDICATIONS & DOSAGE

Agammaglobulinemia or hypogammaglobulinemia –
Adults: 30 to 50 ml I.M. monthly. Alternatively, administer 100 mg/kg I.V. (Gamimune N) monthly. Infuse at 0.01 to 0.02 ml/kg/minute for 30 minutes. For Sandoglobulin, administer 200 mg/kg I.V. monthly. Infuse at 0.5 to 1 ml/minute. After 15 to 30 minutes, increase infusion rate to 1.5 to 2.5 ml/minute.
Children: 20 to 40 ml I.M. monthly.
Hepatitis A exposure –
Adults and children: 0.02 to 0.04 ml/kg I.M. as soon as possible after exposure. Up to 0.1 ml/kg may be given after prolonged or intense exposure.
Post-transfusion hepatitis B –
Adults and children: 10 ml I.M. within 1 week after transfusion and 10 ml I.M. 1 month later.
Measles exposure –
Adults and children: 0.02 ml/kg I.M. within 6 days after exposure.
Modification of measles –
Adults and children: 0.04 ml/kg I.M. within 6 days after exposure.
Measles vaccine complications –
Adults and children: 0.02 to 0.04 ml/kg I.M.
Poliomyelitis exposure –
Adults and children: 0.3 to 0.4 ml/kg I.M. within 7 days after exposure.
Chicken pox exposure –
Adults and children: 0.2 to 1.3 ml/kg I.M. as soon as exposed.
Rubella exposure in first trimester of pregnancy –
Women: 0.2 to 0.4 ml/kg I.M. as soon as exposed.
Prophylaxis in primary immunodeficiencies –
Adults and children: 100 mg/kg by I.V. infusion monthly (Gamimune only). Infusion rate is 0.01 to 0.02 ml/kg/minute for 30 minutes. Rate can then be increased to 0.04 ml/minute for remainder of infusion.
Idiopathic thrombocytopenic purpura –
Adults: 0.4 g/kg Gamimune N or Sandoglobulin I.V. for 5 consecutive days; or 1,000 mg/kg Gammagard. Additional doses may be given based on response. Give up to three doses (every other day) if necessary. Or, give Venoglobulin-I 500 mg/kg daily for 2 to 7 days.

ADVERSE REACTIONS

Common reactions are in italics; life-threatening reactions are in bold italics.
Skin: urticaria.
Systemic: angioedema, headache, malaise, fever, nephrotic syndrome, ***anaphylaxis***.
Local: pain, erythema, muscle stiffness.

INTERACTIONS

Live virus vaccines: don't administer within 3 months after administration of immune globulin.

NURSING CONSIDERATIONS

- *Contraindicated* in patients with hypersensitivity to the drug.
- Most adverse effects are related to a rapid rate of infusion.
- Obtain history of allergies and reaction to immunizations.
- Have drugs available for anaphylactoid reaction.
- When giving I.M., inject into different sites, preferably anterolateral aspect of thigh or deltoid muscle for adults and anterolateral aspect of thigh for neonates and children under 3 years. Do not inject more than 3 ml per injection site.
- Do not give for hepatitis A exposure if 6 weeks or more have elapsed since exposure or after onset of clinical illness.
- **I.V. use:** Know that I.V. products

are not interchangeable. Gamimune-N, Sandoglobulin, and Venoglubulin-I do not require an in-line filter. Gammagard and Iveegam require filters, which are supplied by the manufacturer.

rabies immune globulin, human

Hyperab, Imogam

Pregnancy Risk Category: C

HOW SUPPLIED

Injection: 150 IU/ml in 2-ml, 10-ml vials

MECHANISM OF ACTION

Provides passive immunity to rabies.

INDICATIONS & DOSAGE

Rabies exposure –

Adults and children: 20 IU/kg I.M. at time of first dose of rabies vaccine. Use half of dose to infiltrate wound area. Give remainder I.M. Don't give rabies vaccine and rabies immune globulin in same syringe or at same site.

ADVERSE REACTIONS

Common reactions are in italics; life-threatening reactions are in bold italics.

Local: pain, redness, induration at injection site.

Other: slight fever, ***anaphylaxis, angioedema.***

INTERACTIONS

Corticosteroids and immunosuppressive agents: interferes with response. Avoid during postexposure immunization period.

Live virus vaccines (measles, mumps, rubella, or polio): response to these vaccines may not be reliable because of antibodies present in rabies immune globulin. Don't administer live vaccines within 3 months of rabies immune globulin.

NURSING CONSIDERATIONS

- *Contraindicated* in patients with hypersensitivity to the drug.
- Repeated doses contraindicated after rabies vaccine is started.
- Use only with rabies vaccine and immediate local treatment of wound. Give regardless of interval between exposure and initiation of therapy.
- Obtain history of animal bites, allergies, and reaction to immunizations.
- Don't administer more than 5 ml I.M. at one injection site; divide I.M. doses greater than 5 ml, and administer at different sites.
- This immune serum provides passive immunity.
- Do not confuse this drug with rabies vaccine, which is a suspension of attenuated or killed microorganisms used to confer active immunity. These two drugs are often given together prophylactically after exposure to known or suspected rabid animals.
- Ask the patient when he received his last tetanus immunization, since many doctors order a booster at this time.

Rh_o(D) immune globulin, human

Gamulin Rh, HypRho-D, MICRhoGAM, Mini-Gamulin Rh, Rhesonativ, RhoGAM

Pregnancy Risk Category: C

HOW SUPPLIED

Injection: 300 mcg of Rh_o(D) immune globulin/vial (standard dose); 50 mcg of Rh_o(D) immune globulin/vial (microdose)

MECHANISM OF ACTION

Suppresses the active antibody response and formation of anti-Rh_o(D) in Rh_o(D)-negative, D^u-negative individuals, exposed to Rh-positive blood.

INDICATIONS & DOSAGE

Rh exposure –

Women (postabortion, postmiscarriage, ectopic pregnancy, or postpartum): transfusion unit or blood bank determines fetal packed red blood cell (RBC) volume entering woman's blood, then gives one vial I.M. if fetal packed RBC volume is less than 15 ml. More than one vial I.M. may be required if there is large fetomaternal hemorrhage. Must be given within 72 hours after delivery or miscarriage.

Transfusion accidents –

Adults and children: consult blood bank or transfusion unit at once. Must be given within 72 hours.

Postabortion or postmiscarriage to prevent Rh antibody formation –

Women: consult transfusion unit or blood bank. One microdose vial will suppress immune reaction to 2.5 ml Rh_o(D)-positive RBCs. Ideally should be given within 3 hours, but may be given up to 72 hours after abortion or miscarriage.

ADVERSE REACTIONS

Common reactions are in italics; life-threatening reactions are in bold italics.

Local: discomfort at injection site.

Other: slight fever, ***anaphylaxis***.

INTERACTIONS

Live virus vaccines: may interfere with response. Defer vaccination for 3 months after administration of Rh_o(D) immune globulin.

NURSING CONSIDERATIONS

- *Contraindicated* in Rh_o(D)-positive or D^u-positive patients and those previously immunized to Rh_o(D) blood factor.
- Immediately after delivery, send a sample of infant's cord blood to laboratory for typing and cross matching. Confirm if mother is Rh_o(D)-negative and D^u-negative. Infant must be Rh_o(D)-positive or D^u-positive.
- Obtain history of allergies and reaction to immunization.
- MICRhoGAM is recommended for every woman undergoing abortion or miscarriage up to 12 weeks' gestation unless she is Rh_o(D)-positive or D^u-positive, has Rh antibodies, or the father and/or fetus is Rh-negative.
- Store at 36° to 46° F (2° to 8° C).
- This immune serum provides passive immunity to the woman exposed to Rh_o-positive fetal blood during pregnancy. Prevents formation of maternal antibodies (active immunity), which would endanger future Rh_o-positive pregnancies.
- Explain to the patient how drug protects future Rh_o-positive infants.

tetanus immune globulin, human

Homo-Tet, Hu-Tet, Hyper-Tet†

Pregnancy Risk Category: C

HOW SUPPLIED

Injection: 250 units per vial or syringe

MECHANISM OF ACTION

Provides passive immunity to tetanus.

INDICATIONS & DOSAGE

Tetanus exposure –

Adults and children: 250 to 500 units I.M.

Tetanus treatment –

Adults and children: single doses of 3,000 to 6,000 units I.M. have been used. Optimal dosage schedules have not been established. Don't give at same site as toxoid.

ADVERSE REACTIONS

Common reactions are in italics; life-threatening reactions are in bold italics.

Local: pain, stiffness, erythema.

Other: slight fever, allergy, ***anaphylaxis***.

INTERACTIONS

None significant.

NURSING CONSIDERATIONS

- Use tetanus immune globulin only if wound is over 24 hours old or patient has had less than two previous tetanus toxoid injections.
- Obtain history of injury, tetanus immunizations, last tetanus toxoid injection, allergies, and reaction to immunizations.
- Thoroughly cleanse and remove all foreign matter from wound.
- Antibodies remain at effective levels for 3 weeks or longer, which is several times the duration of antitoxin-induced antibodies. Protects the patient for the incubation period of most tetanus cases.
- Human globulin is not a substitute for tetanus toxoid, which should be given at the same time to produce active immunization.
- Inject into the deltoid muscle for adults and children 3 years and older and into the anterolateral aspect of the thigh in neonates and children under 3 years.
- Do not confuse this drug with tetanus toxoid.

varicella-zoster immune globulin (VZIG)

Pregnancy Risk Category: C

HOW SUPPLIED

Injection: 10% to 18% solution of the globulin fraction of human plasma containing 125 units of varicella-zoster virus antibody (volume is about 1.25 ml)

MECHANISM OF ACTION

Provides passive immunity to varicella-zoster virus.

INDICATIONS & DOSAGE

Passive immunization of susceptible immunodeficient patients after exposure to varicella (chicken pox or herpes zoster) –

Children to 10 kg: 125 units I.M.
Children 10.1 to 20 kg: 250 units I.M.
Children 20.1 to 30 kg: 375 units I.M.
Children 30.1 to 40 kg: 500 units I.M.
Adults and children over 40 kg: 625 units I.M.

ADVERSE REACTIONS

Common reactions are in italics; life-threatening reactions are in bold italics.

Systemic: GI distress, malaise, headache, respiratory distress, ***anaphylaxis.***
Local: discomfort at injection site, rash.

INTERACTIONS

Live virus vaccines: may interfere with response. Defer vaccination for 3 months after administration of VZIG.

NURSING CONSIDERATIONS

- *Contraindicated* in patients with a history of severe reaction to human immune serum globulin or severe thrombocytopenia.
- For maximum benefit, administer as soon as possible after presumed exposure. May be of benefit when given as late as 96 hours after exposure.
- VZIG is not recommended for nonimmunosuppressed patients.
- Although usually restricted to children under 15 years, VZIG may be administered to adolescents and adults if necessary.
- Not commercially distributed. Available only from 20 regional U.S. distribution centers. These centers will distribute to Canada and overseas. Call the CDC for details Monday to Friday, 8 a.m. to 4:30 p.m. (EST), (404) 329-3670; all other times, (404) 329-2888.
- Administer only by deep I.M. injection. Never administer I.V.
- Store vial in refrigerator.

77

Biological response modifiers

aldesleukin
epoetin alfa
filgrastim
interferon alfa-2a, recombinant
interferon alfa-2b, recombinant
interferon alfa-n3
sargramostim

COMBINATION PRODUCTS
None.

aldesleukin (interleukin-2, IL-2)

Proleukin

Pregnancy Risk Category: C

HOW SUPPLIED

Powder for injection: 22 million IU/vial

MECHANISM OF ACTION

A highly purified immunoregulatory protein known as lymphokine synthesized using genetically engineered *Escherichia coli.* The drug produced is similar to human interleukin-2 (IL-2): it enhances lymphocyte mitogenesis, stimulates long-term growth of IL-2-dependent cell lines, enhances lymphocyte cytotoxicity, induces both lymphokine-activated and natural killer cell activity, and induces the production of interferon gamma.

INDICATIONS & DOSAGE

Metastatic renal cell carcinoma –
Adults: 600,000 IU/kg (0.037 mg/kg) I.V. q 8 hours for 5 days (total of 14 doses). After a 9-day rest, repeat the sequence for another 14 doses. Repeat courses may be administered after a rest period of at least 7 weeks from hospital discharge.

ADVERSE REACTIONS

Common reactions are in italics; life-threatening reactions are in bold italics.

Blood: *anemia, thrombocytopenia, leukopenia, coagulation disorders, leukocytosis, eosinophilia.*

CNS: *mental status changes, dizziness, sensory dysfunction, special senses disorders, syncope, motor dysfunction,* ***coma.***

CV: ***hypotension,*** *sinus tachycardia, arrhythmias, bradycardia,* ***premature ventricular contractions,*** *premature atrial contractions, myocardial ischemia,* ***MI, CHF, cardiac arrest,*** myocarditis, endocarditis, ***CVA,*** pericardial effusion, thrombosis.

GI: *nausea, vomiting, diarrhea, stomatitis, anorexia, bleeding, dyspepsia, constipation.*

GU: ***oliguria, anuria,*** *proteinuria, hematuria, dysuria,* urine retention, urinary frequency.

Hepatic: *jaundice; ascites; hepatomegaly; elevated bilirubin, serum transaminase, alkaline phosphatase levels.*

Respiratory: *pulmonary congestion, dyspnea,* ***pulmonary edema, respiratory failure, pleural effusion, apnea, pneumothorax,*** tachypnea.

Skin: *pruritus, erythema, rash, dryness,* ***exfoliative dermatitis,*** purpura, alopecia, petechiae.

Other: *elevated BUN, serum creatinine levels; hypomagnesemia; acidosis; hypocalcemia; hypophosphatemia; hypokalemia; hyperuricemia; hypoalbuminemia;* hypoproteinemia; hyponatremia; hyperkalemia; arthralgia; myalgia; *fever; chills;* abdominal, chest, or back pain; fatigue; weakness; malaise; edema; infections of the catheter tip, urinary tract, or injection site; phlebitis; ***sepsis;*** weight gain; headache; weight loss; conjunctivitis.

INTERACTIONS

Antihypertensives: increased risk of hypotension. Monitor closely.
Corticosteroids: decreased antitumor effectiveness of aldesleukin. Avoid concomitant use.
Hepatotoxic, nephrotoxic, cardiotoxic, or myelotoxic drugs: enhanced toxicity. Avoid concomitant use.
Psychotropic agents: unpredictable interaction. Because aldesleukin can alter CNS function, use cautiously.

NURSING CONSIDERATIONS

- *Contraindicated* in patients with hypersensitivity to the drug or any component of the formulation. Also contraindicated in patients with abnormal cardiac (thallium) stress test or pulmonary function tests. Retreatment is contraindicated in patients who experience any of the following toxicities: pericardial tamponade; disturbances in cardiac rhythm that were uncontrolled or unresponsive to intervention; sustained ventricular tachycardia (five beats or more); chest pain accompanied by ECG changes, indicated MI or angina pectoris; renal dysfunction requiring dialysis for 72 hours or more; coma or toxic psychosis lasting 48 hours or more; seizures that were repetitive or difficult to control; ischemia or perforation of the bowel; GI bleeding requiring surgery.
- Do not use this drug unless the patient has had definitive tests documenting normal cardiac and pulmonary function. *Use with extreme caution* in patients with normal test results if they have a history of cardiac or pulmonary disease and in patients with a history of seizure disorders because the drug may cause seizures.
- *Use cautiously* and with close clinical monitoring because severe adverse effects generally accompany therapy at the recommended dosage. This drug should be used only in a hospital setting under the direction of a doctor experienced in the use of chemotherapeutic agents. An intensive care facility and intensive care or cardiopulmonary specialists must be readily available. Because fluid management or administration of pressor agents may be essential to treat CLS, also use cautiously in patients who require large volumes of fluid (such as patients with hypercalcemia).
- Perform standard hematologic tests, including CBC, differential, and platelet counts; serum electrolytes; and renal and hepatic function tests, before therapy. Also obtain chest x-ray. Repeat daily during drug administration.
- Therapy is associated with impaired neutrophil function, which can lead to disseminated infection. Many studies employed prophylactic antibiotic therapy with oxacillin, nafcillin, ciprofloxacin, or vancomycin; check protocol and administer antibiotics as ordered. Monitor for infection. Patients with bacterial infections should be treated before therapy.
- Hold dose and notify doctor if patient develops moderate to severe lethargy or somnolence because continued administration can result in coma.
- Patients should be neurologically stable with a negative computed tomography scan for CNS metastases. Drug may exacerbate symptoms in patients with unrecognized or undiagnosed CNS metastases.
- Renal and hepatic impairment occurs during treatment. Avoid concurrent use of other hepatotoxic or nephrotoxic drugs because toxicity may be additive. Also, be prepared to adjust dosage of other drugs to compensate for this impairment.
- Dosage modification because of toxicity is usually accomplished by

holding a dose or interrupting therapy rather than by reducing the dose.

- Severe anemia or thrombocytopenia may occur. Administer packed RBCs or platelets, as ordered.
- This drug has been associated with capillary leak syndrome (CLS), a condition that results from the loss of vascular tone in which plasma proteins and fluids escape into the extravascular space. Mean arterial blood pressure begins to drop within 2 to 12 hours of treatment; edema and effusions may be severe, and death can result from hypoperfusion of major organs. Other conditions that accompany CLS include cardiac arrhythmias, MI, angina, mental status changes, renal insufficiency, respiratory distress or failure, and GI bleeding or infarction.
- Treat CLS with careful monitoring of fluid status, pulse, mental status, urine output, and organ perfusion. Central venous pressure monitoring is necessary.
- **I.V. use:** To avoid altering the pharmacologic properties of the drug, reconstitute and dilute carefully, and follow manufacturer's recommendations. Do not mix with other drugs or albumin.
- Reconstitute the vial containing 22 million IU (1.3 mg) with 1.2 ml sterile water for injection. Do not use bacteriostatic water or 0.9% sodium chloride injection because these diluents cause increased aggregation of drug. Direct the stream at the sides of the vial and gently swirl to reconstitute. Do not shake.
- Add the ordered dose of reconstituted drug to 50 ml dextrose 5% in water and infuse over 15 minutes. Do not use an in-line filter. Plastic infusion bags are preferred because they provided consistent drug delivery in early clinical trials.
- The reconstituted solution will have a concentration of 18 million IU (1.1 mg)/ml. The reconstituted drug should be particle-free and colorless to slightly yellow.
- Vials are for single-use only and contain no preservatives. Discard unused drug.
- Store powder for injection or reconstituted solutions in the refrigerator. After reconstitution and dilution, drug must be administered within 48 hours. Be sure that solutions are returned to room temperature before drug is administered to the patient.
- IL-2 has been investigated for a number of cancers, including Kaposi's sarcoma, metastatic melanoma, colorectal cancer and non-Hodgkin's lymphoma.

epoetin alfa (erythropoietin)

Epogen, Procrit

Pregnancy Risk Category: C

HOW SUPPLIED

Injection: 2,000 units/ml, 3,000 units/ml, 4,000 units/ml, 6,000 units/ml

MECHANISM OF ACTION

A naturally occurring hormone, produced by recombinant DNA techniques. Epoetin alfa is one of the factors controlling the rate of red cell production. It acts on the erythroid tissues in the bone marrow stimulating the mitotic activity of erythroid progenitor cells and early precursor cells. It functions as a growth factor and as a differentiating factor.

INDICATIONS & DOSAGE

Anemia due to reduced production of endogenous erythropoietin, end-stage renal disease –

Adults: dosage is individualized. Starting dose is 50 to 100 units/kg I.V. three times weekly. (Nondialysis patients with chronic renal failure or patients receiving continuous peritoneal dialysis may receive the drug by S.C. injection or I.V.) Reduce dosage when target hematocrit is reached or if the hematocrit rises more than 4 points in any 2-week period. Increase dosage if hematocrit does not increase by 5 to 6 points after 8 weeks of therapy. Maintenance dose is usually 25 units/kg three times weekly.

Adjunctive treatment of HIV-infected patients with anemia secondary to zidovudine therapy –
Adults: 100 units/kg I.V. or S.C. three times weekly for 8 weeks or until target hemoglobin is reached.

ADVERSE REACTIONS
Common reactions are in italics; life-threatening reactions are in bold italics.
Blood: iron deficiency, elevated platelet count.
CNS: headache, ***seizures.***
CV: *hypertension,* decreased plasma volume.
GI: nausea, vomiting, diarrhea.
Skin: rash.
Other: increased clotting of arteriovenous grafts.

INTERACTIONS
None reported.

NURSING CONSIDERATIONS
- *Contraindicated* in patients with uncontrolled hypertension. Reduce dosage in patients who exhibit a rapid rise in hematocrit (more than 4 points in any 2-week period) because of the risk of hypertension.
- When used in HIV-infected patients, dosage should be individualized based on responses. Dosage recommendations are for patients with endogenous erythropoetin levels of 500 units/liter or less and cumulative zidovudine doses of 4.2 g/week or less.
- Blood count should be monitored during therapy. Hematocrit may rise and cause excessive clotting.
- Monitor blood pressure before initiating therapy. Up to 80% of patients with chronic renal failure have hypertension. Blood pressure may rise, especially when the hematocrit is increasing in the early part of therapy. Diet restrictions or drug therapy may be required to control blood pressure.
- Patients should avoid hazardous activities, such as driving or operating heavy machinery, during the initiation of therapy. There may be a relationship between excessively rapid hematocrit rise and seizures.
- Patients treated with epoetin alfa may require additional heparin to prevent clotting during dialysis treatments.
- After injection (usually within 2 hours), some patients complain of pain or discomfort in their limbs (long bones) and pelvis. Coldness and sweating may also occur. These symptoms may persist up to 12 hours and then disappear.
- Patients with end-stage renal disease may experience an improved appetite and enhanced well-being as a result of increased hematocrit.
- Epoetin alfa has also been used to correct the hemostatic defect associated with uremia.
- Additional clinical trials are investigating epoetin alfa for treatment of the anemia of AIDS patients receiving zidovudine, of cancer patients undergoing chemotherapy, and of patients with rheumatoid arthritis. It is also being investigated for facilitating autologous transfusion by helping to produce more units of blood before surgery.
- Advise the patient that blood specimens will be drawn weekly for blood counts and, depending on their results, dosage adjustments may be necessary.
- Patient's response to epoetin is probably dependent on amount of endogenous erythropoietin in the plasma. Patients with levels of 500 units/liter or more usually have transfusion-dependent anemia and will probably not respond to the drug; with

levels below 500 units/liter, mild to moderate anemia; and with levels below 100 units/liter, renal failure. Those with levels below 500 units/liter usually respond well.

filgrastim (granulocyte colony stimulating factor; G-CSF)

Neupogen

Pregnancy Risk Category: C

HOW SUPPLIED

Injection: 300 mcg/ml

MECHANISM OF ACTION

A glycoprotein that stimulates proliferation and differentiation of hematopoietic cells. Filgrastim is specific for neutrophils.

INDICATIONS & DOSAGE

To decrease the incidence of infection in patients with nonmyeloid malignancies receiving myelosuppressive antineoplastic agents –
Adults and children: 5 mcg/kg/day I.V. or S.C. as a single dose. Doses may be increased in increments of 5 mcg/kg for each chemotherapy cycle depending on the duration and severity of the nadir of the absolute neutrophil count (ANC).

ADVERSE REACTIONS

Common reactions are in italics; life-threatening reactions are in bold italics.
Blood: ***thrombocytopenia.***
GU: hematuria, proteinuria.
Skin: alopecia, exacerbation of preexisting conditions (such as psoriasis).
Other: *skeletal pain,* fever, splenomegaly, osteoporosis.

INTERACTIONS

Chemotherapeutic agents: rapidly dividing myeloid cells are potentially sensitive to cytotoxic agents. Do not use filgrastim concomitantly with chemotherapy.

NURSING CONSIDERATIONS

- *Contraindicated* in patients hypersensitive to proteins derived from *Escherichia coli.* Although the drug is a growth factor for neutrophils only, the potential exists for stimulation of myeloid tumor growth.
- Do not give the drug within 24 hours of cytotoxic chemotherapy.
- Note that a transiently increased neutrophil count is common 1 or 2 days after initiation of therapy. However, the drug should be given daily for up to 2 weeks or until the ANC has returned to 10,000/mm³ after the expected chemotherapy-induced neutrophil nadir.
- Obtain a CBC and platelet count before therapy and monitor twice weekly during therapy. Note that patients who receive this drug have the potential for receiving higher doses of chemotherapy, which may increase the risk of chemotherapy-induced toxicities.
- Store in the refrigerator at 36° to 46° F (2° to 8° C). Do not freeze; avoid shaking. The drug may be stored at room temperature for a maximum of 6 hours; discard any vial that has been at room temperature for more than 6 hours.
- The vials are intended for single use only and contain no preservatives. Once a dose is withdrawn, do not reenter the vial.
- If the patient is going to self-administer the drug, teach him how to administer it and dispose of used needles, syringes, and drug containers. Give him a copy of the "information for patients" section included with the product information and ensure that he understands the information.

interferon alfa-2a, recombinant (rIFN-A)

Roferon-A

Pregnancy Risk Category: C

HOW SUPPLIED
Injection: 3 million IU/vial; 18 million IU/multiple-dose vial

MECHANISM OF ACTION
Interferon alfa-2a is a sterile protein product produced by recombinant DNA techniques. Its exact mechanism of action is unknown, but appears to involve direct antiproliferative action against tumor cells or viral cells to inhibit replication, and modulation of host immune response by enhancing the phagocytic activity of macrophages and by augmenting specific cytotoxicity of lymphocytes for target cells.

INDICATIONS & DOSAGE
Treatment of hairy-cell leukemia –
Adults: for induction, give 3 million units S.C. or I.M. daily for 16 to 24 weeks. For maintenance, 3 million units S.C. or I.M. three times a week.
Treatment of AIDS-related Kaposi's sarcoma –
Adults: for induction, give 36 million units S.C. or I.M. daily for 10 to 12 weeks. For maintenance, 36 million units S.C. or I.M. three times a week.

ADVERSE REACTIONS
Common reactions are in italics; life-threatening reactions are in bold italics.
Blood: ***leukopenia,*** mild thrombocytopenia.
CNS: *dizziness,* confusion, paresthesias, numbness, lethargy, depression, nervousness, difficulty in thinking or concentrating, insomnia, sedation, apathy, anxiety, irritability, fatigue, vertigo, gait disturbances, poor coordination.
CV: hypotension, chest pain, arrhythmias, palpitations, syncope, ***CHF,*** hypertension, edema.
EENT: visual disturbances, dryness or inflammation of the oropharynx, rhinorrhea, sinusitis, conjunctivitis, earache, eye irritation, rhinitis.
GI: *anorexia, nausea, diarrhea,* vomiting, abdominal fullness, abdominal pain, flatulence and constipation, hypermotility, gastric distress, dysgeusia.
GU: transient impotence.
Hepatic: ***hepatitis.***
Respiratory: ***bronchospasm,*** coughing, dyspnea, tachypnea.
Skin: *rash,* dryness, *pruritus,* partial alopecia, urticaria, flushing.
Local: inflammation at injection site (rare).
Other: *flu-like syndrome (fever, fatigue, myalgia, headache, chills, arthralgia),* diaphoresis, hot flashes, excessive salivation, cyanosis.

INTERACTIONS
Aminophylline: may reduce the clearance of aminophylline.
CNS depressants: enhanced CNS effects.

NURSING CONSIDERATIONS
- *Contraindicated* in patients with hypersensitivity to the drug.
- *Use cautiously* in severe hepatic or renal function impairment, seizure disorders, compromised CNS function, cardiac disease, and myelosuppression.
- Information based on current literature. Dosage, indications, and adverse reactions profile may change with additional clinical experience.
- Neurotoxicity and cardiotoxicity are more common in elderly patients, especially those with underlying CNS or cardiac impairment.
- Use with blood dyscrasia-causing medications, bone marrow suppressant therapy, or radiation therapy may increase bone marrow suppressant effects. Dosage reduction may be required.
- Obtain allergy history. Drug contains phenol as a preservative and serum albumin as a stabilizer.
- S.C. administration route should be used in patients whose platelet count is below 50,000/mm^3.

• Different brands of interferon may not be equivalent and may require different dosage.
• Almost all patients experience flulike symptoms at the beginning of therapy. These effects tend to diminish with continued therapy. Premedication with acetaminophen minimizes flulike symptoms.
• Patients should be well hydrated, especially during initial stages of treatment.
• Administer at bedtime to minimize daytime drowsiness.
• Severe adverse reactions may require reduction of dosage to one-half or discontinuation of therapy until reactions subside.
• Advise patient that laboratory tests will be performed before and periodically during therapy. Such tests will include a CBC with differential, platelet count, blood chemistry and electrolyte studies, liver function tests, and if the patient has a preexisting cardiac disorder or advanced stages of cancer, ECGs.
• Interferons may decrease hemoglobin, hematocrit, leukocytes, platelets, and neutrophils; increase prothrombin and partial thromboplastin time; and increase serum levels of AST (SGOT), ALT (SGPT), LDH, alkaline phosphatase, calcium, phosphorus, and fasting glucose. These effects are dose-related and reversible; recovery occurs within several days or weeks after withdrawal of interferon.
• Monitor for CNS adverse reactions, such as decreased mental status and dizziness. Periodic neuropsychiatric monitoring is recommended during therapy.
• Special precautions required for patients who develop thrombocytopenia: exercise extreme care in performing invasive procedures; inspect injection site and skin frequently for signs of bruising; limit frequency of I.M. injections; test urine, emesis fluid, stool, and secretions for occult blood.
• Instruct patient in proper oral hygiene during treatment, because the bone marrow suppressant effects of interferon may lead to microbial infection, delayed healing, and gingival bleeding. Interferon may also decrease salivary flow.
• Advise patient to check with doctor for further instructions after missing a dose.
• If patient is to self-administer drug, teach patient how to prepare and administer the injection and how to use disposable syringe. Give information on drug stability.
• Store drug in refrigerator.
• Emphasize need to follow doctor's instructions about taking and recording temperature, and how and when to take acetaminophen.
• Concurrent use with a live virus vaccine may potentiate replication of vaccine virus, increase adverse reactions, and decrease patient's antibody response.
• Warn patient not to have any immunization without doctor's approval and to avoid contact with persons who have taken oral polio vaccine. Because interferon may decrease antibody response and potentiate replication of vaccine viruses, the patient is at special risk for infection during therapy.
• Tell patient drug may cause temporary loss of some hair. Normal hair growth should return when drug is withdrawn.

interferon alfa-2b, recombinant (IFN-alpha 2)
Intron A
Pregnancy Risk Category: C

HOW SUPPLIED
Injection: 3 million IU/vial with diluent, 5 million IU/vial with diluent, 10 million IU/vial with diluent, 25 million IU/vial with diluent, 50 million IU/vial with diluent

MECHANISM OF ACTION

Interferon alfa-2b is a sterile protein product produced by recombinant DNA techniques. Its exact mechanism of action is unknown, but appears to involve direct antiproliferative action against tumor cells or viral cells to inhibit replication, and modulation of host immune response by enhancing the phagocytic activity of macrophages and by augmenting specific cytotoxicity of lymphocytes for target cells.

INDICATIONS & DOSAGE

Treatment of hairy-cell leukemia –
Adults: 2 million units/m² I.M. or S.C. three times a week.
Treatment of condylomata acuminata (genital or venereal warts) –
Adults: 1 million units/lesion intralesionally three times a week for 3 weeks.
Treatment of AIDS-related Kaposi's sarcoma –
Adults: 30 million units/m² S.C. or I.M. three times a week.
Treatment of chronic hepatitis B –
Adults: 5 million units S.C. daily for up to 4 months.

ADVERSE REACTIONS

Common reactions are in italics; life-threatening reactions are in bold italics.
Blood: ***leukopenia,*** mild thrombocytopenia.
CNS: dizziness, confusion, paresthesias, lethargy, depression, difficulty in thinking or concentrating, insomnia, sedation, anxiety, *fatigue,* hypoesthesia, amnesia, agitation, weakness.
CV: hypotension, chest pain.
EENT: visual disturbances, hearing disorders, stye, pharyngitis, nasal congestion, sinusitis, rhinitis.
GI: *anorexia, nausea,* diarrhea, vomiting, abdominal pain, dyspepsia, constipation, loose stools, eructation, dry mouth, dysgeusia.
GU: transient impotence, gynecomastia.
Respiratory: dyspnea, coughing.
Skin: rash, dryness, pruritus, partial alopecia, urticaria, moniliasis, flushing, dermatitis.
Other: *flulike symptoms (fever, fatigue, headache, chills, muscle aches), arthralgia,* asthenia, rigors, leg cramps, arthrosis, bone disorders, back pain, increased sweating, stomatitis, gingivitis, decreased libido, hypertonia, migraine, thirst.

INTERACTIONS

CNS depressants: CNS effects enhanced.

NURSING CONSIDERATIONS

- *Contraindicated* in patients with hypersensitivity to the drug.
- *Use cautiously* in history of cardiovascular disease, pulmonary disease, diabetes mellitus, coagulation disorders, and severe myelosuppression.
- Information based upon current literature. Dosage, indications, and adverse reactions profile may change with additional clinical experience.
- Neurotoxicity and cardiotoxicity are more common in elderly patients, especially those with underlying CNS or cardiac impairment.
- Concurrent use with a live virus vaccine may potentiate replication of vaccine virus, increase adverse reactions, and decrease patient's antibody response.
- Use with blood dyscrasia-causing medications, bone marrow suppressant therapy, or radiation therapy may increase bone marrow suppressant effects. Dosage reduction may be required.
- S.C. administration route should be used in patients whose platelet count is below 50,000/mm³.
- Different brands of interferon may not be equivalent and may require different dosage.
- Almost all patients experience flu-

like symptoms at the beginning of therapy. These effects tend to diminish with continued therapy. Premedicate with acetaminophen to minimize flu-like symptoms.
- Patients should be well hydrated, especially during initial stages of treatment.
- Administer at bedtime to minimize daytime drowsiness.
- Severe adverse reactions may require reduction of dosage to one-half or discontinuation of therapy until reactions subside.
- Advise patient that laboratory tests will be performed before and periodically during therapy. Such tests will include a complete blood cell count with differential, platelet count, blood chemistry and electrolyte studies, liver function tests, and if the patient has a preexisting cardiac disorder or advanced stages of cancer, ECGs.
- When administering interferon for condylomata acuminata, use only 10-million-IU vial since dilution of other strengths required for intralesional use results in a hypertonic solution. Do not reconstitute 10-million-IU vial with more than 1 ml diluent. Use tuberculin or similar syringe and 25G to 30G needle. Do not inject too deeply beneath lesion or too superficially. As many as five lesions can be treated at one time. To ease discomfort, administer in evening with acetaminophen.
- Maximum response usually occurs 4 to 8 weeks after initiation of therapy. If results are not satisfactory after 12 to 16 weeks, a second course may be instituted. Patients with six to ten condylomata may receive a second course of treatment; patients with more than ten condylomata may receive additional courses.
- Interferons may decrease hemoglobin, hematocrit, leukocytes, platelets, and neutrophils; increase prothrombin and partial thromboplastin time; and increase serum levels of AST (SGOT), ALT (SGPT), LDH, alkaline phosphatase calcium, phosphorus, and fasting glucose. These effects are dose-related and reversible; recovery occurs within several days or weeks after withdrawal of interferon.
- Monitor for adverse CNS reactions, such as decreased mental status and dizziness. Periodic neuropsychiatric monitoring is recommended during therapy.
- Special precautions required for patients who develop thrombocytopenia: exercise extreme care in performing invasive procedures; inspect injection site and skin frequently for signs of bruising; limit frequency of I.M. injections; test urine, emesis fluid, stool, and secretions for occult blood.
- Instruct patient in proper oral hygiene during treatment, because the bone marrow suppressant effects of interferon may lead to microbial infection, delayed healing, and gingival bleeding. Interferon may also decrease salivary flow.
- Advise patient to check with doctor for instructions after missing a dose.
- If patient is to self-administer drug, teach how to prepare the injection and how to use disposable syringe. Give information on drug stability.
- Store drug in refrigerator.
- Emphasize need to follow doctor's instructions about taking and recording temperature, and how and when to take acetaminophen.
- Warn patient not to have any immunization without doctor's approval, and to avoid contact with persons who have taken oral polio vaccine. Because interferon may decrease antibody response and potentiate replication of vaccine viruses, the patient is at risk for infection during therapy.
- Tell patient drug may cause temporary loss of some hair. Normal hair growth should return when drug is withdrawn.

interferon alfa-n3

Alferon N

Pregnancy Risk Category: C

HOW SUPPLIED

Injection: 5 million units/ml in 1-ml vials

MECHANISM OF ACTION

Interferon alfa-n3 is a naturally occurring antiviral agent derived from human leukocytes. It attaches to membrane receptors and causes cellular changes, including increased protein synthesis.

INDICATIONS & DOSAGE

Treatment of condylomata acuminata (genital or venereal warts) –
Adults: 0.05 ml/wart by intralesional injection. Treatment usually continues twice weekly for 8 weeks. Dosage should not exceed 0.5 ml (2.5 million units)/session.

ADVERSE REACTIONS

Common reactions are in italics; life-threatening reactions are in bold italics.
CNS: dizziness, light-headedness.
GI: dyspepsia, heartburn, vomiting, nausea.
Other: *acute hypersensitivity reaction with mild to moderate flu-like syndrome (myalgia, fever, headache), arthralgia, back pain, malaise.*

INTERACTIONS

None reported.

NURSING CONSIDERATIONS

- *Contraindicated* in patients hypersensitive to interferon alfa and in patients with a history of anaphylactic reactions to murine immunoglobulin, egg protein, or neomycin.
- *Use cautiously* in patients with debilitating illnesses (uncontrolled CHF, unstable angina, severe pulmonary disease, coagulation disorders, seizure disorders, severe myelosuppression, or diabetes mellitus with ketoacidosis) because of the association of interferon with a flu-like syndrome.
- Although anaphylaxis hasn't been reported, be prepared to treat acute hypersensitivity reactions. Teach patients how to recognize symptoms of hypersensitivity (hives or urticaria, tightness of the chest, wheezing, shortness of breath). Tell patients to report such symptoms immediately.
- Flu-like symptoms may be relieved with acetaminophen.
- Explain to the patient that the warts will continue to disappear after the 8 weeks of therapy are complete and the drug has been discontinued.
- The drug should be injected into each lesion at the base of the wart using a 30G needle.
- Do not change brands of interferon during the course of therapy because dosage changes may be necessary.

sargramostim (granulocyte-macrophage colony stimulating factor, GM-CSF)

Leukine, Prokine

Pregnancy Risk Category: C

HOW SUPPLIED

Powder for injection: 250 mcg, 500 mcg

MECHANISM OF ACTION

A glycoprotein containing 127 amino acids manufactured by recombinant DNA technology in a yeast expression system. It differs from the natural human granulocyte-macrophage colony stimulating factor by substitution of leucine for arginine at position 23. The carbohydrate moiety may also be different. Sargramostim induces cellular responses by binding to specific receptors on cell surfaces of target cells.

*Liquid form contains alcohol. **May contain tartrazine.

INDICATIONS & DOSAGE
Acceleration of hematopoietic reconstitution after autologous bone marrow transplantation in patients with non-Hodgkin's lymphoma or acute lymphoblastic leukemia or during autologous bone marrow transplantation in patients with Hodgkin's disease –
Adults: 250 mcg/m² daily for 21 consecutive days given as a 2-hour I.V. infusion beginning 2 to 4 hours after bone marrow transplantation.

ADVERSE REACTIONS
Common reactions are in italics; life-threatening reactions are in bold italics.
CNS: malaise, CNS disorder.
CV: *blood dyscrasias,* hemorrhage.
GI: nausea, vomiting, diarrhea, anorexia, hemorrhage, GI disorder, stomatitis, liver damage.
GU: urinary tract disorder, abnormal kidney function.
Respiratory: dyspnea, lung disorder.
Skin: alopecia, rash.
Other: fever, mucous membrane disorder, asthenia, edema, peripheral edema, ***sepsis***.

INTERACTIONS
Lithium and corticosteroids: may potentiate myeloproliferative effects of sargramostim. Use cautiously.

NURSING CONSIDERATIONS
• *Contraindicated* in patients with excessive leukemic myeloid blasts in bone marrow or peripheral blood; with hypersensitivity to the drug or any of its components or to yeast-derived products.
• *Use cautiously* in patients with preexisting cardiac disease, hypoxia, preexisting fluid retention, pulmonary infiltrates, CHF, or impaired renal or hepatic function because these conditions may be exacerbated.
• Do not administer within 24 hours of last dose of chemotherapy or within 12 hours of last dose of radiotherapy because rapidly dividing progenitor cells may be sensitive to these cytotoxic therapies and drug would be ineffective.
• Reduce dose by half or temporarily discontinue if severe adverse reactions occur. Therapy may be resumed when reactions abate. Transient rashes and local injection site reactions may occur; no serious allergic or anaphylactic reactions have been reported.
• The effect of sargramostim may be limited in patients who have received extensive radiotherapy to hematopoietic sites for treatment of primary disease in the abdomen or chest or who have been exposed to multiple agents (alkylating, anthracycline antibiotics, antimetabolites) before autologous bone marrow transplantation.
• Stimulation of marrow precursors may result in rapid rise of WBC count; biweekly monitoring of CBC with differential, including examination for presence of blast cells, is recommended. If blast cells appear or increase to 10% or more of the WBC count or if progression of the underlying disease occurs, discontinue therapy. If the absolute neutrophil count is above 20,000 cells/mm³ or if platelet counts are above 50,000 cells/mm³, therapy should be discontinued temporarily or the dose reduced by half.
• Blood counts return to normal or baseline levels within 3 to 7 days after stopping treatment.
• Sargramostim is effective in accelerating myeloid recovery in patients receiving bone marrow purged from monoclonal antibodies.
• Sargramostim can act as a growth factor for any tumor type, particularly myeloid malignancies.
• **I.V. use:** Reconstitute with 1 ml sterile water for injection. Do not reenter or reuse the single-dose vial. Discard any unused portion. Direct stream of sterile water against side of vial and *gently swirl* contents to mini-

mize foaming. Avoid excessive or vigorous agitation or shaking. Dilute in 0.9% sodium chloride solution. If final concentration is below 10 mcg/ml, add human albumin at a final concentration of 0.1% to the saline *before* adding sargramostim to prevent adsorption to components of the delivery system. For a final concentration of 0.1% human albumin, add 1 mg human albumin/1 ml sodium chloride. Administer as soon as possible after admixture and no later than 6 hours after reconstitution or dilution because drug has no preservative.

- Refrigerate the sterile powder, reconstituted solution, and diluted solution for injection. Don't freeze or shake. Don't use after expiration date.
- Don't add other medications to infusion solution because no data exists regarding solution compatibility and stability. Discard any unused solution after 6 hours.
- Sargramostim has been used to increase WBC counts in patients with myelodysplastic syndromes and in AIDS patients on zidovudine; to decrease nadir of leukopenia secondary to myelosuppressive chemotherapy; to decrease myelosuppression in preleukemic patients; and to correct neutropenia in aplastic anemia; to decrease transplant-associated organ system damage, particularly of liver and kidneys.

78

Ophthalmic anti-infectives

bacitracin
boric acid
chloramphenicol
ciprofloxacin hydrochloride
erythromycin
gentamicin
gentamicin sulfate
idoxuridine
natamycin
norfloxacin
polymyxin B sulfate
silver nitrate 1%
sulfacetamide sodium 10%
sulfacetamide sodium 15%
sulfacetamide sodium 30%
tetracycline
tetracycline hydrochloride
tobramycin
trifluridine
vidarabine

COMBINATION PRODUCTS

BLEPHAMIDE S.O.P. STERILE OPHTHALMIC OINTMENT: sulfacetamide sodium 10% and prednisolone acetate 0.2%.
CETAPRED OINTMENT: sulfacetamide sodium 10% and prednisolone acetate 0.25%.
CHLOROMYCETIN-HYDROCORTISONE OPHTHALMIC: chloramphenicol 0.25% and hydrocortisone acetate 0.5% (as the prepared solution).
CORTISPORIN OPHTHALMIC OINTMENT: polymyxin B sulfate 10,000 units, bacitracin zinc 400 units, neomycin sulfate 0.35%, and hydrocortisone 1%.
CORTISPORIN OPHTHALMIC SUSPENSION: polymyxin B sulfate 10,000 units, neomycin sulfate 0.35%, and hydrocortisone 1%.
ISOPTO CETAPRED: sulfacetamide sodium 10% and prednisolone acetate 0.25%.
MAXITROL OINTMENT/OPHTHALMIC SUSPENSION: dexamethasone 0.1%, neomycin sulfate 0.35%, and polymyxin B sulfate 10,000 units.
METIMYD OPHTHALMIC OINTMENT/SUSPENSION: sulfacetamide sodium 10% and prednisolone acetate 0.5%.
MYCITRACIN OPHTHALMIC OINTMENT: polymyxin B sulfate 5,000 units, neomycin sulfate 3.5 mg, and bacitracin 500 units.
NEODECADRON OPHTHALMIC OINTMENT: dexamethasone phosphate 0.1% and neomycin sulfate 0.35%.
NEOSPORIN OPHTHALMIC: polymyxin B sulfate 10,000 units, neomycin sulfate 1.75 mg, and gramicidin 0.025 mg.
NEOSPORIN OPHTHALMIC OINTMENT: polymyxin B sulfate 10,000 units, neomycin sulfate 3.5 mg, and bacitracin zinc 400 units/g.
NEOTAL: polymyxin B sulfate 5,000 units, neomycin sulfate 5 mg, and bacitracin zinc 400 units.
OPHTHA P/S OPHTHALMIC SUSPENSION: prednisolone acetate 0.5%, sulfacetamide sodium 10%.
OPHTHOCORT: chloramphenicol 1.0%, polymyxin B sulfate 10,000 units, and hydrocortisone acetate 0.5%.
OPTIMYD: prednisolone phosphate 0.5% and sulfacetamide sodium 10%.
POLYSPORIN OPHTHALMIC OINTMENT: polymyxin B sulfate 10,000 units, and bacitracin zinc 500 units.
POLYTRIM OPHTHALMIC: trimethoprim sulfate 1 mg and polymixin B sulfate 10,000 units/ml.
PRED G: prednisolone acetate 0.6%, gentamicin sulfate equivalent to gentamicin base 0.3%, chlorobutanol 0.5%, petrolatum, white petrolatum, mineral oil, and lanolin alcohol.

STATROL: neomycin sulfate 3.5 mg and polymyxin B sulfate 10,000 units.
SULFAPRED: sulfacetamide sodium 10%, prednisolone acetate 0.25%, and phenylephrine hydrochloride 0.125%.
TOBRADEX: dexamethasone 0.1%, tobramycin 0.3%, chlorobutanol 0.5%, mineral oil, and white petrolatum.
VASOCIDIN OPHTHALMIC OINTMENT: sulfacetamide sodium 10%, prednisolone acetate 0.5%, and phenylephrine hydrochloride 0.125%.
VASOCIDIN OPHTHALMIC SOLUTION: sulfacetamide sodium 10%, prednisolone phosphate 0.25%.
VASOSULF: sulfacetamide sodium 15% and phenylephrine hydrochloride 0.125%.

bacitracin

Pregnancy Risk Category: C

HOW SUPPLIED

Ophthalmic ointment: 500 units/g

MECHANISM OF ACTION

Inhibits protein synthesis. Bactericidal or bacteriostatic, depending on concentration and infection.

INDICATIONS & DOSAGE

Ocular infections –
Adults and children: apply small amount of ointment into conjunctival sac several times daily or p.r.n. until favorable response is observed.

ADVERSE REACTIONS

Common reactions are in italics; life-threatening reactions are in bold italics.
Eye: slowed corneal wound healing, temporary visual haze.
Other: overgrowth of nonsusceptible organisms.

INTERACTIONS

Heavy metals (e.g., silver nitrate): inactivate bacitracin. Don't use together.

NURSING CONSIDERATIONS

- *Contraindicated* in patients with hypersensitivity to the drug.
- *Use cautiously* in patients with hereditary predisposition to antibiotic hypersensitivity.
- Warn patient to avoid sharing washcloths and towels with family members during infection.
- Always wash hands before and after applying ointment.
- Cleanse eye area of excessive exudate before application.
- Tell patient to watch for signs of sensitivity, such as itching lids, swelling, or constant burning. Patient who develops such signs should stop drug and notify doctor immediately.
- Teach patient how to apply. Advise him to wash his hands before and after administering and not to touch tip of tube or dropper to eye or surrounding tissue.
- Stress importance of compliance with recommended therapy.
- Tell patient that only a small amount of ointment is needed and warn him that it may cause blurred vision.
- Solution not commercially available but may be prepared by pharmacy. May be stored up to 3 weeks in refrigerator.
- Store in tightly closed, light-resistant container.
- Tell patient not to share eye medications with family members. If a family member develops the same symptoms, instruct him to contact the doctor.

boric acid

Blinx◇, Collyrium◇, Neo-Flo◇

Pregnancy Risk Category: C

HOW SUPPLIED
Ophthalmic ointment: 5%◊, 10%◊
Ophthalmic solution: 30 ml◊, 120 ml◊, 180 ml◊

MECHANISM OF ACTION
Unknown. However, drug has fungistatic and bacteriostatic properties.

INDICATIONS & DOSAGE
For irrigation following tonometry, gonioscopy, foreign body removal, or use of fluorescein; used to soothe and cleanse the eye –
Adults: apply 5% or 10% ointment, p.r.n.

ADVERSE REACTIONS
Common reactions are in italics; life-threatening reactions are in bold italics.
Note: Toxic if absorbed from abraded skin areas, granulating wounds, or ingestion.

INTERACTIONS
Idoxuridine, polyvinyl alcohol (Liquifilm): may form insoluble complex. Check with pharmacy on contents in other eye drugs and contact lens wetting solutions.

NURSING CONSIDERATIONS
- *Contraindicated* in eye lacerations.
- Don't apply to abraded cornea.
- Always wash hands before and after instilling solution or ointment.
- Not for use with soft contact lenses.
- Tell patient not to share eye solution with family members.
- Avoid contaminating solution container.

chloramphenicol
AK-Chlor, Chloromycetin Ophthalmic, Chloroptic, Chloroptic S.O.P., Chlorsig‡, Fenicol†, Isopto Fenicol†, Ophthoclor Ophthalmic, Pentamycetin†
Pregnancy Risk Category: C

HOW SUPPLIED
Ophthalmic ointment: 1%
Ophthalmic solution: 0.5%

MECHANISM OF ACTION
Inhibits protein synthesis. Bacteriostatic or bacteriocidal, depending upon concentration.

INDICATIONS & DOSAGE
Surface bacterial infection involving conjunctiva or cornea –
Adults and children: instill 1 drop of solution in eye q 1 to 4 hours around the clock until condition improves, or instill q.i.d., depending on severity of infection. Apply small amount of ointment to lower conjunctival sac at bedtime as supplement to drops. May use ointment alone by applying a small amount of ointment to lower conjunctival sac q 3 to 6 hours or more frequently, if necessary. Continue until condition improves.

ADVERSE REACTIONS
Common reactions are in italics; life-threatening reactions are in bold italics.
Note: Systemic adverse reactions have not been reported with short-term topical use.
Blood: ***bone marrow hypoplasia with prolonged use, aplastic anemia.***
Eye: optic atrophy in children, stinging or burning of eye after instillation, blurred vision (with ointment).
Other: overgrowth of nonsusceptible organisms; hypersensitivity, including itching and burning eye, dermatitis, angioedema.

INTERACTIONS
None significant.

NURSING CONSIDERATIONS
- *Contraindicated* in minor infections. Do not use chloramphenicol when less potentially dangerous drugs are available.
- Not for long-term use. Notify doctor if no improvement in 3 days.

†Available in Canada only. ‡Available in Australia only. ◊Available OTC.

• If patient has more than a superficial infection, systemic therapy should also be used.
• One of the safest topical ocular antibiotics, especially for endophthalmitis.
• Warn patient to avoid sharing washcloths and towels with family members during infection.
• Cleanse eye area of excessive exudate before application.
• Tell patient to watch for signs of sensitivity, such as itching lids, swelling, or constant burning. Patient who develops such signs should stop drug and notify doctor immediately.
• Teach patient how to instill. Advise him to wash hands before and after administering ointment or solution, and warn him not to touch tip of applicator to eye or surrounding tissue. Tell him to apply light finger-pressure on lacrimal sac for 1 minute after drops are instilled. Stress importance of compliance with recommended therapy.
• If chloramphenicol drops are to be given q 1 hour, then tapered, follow order closely to ensure adequate anterior chamber levels.
• Store in tightly closed, light-resistant container.
• Tell patient not to share eye medications with family members. If a family member develops the same symptoms, instruct him to contact the doctor.

ciprofloxacin hydrochloride
Ciloxan

Pregnancy Risk Category: C

HOW SUPPLIED
Ophthalmic solution: 0.3% in 2.5- and 5-ml containers

MECHANISM OF ACTION
Inhibits bacterial DNA gyrase, an enzyme necessary for bacterial replication. Bacteriostatic or bactericidal, depending on concentration.

INDICATIONS & DOSAGE
Corneal ulcers caused by Pseudomonas aeruginosa, Staphylococcus aureus, S. epidermidis, Streptococcus pneumoniae, *and possibly* Serratia marcescens *and* Streptococcus viridans –
Adults and children over 12 years: 2 drops in the affected eye q 15 minutes for the first 6 hours, then 2 drops q 30 minutes for the remainder of the first day. On day 2, administer 2 drops hourly. On days 3 to 14, administer 2 drops q 4 hours.
Bacterial conjunctivitis caused by Staphylococcus aureus *and* S. epidermidis *and possibly* Streptococcus pneumoniae –
Adults and children over 12 years: 1 or 2 drops into the conjunctival sac of the affected eye q 2 hours while awake, for the first 2 days. Then 1 or 2 drops q 4 hours while awake, for the next 5 days.

ADVERSE REACTIONS
Common reactions are in italics; life-threatening reactions are in bold italics.
EENT: *local burning or discomfort, white crystalline precipitate* (in the superficial portion of the corneal defect in patients with corneal ulcers), *margin crusting, crystals or scales, foreign body sensation, itching, conjunctival hyperemia.*
Other: bad taste in mouth.

INTERACTIONS
None reported.

NURSING CONSIDERATIONS
• *Contraindicated* in patients with a history of hypersensitivity to ciprofloxacin or other quinolone antibiotics. This drug shouldn't be injected into the eye.
• Serious hypersensitivity reactions, including anaphylaxis, have occurred in patients receiving systemic quinolone therapy. Discontinue drug at the

*Liquid form contains alcohol. **May contain tartrazine.

first sign of hypersensitivity, such as skin rash.
- Prolonged use may result in overgrowth of nonsusceptible organisms, including fungi. Institute appropriate therapy if superinfection occurs.
- If corneal epithelium is still compromised after 14 days of treatment, continue therapy.
- Teach patient how to instill drug correctly. Remind him not to touch the tip of the bottle with his hands and to avoid contact of the tip with the eye or surrounding tissue.
- Remind patient not to share washcloths or towels with other family members to avoid spreading infection. Also tell him not to share the drug with others.
- Advise patient to wash hands before and after instilling solution.
- Safety and efficacy in children under 12 years haven't been established. Because systemic ciprofloxacin has been shown to cause arthropathy in young animals, drug shouldn't be used in children.
- It's unknown if drug is excreted in breast milk after application to the eye; however, systemically administered ciprofloxacin has been detected in human milk. Use caution.

erythromycin

Ilotycin Ophthalmic

Pregnancy Risk Category: C

HOW SUPPLIED
Ophthalmic ointment: 5 mg/g

MECHANISM OF ACTION
Inhibits protein synthesis. Bacteriostatic, but may be bactericidal in high concentrations or against highly susceptible organisms.

INDICATIONS & DOSAGE
Acute and chronic conjunctivitis, trachoma, other eye infections –
Adults and children: apply 0.5% ointment 1 or more times daily, depending upon severity of infection.
Prophylaxis of ophthalmia neonatorum –
Neonates: a ribbon of ointment approximately 0.5 to 1 cm long placed in the lower conjunctival sac of each eye shortly after birth.

ADVERSE REACTIONS
Common reactions are in italics; life-threatening reactions are in bold italics.
Eye: slowed corneal wound healing, blurred vision.
Other: overgrowth of nonsusceptible organisms with long-term use; hypersensitivity, including itching and burning eyes, urticaria, dermatitis, ***angioedema.***

INTERACTIONS
None significant.

NURSING CONSIDERATIONS
- *Contraindicated* in patients with hypersensitivity to the drug.
- Has a limited antibacterial spectrum. Use only when sensitivity studies show it is effective against infecting organisms. Don't use in infections of unknown etiology.
- For prophylaxis of ophthalmia neonatorum, apply ointment no later than 1 hour after birth. Gently massage the eyelids for one minute to spread the ointment.
- Warn patient to avoid sharing washcloths and towels with family members during infection.
- Cleanse eye area of excessive exudate before application.
- Tell patient to watch for signs of sensitivity, such as itching lids, swelling, or constant burning. Patient who develops such signs should stop drug and notify doctor immediately.
- Teach patient how to apply. Advise him to wash hands before and after administering ointment and warn patient not to touch tip of applicator to eye or surrounding tissue. Tell him to

apply light finger-pressure on lacrimal sac for 1 minute after administering. Stress importance of compliance with recommended therapy.

- Warn patient that ointment may cause blurred vision.
- Store at room temperature in tightly closed, light-resistant container.
- Tell patient not to share eye medications with family members. If a family member develops the same symptoms, instruct him to contact the doctor.

gentamicin
Gentacidin

gentamicin sulfate
Garamycin Ophthalmic, Genoptic

Pregnancy Risk Category: C

HOW SUPPLIED
gentamicin

Ophthalmic ointment: 0.3%

gentamicin sulfate

Ophthalmic ointment: 0.3%

Ophthalmic solution: 0.3%

MECHANISM OF ACTION
Inhibits protein synthesis.

INDICATIONS & DOSAGE
External ocular infections (conjunctivitis, keratoconjunctivitis, corneal ulcers, blepharitis, blepharoconjunctivitis, meibomianitis, and dacryocystitis) caused by susceptible organisms, especially Pseudomonas aeruginosa, Proteus, Klebsiella pneumoniae, Escherichia coli, *and other gram-negative organisms –*

Adults and children: instill 1 to 2 drops in eye q 4 hours. In severe infections, may use up to 2 drops q 1 hour. Apply ointment to lower conjunctival sac b.i.d. or t.i.d.

ADVERSE REACTIONS
Common reactions are in italics; life-threatening reactions are in bold italics.

Note: systemic absorption from excessive use may cause systemic toxicities.

Eye: burning, stinging or blurred vision (with ointment), transient irritation (from solution).

Other: hypersensitivity, overgrowth of nonsusceptible organisms with long-term use.

INTERACTIONS
None significant.

NURSING CONSIDERATIONS
- *Contraindicated* in aminoglycoside hypersensitivity. *Use cautiously* in impaired renal function.
- Solution is not for injection in conjunctiva or anterior chamber of the eye.
- Have culture taken before giving drug.
- If ophthalmic gentamicin is administered concomitantly with systemic gentamicin, be sure to carefully monitor serum gentamicin concentration levels.
- Stress importance of following recommended therapy. *Pseudomonas* infections can cause complete vision loss within 24 hours if infection is not controlled.
- Warn patient to avoid sharing washcloths and towels with family members during infection.
- Always wash hands before and after applying ointment or solution.
- Cleanse eye area of excessive exudate before application.
- Tell patient to watch for signs of sensitivity, such as itching lids, swelling, or constant burning. Patient who develops such signs should stop drug and notify doctor immediately.
- Teach patient how to instill. Advise him to wash hands before and after administering ointment or solution, and not to touch tip of tube or dropper to eye or surrounding tissue. Tell him to apply light finger-pressure on lacrimal sac for 1 minute after drops are

instilled. Stress importance of compliance with recommended therapy.
- Store away from heat.
- Tell patient not to share eye medications with family members. If a family member develops the same symptoms, instruct him to contact the doctor.

idoxuridine (IDU)
Herplex, Stoxil

Pregnancy Risk Category: C

HOW SUPPLIED
Ophthalmic ointment: 0.5%
Ophthalmic solution: 0.1%

MECHANISM OF ACTION
Interferes with DNA synthesis.

INDICATIONS & DOSAGE
Herpes simplex keratitis –
Adults and children: instill 1 drop of solution into conjunctival sac q 1 hour during day and q 2 hours at night, or apply ointment to conjunctival sac q 4 hours or 5 times daily, with last dose at bedtime. A response should be seen in 7 days; if not, discontinue and begin alternate therapy. Therapy should not be continued longer than 21 days.

ADVERSE REACTIONS
Common reactions are in italics; life-threatening reactions are in bold italics.
Eye: temporary visual haze; blurred vision (with ointment); irritation, pain, burning, or inflammation of eye; mild edema of eyelid or cornea; photophobia; small punctate defects in corneal epithelium, corneal ulceration; slowed corneal wound healing (with ointment).
Other: hypersensitivity.

INTERACTIONS
Boric acid: precipitate formation; increased risk of ocular toxicity.

NURSING CONSIDERATIONS
- *Contraindicated* in deep ulceration.
- Not for long-term use.
- Idoxuridine should not be mixed with other topical eye medications.
- Don't use old solution; causes ocular burning and has no antiviral activity.
- Warn patient to avoid sharing washcloths and towels with family members during infection.
- Tell patient to watch for signs of sensitivity, such as itching lids, swelling, or constant burning. Patient who develops such signs should stop drug and notify doctor immediately.
- Teach patient how to instill. Advise him to wash hands before and after administering and warn him not to touch dropper or tip to eye or surrounding tissue. Tell him to apply light finger-pressure on lacrimal sac for 1 minute after drops are instilled.
- Cleanse eye area of excessive exudate before application. Stress importance of compliance with recommended therapy.
- Refrigerate idoxuridine 0.1% solution. Store in tightly closed, light-resistant container.
- Tell patient not to share eye medications with family members. If a family member develops the same symptoms, instruct him to contact the doctor.
- If photophobia develops, patient should wear sunglasses. Avoid prolonged exposure to sunlight.

natamycin
Natacyn

Pregnancy Risk Category: C

HOW SUPPLIED
Ophthalmic suspension: 5%
Limited availability requires that orders be placed with manufacturer directly.

MECHANISM OF ACTION
Increases fungal cell-membrane permeability.

INDICATIONS & DOSAGE
Treatment of fungal keratitis –
Adults: initial dosage is 1 drop instilled in conjunctival sac q 1 to 2 hours. After 3 to 4 days, reduce dosage to 1 drop 6 to 8 times daily.
Treatment of blepharitis or fungal conjunctivitis –
Adults: instill 1 drop q 4 to 6 hours.

ADVERSE REACTIONS
Common reactions are in italics; life-threatening reactions are in bold italics.
Eye: ocular edema, hyperemia.

INTERACTIONS
None significant.

NURSING CONSIDERATIONS
- *Contraindicated* in patients with hypersensitivity to the drug.
- Only antifungal available as ophthalmic preparation.
- Treatment of choice for fungal keratitis. May also be used to treat fungal blepharitis and conjunctivitis.
- Therapy should be continued for 14 to 21 days, or until active disease subsides.
- Reduce dosage gradually at 4- to 7-day intervals to ensure that organism has been eliminated.
- If infection does not improve with 7 to 10 days of therapy, clinical and laboratory reevaluation is recommended.
- Warn patient to avoid sharing washcloths and towels with family members during infection.
- Cleanse eye area of excessive exudate before application.
- Teach patient how to instill. Advise him to wash hands before and after administering ointment or solution, to apply light finger-pressure on lacrimal sac for 1 minute after drops are instilled, and not to touch tip of dropper to eye or surrounding tissue. Stress importance of compliance with recommended therapy.
- Tell patient not to share eye medications with family members. If a family member develops the same symptoms, instruct him to contact the doctor.
- Shake well before use. May be kept in refrigerator or at room temperature.

norfloxacin
Chibroxin

Pregnancy Risk Category: C

HOW SUPPLIED
Ophthalmic solution: 0.3% in 5-ml containers

MECHANISM OF ACTION
Inhibits bacterial DNA gyrase, an enzyme necessary for bacterial replication. Bacteriostatic or bactericidal, depending on concentration.

INDICATIONS & DOSAGE
Conjunctivitis caused by susceptible strains of bacteria –
Adults and children 1 year and over: 1 or 2 drops in the affected eye q.i.d. for up to 7 days. If condition warrants, 2 drops may be applied q 2 hours during the waking hours of the first day of treatment.

ADVERSE REACTIONS
Common reactions are in italics; life-threatening reactions are in bold italics.
EENT: local burning or discomfort, itching, chemosis, photophobia, conjunctival hyperemia.
Other: bad taste in mouth.

INTERACTIONS
Oral anticoagulants: systemic norfloxacin enhances the activity of oral anticoagulants. It's unknown if ophthalmic norfloxacin will have this effect. Monitor closely.
Theophylline, caffeine, cyclosporine: systemic norfloxacin impairs metabolism of these drugs. It's unknown if ophthalmic norfloxacin will have this effect. Monitor closely.

NURSING CONSIDERATIONS

- *Contraindicated* in patients with a history of hypersensitivity to norfloxacin or other quinolone antibiotics. Drug shouldn't be injected into the eye.
- *Use cautiously* in breast-feeding women. It's unknown if drug is excreted in breast milk.
- Serious hypersensitivity reactions, including anaphylaxis, have occurred in patients receiving systemic quinolone therapy. Discontinue drug at the first sign of hypersensitivity, such as skin rash.
- Drug is indicated for treatment of conjunctivitis when caused by susceptible bacteria. Known susceptible strains include *Acinetobacter calcoaceticus, Aeromonas hydrophila, Haemophilus influenzae, Proteus mirabilis, Serratia marcescens, Staphylococcus aureus, S. epidermidis, S. warnerii,* and *Streptococcus pneumoniae.*
- Prolonged use may result in overgrowth of nonsusceptible organisms, including fungi. Institute appropriate therapy if superinfection occurs.
- Teach patient how to instill drug correctly. Remind him not to touch the tip of the bottle with his hands and to avoid contact of the tip with the eye or surrounding tissue.
- Remind patient not to share washcloths or towels with other family members to avoid spreading infection. Also tell him not to share the drug with others.
- Advise patient to wash hands before and after instilling solution.
- Although systemically administered quinolones have been shown to cause arthropathy in young animals, ophthalmic norfloxacin has not produced this adverse effect.

polymyxin B sulfate

Pregnancy Risk Category: B

HOW SUPPLIED

Ophthalmic sterile powder for solution: 500,000-unit vials to be reconstituted to 20 to 50 ml

MECHANISM OF ACTION

Inhibits protein synthesis.

INDICATIONS & DOSAGE

Used alone or in combination with other agents for treating corneal ulcers resulting from Pseudomonas *infection or other gram-negative organism infections –*

Adults and children: instill 1 to 3 drops of 0.1% to 0.25% (10,000 to 25,000 units/ml) q 1 hour. Increase interval according to patient response; or up to 10,000 units subconjunctivally daily by doctor. Do not exceed 2,000,000 units daily.

ADVERSE REACTIONS

Common reactions are in italics; life-threatening reactions are in bold italics.

Eye: eye irritation, conjunctivitis.

Other: overgrowth of nonsusceptible organisms, hypersensitivity (local burning, itching).

INTERACTIONS

None significant.

NURSING CONSIDERATIONS

- *Contraindicated* in patients with hypersensitivity to the drug.
- One of the most effective antibiotics against gram-negative organisms, especially *Pseudomonas.*
- Often used in combination with neomycin sulfate.
- In severe, life-threatening *Pseudomonas* infections, polymyxin B may be used as an ocular irrigant.
- Warn patient to avoid sharing washcloths and towels with family members during infection.
- Tell patient to watch for signs of sensitivity, such as itching lids, swelling, or constant burning. Patient who

develops such signs should stop drug and notify doctor immediately.
- Cleanse eye area of excessive exudate before application.
- Teach patient how to instill. Advise him to wash hands before and after administering solution, and warn patient not to touch tip of dropper to eye or surrounding tissue. Apply light finger-pressure on lacrimal sac for 1 minute after drops are instilled. Stress importance of compliance with recommended therapy.
- Reconstitute carefully to ensure correct drug concentration in solution.
- Tell patient not to share eye medications with family members. If a family member develops the same symptoms, instruct him to contact the doctor.

silver nitrate 1%

Pregnancy Risk Category: C

HOW SUPPLIED
Ophthalmic solution: 1%

MECHANISM OF ACTION
Causes protein denaturation, which prevents gonorrheal ophthalmia neonatorum. Bacteriostatic, germicidal, and astringent.

INDICATIONS & DOSAGE
Prevention of gonorrheal ophthalmia neonatorum –
Neonates: cleanse lids thoroughly; instill 2 drops of 1% solution into the lower conjunctival sac of each eye at the angle of the nasal bridge and eyes, no later than 1 hour after delivery.

ADVERSE REACTIONS
Common reactions are in italics; life-threatening reactions are in bold italics.
Eye: periorbital edema, temporary staining of lids and surrounding tissue, conjunctivitis (with concentrations of 1% or greater).

INTERACTIONS
Bacitracin: inactivates silver nitrate. Don't use together.

NURSING CONSIDERATIONS
- Legally required for neonates in most states.
- Don't use repeatedly.
- If 2% solution is accidentally used in eye, prompt irrigation with normal saline solution is advised to prevent eye irritation.
- Solution may stain skin and utensils. Handle carefully.
- May delay instillation slightly to allow neonate to bond with mother.
- Always wash hands before instilling solution.
- Store wax ampules away from light and heat.
- Don't irrigate eyes after instillation.

sulfacetamide sodium 10%

Bleph-10 Liquifilm Ophthalmic, Cetamide Ophthalmic, Sodium Sulamyd 10% Ophthalmic, Sulf-10 Ophthalmic

sulfacetamide sodium 15%

Isopto Cetamide Ophthalmic, Sulfacel-15 Ophthalmic

sulfacetamide sodium 30%

Sodium Sulamyd 30% Ophthalmic

Pregnancy Risk Category: C

HOW SUPPLIED
Ophthalmic ointment: 10%
Ophthalmic solution: 10%, 15%, 30%

MECHANISM OF ACTION
Prevents uptake of para-aminobenzoic acid, a metabolite of bacterial folic-acid synthesis.

INDICATIONS & DOSAGE
Inclusion conjunctivitis, corneal ulcers, trachoma, chlamydial infection –
Adults and children: instill 1 to 2

drops of 10% solution into lower conjunctival sac q 2 to 3 hours during day, less often at night; or instill 1 to 2 drops of 15% solution into lower conjunctival sac q 1 to 2 hours initially, increasing interval as condition responds; or instill 1 drop of 30% solution into lower conjunctival sac q 2 hours. Instill ½″ to 1″ of 10% ointment into conjunctival sac q.i.d. and h.s. May use ointment at night along with drops during the day.

ADVERSE REACTIONS

Common reactions are in italics; life-threatening reactions are in bold italics.

Eye: slowed corneal wound healing (ointment), *pain on instilling eyedrop,* headache or brow pain, photophobia.

Other: hypersensitivity (including itching or burning), overgrowth of nonsusceptible organisms, ***Stevens-Johnson syndrome,*** sensitivity to light.

INTERACTIONS

Gentamicin (ophthalmic): in vitro antagonism. Avoid using together.

Local anesthetics (procaine, tetracaine), para-aminobenzoic acid derivatives: decreased sulfacetamide sodium action. Wait ½ to 1 hour after instilling anesthetic or para-aminobenzoic acid derivative before instilling sulfacetamide.

Silver preparations: precipitate formation. Avoid using together.

NURSING CONSIDERATIONS

- *Contraindicated* in sulfonamide hypersensitivity. Not recommended for children under 2 months.
- Often used with systemic tetracycline in treating trachoma and inclusion conjunctivitis.
- Replaced by other antibiotics in treating major ocular infections; still used in minor ocular infections.
- Purulent exudate interferes with sulfacetamide action. Remove as much exudate as possible from lids before instilling sulfacetamide.
- Incompatible with silver preparations.
- Warn patient eyedrop burns slightly.
- Warn patient to avoid sharing washcloths and towels with family members during infection.
- Tell patient to watch for signs of sensitivity, such as itching lids, swelling, or constant burning. Patient who develops such signs should stop drug and notify doctor immediately.
- Teach patient how to instill. Advise him to wash hands before and after administering ointment or solution, not to touch tip of dropper to eye or surrounding tissues, and to apply light finger-pressure on lacrimal sac for 1 minute after drops are instilled. Stress importance of compliance with recommended therapy.
- Wait at least 5 minutes before administering other eyedrops.
- Warn patient not to touch tip of tube or dropper to eye or surrounding tissue.
- Warn patient that solution may stain clothing.
- Store in tightly closed, light-resistant container away from heat.
- Don't use discolored (dark brown) solution.
- Tell patient not to share eye medications with family members. If a family member develops the same symptoms, instruct him to contact the doctor.
- Tell patient he may minimize photophobia by wearing sunglasses. He should avoid prolonged exposure to sunlight.

tetracycline

Achryomycin Ophthalmic

tetracycline hydrochloride

Achromycin

Pregnancy Risk Category: D

HOW SUPPLIED
tetracycline
Ophthalmic suspension: 1%
tetracycline hydrochloride
Ophthalmic ointment: 1%

MECHANISM OF ACTION
Inhibits protein synthesis. Bactericidal or bacteriostatic, depending upon concentration.

INDICATIONS & DOSAGE
Superficial ocular infections and inclusion conjunctivitis –
Adults and children: instill 1 to 2 drops in eye b.i.d., q.i.d., or more often, depending on severity of infection.
Trachoma –
Adults and children: instill 2 drops in each eye b.i.d., t.i.d., or q.i.d. Continue for 1 to 2 months or longer, or use 1% ointment t.i.d. or q.i.d. for 30 days.
Prophylaxis of ophthalmia neonatorum –
Neonates: 1 to 2 drops into the lower conjunctival sac of each eye shortly after delivery.

ADVERSE REACTIONS
Common reactions are in italics; life-threatening reactions are in bold italics.
Eye: itching, blurred vision (with ointment).
Other: hypersensitivity (eye itching and dermatitis), overgrowth of nonsusceptible organisms with long-term use.

INTERACTIONS
None significant.

NURSING CONSIDERATIONS
- *Contraindicated* in patients with hypersensitivity to the drug.
- Tell patient or family that trachoma therapy should continue for 1 to 2 months or longer. Trachoma may cause blindness if left untreated or if not treated properly.
- Tell patient that gnats and flies are vectors of *Chlamydia trachomatis.* Warn patient with trachoma not to let them settle around eye area. Also explain that infection is spread by direct contact, so handwashing is essential to prevent spread. Severe trachoma may require oral therapy as well.
- For prophylaxis of ophthalmia neonatorum, apply ointment no later than 1 hour after birth.
- Warn patient to avoid sharing washcloths and towels with family members during infection.
- Tell patient to watch for signs of sensitivity, such as itching lids, swelling, or constant burning. Patient who develops such signs should stop drug and notify doctor immediately.
- Cleanse eye area of excessive exudate before application.
- Teach patient how to instill. Advise him to wash hands before and after administering ointment or solution and not to touch tip of dropper to eye or surrounding tissue. Apply light finger-pressure on lacrimal sac for 1 minute after drops are instilled. Stress importance of compliance with recommended therapy.
- Store in tightly closed, light-resistant container.
- Remind patient to shake suspension well before use.
- Tell patient not to share eye medications with family members. If a family member develops the same symptoms, instruct him to contact the doctor.
- Ophthalmic ointment may be used with suspension to provide prolonged drug contact with affected area at night.

tobramycin
Tobrex
Pregnancy Risk Category: B

HOW SUPPLIED
Ophthalmic ointment: 0.3%
Ophthalmic solution: 0.3%

*Liquid form contains alcohol. **May contain tartrazine.

MECHANISM OF ACTION
Inhibits protein synthesis.

INDICATIONS & DOSAGE
Treatment of external ocular infections caused by susceptible gram-negative bacteria –
Adults and children: In mild to moderate infections, instill 1 or 2 drops into the affected eye q 4 hours or a thin strip of ointment q 8 to 12 hours. In severe infections, instill 2 drops into the infected eye hourly until condition improves; then reduce frequency. Or, apply thin strip of ointment q 3 to 4 hours until improvement then reduce frequency.

ADVERSE REACTIONS
Common reactions are in italics; life-threatening reactions are in bold italics.
Eye: burning or stinging upon instillation, lid itching, lid swelling, blurred vision (with ointment).
Other: hypersensitivity.

INTERACTIONS
Tetracycline-containing eye preparations: incompatible with tyloxapol, an ingredient in Tobrex. Don't use together.

NURSING CONSIDERATIONS
- *Contraindicated* in patients with hypersensitivity to the drug.
- Prolonged use may result in overgrowth of nonsusceptible organisms, including fungi.
- If topical ocular tobramycin is administered concomitantly with systemic tobramycin, be sure to carefully monitor serum levels.
- Clinical symptoms of tobramycin overdose include keratitis, erythema, increased lacrimation, edema, and lid itching. Stop drug and notify doctor if any of these occur.
- Warn patient to avoid sharing washcloths and towels with family members during infection.
- Tell patient to watch for signs of sensitivity, such as itching lids, swelling, or constant burning. Patient who develops them should discontinue drug and notify doctor immediately.
- Cleanse eye area of excessive exudate before application.
- Teach patient how to instill. Advise him to wash hands before and after administering ointment or solution and to avoid touching tip of dropper to eye or surrounding tissue. Apply light finger-pressure on lacrimal sac for 1 minute after drops are instilled. Stress importance of compliance with recommended therapy.
- Often used to combat gram-negative organisms that are resistant to gentamicin.
- When two different ophthalmic solutions are used, allow at least 5 minutes before instillation.

trifluridine
Viroptic Ophthalmic Solution 1%

Pregnancy Risk Category: C

HOW SUPPLIED
Ophthalmic solution: 1%

MECHANISM OF ACTION
Interferes with DNA synthesis.

INDICATIONS & DOSAGE
Primary keratoconjunctivitis and recurrent epithelial keratitis caused by herpes simplex virus, types I and II –
Adults: 1 drop of solution q 2 hours while patient is awake, to a maximum of 9 drops daily until re-epithelialization of the corneal ulcer occurs; then 1 drop q 4 hours (minimum 5 drops daily) for an additional 7 days.

ADVERSE REACTIONS
Common reactions are in italics; life-threatening reactions are in bold italics.
Eye: *stinging upon instillation,* edema of eyelids, increased intraocular pressure.
Other: hypersensitivity.

INTERACTIONS
None significant.

NURSING CONSIDERATIONS
- *Contraindicated* in patients with hypersensitivity to the drug.
- Should be prescribed only for those patients with clinical diagnosis of herpetic keratitis.
- Consider another form of therapy if improvement doesn't occur after 7 days' treatment or complete re-epithelialization after 14 days' treatment. Trifluridine shouldn't be used more than 21 days continuously due to potential ocular toxicity.
- Watch for signs of increased intraocular pressure.
- Reassure patient that mild local irritation of the conjunctiva and cornea that occurs when solution is instilled is usually temporary.
- More effective than vidarabine or idoxuridine with fewer adverse reactions.
- Warn patient to avoid sharing washcloths and towels with family members during infection.
- Cleanse eye area of excessive exudate before application.
- Teach patient how to instill. Advise him to wash hands before and after administering solution. Warn patient not to touch tip of dropper to eye or surrounding tissue. Apply light finger-pressure on lacrimal sac for 1 minute after drops are instilled. Stress importance of complying with recommended therapy.
- Tell patient not to share eye medications with family members. A family member who develops the same disease symptoms should contact the doctor.
- Continue trifluridine for several days after steroid therapy.
- Keep refrigerated. Do not use if outdated.

vidarabine
Vira-A Ophthalmic
Pregnancy Risk Category: C

HOW SUPPLIED
Ophthalmic ointment: 3% in 3.5-g tube (equivalent to 2.8% vidarabine)

MECHANISM OF ACTION
Interferes with DNA synthesis.

INDICATIONS & DOSAGE
Acute keratoconjunctivitis, superficial keratitis, and recurrent epithelial keratitis resulting from herpes simplex types I and II –
Adults and children: instill ½″ ointment into lower conjunctival sac 5 times daily at 3-hour intervals.

ADVERSE REACTIONS
Common reactions are in italics; life-threatening reactions are in bold italics.
Eye: temporary burning, itching, mild irritation, pain, lacrimation, foreign body sensation, conjunctival injection, superficial punctate keratitis, photophobia.
Other: hypersensitivity.

INTERACTIONS
None significant.

NURSING CONSIDERATIONS
- *Contraindicated* in patients with hypersensitivity to the drug.
- *Use cautiously* and with close monitoring with steroids. Continue vidarabine for several days after steroid therapy.
- Not for long-term use. Treatment should not exceed 21 days, or 3 to 5 days after healing.
- Warn patient not to exceed recommended frequency or duration of dosage.
- Not effective against RNA virus, adenoviral ocular infections, or bacterial, fungal, or chlamydial infections.
- Warn patient to avoid sharing wash-

*Liquid form contains alcohol. **May contain tartrazine.

cloths and towels with family members during infection.

- Tell patient to watch for signs of sensitivity, such as itching lids, swelling, or constant burning. Patient who develops such signs should stop drug and notify doctor immediately.
- Cleanse eye area of excessive exudate before application.
- Teach patient how to instill. Advise him to wash hands before and after administering ointment and to avoid touching tip of tube to eye or surrounding tissue. Apply light finger-pressure on lacrimal sac for 1 minute after drops are instilled.
- Store in tightly closed, light-resistant container.
- Tell patient not to share eye medications with family members. If a family member develops the same symptoms, instruct him to contact the doctor.
- Explain to patient that the ointment may produce a temporary visual haze.
- If photophobia develops, patient should wear sunglasses and avoid prolonged exposure to sunlight.

79

Ophthalmic anti-inflammatory agents

dexamethasone
dexamethasone sodium phosphate
fluorometholone
flurbiprofen sodium
ketorolac tromethamine
medrysone
prednisolone acetate (suspension)
prednisolone sodium phosphate (solution)
suprofen

COMBINATION PRODUCTS
Corticosteroids for ophthalmic use are commonly combined with antibiotics and sulfonamides. See Chapter 78, OPHTHALMIC ANTI-INFECTIVES.

dexamethasone
Maxidex Ophthalmic Suspension

dexamethasone sodium phosphate
Decadron Phosphate Ophthalmic, Maxidex Ophthalmic

Pregnancy Risk Category: C

HOW SUPPLIED
dexamethasone
Ophthalmic suspension: 0.1%
dexamethasone sodium phosphate
Ophthalmic ointment: 0.05%
Ophthalmic solution: 0.1%

MECHANISM OF ACTION
Decreases the infiltration of leukocytes at the site of inflammation.

INDICATIONS & DOSAGE
Uveitis; iridocyclitis; inflammatory conditions of eyelids, conjunctiva, cornea, anterior segment of globe; corneal injury from chemical or thermal burns, or penetration of foreign bodies; allergic conjunctivitis – **Adults and children:** instill 1 to 2 drops of 0.1% suspension or 0.1% solution into conjunctival sac. In severe disease, drops may be used hourly, tapering to discontinuation as condition improves. In mild conditions, drops may be used up to four to six times daily or ointment applied q.i.d. As condition improves, taper dosage to b.i.d. then once daily. Treatment may extend from a few days to several weeks.

ADVERSE REACTIONS
Common reactions are in italics; life-threatening reactions are in bold italics.
Eye: increased intraocular pressure; thinning of cornea, interference with corneal wound healing, increased susceptibility to viral or fungal corneal infection, corneal ulceration; with excessive or long-term use, glaucoma exacerbations, cataracts, defects in visual acuity and visual field, optic nerve damage; mild blurred vision; burning, stinging, or redness of eyes; watery eyes.
Other: systemic effects and adrenal suppression with excessive or long-term use.

INTERACTIONS
None significant.

NURSING CONSIDERATIONS
• *Contraindicated* in acute superficial herpes simplex (dendritic keratitis), vaccinia, varicella, or other fungal or viral diseases of cornea and conjunctiva; ocular tuberculosis; or any acute, purulent, untreated infection of the eye.
• *Use cautiously* in corneal abrasions, since these may be infected (espe-

cially with herpes); and in glaucoma (any form), because of possibility of increasing intraocular pressure (glaucoma medications may need to be increased to compensate).
- Viral and fungal infections of the cornea may be exacerbated by the application of steroids.
- Warn patient to call doctor immediately and to stop drug if visual acuity changes or visual field diminishes.
- Not for long-term use.
- May use eye pad with ointment.
- Teach patient how to instill. Advise him to wash hands before and after administering and warn him not to touch dropper tip to eye or surrounding tissue. Apply light finger-pressure on lacrimal sac for 1 minute following instillation.
- Watch for corneal ulceration; may require stopping drug.
- Warn patient not to use leftover medication for a new eye inflammation; may cause serious problems.
- Tell patient not to share eye medications with family members. If a family member develops similar symptoms, he should contact the doctor.
- Shake suspension well before use.

fluorometholone

FML Liquifilm Ophthalmic, FML S.O.P.

Pregnancy Risk Category: C

HOW SUPPLIED

Ophthalmic ointment: 0.1%
Ophthalmic suspension: 0.1%, 0.25%

MECHANISM OF ACTION

Decreases the infiltration of leukocytes at the site of inflammation.

INDICATIONS & DOSAGE

Inflammatory and allergic conditions of cornea, conjunctiva, sclera, anterior uvea –
Adults and children: instill 1 to 2 drops in conjunctival sac b.i.d. to q.i.d. May use q hour during first 1 to 2 days if needed. Alternatively, apply thin strip of ointment to conjunctival sac q 4 hours, decreasing to one to three times a day as inflammation subsides.

ADVERSE REACTIONS

Common reactions are in italics; life-threatening reactions are in bold italics.
Eye: increased intraocular pressure, thinning of cornea, interference with corneal wound healing, corneal ulceration, increased susceptibility to viral or fungal corneal infections; with excessive or long-term use, glaucoma exacerbations, cataracts, decreased visual acuity, diminished visual field, optic nerve damage.
Other: systemic effects and adrenal suppression in excessive or long-term use.

INTERACTIONS

None significant.

NURSING CONSIDERATIONS

- *Contraindicated* in vaccinia, varicella, acute superficial herpes simplex (dendritic keratitis), or other fungal or viral eye diseases; ocular tuberculosis; or any acute, purulent, untreated eye infection.
- *Use cautiously* in corneal abrasions since these may be contaminated (especially with herpes).
- Not for long-term use.
- Less likely to cause increased intraocular pressure with long-term use than other ophthalmic anti-inflammatory drugs (except medrysone).
- Store in tightly covered, light-resistant container.
- Warn patient to call doctor immediately and to stop drug if visual acuity decreases or visual field diminishes.
- Shake well before using.
- Teach patient how to instill. Advise him to wash hands before and after administering ointment or solution, and warn him not to touch dropper or

tip to eye or surrounding tissue. Apply light finger-pressure on lacrimal sac for 1 minute following instillation.

- Warn patient not to use leftover medication for a new eye inflammation; may cause serious problems.
- Tell patient not to share eye medications with family members. If a family member develops similar symptoms, instruct him to contact the doctor.

flurbiprofen sodium

Ocufen

Pregnancy Risk Category: C

HOW SUPPLIED

Ophthalmic solution: 0.03%

MECHANISM OF ACTION

Blocks the synthesis of prostaglandins. Constricts the iris sphincter, inhibiting miosis by a mechanism independent of cholinergic action.

INDICATIONS & DOSAGE

Inhibition of intraoperative miosis–
Adults: instill 1 drop into the eye undergoing surgery approximately every ½ hour, beginning 2 hours before surgery. Give a total of 4 drops.

ADVERSE REACTIONS

Common reactions are in italics; life-threatening reactions are in bold italics.

Eye: transient burning and stinging on instillation, ocular irritation.

INTERACTIONS

Acetylcholine, carbachol: may be rendered ineffective.

Epinephrine or other antiglaucoma agents: reduced ability to lower intraocular pressure.

NURSING CONSIDERATIONS

- *Contraindicated* in epithelial herpes simplex keratitis.
- *Use cautiously* in patients who may be allergic to aspirin and other NSAIDs.
- *Use cautiously* in patients with bleeding tendencies and those who are receiving medications that may prolong clotting times.
- Wound healing may be delayed.

ketorolac tromethamine

Acular

Pregnancy Risk Category:

HOW SUPPLIED

Ophthalmic solution: 0.5%

MECHANISM OF ACTION

An NSAID that inhibits the action of cyclooxygenase, an enzyme responsible for the synthesis of prostaglandins. Prostaglandins are mediators of the inflammatory response and also cause miosis.

INDICATIONS & DOSAGE

Relief of ocular itching caused by seasonal allergic conjunctivitis–
Adults: instill 1 drop into the conjunctival sac of each eye q.i.d.

ADVERSE REACTIONS

Common reactions are in italics; life-threatening reactions are in bold italics.

EENT: *transient stinging and burning on instillation,* superficial keratitis, superficial ocular infections.

Other: allergic reactions.

INTERACTIONS

None reported.

NURSING CONSIDERATIONS

- *Contraindicated* in patients with hypersensitivity to any component of the formulation. Because of the risk of serious adverse effects in the infant, don't administer to breast-feeding patients.
- *Use cautiously* in patients who have experienced hypersensitivity reactions to other NSAIDs or aspirin and in patients with bleeding disorders.
- Remind patient to store drug away

from heat in a dark, tightly closed container; protect drug from freezing.
- Teach patient proper instillation technique. Remind him not to touch dropper tip to eye.
- Remind patient to discard drug when it's no longer needed.

medrysone

HMS Liquifilm Ophthalmic

Pregnancy Risk Category: C

HOW SUPPLIED

Ophthalmic suspension: 1%

MECHANISM OF ACTION

Decreases the infiltration of leukocytes at the site of inflammation.

INDICATIONS & DOSAGE

Allergic conjunctivitis, vernal conjunctivitis, episcleritis, ophthalmic epinephrine sensitivity reaction – **Adults and children:** instill 1 drop in conjunctival sac b.i.d. to q.i.d. May use q hour during first 1 to 2 days if needed.

ADVERSE REACTIONS

Common reactions are in italics; life-threatening reactions are in bold italics.

Eye: thinning of cornea, interference with corneal wound healing, increased susceptibility to viral or fungal corneal infection, corneal ulceration; with excessive or long-term use, glaucoma exacerbations, cataracts, visual acuity and visual field defects, optic nerve damage.

Other: systemic effects and adrenal suppression with excessive or long-term use.

INTERACTIONS

None significant.

NURSING CONSIDERATIONS

- *Contraindicated* in vaccinia, varicella, acute superficial herpes simplex (dendritic keratitis), viral diseases of conjunctiva and cornea, ocular tuberculosis, fungal or viral eye diseases, iritis, uveitis, or any acute, purulent, untreated eye infection.
- *Use cautiously* in corneal abrasions since these may be contaminated (especially with herpes).
- Shake well before using. Don't freeze.
- Teach patient how to instill. Advise him to wash hands before and after applying ointment or solution, and warn him not to touch dropper or tip to eye or surrounding tissue. Apply light finger-pressure on lacrimal sac for 1 minute following instillation.
- Warn patient not to use leftover medication for a new eye inflammation; may cause serious problems.
- Tell patient not to share eye medications with family members. If a family member develops similar symptoms, he should contact the doctor.

prednisolone acetate (suspension)

Econopred Ophthalmic, Econopred Plus Ophthalmic, Pred-Forte, Pred Mild Ophthalmic

prednisolone sodium phosphate (solution)

AK-Pred, Hydeltrasol Ophthalmic, Inflamase Forte, Inflamase Ophthalmic, Ocu-Pred, Predsol Eye Drops‡

Pregnancy Risk Category: C

HOW SUPPLIED

prednisolone acetate

Ophthalmic suspension: 0.12%, 0.125%, 1%

prednisolone sodium phosphate

Ophthalmic solution: 0.125%, 0.5%, 1%

MECHANISM OF ACTION

Decreases the infiltration of leukocytes at the site of inflammation.

INDICATIONS & DOSAGE
Inflammation of palpebral and bulbar conjunctiva, cornea, and anterior segment of globe –
Adults and children: instill 1 to 2 drops in eye of 0.12% to 1% suspension (acetate) or 0.125% to 1% solution (phosphate). In severe conditions, may be used hourly, tapering to discontinuation as inflammation subsides. In mild conditions, may be used up to four to six times daily.

ADVERSE REACTIONS
Common reactions are in italics; life-threatening reactions are in bold italics.
Eye: increased intraocular pressure; thinning of cornea, interference with corneal wound healing, increased susceptibility to viral or fungal corneal infection, corneal ulceration; with excessive or long-term use, glaucoma exacerbations, cataracts, visual acuity and visual field defects, optic nerve damage.
Other: systemic effects and adrenal suppression with excessive or long-term use.

INTERACTIONS
None significant.

NURSING CONSIDERATIONS
- *Contraindicated* in acute, untreated, purulent, ocular infections; acute superficial herpes simplex (dendritic keratitis); vaccinia, varicella, or other viral or fungal eye diseases; or ocular tuberculosis.
- *Use cautiously* in corneal abrasions since these may be contaminated (especially with herpes).
- Tell patient on long-term therapy to have frequent tonometric examinations.
- Shake suspension before using, and store in tightly covered container.
- Teach patient how to instill. Advise patient to wash hands before and after applying, and warn him not to touch dropper or tip to eye or surrounding area. Apply light finger-pressure on lacrimal sac for 1 minute following instillation.
- Warn patient not to use leftover medication for a new eye inflammation; may cause serious problems.
- Tell patient not to share eye medications with family members. If a family member develops similar symptoms, instruct him to contact the doctor.
- Check dosage before administering to ensure using the correct strength.

suprofen
Profenal
Pregnancy Risk Category: C

HOW SUPPLIED
Ophthalmic solution: 1%

MECHANISM OF ACTION
An NSAID that inhibits the action of cyclooxygenase, an enzyme responsible for the synthesis of prostaglandins. Prostaglandins are mediators of the inflammatory response and also cause miosis.

INDICATIONS & DOSAGE
Inhibition of intraoperative miosis –
Adults: instill two drops into the conjunctival sac q 4 hours the day before surgery. On the day of surgery, instill two drops 3 hours, 2 hours, and 1 hour before surgery.

ADVERSE REACTIONS
Common reactions are in italics; life-threatening reactions are in bold italics.
EENT: *transient stinging and burning on instillation,* discomfort, itching, redness, iritis, pain, chemosis, photophobia, irritation, punctate epithelial staining.
Other: allergy.

INTERACTIONS
Acetylcholine, carbachol: may be ineffective in patients treated with suprofen.

*Liquid form contains alcohol. **May contain tartrazine.

NURSING CONSIDERATIONS

- *Contraindicated* in patients with hypersensitivity to any component of the formulation and in patients with epithelial herpes simplex keratitis. Because of the risk of serious adverse reactions in the infant, don't administer to breast-feeding patients.
- *Use cautiously* in patients who have experienced hypersensitivity reactions to other NSAIDs or aspirin and in patients with bleeding disorders.
- Remind patient to store drug away from heat in a dark, tightly closed container; protect drug from freezing.
- Teach patient proper instillation technique. Remind him not to touch dropper tip to eye.
- Remind patient to discard drug when it's no longer needed.

80

Miotics

acetylcholine chloride
carbachol (intraocular)
carbachol (topical)
demecarium bromide
echothiophate iodide
isoflurophate
physostigmine
pilocarpine hydrochloride
pilocarpine nitrate

COMBINATION PRODUCTS

E-PILO: epinephrine bitartrate 1% and pilocarpine hydrochloride 1%, 2%, 3%, 4%, or 6%.
ISOPTO P-ES: pilocarpine hydrochloride 2% and physostigmine salicylate 0.25%.
P_1E_1, P_2E_1, P_3E_1, P_4E_1, P_6E_1: epinephrine bitartrate 1% and pilocarpine hydrochloride 1%, 2%, 3%, 4%, or 6%.

acetylcholine chloride

Miochol

Pregnancy Risk Category: C

HOW SUPPLIED

Ophthalmic injection: 1%

MECHANISM OF ACTION

A cholinergic drug that causes contraction of the sphincter muscles of the iris, resulting in miosis. Also produces ciliary spasm, deepening of the anterior chamber, and vasodilation of conjunctival vessels of the outflow tract.

INDICATIONS & DOSAGE

Anterior segment surgery –
Adults and children: doctor instills 0.5 to 2 ml of 1% injection gently in anterior chamber of eye.

ADVERSE REACTIONS

Common reactions are in italics; life-threatening reactions are in bold italics.
Note: None reported with 1% concentration.
Eye: iris atrophy possible (with higher concentrations).

INTERACTIONS

None significant.

NURSING CONSIDERATIONS

- For ophthalmic injection only.
- Reconstitute immediately before using.
- May be instilled before or after securing sutures.
- Shake vial gently until clear solution is obtained.
- Discard any unused solution.
- Complete miosis within seconds.
- Don't gas-sterilize vial. Ethylene oxide may produce formic acid.

carbachol (intraocular)

Miostat

carbachol (topical)

Carbacel, Isopto Carbachol

Pregnancy Risk Category: C

HOW SUPPLIED

Intraocular injection: 0.01%
Topical ophthalmic solution: 0.75%, 1.5%, 2.25%, 3%

MECHANISM OF ACTION

A cholinergic drug that causes contraction of the sphincter muscles of the iris, resulting in miosis. Also produces ciliary spasm, deepening of the anterior chamber, and vasodilation of conjunctival vessels of the outflow tract.

INDICATIONS & DOSAGE

Ocular surgery (to produce pupillary miosis) –

Adults: doctor gently instills 0.5 ml (intraocular form) into the anterior chamber for production of satisfactory miosis. It may be instilled before or after securing sutures.

Open-angle glaucoma –

Adults: instill 1 drop (topical form) into eye daily, b.i.d., t.i.d., or q.i.d.

ADVERSE REACTIONS

Common reactions are in italics; life-threatening reactions are in bold italics.

CNS: headache.

Eye: accommodative spasm, blurred vision, conjunctival vasodilation, eye and brow pain.

GI: abdominal cramps, diarrhea.

Other: sweating, flushing, asthma.

INTERACTIONS

Pilocarpine: additive effect.

NURSING CONSIDERATIONS

- *Contraindicated* in acute iritis and corneal abrasion.
- *Use cautiously* in acute heart failure, bronchial asthma, peptic ulcer, hyperthyroidism, GI spasm, urinary tract obstruction, and Parkinson's disease.
- Miosis occurs within 10 to 20 minutes and lasts 4 to 8 hours.
- Used in open-angle glaucoma, especially when patient is resistant or allergic to pilocarpine hydrochloride or nitrate.
- Teach patient how to instill. Advise him to wash hands before and after administering ointment or solution, and to apply light finger-pressure on lacrimal sac for 1 minute after drops are instilled. Warn him not to exceed recommended dosage.
- Tell glaucoma patient that long-term use may be necessary. Stress compliance. Tell him to remain under medical supervision for periodic tonometric readings.
- In case of toxicity, atropine should be given parenterally.
- Caution patient not to drive for 1 or 2 hours after administration until effect on vision is determined.
- Reassure patient that blurred vision usually diminishes with prolonged use.
- Patients with dark eyes (hazel or brown irides) may require stronger solutions or more frequent instillation to produce the desired reduction of intraocular pressure because the drug may be absorbed by the eye pigment.
- Tolerance to the drug effect may develop, which may be restored by switching to another miotic for a short period of time.

demecarium bromide

Humorsol

Pregnancy Risk Category: X

HOW SUPPLIED

Ophthalmic solution: 0.125%, 0.25%

MECHANISM OF ACTION

An anticholinesterase drug that inhibits the enzymatic destruction of acetylcholine by inactivating cholinesterase. This leaves acetylcholine free to act on the effector cells of the iridic sphincter and ciliary muscles, causing pupillary constriction and accommodation spasm.

INDICATIONS & DOSAGE

Angle-closure glaucoma after iridectomy, primary open-angle glaucoma –

Adults: instill 1 drop of 0.125% or 0.25% solution once or twice/day.

Treatment of convergent strabismus (uncomplicated) –

Adults: instill 1 drop of 0.125% or 0.25% solution q.d for 2 to 3 weeks then reduce to 1 drop q 2 days for 3 to 4 weeks. After reevaluation, 1 drop once or twice/week to once q 2 days as determined by patient's condition.

Reevaluate q 4 to 12 weeks, adjusting dose as needed. Discontinue after 4 months if dose required is 1 drop q 2 days.
Diagnostic use –
Adults: 1 drop q.d. for 2 weeks then 1 drop q 2 days for 2 to 3 weeks.

ADVERSE REACTIONS
Common reactions are in italics; life-threatening reactions are in bold italics.
CNS: browache, unusual fatigue or weakness, headache.
CV: slow or irregular heartbeat.
Eye: eye pain, retinal detachment, iris cysts, conjunctival thickening, lens opacities, paradoxical increase in intraocular pressure, *lacrimation,* obstruction of nasolacrimal canals, burning, redness, stinging, irritation, twitching of eyelids, *blurred vision,* visual disturbances.
GI: nausea, vomiting, diarrhea, stomach cramps or pain.
GU: loss of bladder control.

INTERACTIONS
Anticholinergics, antimyasthenics, other cholinesterase inhibitors: potential for additive toxicity.
Carbamate or organophosphate-type insecticides: increased risk of systemic effects through respiratory tract or skin. Protective measures advised.
Cocaine: increased risk of cocaine toxicity; anticholinesterase effects may last weeks or months.
Edrophonium: worsening of patient's condition.
Local anesthetics, ophthalmic tetracaine: increased risk of systemic toxicity, prolonged ocular anesthetic effect.
Ophthalmic adrenocorticoids: increased intraocular pressure, decreased effectiveness of antiglaucoma agent.
Ophthalmic belladonna alkaloids, cyclopentolate: may antagonize miotic effects.
Succinylcholine: enhanced neuromuscular blockade, possible cardiovascular collapse, prolonged respiratory depression or apnea; effects may occur for several weeks or months after demecarium is discontinued.

NURSING CONSIDERATIONS
- *Contraindicated* in patients with bronchial asthma, pronounced bradycardia and hypotension, Down's syndrome, epilepsy, spastic GI disturbances, angle-closure glaucoma before iridectomy, Parkinson's disease, uveitis, marked vagotonia, myocardial infarction, history of retinal detachment.
- Miosis occurs within 15 to 60 minutes and lasts 3 to 10 days.
- Toxicity is cumulative; toxic systemic symptoms may not appear for weeks or months after start of therapy.
- Phenylephrine may be administered concurrently to reduce incidence of iris cyst formation.
- Tolerance may develop after prolonged use. Restore effectiveness by changing to another miotic for a short time then resuming demecarium.
- Concurrent use with epinephrine has additive effect, resulting in better control and lower dosage of both drugs.
- Regular medical supervision required to check ocular pressure.
- Patient should carry medical alert card or identification at all times during therapy.
- Instruct patient in correct administration techniques and dosages. Warn against using more than prescribed. Instruct patient to wash hands before and after application; avoid touching applicator tip to any surface; remove excess solution around eyes with clean tissue and without touching eye.
- If dose is missed, patient should not double dose. If schedule is every other day, apply as soon as possible if remembered same day; if remembered later, do not apply until next day then

skip a day and resume regular schedule. If once a day, apply as soon as possible. If not remembered until next day, do not double dose; skip previous day's (missed) dose and resume schedule. If more than once daily, apply as soon as possible. If close to time for next dose, skip missed dose and resume regular schedule.

- Atropine sulfate I.V. or I.M. is antidote of choice for systemic cholinergic effects.

echothiophate iodide (ecothiopate iodide)

Phospholine Iodide

Pregnancy Risk Category: C

HOW SUPPLIED

Ophthalmic powder for solution: for reconstitution to make 0.03%, 0.06%, 0.125%, and 0.25% solutions

MECHANISM OF ACTION

An anticholinesterase drug that inhibits the enzymatic destruction of acetylcholine by inactivating cholinesterase. This leaves acetylcholine free to act on the effector cells of the iridic sphincter and ciliary muscles, causing pupillary constriction and accommodation spasm.

INDICATIONS & DOSAGE

Primary open-angle glaucoma, conditions obstructing aqueous outflow – **Adults and children:** instill 1 drop of 0.03% to 0.125% solution into conjunctival sac daily. Maximum 1 drop b.i.d. Use lowest possible dosage to continuously control intraocular pressure.

Diagnosis of convergent strabismus – **Adults:** instill 1 drop of 0.125% solution daily h.s. for 2 to 3 weeks.

Convergent strabismus (treatment) – **Adults:** instill 1 drop of 0.03% to 0.125% solution daily or every other day h.s.

ADVERSE REACTIONS

Common reactions are in italics; life-threatening reactions are in bold italics.

CNS: fatigue, muscle weakness, paresthesias, headache.

CV: bradycardia, hypotension.

Eye: ciliary or accommodative spasm, ciliary or conjunctival injection, nonreversible cataract formation (time- and dose-related), reversible iris cysts, pupillary block, blurred or dimmed vision, eye or brow pain, lid twitching, hyperemia, photophobia, lens opacities, lacrimation, retinal detachment.

GI: diarrhea, nausea, vomiting, abdominal pain, intestinal cramps, salivation.

GU: frequent urination.

Other: flushing, sweating, bronchial constriction.

INTERACTIONS

Anticholinergics, ophthalmic belladonna alkaloids (such as atropine), cyclopentolate: antagonized miotic effects.

Cocaine: increased risk of cocaine toxicity.

Local anesthetics, ophthalmic tetracaine: increased rate of systemic toxicity; prolonged ocular anesthesia.

Ophthalmic adrenocorticoids: increased intraocular pressure and decreased antiglaucoma effect.

Other cholinesterase inhibitors, edrophonium, organophosphorus insecticides (parathion, malathion): may have an additive effect that could cause systemic effects. Warn patient exposed to insecticides of this danger.

Succinylcholine: respiratory and cardiovascular collapse. Don't use together.

Systemic anticholinesterase for myasthenia gravis, pilocarpine: effects may be additive. Monitor patient for signs of toxicity.

NURSING CONSIDERATIONS

- *Contraindicated* in narrow-angle glaucoma, epilepsy, vasomotor instability, parkinsonism, iodide hypersensitivity, active uveal inflammation, bronchial asthma spastic GI conditions, urinary tract obstruction, peptic ulcer, severe bradycardia or hypotension, vascular hypertension, myocardial infarction, history of retinal detachment.
- *Use cautiously* in patients routinely exposed to organophosphorus insecticides. May cause nausea, vomiting, and diarrhea, progressing to muscle weakness and respiratory difficulty. *Use cautiously* in patients with myasthenia gravis receiving anticholinesterase therapy.
- Miosis begins within 10 to 30 minutes and can last for 3 to 4 weeks.
- Toxicity is cumulative. Toxic systemic symptoms don't appear for weeks or months after initiating therapy.
- Reconstitute powder carefully to avoid contamination. Use only diluent provided. Discard refrigerated, reconstituted solution after 6 months; discard solution at room temperature after 1 month.
- Warn patient that transient brow pain or dimmed or blurred vision is common at first but usually disappears within 5 to 10 days.
- Instill at bedtime since drug causes transient blurred vision.
- Tell patient to remain under constant medical supervision. Warn him not to exceed recommended dosage.
- Report salivation, diarrhea, profuse sweating, urinary incontinence, or muscle weakness.
- Stop drug at least 2 weeks preoperatively if succinylcholine is to be used in surgery.
- Atropine sulfate (S.C., I.M., or I.V.) is antidote of choice.
- A potent, long-acting, irreversible drug. Tell patient to carry medical alert card or identification during therapy.
- Teach patient how to instill. Advise him to wash hands before and after administering ointment or solution, and to apply light finger-pressure on lacrimal sac for 1 minute following instillation. Warn him not to touch tip of dropper to eye or surrounding tissue.

isoflurophate

Floropryl

Pregnancy Risk Category: X

HOW SUPPLIED

Ophthalmic ointment: 0.025%

MECHANISM OF ACTION

Inhibits the enzymatic destruction of acetylcholine by inactivating cholinesterase, leaving the acetylcholine free to act on effector cells of iridic sphincter and ciliary muscles, causing pupillary constriction and accommodation spasm.

INDICATIONS & DOSAGE

Antiglaucoma agent –
Adults: apply thin strip of ointment to conjunctiva q 8 to 72 hours.
Treatment of convergent strabismus (uncomplicated); diagnostic –
Adults: apply thin strip of ointment to conjunctiva h.s. for 2 weeks.
Treatment of convergent strabismus –
Adults: apply thin strip of ointment to each eye at h.s. for 2 weeks then once every 2 to 7 days depending on patient's condition, for 2 months. If patient cannot be maintained on q 2 days dosage, discontinue drug.

ADVERSE REACTIONS

Common reactions are in italics; life-threatening reactions are in bold italics.
CNS: headache, browache, unusual fatigue or weakness.
CV: slow or irregular heartbeat.
Eye: eye pain, retinal detachment, iris

*Liquid form contains alcohol. **May contain tartrazine.

cysts, conjunctival thickening, lens opacity, obstruction of nasolacrimal canals, paradoxical increase in intraocular pressure, *burning,* redness, stinging, irritation, twitching of eye lids, *blurred vision,* visual disturbances.
GI: nausea, vomiting, diarrhea, stomach cramps or pain.
GU: loss of bladder control.
Other: sweating, flushing.

INTERACTIONS

Anticholinergics, antimyasthenics, other cholinesterase inhibitors: potential for additive toxicity.
Carbamate or organophosphate-type insecticides: increased risk of systemic effects through respiratory tract or skin. Protective measures advised.
Cocaine: increased risk of cocaine toxicity; anticholinesterase effects may last weeks or months.
Edrophonium: worsening of patient's condition.
Local anesthetics, ophthalmic tetracaine: increased risk of systemic toxicity, prolonged ocular anesthetic effect.
Ophthalmic adrenocorticoids: increased intraocular pressure, decreased effectiveness of antiglaucoma agent.
Ophthalmic belladonna alkaloids, cyclopentolate: may antagonize miotic effects.
Ophthalmic physostigmine: may shorten duration of action.
Succinylcholine: enhanced neuromuscular blockade, possible cardiovascular collapse, prolonged respiratory depression or apnea; effects may occur for several weeks or months after isoflurophate is discontinued.

NURSING CONSIDERATIONS

- *Contraindicated* in patients with bronchial asthma, pronounced bradycardia and hypotension, Down's syndrome, epilepsy, spastic GI disturbances, angle-closure glaucoma before iridectomy, Parkinson's disease, uveitis, marked vagotonia, myocardial infarction, history of retinal detachment.
- Toxicity is cumulative; toxic systemic symptoms may not appear for weeks or months after isoflurophate therapy is discontinued.
- Phenylephrine may be used concurrently to reduce incidence of iris cyst formation.
- Tolerance may develop after prolonged use. Restore effectiveness by changing to another miotic for a short time then resuming isoflurophate.
- Concurrent use with epinephrine has additive effect, resulting in better control and lower dosage of both drugs.
- Regular medical supervision required to check ocular pressure.
- Patient should carry medical alert card or identification at all times during therapy.
- Instruct patient in correct administration techniques and dosages. Warn against using more than prescribed. Instruct patient to wash hands before and after application; avoid touching applicator tip to any surface; avoid washing applicator tip or touching it to moist surface, which will cause medication to lose efficacy; and wipe tip with clean tissue.
- If dose is missed, patient should not double dose. If schedule is every other day, apply as soon as possible if remembered same day; if remembered later, do not apply until next day then skip a day and resume regular schedule. If once a day, apply as soon as possible. If not remembered until next day, skip missed dose and resume schedule. If more than once daily, apply as soon as possible. If close to time for next dose, skip missed dose and resume regular schedule.
- Atropine sulfate I.V. or I.M. is antidote of choice for systemic cholinergic effects.

physostigmine

Eserine, Isopto-Eserine

Pregnancy Risk Category: C

HOW SUPPLIED

Ophthalmic ointment: 0.25%
Ophthalmic solution: 0.25%, 0.5%

MECHANISM OF ACTION

Contraction of iris sphincter muscles results in miosis. Contraction of ciliary muscle increases outflow of aqueous humor and decreases intraocular pressure.

INDICATIONS & DOSAGE

Treatment of open-angle glaucoma – **Adults and children:** 1 drop of 0.25% to 0.5% solution b.i.d. to t.i.d. or thin strip of ointment once daily to t.i.d.

ADVERSE REACTIONS

Common reactions are in italics; life-threatening reactions are in bold italics.
CNS: headache, weakness.
CV: slow or irregular heartbeats.
Eye: blurred vision, eye pain, burning, redness, stinging, eye irritation, twitching of eyelids, watering of eyes.
GI: nausea, vomiting, diarrhea.
GU: loss of bladder control.
Other: increased sweating, muscle weakness, shortness of breath.

INTERACTIONS

Echothiophate, isoflurophate: duration of action may be shortened.
Ophthalmic belladonna alkaloids: may antagonize miotic actions.

NURSING CONSIDERATIONS

- *Contraindicated* in patients with intolerance to physostigmine, active uveitis, or corneal injury.
- Miosis begins within 20 to 30 minutes and usually lasts 12 to 36 hours.
- Instruct patient in correct administration techniques and dosages. Warn patient against using more than prescribed. Instruct patient to wash hands immediately before and after application and avoid touching applicator tip to any surface.
- Tolerance may develop with prolonged use. Restore effectiveness by changing to another miotic for a short time then resuming physostigmine.
- Ointment form may be used at night to prolong contact with medication.

pilocarpine hydrochloride

Adsorbocarpine, Isopto Carpine, Miocarpine†, Ocusert Pilo, Pilocar, Pilocel, Pilomiotin, Pilopine HS, Pilopt‡

pilocarpine nitrate

P.V. Carpine Liquifilm

Pregnancy Risk Category: C

HOW SUPPLIED

hydrochloride
Ophthalmic solution: 0.25%, 0.5%, 1%, 2%, 3%, 4%, 5%, 6%, 8%, 10%
Ophthalmic gel: 4%
Releasing-system insert: 20 mcg/hr, 40 mcg/hr for 7 days
nitrate
Ophthalmic solution: 1%, 2%, 4%

MECHANISM OF ACTION

A cholinergic drug that causes contraction of the sphincter muscles of the iris, resulting in miosis. Also produces ciliary spasm, deepening of the anterior chamber, and vasodilation of conjunctival vessels of the outflow tract.

INDICATIONS & DOSAGE

Primary open-angle glaucoma – **Adults and children:** instill 1 to 2 drops in eye q.d. to q.i.d., as directed by doctor. Or, may apply 4% gel (Pilopine HS) once daily.

Alternatively, apply one Ocusert Pilo system (20 or 40 mcg/hour) q 7 days.

*Liquid form contains alcohol. **May contain tartrazine.

Emergency treatment of acute narrow-angle glaucoma –
Adults and children: 1 drop of 2% solution q 5 minutes for three to six doses, followed by 1 drop q 1 to 3 hours until pressure is controlled.

ADVERSE REACTIONS
Common reactions are in italics; life-threatening reactions are in bold italics.
Eye: suborbital headache, *myopia,* ciliary spasm, *blurred vision,* conjunctival irritation, lacrimation, changes in visual field, *brow pain.*
GI: nausea, vomiting, abdominal cramps, diarrhea, salivation.
Other: bronchiolar spasm, pulmonary edema, hypersensitivity.

INTERACTIONS
Carbachol, echothiophate: additive effect. Don't use together.
Ophthalmic belladonna alkaloids (such as atropine, scopolamine), cyclopentolate: decreased antiglaucoma effects of pilocarpine; mydriatic effects of these agents blocked by pilocarpine.
Phenylephrine: decreased dilation by phenylephrine. Don't use together.

NURSING CONSIDERATIONS
• *Contraindicated* in acute iritis, acute inflammatory disease of anterior segment of eye, secondary glaucoma.
• *Use cautiously* in bronchial asthma and hypertension.
• Miosis starts within 30 minutes and usually lasts 4 to 8 hours.
• Warn patient that vision will be temporarily blurred. Warn patient to avoid hazardous activities until this effect subsides.
• Transient brow pain and myopia are common at first; usually disappear in 10 to 14 days.
• Teach patient how to instill. Advise him to wash hands before and after administering gel or solution, and to apply light finger-pressure on lacrimal sac for 1 minute following instillation of drops. Warn him not to touch dropper to eye or surrounding tissue.
• Widely used drug to treat primary open-angle glaucoma.
• Used to counteract effects of mydriatics and cycloplegics after surgery or ophthalmoscopic examination.
• May be used alternately with atropine to break adhesions.
• In acute narrow-angle glaucoma before surgery, may be used alone or with mannitol, urea, glycerol, or acetazolamide.
• If the Ocusert Pilo system falls out of the eye during sleep, patient should wash hands, rinse the system in cool tap water, and reposition it in the eye. Tell patient not to use it if deformed.
• Instruct patient to apply gel at bedtime, as it will blur vision.

81

Mydriatics

atropine sulfate
cyclopentolate hydrochloride
epinephrine hydrochloride
epinephryl borate
homatropine hydrobromide
phenylephrine hydrochloride
scopolamine hydrobromide
tropicamide

COMBINATION PRODUCTS
CYCLOMYDRIL OPHTHALMIC: cyclopentolate hydrochloride 0.2% and phenylephrine hydrochloride 1%.
MUROCOLL-2: scopolamine hydrobromide 0.3% and phenylephrine hydrochloride 10%.

atropine sulfate

Atropisol, Atropt‡, BufOpto Atropine, Isopto Atropine

Pregnancy Risk Category: C

HOW SUPPLIED
Ophthalmic ointment: 0.5%, 1%
Ophthalmic solution: 0.5%, 1%, 2%, 3%

MECHANISM OF ACTION
Anticholinergic action leaves the pupil under unopposed adrenergic influence, causing it to dilate.

INDICATIONS & DOSAGE
Treatment of acute iritis; treatment of uveitis –
Adults and children: instill 1 drop of 1% solution or small amount of ointment daily to b.i.d.
Cycloplegic refraction –
Adults: instill 1 to 2 drops of 1% solution 1 hour before refracting.
Children: instill 1 to 2 drops of 0.5% to 1% solution in each eye b.i.d. for 1 to 3 days before eye examination and 1 hour before refraction, or instill small amount of ointment into the conjunctival sac daily to t.i.d. or b.i.d. 2 to 3 days before examination.

ADVERSE REACTIONS
Common reactions are in italics; life-threatening reactions are in bold italics.
Eye: ocular congestion in long-term use, conjunctivitis, contact dermatitis, edema, *blurred vision,* eye dryness, *photophobia.*
Systemic: flushing, dry skin and mouth, fever, tachycardia, abdominal distention in infants, ataxia, irritability, confusion, somnolence.

INTERACTIONS
None significant.

NURSING CONSIDERATIONS
- *Contraindicated* in angle-closure glaucoma (narrow-angle).
- *Use cautiously* in infants, children, and elderly or debilitated patients. Children with blond hair and blue eyes, patients with Down's syndrome, or patients with brain damage may be more susceptible to atropine or experience higher incidence of adverse reactions.
- Warn patient vision will be temporarily blurred. Dark glasses ease discomfort of photophobia.
- Not for internal use. Treat drops and ointment as poison. Signs of poisoning are disorientation and confusion. Physostigmine salicylate I.V. or I.M. may be used as an antidote.
- Watch for signs of glaucoma: increased intraocular pressure, ocular pain, headache, progressive blurring of vision.
- Most potent mydriatic and cycloplegic available; long duration.
- Systemic adverse reactions most

commonly occur in children and elderly patients.

- Warn patient to avoid hazardous activities such as operating machinery or driving a car until the temporary visual impairment caused by this drug wears off.
- Teach patient how to instill. Advise him to wash hands before and after administering solution, and to apply light finger-pressure on lacrimal sac for 1 minute following instillation. Warn patient not to touch dropper or tip of tube to eye or surrounding tissue.
- Advise patient to use sugarless hard candy or gum for dry mouth.

cyclopentolate hydrochloride

AK-Pentolate, Cyclogyl

Pregnancy Risk Category: C

HOW SUPPLIED

Ophthalmic solution: 0.5%, 1%, 2%

MECHANISM OF ACTION

Anticholinergic action leaves the pupil under unopposed adrenergic influence, causing it to dilate.

INDICATIONS & DOSAGE

Diagnostic procedures requiring mydriasis and cycloplegia –

Adults: instill 1 drop of 1% solution in eye, followed by 1 more drop in 5 minutes. Use 2% solution in heavily pigmented irises.

Children: instill 1 drop of 0.5%, 1%, or 2% solution in each eye, followed in 5 minutes with 1 drop 0.5% or 1% solution, if necessary.

ADVERSE REACTIONS

Common reactions are in italics; life-threatening reactions are in bold italics.

Eye: burning sensation on instillation, blurred vision, eye dryness, *photophobia,* ocular congestion, contact dermatitis, conjunctivitis.

Systemic: flushing, tachycardia, urine retention, dry skin, fever, ataxia, irritability, confusion, somnolence, hallucinations, ***seizures,*** behavioral disturbances in children.

INTERACTIONS

Carbachol, pilocarpine: may counteract mydriatic effect.

Long-acting cholinergic antiglaucoma agents: Miotic actions may be inhibited.

NURSING CONSIDERATIONS

- *Contraindicated* in narrow-angle glaucoma. *Use cautiously* in elderly patients and in children with spastic paralysis.
- Potent drug with mydriatic and cycloplegic effect; superior to homatropine hydrobromide and has shorter duration of action. Physostigmine is antidote of choice.
- Instruct patient to wear dark glasses to ease discomfort of photophobia.
- Warn patient drug will burn when instilled.
- Warn patient to avoid hazardous activities such as operating machinery or driving until the temporary visual impairment caused by this drug subsides.
- Teach patient how to instill. Advise him to wash hands before and after administering, and to apply light finger-pressure on lacrimal sac for 1 minute following instillation. Warn patient not to touch tip of dropper to eye or surrounding tissue.

epinephrine hydrochloride

Epifrin, Glaucon

epinephryl borate

Epinal, Eppy/N

Pregnancy Risk Category: C

HOW SUPPLIED

epinephrine hydrochloride

Ophthalmic solution: 0.1%, 0.25%, 0.5%, 1%, 2%

epinephryl borate
Ophthalmic solution: 0.5%, 1%, 2%

MECHANISM OF ACTION
An adrenergic that dilates the pupil by contracting the dilator muscle.

INDICATIONS & DOSAGE
Open-angle glaucoma –
Adults: instill 1 drop of 0.5%, 1%, or 2% hydrochloride solution (or 0.5% or 1% epinephryl borate solution) in eye b.i.d. Adjust dosage according to tonometric readings.
During surgery –
Adults: instill 1 or more drops of 0.1% hydrochloride solution up to three times.

ADVERSE REACTIONS
Common reactions are in italics; life-threatening reactions are in bold italics.
Eye: corneal or conjunctival pigmentation or corneal edema in long-term use; follicular hypertrophy; chemosis; conjunctivitis; iritis; hyperemic conjunctiva; maculopapular rash; severe stinging, burning, and tearing on instillation; browache.
Systemic: palpitations, tachycardia.

INTERACTIONS
Cyclopropane or halogenated hydrocarbons: arrhythmias, tachycardia. Use together cautiously, if at all.
Digitalis glycosides: increased risk of cardiac arrhythmias.
Local or systemic sympathomimetics: additive toxic effects.
MAO inhibitors: exaggerated adrenergic effects. Adjust dose of epinephrine carefully.
Topical miotics, beta-adrenergic blocking agents, osmotic agents, systemic carbonic anhydrase inhibitors: additive effect in lowering intraocular pressure. Use together cautiously.
Tricyclic antidepressants, antihistamines (diphenhydramine, dexchlorpheniramine): potentiated cardiac effects of epinephrine.

NURSING CONSIDERATIONS
- *Contraindicated* in shallow anterior chamber or narrow-angle glaucoma.
- *Use cautiously* in diabetes mellitus, hypertension, Parkinson's disease, hyperthyroidism, aphakia (eye without lens), cardiac disease, or cerebral arteriosclerosis; in elderly patients or pregnant women.
- May stain soft contact lenses.
- Monitor blood pressure and other systemic effects.
- Don't use darkened solution.
- Also used during surgery to control local bleeding, or injected into the anterior chamber to produce rapid mydriasis during cataract removal.
- Teach patient how to instill. Advise him to wash hands before and after administering and to apply light finger-pressure on lacrimal sac for 1 minute following instillation. Warn patient not to touch dropper to eye or surrounding tissue.
- Epinephrine salts are not interchangeable. Don't substitute one salt if another one is ordered.

homatropine hydrobromide
Homatrine, Homatropine, Isopto Homatropine

Pregnancy Risk Category: C

HOW SUPPLIED
Ophthalmic solution: 2%, 5%

MECHANISM OF ACTION
Anticholinergic action leaves the pupil under unopposed adrenergic influence, causing it to dilate.

INDICATIONS & DOSAGE
Cycloplegic refraction –
Adults and children: instill 1 to 2 drops of 2% or 1 drop of a 5% solution in eye; repeat in 5 to 10 minutes if needed, for two or three doses.
Uveitis –
Adults and children: instill 1 to 2

*Liquid form contains alcohol. **May contain tartrazine.

drops of 2% or 1 drop of 5% solution in eye up to q 3 to 4 hours.

ADVERSE REACTIONS
Common reactions are in italics; life-threatening reactions are in bold italics.
Eye: irritation, *blurred vision, photophobia.*
Systemic: flushing, dry skin and mouth, fever, tachycardia, ataxia, irritability, confusion, somnolence.

INTERACTIONS
None significant.

NURSING CONSIDERATIONS
- *Contraindicated* in angle-closure glaucoma (narrow-angle).
- *Use cautiously* in infants and elderly or debilitated patients; children with blond hair and blue eyes; patients with cardiac disease; or patients with increased intraocular pressure.
- Patients who are hypersensitive to atropine will also be hypersensitive to homatropine.
- Warn patient that vision will be temporarily blurred after instillation. Tell patient to avoid hazardous activities such as operating machinery or driving a car until blurring subsides. Patient should wear dark glasses to ease discomfort of photophobia.
- May produce symptoms of atropine poisoning, such as severe dryness of mouth, tachycardia.
- Similar to atropine but weaker, with a shorter duration of action.
- Not for internal use.
- Teach patient how to instill. Advise him to wash hands before and after administering and to apply light finger-pressure on lacrimal sac for 1 minute following instillation. Warn patient not to touch dropper tip to eye or surrounding tissue.
- Advise patient to use sugarless hard candy or gum if dry mouth is a problem.

phenylephrine hydrochloride
AK-Dilate, AK-Nefrin Ophthalmic◇, I-Phrine 2.5%, Isopto Frin◇, Mydfrin, Neo-Synephrine, Prefrin Liquifilm

Pregnancy Risk Category: C

HOW SUPPLIED
Ophthalmic solution: 0.12%◇, 2.5%, 10%

MECHANISM OF ACTION
An adrenergic that dilates the pupil by contracting the pupil's dilator muscle.

INDICATIONS & DOSAGE
Mydriasis (without cycloplegia) –
Adults and children: instill 1 drop of 2.5% or 10% solution in eye before examination.
Mydriasis and vasoconstriction –
Adults and adolescents: instill 1 drop of 2.5% or 10% solution in eye; repeat in 1 hour if needed.
Children: instill 1 drop of 2.5% solution in eye; repeat in 1 hour if needed.
To relieve eye redness –
Adults: instill 1 to 2 drops of 0.12% solution in eye daily up to q.i.d.
Chronic mydriasis –
Adults and adolescents: instill 1 drop of 2.5% or 10% solution in eye b.i.d. or t.i.d.
Children: instill 1 drop of 2.5% solution in eye b.i.d. or t.i.d.
Posterior synechia (adhesion of iris) –
Adults and children: instill 1 drop of 10% solution in eye.

Do not use 10% concentration in infants.

ADVERSE REACTIONS
Common reactions are in italics; life-threatening reactions are in bold italics.
CNS: headache, browache.
CV: *hypertension* (with 10% solution), tachycardia, palpitations, ***premature ventricular contractions.***
Eye: transient burning or stinging on

†Available in Canada only. ‡Available in Australia only. ◇Available OTC.

instillation, blurred vision, reactive hyperemia, allergic conjunctivitis, iris floaters, narrow-angle glaucoma, rebound miosis, dermatitis.
Other: pallor, trembling, sweating.

INTERACTIONS
Guanethidine: increased mydriatic and pressor effects of phenylephrine. Use together cautiously.
Levodopa (systemic): reduced mydriatic effect of phenylephrine. Use together cautiously.
MAO inhibitors and beta blockers: may cause arrhythmias due to increased pressor effect. Use together cautiously.
Topically applied atropine, cyclopentolate, homatropine, scopolamine: may increase dilation of pupil. Use together cautiously.
Tricyclic antidepressants: potentiated cardiac effects of epinephrine. Use together cautiously.

NURSING CONSIDERATIONS
• *Contraindicated* in narrow-angle glaucoma, soft contact lens use. Avoid 10% solution and *use cautiously* in marked hypertension, cardiac disorders, in children of low body weight, and elderly patients.
• Should be avoided in patients with idiopathic orthostatic hypotension. May produce high blood pressure.
• Protect from light and heat.
• Warn patient not to exceed recommended dosage. Systemic effects can result. Monitor blood pressure and pulse rate.
• Potential for systemic adverse reactions less severe with 2.5% solution. Adverse reactions and toxicity much more likely with 10% solution.
• Teach patient how to instill. Advise him to wash hands before and after administering and to apply light finger-pressure on lacrimal sac for 1 minute following instillation. Warn patient not to touch dropper tip to eye or surrounding tissue.
• May cause blurred vision. Warn patient to avoid driving or operating machinery until this effect subsides.
• May cause photophobia. Advise patient to wear dark sunglasses and to contact doctor if condition persists longer than 12 hours after discontinuation of the drug.
• Do not use brown solutions or solutions that contain a precipitate.

scopolamine hydrobromide
Isopto Hyoscine

Pregnancy Risk Category: C

HOW SUPPLIED
Ophthalmic solution: 0.25%

MECHANISM OF ACTION
Anticholinergic action leaves the pupil under unopposed adrenergic influence, causing it to dilate.

INDICATIONS & DOSAGE
Cycloplegic refraction –
Adults: instill 1 to 2 drops of 0.25% solution in eye 1 hour before refraction.
Children: instill 1 drop of 0.25% solution or ointment b.i.d. for 2 days before refraction.
Iritis, uveitis –
Adults: instill 1 to 2 drops of 0.25% solution daily b.i.d. or t.i.d.
Children: instill 1 drop once daily to t.i.d.

ADVERSE REACTIONS
Common reactions are in italics; life-threatening reactions are in bold italics.
Eye: ocular congestion with prolonged use, conjunctivitis, *blurred vision,* eye dryness, increased intraocular pressure, *photophobia,* contact dermatitis.
Systemic: flushing, fever, dry skin and mouth, tachycardia, hallucinations, ataxia, irritability, confusion, delirium, somnolence, acute psychotic reactions.

INTERACTIONS
None significant.

NURSING CONSIDERATIONS
- *Contraindicated* in angle-closure glaucoma (shallow anterior chamber or narrow-angle).
- *Use cautiously* in cardiac disease, increased intraocular pressure, and in elderly patients. *Use with extreme caution* (if at all) in infants or small children.
- Observe patient closely for systemic effects (disorientation, delirium).
- Warn patient that vision will be temporarily blurred; tell patient to avoid hazardous activities such as driving or operating machinery until this effect subsides.
- Instruct patient to wear dark glasses to ease discomfort of photophobia.
- May be used when patient is sensitive to atropine. Faster acting and has shorter duration of action and fewer adverse reactions.
- Teach patient how to instill. Advise him to wash hands before and after administering and to apply light finger-pressure on lacrimal sac for 1 minute following instillation. Warn him not to touch dropper tip to eye or surrounding tissue.

tropicamide
Mydriacyl, Tropicacyl

Pregnancy Risk Category: C

HOW SUPPLIED
Ophthalmic solution: 0.5%, 1%

MECHANISM OF ACTION
Anticholinergic action leaves the pupil under unopposed adrenergic influence, causing it to dilate.

INDICATIONS & DOSAGE
Cycloplegic refractions –
Adults: instill 1 drop of 1% solution; repeat in 5 minutes. Additional drop may be instilled in 20 to 30 minutes.
Children: instill 1 drop of 0.5% to 1% solution; may repeat in 5 minutes.
Fundus examinations –
Adults and children: instill 1 to 2 drops of 0.5% solution in each eye 15 to 20 minutes before examination.

ADVERSE REACTIONS
Common reactions are in italics; life-threatening reactions are in bold italics.
Eye: *transient stinging on instillation,* increased intraocular pressure (less than with other mydriatic agents because of shorter duration of action), *blurred vision, photophobia.*
Systemic: flushing, fever, dry skin, dry mouth and throat, ataxia, irritability, confusion, somnolence, hallucinations, behavioral disturbances in children.

INTERACTIONS
None significant.

NURSING CONSIDERATIONS
- *Contraindicated* in narrow-angle and shallow anterior chamber glaucoma.
- *Use cautiously* in elderly patients.
- Shortest-acting cycloplegic, but mydriatic effect greater than cycloplegic effect.
- Causes transient stinging; vision temporarily blurred. Warn patient to avoid driving and other hazardous activities that require good vision.
- Instruct patient to wear dark glasses if photophobia occurs.
- Teach patient how to instill. Advise him to wash hands before and after administering and to apply light finger-pressure on lacrimal sac for 1 minute following instillation. Warn him not to touch dropper to eye or surrounding tissue.

82

Ophthalmic vasoconstrictors

naphazoline hydrochloride
phenylephrine hydrochloride
(See Chapter 81, MYDRIATICS.)
tetrahydrozoline hydrochloride
zinc sulfate

COMBINATION PRODUCTS

ALBALON-A LIQUIFILM: naphazoline hydrochloride 0.05% and antazoline phosphate 0.5%.
BLEPHAMIDE LIQUIFILM SUSPENSION: phenylephrine hydrochloride 0.12%, sulfacetamide sodium 10%, and prednisolone acetate 0.2%. EDTA, 1.4% polyvinyl alcohol, polysorbate 80, sodium thiosulfate, and benzalkonium chloride.
PHENYLZIN◇: zinc sulfate 0.25% and phenylephrine hydrochloride 0.12%.
PREFRIN-A: phenylephrine hydrochloride 0.12%, pyrilamine maleate 0.1%, and antipyrine 0.1%.
VASOCIDIN OPHTHALMIC OINTMENT: phenylephrine hydrochloride 0.125%, sulfacetamide sodium 10%, and prednisolone acetate 0.5%.
VASOCIDIN OPHTHALMIC SOLUTION: phenylephrine hydrochloride 0.125%, sulfacetamide sodium 10%, and prednisolone sodium phosphate 0.25%.
VASOCON-A OPHTHALMIC SOLUTION: naphazoline hydrochloride 0.05% and antazoline phosphate 0.5%.
ZINCFRIN◇: phenylephrine hydrochloride 0.12% and zinc sulfate 0.25%.

naphazoline hydrochloride

AK-Con, Albalon Liquifilm, Allerest◇, Clear Eyes◇, Degest 2◇, Estivin II, Naphcon◇, Naphcon Forte, Optazine‡, Vasoclear◇, Vasocon Regular
Pregnancy Risk Category: C

HOW SUPPLIED

Ophthalmic solution: 0.012%◇, 0.02%, 0.03%, 0.1%

MECHANISM OF ACTION

Produces vasoconstriction by local adrenergic action on the blood vessels of the conjunctiva.

INDICATIONS & DOSAGE

Ocular congestion, irritation, itching–
Adults: instill 1 to 3 drops of 0.1% solution in eye q 3 to 4 hours or 1 to 2 drops of 0.012% to 0.03% solution up to q.i.d.

ADVERSE REACTIONS

Common reactions are in italics; life-threatening reactions are in bold italics.
Eye: transient stinging, pupillary dilation, irritation, photophobia, blurred vision, increased intraocular pressure.
Other: dizziness, headache, increased sweating, nausea, nervousness, weakness.

INTERACTIONS

Tricyclic antidepressants, MAO inhibitors: hypertensive crisis if naphazoline is systemically absorbed. Use together cautiously.

NURSING CONSIDERATIONS
- *Contraindicated* in narrow-angle glaucoma, hypersensitivity to any ingredients.
- *Use cautiously* in patients with hyperthyroidism, cardiac disease, hypertension, and diabetes mellitus, and in elderly patients.
- Not recommended for use in infants and children.
- Can produce marked sedation and coma if ingested by child.
- Photophobia may follow pupil dilation if patient is sensitive to drug. Tell him to report this to the doctor.
- Warn patient not to exceed recommended dosage. Rebound congestion and conjunctivitis may occur with frequent or prolonged use. Patient should not use nonprescription drops for more than 72 hours without the direction of a physician.
- Notify doctor if blurred vision, pain, or lid edema develops.
- Store in tightly closed container.
- Most widely used ocular decongestant.
- Teach patient how to instill. Advise him to wash hands before and after administering, and to apply light finger-pressure on lacrimal sac for 1 minute after instillation. Warn him not to touch tip of dropper to eye or surrounding tissues.

tetrahydrozoline hydrochloride

Murine Plus◇, Optigene◇, Soothe◇, Tetrasine◇, Visine◇

Pregnancy Risk Category: C

HOW SUPPLIED
Ophthalmic solution: 0.05%◇

MECHANISM OF ACTION
Produces vasoconstriction by local adrenergic action on the blood vessels of the conjunctiva.

INDICATIONS & DOSAGE
Ocular congestion, irritation, and allergic conditions –
Adults and children over 2 years: instill 1 to 2 drops of 0.05% solution in eye b.i.d. or t.i.d., or as directed by doctor.

ADVERSE REACTIONS
Common reactions are in italics; life-threatening reactions are in bold italics.
Eye: transient stinging, pupillary dilation, increased intraocular pressure, irritation, iris floaters in elderly.
Systemic: drowsiness, CNS depression, ***cardiac irregularities,*** headache, dizziness, tremors, insomnia.

INTERACTIONS
Tricyclics, guanethidine, MAO inhibitors: hypertensive crisis if tetrahydrozoline is systemically absorbed. Don't use together.

NURSING CONSIDERATIONS
- *Contraindicated* in patients receiving MAO inhibitors and in those with hypersensitivity to any ingredients or narrow-angle glaucoma.
- *Use cautiously* in patients with hyperthyroidism, heart disease, hypertension, and diabetes mellitus and in the elderly.
- Do not exceed recommended dosage. Rebound congestion may occur with frequent or prolonged use.
- Warn patient to stop drug and notify doctor if relief is not obtained within 48 hours, or if redness or irritation persists or increases.
- Teach patient how to instill. Advise him to wash hands before and after administering, and to apply light finger-pressure on lacrimal sac for 1 minute after instillation. Warn patient not to touch dropper tip to eye or surrounding tissues.
- Caution patient not to share eye medications with others.

zinc sulfate

Bufopto Zinc Sulfate◇, Eye-Sed Ophthalmic◇, Op-Thal-Zin◇

Pregnancy Risk Category: C

HOW SUPPLIED

Ophthalmic solution: 0.217%◇

MECHANISM OF ACTION

Produces astringent and weak antiseptic action on the conjunctiva.

INDICATIONS & DOSAGE

Ocular congestion, irritation –
Adults and children: instill 1 to 2 drops of 0.217% solution in eye b.i.d. or t.i.d.

ADVERSE REACTIONS

Common reactions are in italics; life-threatening reactions are in bold italics.
Eye: irritation.

INTERACTIONS

None significant.

NURSING CONSIDERATIONS

- *Use cautiously* in patients with a shallow anterior chamber or predisposition to narrow-angle glaucoma.
- Patient should contact doctor if redness or irritation increases, or if no relief is obtained within 3 days.
- A decongestant astringent.
- Store in tightly closed container.
- Teach patient how to instill. Advise him to wash hands before and after administering, and to apply light finger-pressure on lacrimal sac for 1 minute after instillation. Warn patient not to touch dropper tip to eye or surrounding tissues.

*Liquid form contains alcohol. **May contain tartrazine.

83

Topical ophthalmic anesthetics

proparacaine hydrochloride
tetracaine
tetracaine hydrochloride

COMBINATION PRODUCTS
FLUOROCAINE, I-PARASCEIN: fluorescein sodium 0.25% and proparacaine hydrochloride 0.5%.

proparacaine hydrochloride

Alcaine, Ophthaine, Ophthetic

Pregnancy Risk Category: C

HOW SUPPLIED
Ophthalmic solution: 0.5%

MECHANISM OF ACTION
Produces anesthesia by preventing initiation and transmission of impulses at the nerve-cell membrane.

INDICATIONS & DOSAGE
Anesthesia for tonometry, gonioscopy; suture removal from cornea, removal of corneal foreign bodies –
Adults and children: instill 1 to 2 drops of 0.5% solution in eye just before procedure.
Anesthesia for cataract extraction, glaucoma surgery –
Adults and children: instill 1 drop of 0.5% solution in eye q 5 to 10 minutes for five to seven doses.

ADVERSE REACTIONS
Common reactions are in italics; life-threatening reactions are in bold italics.
Eye: occasional conjunctival redness, transient pain.
Other: hypersensitivity.

INTERACTIONS
None significant.

NURSING CONSIDERATIONS
- *Use cautiously* in patients with cardiac disease and hyperthyroidism.
- *Not* for long-term use; may delay wound healing.
- Warn patient not to rub or touch eye while cornea is anesthetized, since this may cause corneal abrasion and greater discomfort when anesthesia wears off.
- Warn patient with corneal abrasion that pain is relieved only temporarily.
- Systemic reactions unlikely when used in recommended doses.
- Equal in potency to tetracaine, but less irritating.
- Topical ophthalmic anesthetic of choice in diagnostic and minor surgical procedures.
- Don't use discolored solution.
- Store in tightly closed container.
- Ophthaine brand packaged in bottle that looks similar in size and shape to Hemoccult. When taking bottle from shelf, check label carefully.
- Opened containers should be refrigerated.

tetracaine

Pontocaine Eye

tetracaine hydrochloride

Pontocaine

Pregnancy Risk Category: C

HOW SUPPLIED
tetracaine
Ophthalmic ointment: 0.5%
tetracaine hydrochloride
Ophthalmic solution: 0.5%

MECHANISM OF ACTION
Produces anesthesia by preventing initiation and transmission of impulses at the nerve-cell membrane.

INDICATIONS & DOSAGE

Anesthesia for tonometry, gonioscopy; removal of corneal foreign bodies, suture removal from cornea; other diagnostic and minor surgical procedures –

Adults and children: instill 1 to 2 drops of 0.5% solution or a small strip of ointment in eye just before procedure.

ADVERSE REACTIONS

Common reactions are in italics; life-threatening reactions are in bold italics.

Eye: transient stinging in eye 30 seconds after initial instillation, epithelial damage in excessive or long-term use.

Other: sensitization in repeated use (allergic skin rash, urticaria).

INTERACTIONS

Cholinesterase inhibitors: prolonged ocular anesthesia and increased risk of toxicity.

Sulfonamides: interference with sulfonamide antibacterial activity. Wait ½ hour after anesthesia before instilling sulfonamide.

NURSING CONSIDERATIONS

- Systemic absorption unlikely in recommended doses.
- Avoid repeated use.
- Does not dilate the pupil, paralyze accommodation, or increase intraocular pressure.
- Don't use discolored solution. Keep container tightly closed.
- Warn patient not to touch or rub the eye while the cornea is anesthetized. This may cause corneal abrasion and greater discomfort when the anesthetic wears off.

*Liquid form contains alcohol. **May contain tartrazine.

84

Miscellaneous ophthalmics

apraclonidine hydrochloride
artificial tears
betaxolol hydrochloride
botulinum toxin type A
dapiprazole hydrochloride
dipivefrin
eye irrigation solutions
fluorescein sodium
glycerin, anhydrous
isosorbide
levobunolol hydrochloride
metipranolol hydrochloride
sodium chloride, hypertonic
timolol maleate

COMBINATION PRODUCTS
FLURESS: sodium fluorescein 0.25% and benoxinate hydrochloride 0.4%.

apraclonidine hydrochloride
Iopidine

Pregnancy Risk Category: C

HOW SUPPLIED
Ophthalmic solution: 1%

MECHANISM OF ACTION
An alpha-adrenergic agonist that reduces intraocular pressure, possibly by decreasing production of aqueous humor.

INDICATIONS & DOSAGE
Prevention or control of intraocular pressure elevations after argon laser trabeculoplasty or iridotomy –
Adults: instill 1 drop in the eye 1 hour before initiation of laser surgery on the anterior segment, followed by 1 drop immediately after completion of surgery.

ADVERSE REACTIONS
Common reactions are in italics; life-threatening reactions are in bold italics.
CNS: insomnia, irritability, dream disturbances, headache.
CV: bradycardia, vasovagal attack, palpitations, hypotension, orthostatic hypotension.
EENT: upper eyelid elevation, conjunctival blanching, mydriasis, burning, discomfort, foreign body sensation, eye dryness and itching, blurred vision, allergic response, conjunctival microhemorrhage, taste disturbances, dry mouth, nasal burning or dryness, increased pharyngeal secretions.
GI: abdominal pain, discomfort, diarrhea, vomiting.
Skin: pruritus not associated with rash.
Other: sweaty palms, body heat sensation, decreased libido, extremity pain or numbness.

INTERACTIONS
Topical pilocarpine or beta-adrenergic blocking agents: additive effects in lowering intraocular pressure. Use together cautiously.

NURSING CONSIDERATIONS
- *Contraindicated* in patients with hypersensitivity to apraclonidine or clonidine.
- Patients who tend to develop exaggerated decreases in intraocular pressure after drug therapy should be monitored closely.
- Onset of action is usually less than 1 hour, and drug effects usually peak within 4 to 5 hours.
- Systemic effects of the drug (altered heart rate and blood pressure) are uncommon after usual dose, but patients with severe systemic disease, includ-

ing hypertension, should be monitored closely.
• Observe patient closely for vasovagal attack during laser surgery.

artificial tears

Adsorbotear◇, Hypotears◇, Isopto Alkaline◇, Isopto Plain◇, Isopto Tears◇, Lacril◇, Lacrisert, Liquifilm Forte◇, Liquifilm Tears◇, Lyteers◇, Methulose◇, Moisture Drops◇, Neo-Tears◇, Refresh◇, Tearisol◇, Tears Naturale◇, Tears Plus◇, Ultra Tears◇, Visculose◇

Pregnancy Risk Category: C

HOW SUPPLIED
Ophthalmic solution: 2-ml◇, 15-ml◇, 30-ml◇ bottles
Ocular insert: 5-mg (hydroxypropyl cellulose) insert

MECHANISM OF ACTION
Augments insufficient tear production.

INDICATIONS & DOSAGE
Insufficient tear production –
Adults and children: instill 1 to 2 drops of solution in eye t.i.d., q.i.d., or p.r.n.
Moderate to severe dry eye syndromes, including keratoconjunctivitis sicca –
Adults: insert 1 Lacrisert rod daily into inferior cul-de-sac. Some patients may require twice daily use.

ADVERSE REACTIONS
Common reactions are in italics; life-threatening reactions are in bold italics.
Eye: discomfort; burning, pain on instillation; blurred vision (especially with Lacrisert); crust formation on eyelids and eyelashes in products with high viscosity, such as Adsorbotear, Isopto Tears, and Tearisol.

INTERACTIONS
Borate external irrigation solutions: may form gummy deposits on the lid when used with artificial tear products containing polyvinyl alcohol (Liquifilm Forte, Liquifilm Tears). Keep patient's eyelids clean.

NURSING CONSIDERATIONS
• *Contraindicated* in patients with hypersensitivity to the ingredients. Do not use with contact lens in place unless product is designated for this use.
• Teach patient how to instill. Warn him not to touch dropper to eye or surrounding tissue. Advise him to wash hands before and after administration.
• To avoid contamination of solution, warn patient not to touch tip of container to eye, surrounding tissue, or other surface.
• Instruct patient that product should be used by one person only.
• Lacrisert rod should be inserted with special applicator that is included in the package. Familiarize patient with illustrated instructions that are also included.
• If no improvement or condition worsens, discontinue use and contact physician.

betaxolol hydrochloride

Betoptic

Pregnancy Risk Category: C

HOW SUPPLIED
Ophthalmic solution: 0.5%
Ophthalmic suspension: 0.25%

MECHANISM OF ACTION
Reduces formation and possibly increases outflow of aqueous humor. A cardioselective beta-blocker.

INDICATIONS & DOSAGE
Chronic open-angle glaucoma and ocular hypertension –
Adults: instill 1 drop of 0.5% solution or 1 to 2 drops of 0.25% suspension in eyes b.i.d.

*Liquid form contains alcohol. **May contain tartrazine.

ADVERSE REACTIONS
Common reactions are in italics; life-threatening reactions are in bold italics.
CNS: insomnia, confusion.
Eye: *stinging upon instillation,* occasional tearing, photophobia.

INTERACTIONS
Calcium channel blocking agents: AV conduction disturbances, ventricular failure, hypotension if significant systemic absorption occurs.
Cocaine: may inhibit betaxolol's effects.
Digitalis glycosides: excessive bradycardia; may require ECG monitoring if significant systemic absorption occurs.
Dipivefrin, ophthalmic epinephrine: may produce mydriasis.
Inhalational hydrocarbon anesthetics: prolonged severe hypotension if significant systemic absorption occurs.
Insulin, oral hypoglycemics: dosage adjustments or hypoglycemic medication may be necessary because of the risk of hypoglycemia or hyperglycemia if significant systemic absorption occurs.
Phenothiazines: additive hypotensive effects, increased risk of side effects if significant systemic absorption occurs.
Reserpine: excessive beta blockade.
Systemic beta blockers: additive effects.

NURSING CONSIDERATIONS
- *Contraindicated* in sinus bradycardia, greater than first-degree AV block, cardiogenic shock, or patients with overt heart failure.
- *Use cautiously* in patients with a history of heart failure; patients with restricted pulmonary function; patients with diabetes mellitus.
- Betaxolol differs from timolol and levobunolol in that it is a cardioselective beta-adrenergic blocker. Its pulmonary systemic effects are considerably milder.
- Betaxolol is intended for twice-daily dosage. Encourage your patient to comply with this regimen.
- In some patients, a few weeks' treatment may be required to stabilize pressure-lowering response. Determine intraocular pressure after 4 weeks of treatment.
- Teach patient how to instill. Advise him to wash hands before and after administering and to apply light finger-pressure on lacrimal sac for 1 minute following instillation. Warn patient not to touch dropper to eye or surrounding tissue. Be sure he shakes suspension well before administering.
- May cause photophobia. Advise patient to wear dark sunglasses.

botulinum toxin type A
Oculinum
Pregnancy Risk Category: C

HOW SUPPLIED
Powder for injection: 100 units/vial

MECHANISM OF ACTION
Produces a neuromuscular paralysis by binding to acetylcholine receptors on the motor end-plate; it may also inhibit the release of acetylcholine from presynaptic nerve endings.

INDICATIONS & DOSAGE
Treatment of strabismus –
Adults and children 12 years and over: injections should be made only by doctors familiar with the technique, which involves surgical exposure of the region as well as electromyographic guidance of the injection needle.

Dosage varies with the degree of deviation (lower doses are used for small deviations). For vertical muscles and for horizontal strabismus of < 20 prism diopters, the usual dosage is 1.25 to 2.5 units in any one muscle. For horizontal strabismus of 20 to 50 prism diopters, dosage is 2.5 to 5 units injected into any one muscle. For persistent VI nerve palsy of greater than 1 month's duration, dosage is 1.25 to 2.5 units injected into the medial rectus muscle.

Subsequent injections for recurrent or residual strabismus should not be made unless 7 to 14 days have elapsed after the initial dose, and substantial function has returned to the injected and adjacent muscles. Dosage may be increased up to twice the initial dose for patients experiencing incomplete paralysis; subsequent doses in patients with adequate response should not be increased. The maximum single dose for any one muscle is 25 units.

Treatment of blepharospasm –
Adults: initially, 1.25 to 2.5 units injected into the medial and lateral pretarsal orbicularis oculi of the upper lid and into the lateral pretarsal orbicularis oculi of the lower lid. Effects should be apparent within 3 days and peak in 1 to 2 weeks after treatment. At subsequent treatments, dosage may be doubled if inadequate paralysis is achieved; however, exceeding 5 units/site produces no apparent benefit. Each treatment lasts about 3 months and can be repeated indefinitely.

ADVERSE REACTIONS
Common reactions are in italics; life-threatening reactions are in bold italics.
EENT: double vision, blurred vision, spacial disorientation, *ptosis, vertical deviation (after treatment of strabismus), irritation (after treatment of blepharospasm), swelling of eyelid.*
Skin: diffuse skin rash, ecchymosis.

INTERACTIONS
None reported.

NURSING CONSIDERATIONS
- *Contraindicated* in patients hypersensitive to the ingredients (which include human albumin).
- Because the drug is a protein, epinephrine should be readily available in case of an anaphylactic reaction.
- The drug should be stored in the freezer at or below 23° F (−5° C).
- Reconstitute the drug with 0.9% sodium chloride without a preservative. The vacuum in the vial should be noticeable when reconstituting. Inject the diluent into the vial gently, because severe agitation can denature the protein.
- When treating strabismus, injection volume should be 0.05 to 0.15 ml/muscle; when treating blepharospasm, injection volumes are maintained at 0.05 to 0.1 ml/site. Dosage adjustments are made by altering the volume of diluent used to reconstitute the drug.
- Reconstituting with 1 ml of sodium chloride solution produces a concentration of 10 units/0.1 ml, adding 2 ml yields 5 units/0.1 ml. Adding more diluent (such as 4 ml to produce 2.5 units/0.1 ml or 8 ml to yield 1.25 units/0.1 ml) or using different injection volumes are common methods of adjusting dosage.
- Reconstituted drug should be clear, colorless, and free of particulate matter. It must be administered within 4 hours of removal from the freezer. Reconstituted drug should be kept in the refrigerator until use. Be sure to record the date and time of reconstitution.
- When treating strabismus, several drops of an ocular decongestant and a topical anesthetic should be applied before the procedure.
- Prepare the injection by drawing slightly more volume than needed into a sterile 1-ml syringe. Expel air bubbles in the barrel of the syringe, and attach an electromyographic injection needle (if treating strabismus), such as a 1.5-inch, 27G needle. Expel excess drug (into an appropriate waste container) while checking for leakage around the needle. Be sure to

use a new needle and syringe for each injection.
- Muscle paralysis becomes evident 1 or 2 days after injection and increases in intensity over the first week. The paralysis lasts for 2 to 6 weeks and eventually resolves.
- The cumulative dosage of botulinum toxin type A should not exceed 200 units/month.

dapiprazole hydrochloride
Rēv-Eyes

Pregnancy Risk Category: B

HOW SUPPLIED
Ophthalmic powder: 25 mg/vial with 5 ml diluent and dropper supplied

MECHANISM OF ACTION
Blocks alpha adrenergic receptors in smooth muscle, producing miosis through an effect on the dilator muscle of the iris. It has no significant activity on ciliary muscle contraction nor does it significantly alter intraocular pressure in normotensive eyes or in eyes with increased intraocular pressure. Eye color can effect the rate of pupillary constriction, but not the final pupil size.

INDICATIONS & DOSAGE
Iatrogenically induced mydriasis produced by adrenergic or parasympatholytic agents –
Adults: instill 2 drops, followed in 5 minutes by another 2 drops.

ADVERSE REACTIONS
CNS: headache, brow ache.
Eye: *conjunctival injection lasting 20 minutes,* burning on instillation, ptosis, lid erythema, lid edema, chemosis, itching, punctate keratitis, corneal edema, photophobia, dry eyes, tearing, blurry vision.

INTERACTIONS
None reported.

NURSING CONSIDERATIONS
- *Contraindicated* in patients with hypersensitivity to any ingredient and when pupil constriction is undesirable, as in acute iritis.
- Not indicated for reduction of intraocular pressure or to treat open-angle glaucoma.
- To avoid contamination, do not touch dropper to any surface.
- Do not use in same patient more than once per week.
- To prepare: Remove and discard aluminum seals and rubber stoppers from both drug and diluent vials. Pour diluent into drug vial and attach dropper assembly. Shake vial to ensure mixing.
- Store at room temperature for 21 days. Discard any discolored solution.

dipivefrin
Propine

Pregnancy Risk Category: B

HOW SUPPLIED
Ophthalmic solution: 0.1%

MECHANISM OF ACTION
A prodrug of epinephrine (in the eye, dipivefrin is converted to epinephrine). The liberated epinephrine appears to decrease aqueous production and increase aqueous outflow.

INDICATIONS & DOSAGE
To reduce intraocular pressure in chronic open-angle glaucoma –
Adults: for initial glaucoma therapy, 1 drop in eye q 12 hours.

ADVERSE REACTIONS
Common reactions are in italics; life-threatening reactions are in bold italics.
CV: tachycardia, hypertension.
Eye: burning, stinging.

INTERACTIONS
Digitalis glycosides, inhalational hydrocarbon anesthetics, tricyclic anti-

depressants: increased risk of cardiac side effects if significant systemic absorption occurs.
Ophthalmic beta blockers, osmotic agents, systemically administered carbonic anhydrase inhibitors: additive effects in lowering intraocular pressure. Use together cautiously. Monitor for potential adverse effects.
Systemic sympathomimetics: possible additive effects if significant systemic absorption occurs.

NURSING CONSIDERATIONS

- *Contraindicated* in narrow-angle glaucoma.
- *Use cautiously* in patients with aphakia.
- Dipivefrin is a prodrug of epinephrine: It's converted to epinephrine when it enters the eye.
- May have fewer adverse reactions than conventional epinephrine therapy.
- Often used concomitantly with other antiglaucoma drugs.
- Teach patient how to instill. Advise him to wash hands before and after administration. Warn him not to touch dropper to eye or surrounding tissue.

eye irrigation solutions

Blinx◇, Collyrium◇, Dacriose◇, Eye-Stream◇, I-Lite Eye Drops◇, Lauro Eye Wash◇, Lavoptik Eye Wash◇, Murine Eye Drops◇, Neo-Flo◇, Sterile Normal Saline (0.9%)◇

HOW SUPPLIED
Ophthalmic solution: 15 ml◇, 30 ml◇, 120 ml◇, 180 ml◇

MECHANISM OF ACTION
Cleans the eye.

INDICATIONS & DOSAGE
Eye irrigation –
Adults and children: flush eye with 1 to 2 drops of solution t.i.d., q.i.d., or p.r.n.

ADVERSE REACTIONS
None reported.

INTERACTIONS
Products containing polyvinyl alcohol: may form gel and gummy deposits on the eye. Keep eyelids clean.

NURSING CONSIDERATIONS

- *Contraindicated* in patients with hypersensitivity to the ingredients.
- To avoid contamination, don't touch tip of container to eye, surrounding tissue, or other surface.
- Store in tightly closed, light-resistant container. Check expiration date.
- Teach patient how to instill. Advise him to wash hands before and after administration.
- Should be used by one person only.
- When irrigating, have patient turn his head to side and irrigate from inner to outer canthus.

fluorescein sodium

Fluorescite, Fluor-I-Strip, Fluor-I-Strip A.T., Ful-Glo, Funduscein Injections

Pregnancy Risk Category: C

HOW SUPPLIED
Ophthalmic solution: 2%
Ophthalmic strips: 0.6 mg, 1 mg, 9 mg
Parenteral injection: 10%, 25%

MECHANISM OF ACTION
Produces an intense green fluorescence in alkaline solution (pH 5.0 or less) or a bright yellow if viewed under cobalt blue illumination.

INDICATIONS & DOSAGE
Diagnostic in corneal abrasions and foreign bodies; fitting hard contact lenses; lacrimal patency; fundus photography; applanation tonometry –
Topical solution:
Adults and children: instill 1 drop of 2% solution followed by irrigation, or

moisten strip with sterile water. Touch conjunctiva or fornix with moistened tip. Flush eye with irrigating solution. Patient should blink several times after application.
Retinal angiography –
Intravenous:
Adults: 5 ml of 10% solution (500 mg) or 3 ml of 25% solution (750 mg) injected rapidly into antecubital vein, by doctor or a specially trained nurse.
Children: 0.077 ml of 10% solution (7.7 mg/kg body weight) or 0.044 ml of 25% solution (11 mg/kg body weight) injected rapidly into antecubital vein by doctor.

ADVERSE REACTIONS
Common reactions are in italics; life-threatening reactions are in bold italics.
Topical use:
Eye: stinging, burning, yellow streaks from tears.
Intravenous use:
CNS: headache persisting for 24 to 36 hours, dizziness, syncope, seizures.
CV: hypotension, ***shock, cardiac arrest.***
GI: nausea, vomiting.
GU: bright yellow urine (persists for 24 to 36 hours).
Skin: yellow skin discoloration (fades in 6 to 12 hours).
Local: extravasation at injection site, thrombophlebitis.
Other: hypersensitivity, including urticaria and ***anaphylaxis.***

INTERACTIONS
None significant.

NURSING CONSIDERATIONS
- *Use cautiously* in patients with history of allergy or bronchial asthma.
- Never instill while patient is wearing soft contact lens. Drug will ruin it.
- Use topical anesthetic before instilling to relieve burning and irritation.
- Always use aseptic technique. Easily contaminated by *Pseudomonas.*
- Yellow skin discoloration may persist 6 to 12 hours.
- Warn patient that urine will be bright yellow after I.V. injection.
- Routine urinalysis will be abnormal within 1 hour after I.V. injection.
- A water-soluble dye.
- Don't freeze; store below 80° F (26.7° C).
- Defects appear green under normal light, or bright yellow under cobalt blue illumination. Foreign bodies are surrounded by a green ring. Similar lesions of the conjunctiva are delineated in orange-yellow.
- Always keep an emergency tray with an antihistamine, epinephrine, and oxygen available when giving parenterally.

glycerin, anhydrous
Ophthalgan

Pregnancy Risk Category: C

HOW SUPPLIED
Ophthalmic solution: 7.5-ml containers

MECHANISM OF ACTION
Removes excess fluid from the cornea.

INDICATIONS & DOSAGE
Corneal edema before ophthalmoscopy or gonioscopy in acute glaucoma and bullous keratitis –
Adults and children: instill 1 to 2 drops glycerin solution after instilling a local anesthetic.

ADVERSE REACTIONS
Common reactions are in italics; life-threatening reactions are in bold italics.
Eye: pain if instilled without topical anesthetic.

INTERACTIONS
None significant.

NURSING CONSIDERATIONS

- Use topical tetracaine or proparacaine before instilling to prevent discomfort.
- Don't touch tip of dropper to eye, surrounding tissues, or tear-film; glycerin will absorb moisture.
- Used to temporarily restore corneal transparency when cornea is too edematous to permit diagnosis.

isosorbide
Ismotic

Pregnancy Risk Category: C

HOW SUPPLIED

Oral solution: 45% (100 g/225 ml) in 220-ml containers

MECHANISM OF ACTION

Acts as an osmotic agent by promoting redistribution of water and thereby producing diuresis.

INDICATIONS & DOSAGE

Short-term reduction of intraocular pressure due to glaucoma –

Adults: initially, 1.5 g/kg P.O. Usual dosage range is 1 to 3 g/kg.

ADVERSE REACTIONS

Common reactions are in italics; life-threatening reactions are in bold italics.

CNS: vertigo, light-headedness, lethargy, headache, confusion.

GI: gastric discomfort, diarrhea, anorexia, nausea, vomiting.

Metabolic: hypernatremia, hyperosmolality, thirst.

INTERACTIONS

None significant.

NURSING CONSIDERATIONS

- *Contraindicated* in anuria due to severe renal disease, severe dehydration, in acute pulmonary edema, and in hemorrhagic glaucoma.
- Monitor patient closely for 5 to 10 minutes after administration.
- Tell patient that this medication may make him feel thirsty.
- Repetitive doses should be used cautiously, especially in patients with diseases associated with salt retention, such as congestive heart failure. Carefully monitor patient's fluid and electrolyte balance.
- Pour over cracked ice, and tell patient to sip the medication. This improves palatability.
- Especially useful for rapid reduction in intraocular pressure. May be used to interrupt acute attack of glaucoma before laser surgery.

levobunolol hydrochloride
Betagan

Pregnancy Risk Category: C

HOW SUPPLIED

Ophthalmic solution: 0.25%, 0.5%

MECHANISM OF ACTION

Reduces formation and possibly increases outflow of aqueous humor. A nonselective beta-blocker.

INDICATIONS & DOSAGE

Chronic open-angle glaucoma and ocular hypertension –

Adults: instill 1 to 2 drops in eye once daily or b.i.d.

ADVERSE REACTIONS

Common reactions are in italics; life-threatening reactions are in bold italics.

CNS: headache, dizziness, depression.

CV: slight reduction in resting heart rate.

Eye: *transient stinging and burning.* Long-term use may decrease corneal sensitivity.

GI: nausea.

Skin: urticaria.

Other: evidence of beta blockade and systemic absorption (*hypotension, bradycardia, syncope,* ***exacerbation of asthma,*** and ***CHF***).

*Liquid form contains alcohol. **May contain tartrazine.

INTERACTIONS
Propranolol, metoprolol, and other oral beta-adrenergic blockers: increased ocular and systemic effect. Use together cautiously.
Reserpine and other catecholamine-depleting drugs: enhanced hypotensive and bradycardiac effects.
Topical miotics, dipivefrin, epinephrine; systemically administered carbonic anhydrase inhibitors: additive effects in lowering intraocular pressure. Use together cautiously.

NURSING CONSIDERATIONS
- *Contraindicated* in bronchial asthma, a history of bronchial asthma or severe chronic obstructive pulmonary disease; sinus bradycardia; second-degree and third-degree AV block; cardiac failure; cardiogenic shock.
- *Use cautiously* in patients with chronic bronchitis and emphysema, diabetes mellitus, and hyperthyroidism.
- Levobunolol is faster acting than timolol. The onset of action occurs within 1 hour; maximum effect is between 2 and 6 hours.
- Teach patient how to instill. Advise him to wash hands before and after administering and to apply light finger-pressure on lacrimal sac for 1 minute after instillation. Warn patient not to touch dropper to eye or surrounding tissue.

metipranolol hydrochloride
OptiPranolol
Pregnancy Risk Category: C

HOW SUPPLIED
Ophthalmic solution: 0.3% in 5- or 10-ml dropper bottles

MECHANISM OF ACTION
A beta-adrenergic blocker. Exact mechanism of ocular antihypertensive action is unknown but appears to be a reduction of aqueous production. A slight increase in outflow facility has been demonstrated with metipranolol. Like other noncardioselective beta-adrenergic blockers, metipranolol does not have significant local anesthetic (membrane-stabilizing) actions or intrinsic sympathomimetic activity. It reduces elevated and normal intraocular pressure (IOP) with or without glaucoma with little or no effect on pupil size or accommodation. IOP above 24 mm Hg is reduced an average of 20% to 26%.

INDICATIONS & DOSAGE
Ocular conditions in which lowering of IOP would be beneficial, including ocular hypertension and chronic open-angle glaucoma –
Adults: instill 1 drop into affected eye(s) b.i.d. Larger dose or more frequent administration is not known to be of benefit. If IOP is not at a satisfactory level, concomitant therapy to lower it may be instituted.

ADVERSE REACTIONS
Common reactions are in italics; life-threatening reactions are in bold italics.
CNS: headache, anxiety, dizziness, depression, somnolence, nervousness.
CV: hypertension, ***MI,*** atrial fibrillation, angina, palpitation, bradycardia.
EENT: transient local discomfort, tearing, conjunctivitis, eyelid dermatitis, blurred vision, blepharitis, abnormal vision, photophobia, edema, rhinitis, epistaxis.
GI: nausea.
Respiratory: dyspnea, bronchitis, cough.
Skin: rash.
Other: allergic reaction, asthenia, brow ache, myalgia.

INTERACTIONS
Antithyroid agents, antihypertensives: increased risk of systemic toxicity from absorbed drug. Monitor closely.

NURSING CONSIDERATIONS

• *Contraindicated* in patients with hypersensitivity to the drug or any of its components and in patients with bronchial asthma, history of bronchial asthma or severe COPD, second- and third-degree AV block, cardiac failure, and cardiogenic shock.

• *Use cautiously* in patients with nonallergic bronchospasm, chronic bronchitis, emphysema, diabetes mellitus (especially in those subject to spontaneous hypoglycemia), hyperthyroidism, or cerebrovascular insufficiency.

• The normal eye can retain about 10 microliters of fluid, and the average dropper delivers 25 to 50 microliters/drop; therefore, the value of using more than 1 drop is questionable. If multiple drops are needed, the best interval between drops is 5 minutes.

• Concomitant pilocarpine, other miotics, or systemic carbonic anhydrase inhibitors may be administered if IOP is not adequately controlled.

• Instruct patient in correct administration technique, which is essential for optimal therapeutic response. Tell patient to wash hands thoroughly before administration. Tilt head back or lie down and gaze upward. Gently grasp lower eyelid below eyelashes and pull eyelid away from eye to form a pouch. Place dropper directly over eye, avoiding contact of dropper with eye or any surface. Look up just before applying drop; look down for several seconds after applying drop. Slowly release eyelid. Close eyes gently for 1 to 2 minutes; closing them too tightly after instillation may expel medication from "pouch." Apply gentle pressure to inside corner of eye at bridge of nose to retard draining of solution from intended area. Do not rub eye; minimize blinking. Do not rinse dropper.

• If more than one type of drop is used, wait at least 5 minutes between instillations.

• Onset of action occurs in less than 30 minutes, with a maximum effect in about 2 hours; duration of action is 12 to 24 hours.

• Check expiration date on bottle before use. Do not use if eye drops have changed color.

sodium chloride, hypertonic

Adsorbonac Ophthalmic Solution, Muro-128 Ointment, Sodium Chloride Ointment 5%

Pregnancy Risk Category: C

HOW SUPPLIED

Ophthalmic ointment: 5%
Ophthalmic solution: 2%, 5%

MECHANISM OF ACTION

Removes excess fluid from the cornea.

INDICATIONS & DOSAGE

Corneal edema (postoperative) after cataract extraction or corneal transplantation; also in trauma or bullous keratopathy –

Adults and children: instill 1 to 2 drops q 3 to 4 hours, or apply ointment at bedtime.

ADVERSE REACTIONS

Common reactions are in italics; life-threatening reactions are in bold italics.

Eye: slight stinging.
Other: hypersensitivity.

INTERACTIONS

None significant.

NURSING CONSIDERATIONS

• Discontinue immediately if patient experiences severe headache, pain, rapid change in vision, acute redness of eyes, sudden appearance of floating spots, pain on exposure to light, or double vision.

• An osmotic agent used to reduce corneal edema when repeated instillation is indicated.

• May use a few drops of sterile irri-

gation solution inside bottle cap to prevent caking on dropper bottle tip.
- Store in tightly closed container.
- Ointment may cause blurred vision.
- Teach patient how to instill. Advise him to wash hands before and after administering and to apply light finger-pressure on lacrimal sac for 1 minute after drops are instilled. Warn patient not to touch dropper to eye or surrounding tissue.

timolol maleate

Timoptic Solution

Pregnancy Risk Category: C

HOW SUPPLIED

Ophthalmic solution: 0.25%, 0.5%

MECHANISM OF ACTION

Reduces aqueous formation and possibly increases aqueous outflow. A beta-blocker.

INDICATIONS & DOSAGE

Chronic open-angle glaucoma, secondary glaucoma, aphakic glaucoma, ocular hypertension –
Adults: initially, instill 1 drop of 0.25% solution in each eye b.i.d.; reduce to 1 drop daily for maintenance. If patient doesn't respond, instill 1 drop of 0.5% solution in each eye b.i.d. If intraocular pressure is controlled, dosage may be reduced to 1 drop in each eye daily.

ADVERSE REACTIONS

Common reactions are in italics; life-threatening reactions are in bold italics.
CNS: headache, depression, fatigue.
CV: slight reduction in resting heart rate.
Eye: minor irritation. Long-term use may decrease corneal sensitivity.
GI: anorexia.
Other: apnea in infants, *evidence of beta blockade and systemic absorption (hypotension, bradycardia, syncope,* ***exacerbation of asthma,*** *and* ***CHF****).*

INTERACTIONS

Digitalis glycosides, quinidine, calcium channel blockers: increased risk of adverse cardiac effects if significant amounts of timolol are absorbed systemically. Use together cautiously.
General anesthetics, fentanyl: excessive hypotension.
Propranolol, metoprolol tartrate, other oral beta-adrenergic blockers: increased ocular and systemic effect. Use together cautiously.
Reserpine and other catecholamine-depleting drugs: enhanced hypotensive and bradycardiac effects. Avoid concurrent use.

NURSING CONSIDERATIONS

- *Contraindicated* in patients with hypersensitivity to the drug.
- *Use cautiously* in bronchial asthma, sinus bradycardia, second- and third-degree heart block, cardiogenic shock, right ventricular failure resulting from pulmonary hypertension, congestive heart failure, severe cardiac disease, and in infants with congenital glaucoma. Systemic beta blocking effects can mask some signs of hypoglycemia in diabetic patients.
- In some patients, a few weeks may be required to stabilize pressure-lowering response. Determine intraocular pressure after 4 weeks of treatment.
- Can be used safely in patients with glaucoma who wear conventional (PMMA) hard contact lenses.
- Teach patient how to instill. Advise him to wash hands before and after administering and to apply light finger-pressure on lacrimal sac for 1 minute following instillation. Warn him not to touch dropper to eye or surrounding tissue.

85

Otics

acetic acid
boric acid
carbamide peroxide
chloramphenicol
triethanolamine polypeptide oleate-condensate

COMBINATION PRODUCTS

COLY-MYCIN S OTIC: each ml contains neomycin SO_4 3.3 mg, colistin SO_4 3 mg, hydrocortisone acetate 10 mg, and thonzonium bromide 0.05%.
CORTISPORIN OTIC: each ml contains neomycin SO_4 5 mg, polymyxin B 10,000 units, and hydrocortisone 1%.

acetic acid

Domeboro Otic, VoSol Otic

Pregnancy Risk Category: C

HOW SUPPLIED

Otic solution: 2% in aluminum acetate, 2% in propylene glycol, 3%

MECHANISM OF ACTION

Inhibits or destroys bacteria present in the ear canal.

INDICATIONS & DOSAGE

External ear canal infection –
Adults and children: 4 to 6 drops into ear canal t.i.d. or q.i.d., or insert saturated wick for first 24 hours, then continue with instillations.
Prophylaxis of swimmer's ear –
Adults and children: 2 drops in each ear b.i.d.

ADVERSE REACTIONS

Ear: irritation or itching.
Skin: urticaria.
Other: overgrowth of nonsusceptible organisms.

INTERACTIONS

None significant.

NURSING CONSIDERATIONS

- *Use cautiously* in perforated eardrum.
- Has anti-infective, anti-inflammatory, and antipruritic effects.
- *Pseudomonas aeruginosa* particularly sensitive to drug.
- Reculture persistent drainage.
- Avoid touching ear with dropper.

boric acid

Aurocaine 2◇, Auro-Dri◇, Dri/Ear◇, Ear-Dry◇

Pregnancy Risk Category: C

HOW SUPPLIED

Otic solution: 2.75% boric acid in isopropyl alcohol

MECHANISM OF ACTION

Inhibits or destroys bacteria present in the ear canal. Weak bacteriostatic action; also fungistatic agent.

INDICATIONS & DOSAGE

External ear canal infection –
Adults and children: 3 to 6 drops in ear canal and plug with cotton. Repeat t.i.d. or q.i.d.

ADVERSE REACTIONS

Common reactions are in italics; life-threatening reactions are in bold italics.
Ear: irritation or itching.
Skin: urticaria.
Other: overgrowth of nonsusceptible organisms.

INTERACTIONS

None significant.

NURSING CONSIDERATIONS
- *Contraindicated* in perforated eardrum or excoriated membranes in ear.
- Watch for signs of superinfection (continual pain, inflammation, fever).
- If cotton plug used, always moisten with medication.
- Avoid touching ear with dropper.

carbamide peroxide
Debrox◇

Pregnancy Risk Category: C

HOW SUPPLIED
Otic solution: 6.5% carbamide in glycerin or glycerin and propylene glycol

MECHANISM OF ACTION
Emulsifies and disperses accumulated cerumen. A ceruminolytic.

INDICATIONS & DOSAGE
Impacted cerumen –
Adults and children: 5 to 10 drops into ear canal b.i.d. Allow solution to remain in ear canal for 15 to 30 minutes; remove with warm water.

ADVERSE REACTIONS
None reported.

INTERACTIONS
None significant.

NURSING CONSIDERATIONS
- *Contraindicated* in perforated eardrum. Use in children under 12 years should be under the direction of a doctor.
- Tell patient to call doctor if redness, pain, or swelling persists.
- Irrigation of ear with warm tap water using a rubber bulb syringe may be necessary to aid in removal of cerumen.
- Avoid touching ear with dropper.

chloramphenicol
Chloromycetin Otic, Sopamycetin†

Pregnancy Risk Category: C

HOW SUPPLIED
Otic solution: 0.5%

MECHANISM OF ACTION
Inhibits or destroys bacteria present in the ear canal.

INDICATIONS & DOSAGE
External ear canal infection –
Adults and children: 2 to 3 drops into ear canal t.i.d.

ADVERSE REACTIONS
Common reactions are in italics; life-threatening reactions are in bold italics.
Ear: itching or burning.
Local: pruritus, burning, urticaria, vesicular or maculopapular dermatitis.
Systemic: sore throat, angioedema.
Other: overgrowth of nonsusceptible organisms.

INTERACTIONS
None significant.

NURSING CONSIDERATIONS
- *Contraindicated* in patients with a perforated eardrum.
- Avoid prolonged use.
- Obtain history of use and reaction to drug.
- Watch for signs of superinfection (continued pain, inflammation, fever).
- Reculture persistent drainage.
- Watch for signs of sore throat (early sign of toxicity).
- Avoid touching ear with dropper.

triethanolamine polypeptide oleate-condensate

Cerumenex

Pregnancy Risk Category: C

HOW SUPPLIED

Otic solution: 10% in 6-ml, 12-ml bottles with droppers

MECHANISM OF ACTION

Emulsifies and disperses accumulated cerumen. A ceruminolytic.

INDICATIONS & DOSAGE

Impacted cerumen –

Adults and children: fill ear canal with solution and insert cotton plug. After 15 to 30 minutes, flush ear with warm water.

ADVERSE REACTIONS

Common reactions are in italics; life-threatening reactions are in bold italics.

Ear: erythema, pruritus.

Skin: severe eczema.

INTERACTIONS

None significant.

NURSING CONSIDERATIONS

- *Contraindicated* in perforated eardrum, otitis media, otitis externa, and allergies. Advise patient to discontinue the drug if adverse reactions occur and to contact the doctor immediately.
- If hypersensitivity is suspected, do patch test by placing 1 drop of drug on inner forearm; cover with small bandage. Read results in 24 hours. If any reaction (redness, swelling) occurs, don't use drug.
- Warn patient that this medication is for use only in the ears.
- Tell patient not to use drops more often than prescribed.
- Teach patient how to apply the drug. Moisten cotton plug with medication before insertion. Leave cotton in place for a maximum of 30 minutes. Flush ear gently with warm water, using soft rubber bulb ear syringe.
- Keep container tightly closed and away from moisture.

86

Nasal agents

beclomethasone dipropionate
dexamethasone sodium phosphate
ephedrine hydrochloride
ephedrine sulfate
epinephrine hydrochloride
flunisolide
naphazoline hydrochloride
oxymetazoline hydrochloride
phenylephrine hydrochloride
tetrahydrozoline hydrochloride
xylometazoline hydrochloride

COMBINATION PRODUCTS

4-WAY NASAL SPRAY◇: phenylephrine hydrochloride 0.5%, naphazoline hydrochloride 0.05%, and pyrilamine maleate 0.2%.

beclomethasone dipropionate

Aldecin Aqueous Nasal Spray, Beconase AQ Nasal Spray, Beconase Nasal Inhaler, Vancenase AQ Nasal Spray, Vancenase Nasal Inhaler

Pregnancy Risk Category: C

HOW SUPPLIED

Nasal aerosol: 42 mcg/metered spray, 50 mcg/metered spray‡
Nasal spray: 0.042%, 50 mcg/metered spray‡

MECHANISM OF ACTION

Decreases inflammation, mainly by stabilizing leukocyte lysosomal membranes.

INDICATIONS & DOSAGE

Relief of symptoms of seasonal or perennial rhinitis; prevention of recurrence of nasal polyps after surgical removal—

Adults and children over 12 years: usual dosage is 1 spray (42 mcg) in each nostril b.i.d. to q.i.d. (total dosage 168 to 336 mcg daily). Most patients require 1 spray in each nostril t.i.d. (252 mcg daily).

Not recommended for children under 12 years.

ADVERSE REACTIONS

Common reactions are in italics; life-threatening reactions are in bold italics.

CNS: headache.
EENT: *mild transient nasal burning and stinging,* nasal congestion, sneezing, epistaxis, watery eyes.
GI: nausea and vomiting.
Other: development of nasopharyngeal fungal infections.

INTERACTIONS

None reported.

NURSING CONSIDERATIONS

- *Use cautiously,* if at all, in patients with active or quiescent respiratory tract tubercular infections or in untreated fungal, bacterial, or systemic viral or ocular herpes simplex infections. Also *use cautiously* in patients who have recently had nasal septal ulcers or nasal surgery or trauma.
- Recommended dosages will not suppress hypothalamic-pituitary-adrenal (HPA) function. Warn patient not to exceed this dosage.
- Beclomethasone is not effective for active exacerbations. Decongestants or antihistamines may be needed.
- Advise patients to use drug regularly, as prescribed; its effectiveness depends on regular use.
- Explain that the therapeutic effects of this corticosteroid, unlike those of decongestants, are not immediate. Most patients achieve benefit within a

few days, but some may need 2 to 3 weeks for maximum benefit.
• If symptoms don't improve within 3 weeks or if nasal irritation persists, patient should notify doctor.
• Observe for fungal infections.
• Teach patient good nasal and oral hygiene.
• Teach patient how to use. Shake container and invert. After clearing nasal passages, tilt head slightly forward and insert nozzle into nostril, pointing away from septum. While holding other nostril closed, inspire gently and spray. Shake container again and repeat in other nostril.
• The nasal spray pump should be primed with three or four activators before the first use, and one or two activators before first use each day. The cap and nosepiece of the activator should be cleaned in warm water every day; allow to air dry.

dexamethasone sodium phosphate

Decadron Phosphate Turbinaire

Pregnancy Risk Category: C

HOW SUPPLIED

Nasal aerosol: 100 mcg/metered spray, 170 doses/canister

MECHANISM OF ACTION

Decreases inflammation, mainly by stabilizing leukocyte lysosomal membranes.

INDICATIONS & DOSAGE

Allergic or inflammatory conditions, nasal polyps –

Adults: 2 sprays in each nostril b.i.d. or t.i.d. Maximum 12 sprays daily.

Children 6 to 12 years: 1 or 2 sprays in each nostril b.i.d. Maximum 8 sprays daily.

Each spray delivers 0.1 mg dexamethasone sodium phosphate equal to 0.084 mg dexamethasone.

ADVERSE REACTIONS

Common reactions are in italics; life-threatening reactions are in bold italics.

EENT: nasal irritation, dryness, rebound nasal congestion.

Other: hypersensitivity, systemic effects with prolonged use (pituitary-adrenal suppression, sodium retention, ***CHF,*** hypertension, hypokalemia, headaches, ***seizures,*** peptic ulcer, ecchymoses, petechiae, masking of infection).

INTERACTIONS

None significant.

NURSING CONSIDERATIONS

• *Contraindicated* in cutaneous tuberculosis, fungal and herpetic lesions.
• *Use cautiously* in diabetes mellitus, peptic ulcer, or tuberculosis, as systemic absorption can activate disease.
• Mothers should not breast-feed, as systemic absorption can occur.
• Control underlying bacterial infection with anti-infectives.
• Irritation or sensitivity may require stopping drug.
• Don't break, incinerate, or store in extreme heat; contents under pressure.
• Gradually reduce dose as nasal condition improves.
• Fluid retention can occur as a result of systemic absorption.
• Teach patient how to use according to directions in package. Patient should shake container. After cleaning nasal passages, tilt head slightly forward and insert nozzle into nostril, pointing away from septum. While holding other nostril closed, inspire gently and spray. Shake container again and repeat in other nostril.
• Only one person should use nasal spray.
• Hypertension and hypokalemia can occur with systemic absorption. Frequently monitor blood pressure and serum potassium level. A patient who experiences fever, joint or muscle

aches, or extreme tiredness should contact the doctor.
- Prolonged use should be avoided because of the risk of hypothalamic-pituitary-adrenal-axis suppression.
- Teach patient good nasal and oral hygiene.

ephedrine hydrochloride
Efedron Nasal Jelly◊

ephedrine sulfate
Va-tro-nol Nose Drops◊

Pregnancy Risk Category: C

HOW SUPPLIED
hydrochloride
Nasal jelly: 0.5%◊
sulfate
Nasal solution: 0.5%◊

MECHANISM OF ACTION
Produces local vasoconstriction of dilated arterioles to reduce blood flow and nasal congestion.

INDICATIONS & DOSAGE
Nasal congestion –
Adults and children: apply 3 to 4 drops of 0.5% solution or apply a small amount of jelly to nasal mucosa. Use no more frequently than q 4 hours.

ADVERSE REACTIONS
Common reactions are in italics; life-threatening reactions are in bold italics.
CNS: nervousness, excitation.
CV: *tachycardia.*
EENT: rebound nasal congestion with long-term or excessive use.
Local: mucosal irritation.

INTERACTIONS
MAO inhibitors: hypertensive crisis if ephedrine is absorbed. Don't use together.

NURSING CONSIDERATIONS
- *Use cautiously* in hyperthyroidism, coronary artery disease, hypertension, or diabetes mellitus, as systemic absorption can occur.
- Tell patient not to exceed recommended dose. Use only when needed.
- Teach patient how to apply. Only one person should use dropper bottle.

epinephrine hydrochloride
Adrenalin Chloride

Pregnancy Risk Category: C

HOW SUPPLIED
Nasal solution: 0.1%

MECHANISM OF ACTION
Produces local vasoconstriction of dilated arterioles to reduce blood flow and nasal congestion.

INDICATIONS & DOSAGE
Nasal congestion, local superficial bleeding –
Adults and children: apply 0.1% solution to oral or nasal mucosa.

ADVERSE REACTIONS
Common reactions are in italics; life-threatening reactions are in bold italics.
CNS: nervousness, excitation.
CV: *tachycardia.*
EENT: rebound nasal congestion, slight sting upon application.

INTERACTIONS
None significant.

NURSING CONSIDERATIONS
- *Use cautiously* in hyperthyroidism, coronary artery disease, hypertension, or diabetes mellitus, as systemic absorption can occur.
- Tell patient not to exceed recommended dose. Use only when needed.
- Teach patient how to apply. Only one person should use dropper bottle.

flunisolide

Nasalide, Rhinalar Nasal Mist‡

Pregnancy Risk Category: C

HOW SUPPLIED

Nasal inhalant: 25 mcg/metered spray, 200 doses/bottle‡

Nasal solution: 0.25 mg/ml in pump spray bottle

MECHANISM OF ACTION

Decreases inflammation, mainly by stabilizing leukocyte lysosomal membranes.

INDICATIONS & DOSAGE

Relief of symptoms of seasonal or perennial rhinitis –

Adults: starting dose is 2 sprays (50 mcg) in each nostril b.i.d. Total daily dosage is 200 mcg. If necessary, dose may be increased to 2 sprays in each nostril t.i.d. Maximum total daily dosage is 8 sprays in each nostril (400 mcg daily).

Children 6 to 14 years: starting dose is 1 spray (25 mcg) in each nostril t.i.d. or 2 sprays (50 mcg) in each nostril b.i.d. Total daily dosage is 150 to 200 mcg. Maximum total daily dosage is 4 sprays in each nostril (200 mcg daily).

Not recommended for children under age 6.

ADVERSE REACTIONS

Common reactions are in italics; life-threatening reactions are in bold italics.

CNS: headache.

EENT: *mild, transient nasal burning and stinging,* nasal congestion, sneezing, epistaxis, watery eyes.

GI: nausea, vomiting.

Other: development of nasopharyngeal fungal infections.

INTERACTIONS

None reported.

NURSING CONSIDERATIONS

- *Contraindicated* in patients with hypersensitivity to the drug.
- *Use cautiously,* if at all, in patients with active or quiescent respiratory tract tubercular infections or in untreated fungal, bacterial, or systemic viral or ocular herpes simplex infections. Also *use cautiously* in patients who have recently had nasal septal ulcers or nasal surgery or trauma.
- Recommended dosages will not suppress hypothalamic-pituitary-adrenal (HPA) function. Warn patient not to exceed this dosage.
- Flunisolide is not effective for acute exacerbations. Decongestants or antihistamines may be needed.
- Advise patient to use drug regularly, as prescribed; its effectiveness depends on regular use.
- Explain that the therapeutic effects of this corticosteroid, unlike those of decongestants, are not immediate. Most patients achieve benefit within a few days, but some may need 2 to 3 weeks for maximum benefit.
- Patients with dryness and crusting of the nasal mucosa may prefer the liquid spray of flunisolide to the aerosolized powder of beclomethasone.
- If symptoms don't improve within 3 weeks or if nasal irritation persists, patient should stop drug and notify doctor.
- Teach patient how to apply. Clear nasal passages. After priming inhaler, tilt head slightly forward, insert spray tip into nostril pointing away from septum. While holding other nostril closed, inspire gently and spray. Repeat in other nostril.
- The nosepiece should be cleaned with warm water if it becomes clogged.

naphazoline hydrochloride

Privine◊

Pregnancy Risk Category: C

HOW SUPPLIED
Nasal drops: 0.05% solution
Nasal spray: 0.05% solution

MECHANISM OF ACTION
Produces local vasoconstriction of dilated arterioles to reduce blood flow and nasal congestion.

INDICATIONS & DOSAGE
Nasal congestion –
Adults: apply 2 drops or sprays of 0.05% solution to nasal mucosa q 3 to 4 hours.
Children 6 to 12 years: 1 to 2 drops or sprays of 0.05% solution. Repeat q 3 to 6 hours, p.r.n. Use no longer than 3 to 5 days.

ADVERSE REACTIONS
Common reactions are in italics; life-threatening reactions are in bold italics.
EENT: rebound nasal congestion with excessive or long-term use, sneezing, stinging, dryness of mucosa.
Other: systemic effects in children after excessive or long-term use; marked sedation.

INTERACTIONS
None significant.

NURSING CONSIDERATIONS
• *Contraindicated* in narrow-angle glaucoma. *Use cautiously* in hyperthyroidism, heart disease, hypertension, or diabetes mellitus, as systemic absorption can occur.
• Warn patient not to exceed recommended dosage.
• Tell patient to notify doctor if nasal congestion persists after 5 days.
• Teach patient how to apply. For nasal drops, instruct patient to tilt head back as far as possible, instill drops, then lean head forward while inhaling. Repeat procedure for other nostril. For nasal spray, instruct patient to hold spray container and head upright. Only one person should use dropper bottle or nasal spray.
• Do not shake container.

oxymetazoline hydrochloride
Afrin◇, Afrin Children's Strength Nose Drops◇, Allerest 12-Hour Nasal◇, Chlorphed-LA◇, Coricidin Nasal Mist◇, Dristan Long Lasting◇, Drixine Nasal‡, Duramist Plus◇, Duration◇, 4-Way Long-Acting Nasal, Genasal Spray◇, Neo-Synephrine 12 Hour◇, Nostrilla◇, NTZ Long Acting Nasal◇, Sinarest 12-Hour◇, Sinex Long-Acting◇, Twice-A-Day Nasal◇

Pregnancy Risk Category: C

HOW SUPPLIED
Nasal solution: 0.025%◇, 0.05%◇

MECHANISM OF ACTION
Produces local vasoconstriction of dilated arterioles to reduce blood flow and nasal congestion.

INDICATIONS & DOSAGE
Nasal congestion –
Adults and children over 6 years: apply 2 to 4 drops or sprays of 0.05% solution to nasal mucosa b.i.d.
Children 2 to 6 years: apply 2 to 3 drops 0.025% solution to nasal mucosa b.i.d. Use no longer than 3 to 5 days. Dosage for younger children has not been established.

ADVERSE REACTIONS
Common reactions are in italics; life-threatening reactions are in bold italics.
CNS: headache, drowsiness, dizziness, insomnia, possible sedation.
CV: palpitations, ***hypotension with cardiovascular collapse,*** hypertension.
EENT: rebound nasal congestion or irritation with excessive or long-term use, dryness of nose and throat, in-

creased nasal discharge, stinging, sneezing.
Other: systemic effects in children with excessive or long-term use.

INTERACTIONS
None significant.

NURSING CONSIDERATIONS
- *Use cautiously* in hyperthyroidism, cardiac disease, hypertension, or diabetes mellitus, as systemic absorption can occur.
- Tell patient not to exceed recommended dose. Use only when needed.
- Warn patient that excessive use may cause bradycardia, hypotension, dizziness, and weakness.
- Teach patient how to apply. Have patient hold head upright and sniff spray briskly. Only one person should use dropper bottle or nasal spray.

phenylephrine hydrochloride
Alconefrin 12◇, Alconefrin 25◇, Alconefrin 50◇, Doktors◇, Duration◇, Neo-Synephrine◇, Nostril◇, Rhinall◇, Rhinall-10◇, Sinex◇, St. Joseph Measured Dose Nasal Decongestant◇
Pregnancy Risk Category: C

HOW SUPPLIED
Nasal jelly: 0.5%
Nasal solution: 0.125%, 0.16%, 0.2%, 0.25%, 0.5%, 1%

MECHANISM OF ACTION
Produces local vasoconstriction of dilated arterioles to reduce blood flow and nasal congestion.

INDICATIONS & DOSAGE
Nasal congestion –
Adults: 1 to 2 drops or sprays of 0.125% to 1% solution; apply jelly or spray to nasal mucosa.
Children 6 to 12 years: apply 1 to 2 drops or sprays of 0.25% solution.
Children under 6 years: apply 2 to 3 drops or sprays of 0.125% solution.
Drops, spray, or jelly can be given q 4 hours, p.r.n.

ADVERSE REACTIONS
Common reactions are in italics; life-threatening reactions are in bold italics.
CNS: headache, tremors, dizziness, nervousness.
CV: *palpitations, tachycardia,* ***premature ventricular contractions,*** hypertension, pallor.
EENT: transient burning, stinging; dryness of nasal mucosa; rebound nasal congestion may occur with continued use.
GI: nausea.

INTERACTIONS
None significant.

NURSING CONSIDERATIONS
- *Contraindicated* in narrow-angle glaucoma.
- *Use cautiously* in hyperthyroidism, hypertension, diabetes mellitus, or ischemic cardiac disease, as systemic absorption may occur.
- Tell patient not to exceed recommended dose. Use only when needed.
- Advise patient to contact the doctor if symptoms persist beyond 3 days.
- Teach patient how to apply. Have patient hold head erect to minimize swallowing of medication. Only one person should use dropper bottle or nasal spray.

tetrahydrozoline hydrochloride
Tyzine Drops, Tyzine Pediatric Drops
Pregnancy Risk Category: C

HOW SUPPLIED
Nasal solution: 0.05%, 0.1%

*Liquid form contains alcohol. **May contain tartrazine.

MECHANISM OF ACTION
Produces local vasoconstriction of dilated arterioles to reduce blood flow and nasal congestion.

INDICATIONS & DOSAGE
Nasal congestion –
Adults and children over 6 years: apply 2 to 4 drops of 0.1% solution or spray to nasal mucosa q 4 to 6 hours, p.r.n.
Children 2 to 6 years: apply 2 to 3 drops of 0.05% solution to nasal mucosa q 4 to 6 hours, p.r.n.

ADVERSE REACTIONS
Common reactions are in italics; life-threatening reactions are in bold italics.
EENT: transient burning, stinging; sneezing, rebound nasal congestion in excessive or long-term use.

INTERACTIONS
None significant.

NURSING CONSIDERATIONS
- *Contraindicated* in children under 2 years and in narrow-angle glaucoma.
- *Use cautiously* in hyperthyroidism, hypertension, diabetes mellitus.
- Don't use 0.1% solution in children under 6 years.
- Tell patient not to exceed recommended dose. Use only as needed for 3 to 5 days.
- Show patient how to apply. Only one person should use dropper or nasal spray.

xylometazoline hydrochloride
4-Way Long Acting, Neo-Synephrine II, Otrivin, Sine-Off Nasal Spray, Sinex-L.A.

Pregnancy Risk Category: C

HOW SUPPLIED
Nasal solution: 0.05%, 0.1%

MECHANISM OF ACTION
Produces local vasoconstriction of dilated arterioles to reduce blood flow and nasal congestion.

INDICATIONS & DOSAGE
Nasal congestion –
Adults and children over 12 years: apply 2 to 3 drops or 1 to 2 sprays of 0.1% solution to nasal mucosa q 8 to 10 hours.
Children 6 months to 12 years: apply 2 to 3 drops or 1 spray of 0.05% solution to nasal mucosa q 8 to 10 hours.
Infants under 6 months: 1 drop of 0.05% solution into each nostril q 6 hours p.r.n.

ADVERSE REACTIONS
Common reactions are in italics; life-threatening reactions are in bold italics.
EENT: rebound nasal congestion or irritation with excessive or long-term use; transient burning, stinging; dryness or ulceration of nasal mucosa; sneezing.

INTERACTIONS
None significant.

NURSING CONSIDERATIONS
- *Contraindicated* in narrow-angle glaucoma.
- *Use cautiously* in hyperthyroidism, cardiac disease, hypertension, diabetes mellitus, and advanced arteriosclerosis, as systemic absorption can occur. Use in infants under 6 months only under the direction of a doctor.
- Tell patient not to exceed recommended dose, and to use only for 3 to 5 days.
- Teach patient how to apply. Have patient hold head upright and sniff spray briskly. Only one person should use dropper bottle or nasal spray.

87
Local anti-infectives

- acyclovir
- amphotericin B
- bacitracin
- butoconazole nitrate
- carbol-fuchsin solution
- chloramphenicol
- chlortetracycline hydrochloride
- ciclopirox olamine
- clindamycin phosphate
- clotrimazole
- econazole nitrate
- erythromycin
- gentamicin sulfate
- gentian violet
- haloprogin
- iodochlorhydroxyquin
- ketoconazole
- mafenide acetate
- metronidazole (topical)
- miconazole nitrate
- mupirocin
- naftifine
- neomycin sulfate
- nitrofurazone
- nystatin
- oxiconazole nitrate
- podofilox
- silver sulfadiazine
- sulconazole nitrate
- terbinafine hydrochloride
- terconazole
- tetracycline hydrochloride
- tioconazole
- tolnaftate
- undecylenic acid and zinc undecylenate

COMBINATION PRODUCTS

BENZAMYCIN GEL: erythromycin 3% and benzoyl peroxide 5%.
CORDRAN-N CREAM, OINTMENT: flurandrenolide 0.05% and neomycin sulfate 0.5%.
LANABIOTIC◇: polymyxin B sulfate 5,000 units, neomycin sulfate 5 mg, bacitracin 500 units, and lidocaine 40 mg/g.
LOTRISONE CREAM: clotrimazole 1% and betamethasone dipropionate 0.05%.
MYCITRACIN OINTMENT◇: polymyxin B sulfate 5,000 units, bacitracin 500 units, and neomycin sulfate 3.5 mg/g.
MYCOLOG II CREAM, OINTMENT: triamcinolone acetonide 0.1%, and nystatin 100,000 units/g.
NEO-CORTEF OINTMENT: hydrocortisone acetate 1% and neomycin sulfate 0.5%.
NEODECADRON CREAM: dexamethasone phosphate 0.1% and neomycin sulfate 0.5%.
NEO-POLYCIN OINTMENT◇: polymyxin B sulfate 5,000 units, neomycin sulfate 5 mg, and zinc bacitracin 400 units/g.
NEOSPORIN CREAM†◇: polymyxin B sulfate 10,000 units, neomycin sulfate 5 mg.
NEOSPORIN OINTMENT◇: polymyxin B sulfate 5,000 units, bacitracin zinc 400 units, and neomycin sulfate 5 mg/g.
POLYSPORIN OINTMENT◇: polymyxin B sulfate 10,000 units and zinc bacitracin 500 units/g.
SULFACET-R LOTION: sulfacetamide sodium 10% and sulfur 5%.
VIOFORM-HYDROCORTISONE MILD CREAM, RACET CREAM: iodochlorhydroxyquin 3% and hydrocortisone 0.5%.
VYTONE CREAM: hydrocortisone 1% and iodoquinol 1%

acyclovir
Zovirax

Pregnancy Risk Category: C

HOW SUPPLIED
Ointment: 5%

MECHANISM OF ACTION
Inhibits herpes virus DNA synthesis by interfering with the action of viral DNA polymerase.

INDICATIONS & DOSAGE
Initial herpes genitalis; limited, non-life-threatening mucocutaneous herpes simplex virus infections in immunocompromised patients –
Adults and children: apply sufficient quantity to adequately cover all lesions q 3 hours six times daily for 7 days.

ADVERSE REACTIONS
Common reactions are in italics; life-threatening reactions are in bold italics.
Skin: transient burning and stinging, rash, pruritus.

INTERACTIONS
None reported.

NURSING CONSIDERATIONS
- *Contraindicated* in patients with hypersensitivity to the drug.
- For cutaneous use only. Don't apply to the eye. For information on systemic use, see Chapter 17, Antivirals.
- Although the dose size for each application will vary depending upon the total lesion area, use approximately a ½" ribbon of ointment on each 4-inch square of surface area.
- Ointment must thoroughly cover all lesions.
- Apply with a finger cot or rubber glove to prevent autoinoculation of other body sites and transmission of infection to other persons.
- Therapy should be initiated as early as possible following onset of signs and symptoms of herpes.
- Most studies show that acyclovir is not effective when used to treat *recurrent* genital herpes.
- Emphasize importance of compliance for successful therapy.
- Teach patient that he may transmit the virus even during treatment.

amphotericin B
Fungizone
Pregnancy Risk Category: B

HOW SUPPLIED
Cream: 3%
Lotion: 3%
Ointment: 3%

MECHANISM OF ACTION
Alters the permeability of the cell membrane of fungi. Fungistatic.

INDICATIONS & DOSAGE
Cutaneous or mucocutaneous candidal infections –
Adults and children: apply liberally b.i.d., t.i.d., or q.i.d. for 1 to 3 weeks; up to several months for interdigital lesions and paronychias.

ADVERSE REACTIONS
Common reactions are in italics; life-threatening reactions are in bold italics.
Skin: possible drying, contact sensitivity, erythema, burning, pruritus.

INTERACTIONS
None significant.

NURSING CONSIDERATIONS
- *Contraindicated* in patients with hypersensitivity to the drug.
- Cleanse area before applying.
- Cream or lotion preferred for such areas as folds of groin, armpit, and neck creases.
- Cream discolors skin slightly when rubbed in; lotion or ointment doesn't. Lotion may stain nail lesions.
- Watch for and report signs of local irritation. Cream may have a drying effect on the skin; ointment may irritate if applied to moist hairy areas.
- Avoid occlusive dressings.

- Store at room temperature; avoid freezing.
- Well tolerated, even by infants, for long periods.
- Tell patient to continue using medication for full length of time prescribed, even if condition has improved.
- Discoloration of fabric caused by cream or lotion can usually be removed by ordinary washing. Discoloration caused by ointment requires removal with cleaning fluid.
- Drug should be discontinued if irritation or hypersensitivity occurs.

bacitracin

Baciguent◇, Bacitin†

Pregnancy Risk Category: C

HOW SUPPLIED

Ointment: 500 units/g

MECHANISM OF ACTION

Inhibits bacterial cell-wall synthesis. Effective mainly against gram-positive organisms, such as staphylococci and streptococci.

INDICATIONS & DOSAGE

Topical infections, impetigo, abrasions, cuts, and minor burns or wounds –

Adults and children: apply thin film b.i.d. or t.i.d. or more often, depending on severity of condition.

ADVERSE REACTIONS

Common reactions are in italics; life-threatening reactions are in bold italics.

Skin: stinging, rashes, and other allergic reactions; itching, burning, swelling of lips or face.

Other: *possible systemic adverse reactions when used over large areas for prolonged periods: potentially nephrotoxic and ototoxic; allergic reactions;* tightness in chest, hypotension.

INTERACTIONS

None significant.

NURSING CONSIDERATIONS

- *Contraindicated* in patients with hypersensitivity to the drug and for application in the external ear canal if the eardrum is perforated.
- *Use cautiously.* Overgrowth of nonsusceptible organisms (particularly *Candida* species) can occur.
- Cleanse area before applying, especially in areas with crusted or suppurative lesions.
- Patients allergic to neomycin may also be allergic to bacitracin.
- Consider alternative treatment for burns that cover more than 20% of body surface, especially if patient suffers impaired renal function.
- If no improvement or if condition worsens, stop using and notify doctor.
- Prolonged use may result in overgrowth of nonsusceptible organisms.

butoconazole nitrate

Femstat

Pregnancy Risk Category: C

HOW SUPPLIED

Vaginal cream: 2% supplied with applicators

MECHANISM OF ACTION

Controls or destroys fungus by disrupting cell membrane permeability and reducing osmotic resistance.

INDICATIONS & DOSAGE

Local treatment of vulvovaginal mycotic infections caused by Candida *species –*

Adults (nonpregnant): one applicatorful intravaginally at bedtime for 3 days.

Adults (pregnant): one applicatorful intravaginally at bedtime for 6 days. Use only during second and third trimester.

ADVERSE REACTIONS
Common reactions are in italics; life-threatening reactions are in bold italics.
Skin: vulvar itching, soreness, and swelling; itching of the fingers.

INTERACTIONS
None significant.

NURSING CONSIDERATIONS
- *Contraindicated* in patients with hypersensitivity to the drug and during the first trimester of pregnancy.
- Butoconazole may be used with oral contraceptive and antibiotic therapy.
- Diagnosis of *Candida* vulvovaginal infection should be confirmed by smears or cultures.
- Symptom resolution comparable to 7-day miconazole cream therapy. Antifungal effect of butoconazole therapy is apparent after only 3 days of therapy.
- Teach patient how to apply. Tell patient not to use tampons during treatment.
- The patient's sexual partner should wear a condom during intercourse until treatment is complete. He should consult his doctor if he experiences penile itching, redness, or discomfort.
- Advise patient to do the following to prevent reinfection: Keep cool and dry, wear loose-fitting cotton clothing, avoid feminine hygiene sprays, wash daily with unscented soap, dry thoroughly with clean towel, and maintain proper bowel hygiene by wiping from front to back.

carbol-fuchsin solution (Castellani's paint; Magenta paint)
Castaderm

Pregnancy Risk Category: C

HOW SUPPLIED
Topical solution: 0.3% basic fuchsin, 4.5% phenol, 10% resorcinol, 5% acetone, and 10% alcohol.

MECHANISM OF ACTION
Disrupts protein synthesis. A fungicidal and bactericidal agent.

INDICATIONS & DOSAGE
Tinea, dermatophytosis, skin infections –
Adults and children: apply liberally once daily to b.i.d.

ADVERSE REACTIONS
Common reactions are in italics; life-threatening reactions are in bold italics.
Blood: possibility of bone marrow hypoplasia with use over long periods or at frequent intervals.
Skin: *contact dermatitis.*

INTERACTIONS
None significant.

NURSING CONSIDERATIONS
- *Contraindicated* in patients with hypersensitivity to the drug.
- Warn patient to expect a stinging sensation, which is usually followed by the drug's local anesthetic effect.
- An initial test application over a small area is recommended. If contact dermatitis or sensitivity occurs, discontinue use.
- Discontinue use after 1 week if no improvement shown; consult doctor. Toxicities may develop in long-term use.
- Poisonous; warn against swallowing. Store in tight, light-resistant container.
- Instruct patient to continue using for full treatment period prescribed, even if condition has improved.
- Useful in treating moist eczematous dermatitis, especially in hairy areas.
- Don't apply to eroded skin or over extensive areas.
- Will stain clothing.
- Clean skin with soap and water before application.

chloramphenicol

Chloromycetin

Pregnancy Risk Category: C

HOW SUPPLIED

Cream: 1%

MECHANISM OF ACTION

Disrupts protein synthesis.

INDICATIONS & DOSAGE

Superficial skin infections caused by susceptible bacteria –
Adults and children: after thorough cleansing, apply t.i.d. or q.i.d.

ADVERSE REACTIONS

Common reactions are in italics; life-threatening reactions are in bold italics.
Skin: possible contact sensitivity; itching, burning, urticaria, angioneurotic edema in patients hypersensitive to any of the components.
Other: ***blood dyscrasias*** (including ***bone marrow hypoplasia*** and ***aplastic anemia***).

INTERACTIONS

None significant.

NURSING CONSIDERATIONS

- *Contraindicated* in patients with hypersensitivity to the drug.
- If no improvement or if condition worsens, stop using and report to doctor.
- Prolonged use may result in overgrowth of nonsusceptible organisms.
- For all but very superficial infections, topical use of this drug should be supplemented by appropriate systemic medication.
- Discontinue if signs of hypersensitivity develop.
- Tell patient to continue using for full treatment period prescribed, even if condition has improved.

chlortetracycline hydrochloride

Aureomycin 3%◊

Pregnancy Risk Category: D

HOW SUPPLIED

Ointment: 3% in 14.2-g, 30-g tubes◊

MECHANISM OF ACTION

Disrupts protein synthesis.

INDICATIONS & DOSAGE

Superficial infections of the skin caused by susceptible bacteria –
Adults and children: rub into affected area b.i.d. or t.i.d.

ADVERSE REACTIONS

Common reactions are in italics; life-threatening reactions are in bold italics.
Skin: *dermatitis,* drying.

INTERACTIONS

None significant.

NURSING CONSIDERATIONS

- *Contraindicated* in patients with hypersensitivity to the drug.
- Drug has lanolin base. Don't use in persons allergic to wool.
- Prolonged use may result in overgrowth of nonsusceptible organisms.
- If no improvement or if condition worsens, stop using and report to doctor.
- Treated skin fluoresces under ultraviolet light.

ciclopirox olamine

Loprox

Pregnancy Risk Category: B

HOW SUPPLIED

Cream: 1%
Lotion: 1%

MECHANISM OF ACTION

Depletes essential intracellular substrates of fungi.

INDICATIONS & DOSAGE
Treatment of tinea pedis, tinea cruris, tinea corporis, and tinea versicolor; cutaneous candidiasis –
Adults and children over 10 years: massage gently into the affected and surrounding areas b.i.d., in the morning and evening.

ADVERSE REACTIONS
Common reactions are in italics; life-threatening reactions are in bold italics.
Local: pruritus, burning.

INTERACTIONS
None reported.

NURSING CONSIDERATIONS
- *Contraindicated* in patients with hypersensitivity to the drug.
- If sensitivity or chemical irritation occurs, discontinue treatment.
- Use the drug for the full treatment period even though symptoms may have improved (usually continued for 1 week after clearing). Notify doctor if there's no improvement after 4 weeks.
- Don't use occlusive dressings.
- Hypopigmentation from *tinea versicolor* will resolve gradually.

clindamycin phosphate
Cleocin T Gel, Lotion, Solution; Cleocin Vaginal Cream

Pregnancy Risk Category: B

HOW SUPPLIED
Gel: 1%
Lotion: 1%
Topical solution: 1%
Vaginal cream: 2%

MECHANISM OF ACTION
Suppresses growth of susceptible organisms in sebaceous glands.

INDICATIONS & DOSAGE
Acne vulgaris, grades II and III –
Adults and adolescents: apply to skin b.i.d., morning and evening; solutions have been used once daily to q.i.d.
Bacterial vaginosis –
Women: 1 applicator full intravaginally h.s. for 7 consecutive days.

ADVERSE REACTIONS
Common reactions are in italics; life-threatening reactions are in bold italics.
GI: GI disturbance, diarrhea, bloody diarrhea, abdominal pain, colitis (including pseudomembranous colitis).
GU: *cervicitis or vaginitis,* Candida albicans *overgrowth, vulvar irritation.*
Skin: *dryness,* rash, redness, itching, swelling, irritation.

INTERACTIONS
Abrasive or medicated soaps or cleansers; acne preparations or any containing a peeling agent (benzoyl peroxide, salicylic acid, sulfur, resorcinol, tretinoin); alcohol-containing products (after-shave, perfumed toiletries, shaving creams or lotions, cosmetics); soaps or cosmetics with strong drying effect; isotretinoin; medicated cosmetics or "cover-ups": may cause cumulative drying or irritation, resulting in excessive skin irritation.

NURSING CONSIDERATIONS
- *Contraindicated* in patients with hypersensitivity to the drug and in patients with a history of ulcerative colitis, regional enteritis, or antibiotic-associated colitis.
- When used intravaginally, be sure the patient understands how to use the applicator that comes with the drug. Seven plastic applicators are dispensed with the drug; each is for one-time use only.
- May be used concurrently with tretinoin or benzoyl peroxide as well as systemic antibiotics. Caution patient to notify doctor if skin becomes excessively dry.
- When used topically, noticeable improvement is usually seen within 6

weeks; however, 8 to 12 weeks may be required for maximum benefit.
• Instruct patient to wash area with warm water and soap, rinse and pat dry before application; and allow 30 minutes after washing or shaving to apply. Warn patient to avoid too frequent washing of area. Tell patient to cover entire affected area, but to avoid contact with eyes, nose, mouth, and other mucous membranes.
• Patient should not smoke while applying topical solution.
• Use only as prescribed.
• Tell patient to check with doctor or pharmacist before using antidiarrheal if diarrhea occurs.
• Use with caution in patients with GI disease, especially ulcerative colitis, regional enteritis, or antibiotic-related colitis.
• Explain correct use of applicator-tip bottle: use dabbing motion rather than rolling action. If tip becomes dry, invert bottle and depress tip several times to moisten.

clotrimazole

Canesten†, Gyne-Lotrimin◊, Lotrimin (1% clotrimazole), Mycelex, Mycelex-7◊, Mycelex-G, Mycelex-OTC◊

Pregnancy Risk Category: B

HOW SUPPLIED

Lozenges: 1%
Cream: 1%
Topical lotion: 1%
Topical solution: 1%
Vaginal cream: 1%◊
Vaginal tablets: 100 mg◊, 500 mg

MECHANISM OF ACTION

Alters fungal cell wall permeability.

INDICATIONS & DOSAGE

Superficial fungal infections (tinea pedis, tinea cruris, tinea corporis, tinea versicolor, candidiasis) –
Adults and children: apply thinly and massage into affected and surrounding area, morning and evening, 2 to 8 weeks.
Candidal vulvovaginitis –
Women: insert 1 applicator full or 1 tablet intravaginally daily h.s. for 7 days. Alternatively, insert two 100-mg tablets daily h.s. for 3 consecutive days, or one 500-mg tablet as a single dose at bedtime.
Oropharyngeal candidiasis –
Adults and children: dissolve lozenge in mouth five times daily for 14 consecutive days.

ADVERSE REACTIONS

Common reactions are in italics; life-threatening reactions are in bold italics.
GI: nausea and vomiting (with lozenges).
GU: (with vaginal use) *mild vaginal burning, irritation.*
Hepatic: elevated AST (SGOT) levels (from lozenges).
Skin: blistering, *erythema,* edema, pruritus, burning, stinging, peeling, urticaria, skin fissures, general irritation.

INTERACTIONS

None significant.

NURSING CONSIDERATIONS

• *Contraindicated* in patients with hypersensitivity to the drug.
• Not for ophthalmic use.
• Clean area before applying.
• Watch for and report irritation or sensitivity. Discontinue use if irritation occurs.
• Improvement usually within a week; if no improvement in 4 weeks, diagnosis should be reviewed.
• Make sure patient understands that frequent or persistent yeast infections may be a symptom of a more serious medical problem, such as immunodeficiency or AIDS.
• Emphasize the need to continue treatment for full course even if symptoms have improved.

• Warn patients not to use occlusive wrappings or dressings.
• Shortened dosage schedule with tablets may be used when compliance is a problem.
• Hypopigmentation from *tinea versicolor* will resolve gradually.
• Topical preparation may stain clothing.

econazole nitrate

Ecostatin, Spectazole

Pregnancy Risk Category: C

HOW SUPPLIED

Cream: 1%

MECHANISM OF ACTION

Alters fungal cell wall permeability.

INDICATIONS & DOSAGE

Treatment of tinea pedis, tinea cruris, and tinea corporis; cutaneous candidiasis –
Adults and children: apply sufficient quantity to cover affected areas b.i.d., in the morning and evening for at least 2 weeks.
Tinea versicolor –
Adults and children: apply once daily.

ADVERSE REACTIONS

Common reactions are in italics; life-threatening reactions are in bold italics.
Local: burning, itching, stinging, erythema.

INTERACTIONS

Topical corticosteroids: may inhibit antifungal effect.

NURSING CONSIDERATIONS

• *Contraindicated* in patients with hypersensitivity to the drug.
• If condition persists or worsens or if irritation (burning, itching, stinging, redness) occurs, discontinue use and report this to doctor.
• Use medication for entire treatment period, even though symptoms may have improved. Notify doctor if there is no improvement; after 2 weeks (tinea cruris, corporis and versicolor) or 4 weeks (tinea pedis).
• Clean affected area before applying.
• Don't use occlusive dressings.
• Hypopigmentation from *tinea versicolor* will resolve gradually.
• May stain clothing.

erythromycin

Akne-mycin, A/T/S, Erycette, EryDerm, EryGel, Ery-Sol†, ETS†, Sans-Acne†, T-Stat†, Staticin

Pregnancy Risk Category: B

HOW SUPPLIED

Ointment: 2%
Topical gel: 2%
Pledgets: 2%
Topical solution: 1.5%*, 2%*

MECHANISM OF ACTION

Disrupts protein synthesis.

INDICATIONS & DOSAGE

Superficial skin infections due to susceptible organisms, acne vulgaris –
Adults and children: clean affected area; apply b.i.d.

ADVERSE REACTIONS

Common reactions are in italics; life-threatening reactions are in bold italics.
Skin: sensitivity reactions, erythema, burning, *dryness, pruritus.*

INTERACTIONS

None significant.

NURSING CONSIDERATIONS

• *Contraindicated* in patients with hypersensitivity to the drug.
• Prolonged use may result in overgrowth of nonsusceptible organisms.
• If no improvement or if condition worsens, stop using and notify doctor.
• Wash, rinse, and dry affected areas before application.

• Don't use near eyes, nose, mouth, or other mucous membranes.

gentamicin sulfate

Garamycin, G-Myticin

Pregnancy Risk Category: C

HOW SUPPLIED

Cream: 0.1%
Ointment: 0.1%

MECHANISM OF ACTION

Disrupts protein synthesis.

INDICATIONS & DOSAGE

Primary and secondary bacterial infections, superficial burns, skin ulcers, infected insect bites and stings, infected lacerations and abrasions, wounds from minor surgery –
Adults and children over 1 year: rub in small amount gently t.i.d. or q.i.d., with or without gauze dressing.

ADVERSE REACTIONS

Common reactions are in italics; life-threatening reactions are in bold italics.
Skin: minor skin irritation; possible photosensitivity; allergic contact dermatitis.

INTERACTIONS

None reported.

NURSING CONSIDERATIONS

• *Contraindicated* in patients with hypersensitivity to the drug. May exhibit cross-sensitivity with other aminoglycosides, such as neomycin.
• Clean affected area before applying.
• If no improvement or if condition worsens, stop using and report to doctor.
• Should be used in selected patients. Widespread use may lead to resistant organisms.
• Avoid use on large skin lesions or over a wide area because of possible systemic toxic effects.
• Prolonged use may result in overgrowth of nonsusceptible organisms.
• May treat bacterial infections that have not responded to other antibacterial agents.
• Store in cool place.
• Remove crusts before application of gentamicin in impetigo contagiosa.

gentian violet (methylrosaniline chloride, crystal violet)

Genapax

Pregnancy Risk Category: C

HOW SUPPLIED

Tampons: 5 mg
Topical solution: 1%◇, 2%◇

MECHANISM OF ACTION

Fungistatic and antibacterial activity.

INDICATIONS & DOSAGE

Superficial infections of skin; lesions, except ulcerative lesions of face, particularly Candida albicans –
Adults and children: apply with swab b.i.d. or t.i.d. Keep affected area clean, dry, and exposed to air to prevent spread of infection.
Vaginal fungal infections –
Adults: insert 1 tampon intravaginally for 3 to 4 hours once daily to b.i.d. for 12 days. An additional tampon may be used overnight for resistant infections.

ADVERSE REACTIONS

Common reactions are in italics; life-threatening reactions are in bold italics.
Skin: *permanent discoloration if applied to granulation tissue;* irritation or ulceration of mucous membranes.

INTERACTIONS

None significant.

NURSING CONSIDERATIONS

• *Contraindicated* in patients with hypersensitivity to the drug.

*Liquid form contains alcohol. **May contain tartrazine.

- Do not use on ulcerative lesions of the face.
- Apply carefully to avoid undue staining. Will stain skin and clothing.
- Do not use occlusive dressings.
- Tattooing of the skin may occur if applied to granulation tissue.

haloprogin

Halotex

Pregnancy Risk Category: B

HOW SUPPLIED

Cream: 1%
Topical solution: 1%

MECHANISM OF ACTION

Fungistatic and fungicidal activity.

INDICATIONS & DOSAGE

Superficial fungal infections (tinea pedis, tinea cruris, tinea corporis, tinea manuum, and tinea versicolor) –
Adults: apply liberally b.i.d. for 2 to 3 weeks.

ADVERSE REACTIONS

Common reactions are in italics; life-threatening reactions are in bold italics.
Skin: burning sensation, irritation, vesicle formation, increased maceration, *pruritus or exacerbation of preexisting lesions.*

INTERACTIONS

None significant.

NURSING CONSIDERATIONS

- *Contraindicated* in patients with hypersensitivity to the drug.
- Diagnosis should be reconsidered if no improvement in 4 weeks.
- Tell patient to continue using for full treatment period prescribed, even if condition has improved.
- Tell patient to notify doctor if increased irritation occurs.
- Don't allow drug to come in contact with the eyes.

iodochlorhydroxyquin (clioquinol)

Ala-Quin, Corque, Cortin, Torofor◊, Vioform◊

Pregnancy Risk Category: C

HOW SUPPLIED

Cream: 0.5%, 1%, 3%
Ointment: 0.5%, 1%, 3%
Lotion: 1%, 3%

MECHANISM OF ACTION

Fungistatic and fungicidal activity.

INDICATIONS & DOSAGE

Inflamed skin conditions, including eczema, athlete's foot, and other fungal infections; cutaneous or mucocutaneous mycotic infections caused by Candida *species* (monilia) –
Adults and children over 2 years: apply a thin layer b.i.d. or t.i.d., or as directed. Continue for 1 week after cessation of symptoms.

ADVERSE REACTIONS

Common reactions are in italics; life-threatening reactions are in bold italics.
CNS: neurotoxicity (with systemic absorption).
Metabolic: altered protein-bound iodine levels (with systemic absorption).
Skin: *possible burning, itching, acneiform eruptions,* allergic contact dermatitis.

INTERACTIONS

Systemic corticosteroids: possible increased absorption. Use together cautiously.

NURSING CONSIDERATIONS

- *Contraindicated* in patients with hypersensitivity to the drug or to iodine or iodine-containing preparations and in those with tuberculosis, vaccinia, and varicella.
- Don't use to treat diaper rash.
- Note all adverse reactions and pre-

cautions of each component in the combination antifungals.

- Presence in urine may cause false-positive result for phenylketonuria (PKU) or inaccurate thyroid function tests. Discontinue at least 1 month before thyroid function tests.
- Drug will stain fabric and hair.

ketoconazole

Nizoral

Pregnancy Risk Category: C

HOW SUPPLIED

Cream: 2%
Shampoo: 2%

MECHANISM OF ACTION

Inhibits yeast growth by altering the permeability of the cell membrane.

INDICATIONS & DOSAGE

Tinea corporis, tinea pedis, tinea cruris, and tinea versicolor caused by susceptible organisms; seborrheic dermatitis –
Adults: apply once daily to cover the affected and immediate surrounding area. Apply twice daily, if necessary, in the more resistant cases.

ADVERSE REACTIONS

Common reactions are in italics; life-threatening reactions are in bold italics.
Skin: severe irritation, pruritus, stinging.
Systemic: localized allergic reaction.

INTERACTIONS

None reported.

NURSING CONSIDERATIONS

- Discontinue if sensitivity or chemical irritation occurs.
- Most patients show improvement soon after treatment begins. However, treatment of tinea cruris or tinea corporis should continue for at least 2 weeks to reduce the possibility of recurrence.
- Check with doctor if condition worsens. The drug may have to be discontinued and diagnosis redetermined.

mafenide acetate

Sulfamylon

Pregnancy Risk Category: C

HOW SUPPLIED

Cream: 8.5%

MECHANISM OF ACTION

Interferes with bacterial cellular metabolism.

INDICATIONS & DOSAGE

Adjunctive treatment of second- and third-degree burns to prevent infection caused by susceptible organisms (especially Pseudomonas aeruginosa) –
Adults and children: apply 1/16″ thickness of cream daily or b.i.d. to cleansed, debrided wounds. Reapply p.r.n. to keep burned area covered.

ADVERSE REACTIONS

Common reactions are in italics; life-threatening reactions are in bold italics.
Blood: eosinophilia.
Skin: pain, *burning sensation,* rash, itching, swelling, hives, blisters, erythema, facial edema.
Other: *metabolic acidosis.*

INTERACTIONS

None significant.

NURSING CONSIDERATIONS

- *Contraindicated* in patients with hypersensitivity to the drug.
- *Use cautiously* in acute renal failure and in patients with known hypersensitivity to sulfonamides.
- Closely monitor acid-base balance, especially in the presence of pulmonary and renal dysfunction.
- Using reverse isolation technique with sterile gloves and instruments to

*Liquid form contains alcohol. **May contain tartrazine.

apply cream minimizes risk of further wound contamination.
- If acidosis occurs, discontinue use for 24 to 48 hours.
- Can cause pain and burning at application site; if they occur, notify doctor. Severe and prolonged pain may indicate allergy. If other allergic reactions occur, treatment may have to be temporarily discontinued.
- Sometimes difficult to distinguish between adverse reactions and effects of severe burn.
- Cleanse area before applying. Mafenide washes off with water.
- Keep burn areas medicated at all times.
- Bathe patient daily, if possible.

metronidazole (topical)
MetroGel, MetroGel-Vaginal
Pregnancy Risk Category: B

HOW SUPPLIED
Topical gel: 0.75%
Vaginal gel: 0.75%

MECHANISM OF ACTION
Exact mechanism of action is unknown. May cause a bactericidal effect by an interaction with bacterial DNA.

INDICATIONS & DOSAGE
Topical treatment of acne rosacea –
Adults: apply a thin film b.i.d. to affected area during the morning and evening. Significant results should appear within 3 weeks and continue for the first 9 weeks of therapy.
Treatment of bacterial vaginosis –
Adults: 1 applicatorful b.i.d., in the morning and evening, for 5 days.

ADVERSE REACTIONS
Common reactions are in italics; life-threatening reactions are in bold italics.
Topical form
EENT: lacrimation (if drug applied in area around the eyes).
Vaginal form
CNS: dizziness, light-headedness, headache.
GI: cramps, pain, nausea, diarrhea, constipation.
GU: *cervicitis, vaginitis.*
Skin: rash.
Other: overgrowth of nonsusceptible organisms, metallic or bad taste in mouth, decreased appetite.

INTERACTIONS
Oral anticoagulants: may potentiate anticoagulant effect. Monitor patient for potential adverse reactions.

NURSING CONSIDERATIONS
- *Contraindicated* in patients with hypersensitivity to metronidazole or its other ingredients (such as parabens).
- *Use cautiously* in patients with history or evidence of blood dyscrasias because chemically related compounds are associated with blood dyscrasias.
- For vaginal formulation, *use cautiously* in patients with CNS diseases. Because oral form has been associated with the development of seizures and peripheral neuropathy in a few patients, a theoretical risk exists for patients using the vaginal form. However, plasma levels after typical doses of the vaginal form are usually less than 5% of those seen after a 500-mg oral dose of metronidazole.
- Instruct patient using topical form to avoid use of drug around the eyes. Also advise the patient to clean area thoroughly before use. Cosmetics may be used after applying drug.
- If local reactions occur, advise patient to apply less frequently or to discontinue and contact doctor.
- Topical metronidazole therapy has not been associated with the adverse effects observed with parenteral or oral metronidazole therapy (including disulfiram-like reactions after alcohol ingestion). However, some of the drug can be absorbed after topical use.

Limited clinical experience hasn't shown any of these adverse effects.

miconazole nitrate

Micatin◊, Monistat-Derm Cream and Lotion, Monistat 7 Vaginal Cream◊, Monistat 7 Vaginal Suppository◊, Monistat 3 Vaginal Suppository

Pregnancy Risk Category: C

HOW SUPPLIED

Cream: 2%◊
Lotion: 2%◊
Powder: 2%◊
Spray: 2%◊
Vaginal cream: 2%◊
Vaginal suppositories: 100 mg◊, 200 mg

MECHANISM OF ACTION

Controls or destroys fungus by disrupting fungal cell membrane permeability.

INDICATIONS & DOSAGE

Tinea pedis, tinea cruris, tinea corporis, tinea versicolor, cutaneous candidiasis (moniliasis), infections from common dermatophytes –
Adults and children: apply or spray sparingly b.i.d. for 2 to 4 weeks.
Vulvovaginal candidiasis –
Women: insert 1 applicatorful or suppository (Monistat 7) intravaginally for 7 days at bedtime; repeat course if necessary. Alternatively, insert suppository (Monistat 3) intravaginally for 3 days at bedtime.

ADVERSE REACTIONS

Common reactions are in italics; life-threatening reactions are in bold italics.
Skin: isolated reports of irritation, burning, maceration.
Other: (with vaginal cream) vulvovaginal burning, itching, or irritation.

INTERACTIONS

None significant.

NURSING CONSIDERATIONS

- *Contraindicated* in patients with hypersensitivity to the drug.
- For perineal or intravaginal use only. Keep out of eyes.
- Discontinue if sensitivity or chemical irritation occurs.
- Tell patient to continue using for full treatment period prescribed, even if condition has improved.
- Make sure that patient understands that frequent or persistent yeast infections may be a symptom of a more serious medical problem, such as immunodeficiency or AIDS.
- Do not use occlusive dressings.
- When using intravaginal forms, tell patient to cautiously insert high into the vagina with applicator provided.
- May stain clothing.
- Concurrent use of intravaginal forms and certain latex products, such as vaginal contraceptive diaphragms, are not recommended because of possible interaction.

mupirocin

Bactroban

Pregnancy Risk Category: C

HOW SUPPLIED

Ointment: 2%

MECHANISM OF ACTION

Inhibits bacterial protein and RNA synthesis.

INDICATIONS & DOSAGE

Treatment of common bacterial skin infections caused by susceptible bacteria; treatment of impetigo caused by Staphylococcus aureus *or group A beta-hemolytic streptococci –*
Adults and children: apply to affected areas t.i.d.

ADVERSE REACTIONS

Common reactions are in italics; life-threatening reactions are in bold italics.

*Liquid form contains alcohol. **May contain tartrazine.

Local: burning, itching, stinging, rash.

INTERACTIONS
None reported.

NURSING CONSIDERATIONS
• *Contraindicated* in patients with a history of hypersensitivity to the drug.
• Local reactions appear to be from the polyethylene glycol vehicle.
• If no improvement or condition worsens, notify doctor immediately.
• Prolonged use may cause overgrowth of nonsusceptible bacteria and fungi.
• Not intended for use on burns.
• Do not use in eye.

naftifine
Naftin

Pregnancy Risk Category: B

HOW SUPPLIED
Cream: 1%
Gel: 1%

MECHANISM OF ACTION
Inhibits sterol biosynthesis in susceptible fungi by blocking the actions of the enzyme squalene 2,3 epoxidase. A broad spectrum fungicidal agent.

INDICATIONS & DOSAGE
Treatment of tinea corporis and tinea cruris –
Adults: Apply to affected area b.i.d.

ADVERSE REACTIONS
Common reactions are in italics; life-threatening reactions are in bold italics.
Local: burning, dryness, itching, stinging, local irritation.

INTERACTIONS
None significant.

NURSING CONSIDERATIONS
• *Contraindicated* in patients with hypersensitivity to the drug.
• Not for ophthalmic use. Instruct patient to keep cream away from mucous membranes (eyes, nose, and mouth).
• Instruct patient to wash hands after application.
• Therapy should be reevaluated if there is not improvement after 4 weeks.
• Instruct patient to discontinue therapy and notify doctor if irritation or sensitivity develops.
• Cultures should be done to confirm diagnosis before therapy.

neomycin sulfate
Mycifradin†, Myciguent◇, Neo-Rx

Pregnancy Risk Category: C

HOW SUPPLIED
Cream: 0.5%◇
Ointment: 0.5%◇

MECHANISM OF ACTION
Disrupts protein synthesis.

INDICATIONS & DOSAGE
Topical bacterial infections, minor burns, wounds, skin grafts, following surgical procedure, primary pyodermas, pruritus, trophic ulcerations, otitis externa –
Adults and children: rub in small quantity gently b.i.d., t.i.d., or as directed.

ADVERSE REACTIONS
Common reactions are in italics; life-threatening reactions are in bold italics.
Skin: *rashes, contact dermatitis,* urticaria.
Other: *possible nephrotoxicity, ototoxicity, and* ***neuromuscular blockade;*** *possible systemic absorption when used on extensive areas of the body.*

INTERACTIONS
None significant.

NURSING CONSIDERATIONS
- *Contraindicated* in patients with hypersensitivity to the drug.
- If no improvement or if condition worsens, stop using and report to doctor.
- Don't use on more than 20% of the body surface and on patient with impaired renal function unless risk to benefit ratio has been assessed.
- Prolonged use may result in overgrowth of nonsusceptible organisms.
- In those combination products that contain corticosteroids, use of occlusive dressings increases corticosteroid absorption and the likelihood of systemic effects.
- Enhanced systemic absorption occurs on denuded or abraded areas.
- Watch for signs of hypersensitivity and contact dermatitis.
- Evaluate patient for signs of ototoxicity with prolonged or extended use.

nitrofurazone
Furacin

Pregnancy Risk Category: C

HOW SUPPLIED
Cream: 0.2%
Ointment: 0.2% (soluble dressing)
Topical solution: 0.2%

MECHANISM OF ACTION
Inhibits bacterial enzymes.

INDICATIONS & DOSAGE
Adjunctive treatment of second- and third-degree burns (especially when resistance to other antibiotics and sulfonamides occurs); prevention of skin allograft rejection –
Adults and children: apply directly to lesion daily or every few days, depending on severity of burn.

ADVERSE REACTIONS
Common reactions are in italics; life-threatening reactions are in bold italics.
GU: possible renal toxicity.
Skin: *erythema, pruritus,* burning, edema, severe reactions (vesiculation, denudation, ulceration), *allergic contact dermatitis.*

INTERACTIONS
None significant.

NURSING CONSIDERATIONS
- *Contraindicated* in patients with hypersensitivity to the drug.
- *Use cautiously* in patients with known or suspected renal impairment. Monitor serum creatinine regularly.
- If irritation, sensitization, or infection occurs, discontinue use.
- When using wet dressing, protect skin around wound with zinc oxide ointment.
- Cleanse wound as indicated by doctor before reapplying dressings.
- Solution should be stored in tight, light-resistant containers (brown bottles). Avoid exposure of solution at all times to direct light, prolonged heat, and alkaline materials.
- Drug may discolor in light but is still usable because it retains its potency.
- Discard cloudy solutions if warming to 55° to 60° C (131° to 140° F) does not restore clarity.
- Use reverse isolation and/or sterile application technique to prevent further wound contamination.

nystatin
Mycostatin, Nadostine†, Nilstat

Pregnancy Risk Category: B

HOW SUPPLIED
Cream: 100,000 units/g
Ointment: 100,000 units/g
Powder: 100,000 units/g
Vaginal tablets: 100,000 units

MECHANISM OF ACTION
Alters the permeability of the cell membrane of fungi.

INDICATIONS & DOSAGE
Infant eczema, pruritus ani and vulvae, localized forms of candidiasis –
Adults and children: apply to affected area b.i.d. for 2 weeks.
Vulvovaginal candidiasis –
Adults: one vaginal tablet daily or b.i.d. for 14 days.

ADVERSE REACTIONS
Common reactions are in italics; life-threatening reactions are in bold italics.
Skin: occasional contact dermatitis from preservatives present in some formulations.

INTERACTIONS
None significant.

NURSING CONSIDERATIONS
- *Contraindicated* in patients with hypersensitivity to the drug.
- Generally well tolerated by all age-groups, including debilitated infants.
- Preparation does not stain skin or mucous membranes.
- Cream is recommended for intertriginous areas; powder, for very moist areas; ointment, for dry areas.
- Tell patient to continue using for full treatment period prescribed, even if condition has improved. Immunosuppressed patients may use the drug chronically.
- Do not use occlusive dressings.
- Store vaginal tablets in the refrigerator.

oxiconazole nitrate
Oxistat

Pregnancy Risk Category: B

HOW SUPPLIED
Cream: 1%
Lotion: 1%

MECHANISM OF ACTION
Inhibits ergosterol synthesis in fungal cell walls, causing osmotic instability and cell lysis.

INDICATIONS & DOSAGE
Topical treatment of tinea pedis, tinea cruris, and tinea corporis caused by Trichophyton rubrum, T. mentagrophytes, *and* Epidermophyton floccosum –
Adults: apply to affected area daily or b.i.d. Treat tinea cruris and tinea corporis for 2 weeks and tinea pedis for 1 month to minimize risk of recurrence.

ADVERSE REACTIONS
Common reactions are in italics; life-threatening reactions are in bold italics.
Skin: pruritus, burning, scaling, contact dermatitis, irritation, scaling, tingling, pain, dyshidrotic eczema, folliculitis, erythema, papules, rash, stinging, nodules, maceration, fissuring.

INTERACTIONS
None reported.

NURSING CONSIDERATIONS
- *Contraindicated* in patients with hypersensitivity to the drug or any component of the formulation.
- *Use cautiously* in breast-feeding patients. Oxiconazole is excreted in breast milk.
- Tell patient to discontinue drug and contact doctor if local irritation occurs.
- Be sure patient understands that drug is for external use only. Drug shouldn't come into contact the eyes or vagina.

podofilox
Condylox*

Pregnancy Risk Category: C

HOW SUPPLIED
Topical solution: 0.5%*

MECHANISM OF ACTION
Exact mechanism of action unknown. A keratolytic agent that causes local necrosis of wart tissue.

INDICATIONS & DOSAGE
Topical treatment of external genital warts (condylomata acuminata) –
Adults: apply to affected areas once q 12 hours for 3 consecutive days, then withhold for 4 consecutive days. Repeat this 1-week cycle as needed up to four times until warts disappear.

ADVERSE REACTIONS
Common reactions are in italics; life-threatening reactions are in bold italics.
CNS: insomnia, dizziness.
GI: vomiting.
GU: foreskin irretraction, dyspareunia, hematuria.
Local: burning, pain, inflammation, erosion, itching, tingling, *tenderness*, chafing, scarring, vesicle formation, crusting edema, dryness and peeling.

INTERACTIONS
None reported.

NURSING CONSIDERATIONS
- *Contraindicated* in patients hypersensitive to or intolerant of any component of the medication (the solution contains 95% alcohol).
- Drug should not be used to treat genital warts in the perianal area or on mucus membranes of the genital area (including the urethra, rectum, and vagina).
- If there is no response after 4 weeks of therapy, alternate therapy should be considered.
- Tell patient that the drug is for external use only. Systemic administration has caused hematologic toxicity, hematuria, seizures, and GI disturbances.
- Tell patient that additional applications will not improve efficacy but can increase adverse reactions and the risk of systemic absorption. He should understand that systemic absorption is associated with substantial toxicity.
- Teach patient how to apply the drug:
  – Apply with the supplied cotton-tipped applicator.
  – Dampen the applicator with drug and touch it to the wart.
  – Apply only the least amount that covers the lesion.
  – Limit applications to 0.5 ml or less and to less than 10 cm² (4″) of wart tissue.
  – Allow the area to dry before allowing skin to retract.
  – Dispose of used applicator properly and wash hands thoroughly afterward.
- Tell patient to avoid contact with the eyes. If eye contact occurs, the patient should flush the area with plenty of water and contact his doctor immediately.

silver sulfadiazine
Flamazine†, Flint SSD, Silvadene, SSD-AF, Thermazene
Pregnancy Risk Category: C

HOW SUPPLIED
Cream: 1%

MECHANISM OF ACTION
Acts on cell membrane and cell wall. Broad spectrum; bactericidal for many gram-positive and gram-negative organisms. Also effective against yeasts.

INDICATIONS & DOSAGE
Prevention and treatment of wound infection, especially for second- and third-degree burns –
Adults and children: apply 1/16″ thickness of cream to cleansed and debrided burn wound, then apply daily or b.i.d.

ADVERSE REACTIONS
Common reactions are in italics; life-threatening reactions are in bold italics.

*Liquid form contains alcohol. **May contain tartrazine.

Blood: ***neutropenia*** *(in 3% to 5%) of those receiving extensive applications.*
Skin: pain, burning, rashes, itching.

INTERACTIONS
Topical proteolytic enzymes: inactivity of enzymes when used together. Do not use together.

NURSING CONSIDERATIONS
- *Contraindicated* in premature and newborn infants during first month of life. (Drug may increase possibility of kernicterus.) Use with caution in hypersensitivity to sulfonamides.
- Reverse isolation or sterile application technique recommended to prevent wound contamination.
- If hepatic or renal dysfunction occurs, consider discontinuing drug.
- Inspect patient's skin daily, and note any changes. Notify doctor if burning or excessive pain develops.
- Use only on affected areas. Keep medicated at all times.
- For patients with extensive burns, monitor serum sulfadiazine concentrations and renal function, and check urine for sulfa crystals.
- Bathe patient daily, if possible.
- Discard darkened cream.

sulconazole nitrate
Exelderm

Pregnancy Risk Category: C

HOW SUPPLIED
Topical solution: 1%
Cream: 1%

MECHANISM OF ACTION
Unknown. An imidazole derivative that inhibits the growth of both fungi and yeast.

INDICATIONS & DOSAGE
Treatment of tinea cruris and tinea corporis caused by Trichophyton mentagrophytes, Epidermophyton floccosum, *and* Microsporum canis; *treatment of tinea versicolor caused by* Malassezia furfur –
Adults: massage a small amount of solution or cream into affected area daily to b.i.d.

ADVERSE REACTIONS
Common reactions are in italics; life-threatening reactions are in bold italics.
Local: itching, burning, stinging.

INTERACTIONS
None reported.

NURSING CONSIDERATIONS
- *Contraindicated* in patients hypersensitive to any component of the product.
- Treatment should continue for at least 3 weeks. If irritation develops during treatment, drug should be discontinued and patient should contact the doctor. If no improvement after 4 weeks, diagnosis should be reconsidered.
- Clinical improvement is usually apparent within a week, with symptomatic relief in just a few days. Explain to the patient that he should complete the full course of therapy, even after symptoms subside, to prevent recurrence.
- Efficacy against athlete's foot (tinea pedis) has not been proven.
- Patient should avoid contact with the eyes and should wash hands thoroughly after applying.

terbinafine hydrochloride
Lamisil

Pregnancy Risk Category: B

HOW SUPPLIED
Cream: 1%

MECHANISM OF ACTION
Selectively inhibits an early step in the synthesis of sterols used by fungi for cell wall synthesis. Fungicidal.

INDICATIONS & DOSAGE
Interdigital tinea pedis, tinea cruris, and tinea corporis caused by Trichophyton mentagrophytes, T. rubrum, *and* Epidermophyton floccosum –
Adults: apply sufficient cream to cover the affected area and the immediate surrounding area, b.i.d., for at least 1 week.

ADVERSE REACTIONS
Common reactions are in italics; life-threatening reactions are in bold italics.
Skin: irritation, burning, itching, dryness.

INTERACTIONS
None reported.

NURSING CONSIDERATIONS
• *Contraindicated* in patients with hypersensitivity to the drug.
• Tell patient to discontinue drug and contact doctor if irritation or sensitivity develops.
• Duration of drug therapy shouldn't exceed 4 weeks.
• Teach patient proper use of drug. He should use it only as directed and shouldn't apply it near the eyes, mouth, or mucous membranes; should use it for the full treatment course recommended by the doctor, even if symptoms disappear; and shouldn't use occlusive dressings unless otherwise directed by the doctor.
• In clinical trials, many patients continued to improve for 2 to 4 weeks after therapy was discontinued. Consequently, patients should be observed for 2 to 4 weeks after therapy is complete before determining whether or not therapy was successful. Review the diagnosis if the condition persists beyond this observation period.

terconazole
Terazol 3 Vaginal Suppositories, Terazol 7 Vaginal Cream
Pregnancy Risk Category: C

HOW SUPPLIED
Vaginal cream: 0.4%, 0.8%
Vaginal suppositories: 80 mg

MECHANISM OF ACTION
Exact mechanism unknown; may increase fungal cell membrane permeability (*Candida* species only).

INDICATIONS & DOSAGE
Local treatment of vulvovaginal candidiasis –
Adults: insert 1 applicatorful of cream into vagina h.s. for 7 days; or 1 suppository intravaginally h.s. for 3 days; may repeat course if necessary after reconfirmation by smear and/or culture

ADVERSE REACTIONS
Common reactions are in italics; life-threatening reactions are in bold italics.
CNS: headache.
Skin: vulvovaginal burning, irritation.
Other: fever, chills, body aches.

INTERACTIONS
None.

NURSING CONSIDERATIONS
• *Contraindicated* in patients with known sensitivity to terconazole or any inactive ingredients in formulations.
• Discontinue and do not retreat if patient develops fever, chills, other flu-like symptoms, or sensitivity.
• Some photosensitivity reactions were observed after dermal use; none observed with vaginal use.
• Vaginal burning or itching is reportedly less frequent with terconazole than with miconazole or clotrimazole.
• Therapeutic effect of terconazole is

unaffected by menstruation. However, tell patient not to use tampons during treatment.
• Tell patient to use for full treatment period prescribed. Explain how to prevent reinfection.

tetracycline hydrochloride

Achromycin, Topicycline

Pregnancy Risk Category: D

HOW SUPPLIED

Ointment: 3%
Topical solution: 2.2 mg/ml

MECHANISM OF ACTION

Disrupts protein synthesis.

INDICATIONS & DOSAGE

Acne vulgaris –
Adults and children over 12 years: apply generously to affected areas b.i.d. until skin is thoroughly covered.
Prevention or treatment of superficial skin infections caused by susceptible bacteria –
Adults: apply a sufficient amount to affected area b.i.d. to t.i.d.

ADVERSE REACTIONS

Common reactions are in italics; life-threatening reactions are in bold italics.
Skin: temporary stinging or burning on application; slight yellowing of treated skin, especially in patients with light complexions; severe dermatitis.

INTERACTIONS

None significant.

NURSING CONSIDERATIONS

• *Contraindicated* in patients with hypersensitivity to the drug.
• Wash area before applying.
• If no improvement or if condition worsens, stop using and notify doctor.
• Prolonged use may result in overgrowth of nonsusceptible organisms.
• Patient may continue normal use of cosmetics.
• Store at room temperature, away from excessive heat.
• Medication to be used by one person only. Tell patient not to share with family members.
• Apply in morning and evening. Warn that drug should be used or discarded within 2 months.
• Explain that floating plug in bottle of Topicycline – an inert and harmless result of proper reconstitution of the preparation – shouldn't be removed.
• Serum levels with topical tetracycline hydrochloride are much lower than those for orally administered drug, so significant systemic effects are unlikely.
• To control flow rate of solution, increase or decrease pressure of the applicator against the skin.

tioconazole

Vagistat

Pregnancy Risk Category: C

HOW SUPPLIED

Vaginal ointment: 6.5%

MECHANISM OF ACTION

A fungicidal imidazole that alters cell wall permeability.

INDICATIONS & DOSAGE

Treatment of vulvovaginal candidiasis –
Women: insert 1 applicatorful (about 4.6 g) intravaginally h.s.

ADVERSE REACTIONS

Common reactions are in italics; life-threatening reactions are in bold italics.
GU: *burning, itching,* discharge, vulvar edema and swelling, irritation.

INTERACTIONS

None reported.

NURSING CONSIDERATIONS

• *Contraindicated* in patients with hypersensitivity to the drug or other imidazole antifungal agents (miconazole, ketoconazole).
• To avoid contamination of the ointment, open the applicator just before using it.
• Review proper use of the drug with the patient. Instruct the patient to insert drug high into the vagina. Written instructions for the patient are available with the product.
• Watch for irritation or sensitivity. If it occurs, discontinue drug and report adverse reaction to the doctor.
• Emphasize to the patient the need to complete the full course of therapy, even after symptoms have improved. The patient should continue using the drug even during her menstrual period.
• Patient should use a sanitary napkin to avoid staining of clothing.
• Patient should avoid sexual intercourse during therapy or advise partner to use a condom to prevent reinfection.

tolnaftate

Aftate for Athlete's Foot◇, Aftate for Jock Itch◇, Dr. Scholl's Athlete's Foot Powder◇, Dr. Scholl's Athlete's Foot Spray◇, Footwork◇, Fungatin◇, Genaspor◇, NP-27◇, Tinactin◇, Ting◇, Zeasorb-AF◇

Pregnancy Risk Category: C

HOW SUPPLIED

Aerosol liquid: 1% (with 36% alcohol)◇
Aerosol powder: 1% (with 14% alcohol)◇
Cream: 1%◇
Gel: 1%◇
Powder: 1%◇
Pump spray liquid: 1% (with 36% alcohol)◇
Topical solution: 1%◇

MECHANISM OF ACTION

Fungistatic and fungicidal activity.

INDICATIONS & DOSAGE

Superficial fungal infections of the skin, infections due to common pathogenic fungi, tinea pedis, tinea cruris, tinea corporis, tinea versicolor–
Adults and children: ¼″ to ½″ ribbon of cream or 3 drops of lotion to cover about the size of one hand; same amount of cream or 3 drops of lotion to cover the toes and interdigital webs of one foot; or an amount of gel, powder, or spray to cover affected area. Apply and massage gently into skin b.i.d. for 2 to 6 weeks.

ADVERSE REACTIONS

Common reactions are in italics; life-threatening reactions are in bold italics.
Skin: possible irritation in hypersensitive person.

INTERACTIONS

None significant.

NURSING CONSIDERATIONS

• *Contraindicated* in patients with hypersensitivity to the drug.
• Discontinue if condition worsens. Check with doctor.
• Odorless, greaseless. Won't stain or discolor skin, hair, nails, or clothing.
• Use only a small quantity of cream or lotion; treated area should not be wet with solution.
• Commonly used to treat athlete's foot (tinea pedis). If no improvement after 10 days, consult doctor.
• Tell patient to continue using for full treatment period prescribed, even if condition has improved.
• Don't use as a side agent to treat hair or nail infections. Will not eradicate fungus from these structures.
• Powder or aerosol may continue to be used inside socks and shoes of persons susceptible to tinea infections.

undecylenic acid and zinc undecylenate

Cruex◇, Desenex◇, Desenex Aerosol◇, Quinsana Plus◇

Pregnancy Risk Category: C

HOW SUPPLIED

Powder: 2% undecylenic acid and 20% zinc undecylenate◇

MECHANISM OF ACTION

Fungistatic and fungicidal activity.

INDICATIONS & DOSAGE

Athlete's foot and ringworm of the body except nails and hairy areas –
Adults and children: apply b.i.d. to thoroughly cleansed area.

ADVERSE REACTIONS

Common reactions are in italics; life-threatening reactions are in bold italics.
Skin: possible irritation in hypersensitive person.

INTERACTIONS

None significant.

NURSING CONSIDERATIONS

- *Contraindicated* in patients with hypersensitivity to the drug.
- Tell patient to continue using for full treatment period prescribed, even if condition has improved.
- Apply for at least 2 weeks to minimize risk of relapse.
- Liquids are preferable for hairy areas; powders in moist areas, for example, between skin folds.

Scabicides and pediculicides

benzyl benzoate lotion
crotamiton
lindane
permethrin
pyrethrins

COMBINATION PRODUCTS
None.

benzyl benzoate lotion

Scabanca†

Pregnancy Risk Category: C

HOW SUPPLIED
Lotion: 14% (with benzocaine 2%)
Emulsion: 50%

MECHANISM OF ACTION
Unknown.

INDICATIONS & DOSAGE
Parasitic infestation (scabies, Phthirus pubis, Pediculus capitis) –
Adults and children: first, scrub entire body with soap and water. Remove scales or crusts. Then apply the lotion undiluted over entire body, except the face and scalp, while still damp. Be sure to apply around nails. Let dry. Apply second coat on the most involved areas. Bathe after 24 hours.

ADVERSE REACTIONS
Common reactions are in italics; life-threatening reactions are in bold italics.
Skin: *irritation, itching; contact dermatitis with repeated applications.*

INTERACTIONS
None significant.

NURSING CONSIDERATIONS
- *Contraindicated* when skin is raw or inflamed. Notify doctor immediately if skin irritation or hypersensitivity develops; tell patient to discontinue drug and to wash it off skin.
- If live mites or new lesions occur, retreatment may be indicated in 7 to 10 days.
- Preferred over lindane for treatment of infants, young children, and pregnant or breast-feeding women.
- Do not apply to face, eyes, mucous membranes, or urethral meatus. If accidental contact with eyes does occur, flush with water and notify doctor.
- Instruct patient to change and sterilize (boil, launder, dry clean, or apply very hot iron) all clothing and bed linen after drug is washed off.
- Itching may continue for several weeks; this does not indicate that therapy is ineffective. Reassure patient that itching will cease.
- Topical corticosteroids may be needed if dermatitis develops from scratching.
- After application for lice infestation, use a fine-tooth comb dipped in white vinegar on hair to remove nits from hairy areas.
- Instruct patient to reapply if drug is washed off during treatment time.
- Don't apply to infant's or small children's hands because they will put hands in their mouths.
- Hospitalized patients should be placed in isolation with linen-handling precautions until treatment is completed.
- Store drug in light-resistant container; avoid exposure to excessive heat.

crotamiton

Eurax

Pregnancy Risk Category: C

HOW SUPPLIED
Cream: 10%

MECHANISM OF ACTION
Unknown.

INDICATIONS & DOSAGE
Parasitic infestation (scabies) –
Adults and children: first, scrub entire body with soap and water. Remove scales or crusts. Then, apply a thin layer of cream over entire body, from chin down (with special attention to folds, creases, interdigital spaces, and genital area). Apply second coat in 24 hours. Wait additional 48 hours, then wash off.
Itching –
Adults and children: apply locally b.i.d. or t.i.d.

ADVERSE REACTIONS
Common reactions are in italics; life-threatening reactions are in bold italics.
Skin: *irritation.*

INTERACTIONS
None significant.

NURSING CONSIDERATIONS
- *Contraindicated* when skin is raw or inflamed. Notify doctor immediately if skin irritation or hypersensitivity develops; tell patient to discontinue drug and to wash it off skin.
- Do not apply to face, eyes, mucous membranes, or urethral meatus. If accidental contact with eyes does occur, flush with water and notify doctor.
- Instruct patient to change and sterilize (boil, launder, dry clean, or apply very hot iron) all clothing and bed linen after drug is washed off.
- After application for lice infestation, use a fine-tooth comb dipped in white vinegar on hair to remove nits from hairy areas.
- Topical corticosteroids may be needed if dermatitis develops from scratching.
- Tendency to overuse scabicides. Estimate amount needed.
- Question other family members and sexual contacts about infestation.
- Instruct patient to reapply if drug is washed off during treatment time.
- Hospitalized patients should be placed in isolation with special linen-handling precautions until treatment is completed.

lindane
Gamma Benzene, gBh†, Kildane, Kwell, Kwellada†, Scabene
Pregnancy Risk Category: C

HOW SUPPLIED
Cream: 1%
Lotion: 1%
Shampoo: 1%

MECHANISM OF ACTION
Appears to inhibit neuronal membrane function in arthropods.

INDICATIONS & DOSAGE
Parasitic infestation (scabies, pediculosis) –
Adults and children: scrub entire body with soap and water.
Cream or lotion – apply thin layer over entire skin surface (with special attention to folds, creases, interdigital spaces, and genital area) for scabies, or to hairy areas for pediculosis. After 12 hours, wash off drug. If second application is needed, wait 1 week before repeating, but never more than twice in a week.
Shampoo – apply 30 ml undiluted to affected area and work into lather for 4 to 5 minutes. Rinse thoroughly and rub with dry towel.

ADVERSE REACTIONS
Common reactions are in italics; life-threatening reactions are in bold italics.
CNS: dizziness, ***seizures.***
Skin: irritation with repeated use.

INTERACTIONS
None significant.

NURSING CONSIDERATIONS
• *Contraindicated* in patients with hypersensitivity to the drug and when skin is raw or inflamed. Notify doctor immediately if skin irritation or hypersensitivity develops; tell patient to discontinue drug and to wash it off skin.
• *Use cautiously* in infants and young children as there's a greater risk for CNS toxicity in this group.
• Do not apply to open areas or acutely inflamed skin, or to face, eyes, mucous membranes, or urethral meatus. If accidental contact with eyes does occur, flush with water and notify doctor. Avoid inhaling vapors.
• Discourage repeated use, which can lead to skin irritation and systemic toxicity. Repeat use only if live lice or nits are found after 1 week.
• Warn patient that itching may continue for several weeks after effective treatment, especially in scabies.
• Topical corticosteroids or oral antihistamines may be needed for itching.
• Instruct patient to change and sterilize (boil, launder, dry clean, or apply very hot iron) all clothing and bed linen after drug is washed off.
• After application, use a fine-tooth comb dipped in white vinegar on hair to remove nits.
• Lindane shampoo can be used to clean combs or brushes; wash them thoroughly afterward. Warn patient not to use routinely.
• Instruct patient to reapply if drug is washed off during treatment time.
• Hospitalized patients should be placed in isolation with special linen-handling precautions until treatment is completed.
• Extremely toxic to CNS if accidentally swallowed.

permethrin
Elimite, Nix
Pregnancy Risk Category: B

HOW SUPPLIED
Cream: 5%
Topical liquid: 1%

MECHANISM OF ACTION
Acts on the parasites' nerve cells to disrupt the sodium channel current, causing paralysis of the parasite.

INDICATIONS & DOSAGE
Treatment of infestation with Pediculus humanus capitis *(head lice) and its nits –*
Adults and children: use after hair has been washed with shampoo, rinsed with water, and towel-dried. Apply a sufficient amount (25 to 50 ml) of liquid to saturate the hair and scalp. Allow to remain on hair for 10 minutes before rinsing off with water.
Treatment of scabies (Sarcoptes scabiei) –
Adults and children: massage cream into the skin, from the head to the soles of the feet. Remove cream by washing (shower or bath) in 8 to 14 hours.

ADVERSE REACTIONS
Common reactions are in italics; life-threatening reactions are in bold italics.
Skin: itching, burning, stinging, tingling, numbness or scalp discomfort, mild erythema, rash on the scalp.

INTERACTIONS
None reported.

NURSING CONSIDERATIONS
• *Contraindicated* in patients with hypersensitivity to pyrethrins or chrysanthemums. Don't use in infants because their skin is more permeable than that of children or adults.
• A single treatment is usually all that is necessary. Combing of nits is not

*Liquid form contains alcohol. **May contain tartrazine.

required for effectiveness, but drug package supplies a fine-tooth comb for cosmetic use as desired.
- A second application may be necessary if lice are observed 7 days after the initial application.
- Head lice infestation is frequently accompanied by pruritus, erythema, and edema. Explain to the patient that treatment with permethrin may temporarily worsen these symptoms.
- Permethrin has been shown to be at least as effective as lindane (Kwell) in treating head lice.

pyrethrins

A-200 Pyrinate◇, Barc◇, Blue Gel, R&C, Pronto, Pyrinyl◇, RID◇, TISIT◇, Triple X◇

Pregnancy Risk Category: C

HOW SUPPLIED

Shampoo: pyrethrins 0.17% and piperonyl butoxide 2%; pyrethrins 0.3% and piperonyl butoxide 3%
Topical gel: pyrethrins 0.18% and piperonyl butoxide 2.2%; pyrethrins 0.33% and piperonyl butoxide 3%; pyrethrins 0.3% and piperonyl butoxide 4%
Topical solution: pyrethrins 0.18% and piperonyl butoxide 2%; pyrethrins 0.2%, piperonyl butoxide 2%, and deodorized kerosene 0.8%; pyrethrins 0.3% and piperonyl butoxide 3%

MECHANISM OF ACTION

Acts as contact poison that disrupts the parasite's nervous system, causing the parasite's paralysis and death.

INDICATIONS & DOSAGE

Treatment of infestations of head, body, and pubic (crab) lice and their eggs –
Adults and children: apply to hair, scalp, or other infested area until entirely wet. Allow to remain for 10 minutes, but no longer. Wash thoroughly with warm water and soap, or shampoo. Remove dead lice and eggs with fine-tooth comb. Treatment may be repeated, if necessary, but don't exceed two applications within 24 hours. May repeat in 7 to 10 days to kill newly hatched lice.

ADVERSE REACTIONS

Common reactions are in italics; life-threatening reactions are in bold italics.
Skin: *irritation with repeated use.*

INTERACTIONS

None significant.

NURSING CONSIDERATIONS

- *Contraindicated* in hypersensitivity to the drug or when skin is raw or inflamed. Notify doctor immediately if skin irritation develops; tell patient to discontinue drug and to wash it off skin. All preparations contain petroleum distillates. Also *contraindicated* in patients allergic to ragweed.
- *Use cautiously* in infants and small children.
- Do not apply to open areas or acutely inflamed skin, or to face, eyes, mucous membranes, or urethral meatus. If accidental contact with eyes does occur, flush with water and notify doctor.
- Discourage repeated use, which can lead to skin irritation and possible systemic toxicity.
- Topical corticosteroids or oral antihistamines may be needed if dermatitis develops from scratching.
- Instruct patient to change and sterilize (boil, launder, dry clean, or apply very hot iron) all clothing and bed linen after drug is washed off.
- Some authorities believe pyrethrins and lindane (Kwell) are equally effective for lice infestation and that pyrethrins are less hazardous.
- Teach patient to remove dead parasites with a fine-tooth comb.
- Not effective against scabies.

89
Topical corticosteroids

alclometasone dipropionate
amcinonide
betamethasone benzoate
betamethasone dipropionate
betamethasone valerate
clobetasol propionate
clocortolone pivalate
desonide
desoximetasone
dexamethasone
dexamethasone sodium phosphate
diflorasone diacetate
fluocinolone acetonide
fluocinonide
flurandrenolide
fluticasone propionate
halcinonide
halobetasol propionate
hydrocortisone
hydrocortisone acetate
hydrocortisone butyrate
hydrocortisone valerate
methylprednisolone acetate
mometasone furoate
triamcinolone acetonide

COMBINATION PRODUCTS
Corticosteroids for topical use are commonly combined with antibiotics and antifungals. (See Chapter 87, LOCAL ANTI-INFECTIVES.)

alclometasone dipropionate
Alclovate, Logoderm‡
Pregnancy Risk Category: C

HOW SUPPLIED
Cream: 0.05%
Ointment: 0.05%

MECHANISM OF ACTION
Diffuses across cell membranes to form complexes with specific cytoplasmic receptors.

INDICATIONS & DOSAGE
Inflammation of corticosteroid-responsive dermatoses—
Adults: apply a thin film to affected areas b.i.d. or t.i.d. Gently massage until the medication disappears.

ADVERSE REACTIONS
Common reactions are in italics; life-threatening reactions are in bold italics.
Skin: burning, itching, irritation, dryness, folliculitis, striae, acneiform eruptions, perioral dermatitis, hypopigmentation, hypertrichosis, allergic contact dermatitis. With occlusive dressings: *secondary infection, maceration, atrophy, striae, miliaria.*

INTERACTIONS
None significant.

NURSING CONSIDERATIONS
- *Use cautiously* in viral skin diseases, such as varicella, vaccinia, and herpes simplex; in fungal infections; and in bacterial skin infections.
- Warn patient not to use for more than 14 consecutive days because of the potential for systemic absorption and suppression of hypothalamic-pituitary-adrenal axis.
- Avoid application near eyes or mucous membranes. Do not apply to face, armpits, groin, or under breasts unless specifically ordered.
- Systemic absorption especially likely with occlusive dressings, prolonged treatment, or application to extensive body surface.
- Stop drug and notify doctor if patient develops signs of systemic ab-

sorption, skin irritation or ulceration, hypersensitivity, or infection. (If antifungals or antibiotics are being used concurrently, and infection does not respond immediately, corticosteroids should be discontinued until infection is controlled.)

- Before applying, wash skin gently. To prevent damage to skin, rub medication in gently, leaving a thin coat. When treating hairy sites, part hair and apply directly to lesion.
- Occlusive dressing (if ordered): Apply cream, then cover with a thin, pliable, nonflammable plastic film; seal to adjacent normal skin with hypoallergenic tape. Minimize adverse reactions by using occlusive dressing intermittently. Don't leave in place longer than 16 hours each day. Occlusive dressings should not be used in presence of infections or with weeping or exudative lesions.
- Notify doctor and remove occlusive dressing if fever develops.
- Change dressings as ordered by doctor. Inspect skin for infection, striae, and atrophy. Discontinue drug and notify doctor if these occur.
- Treatment should be continued for a few days after clearing of lesions to prevent recurrence.
- Repeated application can result in diminished effectiveness.

amcinonide

Cyclocort

Pregnancy Risk Category: C

HOW SUPPLIED

Cream: 0.1%
Lotion: 0.1%
Ointment: 0.1%

MECHANISM OF ACTION

Diffuses across cell membranes and complexes with specific cytoplasmic receptors.

INDICATIONS & DOSAGE

Inflammation of corticosteroid-responsive dermatoses –

Adults and children: apply a light film to affected areas b.i.d. or t.i.d. Cream should be rubbed in gently and thoroughly until it disappears.

ADVERSE REACTIONS

Common reactions are in italics; life-threatening reactions are in bold italics.

Skin: burning, itching, irritation, dryness, folliculitis, striae, acneiform eruptions, perioral dermatitis, hypopigmentation, hypertrichosis, allergic contact dermatitis. With occlusive dressings: *secondary infection, maceration, atrophy, striae, miliaria.*

INTERACTIONS

None significant.

NURSING CONSIDERATIONS

- *Use cautiously* in viral diseases of skin, such as varicella, vaccinia, herpes simplex; fungal infections; bacterial skin infections.
- Avoid application near eyes or mucous membranes. Do not use on face, armpits, groin, in ear canal, or under breasts unless specifically ordered.
- Systemic absorption especially likely with occlusive dressings, prolonged treatment, or extensive body-surface treatment.
- When used in young children, avoid the use of plastic pants or tight-fitting diapers in treated areas.
- Stop drug and notify doctor if patient develops signs of systemic absorption, skin irritation or ulceration, hypersensitivity, or infection. (If antifungals or antibiotics are being used with corticosteroids and infection does not respond immediately, corticosteroids should be stopped until infection is controlled.)
- Before applying, gently wash skin. To prevent damage to skin, rub medication in gently, leaving a thin coat.

When treating hairy sites, part hair and apply directly to lesion.
- Occlusive dressing (if ordered): apply cream, then cover with a thin, pliable, nonflammable plastic film; seal to adjacent normal skin with hypoallergenic tape. Minimize adverse reactions by using occlusive dressing intermittently. Don't leave in place longer than 16 hours each day. Occlusive dressings should not be used in presence of infections or with weeping or exudative lesions.
- For patient with eczematous dermatitis who may develop irritation with adhesive material, hold dressing in place with gauze, elastic bandages, stockings, or stockinette.
- Notify doctor and remove occlusive dressing if fever develops.
- Change dressings as ordered by doctor. Inspect skin for infection, striae, and atrophy. Discontinue drug and notify doctor if these occur.
- Treatment should be continued for a few days after clearing of lesions to prevent recurrence.

betamethasone benzoate
Benisone, Uticort

betamethasone dipropionate
Alphatrex, Diprolene, Diprolene AF, Diprosone, Maxivate, Psorion

betamethasone valerate
Betatrex, Beta-Val, Betnovate†‡, Valisone

Pregnancy Risk Category: C

HOW SUPPLIED
benzoate
Cream: 0.025%
Gel: 0.025%
Lotion: 0.025%
Ointment: 0.025%
dipropionate
Aerosol: 0.1%
Cream: 0.05%
Lotion: 0.05%
Ointment: 0.05%
valerate
Aerosol: 0.1%
Cream: 0.01%, 0.1%
Lotion: 0.1%
Ointment: 0.1%

MECHANISM OF ACTION
Diffuses across cell membranes and complexes with specific cytoplasmic receptors.

INDICATIONS & DOSAGE
Inflammation of corticosteroid-responsive dermatoses –
Adults and children: clean area; apply cream, lotion, spray, or gel sparingly daily to q.i.d.

ADVERSE REACTIONS
Common reactions are in italics; life-threatening reactions are in bold italics.
Skin: burning, itching, irritation, dryness, folliculitis, striae, acneiform eruptions, perioral dermatitis, hypopigmentation, hypertrichosis, allergic contact dermatitis. With occlusive dressings: *secondary infection, maceration, atrophy, striae, miliaria.*

INTERACTIONS
None significant.

NURSING CONSIDERATIONS
- *Use cautiously* in viral diseases of skin, such as varicella, vaccinia, herpes simplex; fungal infections; bacterial skin infections.
- Avoid application near eyes, mucous membranes, or in ear canal.
- Due to alcohol content of vehicle, gel preparations may cause mild, transient stinging, especially if used on or near excoriated skin.
- Systemic absorption especially likely with occlusive dressings, prolonged treatment, or extensive body-surface treatment.
- When used in young children, avoid

*Liquid form contains alcohol. **May contain tartrazine.

the use of plastic pants or tight-fitting diapers in treated areas.

- Stop drug and notify doctor if patient develops signs of systemic absorption, skin irritation or ulceration, hypersensitivity, or infection. (If antifungals or antibiotics are being used with corticosteroids and infection does not respond immediately, corticosteroids should be stopped until infection is controlled.)
- Before applying, gently wash skin. To prevent damage to skin, rub medication in gently, leaving a thin coat. When treating hairy sites, part hair and apply directly to lesion.
- Occlusive dressing (if ordered): Apply cream, then cover with a thin, pliable, nonflammable plastic film; seal to adjacent normal skin with hypoallergenic tape. Minimize adverse reactions by using occlusive dressing intermittently. Don't leave in place longer than 16 hours each day. Occlusive dressings should not be used in presence of infections or with weeping or exudative lesions.
- For patient with eczematous dermatitis who may develop irritation with adhesive material, hold dressing in place with gauze, elastic bandages, stockings, or stockinette.
- Notify doctor and remove occlusive dressing if fever develops.
- Change dressings as ordered by doctor. Inspect skin for infection, striae, and atrophy. Discontinue drug and notify doctor if these occur.
- Treatment should be continued for a few days after clearing of lesions to prevent recurrence.
- Note that Diprolene and Diprolene AF may not be substituted generically because other products have different potencies.

clobetasol propionate

Dermovate†, Temovate

Pregnancy Risk Category: C

HOW SUPPLIED

Cream: 0.05%
Lotion: 0.05%
Ointment: 0.05%

MECHANISM OF ACTION

Diffuses across cell membranes and forms complexes with specific cytoplasmic receptors.

INDICATIONS & DOSAGE

Inflammation of corticosteroid-responsive dermatoses –

Adults: apply a thin layer to affected skin areas b.i.d., once in the morning and once at night. Do not use more than 50 g of cream or ointment/week. Therapy should be limited to a maximum of 14 days.

ADVERSE REACTIONS

Common reactions are in italics; life-threatening reactions are in bold italics.

Skin: burning, itching, irritation, dryness, folliculitis, perioral dermatitis, allergic contact dermatitis, hypopigmentation, hypertrichosis, acneiform eruptions.

INTERACTIONS

None significant.

NURSING CONSIDERATIONS

- *Use cautiously* in viral skin diseases, such as varicella, vaccinia, herpes simplex; fungal infections; bacterial skin infections. Not recommended for children under 12 years.
- Clobetasol is a potent, fluoridated corticosteroid. Warn patient not to use for longer than 14 consecutive days because of the risk of systemic absorption and suppression of hypothalamic-pituitary-adrenal axis.
- Avoid application near eyes, mucous membranes, or in ear canal.
- Occlusive dressings should not be used. Treated areas of skin should not be bandaged, covered, or wrapped.
- Stop drug and notify doctor if patient develops signs of systemic ab-

sorption, skin irritation or ulceration, hypersensitivity, or infection. (If antifungals or antibiotics are being used with corticosteroids and infection does not respond immediately, corticosteroids should be stopped until infection is controlled.)
- Before applying, gently wash skin. To prevent damage to skin, rub medication in gently, leaving a thin coat. When treating hairy sites, part hair and apply directly to lesions.
- Inspect skin for infection, striae, and atrophy. Discontinue drug and notify doctor if these occur.
- Repeated application can result in diminished effectiveness.
- Do not refrigerate.

clocortolone pivalate
Cloderm

Pregnancy Risk Category: C

HOW SUPPLIED
Cream: 0.1%

MECHANISM OF ACTION
Diffuses across cell membranes and complexes with specific cytoplasmic receptors.

INDICATIONS & DOSAGE
Inflammation of corticosteroid-responsive dermatoses –
Adults and children: apply cream sparingly to affected areas once daily to q.i.d. and rub in gently.

ADVERSE REACTIONS
Common reactions are in italics; life-threatening reactions are in bold italics.
Skin: burning, itching, irritation, dryness, folliculitis, striae, acneiform eruptions, perioral dermatitis, hypertrichosis, hypopigmentation, allergic contact dermatitis. With occlusive dressings: *secondary infection, maceration, atrophy, striae, miliaria.*

INTERACTIONS
None significant.

NURSING CONSIDERATIONS
- *Use cautiously* in viral diseases of skin, such as varicella, vaccinia, herpes simplex; fungal infections; bacterial skin infections.
- Avoid application near eyes or mucous membranes.
- Systemic absorption especially likely with occlusive dressings, prolonged treatment, or extensive body-surface treatment.
- When used in young children, avoid the use of plastic pants or tight-fitting diapers in treated areas.
- Stop drug and notify doctor if patient develops signs of systemic absorption, skin irritation or ulceration, hypersensitivity, or infection. (If antifungals or antibiotics are being used with corticosteroids and infection does not respond immediately, corticosteroids should be stopped until infection is controlled.)
- Before applying, gently wash skin. To prevent damage to skin, rub medication in gently, leaving a thin coat. When treating hairy sites, part hair and apply directly to lesion.
- Occlusive dressing (if ordered): Apply cream, then cover with a thin, pliable, nonflammable plastic film; seal to adjacent normal skin with hypoallergenic tape. Minimize adverse reactions by using occlusive dressing intermittently. Don't leave in place longer than 16 hours each day. Occlusive dressings should not be used in presence of infections or with weeping or exudative lesions.
- For patient with eczematous dermatitis who may develop irritation with adhesive material, hold dressing in place with gauze, elastic bandages, or stockinette.
- Notify doctor and remove occlusive dressing if fever develops.
- Change dressings as ordered by doctor. Inspect skin for infection,

striae, and atrophy. Discontinue drug and notify doctor if these occur.
• Treatment should be continued for a few days after clearing of lesions to prevent recurrence.

desonide

DesOwen, Tridesilon

Pregnancy Risk Category: C

HOW SUPPLIED

Cream: 0.05%
Ointment: 0.05%

MECHANISM OF ACTION

Diffuses across cell membranes and complexes with specific cytoplasmic receptors.

INDICATIONS & DOSAGE

Adjunctive therapy for inflammation in acute and chronic corticosteroid-responsive dermatoses –
Adults and children: clean area; apply cream or lotion sparingly b.i.d. to q.i.d.

ADVERSE REACTIONS

Common reactions are in italics; life-threatening reactions are in bold italics.
Skin: burning, itching, irritation, dryness, folliculitis, perioral dermatitis, allergic contact dermatitis, hypertrichosis, hypopigmentation, acneiform eruptions. With occlusive dressings: *maceration of skin, secondary infection, atrophy, striae, miliaria.*

INTERACTIONS

None significant.

NURSING CONSIDERATIONS

• *Use cautiously* in viral diseases of skin, such as varicella, vaccinia, herpes simplex; fungal infections; bacterial skin infections.
• Avoid application near eyes, mucous membranes, or in ear canal.
• Systemic absorption especially likely with occlusive dressings, prolonged treatment, or extensive body-surface treatment.
• When used in young children, avoid the use of plastic pants or tight-fitting diapers in treated areas.
• Stop drug and notify doctor if patient develops signs of systemic absorption, skin irritation or ulceration, hypersensitivity, or infection. (If antifungals or antibiotics are being used with corticosteroids and infection does not respond immediately, corticosteroids should be stopped until infection is controlled.)
• Before applying, gently wash skin. To prevent damage to skin, rub medication in gently, leaving a thin coat. When treating hairy sites, part hair and apply directly to lesion.
• Occlusive dressing (if ordered): Apply cream or ointment, then cover with a thin, pliable, nonflammable plastic film; seal to adjacent normal skin with hypoallergenic tape. Minimize adverse reactions by using occlusive dressing intermittently. Don't leave in place longer than 16 hours each day. Occlusive dressings should not be used in presence of infection or with weeping or exudative lesions.
• For patient with eczematous dermatitis who may develop irritation with adhesive material, hold dressing in place with gauze, elastic bandages, stockings, or stockinette.
• Notify doctor and remove occlusive dressing if fever develops.
• Change dressing as ordered by doctor. Inspect skin for infection, striae, and atrophy. Discontinue drug and notify doctor if these occur.
• Treatment should be continued for a few days after clearing of lesions to prevent recurrence.

desoximetasone

Topicort

Pregnancy Risk Category: C

HOW SUPPLIED
Cream: 0.05%, 0.25%
Gel: 0.05%
Ointment: 0.25%

MECHANISM OF ACTION
Diffuses across cell membranes and complexes with specific cytoplasmic receptors.

INDICATIONS & DOSAGE
Inflammation of corticosteroid-responsive dermatoses –
Adults and children: clean area; apply cream, gel, or ointment sparingly once daily to b.i.d.

ADVERSE REACTIONS
Common reactions are in italics; life-threatening reactions are in bold italics.
Skin: burning, itching, irritation, dryness, folliculitis, hypertrichosis, acneiform eruptions, perioral dermatitis, hypopigmentation, allergic contact dermatitis. With occlusive dressings: *maceration of skin, secondary infection, atrophy, striae, miliaria.*

INTERACTIONS
None significant.

NURSING CONSIDERATIONS
- *Use cautiously* in viral diseases of skin, such as varicella, vaccinia, herpes simplex; fungal infections; bacterial skin infections.
- Avoid application near eyes, mucous membranes, or in ear canal.
- Systemic absorption especially likely with occlusive dressings, prolonged treatment, or extensive body-surface treatment.
- When used in young children, avoid the use of plastic pants or tight-fitting diapers in treated areas.
- Stop drug and notify doctor if patient develops signs of systemic absorption, skin irritation or ulceration, hypersensitivity, or infection. (If antifungals or antibiotics are being used with corticosteroids and infection does not respond immediately, corticosteroids should be stopped until infection is controlled.)
- Before applying, gently wash skin. To prevent damage to skin, rub medication in gently, leaving a thin coat. When treating hairy sites, part hair and apply directly to lesions.
- Occlusive dressing (if ordered): Apply cream, then cover with a thin, pliable, nonflammable plastic film; seal to adjacent normal skin with hypoallergenic tape. To minimize adverse reactions, use occlusive dressing intermittently. Don't leave in place longer than 16 hours each day. Occlusive dressings should not be used in presence of infection or with weeping or exudative lesions.
- For patient with eczematous dermatitis who may develop irritation with adhesive material, hold dressing in place with gauze, elastic bandages, stockings, or stockinette.
- Notify doctor and remove occlusive dressing if fever develops.
- Change dressing as ordered by doctor. Inspect skin for infection, striae, and atrophy. Discontinue drug and notify doctor if these occur.
- Treatment should be continued for a few days after clearing of lesions to prevent recurrence.
- Gel contains alcohol and may cause burning or irritation in open lesions.
- Store in tightly sealed containers.

dexamethasone
Aeroseb-Dex, Decaderm, Decaspray

dexamethasone sodium phosphate
Decadron Phosphate

Pregnancy Risk Category: C

HOW SUPPLIED
dexamethasone
Aerosol: 0.01%, 0.04%
Gel: 0.1%

*Liquid form contains alcohol. **May contain tartrazine.

dexamethasone sodium phosphate
Cream: 0.1%

MECHANISM OF ACTION
Diffuses across cell membranes and complexes with specific cytoplasmic receptors.

INDICATIONS & DOSAGE
Inflammation of corticosteroid-responsive dermatoses –
Adults and children: clean area; apply cream, gel, or aerosol sparingly b.i.d. to q.i.d.

Aerosol use on scalp – shake can well and apply to dry scalp after shampooing. Hold can upright. Slide applicator tube under hair so that it touches scalp. Spray while moving tube to all affected areas, keeping tube under hair and in contact with scalp throughout spraying, which should take about 2 seconds. Inadequately covered areas may be spot sprayed. Slide applicator tube through hair to touch scalp, press and immediately release spray button. Don't massage medication into scalp or spray forehead or eyes.

ADVERSE REACTIONS
Common reactions are in italics; life-threatening reactions are in bold italics.
Skin: burning, itching, irritation, dryness, folliculitis, hypertrichosis, acneiform eruptions, perioral dermatitis, hypopigmentation, allergic contact dermatitis. With occlusive dressings: *maceration of skin, secondary infection, atrophy, striae, miliaria.*

INTERACTIONS
None significant.

NURSING CONSIDERATIONS
- *Use cautiously* in viral diseases of skin, such as varicella, vaccinia, herpes simplex; fungal infections; and bacterial skin infections.
- Avoid application near eyes, mucous membranes, or in ear canal.
- Systemic absorption especially likely with occlusive dressings, prolonged treatment, or extensive body-surface treatment.
- When used in young children, avoid the use of plastic pants or tight-fitting diapers in treated areas.
- Stop drug and notify doctor if patient develops signs of systemic absorption, skin irritation or ulceration, hypersensitivity, or infection. (If antifungals or antibiotics are being used with corticosteroids and infection does not respond immediately, corticosteroids should be stopped until infection is controlled.)
- Before applying, gently wash skin. To prevent damage to skin, rub medication in gently, leaving a thin coat. When treating hairy sites, part hair and apply directly to lesions.
- For patient with eczematous dermatitis who may develop irritation with adhesive material, hold dressing in place with gauze, elastic bandages, stockings, or stockinette.
- Notify doctor and remove occlusive dressing if fever develops.
- Change dressing as ordered by doctor. Inspect skin for infection, striae, and atrophy. Discontinue drug and notify doctor if these occur.
- Occlusive dressings should not be used in presence of infection or with weeping or exudative lesions.
- Aerosol preparation contains alcohol and may produce irritation or burning in open lesions. When using about the face, cover patient's eyes and warn against inhalation of the spray. To avoid freezing tissues, do not spray longer than 3 seconds or closer than 6″ (15 cm).
- Treatment should be continued for a few days after clearing of lesions to prevent recurrence.

diflorasone diacetate

Florone, Flutone, Maxiflor, Psorcon

Pregnancy Risk Category: C

HOW SUPPLIED

Cream: 0.05%
Ointment: 0.05%

MECHANISM OF ACTION

Diffuses across cell membranes and complexes with specific cytoplasmic receptors.

INDICATIONS & DOSAGE

Inflammation of corticosteroid-responsive dermatoses –
Adults and children: clean area; apply ointment daily to t.i.d.; apply cream b.i.d. to q.i.d. Apply sparingly in a thin film.

ADVERSE REACTIONS

Common reactions are in italics; life-threatening reactions are in bold italics.
Skin: burning, itching, irritation, dryness, folliculitis, perioral dermatitis, hypertrichosis, hypopigmentation, acneiform eruptions. With occlusive dressings: *maceration, secondary infection, atrophy, striae, miliaria.*

INTERACTIONS

None significant.

NURSING CONSIDERATIONS

- *Use cautiously* in viral diseases of skin, such as varicella, vaccinia, herpes simplex; fungal infections; and bacterial skin infections.
- *Use very cautiously* in young children. A high-potency corticosteroid.
- Avoid application near eyes, mucous membranes, or in ear canal.
- Systemic absorption especially likely with occlusive dressings, prolonged treatment, or extensive body-surface treatment.
- When used in young children, avoid the use of plastic pants or tight-fitting diapers in treated areas.
- Stop drug and notify doctor if patient develops signs of systemic absorption, skin irritation or ulceration, hypersensitivity, or infection. (If antifungals or antibiotics are being used concomitantly, corticosteroids should be stopped until infection is controlled.)
- Before applying, gently wash skin. To prevent damage to skin, rub medication in gently, leaving a thin coat. When treating hairy sites, part hair and apply directly to lesion.
- Occlusive dressing (if ordered): Apply cream or ointment, then cover with a thin, pliable, nonflammable plastic film; seal to adjacent normal skin with hypoallergenic tape. Minimize adverse reactions by using occlusive dressing intermittently. Don't leave in place longer than 16 hours each day. Occlusive dressings should not be used in presence of infection or with weeping or exudative lesions.
- For patient with eczematous dermatitis who may develop irritation with adhesive material, hold dressing in place with gauze, elastic bandages, stockings, or stockinette.
- Notify doctor and remove occlusive dressing if fever develops.
- Change dressing as ordered by doctor. Inspect skin for infection, striae, and atrophy. Discontinue drug and notify doctor if these occur.
- Occlusive dressings should not be used with Psorcon.
- Diflorasone is often effective with once-daily application.

fluocinolone acetonide

Fluocet, Fluonid, Flurosyn, Synalar, Synemol

Pregnancy Risk Category: C

HOW SUPPLIED

Cream: 0.01%, 0.025%, 0.2%
Ointment: 0.025%
Topical solution: 0.01%

*Liquid form contains alcohol. **May contain tartrazine.

MECHANISM OF ACTION
Diffuses across cell membranes and complexes with specific cytoplasmic receptors.

INDICATIONS & DOSAGE
Inflammation of corticosteroid-responsive dermatoses –
Adults and children over 2 years: clean area; apply cream, ointment, or solution sparingly b.i.d. to q.i.d. Treat multiple or extensive lesions sequentially, applying to only small areas at any one time.

ADVERSE REACTIONS
Common reactions are in italics; life-threatening reactions are in bold italics.
Skin: burning, itching, irritation, dryness, folliculitis, hypertrichosis, hypopigmentation, acneiform eruptions, perioral dermatitis, allergic contact dermatitis. With occlusive dressings: *maceration of skin, secondary infection, atrophy, striae, miliaria.*

INTERACTIONS
None significant.

NURSING CONSIDERATIONS
- *Use cautiously* in viral diseases of skin, such as varicella, vaccinia, herpes simplex; fungal infections; and bacterial skin infections.
- Avoid application near eyes, mucous membranes, or in ear canal.
- Systemic absorption especially likely with occlusive dressings, prolonged treatment, or extensive body-surface treatment.
- When used in young children, avoid the use of plastic pants or tight-fitting diapers in treated areas.
- Stop drug and notify doctor if patient develops signs of systemic absorption, skin irritation or ulceration, hypersensitivity, or infection. (If antifungals or antibiotics are being used with corticosteroids and infection does not respond immediately, corticosteroids should be stopped until infection is controlled.)
- Before applying, gently wash skin. To prevent damage to skin, rub medication in gently, leaving a thin coat. When treating hairy sites, part hair and apply directly to lesion.
- Occlusive dressing (if ordered): Apply gently and sparingly to the lesion until cream disappears. Then reapply, leaving a thin coat. Cover with a thin, pliable, nonflammable plastic film; seal to adjacent normal skin with hypoallergenic tape. To minimize adverse reactions, use occlusive dressing intermittently. Don't leave in place longer than 16 hours each day. Occlusive dressings should not be used in presence of infection or with weeping or exudative lesions.
- For patient with eczematous dermatitis who may develop irritation with adhesive material, hold dressing in place with gauze, elastic bandages, stockings, or stockinette.
- Notify doctor and remove occlusive dressing if fever develops.
- Change dressing as ordered by doctor. Inspect skin for infection, striae, and atrophy. Discontinue drug and notify doctor if these occur.
- Fluonid solution on dry lesions may increase dryness, scaling, or itching; on denuded or fissured areas, may produce burning or stinging. If burning or stinging persists and dermatitis has not improved, solution should be discontinued.

fluocinonide
Lidemol†, Lidex, Lidex-E, Topsyn
Pregnancy Risk Category: C

HOW SUPPLIED
Cream: 0.05%
Gel: 0.05%
Ointment: 0.05%
Topical solution: 0.05%

MECHANISM OF ACTION
Diffuses across cell membranes and complexes with specific cytoplasmic receptors.

INDICATIONS & DOSAGE
Inflammation of corticosteroid-responsive dermatoses –
Adults and children: clean area; apply cream, ointment, solution, or gel sparingly t.i.d. or q.i.d.

ADVERSE REACTIONS
Common reactions are in italics; life-threatening reactions are in bold italics.
Skin: burning, itching, irritation, dryness, folliculitis, hypertrichosis, hypopigmentation, acneiform eruptions, perioral dermatitis, allergic contact dermatitis. With occlusive dressings: *maceration of skin, secondary infection, atrophy, striae, miliaria.*

INTERACTIONS
None significant.

NURSING CONSIDERATIONS
- *Use cautiously* in viral diseases of skin, such as varicella, vaccinia, and herpes simplex; untreated purulent bacterial skin infections; fungal infections; and bacterial skin infections.
- Avoid application near eyes, mucous membranes, or in ear canal.
- Systemic absorption especially likely with occlusive dressings, prolonged treatment, or extensive body-surface treatment.
- When used in young children, avoid the use of plastic pants or tight-fitting diapers in treated areas.
- Stop drug and notify doctor if patient develops signs of systemic absorption, skin irritation or ulceration, hypersensitivity, or infection. (If antifungals or antibiotics are being used with corticosteroids and infection does not respond immediately, corticosteroids should be stopped until infection is controlled.)
- Before applying, gently wash skin. To prevent damage to skin, rub medication in gently, leaving a thin coat. When treating hairy sites, part hair and apply directly to lesion.
- Occlusive dressing (if ordered): Apply cream or ointment heavily, then cover with a thin, pliable, nonflammable plastic film; seal to adjacent normal skin with hypoallergenic tape. To minimize adverse reactions, use occlusive dressing intermittently. Don't leave in place longer than 16 hours each day. Occlusive dressings should not be used in presence of infection or with weeping or exudative lesions.
- For patient with eczematous dermatitis who may develop irritation with adhesive material, hold dressing in place with gauze, elastic bandages, stockings, or stockinette.
- Notify doctor and remove occlusive dressing if fever develops.
- Change dressing as ordered by doctor. Inspect skin for infection, striae, and atrophy. Discontinue drug and notify doctor if these occur.
- Treatment should be continued for a few days after clearing of lesions to prevent recurrence.

flurandrenolide
Cordran, Cordran SP, Cordran Tape, Drenison†, Drenison 1/4†, Drenison Tape†

Pregnancy Risk Category: C

HOW SUPPLIED
Cream: 0.025%, 0.05%
Lotion: 0.05%
Ointment: 0.025%, 0.05%
Tape: 4 mcg/cm²

MECHANISM OF ACTION
Diffuses across cell membranes and complexes with specific cytoplasmic receptors.

INDICATIONS & DOSAGE
Inflammation of corticosteroid-responsive dermatoses –

*Liquid form contains alcohol. **May contain tartrazine.

Adults and children: clean area; apply cream, lotion, or ointment sparingly b.i.d. or t.i.d. Apply tape q 12 to 24 hours. Before applying tape, cleanse skin carefully, removing scales, crust, and dried exudates. Allow skin to dry for 1 hour before applying new tape. Shave or clip hair to allow good contact with skin and comfortable removal. If tape ends loosen prematurely, trim off and replace with fresh tape. Lowest incidence of adverse reactions if tape is replaced q 12 hours, but may be left in place for 24 hours if well tolerated and adheres satisfactorily. Drenison 1/4 – for maintenance therapy of widespread or chronic lesions.

ADVERSE REACTIONS

Common reactions are in italics; life-threatening reactions are in bold italics.

Skin: burning, itching, irritation, dryness, folliculitis, hypertrichosis, hypopigmentation, acneiform eruptions, allergic contact dermatitis. With occlusive dressings: *maceration of skin, secondary infection, atrophy, striae, miliaria.* With tape: purpura, stripping of epidermis, furunculosis.

INTERACTIONS

None significant.

NURSING CONSIDERATIONS

- *Use cautiously* in viral diseases of skin, such as varicella, vaccinia, herpes simplex; fungal infections; and bacterial skin infections.
- Tape not advised for exudative lesions or those in intertriginous areas.
- Tape should be cut with scissors. Don't tear.
- Avoid application near eyes, mucous membranes, or in ear canal.
- Systemic absorption especially likely with occlusive dressings, prolonged treatment, or extensive body-surface treatment.
- When used in young children, avoid the use of plastic pants or tight-fitting diapers in treated areas.
- Stop drug and notify doctor if patient develops signs of systemic absorption, skin irritation or ulceration, hypersensitivity, or infection. (If antifungals or antibiotics are being used with corticosteroids and infection does not respond immediately, corticosteroids should be stopped until infection is controlled.)
- Before applying, gently wash skin. To prevent damage to skin, rub medication in gently, leaving a thin coat. When treating hairy sites, part hair and apply directly to lesion.
- Occlusive dressing (if ordered): Apply cream heavily, then cover with a thin, pliable, nonflammable plastic film; seal to adjacent normal skin with hypoallergenic tape. To minimize adverse reactions, use occlusive dressing intermittently. Don't leave in place longer than 16 hours each day. Occlusive dressings should not be used in presence of infection or with weeping or exudative lesions.
- For patient with eczematous dermatitis who may develop irritation with adhesive material, hold dressing in place with gauze, elastic bandages, stockings, or stockinette.
- Notify doctor and remove occlusive dressing if fever develops.
- Inspect skin for infection, striae, and atrophy. Discontinue drug and notify doctor if these occur.
- Treatment should be continued for a few days after clearing of lesions to prevent recurrence.

fluticasone propionate

Cutivate

Pregnancy Risk Category: C

HOW SUPPLIED

Cream: 0.05%
Ointment: 0.005%

MECHANISM OF ACTION

A synthetic corticosteroid that stimulates the synthesis of enzymes needed to decrease inflammation. May also exhibit some vasoconstrictive properties.

INDICATIONS & DOSAGE

Relief of inflammation and pruritus of corticosteroid-responsive dermatoses –

Adults: apply sparingly to affected area b.i.d. and rub in gently and completely. Treatment beyond 2 consecutive weeks is not recommended; total dose should not exceed 50 g weekly.

ADVERSE REACTIONS

Common reactions are in italics; life-threatening reactions are in bold italics.

Skin: stinging, burning, itching, irritation, dryness, folliculitis, erythema, skin atrophy, leukoderma, vesicles, rash, hypertrichosis, acneiform eruptions, hypopigmentation, perioral dermatitis, allergic contact dermatitis, secondary infection, striae, miliaria.

Significant systemic absorption can produce the following reactions –

CNS: euphoria, insomnia, headache, psychotic behavior, pseudotumor cerebri, mental changes, nervousness, restlessness.

CV: ***CHF,*** hypertension, edema.

EENT: cataracts, glaucoma, thrush.

GI: peptic ulcer, irritation, increased appetite.

Other: immunosuppression, increased susceptibility to infection, hypokalemia, sodium retention, fluid retention, weight gain, hyperglycemia, osteoporosis, muscle atrophy, growth suppression in children, withdrawal syndrome.

Note: Drug should be discontinued if local irritation, systemic infection, systemic absorption, or hypersensitivity reactions occur.

INTERACTIONS

None reported.

NURSING CONSIDERATIONS

- *Contraindicated* in patients with hypersensitivity to the drug or any of its components and in patients with viral, fungal, herpetic, or tubercular skin lesions.
- *Use cautiously* in pediatric patients because higher ratio of skin surface to body mass increases susceptibility to systemic absorption and toxicity. Children may be more susceptible to topical steroid-induced hypothalamic-pituitary-adrenal-axis suppression because they may absorb proportionally larger amounts of the drug. Do not exceed 15 g weekly.
- It is unknown if topically applied corticosteroids appear in breast milk; however, cautious use is recommended is breast-feeding women because systemically administered corticosteroids appear in breast milk and could suppress growth.
- Do not use to treat rosacea, perioral dermatitis, or acne.
- Mixing drug with other bases or vehicles may affect potency far beyond expectations.
- The risk of adverse reactions may be minimized by changing to a less potent agent.
- To cover the adult body once requires 12 to 26 g. Use of more than 50 g weekly is not recommended.
- Tell patient to apply drug sparingly and rub in lightly. Washing the area before application may increase drug penetration.
- Tell patient to notify doctor if the condition persists or worsens or if burning or irritation develops.
- Avoid prolonged use; contact with eyes; and use around eyes, genitals, or rectum; on face, and in skin creases.

halcinonide

Halciderm, Halog

Pregnancy Risk Category: C

HOW SUPPLIED
Cream: 0.025%, 0.1%
Ointment: 0.1%
Topical solution: 0.1%

MECHANISM OF ACTION
Diffuses across cell membranes and complexes with specific cytoplasmic receptors.

INDICATIONS & DOSAGE
Inflammation of acute and chronic corticosteroid-responsive dermatoses –
Adults and children: clean area; apply cream, ointment, or solution sparingly b.i.d. or t.i.d.

ADVERSE REACTIONS
Common reactions are in italics; life-threatening reactions are in bold italics.
Skin: burning, itching, irritation, dryness, folliculitis, hypertrichosis, hypopigmentation, acneiform eruptions, allergic contact dermatitis. With occlusive dressings: *maceration of skin, secondary infection, atrophy, striae, miliaria.*

INTERACTIONS
None significant.

NURSING CONSIDERATIONS
• *Use cautiously* in viral diseases of skin, such as varicella, vaccinia, herpes simplex; fungal infections; and bacterial skin infections.
• Avoid application near eyes, mucous membranes, or in ear canal.
• Systemic absorption especially likely with occlusive dressings, prolonged treatment, or extensive body-surface treatment.
• When used in young children, avoid the use of plastic pants or tight-fitting diapers in treated areas.
• Stop drug and notify doctor if patient develops signs of systemic absorption, skin irritation or ulceration, hypersensitivity, or infection. (If antifungals or antibiotics are being used with corticosteroids and infection does not respond immediately, corticosteroids should be stopped until infection is controlled.)
• Before applying, gently wash skin. To prevent damage to skin, rub medication in gently, leaving a thin coat. When treating hairy sites, part hair and apply directly to lesion.
• Occlusive dressing with cream: Gently rub small amount into lesion until it disappears. Reapply, leaving a thin coating on lesion, and cover with occlusive dressing. With ointment: Apply to lesion and cover with occlusive dressing. Cover with a thin, pliable, nonflammable plastic film; seal to adjacent normal skin with hypoallergenic tape. To minimize adverse reactions, use occlusive dressing intermittently. Don't leave in place longer than 16 hours each day.
• Good results have been obtained by applying occlusive dressings in the evening and removing them in the morning (that is, 12-hour occlusion). Medication should then be reapplied in the morning, without using the occlusive dressings during the day.
• For patient with eczematous dermatitis who may develop irritation with adhesive material, hold dressing in place with gauze, elastic bandages, stockings, or stockinette.
• Notify doctor and remove occlusive dressing if fever develops.
• Occlusive dressings should not be used in presence of infection or with weeping or exudative lesions.
• Change dressing as ordered by doctor. Inspect skin for infection, striae, and atrophy. Discontinue drug and notify doctor if these occur.
• Treatment should be continued for a few days after clearing of lesions to prevent recurrence.

halobetasol propionate

Ultravate

Pregnancy Risk Category: C

HOW SUPPLIED

Cream: 0.05%
Ointment: 0.05%

MECHANISM OF ACTION

A super high potency (group I) corticosteroid. Drug's anti-inflammatory response is related to the stimulation of synthesis of enzymes needed to decrease inflammation.

INDICATIONS & DOSAGE

Relief of inflammation and pruritus of corticosteroid-responsive dermatoses –

Adults: apply sparingly to affected area b.i.d. and rub in gently and completely. Treatment beyond 2 consecutive weeks is not recommended; total dose should not exceed 50 g weekly.

ADVERSE REACTIONS

Common reactions are in italics; life-threatening reactions are in bold italics.

Skin: stinging, burning, itching, irritation, dryness, folliculitis, erythema, skin atrophy, leukoderma, vesicles, rash, hypertrichosis, acneiform eruptions, hypopigmentation, perioral dermatitis, allergic contact dermatitis, secondary infection, striae, miliaria.

Significant systemic absorption can produce the following reactions –

CNS: euphoria, insomnia, headache, mental changes, nervousness, psychotic behavior, restlessness, pseudotumor cerebri, fatigue, dizziness, syncope.

CV: *CHF, hypertension, hypotension.*

EENT: cataracts, glaucoma, thrush.

GI: peptic ulcer, GI irritation, increased appetite, nausea, anorexia.

Other: edema, hypokalemia, weight gain, hyperglycemia, fluid retention, osteoporosis, muscle atrophy, myalgia, arthralgia, fever, growth suppression of children.

INTERACTIONS

None reported.

NURSING CONSIDERATIONS

- *Contraindicated* in patients with hypersensitivity to the drug or any of its components and in patients with viral, fungal, herpetic, or tubercular skin lesions.
- *Use cautiously* in pediatric patients because their higher ratio of skin surface to body mass increases susceptibility to systemic absorption and toxicity.
- It is unknown if topically applied corticosteroids appear in breast milk; however, cautious use is recommended in breast-feeding women because systemically administered corticosteroids appear in breast milk and could suppress growth.
- Some systemic absorption usually occurs. Amount absorbed depends on amount applied, application site, vehicle used, use of occlusive dressing, and integrity of epidural barrier. Sufficient amounts can be absorbed to produce systemic effects (specifically, hypothalamic-pituitary-adrenal-axis [HPA-axis] suppression, Cushing's syndrome, hyperglycemia, and glucosuria) and are reversible after discontinuation of therapy.
- Corticotropin stimulation, morning plasma cortisol, and urinary cortisol tests are useful in determining the extent of HPA-axis suppression.
- If HPA-axis suppression occurs, discontinue drug, reduce frequency of application, or substitute a less potent corticosteroid.
- Treatment should be limited to 2 weeks in amounts below 50 g weekly.
- Do not use occlusive dressings.
- Do not use drug to treat rosacea or perioral dermatitis. Discontinue if infection occurs.
- Avoid use on face, groin, or axilla.

• Tell patient that drug is for external use only as directed by doctor. Avoid contact with eyes. Do not cover, bandage, or wrap treated area unless directed by doctor. Do not use more often or for any condition other than prescribed.
• Tell patient to notify doctor of any signs of stinging, burning, or irritation.

hydrocortisone

Acticort, Aeroseb-HC, Bactine HC◇, CaldeCort, Carmol HC, Cetacort, Cort-Dome, Cortef◇, Cortenema, Cortinal, Cortizone 5◇, Cortril, Cremesone, Delacort, DermaCort◇, Dermolate◇, Dermtex HC, Durel-Cort, Ecosone, HC Cream, HI-Cor-2.5, Hycortole, Hydrocortex, HydroTex, Hytone, Ivocort, Maso-Cort, Microcort, Nutracort, Orabase HCA, Penecort, Proctocort, Rhus Tox HC, Rocort, Squibb-HC‡, Synacort, Unicort

hydrocortisone acetate

CortaGel, Cortaid◇, Cortamed†, Cortef, Corticaine, Corticreme†, Cortifoam, Dermacort‡, Dermacort Ointment‡, Epifoam, Gynecort, Hydrocortisone Acetate, Lanacort, MyCort Lotion, Proctofoam-HC

hydrocortisone butyrate

Locoid

hydrocortisone valerate

Westcort Cream

Pregnancy Risk Category: C

HOW SUPPLIED

hydrocortisone
Aerosol: 0.5%
Cream: 0.25%◇, 0.5%◇, 1%◇, 2.5%
Gel: 1%
Lotion: 0.125%, 0.25%, 0.5%◇, 1%, 2%, 2.5%
Ointment: 0.5%◇, 1%◇, 2.5%
Topical solution: 1%
hydrocortisone acetate
Cream: 0.5%◇
Lotion: 0.5%◇
Ointment: 0.5%◇, 1%
Rectal foam: 90 mg/application
hydrocortisone butyrate
Cream: 0.1%
Ointment: 0.1%
hydrocortisone valerate
Cream: 0.2%
Ointment: 0.2%

MECHANISM OF ACTION

Diffuses across cell membranes and complexes with specific cytoplasmic receptors.

INDICATIONS & DOSAGE

Inflammation of corticosteroid-responsive dermatoses; adjunctive topical management of seborrheic dermatitis of scalp; may be safely used on face, groin, armpits, and under breasts –
Adults and children: clean area; apply cream, gel, lotion, ointment, topical solution, or aerosol sparingly daily to q.i.d.
Aerosol – shake can well. Direct spray onto affected area from a distance of 6″ (15 cm). Apply for only 3 seconds (to avoid freezing tissues). Apply to dry scalp after shampooing; no need to massage or rub medication into scalp after spraying. Apply daily until acute phase is controlled, then reduce dosage to 1 to 3 times a week as needed to maintain control.
Rectal form – shake can well. One applicatorful daily to b.i.d. for 2 to 3 weeks, then every other day as necessary.

ADVERSE REACTIONS

Common reactions are in italics; life-threatening reactions are in bold italics.
Skin: burning, itching, irritation, dryness, folliculitis, hypertrichosis, hypopigmentation, acneiform eruptions, allergic contact dermatitis. With occlusive dressings: *maceration of skin,*

†Available in Canada only. ‡Available in Australia only. ◇Available OTC.

secondary infection, atrophy, striae, miliaria.

INTERACTIONS
None significant.

NURSING CONSIDERATIONS
- *Use cautiously* in viral diseases of skin, such as varicella, vaccinia, herpes simplex; fungal infections; and bacterial skin infections.
- Avoid application near eyes, mucous membranes, or in ear canal.
- Systemic absorption especially likely with occlusive dressings, prolonged treatment, or extensive body-surface treatment.
- When used in young children, avoid the use of plastic pants or tight-fitting diapers in treated areas.
- Stop drug and notify doctor if patient develops signs of systemic absorption, skin irritation or ulceration, hypersensitivity, or infection. (If antifungals or antibiotics are being used with corticosteroids and infection does not respond immediately, corticosteroids should be stopped until infection is controlled.)
- Before applying, gently wash skin. To prevent damage to skin, rub medication in gently, leaving a thin coat. When treating hairy sites, part hair and apply directly to lesion.
- Occlusive dressing (if ordered): Apply cream heavily, then cover with a thin, pliable, nonflammable plastic film; seal to adjacent normal skin with hypoallergenic tape. To minimize adverse reactions, use occlusive dressing intermittently. Don't leave in place longer than 16 hours each day. Occlusive dressings should not be used in presence of infection or with weeping or exudative lesions.
- For patient with eczematous dermatitis who may develop irritation with adhesive material, it may be helpful to hold dressing in place with gauze, elastic bandages, stockings, or stockinette.
- Notify doctor and remove occlusive dressing if fever develops.
- Aerosol preparation contains alcohol and may produce irritation or burning in open lesions. When using about the face, cover patient's eyes and warn against inhalation of the spray. To avoid freezing tissues, do not spray longer than 3 seconds or closer than 6″ (15 cm).
- Change dressing as ordered by doctor. Inspect skin for infection, striae, and atrophy. Discontinue drug and notify doctor if these occur.
- Treatment should be continued for a few days following clearing of lesions to prevent recurrence.

methylprednisolone acetate
Medrol

Pregnancy Risk Category: C

HOW SUPPLIED
Ointment: 0.25%, 1%

MECHANISM OF ACTION
Diffuses across cell membranes and complexes with specific cytoplasmic receptors.

INDICATIONS & DOSAGE
Inflammation of corticosteroid-responsive dermatoses –
Adults and children: clean area; apply ointment daily to q.i.d.

ADVERSE REACTIONS
Common reactions are in italics; life-threatening reactions are in bold italics.
Skin: burning, itching, irritation, dryness, folliculitis, hypertrichosis, hypopigmentation, acneiform eruptions, allergic contact dermatitis. With occlusive dressings: *maceration of skin, secondary infection, atrophy, striae, miliaria.*

INTERACTIONS
None significant.

*Liquid form contains alcohol. **May contain tartrazine.

NURSING CONSIDERATIONS

- *Use cautiously* in viral diseases of skin, such as varicella, vaccinia, herpes simplex; fungal infections; and bacterial skin infections.
- Avoid application near eyes, mucous membranes, or in ear canal.
- Systemic absorption especially likely with occlusive dressings, prolonged treatment, or extensive body-surface treatment.
- When used in young children, avoid the use of plastic pants or tight-fitting diapers in treated areas.
- Stop drug and notify doctor if patient develops signs of systemic absorption, skin irritation or ulceration, hypersensitivity, or infection. (If antimicrobials are being used concomitantly, corticosteroids should be stopped until infection is controlled.)
- Before applying, gently wash skin. To prevent damage to skin, rub medication in gently, leaving a thin coat. When treating hairy sites, part hair and apply directly to lesion.
- Occlusive dressing (if ordered): Apply ointment heavily, then cover with a thin, pliable, nonflammable plastic film; seal to adjacent normal skin with hypoallergenic tape. To minimize adverse effects, use occlusive dressing intermittently. Don't leave in place longer than 16 hours each day. Occlusive dressings should not be used in presence of infection or with weeping or exudative lesions.
- For patient with eczematous dermatitis who may develop irritation with adhesive material, hold dressing in place with gauze, elastic bandages, stockings, or stockinette.
- Notify doctor and remove occlusive dressing if fever develops.
- Change dressing as ordered by doctor. Inspect skin for infection, striae, and atrophy.
- Treatment should be continued for a few days after clearing of lesions to prevent recurrence.

mometasone furoate

Elocon

Pregnancy Risk Category: C

HOW SUPPLIED

Cream: 0.1%
Ointment: 0.1%

MECHANISM OF ACTION

Diffuses across cell membranes and complexes with specific cytoplasmic receptors.

INDICATIONS & DOSAGE

Inflammatory and pruritic manifestations of corticosteroid-responsive dermatoses –
Adults: apply cream or ointment to affected areas once daily. Do not use occlusive dressings.

ADVERSE REACTIONS

Common reactions are in italics; life-threatening reactions are in bold italics.
Skin: burning, pruritus, atrophy, irritation, acneiform eruptions, hypopigmentation, allergic contact dermatitis.
Other: ***HPA-axis suppression,*** Cushing's syndrome.

INTERACTIONS

None reported.

NURSING CONSIDERATIONS

- *Use cautiously* in viral diseases of skin, such as varicella, vaccinia, herpes simplex; fungal infections; and bacterial skin infections. Also *use very cautiously* in young children. A high-potency corticosteroid.
- Avoid application near eyes, mucous membranes, or in ear canal.
- Systemic absorption especially likely with occlusive dressings, prolonged treatment, or extensive body-surface treatment.
- Stop drug and notify doctor if patient develops signs of systemic absorption, skin irritation or ulceration, hypersensitivity, or infection. (If anti-

microbials are being used concomitantly, corticosteroids should be stopped until infection is controlled.)
• Before applying, gently wash skin. To prevent damage to skin, rub medication in gently, leaving a thin coat. When treating hairy sites, part hair and apply directly to lesion.

triamcinolone acetonide
Aristocort, Flutex, Kenalog, Kenalone‡, Triacet

Pregnancy Risk Category: C

HOW SUPPLIED
Aerosol: 0.2 mg/2-second spray
Cream: 0.02%‡, 0.025%, 0.1%, 0.5%
Lotion: 0.025%, 0.1%
Ointment: 0.02%‡, 0.025%, 0.1%, 0.5%

MECHANISM OF ACTION
Diffuses across cell membranes and complexes with specific cytoplasmic receptors.

INDICATIONS & DOSAGE
Inflammation of corticosteroid-responsive dermatoses –
Adults and children: clean area; apply aerosol, cream, lotion, or ointment sparingly b.i.d. to q.i.d.
Aerosol – shake can well. Direct spray onto affected area from a distance of approximately 6″ (15 cm) and apply for only 3 seconds.

ADVERSE REACTIONS
Common reactions are in italics; life-threatening reactions are in bold italics.
Skin: burning, itching, irritation, dryness, folliculitis, hypertrichosis, hypopigmentation, acneiform eruptions, perioral dermatitis, allergic contact dermatitis. With occlusive dressings: *maceration of skin, secondary infection, atrophy, striae, miliaria.*

INTERACTIONS
None significant.

NURSING CONSIDERATIONS
• *Use cautiously* in viral diseases of skin, such as varicella, vaccinia, herpes simplex; fungal infections; and bacterial skin infections.
• Avoid application near eyes, mucous membranes, or in ear canal.
• Systemic absorption especially likely with occlusive dressings, prolonged treatment, or extensive body-surface treatment.
• When used in young children, avoid the use of plastic pants or tight-fitting diapers in treated areas.
• Stop drug and notify doctor if patient develops signs of systemic absorption, skin irritation or ulceration, hypersensitivity, or infection. (If antifungals or antibiotics are being used with corticosteroids and infection does not respond immediately, corticosteroids should be stopped until infection is controlled.)
• Before applying, gently wash skin. To prevent damage to skin, rub medication in gently, leaving a thin coat. When treating hairy sites, part hair and apply directly to lesion.
• Aerosol preparation contains alcohol and may produce irritation or burning in open lesions. When using about the face, cover patient's eyes and warn against inhalation of the spray. To avoid freezing tissues, do not spray longer than 3 seconds or closer than 6″ (15 cm).
• Occlusive dressing (if ordered): Apply cream or ointment heavily, then cover with a thin, pliable, nonflammable plastic film; seal to adjacent normal skin with hypoallergenic tape. To minimize adverse reactions, use occlusive dressing intermittently. Don't leave in place longer than 16 hours each day.
• Change dressing as ordered by doctor. Inspect skin for infection, striae, and atrophy.

*Liquid form contains alcohol. **May contain tartrazine.

90

Local anesthetics

bupivacaine hydrochloride
chloroprocaine hydrochloride
etidocaine hydrochloride
lidocaine hydrochloride
mepivacaine hydrochloride
procaine hydrochloride
tetracaine hydrochloride

COMBINATION PRODUCTS
EMLA CREAM: lidocaine 2.5% and prilocaine 2.5%.

bupivacaine hydrochloride

Marcain‡, Marcaine, Sensorcaine
Pregnancy Risk Category: C

HOW SUPPLIED
Injection: 0.25%, 0.5%, 0.75%; also available with epinephrine 1:200,000

MECHANISM OF ACTION
A local anesthetic of the amide type. Blocks depolarization by interfering with sodium-potassium exchange across the nerve cell membrane, preventing generation and conduction of the nerve impulse. When combined with epinephrine, action is prolonged.

INDICATIONS & DOSAGE
Dosages given are for the drug without epinephrine and for adults.

Epidural–

Sol.	Vol. (ml)	Dose (mg)
0.25%	10 to 20	25 to 50
0.5%	10 to 20	50 to 100

Caudal–

Sol.	Vol. (ml)	Dose (mg)
0.25%	15 to 30	37.5 to 75
0.5%	15 to 30	75 to 150

Spinal–

Sol.	Vol. (ml)	Dose (mg)
0.75 (in dextrose 8.25%)	0.8 to 1.6	6 to 12

Peripheral nerve block–

Sol.	Vol. (ml)	Dose (mg)
0.25%	5	12.5
0.5%	5	25
		(400 max.)

May repeat dose q 3 hours. Dosage and interval may be increased with epinephrine. Maximum 400 mg daily.

ADVERSE REACTIONS
Common reactions are in italics; life-threatening reactions are in bold italics.
Skin: dermatologic reactions.
Other: edema, ***status asthmaticus, anaphylaxis, anaphylactoid reactions.***

The following systemic effects may result from high blood levels of the drug:
CNS: anxiety, nervousness, ***seizures*** followed by drowsiness, unconsciousness, tremors, twitches, shivering, ***respiratory arrest.***
CV: bradycardia, hypotension, myocardial depression, ***arrhythmias, cardiac arrest.***
EENT: blurred vision, tinnitus.
GI: nausea, vomiting.

INTERACTIONS
Beta adrenergic blockers: enhanced sympathomimetic adverse effects. Avoid concomitant use.
Chloroprocaine: may lessen bupivacaine's action. Don't use together.
Enflurane, halothane, isoflurane, and related drugs: cardiac arrhythmias when used with bupivacaine *with* epinephrine. Use with extreme caution.
MAO inhibitors, cyclic antidepressants: severe, sustained hypertension when used with bupivacaine *with* epinephrine. Use with extreme caution.

NURSING CONSIDERATIONS

- *Contraindicated* in children under 12 years and for spinal or topical anesthesia or paracervical block. Some solutions contain sulfites and should be avoided in patients with sulfite allergy.
- *Use cautiously* in debilitated, elderly, or acutely ill patients and in patients with severe hepatic disease or drug allergies.
- Bupivacaine should not be used for I.V. regional anesthesia (Bier's anesthesia).
- Although the 0.75% solution is still available, it is not to be used for obstetrical surgery. According to the FDA, lower concentrations are effective and much less hazardous.
- Drug should be administered only by persons who know how to recognize and manage adverse effects caused by epidural anesthetics.
- For epidural use, test doses are administered to verify needle or catheter placement. Initially, 2 to 3 ml is given to check for subarachnoid injection (which would cause extensive motor paralysis of the lower limbs and excessive sensory deficit). After about 5 minutes and in the absence of symptoms, a second, larger test dose of about 5 ml is given to check for intravascular injection (which would cause tinnitus, numbness around the lips, metallic taste, dysphoria, lethargy, or hypotension).
- Use solutions with epinephrine cautiously in cardiovascular disorders and in body areas with limited blood supply (ears, nose, fingers, toes).
- Keep resuscitation equipment and drugs available.
- Don't use solution with preservatives for caudal or epidural block.
- Onset in 4 to 17 minutes; duration is 3 to 6 hours.
- Discard partially used vials without preservatives.
- Check solution for particles.
- Protect solutions containing epinephrine from light.

chloroprocaine hydrochloride

Nesacaine, Nesacaine MPF

Pregnancy Risk Category: C

HOW SUPPLIED

Nesacaine

Injection (for infiltration and regional anesthesia): 1%, 2%

Nesacaine MPF

Injection (preservative-free, for caudal and epidural anesthesia): 2%, 3%

MECHANISM OF ACTION

A local anesthetic of the ester type. Blocks depolarization by interfering with sodium-potassium exchange across the nerve cell membrane, preventing generation and conduction of the nerve impulse.

INDICATIONS & DOSAGE

Infiltration and nerve block –

Adults: dosage limit is 800 mg or 11 mg/kg (1,000 mg or 14 mg/kg when used with epinephrine).

Sol.	Vol. (ml)	Dose (mg)
1%	3 to 20	30 to 200
2%	2 to 40	40 to 800

Caudal and epidural –

Sol.	Vol. (ml)	Dose (mg)
2% to 3%	15 to 25	300 to 750

May repeat with smaller doses q 40 to 50 minutes. Dose and interval may be increased with epinephrine. Maximum adult dosage is 800 mg, or 1 g when mixed with epinephrine.

ADVERSE REACTIONS

Common reactions are in italics; life-threatening reactions are in bold italics.

Skin: dermatologic reactions.

Other: edema, ***status asthmaticus, anaphylaxis, anaphylactoid reactions.***

The following systemic effects may

*Liquid form contains alcohol. **May contain tartrazine.

result from high blood levels of the drug:
CNS: anxiety, nervousness, ***seizures*** followed by drowsiness, unconsciousness, tremors, twitches, shivering, ***respiratory arrest.***
CV: myocardial depression, hypotension, ***arrhythmias, cardiac arrest.***
EENT: blurred vision, tinnitus.
GI: nausea, vomiting.

INTERACTIONS
None significant.

NURSING CONSIDERATIONS
- *Contraindicated* in hypersensitivity to procaine, tetracaine, or other para-aminobenzoic acid derivatives, and for spinal or topical anesthesia. Epidural and caudal blocks are contraindicated in CNS disease.
- *Use cautiously* in debilitated, elderly, or acutely ill patients; in children; and in patients with drug allergies, paracervical block, or cardiovascular disease.
- For epidural use, test doses are administered to verify needle or catheter placement. Initially, 2 to 3 ml is given to check for subarachnoid injection (which would cause extensive motor paralysis of the lower limbs and excessive sensory deficit). After about 5 minutes and in the absence of symptoms, a second, larger test dose of about 5 ml is given to check for intravascular injection (which would cause tinnitus, numbness around the lips, metallic taste, dysphoria, lethargy, or hypotension).
- Repeat the test dose if patient is moved in a way that might displace the epidural catheter.
- At least 5 minutes should elapse after each test before proceeding further.
- Don't use solution with preservatives for caudal or epidural block.
- Don't use discolored solution.
- Keep resuscitation equipment and drugs available.
- Duration is 30 to 60 minutes.
- Discard partially used vials without preservatives.
- Check solution for particles.

etidocaine hydrochloride
Duranest
Pregnancy Risk Category: B

HOW SUPPLIED
Injection: 1%; also available with epinephrine 1:200,000 as a 1% or 1.5% solution

MECHANISM OF ACTION
A local anesthetic of the amide type. Blocks depolarization by interfering with sodium-potassium exchange across the nerve cell membrane, preventing generation and conduction of the nerve impulse. When combined with epinephrine, action is prolonged.

INDICATIONS & DOSAGE
Doses cited are for the drug *with* epinephrine. Dose and interval are decreased without epinephrine.
Adults: Dose limit is 4 mg/kg or 300 mg per injection. When combined with epinephrine, dose limit is 5.5 mg/kg or 400 mg/injection. May be repeated q 2 to 3 hours.

Peripheral nerve block –

Sol.	Vol. (ml)	Dose (mg)
0.5%	5 to 40	25 to 200
1%	5 to 40	50 to 400

Central neural block –
Lower limbs, cesarean section, lumbar peridural

Sol.	Vol. (ml)	Dose (mg)
1%	10 to 30	100 to 300
1.5%	10 to 20	150 to 300

Vaginal –

Sol.	Vol. (ml)	Dose (mg)
1%	5 to 20	50 to 200

Caudal –

Sol.	Vol. (ml)	Dose (mg)
1%	10 to 30	100 to 300

ADVERSE REACTIONS
Common reactions are in italics; life-threatening reactions are in bold italics.
Skin: dermatologic reactions.
Other: edema, ***status asthmaticus, anaphylaxis, anaphylactoid reactions.***

The following systemic effects may result from high blood levels of the drug:
CNS: anxiety, apprehension, nervousness, ***seizures*** followed by drowsiness, unconsciousness, tremors, twitches, shivering, and ***respiratory arrest.***
CV: myocardial depression, hypotension, ***arrhythmias, cardiac arrest.***
EENT: blurred vision, tinnitus.
GI: nausea, vomiting.

INTERACTIONS
Enflurane, halothane, isoflurane, and related drugs: cardiac arrhythmias when used with etidocaine *with* epinephrine. Use with extreme caution.
MAO inhibitors, cyclic antidepressants, phenothiazines: severe, sustained hypertension or hypotension when used with etidocaine solution *with* epinephrine. Use with extreme caution.

NURSING CONSIDERATIONS
- *Contraindicated* in inflammation or infection in puncture region, children under 14 years, septicemia, severe hypertension, spinal deformities, neurologic disorders, and spinal anesthesia. Some solutions contain sulfites and should be avoided in patients with sulfite hypersensitivity.
- *Use cautiously* in debilitated, elderly, or acutely ill patients; severe shock; heart block; epidural block in obstetrics; general drug allergies; and hepatic and renal disease.
- Drug should be administered only by persons who know how to recognize and manage adverse effects caused by epidural anesthetics.
- For epidural use, test doses are administered to verify needle or catheter placement. Initially, 2 to 3 ml is given to check for subarachnoid injection (which would cause extensive motor paralysis of the lower limbs and excessive sensory deficit). After about 5 minutes and in the absence of symptoms, a second, larger test dose of about 5 ml is given to check for intravascular injection (which would cause tinnitus, numbness around the lips, metallic taste, dysphoria, lethargy, or hypotension).
- Use solutions with epinephrine cautiously in cardiovascular disease and in body areas with limited blood supply (ears, nose, fingers, toes).
- Don't use solution with preservatives for caudal or epidural block.
- Keep resuscitation equipment and drugs available.
- Onset in 2 to 8 minutes; duration is 3 to 6 hours.
- Check solution for particles.

lidocaine hydrochloride (lignocaine hydrochloride)
Caine-2, Dalcaine, Dilocaine, Duo-Trach Kit, Lidoject-2, Nervocaine 2%, Octocaine, Xylocaine
Pregnancy Risk Category: B

HOW SUPPLIED
Injection: 2%, 4%, 10%, 20%
Injection (with dextrose 7.5%): 1.5%, 5%
Injection (with epinephrine 1:50,000): 2% (for dental use)
Injection (with epinephrine 1:100,000): 1%, 2%
Injection (with epinephrine 1:200,000): 1%, 1.5%, 2%

MECHANISM OF ACTION
A local anesthetic of the amide type. Blocks depolarization by interfering with sodium-potassium exchange across the nerve cell membrane, preventing generation and conduction of

the nerve impulse. When combined with epinephrine, action is prolonged.

INDICATIONS & DOSAGE

Doses cited are for the drug *without* epinephrine except where indicated and are for adults.

For anesthesia other than spinal – Maximum single dose is 4.5 mg/kg or 300 mg. When used with epinephrine, the maximum dose is 7 mg/kg or 500 mg.

Caudal (obstetrics) or epidural (thoracic) –

Sol.	Vol. (ml)	Dose (mg)
1%	20 to 30	200 to 300

Epidural (lumbar anesthesia) –

Sol.	Vol. (ml)	Dose (mg)
1.5%	15 to 20	225 to 300
2%	10 to 15	200 to 300

Spinal surgical anesthesia –

Sol.	Vol. (ml)	Dose (mg)
5% with 7.5% dextrose	1.5 to 2	75 to 100

Caudal (surgery) –

Sol.	Vol. (ml)	Dose (mg)
1.5%	15 to 20	225 to 300

ADVERSE REACTIONS

Common reactions are in italics; life-threatening reactions are in bold italics.

Skin: dermatologic reactions.

Other: edema, ***status asthmaticus, anaphylaxis, anaphylactoid reactions.***

The following systemic effects may result from high blood levels:

CNS: anxiety, nervousness, ***seizures*** followed by drowsiness, unconsciousness, tremors, twitches, shivering, ***respiratory arrest.***

CV: myocardial depression, hypotension, ***arrhythmias, cardiac arrest.***

EENT: blurred vision, tinnitus.

GI: nausea, vomiting.

INTERACTIONS

Enflurane, halothane, isoflurane, and related drugs: cardiac arrhythmias when used with lidocaine *with* epinephrine. Use with extreme caution.

MAO inhibitors, cyclic antidepressants: severe, sustained hypertension when used with lidocaine *with* epinephrine. Use with extreme caution.

NURSING CONSIDERATIONS

- *Contraindicated* in inflammation or infection in puncture region, septicemia, severe hypertension, spinal deformities, and neurologic disorders.
- *Use cautiously* in debilitated, elderly, or acutely ill patients; severe shock; heart block; obstetrics; general drug allergies; and paracervical block.
- Dosage and interval are increased with epinephrine.
- For epidural use, test doses are administered to verify needle or catheter placement. Initially, 2 to 3 ml is given to check for subarachnoid injection (which would cause extensive motor paralysis of the lower limbs and excessive sensory deficit). After about 5 minutes and in the absence of symptoms, a second, larger test dose of about 5 ml is given to check for intravascular injection (which would cause tinnitus, numbness around the lips, metallic taste, dysphoria, lethargy, or hypotension).
- Use solutions with epinephrine cautiously in cardiovascular disorders and in body areas with limited blood supply (ears, nose, fingers, toes). Do not use solutions with preservatives for spinal, epidural, or caudal block.
- Keep resuscitation equipment and drugs available.
- Discard partially used vials without preservatives.
- Check solution for particles.

mepivacaine hydrochloride

Carbocaine, Cavacaine, Isocaine

Pregnancy Risk Category: C

HOW SUPPLIED

Injection: 1%, 1.5%, 2%, 3% (dental injection); 2% injection also available with levonordefrin 1:200,000

MECHANISM OF ACTION

A local anesthetic of the amide type. Blocks depolarization by interfering with sodium-potassium exchange across the nerve cell membrane, preventing generation and conduction of the nerve impulse. When combined with levonordefrin, action is prolonged.

INDICATIONS & DOSAGE

Doses cited are for the drug *without* levonordefrin and for adults.

Nerve block–

Sol.	Vol. (ml)	Dose (mg)
1%	5 to 20	50 to 200
2%	5 to 20	100 to 400

Transvaginal block or infiltration (maximum dose)–

Sol.	Vol. (ml)	Dose (mg)
1%	20	200

Paracervical block (obstetrics)–

Sol.	Vol. (ml)	Dose (mg)
1%	10	100

Give on each side (200 mg total) per 90-minute period.

Caudal and epidural–

Sol.	Vol. (ml)	Dose (mg)
1%	15 to 30	150 to 300
1.5%	10 to 25	150 to 375
2%	10 to 20	200 to 400

Therapeutic block (pain management)–

Sol.	Vol. (ml)	Dose (mg)
1%	1 to 5	10 to 50
2%	1 to 5	20 to 100

Adults: maximum single dose 7 mg/kg up to 550 mg. Don't repeat more often than q 90 minutes. Maximum dosage 1,000 mg daily.

Children: maximum dose 5 to 6 mg/kg. In children under 3 years or weighing less than 14 kg, use 0.5% or 1.5% solution only. Dose and interval may be increased with levonordefrin.

ADVERSE REACTIONS

Common reactions are in italics; life-threatening reactions are in bold italics.

Skin: dermatologic reactions.

Other: edema, ***status asthmaticus, anaphylaxis, anaphylactoid reactions.***

The following systemic effects may result from high blood levels of the drug:

CNS: anxiety, nervousness, ***seizures*** followed by drowsiness, unconsciousness, tremors, twitches, shivering, ***respiratory arrest.***

CV: myocardial depression, hypotension, ***arrhythmias, cardiac arrest.***

EENT: blurred vision, tinnitus.

GI: nausea, vomiting.

INTERACTIONS

Enflurane, halothane, isoflurane, and related drugs: cardiac arrhythmias when used with mepivacaine *with* levonordefrin. Use with extreme caution.

MAO inhibitors, cyclic antidepressants: severe, sustained hypertension when used with mepivacaine *with* levonordefrin. Use with extreme caution.

NURSING CONSIDERATIONS

- *Contraindicated* in sensitivity to methylparaben, in heart block, or for spinal anesthesia.
- *Use cautiously* in debilitated, elderly, or acutely ill patients, and for paracervical block.
- For epidural use, test doses are administered to verify needle or catheter placement. Initially, 2 to 3 ml is given to check for subarachnoid injection (which would cause extensive motor paralysis of the lower limbs and excessive sensory deficit). After about 5 minutes and in the absence of symptoms, a second, larger test dose of about 5 ml is given to check for intravascular injection (which would cause tinnitus, numbness around the lips,

*Liquid form contains alcohol. **May contain tartrazine.

metallic taste, dysphoria, lethargy, or hypotension).
- Drug should be administered only by persons who know how to recognize and manage adverse effects caused by epidural anesthetics.
- Use solutions with levonordefrin cautiously in cardiovascular disease and in body areas with limited blood supply (ears, nose, fingers, toes).
- Monitor fetal heart rate when paracervical block is used in delivery.
- Keep resuscitation equipment and drugs available.
- Don't use solutions with preservatives for caudal or epidural block.
- Onset in 15 minutes; duration is 3 hours.
- Discard partially used vials without preservatives.
- Check solution for particles.

procaine hydrochloride

Novocain

Pregnancy Risk Category: C

HOW SUPPLIED

Injection: 1%, 2%, 10%

MECHANISM OF ACTION

A local anesthetic of the ester type. Blocks depolarization by interfering with sodium-potassium exchange across the nerve cell membrane, preventing generation and conduction of the nerve impulse.

INDICATIONS & DOSAGE

Spinal anesthesia –

Adults: maximum dose is 11 mg/kg (14 mg/kg when mixed with epinephrine).

Before using, dilute 10% solution with 0.9% sodium chloride injection, sterile distilled water, or cerebrospinal fluid.

For hyperbaric technique, use dextrose solution.

Perineum: use 0.5 ml 10% solution and 0.5 ml diluent injected at fourth lumbar interspace.

Perineum and lower extremities: use 1 ml 10% solution and 1 ml diluent injected at third or fourth lumbar interspace.

Up to costal margin: use 2 ml 10% solution and 1 ml diluent injected at second, third, or fourth lumbar interspace.

Epidural block –

Sol.	Vol. (ml)	Dose (mg)
1.5%	25	375

Peripheral nerve block –

Sol.	Vol. (ml)	Dose (mg)
1%	50	500
2%	25	500

Infiltration: use 250 to 600 mg 0.25% to 0.5% solution. Maximum initial dose 1 g. Dose and interval may be increased with epinephrine. Maximum dosage 11 mg/kg to 14 mg/kg or epinephrine.

ADVERSE REACTIONS

Common reactions are in italics; life-threatening reactions are in bold italics.

Skin: dermatologic reactions.

Other: edema, ***status asthmaticus, anaphylaxis, anaphylactoid reactions.***

The following systemic effects may result from high blood levels of the drug:

CNS: anxiety, nervousness, ***seizures*** followed by drowsiness, unconsciousness, tremors, twitches, shivering, ***respiratory arrest.***

CV: myocardial depression, hypotension, ***arrhythmias, cardiac arrest.***

EENT: blurred vision, tinnitus.

GI: nausea, vomiting.

INTERACTIONS

Echothiophate iodide: reduced hydrolysis of procaine. Use together cautiously.

Succinylcholine: prolonged neuromuscular blockade. Use together cautiously.

NURSING CONSIDERATIONS

- *Contraindicated* in traumatized urethra and in hypersensitivity to chloroprocaine, tetracaine, or other para-aminobenzoic acid derivatives.
- *Use cautiously* in hyperexcitable patients and in CNS diseases, infection at puncture site, shock, profound anemia, cachexia, sepsis, hypertension, hypotension, GI hemorrhage, bowel perforation or strangulation, peritonitis, cardiac decompensation, massive pleural effusions, obstetrics, and increased intraabdominal pressure.
- Contraindications in obstetric use are pelvic disproportion, placenta previa, abruptio placentae, floating fetal head, and intrauterine manipulation.
- Keep resuscitation equipment and drugs available.
- For epidural use, test doses are administered to verify needle or catheter placement. Initially, 2 to 3 ml is given to check for subarachnoid injection (which would cause extensive motor paralysis of the lower limbs and excessive sensory deficit). After about 5 minutes and in the absence of symptoms, a second, larger test dose of about 5 ml is given to check for intravascular injection (which would cause tinnitus, numbness around the lips, metallic taste, dysphoria, lethargy, or hypotension).
- Use solution without preservatives for epidural block.
- Onset in 2 to 5 minutes; duration 60 minutes.
- Discard partially used vials without preservatives.
- Check solution for particles.

tetracaine hydrochloride

Pontocaine

Pregnancy Risk Category: C

HOW SUPPLIED

Injection: 1%
Injection (with dextrose, 6%): 0.2%, 0.3%
Powder for reconstitution: 20 mg/ampule

MECHANISM OF ACTION

A local anesthetic of the ester type. Blocks depolarization by interfering with sodium-potassium exchange across the nerve cell membrane, preventing generation and conduction of the nerve impulse.

INDICATIONS & DOSAGE

Dosage for adults varies according to the extent of the block as follows.
Low spinal (saddle block) in vaginal delivery –
give 2 to 5 mg as hyperbaric solution (in 10% dextrose).
Perineum and lower extremities: give 5 to 10 mg.
Up to costal margin: give 15 to 20 mg.

ADVERSE REACTIONS

Common reactions are in italics; life-threatening reactions are in bold italics.
Skin: dermatologic reactions.
Other: edema, ***status asthmaticus, anaphylaxis, anaphylactoid reactions.***

The following systemic effects may result from high blood levels of the drug:
CNS: anxiety, nervousness, seizures followed by drowsiness, unconsciousness, tremors, twitches, shivering, and ***respiratory arrest.***
CV: myocardial depression, hypotension, ***arrhythmias, cardiac arrest.***
EENT: blurred vision, tinnitus.
GI: nausea, vomiting.

INTERACTIONS

None significant.

NURSING CONSIDERATIONS

- *Contraindicated* in infection at injection site, CNS diseases, hypersensitivity to procaine, chloroprocaine, tetracaine, or related agents.
- Saddle block is contraindicated in cephalopelvic disproportion, placenta

previa, abruptio placentae, intrauterine manipulation, and floating fetal head.

- *Use cautiously* in shock, profound anemia, cachexia, hypertension, hypotension, peritonitis, cardiac decompensation, massive pleural effusion, increased intracranial pressure, infection, and in nervous patients.
- Don't use cloudy, discolored, or crystallized solutions.
- Keep resuscitation equipment and drugs available.
- 10 times as strong as procaine hydrochloride.
- Onset in 15 minutes; duration up to 3 hours.
- When cerebrospinal fluid is added to powdered drug or drug solution during spinal anesthesia, solution may be cloudy.
- Protect from light; store refrigerated.

91
General anesthetics

droperidol
etomidate
fentanyl citrate with droperidol
ketamine hydrochloride
methohexital sodium
propofol
thiopental sodium

COMBINATION PRODUCTS
None.

droperidol
Droleptan‡, Inapsine
Pregnancy Risk Category: C

HOW SUPPLIED
Tablets: 10 mg‡
Oral solution: 1 mg/ml‡
Injection: 2.5 mg/ml, 5 mg/ml‡

MECHANISM OF ACTION
Acts at subcortical levels to produce sedation.

INDICATIONS & DOSAGE
Premedication –
Adults: 2.5 to 10 mg (1 to 4 ml) I.M. 30 to 60 minutes preoperatively.
Children 2 to 12 years: 0.088 to 0.165 mg/kg or 1 to 1.5 mg (0.4 to 0.6 ml)/20 to 25 lb body weight I.M.
As an induction agent –
Adults: 0.22 to 0.275 mg/kg or 2.5 mg (1 ml)/20 to 25 lb body weight I.V. with analgesic or general anesthetic.
Children 2 to 12 years: 0.088 to 0.165 mg/kg or 1 to 1.5 mg (0.4 to 0.6 ml)/20 to 25 lb I.V. Dosage should be titrated.
Elderly and debilitated patients: initial dose should be decreased.
Maintenance dosage in general anesthesia –
Adults: 1.25 to 2.5 mg I.V.
To suppress nystagmus, nausea, vomiting, and vertigo associated with an acute attack of Ménière's disease –
Adults: 5 mg I.M. as a single dose.
Management of severe agitation of psychotic disorders‡ –
Adults: 10 to 25 mg P.O. daily in divided doses.

ADVERSE REACTIONS
Common reactions are in italics; life-threatening reactions are in bold italics.
Blood: ***agranulocytosis.***
CNS: extrapyramidal reactions (dystonia, akathisia), upward rotation of eyes and oculogyric crises, extended neck, flexed arms, fine tremor of limbs, dizziness, chills or shivering, facial sweating, restlessness, decreased seizure threshold.
CV: *hypotension,* tachycardia.
Respiratory: ***laryngospasm, bronchospasm.***

INTERACTIONS
Epinephrine: may cause hypotension. Avoid concomitant use.

NURSING CONSIDERATIONS
- *Use cautiously* in elderly or debilitated patients and in patients with hypotension or other cardiovascular disease, impaired hepatic or renal function, and Parkinson's disease.
- Watch for extrapyramidal reactions. Call doctor at once if any occur.
- A butyrophenone compound, related to haloperidol; has greater tendency to cause extrapyramidal reactions than other antipsychotics.
- Droperidol has been used as an I.V. antiemetic in cancer chemotherapy.
- **I.V. use:** Give I.V. injections slowly.
- Keep I.V. fluids and vasopressors

*Liquid form contains alcohol. **May contain tartrazine.

available for treatment of hypotension.
• Monitor vital signs frequently; notify doctor of any changes immediately.
• Do not place patient in Trendelenburg's position; severe hypotension and deeper anesthesia may result, causing respiratory arrest.
• If hypotension occurs, do not treat with epinephrine; it may worsen hypotension.

etomidate

Amidate, Hypnomidate

Pregnancy Risk Category: C

HOW SUPPLIED
Injection: 2 mg/ml

MECHANISM OF ACTION
Inhibits the firing rate of neurons within the ascending reticular-activating system.

INDICATIONS & DOSAGE
Induction of general anesthesia – **Adults and children over 10 years:** 0.2 to 0.6 mg/kg I.V. over a period of 30 to 60 seconds.

ADVERSE REACTIONS
Common reactions are in italics; life-threatening reactions are in bold italics.
CNS: myoclonic movements, averting movements, tonic movements, transient apnea, hyperventilation, hypoventilation.
CV: hypertension, hypotension, tachycardia, bradycardia.
EENT: *eye movements, **laryngospasm.***
GI: nausea or vomiting following induction of anesthesia.
Local: *transient venous pain.*
Other: hiccups, snoring, inhibition of adrenal steroid production.

INTERACTIONS
None significant.

NURSING CONSIDERATIONS
• *Contraindicated* during labor and delivery, including cesarean sections.
• Smaller increments of I.V. etomidate may be administered to adults during short operations to supplement subpotent anesthetic agents, such as nitrous oxide.
• Other commonly used preanesthesia drugs may be given before etomidate is used.
• **I.V. use:** Inject drug into I.V. tubing containing a free-flowing compatible solution over 30 to 60 seconds. Intermittent or continuous infusion is not recommended.
• Etomidate has a rapid onset of action (about 1 minute). Duration of effect is short (3 to 5 minutes).
• Transient muscle movements can be decreased by first administering 0.1 mg of fentanyl.
• Muscle movements seem more common in patients who feel transient venous pain after injection.
• Monitor vital signs before, during, and after anesthesia.
• Have resuscitation equipment and drugs ready. Maintain airway.
• Etomidate has a much lower incidence of cardiovascular and respiratory effects; therefore, it is advantageous for inducing anesthesia in high-risk surgical patients.

fentanyl citrate with droperidol

Innovar

Controlled Substance Schedule II

Pregnancy Risk Category: C

HOW SUPPLIED
Injection: 0.5 mg fentanyl and 2.5 mg droperidol per ml

MECHANISM OF ACTION
Acts as a CNS depressant to produce a general calming effect, reduced motor activity, and analgesia.

INDICATIONS & DOSAGE

Dosages vary depending on application; use of other agents; and patient's age, body weight, and clinical status.

Anesthesia –

Adults: premedication with 0.5 to 2 ml I.M. 45 to 60 minutes before surgery.

Children: premedication with 0.25 ml/20 lb body weight I.M. 45 to 60 minutes before surgery

Adjunct to general anesthesia –

Adults: induction with 0.1 ml/kg or 1 ml/20 to 25 lb body weight by slow I.V. to produce neuroleptanalgesia; not indicated as sole agent for maintenance of surgical anesthesia. Used in combination with other agents. To prevent excessive accumulation of the relatively long-acting droperidol component, fentanyl alone should be used in increments of 0.025 to 0.05 mg (0.5 to 1 ml) for maintenance of analgesia. However, during prolonged surgery, additional 0.5- to 1-ml amounts of Innovar may be given with caution.

Children: 0.05 ml/kg or 0.5 ml/20 lb body weight I.V. (total combined dose for induction and maintenance). Following induction with Innovar, fentanyl alone in a dose of ¼ to ⅓ of adult dosage should be used to avoid accumulation of droperidol. However, during prolonged surgery, additional Innovar may be administered with caution. Safe use in children under 2 years has not been established.

Adjunct in regional anesthesia –

Adults: 1 to 2 ml I.M. or slow I.V.

Diagnostic procedures –

Adults: 0.5 to 2 ml I.M. 45 to 60 minutes before procedure. In prolonged procedure, give 0.5 to 1 ml I.V. with caution and without a general anesthetic.

ADVERSE REACTIONS

Common reactions are in italics; life-threatening reactions are in bold italics.

CNS: emergence delirium and hallucinations, postoperative drowsiness.

CV: vasodilation, *hypotension,* decreased pulmonary arterial pressure, bradycardia, tachycardia.

EENT: blurred vision, ***laryngospasm.***

GI: *nausea, vomiting.*

Respiratory: ***respiratory depression, apnea, or arrest.***

Other: drug dependence, muscle rigidity, chills, *shivering,* diaphoresis.

INTERACTIONS

CNS depressants (such as barbiturates, tranquilizers, narcotics, and general anesthetics): additive effect. Dosage should be reduced.

Epinephrine: may worsen hypotension. Avoid concomitant use.

MAO inhibitors: increased adverse effects. Do not use within 2 weeks of MAO inhibitor therapy.

NURSING CONSIDERATIONS

- *Contraindicated* in intolerance to either component.
- *Use cautiously* in patients with head injuries and increased intracranial pressure, chronic obstructive pulmonary disease, hepatic and renal dysfunction, bradyarrhythmias, and in elderly or debilitated patients.
- **I.V. use:** Inject undiluted drug directly into vein or into I.V. tubing containing a free-flowing compatible solution. Alternatively, rapidly infuse diluted drug until onset of drowsiness. Then slow infusion or stop drip and administer general anesthetic, as appropriate. Intermittent infusion is not recommended.
- Hypotension is a common adverse reaction. However, if blood pressure drops, also consider hypovolemia as a possible cause. Use appropriate parenteral fluids to help restore blood pressure. Do not treat with epinephrine; it may worsen hypotension.
- Vital signs should be monitored frequently.
- Be aware that respiratory depression, rigidity of respiratory muscles,

and respiratory arrest can occur. Have narcotic antagonist and resuscitative equipment available.
- Maintain airway.
- Postoperative EEG pattern may return to normal slowly.
- If narcotic analgesics are required postoperatively, use initially in reduced doses, as low as ¼ to ⅓ those usually recommended.
- When Innovar is given for anesthesia induction, fentanyl (Sublimaze) should be used for maintenance analgesia during procedure.

ketamine hydrochloride
Ketalar

Pregnancy Risk Category: C

HOW SUPPLIED
Injection: 10 mg/ml, 50 mg/ml, 100 mg/ml

MECHANISM OF ACTION
Interrupts association pathways in the brain, causing dissociative anesthesia, a feeling of dissociation from the environment.

INDICATIONS & DOSAGE
Induce anesthesia for procedures, especially short-term diagnostic or surgical, not requiring skeletal muscle relaxation; before giving other general anesthetics or to supplement low-potency agents, such as nitrous oxide –
Adults and children: 1 to 4.5 mg/kg I.V., administered over 60 seconds; or 6.5 to 13 mg/kg I.M. To maintain anesthesia, repeat in increments of half to full initial dose.

ADVERSE REACTIONS
Common reactions are in italics; life-threatening reactions are in bold italics.
CNS: *tonic and clonic movements resembling seizures, dream-like states, hallucinations, confusion, excitement,* irrational behavior, psychic abnormalities, *emergence delirium.*
CV: *increased blood pressure and pulse rate,* hypotension, bradycardia.
EENT: diplopia, nystagmus, slight increase in intraocular pressure, ***laryngospasm,*** *salivation.*
GI: mild anorexia, nausea, vomiting.
Respiratory: ***respiratory depression, apnea when administered too rapidly.***
Skin: transient erythema, measles-like rash.

INTERACTIONS
Barbiturates, opiates, other CNS depressants: may prolong recovery time. Monitor closely.
Halothane: increased risk of adverse cardiac effects. Monitor closely.
Thyroid hormones: may elevate blood pressure and cause tachycardia. Give cautiously.

NURSING CONSIDERATIONS
- *Contraindicated* in patients with history of CVA; patients who would be endangered by a significant rise in blood pressure (including those with increased intracranial pressure and increased intraocular pressure); and in severe hypertension, severe cardiac decompensation, or surgery of the pharynx, larynx, or bronchial tree (unless used with muscle relaxants).
- *Use cautiously* in chronic alcoholism, alcohol-intoxicated patients, and in patients with cerebrospinal fluid pressure elevated before anesthesia.
- Because of rapid induction, patient should be physically supported during administration.
- **I.V. use:** Over 1 minute, inject initial dose directly into vein or into I.V. tubing containing a free-flowing compatible solution. Intermittent infusion is not recommended. For continuous infusion, infuse diluted drug at a rate of 1 to 2 mg/minute.
- Do not inject barbiturates and ketamine from same syringe, as they are chemically incompatible.

• Monitor vital signs before, during, and after anesthesia.
• Maintain airway.
• Resuscitation equipment should be available and ready for use.
• Start supportive respiration if respiratory depression occurs. Use mechanical support if possible rather than administering analeptics.
• Keep verbal, tactile, and visual stimulation at a minimum during recovery phase to reduce incidence of emergent reactions.
• Hallucinations and excitement can occur on emergence from anesthesia; they can be abated by administering diazepam.
• A potent hallucinogen that can readily produce dissociative anesthesia (patient feels detached from environment). Dissociative effect and hallucinatory adverse reactions have made this a popular drug of abuse.

methohexital sodium (methohexitone sodium)

Brevital Sodium, Brietal Sodium†‡
Controlled Substance Schedule IV
Pregnancy Risk Category: D

HOW SUPPLIED
Powder for injection: 500 mg, 2.5 g, 5 g

MECHANISM OF ACTION
Inhibits the firing rate of neurons within the ascending reticular-activating system.

INDICATIONS & DOSAGE
General anesthetic for short-term procedures (oral surgery, gynecologic and genitourinary examinations); reduction of fractures; before electroconvulsive therapy; for prolonged anesthesia when used with gaseous anesthetics –
Adults and children: 5 to 12 ml 1% solution (50 to 120 mg) I.V. at 1 ml/5 seconds. Dose required for induction may vary from 50 to 120 mg or more; average about 70 mg. Induction dose provides anesthesia for 5 to 7 minutes.
Maintenance –
Intermittent injection: 2 to 4 ml 1% solution (20 to 40 mg) q 4 to 7 minutes.
Continuous I.V. drip: administer 0.2% solution (1 drop/second).

ADVERSE REACTIONS
Common reactions are in italics; life-threatening reactions are in bold italics.
CNS: *muscular twitching,* headache, emergence delirium.
CV: *transient hypotension, tachycardia,* circulatory depression, ***peripheral vascular collapse.***
GI: excessive salivation, *nausea, vomiting.*
Respiratory: ***laryngospasm, bronchospasm, respiratory depression, apnea.***
Skin: tissue necrosis with extravasation.
Local: thrombophlebitis, pain at injection site, injury to nerves adjacent to injection site.
Other: hiccups, coughing, acute allergic reactions. Extended use may cause cumulative effect.

INTERACTIONS
None significant.

NURSING CONSIDERATIONS
• *Contraindicated* in severe hepatic dysfunction, hypersensitivity to barbiturates, or porphyria; in shock or impending shock; and in patients for whom general anesthetics would be hazardous.
• *Use cautiously* in debilitated patients; in asthma, respiratory obstruction, severe hypertension or hypotension, myocardial disease, CHF, severe anemia, and extreme obesity.
• Maintain pulmonary ventilation.
• Monitor vital signs before, during, and after anesthesia.

*Liquid form contains alcohol. **May contain tartrazine.

- Have resuscitation equipment and drugs ready.
- Reduce postoperative nausea by having patient fast before administration.
- **I.V. use:** Ensure that catheter is in a vein before injection. Discontinue immediately if extravasation occurs.
- Incompatible with lactated Ringer's solution.
- Do not mix with acid solutions, such as atropine sulfate.
- Do not use distilled water or diluents that contain bacteriostatic agents. Alternative diluents are 5% dextrose solution or 0.9% sodium chloride solution.
- Rate of flow must be individualized for each patient.
- Solutions may be stored and used as long as they remain clear and colorless. Solutions cannot be heated for sterilization.
- Incompatible with silicone; avoid contact with rubber stoppers or parts of syringes that have been treated with silicone.
- Has potential for abuse.

propofol

Diprivan

Pregnancy Risk Category: D

HOW SUPPLIED

Injection: 10 mg/ml in 20-ml ampules

MECHANISM OF ACTION

Propofol produces a dose-dependent CNS depression similar to benzodiazepines and barbiturates. However, it can be used to maintain anesthesia through careful titration of infusion rate.

INDICATIONS & DOSAGE

Induction of anesthesia –

Adults: doses must be individualized according to patient's condition and age. Most patients classified as American Society of Anesthesiologists (ASA) Physical Status category (PS) I or II under 55 years require 2 to 2.5 mg/kg I.V. The drug is usually administered in 40-mg boluses q 10 seconds until the desired response is obtained.

Elderly, debilitated, or hypovolemic patients, or patients in ASA PS III or IV should receive half of the usual induction dose (20 mg-boluses q 10 seconds).

Maintenance of anesthesia –

Adults: propofol may be given as a variable-rate infusion, titrated to clinical effect. Most patients may be maintained with 0.1 to 0.2 mg/kg/minute (6 to 12 mg/kg/hr).

Elderly, debilitated, or hypovolemic patients, or patients in ASA PS III or IV should receive half of the usual maintenance dose (0.05 to 0.1 mg/kg/minute, or 3 to 6 mg/kg/hr).

ADVERSE REACTIONS

Common reactions are in italics; life-threatening reactions are in bold italics.

CNS: headache, dizziness, twitching, clonic or myoclonic movement.

CV: hypotension, bradycardia, hypertension.

GI: nausea, vomiting, abdominal cramping.

Respiratory: ***apnea,*** cough.

Skin: flushing.

Local: burning or stinging, pain, tingling or numbness, and coldness at injection site.

Other: fever, hiccups.

INTERACTIONS

Inhalational anesthetics (such as enflurane, isoflurane, and halothane) or supplemental anesthetics (such as nitrous oxide and opiates): can be expected to enhance the anesthetic and cardiovascular actions of propofol.

Opiate analgesics, sedatives: may cause a more pronounced decrease of systolic, diastolic, and mean arterial pressure and of cardiac output; may also decrease the induction dose requirements.

NURSING CONSIDERATIONS

- *Contraindicated* in patients hypersensitive to propofol or any components of the emulsion, including soybean oil, egg lecithin, and glycerol.
- *Use cautiously* in patients with a history of disorders of lipid metabolism, such as pancreatitis or primary hyperlipoproteinemia, and in patients with diabetic hyperlipidemia, because the drug is administered as an emulsion.
- *Use cautiously* in patients who are elderly or debilitated and in patients with circulatory disorders. Although the hemodynamic effects of the drug can vary, its major effect in patients maintaining spontaneous ventilation is arterial hypotension (arterial pressure can decrease as much as 30%) with little or no change in heart rate and cardiac output. Cardiac output may be markedly depressed in patients undergoing assisted or controlled positive-pressure ventilation.
- Propofol is not recommended for use in obstetric anesthesia because the safety to the fetus has not been established. It is not recommended for use in patients with increased intracranial pressure or impaired cerebral circulation because the drug's effect in reducing systemic arterial pressure may substantially reduce cerebral perfusion pressure.
- Propofol should be administered under direct medical supervision by persons familiar with airway management and the administration of I.V. anesthetics.
- Patients should be closely monitored for signs of significant hypotension or bradycardia. Treatment of such effects may include increased rate of fluid administration, pressor agents, elevation of lower extremities, or atropine. Apnea, which may occur during induction, may persist for longer than 60 seconds and require ventilatory support.
- Pharmacokinetics of propofol are not altered by chronic hepatic cirrosis, chronic renal failure, or gender.
- Propofol has no vagolytic activity. Premedication with anticholinergics such as glycopyrrolate or atropine may help manage potential increases in vagal tone caused by other drugs or surgical manipulations.
- Prepare under strict aseptic technique. The vehicle for propofol is fat emulsion, and it contains no preservatives. Rapid microbial growth is possible if the solution is contaminated. It is intended for single use, and unused solution should be discarded at the end of the procedure. Postoperative fevers have been linked to the use of contaminated solutions.
- Propofol should not be mixed with other drugs or blood products. If it is to be diluted before infusion, use only 5% dextrose in water, and do not dilute to a concentration less than 2 mg/ml. After dilution, it appears to be more stable in glass containers as compared to plastic.
- **I.V. use:** When administered into a running I.V. catheter, propofol emulsion is compatible with 5% dextrose in water, lactated Ringer's injection, lactated Ringer's and 5% dextrose injection, 5% dextrose and 0.45% sodium chloride injection, and 5% dextrose and 0.2% sodium chloride injection.
- Propofol emulsion should be stored above 40° F (4° C) and below 72° F (22° C). Do not refrigerate.
- Propofol is excreted in breast milk and is not recommended for use by breast-feeding mothers.

thiopental sodium (thiopentone sodium)

Intraval Sodium‡, Pentothal Sodium

Controlled Substance Schedule III

Pregnancy Risk Category: C

HOW SUPPLIED

Injection: 250-mg, 400-mg, 500-mg syringes; 500-mg/1-g vial with diluent; 1-g (2.5%), 2.5-g (2.5%), 5-g (2.5%), 2.5-g (2%), and 5-g (2%) kits
Rectal suspension: 2-g disposable syringe (400 mg/g of suspension)

MECHANISM OF ACTION

Inhibits the firing rate of neurons within the ascending reticular-activating system.

INDICATIONS & DOSAGE

Induce anesthesia before administering other anesthetics –
Adults: administer a test dose of 25 to 75 mg I.V. to assess patient for tolerance or unusual sensitivity. Monitor for 60 seconds. Then give 210 to 280 mg (3 to 4 ml/kg) I.V., which is usually required for average adult (70 kg).
General anesthetic for short-term procedures –
Adults: 2 to 3 ml 2.5% solution (50 to 75 mg) administered I.V. only at intervals of 20 to 40 seconds, depending on reaction. Dose may be repeated with caution, if necessary.
Seizures following anesthesia –
Adults: 75 to 125 mg (3 to 5 ml of 2.5% solution) immediately.
Psychiatric disorders (narcoanalysis, narcosynthesis) –
Adults: 100 mg/minute (4 ml/minute 2.5% solution) until confusion occurs and before sleep.
Basal anesthesia by rectal administration –
Adults and children: administer up to 1 g/22.5 kg (50 lb) body weight, or 0.5 ml 10% solution/kg body weight. Maximum 1 to 1.5 g (children weighing 34 kg or more) and 3 to 4 g (adults weighing 91 kg or more).

Note: Thiopental is rarely administered rectally for basal sedation or anesthesia because of variable absorption from the rectum.

ADVERSE REACTIONS

Common reactions are in italics; life-threatening reactions are in bold italics.
CNS: *prolonged somnolence,* retrograde amnesia, emergence delirium.
CV: myocardial depression, ***arrhythmias.***
Skin: tissue necrosis with extravasation.
Respiratory: ***respiratory depression*** *(momentary apnea following each injection is typical),* ***bronchospasm, laryngospasm.***
Local: pain at injection site.
Other: sneezing, coughing, *shivering.*

INTERACTIONS

None significant.

NURSING CONSIDERATIONS

- *Contraindicated* in absence of suitable veins for I.V. administration, hypersensitivity to barbiturates, status asthmaticus, porphyria, respiratory depression or obstruction, decompensated cardiac disease, severe anemia, hepatic cirrhosis, shock, renal dysfunction, myxedema.
- When used as general anesthetic, give atropine sulfate as premedication to diminish laryngeal reflexes and to prevent laryngospasm.
- **I.V. use:** Inject ordered dose through I.V. tubing containing a free-flowing compatible solution.
- Have resuscitation equipment and oxygen available. Maintain airway.
- Avoid extravasation.
- Monitor vital signs before, during, and after anesthesia.
- Solutions of atropine sulfate, *d*-tubocurarine, or succinylcholine may be given concurrently.
- Do not heat solutions for sterilization. Solutions should be used within 24 hours.

92

Vitamins and minerals

vitamin A

vitamin B complex
cyanocobalamin
hydroxocobalamin
folic acid
leucovorin calcium
niacin
niacinamide
pyridoxine hydrochloride
riboflavin
thiamine hydrochloride

vitamin C
vitamin D
cholecalciferol
ergocalciferol
vitamin E

vitamin K analogs
menadione/menadiol sodium diphosphate
phytonadione
sodium fluoride
sodium fluoride, topical

trace elements
chromium
copper
iodine
manganese
selenium
zinc

COMBINATION PRODUCTS

M.T.E.-4: zinc sulfate 1 mg, copper sulfate 0.4 mg, manganese sulfate 0.1 mg, and chromium chloride 4 mcg per ml.

M.T.E.-4 CONCENTRATED: zinc sulfate 5 mg, copper sulfate 1 mg, manganese sulfate 0.5 mg, and chromium chloride 10 mcg per ml.

M.T.E.-5: zinc sulfate 1 mg, copper sulfate 0.4 mg, manganese sulfate 0.1 mg, chromium chloride 4 mcg, and selenium (as selenious acid) 20 mcg per ml.

M.T.E.-5 CONCENTRATED: zinc sulfate 5 mg, copper sulfate 1 mg, manganese sulfate 0.5 mg, chromium chloride 10 mcg, and selenium (as selenious acid) 60 mcg per ml.

M.T.E.-6: zinc sulfate 1 mg, copper sulfate 0.4 mg, manganese sulfate 0.1 mg, chromium chloride 4 mcg, selenium (as selenious acid) 20 mcg, and sodium iodide 25 mcg per ml.

M.T.E.-6 CONCENTRATED: zinc sulfate 5 mg, copper sulfate 1 mg, manganese sulfate 0.5 mg, chromium chloride 10 mcg, selenium (as selenious acid) 60 mcg, and sodium iodide 75 mcg per ml.

M.T.E.-7: zinc sulfate 1 mg, copper sulfate 0.4 mg, manganese sulfate 0.1 mg, chromium chloride 4 mcg, selenium (as selenious acid) 20 mcg, and sodium iodide 25 mcg per ml.

MULTIPLE TRACE ELEMENT: zinc sulfate 1 mg, copper sulfate 0.4 mg, manganese sulfate 0.1 mg, and chromium chloride 4 mcg per ml.

MULTIPLE TRACE ELEMENT CONCENTRATED: zinc sulfate 5 mg, copper sulfate 1 mg, manganese sulfate 0.5 mg, and chromium chloride 10 mcg per ml.

MULTITRACE: zinc chloride 1 mg, copper chloride 0.4 mg, manganese chloride 0.1 mg, and chromium chloride 4 mcg per ml.

MULTITRACE 5: zinc sulfate 1 mg, copper sulfate 0.4 mg, manganese sulfate 0.1 mg, chromium chloride 4 mcg, and selenium (as selenious acid) 20 mcg per ml.

MULTITRACE CONCENTRATE: zinc chloride 5 mg, copper chloride 1 mg, manganese chloride 0.5 mg, and chromium chloride 10 mcg per ml.

MULTITRACE PEDIATRIC: zinc sul-

*Liquid form contains alcohol. **May contain tartrazine.

fate 1 mg, copper sulfate 0.1 mg, manganese sulfate 0.025 mg, and chromium chloride 1 mcg per ml.
NEOTRACE-4: zinc sulfate 1.5 mg, copper sulfate 0.1 mg, manganese sulfate 0.025 mg, and chromium chloride 0.85 mcg per ml.
PEDIATRIC MULTIPLE TRACE ELEMENT: zinc sulfate 0.5 mg, copper sulfate 0.1 mg, manganese sulfate 0.03 mg, and chromium chloride 1 mcg per ml.
PEDTRACE-4: zinc sulfate 0.5 mg, copper sulfate 0.1 mg, manganese sulfate 0.025 mg, and chromium chloride 0.85 mcg per ml.
P.T.E.-4: zinc sulfate 1 mg, copper sulfate 0.1 mg, manganese sulfate 0.025 mg, and chromium chloride 1 mcg per ml.
P.T.E.-5: zinc sulfate 1 mg, copper sulfate 0.1 mg, manganese sulfate 0.025 mg, chromium chloride 1 mcg, and selenium (as selenious acid) 15 mcg per ml.
T.E.C.: zinc sulfate 1 mg, copper sulfate 0.4 mg, manganese sulfate 0.1 mg, and chromium chloride 4 mcg per ml.
TRACE METALS ADDITIVE: zinc chloride 0.8 mg, copper chloride 0.2 mg, manganese chloride 0.16 mg, and chromium chloride 2 mcg per ml.
B complex vitamins◊
B complex vitamins with iron◊
B complex with vitamin C◊
B vitamin combinations◊
Calcium and vitamin products◊
Fluoride with vitamins◊
Geriatric supplements with multivitamins and minerals◊
Miscellaneous vitamins and minerals◊
Multivitamins◊
Multivitamins and minerals with hormones◊
Multivitamins with B_{12}◊
Vitamin A and D combinations◊

vitamin A (retinol)

Acon, Aquasol A, Del-Vi-A

Pregnancy Risk Category: A (X if > RDA)

HOW SUPPLIED

Tablets: 10,000 IU
Capsules: 10,000 IU◊, 25,000 IU, 50,000 IU
Drops: 30 ml with dropper (5,000 IU/0.1 ml)
Injection: 2-ml vials (5,000 IU/ml with 0.5% chlorobutanol, polysorbate 80, butylated hydroxyanisol, and butylated hydroxytoluene)

MECHANISM OF ACTION

Coenzyme necessary for retinal function, bone growth, and differentiation of epithelial tissues.

INDICATIONS & DOSAGE

Recommended daily allowance (RDA) –
Note: RDAs have been converted to IU for convenience. Vitamin A activity is expressed as retinol equivalents (RE). One RE has the activity of 0.3 mcg all-*trans* retinal, 6 mcg beta carotene, or 12 mcg carotenoid provitamins.
Neonates and infants to 1 year: 1,875 IU.
Children over 1 year to 3 years: 2,000 IU.
Children 4 to 6 years: 2,500 IU.
Children 7 to 10 years: 3,500 IU.
Males over 11 years: 5,000 IU.
Females over 11 years: 4,000 IU.
Pregnant women: 5,000 IU.
Lactating women (first 6 months): 6,500 IU.
Lactating women (second 6 months): 6,000 IU.
Severe vitamin A deficiency –
Adults and children over 8 years: 50,000 to 100,000 IU I.M. or 100,000 to 500,000 IU P.O. for 3 days, followed by 50,000 IU I.M. or P.O. for 2 weeks; then 10,000 to

20,000 IU P.O. for 2 months. Follow with adequate dietary nutrition and RDA vitamin A supplements.
Children 1 to 8 years: 17,500 to 35,000 IU I.M. daily for 10 days.
Infants under 1 year: 7,500 to 15,000 IU I.M. daily for 10 days.
Maintenance only –
Children 4 to 8 years: 15,000 IU I.M. daily for 2 months, then adequate dietary nutrition and RDA vitamin A supplements.
Children under 4 years: 10,000 IU I.M. daily for 2 months, then adequate dietary nutrition and RDA vitamin A supplements.

ADVERSE REACTIONS
Common reactions are in italics; life-threatening reactions are in bold italics. Adverse reactions are usually seen only with toxicity.
Blood: hypoplastic anemia, leukocytosis, thrombocytopenia.
CNS: irritability, headache, ***increased intracranial pressure,*** fatigue, lethargy, malaise, vertigo, visual disturbances.
EENT: miosis, papilledema, exophthalmos.
GI: anorexia, epigastric pain, diarrhea, nausea, vomiting.
GU: hypomenorrhea.
Hepatic: jaundice, hepatomegaly, ***cirrhosis,*** elevated liver enzymes.
Skin: alopecia; drying, cracking, scaling of skin; pruritus; lip fissures; massive desquamation; increased pigmentation; night sweating; brittle nails.
Other: skeletal – slow growth, decalcification of bone, hypercalcemia, hypercalciuria, fractures, hyperostosis, periostitis, premature closure of epiphyses, migratory arthralgia, cortical thickening over the radius and tibia, bulging fontanelles; splenomegaly.

INTERACTIONS
Mineral oil, cholestyramine resin: reduced GI absorption of fat-soluble vitamins. If needed, give mineral oil at bedtime.
Multiple vitamins containing vitamin A: risk of toxicity. Avoid concomitant use.
Warfarin: increased risk of bleeding. Monitor prothrombin time closely.

NURSING CONSIDERATIONS
- *Contraindicated* for oral administration in malabsorption syndrome; if malabsorption is from inadequate bile secretion, oral route may be used with concurrent administration of bile salts (dehydrocholic acid). Also contraindicated in hypervitaminosis A. I.V. administration contraindicated except for special water-miscible forms intended for infusion with large parenteral volumes. I.V. push of vitamin A of any type is also contraindicated (anaphylaxis or anaphylactoid reactions and death have resulted).
- *Use cautiously* in pregnant women. Avoid doses exceeding RDA.
- Evaluate patient's vitamin A intake from fortified foods, dietary supplements, self-administered drugs, and prescription drug sources.
- To avoid toxicity, discourage patient self-administration of megavitamin doses without specific indications. Also stress that the patient should not share prescribed vitamins with family members or others. If family member feels vitamin therapy may be of value, have him contact his doctor.
- Watch for adverse reactions if dosage is high.
- Acute toxicity has resulted from single doses of 25,000 IU/kg of body weight; 350,000 IU in infants and over 2,000,000 IU in adults have also proved acutely toxic.
- Chronic toxicity in infants (3 to 6 months) has resulted from doses of 18,500 IU daily for 1 to 3 months. In adults, chronic toxicity has resulted

from doses of 50,000 IU daily for over 8 months; 500,000 IU daily for 2 months, and 1,000,000 IU daily for 3 days.

- Monitor patient closely during vitamin A therapy for skin disorders since high dosages may induce chronic toxicity.
- Liquid preparations available if nasogastric administration is necessary. May be mixed with cereal or fruit juice.
- Record eating and bowel habits. Report abnormalities to doctor.
- Adequate vitamin A absorption requires suitable protein intake, bile (give supplemental salts if necessary), concurrent RDA doses of vitamin E, and zinc (multivitamins usually supply zinc, but supplements may be necessary in long-term total parenteral nutrition).
- Absorption is fastest and most complete with water-miscible preparations, intermediate with emulsions, and slowest with oil suspensions.
- Because of the potential for toxicity, vitamin supplements containing vitamin A should be used cautiously in patients taking isotretinoin (Accutane).
- Protect from light and heat.

cyanocobalamin (vitamin B_{12})

Anacobin†, Bedoce, Bedoz†, Betalin 12, Bioglan B_{12} Plus‡, Crysti-12, Crystamine, Cyanabin†, Cyanocobalamin, Cyano-Gel, Cyanoject, Cyomin, Dodex, Ener-B◊, Kaybovite, Poyamin, Redisol, Rubesol-1000, Rubion†, Rubramin, Sigamine

hydroxocobalamin (vitamin B_{12a})

Alpha-Ruvite, Codroxomin, Droxomin, Hydrobexan, Hydro-Cobex, Hydro-Crysti-12, LA-12, Rubesol-L.A.

Pregnancy Risk Category: A (C if > RDA)

HOW SUPPLIED

cyanocobalamin
Tablets: 500 mcg◊, 1,000 mcg◊
Injection: 30 mcg/ml, 100 mcg/ml, 1,000 mcg/ml
hydroxocobalamin
Injection: 30-ml vials (30 mcg/ml, 100 mcg/ml, 120 mcg/ml with benzyl alcohol, 1,000 mcg/ml, 1,000 mcg/ml with benzyl alcohol), 10-ml vials (100 mcg/ml, 100 mcg/ml with benzyl alcohol, 1,000 mcg/ml, 1,000 mcg/ml with benzyl alcohol, 1,000 mcg/ml with methyl and propyl parabens), 5-ml vials (1,000 mcg/ml with benzyl alcohol), 1-ml vials (1,000 mcg/ml with benzyl alcohol), 1-ml unimatic (1,000 mcg/ml with benzyl alcohol)

MECHANISM OF ACTION

Coenzyme for various metabolic functions. Necessary for cell replication and hematopoiesis.

INDICATIONS & DOSAGE

Recommended daily allowance (RDA) for cyanocobalamin –
Neonates and infants to 6 months: 0.3 mcg.
Infants 6 months to 1 year: 0.5 mcg.
Children over 1 year to 3 years: 0.7 mcg.
Children 4 to 6 years: 1 mcg.
Adults and children 11 years and over: 2 mcg.
Pregnant women: 2.2 mcg.
Lactating women: 2.6 mcg.
Vitamin B_{12} deficiency caused by inadequate diet, subtotal gastrectomy, or any other condition, disorder, or disease except malabsorption related to

pernicious anemia or other GI disease –
Adults: 30 to 100 mcg hydroxocobalamin S.C. or I.M. daily for 5 to 10 days, depending on severity of deficiency. Maintenance dosage is 100 to 200 mcg I.M. once monthly. For subsequent prophylaxis, advise adequate nutrition and daily RDA vitamin B_{12} supplements.
Children: 30 to 100 mcg hydroxocobalamin S.C. or I.M. daily for 5 to 10 days, depending on severity of deficiency. Maintenance dosage is at least 60 mcg/month I.M. or S.C. For subsequent prophylaxis, advise adequate nutrition and daily RDA vitamin B_{12} supplements.
Pernicious anemia or vitamin B_{12} malabsorption –
Adults: initially, 100 to 1,000 mcg hydroxocobalamin I.M. daily for 2 weeks, then 100 to 1,000 mcg I.M. once monthly for life. If neurologic complications are present, follow initial therapy with 100 to 1,000 mcg I.M. once q 2 weeks before starting monthly regimen.
Children: 1,000 to 5,000 mcg hydroxocobalamin I.M. or S.C. given over 2 or more weeks in 100-mcg increments; then 60 mcg I.M. or S.C. monthly for life.
Methylmalonic aciduria –
Neonates: 1,000 mcg hydroxocobalamin I.M. daily for 11 days with a protein-restricted diet.
Schilling test flushing dose –
Adults and children: 1,000 mcg hydroxocobalamin I.M. in a single dose.

ADVERSE REACTIONS

Common reactions are in italics; life-threatening reactions are in bold italics.
CV: peripheral vascular thrombosis.
GI: transient diarrhea.
Skin: itching, transitory exanthema, urticaria.
Local: pain, burning at S.C. or I.M. injection sites.
Other: ***anaphylaxis, anaphylactoid reactions with parenteral administration.***

INTERACTIONS

Aminoglycosides, colchicine, para-aminosalicylic acid and salts, chloramphenicol: malabsorption of vitamin B_{12}. Don't use together.
Ascorbic acid, chlorpromazine, dextrose, phytonadione, prochlorperazine, warfarin, oxidizing or reducing agents, heavy metals, alkaline or additive solutions: incompatible; precipitate may form. Don't mix together.

NURSING CONSIDERATIONS

- *Contraindicated* for parenteral administration in hypersensitivity to vitamin B_{12} or cobalt. Alternative use of large oral doses of vitamin B_{12} is controversial and should not be considered routine; combined with intrinsic factor increases risk of hypersensitive reactions and should be avoided. Therapeutic dosage contraindicated before proper diagnosis; vitamin B_{12} therapy may mask folate deficiency.
- *Use cautiously* in anemic patients with coexisting cardiac, pulmonary, or hypertensive disease; in early Leber's disease; in severe vitamin B_{12}-dependent deficiencies, especially those receiving cardiotonic glycosides (monitor closely the first 2 to 3 days for hypokalemia, fluid overload, pulmonary edema, CHF, and hypertension); and in gouty conditions (monitor serum uric acid for hyperuricemia).
- **I.V. use:** I.V. administration may cause anaphylactoid reactions. Use cautiously and only if other routes are ruled out.
- Don't mix parenteral liquids in same syringe with other medications.
- Protect from light and heat.
- Infection, tumors, or renal, hepatic, and other debilitating diseases may reduce therapeutic response.
- Deficiencies are more common in

strict vegetarians and their breast-fed infants.
- Stress need for patients with pernicious anemia to return for monthly injections. Although total body stores may last 3 to 6 years, anemia will recur if not treated monthly.
- May cause false-positive intrinsic factor antibody test.
- Hydroxocobalamin is approved for I.M. use only. Only advantage of hydroxocobalamin over vitamin B_{12} is its longer duration.
- 50% to 98% of injected dose may appear in urine within 48 hours. Major portion of drug is excreted within first 8 hours after injection.
- Closely monitor serum potassium for first 48 hours. Give potassium if necessary.
- Physically incompatible with dextrose solutions, alkaline or strongly acidic solutions, oxidizing and reducing agents, and many other drugs.

folic acid (vitamin B_9)

Folvite, Novofolacid†

Pregnancy Risk Category: A (C if > RDA)

HOW SUPPLIED

Tablets: 0.1 mg, 0.4 mg, 0.8 mg, 1 mg
Injection: 10-ml vials (5 mg/ml with 1.5% benzyl alcohol or 10 mg/ml with 1.5% benzyl alcohol and 0.2% EDTA)

MECHANISM OF ACTION

Necessary for normal erythropoiesis and nucleoprotein synthesis.

INDICATIONS & DOSAGE

Recommended daily allowance (RDA) –
Neonates and infants to 6 months: 25 mcg.
Infants 6 months to 1 year: 35 mcg.
Children over 1 year to 3 years: 50 mcg.
Children 4 to 6 years: 75 mcg.
Children 7 to 11 years: 100 mcg.
Children 11 to 14 years: 150 mcg.
Males 15 years and over: 200 mcg.
Females 15 years and over: 180 mcg.
Pregnant women: 400 mcg.
Lactating women (first 6 months): 280 mcg.
Lactating women (second 6 months): 260 mcg.

Megaloblastic or macrocytic anemia secondary to folic acid or other nutritional deficiency, hepatic disease, alcoholism, intestinal obstruction, excessive hemolysis –
Pregnant and lactating women: 0.8 mg P.O., S.C., or I.M. daily.
Adults and children over 4 years: 1 mg P.O., S.C., or I.M. daily for 4 to 5 days. After anemia secondary to folic acid deficiency is corrected, proper diet and RDA supplements are necessary to prevent recurrence.
Children under 4 years: up to 0.3 mg P.O., S.C., or I.M. daily.

Prevention of megaloblastic anemia of pregnancy and fetal damage –
Women: 1 mg P.O., S.C., or I.M. daily throughout pregnancy.

Nutritional supplement –
Adults: 0.1 mg P.O., S.C., or I.M. daily.
Children: 0.05 mg P.O. daily.

Treatment of tropical sprue –
Adults: 3 to 15 mg P.O. daily.

Test of megaloblastic anemia patients to detect folic acid deficiency without masking pernicious anemia –
Adults and children: 0.1 to 0.2 mg P.O. or I.M. for 10 days while maintaining a diet low in folate and vitamin B_{12}.
(Reticulosis, reversion to normoblastic hematopoiesis, and return to normal hemoglobin indicate folic acid deficiency.)

ADVERSE REACTIONS

Common reactions are in italics; life-threatening reactions are in bold italics.

Skin: allergic reactions (rash, pruritus, erythema).
Other: ***allergic bronchospasms,*** general malaise.

INTERACTIONS
Anticonvulsants (such as phenobarbital and phenytoin): increased anticonvulsant metabolism and decreased blood levels. Monitor closely.
Chloramphenicol: antagonism of folic acid. Monitor for decreased folic acid effect. Use together cautiously.
Fluorouracil: increased toxicity. Dosage adjustments are necessary.

NURSING CONSIDERATIONS
- *Contraindicated* in normocytic, refractory, or aplastic anemias; as sole agent in treating pernicious anemia (because it may mask neurologic effects); in treating methotrexate, pyrimethamine, or trimethoprim overdose; and in undiagnosed anemia (because it may mask pernicious anemia).
- Patients with small-bowel resections and intestinal malabsorption may require parenteral administration routes.
- Don't mix with other medications in same syringe for I.M. injections.
- Protect from light and heat.
- May use concurrent folic acid and vitamin B_{12} therapy if supported by diagnosis.
- Proper nutrition is necessary to prevent recurrence of anemia.
- Peak folate activity occurs in the blood in 30 to 60 minutes.
- Patients with pernicious anemia should avoid multivitamins containing folic acid.
- Hematologic response to folic acid in patients receiving chloramphenicol concurrently with folic acid should be carefully monitored.

leucovorin calcium (citrovorum factor or folinic acid)
Wellcovorin
Pregnancy Risk Category: C

HOW SUPPLIED
Tablets: 5 mg, 10 mg, 15 mg, 25 mg
Injection: 1-ml ampule (3 mg/ml with 0.9% benzyl alcohol or 5 mg/ml, with methyl and propyl parabens)
Powder for injection: 25 mg/vial, 50 mg/vial, 100 mg/vial, 350 mg/vial

MECHANISM OF ACTION
A reduced form of folic acid that is readily converted to other folic acid derivatives.

INDICATIONS & DOSAGE
Overdose of folic acid antagonist –
Adults and children: P.O., I.M., or I.V. dose equivalent to the weight of the antagonist given.
Leucovorin rescue after high methotrexate dose in treatment of malignancy –
Adults and children: dose at doctor's discretion within 6 to 36 hours of last dose of methotrexate.
Toxic effects of methotrexate used to treat severe psoriasis –
Adults and children: 4 to 8 mg I.M. 2 hours after methotrexate dose.
Hematologic toxicity caused by pyrimethamine therapy –
Adults and children: 5 mg P.O. or I.M. daily.
Hematologic toxicity caused by trimethoprim therapy –
Adults and children: 400 mcg to 5 mg P.O. or I.M. daily.
Megaloblastic anemia caused by congenital enzyme deficiency –
Adults and children: 3 to 6 mg I.M. daily, then 1 mg P.O. daily for life.
Folate-deficient megaloblastic anemia –
Adults and children: up to 1 mg of leucovorin I.M daily. Duration of

treatment depends on hematologic response.

ADVERSE REACTIONS
Common reactions are in italics; life-threatening reactions are in bold italics.
Skin: allergic reactions (rash, pruritus, erythema).
Other: ***allergic bronchospasms.***

INTERACTIONS
None significant.

NURSING CONSIDERATIONS
- *Contraindicated* in treating undiagnosed anemia, since it may mask pernicious anemia.
- *Use cautiously* in pernicious anemia; a hemolytic remission may occur while neurologic manifestations remain progressive.
- Do not confuse leucovorin (folinic acid) with folic acid.
- Follow leucovorin rescue schedule and protocol closely to maximize therapeutic response. Generally, leucovorin should not be administered simultaneously with systemic methotrexate.
- Treat overdosage of folic acid antagonists; administer within 1 hour if possible; usually ineffective after 4-hour delay.
- Protect from light and heat, especially reconstituted parenteral preparations.
- Since allergic reactions have been reported with folic acid, the possibility of allergic reactions to leucovorin should be considered.

niacin (vitamin B_3, nicotinic acid)

Niac, Niacor, Nico-400, Nicobid◊, Nicolar**, Nicotinex, Ni-Span◊

niacinamide (nicotinamide)◊

Pregnancy Risk Category: A (C if > RDA)

HOW SUPPLIED
niacin
Tablets: 25 mg◊, 50 mg◊, 100 mg◊, 250 mg◊, 500 mg
Tablets (timed-release): 150 mg◊, 250 mg◊, 500 mg◊, 750 mg◊
Capsules (timed-release): 125 mg◊, 250 mg◊, 300 mg◊, 400 mg◊, 500 mg
Elixir: 50 mg/5 ml◊
Injection: 30-ml vials, 100 mg/ml
niacinamide
Tablets: 50 mg◊, 100 mg◊, 500 mg◊
Tablets (timed-release): 1,000 mg◊
Injection: 100 mg/ml

MECHANISM OF ACTION
Necessary for lipid metabolism, tissue respiration, and glycogenolysis. Also (niacin only) decreases synthesis of low-density lipoproteins and inhibits lipolysis in adipose tissue.

INDICATIONS & DOSAGE
Recomended daily allowance (RDA) –
Neonates and infants to 6 months: 5 mg.
Infants 6 months to 1 year: 6 mg.
Children 1 to 3 years: 9 mg.
Children 4 to 6 years: 12 mg.
Children 7 to 10 years: 13 mg.
Males 11 to 14 years: 17 mg.
Males 15 to 18 years: 20 mg.
Males 19 to 50 years: 19 mg.
Males 51 years and over: 15 mg.
Females 11 to 50 years: 15 mg.
Females 51 years and over: 13 mg.
Pregnant women: 17 mg.
Lactating women: 20 mg.
Pellagra –
Adults: 10 to 20 mg P.O., S.C., I.M., or I.V. infusion daily, depending on severity of niacin deficiency. Maximum daily dosage recommended is 500 mg; should be divided into 10 doses, 50 mg each.

Children: up to 300 mg P.O. or 100 mg I.V. infusion daily, depending on severity of niacin deficiency.

After symptoms subside, advise adequate nutrition and RDA supplements to prevent recurrence.

Peripheral vascular disease and circulatory disorders –

Adults: 250 to 800 mg P.O. daily in divided doses.

Adjunctive treatment of hyperlipidemias, especially with hypercholesterolemia –

Adults: 1.5 to 3 g P.O. daily in three divided doses with or after meals, increased at intervals to 6 g daily.

ADVERSE REACTIONS

Common reactions are in italics; life-threatening reactions are in bold italics. Most adverse reactions are dose-dependent.

CNS: dizziness, transient headache.

CV: *excessive peripheral vasodilation (especially niacin).*

GI: *nausea, vomiting, diarrhea,* possible activation of peptic ulcer, epigastric or substernal pain.

Hepatic: ***hepatic dysfunction.***

Metabolic: hyperglycemia, hyperuricemia.

Skin: *flushing,* pruritus, dryness.

INTERACTIONS

Antihypertensive drugs (sympathetic blocking type): may have an additive vasodilating effect and cause postural hypotension. Use together cautiously. Warn patient about postural hypotension.

NURSING CONSIDERATIONS

- *Contraindicated* in hepatic dysfunction, active peptic ulcer disease, severe hypotension, or arterial hemorrhage.
- *Use cautiously* in gallbladder disease, diabetes mellitus, and gout.
- Monitor hepatic function and blood glucose early in therapy.
- Give with meals to minimize GI side effects.
- Aspirin (80 to 325 mg P.O. 30 minutes before niacin dose) may reduce the flushing response to niacin.
- Timed-release niacin or niacinamide may avoid excessive flushing effects with large doses. However, timed-release niacin has been associated with hepatic failure, even at doses as low as 1 g per day.
- **I.V. use:** Give slow I.V. (no faster than 2 mg/minute). Explain harmlessness of flushing syndrome to ease anxiety.
- Stress that medication used to treat hyperlipoproteinemia or to dilate peripheral vessels is not "just a vitamin." Explain importance of adhering to therapeutic regimen.
- Advise patient against self-medicating for hyperlipidemia.

pyridoxine hydrochloride (vitamin B_6)

Beesix, Hexa-Betalin, Hexacrest, Nestrex◇, Rodex

Pregnancy Risk Category: A (C if > RDA)

HOW SUPPLIED

Tablets◇: 10 mg, 25 mg, 50 mg, 100 mg, 200 mg, 250 mg, 500 mg

Tablets (timed-release): 500 mg

Injection: 100 mg/ml

MECHANISM OF ACTION

Acts as coenzyme for various metabolic functions. Required for amino acid metabolism.

INDICATIONS & DOSAGE

Recommended daily allowance (RDA) –

Neonates and infants to 6 months: 0.3 mg.

Infants 6 months to 1 year: 0.6 mg.

Children over 1 year to 3 years: 1 mg.

Children 4 to 6 years: 1.1 mg.

Children 7 to 10 years: 1.4 mg.
Males 11 to 14 years: 1.7 mg.
Males 15 years and over: 2 mg.
Females 11 to 14 years: 1.4 mg.
Females 15 to 18 years: 1.5 mg.
Females 19 years and over: 1.6 mg.
Pregnant women: 2.2 mg.
Lactating women: 2.1 mg.
Dietary vitamin B_6 deficiency –
Adults: 10 to 20 mg P.O., I.M., or I.V. daily for 3 weeks, then 2 to 5 mg daily as a supplement to a proper diet.
Children: 100 mg P.O., I.M., or I.V. to correct deficiency, then an adequate diet with supplementary RDA doses to prevent recurrence.
Seizures related to vitamin B_6 deficiency or dependency –
Adults and children: 100 mg I.M. or I.V. in single dose.
Vitamin B_6-responsive anemias or dependency syndrome (inborn errors of metabolism) –
Adults: up to 600 mg P.O., I.M., or I.V. daily until symptoms subside, then 50 mg daily for life.
Children: 100 mg I.M. or I.V., then 2 to 10 mg I.M. or 10 to 100 mg P.O. daily.
Prevention of vitamin B_6 deficiency during isoniazid therapy –
Adults: 25 to 50 mg P.O. daily.
Children: at least 0.5 to 1.5 mg P.O. daily.
Infants: at least 0.1 to 0.5 mg P.O. daily.
If neurologic symptoms develop in pediatric patients, increase dosage as necessary.
Treatment of vitamin B_6 deficiency secondary to isoniazid –
Adults: 100 mg P.O. daily for 3 weeks, then 50 mg daily.

ADVERSE REACTIONS
Common reactions are in italics; life-threatening reactions are in bold italics.
CNS: drowsiness, paresthesias.

INTERACTIONS
Levodopa: decreased levodopa effect. Avoid concomitant use.
Phenobarbital, phenytoin: decreased anticonvulsant serum levels, with increased risk of seizures. Avoid concomitant use.

NURSING CONSIDERATIONS
- *Contraindicated* in hypersensitivity to parenteral pyridoxine and in doses larger than 5 mg for patients also receiving levodopa. Caution patient to check dosage, especially in multivitamins. Patients receiving levodopa alone (not with carbidopa) shouldn't take pyridoxine.
- Protect from light. Do not use injection solution if it contains a precipitate. Slight darkening is acceptable.
- Excessive protein intake increases daily pyridoxine requirements.
- If sodium bicarbonate is required to control acidosis in isoniazid toxicity, do not mix in same syringe with pyridoxine.
- If prescribed for maintenance therapy to prevent deficiency recurrence, stress importance of compliance and of good nutrition. Explain that pyridoxine in combination therapy with isoniazid has a specific therapeutic purpose and is not "just a vitamin." Explain importance of adhering to therapeutic regimen.
- Used to treat seizures and coma as a result of acute isoniazid overdosage. Dosage equal to amount of isoniazid ingested.
- Patients taking high doses (2 to 6 g/day) may experience difficulty in walking because of a diminished proprioceptive and sensory function.
- **I.V. use:** Inject undiluted drug into I.V. line containing a free-flowing compatible solution. Alternatively, infuse diluted drug over prescribed duration for intermittent infusions. Continuous infusion is not used.

riboflavin (vitamin B_2)◊

Pregnancy Risk Category: A (C if > RDA)

HOW SUPPLIED
Tablets: 10 mg◊, 25 mg◊, 50 mg◊, 100 mg◊
Tablets (sugar-free): 50 mg◊, 100 mg◊

MECHANISM OF ACTION
Converted to two other coenzymes that are necessary for normal tissue respiration.

INDICATIONS & DOSAGE
Recommended daily allowance (RDA):
Neonates and infants to 6 months: 0.4 mg.
Infants 6 months to 1 year: 0.5 mg.
Children over 1 year to 3 years: 0.8 mg.
Children 4 to 6 years: 1.1 mg.
Children 7 to 10 years: 1.2 mg.
Males 11 to 14 years: 1.5 mg.
Males 15 to 18 years: 1.8 mg.
Males 19 to 50 years: 1.7 mg.
Males 51 years and over: 1.4 mg.
Females 11 to 50 years: 1.3 mg.
Females 51 years and over: 1.2 mg.
Pregnant women: 1.6 mg.
Lactating women (first 6 months): 1.8 mg.
Lactating women (second 6 months): 1.7 mg.
Riboflavin deficiency or adjunct to thiamine treatment for polyneuritis or cheilosis secondary to pellagra –
Adults and children over 12 years: 5 to 50 mg P.O. daily, depending on severity.
Children under 12 years: 2 to 10 mg P.O. daily, depending on severity.
For maintenance, increase nutritional intake and supplement with vitamin B complex.

ADVERSE REACTIONS
Common reactions are in italics; life-threatening reactions are in bold italics.
GU: high doses turn urine bright yellow.

INTERACTIONS
Propantheline, other anticholinergics: decreased rate and extent of absorption. Avoid concomitant use.

NURSING CONSIDERATIONS
- Protect from light.
- Stress proper nutritional habits to prevent recurrence of deficiency.
- Riboflavin deficiency usually accompanies other vitamin B complex deficiencies and may require multivitamin therapy.
- Since food increases absorption of riboflavin, encourage patient to take with meals.
- May be given I.M. or I.V. as a component of multiple vitamins.

thiamine hydrochloride (vitamin B_1)

Apatate Drops, Betalin S◊, Betamin‡, Beta-Sol‡, Biamine, Thia

Pregnancy Risk Category: A (C if > RDA)

HOW SUPPLIED
Tablets◊: 5 mg, 10 mg, 25 mg, 50 mg, 100 mg, 250 mg, 500 mg
Elixir: 2.25 mg/5 ml (with alcohol 10%)◊
Injection: 100 mg/ml

MECHANISM OF ACTION
Combines with adenosine triphosphate to form a coenzyme necessary for carbohydrate metabolism.

INDICATIONS & DOSAGE
Recommended daily allowance (RDA) –
Neonates and infants to 6 months: 0.3 mg.
Infants 6 months to 1 year: 0.4 mg.
Children over 1 year to 3 years: 0.7 mg.

Children 4 to 6 years: 0.9 mg.
Children 7 to 10 years: 1 mg.
Males 11 to 14 years: 1.3 mg.
Males 15 to 50 years: 1.5 mg.
Males 51 years and over: 1.2 mg.
Females 11 to 50 years: 1.1 mg.
Females 51 years and over: 1 mg.
Pregnant women: 1.5 mg.
Lactating women: 1.6 mg.
Beriberi –
Adults: 10 to 500 mg, depending on severity, I.M. t.i.d. for 2 weeks, followed by dietary correction and multivitamin supplement containing 5 to 100 mg thiamine daily for 1 month.
Children: 10 to 50 mg, depending on severity, I.M. daily for several weeks with adequate dietary intake.
Anemia secondary to thiamine deficiency; polyneuritis secondary to alcoholism, pregnancy, or pellagra –
Adults: 100 mg P.O. daily.
Children: 10 to 50 mg P.O. daily in divided doses.
Wernicke's encephalopathy –
Adults: up to 500 mg to 1 g I.V. for crisis therapy, followed by 100 mg b.i.d. for maintenance; or 50 mg I.V. bolus followed by 50 mg I.M. daily until symptoms improve.
"Wet beriberi," with myocardial failure –
Adults and children: 100 to 500 mg I.V. for emergency treatment.

ADVERSE REACTIONS
Common reactions are in italics; life-threatening reactions are in bold italics.
CNS: restlessness.
CV: ***hypotension after rapid I.V. injection, angioneurotic edema,*** cyanosis.
EENT: tightness of throat (allergic reaction).
GI: nausea, hemorrhage, diarrhea.
Skin: feeling of warmth, pruritus, urticaria, sweating.
Other: *anaphylactoid reactions,* weakness, pulmonary edema.

INTERACTIONS
Neuromuscular blockers: enhanced neuromuscular blockade. Clinical significance unknown.

NURSING CONSIDERATIONS
- *Contraindicated* in hypersensitivity to thiamine products. I.V. push is contraindicated, except when treating life-threatening myocardial failure in "wet beriberi."
- *Use cautiously* in I.V. administration of large doses; give patient skin test if he has a history of hypersensitivity before therapy. Have epinephrine on hand to treat anaphylaxis should it occur after a large parenteral dose.
- Thiamine malabsorption is most likely in alcoholism, cirrhosis, or GI disease.
- Use parenteral administration only when P.O. route is not feasible.
- Clinically significant deficiency can occur in approximately 3 weeks of totally thiamine-free diet. Thiamine deficiency usually requires concurrent treatment for multiple deficiencies.
- Doses larger than 30 mg t.i.d. may not be fully utilized. After tissue saturation with thiamine, it is excreted in urine as pyrimidine.
- If beriberi occurs in a breast-fed infant, both mother and child should be treated with thiamine.
- Unstable in alkaline solutions; should not be used with materials that yield alkaline solutions.

vitamin C (ascorbic acid)
Ascorbicap◊, Cebid Timecelles◊, Cecon◊, Cee-1000 T.D.◊, Cenolate◊, Cetane, Cevalin◊, Cevi-Bid, Ce-Vi-Sol*, Cevita◊, C-Span◊, Dull-C◊, Flavettes‡, Redoxon†, Solucap C, Vita C Crystals◊

Pregnancy Risk Category: A (C if > RDA)

HOW SUPPLIED
Tablets◇: 25 mg, 50 mg, 100 mg, 250 mg, 500 mg, 1,000 mg
Tablets (chewable): 100 mg◇, 250 mg◇, 500 mg◇, 1,000 mg◇
Tablets (effervescent): 1,000 mg sugar-free◇
Tablets (timed-release): 500 mg◇, 750 mg◇, 1,000 mg◇, 1,500 mg
Capsules (timed-release): 500 mg◇
Crystals: 100 g (4 g/tsp)◇, 1,000 g (4 g/tsp, sugar-free)◇
Lozenges: 60 mg◇
Oral liquid: 50 ml (35 mg/0.6 ml)*◇
Oral solution: 60 mg/ml◇, 100 mg/ml◇
Powder: 100 g (4 g/tsp)◇, 500 g (4 g/tsp)◇, 1,000 g (4 g/tsp, sugar-free)◇
Syrup: 20 mg/ml in 120 ml, 480 ml◇; 500 mg/5 ml in 5 ml◇, 10 ml◇, 120 ml◇, 473 ml◇
Injection: 100 mg/ml in 2-ml, 10-ml ampules; 250 mg/ml in 10-ml ampules and 10-ml, 30-ml, 50-ml vials; 500 mg/ml in 2-ml, 5-ml ampules and 50-ml vials; 500 mg/ml (with monothioglycerol) in 1-ml ampules

MECHANISM OF ACTION
Necessary for collagen formation and tissue repair; involved in oxidation-reduction reactions throughout the body.

INDICATIONS & DOSAGE
Recommended daily allowance (RDA) –
Neonates and infants to 6 months: 30 mg.
Infants 6 months to 1 year: 35 mg.
Children 1 to 3 years: 40 mg.
Children 4 to 10 years: 45 mg.
Children 11 to 14 years: 50 mg.
Children 15 years and over and adults: 60 mg.
Pregnant women: 70 mg.
Lactating women (first 6 months): 95 mg.
Lactating women (second 6 months): 90 mg.
Frank and subclinical scurvy –
Adults: 100 mg to 2 g, depending on severity, P.O., S.C., I.M., or I.V. daily, then at least 50 mg daily for maintenance.
Children: 100 to 300 mg, depending on severity, P.O., S.C., I.M., or I.V. daily, then at least 35 mg daily for maintenance.
Infants: 50 to 100 mg P.O., I.M., I.V., or S.C. daily.
Extensive burns, delayed fracture or wound healing, postoperative wound healing, severe febrile or chronic disease states –
Adults: 200 to 500 mg S.C., I.M., or I.V. daily.
Children: 100 to 200 mg P.O., S.C., I.M., or I.V. daily.
Prevention of vitamin C deficiency in those with poor nutritional habits or increased requirements –
Adults: 45 to 60 mg P.O., S.C., I.M., or I.V. daily.
Pregnant and lactating women: at least 60 mg P.O., S.C., I.M., or I.V. daily.
Children: at least 40 mg P.O., S.C., I.M., or I.V. daily.
Infants: at least 35 mg P.O., S.C., I.M., or I.V. daily.
Potentiation of methenamine in urine acidification –
Adults: 4 to 12 g P.O. daily in divided doses.

ADVERSE REACTIONS
Common reactions are in italics; life-threatening reactions are in bold italics.
CNS: faintness or dizziness with fast I.V. administration.
GI: nausea, vomiting, diarrhea, epigastric burning.
GU: acid urine, oxaluria, renal calculi, ***renal failure.***
Skin: discomfort at injection site.

INTERACTIONS
Aspirin, acidic drugs: decreased excretion and risk of toxicity in patients taking large doses of vitamin C. Avoid concomitant use.

*Liquid form contains alcohol. **May contain tartrazine.

Oral iron supplements: increased iron absorption. A beneficial drug interaction.
Warfarin: decreased anticoagulant effect. Avoid concomitant use.

NURSING CONSIDERATIONS
- *Use cautiously* in G6PD deficiency.
- **I.V. use:** Administer I.V. infusion cautiously in patients with renal insufficiency.
- Avoid rapid I.V. administration.
- When administering for urine acidification, check urine pH to ensure efficacy.
- Protect solution from light.

vitamin D

cholecalciferol (vitamin D_3)
Delta-D◇, Vitamin D_3◇

ergocalciferol (vitamin D_2)
Calciferol, Drisdol, Radiostol†, Radiostol Forte†, Vitamin D

Pregnancy Risk Category: A (D if > RDA)

HOW SUPPLIED
Tablets: 1.25 mg (50,000 IU)
Capsules: 0.625 mg (25,000 IU), 1.25 mg (50,000 IU)
Oral liquid: 8,000 IU/ml in 60-ml dropper bottle◇
Injection: 12.5 mg (500,000 IU)/ml

MECHANISM OF ACTION
Promotes absorption and utilization of calcium and phosphate. Helps to regulate calcium homeostasis.

INDICATIONS & DOSAGE
Recommended daily allowance (RDA) for cholecalciferol –
Neonates and infants to 6 months: 300 IU.
Infants 6 months to adults 24 years: 400 IU.
Adults 25 years and over: 200 IU.
Pregnant or lactating women: 400 IU.
Rickets and other vitamin D deficiency diseases; renal osteodystrophy –
Adults: initially, 12,000 IU P.O. or I.M. daily, increased as indicated by response up to 500,000 IU daily in most cases and up to 800,000 IU daily for vitamin D-resistant rickets.
Children: 1,500 to 5,000 IU P.O. or I.M. daily for 2 to 4 weeks, repeated after 2 weeks, if necessary. Alternatively, a single dose of 600,000 IU may be given.

Monitor serum calcium daily to guide dosage. After correction of deficiency, maintenance includes adequate dietary nutrition and RDA supplements.
Hypoparathyroidism –
Adults and children: 50,000 to 200,000 IU P.O. or I.M. daily, with 4-g calcium supplement.

ADVERSE REACTIONS
Common reactions are in italics; life-threatening reactions are in bold italics. Adverse reactions listed are usually seen only in vitamin D toxicity.
CNS: headache, dizziness, ataxia, weakness, somnolence, decreased libido, overt psychosis, ***seizures***.
CV: ***calcifications of soft tissues, including the heart.***
EENT: dry mouth, metallic taste, rhinorrhea, conjunctivitis (calcific), photophobia, tinnitus.
GI: anorexia, nausea, constipation, diarrhea.
GU: polyuria, albuminuria, hypercalciuria, nocturia, ***impaired renal function,*** renal calculi.
Metabolic: ***hypercalcemia,*** hyperphosphatemia.
Skin: pruritus.
Other: bone and muscle pain, bone demineralization, weight loss.

INTERACTIONS
Corticosteroids: antagonized effect of vitamin D. Monitor closely.

Digitalis glycosides: increased risk of cardiac arrhythmias. Monitor closely.
Mineral oil, cholestyramine resin: inhibited GI absorption of oral vitamin D. Space doses. Use together cautiously.
Phenobarbital, phenytoin: increased vitamin D metabolism and decreased effectiveness. Monitor closely.
Thiazide diuretics: may cause hypercalcemia in patients with hypoparathyroidism. Monitor closely.

NURSING CONSIDERATIONS

- *Contraindicated* in hypercalcemia, hypervitaminosis A, or renal osteodystrophy with hyperphosphatemia.
- *Use cautiously* in cardiac patients, especially those receiving digitalis glycosides.
- Monitor eating and bowel habits; dry mouth, nausea, vomiting, metallic taste, and constipation may be early signs and symptoms of toxicity.
- Patients with hyperphosphatemia require dietary phosphate restrictions and binding agents to avoid metastatic calcifications and renal calculi.
- When high therapeutic dosages are used, serum and urine calcium, potassium, and urea should be monitored frequently.
- Malabsorption from inadequate bile or hepatic dysfunction may require addition of exogenous bile salts to oral vitamin D.
- I.M. injection of vitamin D dispersed in oil is preferable in patients who are unable to absorb the oral form.
- This vitamin is fat-soluble. Warn patient of the dangers of increasing dosage without consulting the doctor.
- Dosages of 60,000 IU/day can cause hypercalcemia.
- Patients taking vitamin D should restrict their intake of magnesium-containing antacids.

vitamin E

Aquasol E◇, Eprolin◇, Pertropin◇, Solucap E◇, Tocopher◇

Pregnancy Risk Category: A (C if > RDA)

HOW SUPPLIED

Tablets◇: 100 IU, 200 IU, 400 IU, 500 IU, 600 IU, 1,000 IU
Tablets (chewable): 100 IU◇, 200 IU◇, 400 IU◇
Capsules◇: 50 IU, 100 IU, 200 IU, 400 IU, 600 IU, 1,000 IU
Oral solution: 50 IU/ml◇

MECHANISM OF ACTION

Acts as a cofactor and an antioxidant.

INDICATIONS & DOSAGE

Recommended daily allowance (RDA) –
Neonates and infants to 6 months: 4 IU.
Infants 6 months to 1 year: 6 IU.
Children over 1 year to 3 years: 9 IU.
Children 4 to 10 years: 10 IU.
Males 11 years and over: 15 IU.
Females 11 years and over: 12 IU.
Pregnant women: 15 IU.
Lactating women (first 6 months): 18 IU.
Lactating women (second 6 months): 16 IU.
Vitamin E deficiency in premature infants and in patients with impaired fat absorption –
Adults: 60 to 75 IU, depending on severity, P.O. or I.M. daily.
Children: 1 mg equivalent/0.6 g of dietary unsaturated fat P.O. or I.M. daily.

ADVERSE REACTIONS

None reported.

INTERACTIONS

Mineral oil, cholestyramine resin: inhibited GI absorption of oral vitamin

E. Space doses. Use together cautiously.
Vitamin K: large doses of vitamin E may antagonize the effects of vitamin K. Avoid use.

NURSING CONSIDERATIONS
- Water-miscible forms more completely absorbed in GI tract than other forms.
- Adequate bile is essential for absorption.
- Requirements increase with rise in dietary polyunsaturated acids.
- May protect other vitamins against oxidation.
- Megadoses can cause thrombophlebitis.
- This vitamin is fat-soluble. Discourage patient from self-medication with megadoses.

menadione/menadiol sodium diphosphate (vitamin K_3)
Synkavite†, Synkayvite

Pregnancy Risk Category: C (X near term)

HOW SUPPLIED
Tablets: 10 mg‡
Injection: 5 mg/ml, 10 mg/ml, 37.5 mg/ml

MECHANISM OF ACTION
Promotes hepatic formation of active prothrombin.

INDICATIONS & DOSAGE
Hypoprothrombinemia secondary to vitamin K malabsorption or drug therapy, or when oral administration is desired and bile secretion is inadequate –
Adults: 5 to 15 mg P.O. or parenterally, titrated to patient's requirements.

ADVERSE REACTIONS
Common reactions are in italics; life-threatening reactions are in bold italics.
CNS: headache, ***kernicterus.***
GI: nausea, vomiting.
Skin: allergic rash, pruritus, urticaria.
Local: pain, hematoma at injection site.

INTERACTIONS
Mineral oil, cholestyramine resin: inhibited GI absorption of oral vitamin K. Space doses. Use together cautiously.
Oral anticoagulants: impaired effectiveness. Don't use together.

NURSING CONSIDERATIONS
- *Contraindicated* in treatment of hereditary hypoprothrombinemia (because vitamin K_3 can paradoxically worsen it); in hepatocellular disease, unless it is caused by biliary obstruction; in treatment of heparin-induced bleeding; and during last weeks of pregnancy to avoid toxic reactions in neonates.
- *Use cautiously* in G6PD deficiency to avoid hemolysis. In severe bleeding, do not delay other measures, such as giving fresh frozen plasma or whole blood. Use large dosages cautiously in severe hepatic disease.
- Never use in neonates (especially in premature neonates) because it can cause hemolytic anemia, hyperbilirubinemia, kernicterus, brain damage, and death.
- Do not use to treat hypoprothrombinemia induced by oral anticoagulant. Phytonadione (vitamin K_1) is the drug of choice.
- Failure to respond to vitamin K_3 may indicate coagulation defects.
- Excessive use of vitamin K_3 may temporarily defeat oral anticoagulant therapy. Higher doses of oral anticoagulant or interim use of heparin may be required.
- Protect parenteral products from light.
- **I.V. use:** When I.V. route must be

used, infusion rate shouldn't exceed 1 mg/minute.
- Effects of I.V. injections are more rapid but shorter lived than S.C. or I.M. injections.
- Monitor prothrombin time to determine dosage effectiveness.
- Observe for signs of adverse reactions and report them to doctor.
- Use caution in handling bulk menadione powder. It is irritating to the skin and the respiratory tract.
- This vitamin is fat-soluble.

phytonadione (vitamin K_1)

AquaMEPHYTON, Konakion, Mephyton

Pregnancy Risk Category: C

HOW SUPPLIED

Tablets: 5 mg
Injection (aqueous colloidal solution): 2 mg/ml, 10 mg/ml
Injection (aqueous dispersion): 2 mg/ml, 10 mg/ml

MECHANISM OF ACTION

Promotes hepatic formation of active prothrombin.

INDICATIONS & DOSAGE

Recommended daily allowance (RDA) –
Neonates and infants to 6 months: 5 mcg.
Infants 6 months to 1 year: 10 mcg.
Children over 1 year to 3 years: 15 mcg.
Children 4 to 6 years: 20 mcg.
Children 7 to 10 years: 30 mcg.
Children 11 to 14 years: 45 mcg.
Males 15 to 18 years: 65 mcg.
Males 19 to 24 years: 70 mcg.
Males 25 years and over: 80 mcg.
Females 15 to 18 years: 55 mcg.
Females 19 to 24 years: 60 mcg.
Females 25 years and over; pregnant or lactating women: 65 mcg.
Hypoprothrombinemia secondary to vitamin K malabsorption, drug therapy, or excess vitamin A –
Adults: 2.5 to 25 mg, depending on severity, P.O. or parenterally, repeated and increased up to 50 mg, if necessary.
Children: 5 to 10 mg P.O. or parenterally.
Infants: 2 mg P.O. or parenterally.
I.V. injection rate for children and infants should not exceed 3 mg/m²/minute or a total of 5 mg.
Hypoprothrombinemia secondary to effect of oral anticoagulants –
Adults: 2.5 to 10 mg P.O., S.C., or I.M., based on prothrombin time, repeated, if necessary, within 12 to 48 hours after oral dose or within 6 to 8 hours after parenteral dose. In emergency, give 10 to 50 mg slow I.V., rate not to exceed 1 mg/minute, repeated q 4 hours, p.r.n.
Prevention of hemorrhagic disease in neonates –
Neonates: 0.5 to 1 mg S.C. or I.M. immediately after birth, repeated within 6 to 8 hours, if needed, especially if mother received oral anticoagulants or long-term anticonvulsant therapy during pregnancy.
Differentiation between hepatocellular disease or biliary obstruction as source of hypoprothrombinemia –
Adults and children: 10 mg I.M. or S.C.
Prevention of hypoprothrombinemia related to vitamin K deficiency in long-term parenteral nutrition –
Adults: 5 to 10 mg S.C. or I.M. weekly.
Children: 2 to 5 mg S.C. or I.M. weekly.
Prevention of hypoprothrombinemia in infants receiving less than 0.1 mg/liter vitamin K in breast milk or milk substitutes –
Infants: 1 mg S.C. or I.M. monthly.

ADVERSE REACTIONS

Common reactions are in italics; life-threatening reactions are in bold italics.

CNS: dizziness, seizure-like movements.
CV: transient hypotension after I.V. administration, rapid and weak pulse, cardiac irregularities.
GI: nausea, vomiting.
Skin: sweating, flushing, erythema.
Local: pain, swelling, and hematoma at injection site.
Other: ***bronchospasms,*** dyspnea, cramp-like pain, ***anaphylaxis and anaphylactoid reactions (usually after rapid I.V. administration).***

INTERACTIONS
Mineral oil, cholestyramine resin: inhibited GI absorption of oral vitamin K. Space doses. Use together cautiously.

NURSING CONSIDERATIONS
- *Contraindicated* in hereditary hypoprothrombinemia; bleeding secondary to heparin therapy or overdose; hepatocellular disease, unless caused by biliary obstruction (vitamin K can paradoxically worsen the hypoprothrombinemia). Oral administration is contraindicated if bile secretion is inadequate, unless supplemented with bile salts.
- *Use cautiously,* if at all, during last weeks of pregnancy to avoid toxic reactions in neonates and in G6PD deficiency to avoid hemolysis. Use large dosages cautiously in severe hepatic disease.
- Failure to respond to vitamin K may indicate coagulation defects.
- In severe bleeding, don't delay other measures, such as fresh frozen plasma or whole blood.
- **I.V. use:** Administer I.V. by slow infusion (over 2 to 3 hours). Mix in normal saline solution, dextrose 5% in water, or dextrose 5% in normal saline solution. Observe patient closely for signs of flushing, weakness, tachycardia, and hypotension; may progress to shock.
- Effects of I.V. injections more rapid but shorter lived than S.C. or I.M. injections.
- Protect parenteral products from light. Wrap infusion container with aluminum foil.
- Monitor prothrombin time to determine dosage effectiveness.
- Observe for signs of adverse reactions and report them to the doctor.
- Phytonadione therapy for hemorrhagic disease in infants causes fewer adverse reactions than do other vitamin K analogs.
- Check brand name labels for administration route restrictions.
- This vitamin is fat-soluble.
- Weekly addition of 5 to 10 mg to TPN solutions may be ordered.

sodium fluoride
Fluor-A-Day†, Fluoritab, Flura, Flura-Drops, Karidium, Luride, Pediaflor, Phos-Flur

sodium fluoride, topical
ACT◇, Checkmate, Fluorigard◇, Fluorinse, Flura-Drops, Gel II, Gel-Kam, Gel-Tin, Home Treatment Fluoride Gelution, Karigel, Karigel-N, Listermint with Fluoride◇, Minute-Gel, Point-Two, PreviDent, Stop, Thera-Flur, Thera-Flur N

Pregnancy Risk Category: C

HOW SUPPLIED
sodium fluoride
Tablets: 0.5 mg, 1 mg (sugar-free)
Tablets (chewable): 0.25 mg (sugar-free)
Drops: 0.125 mg/drop (30 ml), 0.125 mg/drop (60 ml, sugar-free), 0.25 mg/drop (19 ml), 0.25 mg/drop (24 ml, sugar-free), 0.5 mg/ml (50 ml)
Rinse: 0.01%◇ (180 ml, 260 ml, 540 ml, 720 ml); 0.02%◇ 180 ml, 300 ml, 360 ml, 480 ml); 0.09%◇ (240 ml)
sodium fluoride, topical
Gel: 0.1% (60 g, 65 g, 105 g, 120 g, 122 g) 0.5% (24 g, 30 g, 60 g, 120 g,

125 g, 130 g), 0.5% (250 g, sugar-free), 1.23% (480 ml)
Gel drops: 0.5% (24 ml, 60 ml)
Rinse: 0.02%◊ (250 ml, 480 ml, 500 ml), 0.09% (250 ml, 480 ml), 0.09% (480 ml, sugar-free)

MECHANISM OF ACTION
May catalyze bone remineralization.

INDICATIONS & DOSAGE
Aid in the prevention of dental caries –
Children over 3 years: 1 mg P.O. (tablet) daily.
Children under 3 years: 0.5 mg P.O. (tablet or drops) daily.
Adults and children over 12 years: 10 ml of solution (rinse) or thin ribbon of gel.
Children 6 to 12 years: 5 to 10 ml of solution (rinse) or thin ribbon of gel.

ADVERSE REACTIONS
Common reactions are in italics; life-threatening reactions are in bold italics.
CNS: headaches, weakness.
GI: gastric distress, nausea, vomiting.
Skin: hypersensitivity reactions, such as atopic dermatitis, eczema, and urticaria.
Other: *bad taste (salty, soapy);* staining of teeth.

INTERACTIONS
None significant.

NURSING CONSIDERATIONS
- *Contraindicated* when fluoride intake from drinking water exceeds 0.7 ppm.
- Chronic toxicity (fluorosis) may result from prolonged use of higher-than-recommended doses.
- Advise patient to notify dentist if tooth mottling occurs.
- Tablets may be dissolved in mouth, chewed, or swallowed whole.
- Drops may be administered orally undiluted or mixed with fluids or food.
- Topical forms (rinses and gels) should not be swallowed. Most effective when used immediately after brushing teeth. Tell patient to rinse around and between teeth for 1 minute, then spit out.
- Tell patient to dilute drops or rinses in plastic containers rather than glass.
- The presence of fluoride in prenatal vitamins has been shown to produce healthier teeth in infants.
- Used investigationally in treating osteoporosis.

trace elements

chromium (chromic chloride)
Chrometrace

copper (cupric chloride, cupric sulfate)
Coppertrace

iodine (sodium iodide)
Iodopen

manganese (manganese chloride, manganese sulfate)
Mangatrace

selenium (selenious acid)
Selenitrace

zinc (zinc chloride, zinc sulfate)
Zinctrace

Pregnancy Risk Category: C

HOW SUPPLIED
chromium
Injection: 4 mcg/ml
copper
Injection: 0.4 mg/ml
iodine
Injection: 100 mcg/ml

*Liquid form contains alcohol. **May contain tartrazine.

manganese
Injection: 0.1 mg/ml, 0.5 mg/ml
selenium
Injection: 40 mcg/ml, 50 mcg/ml
zinc
Injection: 1 mg/ml, 5 mg/ml

MECHANISM OF ACTION
Participate in synthesis and stabilization of proteins and nucleic acids in subcellular and membrane transport systems.

INDICATIONS & DOSAGE
Prevention of individual trace element deficiencies in patients receiving long-term total parenteral nutrition –
Chromium –
Adults: 10 to 15 mcg I.V. daily.
Children: 0.14 to 0.20 mcg/kg I.V. daily.
Copper –
Adults: 0.5 to 1.5 mg I.V. daily.
Children: 20 mcg/kg I.V. daily.
Iodine –
Adults: 1 mcg/kg I.V. daily.
Manganese –
Adults: 0.15 to 0.8 mcg I.V. daily.
Children: 2 to 10 mcg/kg I.V. daily.
Selenium –
Adults: 40 to 120 mcg I.V. daily.
Children: 3 mcg/kg I.V. daily.
Zinc –
Adults: 2 to 4 mg I.V. daily.
Children: 0.05 to 0.1 mg/kg I.V. daily.

ADVERSE REACTIONS
None reported.

INTERACTIONS
None significant at recommended dosages.

NURSING CONSIDERATIONS
- Check serum levels of trace elements in patients who have received total parenteral nutrition for 2 months or longer. Give supplement if ordered. Call doctor's attention to low serum levels of these elements.
- Normal serum levels are 0.07 to 0.15 mg/ml copper; 0.05 to 0.15 mg/100 ml zinc; 4 to 20 mcg/100 ml manganese; selenium 0.1 to 0.19 mcg/ml.
- Solutions of trace elements are compounded by pharmacy for addition to total parenteral nutrition solutions according to various formulas. One common trace element solution is Shil's solution, which contains copper 1 mg/ml, iodide 0.06 mg/ml, manganese 0.4 mg/ml, and zinc 2 mg/ml.
- **I.V. use:** Cautiously infuse diluted solution through a patent I.V. line over the ordered duration. Direct injection and intermittent infusion are not recommended.

93

Calorics

amino acid infusions, crystalline
amino acid infusions in dextrose
amino acid infusions with electrolytes
amino acid infusions with electrolytes in dextrose
amino acid infusions for hepatic failure
amino acid infusions for high metabolic stress
amino acid infusions for renal failure
corn oil
dextrose
fat emulsions
fructose
invert sugar
medium-chain triglycerides

COMBINATION PRODUCTS
Various products contain dextrose, fructose, or invert sugar in combination with electrolytes.

amino acid infusions, crystalline
Aminosyn, Aminosyn II, Aminosyn-PF, FreAmine III, Novamine, Travasol, TrophAmine

amino acid infusions in dextrose
Aminosyn II with dextrose

amino acid infusions with electrolytes
Aminosyn with electrolytes, Aminosyn II with electrolytes, FreAmine III with electrolytes, ProcalAmine with electrolytes, Travasol with electrolytes

amino acid infusions with electrolytes in dextrose
Aminosyn II with electrolytes in dextrose

amino acid infusions for hepatic failure
HepatAmine

amino acid infusions for high metabolic stress
Aminosyn-HBC, BranchAmin, FreAmine HBC

amino acid infusions for renal failure
Aminess, Aminosyn-RF, NephrAmine, RenAmin

Pregnancy Risk Category: C

HOW SUPPLIED
Injection: 250 ml, 500 ml, 1,000 ml, 2,000 ml containing amino acids in varying concentrations
amino acid infusions, crystalline
Aminosyn: 3.5%, 5%, 7%, 8.5%, 10%
Aminosyn II: 3.5%, 5%, 7%, 8.5%, 10%
Aminosyn-PF: 7%, 10%
FreAmine III: 8.5%, 10%
Novamine: 11.4%, 15%
Travasol: 5.5%, 8.5%, 10%
TrophAmine: 6%, 10%
amino acid infusions in dextrose
Aminosyn II: 3.5% in 5% dextrose, 3.5% in 25% dextrose, 4.25% in 10% dextrose, 4.25% in 20% dextrose, 4.25% in 25% dextrose, 5% in 25% dextrose
amino acid infusions with electrolytes
Aminosyn: 3.5%, 7%, 8.5%
Aminosyn II: 3.5%, 7%, 8.5%, 10%
FreAmine III: 3%, 8.5%
ProcalAmine: 3%

*Liquid form contains alcohol. **May contain tartrazine.

Travasol: 3.5%, 5.5%, 8.5%
amino acid infusions with electrolytes in dextrose
Aminosyn II: 3.5% with electrolytes in 5% dextrose, 4.25% with electrolytes in 10% dextrose
amino acid infusions for hepatic failure
HepatAmine: 8%
amino acid infusions for high metabolic stress
Aminosyn-HBC: 7%
BranchAmin: 4%
FreAmine HBC: 6.9%
amino acid infusions for renal failure
Aminess: 5.2%
Aminosyn-RF: 5.2%
NephrAmine: 5.4%
RenAmin: 6.5%

MECHANISM OF ACTION

Provides a substrate for protein synthesis or enhances conservation of existing body protein.

Formulation for hepatic failure and high metabolic stress contain essential and nonessential amino acids, with high concentrations of the branched chain amino acids isoleucine, leucine, and valine. Formulations for patients in renal failure contain histidine and minimal amounts of essential amino acids; nonessential amino acids are synthesized from excess ammonia in the blood of the uremic patient, thus lowering azotemia.

INDICATIONS & DOSAGE

Total parenteral nutrition (TPN) in patients who cannot or will not eat –
Adults: 1 to 1.5 g/kg I.V. daily.
Children over 10 kg: 20 to 25 g/kg I.V. daily for the first 10 kg, then 1 to 1.25 g/kg I.V. daily for each kg over 10 kg.
Children under 10 kg: 2 to 4 g/kg I.V. daily.
Nutritional support in patients with cirrhosis, hepatitis, and hepatic encephalopathy –
Adults: 80 to 120 g of amino acids (12 to 18 g of nitrogen) I.V. daily of the formulation for hepatic failure.
Nutritional support in patients with high metabolic stress –
Adults: 1.5 g/kg I.V. daily of the formulation for high metabolic stress.
Nutritional support in patients with renal failure –
Adults: 0.3 to 0.5 g/kg I.V. daily (up to total of 26 g daily). Patients on dialysis may require 1 to 1.2 g/kg daily.

ADVERSE REACTIONS

Common reactions are in italics; life-threatening reactions are in bold italics.
CNS: mental confusion, unconsciousness, headache, dizziness.
CV: hypervolemia, ***CHF*** (in susceptible patients), ***pulmonary edema,*** exacerbation of hypertension (in predisposed patients).
GI: nausea, vomiting.
GU: glycosuria, osmotic diuresis.
Hepatic: fatty liver.
Metabolic: *rebound hypoglycemia* (when long-term infusions are abruptly stopped), hyperglycemia, metabolic acidosis, alkalosis, hypophosphatemia, ***hyperosmolar nonketotic syndrome,*** hyperammonemia, ***electrolyte imbalances,*** dehydration (if hyperosmolar solutions are used).
Skin: chills, flushing, feeling of warmth.
Local: tissue sloughing at infusion site due to extravasation, *catheter sepsis, thrombophlebitis,* thrombosis.
Other: allergic reactions.

INTERACTIONS

None significant.

NURSING CONSIDERATIONS

- *Contraindicated* in anuria and in those with inborn errors of amino acid metabolism, especially involving branched-chain amino acid metabolism, such as maple syrup urine disease and isovaleric acidemia. Also contraindicated in severe uncorrected electrolyte or acid-base imbalances, hyperammonemia, and decreased circulating blood volume.

- *Use cautiously* in renal insufficiency or failure, cardiac disease, or hepatic impairment.
- *Use extra caution* in pediatric patients and in neonates, especially those with low birth weight.
- *Administer cautiously* to diabetic patients. To prevent hyperglycemia, insulin may be required. Administer cautiously in cardiac insufficiency. May cause circulatory overload. Patients with fluid restriction may tolerate only 1 to 2 liters.
- Safe and effective use of parenteral nutrition requires a knowledge of nutrition as well as clinical expertise in the recognition and treatment of potential complications. Frequent evaluation of the patient and laboratory determinations are necessary.
- Monitor serum electrolytes, glucose, BUN, and renal and hepatic function. Check serum calcium frequently.
- Individualize dosage to metabolic and clinical response as determined by nitrogen balance and body weight corrected for fluid balance.
- Add vitamins, electrolytes, and trace elements as ordered.
- Monitor for extraordinary electrolyte losses that may occur during nasogastric suction, vomiting, or drainage from GI fistula.
- **I.V. use:** Control infusion rate carefully with infusion pump. If infusion rate falls behind, do not attempt to catch up. Notify doctor.
- Peripheral infusions should be limited to 2.5% amino acids and dextrose 10%. Check infusion site frequently for erythema, inflammation, irritation, tissue sloughing, necrosis, and phlebitis. Change peripheral I.V. sites routinely to prevent irritation and infection. If a subclavian catheter is used, the solution is administered into the midsuperior vena cava.
- Protect bottles from light until use.
- Check fractional urine every 6 hours for glycosuria initially, then every 12 to 24 hours in stable patients. Abrupt onset of glycosuria may be an early sign of impending sepsis.
- Assess body temperature every 4 hours; elevation may indicate sepsis or infection.
- If patient has chills, fever, or other signs of sepsis, replace I.V. tubing and bottle, and send them to the laboratory to be cultured.

corn oil

Lipomul

Pregnancy Risk Category: C

HOW SUPPLIED

Liquid: 473-ml container with 10 g corn oil/15 ml (sugar-free)

MECHANISM OF ACTION

Source of calories and fatty acids.

INDICATIONS & DOSAGE

To increase caloric intake –
Adults: 45 ml P.O. b.i.d. to q.i.d. after or between meals, alone or with proteins, milk, or other energy sources.
Children: 30 ml P.O. daily to q.i.d. after or between meals, alone or with proteins, milk, or other energy sources.

ADVERSE REACTIONS

Common reactions are in italics; life-threatening reactions are in bold italics.
GI: nausea, vomiting, diarrhea.

INTERACTIONS

Griseofulvin: increased GI absorption of griseofulvin. A beneficial interaction.

NURSING CONSIDERATIONS

- *Contraindicated* in gallbladder calculi or complete GI obstructions.
- *Use cautiously* in steatorrhea, par-

tial GI obstruction, and enterostomies.

- To minimize nausea, diarrhea, and vomiting, give more frequent, smaller doses with meals or mixed with milk.
- The dosage varies greatly with individual requirements; 30 ml of the emulsion provides 180 calories.

dextrose (D-glucose)

Pregnancy Risk Category: C

HOW SUPPLIED

Injection: 1,000 ml (2.5%, 5%, 10%, 20%, 30%, 40%, 50%, 60%, 70%); 650 ml (38.5%); 500 ml (5%, 10%, 20%, 30%, 40%, 50%, 60%, 70%); 400 ml (5%); 250 ml (5%, 10%); 100 ml (5%); 70-ml pin-top vial (70% for additive use only); 50 ml (5% and 50% available in vial, ampule, and Bristoject); 10 ml (25%); 5-ml ampule (10%); 3-ml ampule (10%)

MECHANISM OF ACTION

Minimizes glyconeogenesis and promotes anabolism in patients who can't receive sufficient oral caloric intake.

INDICATIONS & DOSAGE

Fluid replacement and caloric supplementation in patient who can't maintain adequate oral intake or who is restricted from doing so –

Adults and children: dosage depends on fluid and caloric requirements. Use peripheral I.V. infusion of 2.5%, 5%, or 10% solution, central I.V. infusion of 20% solution for minimal fluid needs. Use 50% solution to treat insulin-induced hypoglycemia. Solutions from 40% to 70% are used diluted in admixtures, normally with amino acid solutions, for total parenteral nutrition given through a central vein.

ADVERSE REACTIONS

Common reactions are in italics; life-threatening reactions are in bold italics.

CNS: mental confusion, unconsciousness in hyperosmolar nonketotic syndrome.

CV: ***(with fluid overload) pulmonary edema, exacerbated hypertension, and CHF*** in susceptible patients. *Prolonged or concentrated infusions may cause phlebitis and venous sclerosis, especially with peripheral route of administration.*

GU: glycosuria, osmotic diuresis.

Metabolic: (with rapid infusion of concentrated solution or prolonged infusion) hyperglycemia, hypervolemia, hyperosmolarity. Rapid termination of long-term infusions may cause hypoglycemia from rebound hyperinsulinemia.

Skin: sloughing and tissue necrosis, if extravasation occurs with concentrated solutions.

INTERACTIONS

None significant.

NURSING CONSIDERATIONS

- *Contraindicated* in hyperglycemia, diabetic coma, intracranial or intraspinal hemorrhage, or delirium tremens.
- *Use cautiously* in cardiac or pulmonary disease, hypertension, renal insufficiency, urinary obstruction, and hypovolemia.
- **I.V. use:** Control infusion rate carefully. Maximal rate for dextrose infusion is 0.5 g/kg hourly. Use infusion pump when infusing dextrose with amino acids for total parenteral nutrition. Never infuse concentrated solutions rapidly; may cause hyperglycemia and fluid shift.
- Monitor serum glucose carefully. Prolonged therapy with dextrose 5% in water solution can cause depletion of pancreatic insulin production and secretion. If blood glucose level exceeds 200 mg/dl for more than 3 days, infusion should be discontinued.
- Never stop hypertonic solutions abruptly. If necessary, have dextrose 10% in water solution available to

treat hypoglycemia if rebound hyperinsulinemia occurs.

- Don't give dextrose solutions without saline solution in blood transfusions; may cause clumping of red blood cells. Use central veins to infuse dextrose solutions with concentrations greater than 10%.
- Take care to prevent extravasation. Check injection site frequently to prevent irritation, tissue sloughing, necrosis, and phlebitis.
- Watch closely for signs of fluid overload, especially if fluid intake is restricted.
- Monitor intake and output and weight carefully, especially when renal function is impaired.
- Check vital signs frequently. Report adverse effects promptly.

fat emulsions

Intralipid 10%, Intralipid 20%, Liposyn 10%, Liposyn 20%, Liposyn III 10%, Liposyn III 20%, Soyacal 10%, Soyacal 20%, Travamulsion 10%, Travamulsion 20%

Pregnancy Risk Category: B for Soyacal 10%; C for all others

HOW SUPPLIED

Injection: 50 ml (10%, 20%), 100 ml (10%, 20%), 200 ml (10%, 20%), 250 ml (10%, 20%), 500 ml (10%, 20%); 50 ml (20%)

MECHANISM OF ACTION

Provides neutral triglycerides, predominantly unsaturated fatty acids. Acts as a source of calories and prevents fatty acid deficiency. When substituted for dextrose as a source of calories, fat emulsions decrease carbon dioxide production.

INDICATIONS & DOSAGE

Intralipid:

Source of calories adjunctive to total parenteral nutrition –

Adults: 1 ml/minute I.V. for 15 to 30 minutes (10% emulsion); 0.5 ml/minute I.V. for 15 to 30 minutes (20% emulsion). If no adverse reactions, increase rate to deliver 500 ml over 4 to 8 hours. Total daily dosage should not exceed 2.5 g/kg.

Children: 0.1 ml/minute for 10 to 15 minutes (10% emulsion), 0.05 ml/minute I.V. for 10 to 15 minutes (20% emulsion). If no adverse reactions, increase rate to deliver 1 g/kg over 4 hours. Daily dosage should not exceed 4 g/kg. Equals 60% of daily caloric intake. Protein-carbohydrate total parenteral nutrition should supply remaining 40%.

Fatty acid deficiency –

Adults and children: 8% to 10% of total caloric intake I.V.

Liposyn:

Prevention of fatty acid deficiency –

Adults: 500 ml (10% emulsion) I.V. twice weekly. Infuse initially at a rate of 1 ml/minute for 30 minutes. Rate may be increased but should not exceed 500 ml over 4 to 6 hours.

Children: 5 to 10 ml/kg (10% emulsion) I.V. daily. Infuse initially at a rate of 0.1 ml/minute for 30 minutes. Rate may be increased but should not exceed 100 ml/hour.

ADVERSE REACTIONS

Common reactions are in italics; life-threatening reactions are in bold italics.

Early reactions of fat overload:

Blood: hyperlipemia, ***hypercoagulability, thrombocytopenia in neonates*** (rare).

CNS: headache, sleepiness, dizziness.

EENT: pressure over eyes.

GI: nausea, vomiting.

Skin: flushing, diaphoresis.

Local: irritation at infusion site.

Other: fever, dyspnea, chest and back pains, cyanosis, allergic reactions, deposition of I.V. fat.

Delayed reactions:

Blood: thrombocytopenia, leukopenia, leukocytosis.
CNS: focal seizures.
CV: ***shock.***
Hepatic: transient increased liver function test, hepatomegaly.
Other: fever, splenomegaly, ***fat accumulation in lungs.***

INTERACTIONS

None significant.

NURSING CONSIDERATIONS

- *Contraindicated* in hyperlipemia, lipid nephrosis, or acute pancreatitis accompanied by hyperlipemia.
- *Use cautiously* in severe hepatic disease, pulmonary disease, anemia, blood coagulation disorders, including thrombocytopenia, and in patients at risk for fat embolism.
- *Use cautiously* also in premature infants because they are susceptible to I.V. fat overload.
- **I.V. use:** Avoid rapid infusion. Use an infusion pump to regulate rate.
- Watch closely for adverse reactions, especially during first half hour of infusion.
- Check platelet count frequently in neonates receiving fat emulsions I.V.
- Lipids support bacterial growth. Change all I.V. tubing at each infusion. Check injection site daily. Report signs of inflammation or infection promptly.
- Carefully monitor triglycerides and free fatty acids in infants.
- May be mixed with amino acid solution, dextrose, electrolytes, and vitamins in the same I.V. container. Check with pharmacist for acceptable proportions and compatibility information.
- Manufacturers do not recommend using an in-line filter for administering fat emulsions because fat particles are larger than the pores of a standard 0.22-micron cellulose filter. However, an in-line filter with pores of 1.2 micron or larger is sometimes used to remove particulate matter.
- Do not use fat emulsion if it separates or becomes oily.
- Refrigeration is not necessary.
- Monitor serum lipids closely when patient is receiving fat emulsion therapy. Lipemia must clear between dosing.
- Monitor hepatic function carefully in long-term use.
- Intralipid, Travamulsion, and Liposyn differ mainly by their fatty acid components.

fructose (levulose)

Pregnancy Risk Category: C

HOW SUPPLIED

Injection: 1,000 ml (10% or 100 g/liter)

MECHANISM OF ACTION

Minimizes glyconeogenesis and promotes anabolism in patients who can't receive sufficient oral caloric intake.

INDICATIONS & DOSAGE

Source of carbohydrate calories primarily when fluid replacement is also indicated and as a dextrose substitute for patients with diabetes –
Adults and children: dosage depends on caloric needs. I.V. infusion rate should not exceed 1 g/kg hourly. Single liter 10% solution yields 375 calories.

ADVERSE REACTIONS

Common reactions are in italics; life-threatening reactions are in bold italics.
CV: increased pulse rate, precipitation or exacerbation of ***CHF*** in susceptible patients, ***pulmonary edema.***
Hepatic: hepatomegaly.
Metabolic: metabolic acidosis, hypervolemia.
Local: extravasation at infusion site may cause sloughing of skin, thrombophlebitis.

Other: increased respiratory rate.

INTERACTIONS
None significant.

NURSING CONSIDERATIONS
- *Contraindicated* in hereditary fructose intolerance, in gout, or in patients receiving therapy for hypoglycemia.
- *Use cautiously* in cardiac disease, hypertension, pulmonary disease, hypervolemia, renal insufficiency, and urinary tract obstructions.
- **I.V. use:** Control infusion rate carefully. Make sure rate does not exceed 1 g/kg hourly for infants. Direct injection or intermittent infusion is not recommended.
- Change infusion sites regularly to avoid irritation with prolonged therapy. Take care to avoid extravasation.
- Don't use unless the solution is clear and the seal is intact.
- Watch closely for signs of fluid overload, pulmonary edema, or CHF.

invert sugar
Travert

Pregnancy Risk Category: C

HOW SUPPLIED
Injection: 5%, 10%, 10% with electrolytes

MECHANISM OF ACTION
Minimizes glyconeogenesis and promotes anabolism in patients who can't receive sufficient oral caloric intake. Composed of equal amounts of dextrose and fructose.

INDICATIONS & DOSAGE
Nonelectrolyte fluid replacement and caloric supplementation solution – **Adults and children:** dosage depends on patient's age, weight, and clinical need. I.V. infusion rate should not exceed 1 g/kg hourly. A single liter of 5% invert sugar yields 375 calories. Most patients receive 1 to 3 liters of 10% solution daily.

ADVERSE REACTIONS
Common reactions are in italics; life-threatening reactions are in bold italics.
CNS: mental confusion, unconsciousness in ***hyperosmolar nonketotic syndrome.***
CV: increased pulse rate, precipitation or exacerbation of ***CHF*** in susceptible patients, ***pulmonary edema,*** hypertension.
GU: glycosuria, osmotic diuresis.
Local: extravasation at infusion site may cause sloughing of skin, thrombophlebitis.
Metabolic: hypervolemia, hyperglycemia, hyperosmolarity. Rapid termination of long-term infusions may cause ***hypoglycemia*** from rebound hyperinsulinemia.

INTERACTIONS
None significant.

NURSING CONSIDERATIONS
- *Contraindicated* in hereditary fructose intolerance, hyperglycemia, diabetic coma, intracranial or intraspinal hemorrhage, or delirium tremens.
- *Use cautiously* in cardiac disease, hypertension, pulmonary disease, hypervolemia, renal insufficiency, and urinary tract obstructions.
- **I.V. use:** Control infusion rate carefully. Make sure rate does not exceed 1 g/kg hourly for infants. Change infusion sites regularly to avoid irritation with prolonged therapy. Take care to avoid extravasation.
- Watch closely for signs of fluid overload, pulmonary edema, or CHF. Monitor blood pressure frequently.
- Monitor serum glucose closely. Prolonged therapy can cause depletion of pancreatic insulin production and secretion.
- Monitor intake and output and weight closely, especially if renal function is impaired.

• Check vital signs frequently. Tell doctor promptly if adverse reactions occur.

medium-chain triglycerides

M.C.T.◊

Pregnancy Risk Category: C

HOW SUPPLIED
Oil: 960 ml (115 calories/15 ml)◊

MECHANISM OF ACTION
Source of rapidly hydrolyzable lipid.

INDICATIONS & DOSAGE
Inadequate digestion or absorption of food fats –
Adults: 15 ml P.O. t.i.d. or q.i.d. Maximum of 100 ml/day.

ADVERSE REACTIONS
Common reactions are in italics; life-threatening reactions are in bold italics.
CNS: reversible *coma* in susceptible patients (such as those with advanced hepatic cirrhosis).
GI: *nausea, vomiting, diarrhea, abdominal distention, cramps.*

INTERACTIONS
None significant.

NURSING CONSIDERATIONS
• *Contraindicated* in advanced hepatic disease or abetalipoproteinemia.
• *Use cautiously* in patients with portacaval shunts.
• To minimize GI adverse reactions, give smaller doses more frequently with meals or mixed with salad dressing or chilled fruit juice.
• More easily absorbed than long-chain fats; not dependent on bile salts for emulsification.
• Rapid metabolism provides quick energy.
• May be useful in lowering cholesterol levels. Also used in patients with short-bowel syndrome.
• Provides 7.7 calories/ml. No essential fatty acids are provided.

94
Antigout agents

allopurinol
colchicine
probenecid
sulfinpyrazone

COMBINATION PRODUCTS
COLBENEMID, PROBEN-C, PROBENECID WITH COLCHICINE: probenecid 500 mg and colchicine 0.5 mg.

allopurinol
Alloremed‡, Capurate‡, Lopurin, Zyloprim

Pregnancy Risk Category: C

HOW SUPPLIED
Tablets (scored): 100 mg, 300 mg
Capsules: 100 mg‡, 300 mg‡

MECHANISM OF ACTION
Reduces uric acid production by inhibiting the biochemical reactions preceding its formation.

INDICATIONS & DOSAGE
Gout, primary or secondary to hyperuricemia; secondary to diseases such as acute or chronic leukemia, polycythemia vera, multiple myeloma, and psoriasis –
Dosage varies with severity of disease; can be given as single dose or divided, but doses larger than 300 mg should be divided.
Adults: mild gout, 200 to 300 mg P.O. daily; severe gout with large tophi, 400 to 600 mg P.O. daily. Same dosage for maintenance in secondary hyperuricemia.
Hyperuricemia secondary to malignancies –
Children 6 to 10 years: 300 mg P.O. daily or divided t.i.d.
Children under 6 years: 50 mg P.O. t.i.d.
Impaired renal function –
Adults: 200 mg P.O. daily if creatinine clearance is 10 to 20 ml/minute; 100 mg P.O. daily if creatinine is less than 10 ml/minute; 100 mg P.O. more than 24 hours apart if clearance is less than 3 ml/minute.
To prevent acute gouty attacks –
Adults: 100 mg P.O. daily; increase at weekly intervals by 100 mg without exceeding maximum dose (800 mg), until serum uric acid falls to 6 mg/100 ml or less.
To prevent uric acid nephropathy during cancer chemotherapy –
Adults: 600 to 800 mg P.O. daily for 2 to 3 days, with high fluid intake.
Recurrent calcium oxalate calculi –
Adults: 200 to 300 mg P.O. daily in single dose or divided doses.

ADVERSE REACTIONS
Common reactions are in italics; life-threatening reactions are in bold italics.
Blood: ***agranulocytosis,*** anemia, ***aplastic anemia.***
CNS: drowsiness, headache.
EENT: cataracts, retinopathy.
GI: nausea, vomiting, diarrhea, abdominal pain.
Hepatic: altered liver function studies, ***hepatitis.***
Skin: *rash, usually maculopapular;* ***exfoliative,*** urticarial, and purpuric lesions; ***erythema multiforme;*** severe furunculosis of nose; ichthyosis, ***toxic epidermal necrolysis.***

INTERACTIONS
Alcohol, diazoxide, diuretics, mecamylamine, pyrazinamide: increased serum acid concentration. Adjust dosage of allopurinol.
Amoxicillin, ampicillin, bacampicil-

lin: increased possibility of skin rash. Avoid concomitant use.
Anticoagulants: potentiation of anticoagulant effect. Dosage adjustments may be necessary.
Antineoplastic agents: increased potential for bone marrow suppression. Monitor patient carefully.
Chlorpropamide: possible increased hypoglycemic effect. Avoid concomitant use.
Ethacrynic acid, thiazide diuretics: increased risk of allopurinol toxicity. Reduce dosage of allopurinol and closely monitor renal function.
Uricosuric agents: additive effect. May be used to therapeutic advantage.
Urinary acidifying agents (ammonium chloride, ascorbic acid, potassium or sodium phosphate): may increase the possibility of kidney stone formation.
Xanthines: increased serum theophylline. Adjust dosage of theophyllines.

NURSING CONSIDERATIONS

- *Contraindicated* in hypersensitivity to the drug and in idiopathic hemochromatosis.
- *Use cautiously* in cataracts and hepatic or renal disease.
- Obtain accurate patient history.
- Discontinue at first sign of rash, which may precede severe hypersensitivity reaction or any other adverse reaction. Tell patient to report all adverse reactions immediately. Skin rash is more common in patients taking diuretics and in those with renal disorders.
- Monitor intake and output; daily urine output of at least 2 liters and maintenance of neutral or slightly alkaline urine are desirable. Patient should be encouraged to drink plenty of fluids while taking this drug unless otherwise contraindicated.
- If renal insufficiency exists at any time during treatment, allopurinol dosage should be reduced.
- Periodically check CBC and hepatic and renal function, especially at start of therapy.
- If patient is taking allopurinol for treatment of recurrent calcium oxalate stones, advise him to also reduce his dietary intake of animal protein, sodium, refined sugars, oxalate-rich foods, and calcium.
- Optimal benefits of therapy may require 2 to 6 weeks of therapy. Because acute gouty attacks may occur during this time, concurrent use of colchicine may be prescribed prophylactically.
- Minimize GI adverse reactions by administering with meals or immediately after.
- Evaluate effectiveness, using serum uric acid level.
- Allopurinol may predispose patient to amoxicillin or ampicillin-induced rash.
- Allopurinol may cause rash even weeks after discontinuation.
- Since drug may cause drowsiness, advise patient to refrain from driving car or performing tasks requiring mental alertness until CNS effects of the drug are known.

colchicine

Colchicine MR‡, Colgout‡,
Colsalide, Novocolchicine†

Pregnancy Risk Category: D

HOW SUPPLIED

Tablets: 0.5 mg (1/120 grain), 0.6 mg (1/100 grain) as sugar-coated granules
Injection: 1 mg (1/60 grain)/2 ml

MECHANISM OF ACTION

As antigout agent, apparently decreases leukocyte motility, phagocytosis, and lactic acid production, thus decreasing urate crystal deposits and reducing inflammation. As antiosteolytic agent, apparently inhibits mitosis of osteoprogenitor cells and decreases the activity of osteoclasts.

INDICATIONS & DOSAGE

To prevent acute attacks of gout as prophylactic or maintenance therapy –
Adults: 0.5 or 0.6 mg P.O. daily. Patients who normally have one attack per year or less should receive the drug only 3 or 4 days per week. Patients who have more than one attack per year should receive the drug daily. In severe cases, give 1 to 1.8 mg daily.
To prevent attacks of gout in patients undergoing surgery –
Adults: 0.5 to 0.6 mg P.O. t.i.d. 3 days before and 3 days after surgery.
To treat acute gout, acute gouty arthritis –
Adults: initially, 1 to 1.2 mg P.O., then 0.5 or 0.6 mg q hour, or 1 to 1.2 mg q 2 hours until pain is relieved; nausea, vomiting, or diarrhea ensues; or the maximum dose of 10 mg is reached. Alternatively, give 2 mg I.V. followed by 0.5 mg I.V. q 6 hours if necessary. (Note that some clinicians prefer to give a single I.V. injection of 3 mg.) Total I.V. dosage over 24 hours (one course of treatment) not to exceed 4 mg.

Note: Colchicine is a toxic drug and fatalities have resulted from overdose. After a full course of I.V. colchicine (4 mg), don't give any more colchicine by any route for at least 7 days.
Familial Mediterranean fever suppression –
Adults: acute attack – 0.6 mg P.O. hourly for four doses, then q 2 hours for four doses on the first day. Then, give 1.2 mg P.O. q 12 hours for 2 days. Maintenance dosage is 0.5 to 0.6 mg P.O. b.i.d. to t.i.d.

ADVERSE REACTIONS

Common reactions are in italics; life-threatening reactions are in bold italics.
Blood: ***aplastic anemia and agranulocytosis with prolonged use;*** nonthrombocytopenic purpura.
CNS: peripheral neuritis.
GI: *nausea, vomiting, abdominal pain, diarrhea.*
Skin: urticaria, dermatitis.
Local: severe local irritation if extravasation occurs.
Other: alopecia.

INTERACTIONS

Alcohol: may impair efficacy of colchicine prophylaxis.
Loop diuretics: may decrease efficacy of colchicine prophylaxis.
Phenylbutazone: may increase risk of leukopenia or thrombocytopenia.
Vitamin B_{12}: impaired absorption of vitamin B_{12}.

NURSING CONSIDERATIONS

- *Use cautiously* in hepatic dysfunction, cardiac disease, blood dyscrasias, renal disease, GI disorders, and in elderly or debilitated patients.
- Reduce dosage if weakness, anorexia, nausea, vomiting, or diarrhea appears. First sign of acute overdosage may be GI symptoms, followed by vascular damage, muscle weakness, and ascending paralysis. Delirium and seizures may occur without the patient losing consciousness.
- Discontinue drug as soon as gout pain is relieved or at the first sign of GI symptoms.
- Colchicine has no effect on nongouty arthritis.
- **I.V. use:** Give by slow I.V. push over 2 to 5 minutes. Be sure to avoid extravasation because colchicine is very irritating to tissues. Don't dilute colchicine injection with dextrose 5% injection or any other fluid that might change pH of colchicine solution. If lower concentration of colchicine injection is needed, dilute with 0.9% sodium chloride solution or sterile water for injection and administer over 2 to 5 minutes by direct injection. Preferably, inject into the tubing of a free-flowing I.V. solution. However, if diluted solution becomes turbid, don't inject.

*Liquid form contains alcohol. **May contain tartrazine.

- Do not administer I.M. or S.C.; severe local irritation occurs.
- As maintenance therapy, give with meals to reduce GI effects. May be used with uricosuric agents.
- Baseline laboratory studies, including CBC, should precede therapy and be repeated periodically.
- Monitor fluid intake and output. Keep output at 2,000 ml daily.
- Store in tightly closed, light-resistant container.

probenecid

Benemid, Benn, Benuryl†, Probalan, Robenecid

Pregnancy Risk Category: B

HOW SUPPLIED

Tablets: 500 mg

MECHANISM OF ACTION

Blocks renal tubular reabsorption of uric acid, increasing excretion. Also inhibits active renal tubular secretion of many weak organic acids (for example, penicillins and cephalosporins).

INDICATIONS & DOSAGE

Adjunct to penicillin or cephalosporin therapy –

Adults and children over 50 kg: 500 mg P.O. q.i.d.

Children 2 to 14 years or under 50 kg: initially, 25 mg/kg P.O., then 40 mg/kg divided q.i.d.

Single-dose treatment of gonorrhea –

Adults: 3.5 g ampicillin P.O. with 1 g probenecid P.O. given together; or 1 g probenecid P.O. 30 minutes before dose of 4.8 million units of aqueous penicillin G procaine I.M., injected at two different sites.

Treatment of hyperuricemia of gout, gouty arthritis –

Adults: 250 mg P.O. b.i.d. for first week, then 500 mg b.i.d., to maximum of 2 g daily. Maintenance dosage is 500 mg daily for 6 months.

ADVERSE REACTIONS

Common reactions are in italics; life-threatening reactions are in bold italics.

Blood: ***hemolytic anemia.***

CNS: *headache,* dizziness.

CV: hypotension.

GI: anorexia, nausea, vomiting, *gastric distress.*

GU: urinary frequency, renal colic.

Skin: dermatitis, pruritus, alopecia.

Other: flushing, sore gums, fever.

INTERACTIONS

Indomethacin: decreased indomethacin excretion. Lower indomethacin dosages may be required.

Methotrexate: decreased methotrexate excretion. Lower methotrexate dosage may be required. Serum levels should be determined.

Oral hypoglycemic agents: enhanced hypoglycemic effect. Monitor blood glucose levels closely. Dosage adjustment may be required.

Salicylates: inhibited uricosuric effect of probenecid, causing urate retention. Do not use together.

NURSING CONSIDERATIONS

- *Contraindicated* in blood dyscrasias; acute gout attack; penicillin therapy in presence of known renal impairment; gouty nephropathy; urinary tract stones or obstruction; and azotemia or hyperuricemia secondary to cancer chemotherapy, radiation, or myeloproliferative neoplastic diseases.
- *Use cautiously* in peptic ulcer and renal impairment.
- Usually preferred over sulfinpyrazone because probenecid produces fewer and less severe GI and hematologic adverse reactions.
- Contains no analgesic or anti-inflammatory agent, and is of no value during acute gout attacks. Don't initiate therapy until acute attack subsides.
- Suitable for long-term use; no cumulative effects or tolerance.

†Available in Canada only. ‡Available in Australia only. ◇Available OTC.

- Not effective with chronic renal insufficiency (glomerular filtration rate less than 30 ml/minute).
- Periodic BUN and renal function tests recommended in long-term therapy.
- May increase frequency, severity, and length of acute gout attacks during first 6 to 12 months of therapy. Prophylactic colchicine or another anti-inflammatory agent is given during first 3 to 6 months.
- Tell patient with gout to avoid alcohol; it increases urate level.
- Patient with gout should avoid all medications that contain aspirin. These may precipitate gout. Acetaminophen may be used for pain.
- Force fluids to maintain minimum daily output of 2 to 3 liters. Alkalinize urine with sodium bicarbonate or potassium citrate as ordered by doctor. These measures will prevent hematuria, renal colic, urate stone development, and costovertebral pain.
- Give with milk, food, or antacids to minimize GI distress. Continued disturbances might indicate need to lower dosage.
- Patients with gout should restrict foods high in purine: anchovies, liver, sardines, kidneys, sweetbreads, peas, and lentils.
- Instruct patient and his family that drug must be taken regularly as ordered or gout attacks may result. Tell him to visit doctor regularly so uric acid can be monitored and dosage can be adjusted if necessary. Lifelong therapy may be required in patients with hyperuricemia.
- May produce false-positive glucose tests with Benedict's solution or Clinitest, but not with glucose oxidase method (Clinistix, Diastix, Tes-Tape).
- Decreases urinary excretion of 17-ketosteroids, Bromsulphalein (BSP), aminohippuric acid, and iodine-related organic acids, interfering with laboratory procedures.

sulfinpyrazone

Anturan†, Anturane

Pregnancy Risk Category: C

HOW SUPPLIED

Tablets: 100 mg
Capsules: 200 mg

MECHANISM OF ACTION

Blocks renal tubular reabsorption of uric acid, increasing excretion. Also inhibits platelet aggregation.

INDICATIONS & DOSAGE

Inhibition of platelet aggregation, increase of platelet survival time in treatment of thromboembolic disorders, angina, myocardial infarction, transient cerebral ischemic attacks, peripheral arterial atherosclerosis –
Adults: 200 mg P.O. q.i.d.
Maintenance therapy for common gout: reduction, prevention of joint changes and tophi formation –
Adults: 100 to 200 mg P.O. b.i.d. first week, then 200 to 400 mg P.O. b.i.d. Maximum dosage is 800 mg daily.

ADVERSE REACTIONS

Common reactions are in italics; life-threatening reactions are in bold italics.
Blood: ***agranulocytosis, blood dyscrasias (rare).***
CNS: dizziness, vertigo, tinnitus.
GI: *nausea, dyspepsia,* epigastric pain, blood loss, reactivation of peptic ulcers.
Skin: rash.

INTERACTIONS

Oral anticoagulants: increased anticoagulant effect and risk of bleeding. Use together cautiously.
Oral antidiabetic agents, anticoagulants: increased effects. Monitor closely.
Probenecid: inhibited renal excretion of sulfinpyrazone. Use together cautiously.

*Liquid form contains alcohol. **May contain tartrazine.

Salicylates: inhibited uricosuric effect of sulfinpyrazone. Do not use together.

NURSING CONSIDERATIONS

- *Contraindicated* in hypersensitivity to pyrazole derivatives (including oxyphenbutazone and phenylbutazone); active peptic ulcer; gouty nephropathy; urolithiasis or urinary obstruction; bone marrow suppression; azotemia, hyperuricemia secondary to cancer chemotherapy, radiation, or myeloproliferative neoplastic diseases; blood dyscrasias; and during or within 2 weeks after gout attack.
- *Use cautiously* in diminished hepatic or renal function.
- Use in treating thromboembolic conditions is investigational and is most often directed at prevention of recurrent myocardial infarction.
- Recommended for patients unresponsive to probenecid. Suitable for long-term use; neither cumulative effects nor tolerance develops.
- Contains no analgesic or anti-inflammatory agent and is of no value during acute gout attacks.
- Periodic BUN, CBC, and renal function studies advised during long-term use.
- May increase frequency, severity, and length of acute gout attacks during first 6 to 12 months of therapy. Prophylactic colchicine or another anti-inflammatory agent is given during first 3 to 6 months.
- Therapy, especially at start, may lead to renal colic and formation of uric acid stones. Until acid levels are normal (about 6 mg/100 ml), monitor intake and output closely.
- Force fluids to maintain minimum daily output of 2 to 3 liters. Alkalinize urine with sodium bicarbonate or other agent ordered by doctor.
- Give with milk, food, or antacids to minimize GI disturbances.
- Patients with gout should restrict foods high in purine: anchovies, liver, sardines, kidneys, sweetbreads, peas, and lentils.
- Instruct patient and his family that drug must be taken regularly as ordered or gout attacks may result. Tell him to visit doctor regularly so blood levels can be monitored and dosage adjusted if necessary.
- Lifelong therapy may be required in patients with hyperuricemia.
- Decreases urinary excretion of aminohippuric acid, interfering with laboratory test results.
- Alkalinizing agents are used therapeutically to increase sulfinpyrazone activity, preventing urolithiasis.
- Warn patients with gout not to take any aspirin-containing medications since these may precipitate gout. Acetaminophen may be used for pain.

95
Enzymes

chymopapain
fibrinolysin and desoxyribonuclease
hyaluronidase

COMBINATION PRODUCTS

CHYMORAL-100: 100,000 units enzymatic activity; trypsin and chymotrypsin in ratio of 6:1.
GRANULEX AEROSOL: trypsin 0.1 mg, balsam Peru 72.5 mg, and castor oil 650 mg/0.82 ml.
ORENZYME BITABS ENTERIC-COATED TABLETS: 100,000 units trypsin and 8,000 units chymotrypsin.

chymopapain

Chymodiactin, Discase

Pregnancy Risk Category: C

HOW SUPPLIED

Powder for injection: 4,000 units/vial, 10,000 units/vial; each unit of chymopapain is also referred to as 1 picoKatal (pKat)

MECHANISM OF ACTION

Hydrolyzes noncollagenous proteins in the chondromucoprotein of the nucleus pulposus.

INDICATIONS & DOSAGE

Treatment of herniated lumbar intervertebral disk –
Adults: 2,000 to 4,000 pKat units/disk injected intradiskally. Maximum dosage in a single patient with multiple disk herniation is 10,000 units.

ADVERSE REACTIONS

Common reactions are in italics; life-threatening reactions are in bold italics.
Systemic: ***anaphylaxis, paraplegia, cerebral hemorrhage, acute transverse myelitis,*** nausea, headache, dizziness, leg weakness, paresthesias, numbness of legs and toes.
Local: *back pain, stiffness, back spasm.*

INTERACTIONS

None significant.

NURSING CONSIDERATIONS

- *Contraindicated* in patients with history of allergy to papaya or meat tenderizer; patients who have previously received an injection of chymopapain; severe spondylolisthesis in addition to spinal stenosis; severe progressing paralysis; or evidence of spinal cord tumor or a cauda equina lesion. Most clinicians advocate pretreatment with antihistamine (both H_1 and H_2 blockers).
- Should be used only by doctors qualified by training and experience to perform laminectomy, diskectomy or other spinal procedures, and who have received specialized training in chemonucleolysis. Drug shouldn't be injected in any region other than the lumbar spine. Chymopapain is extremely toxic if injected into the subarachnoid space.
- A new test (ChymoFAST) can detect allergic sensitivity to chymopapain.
- Monitor very closely for anaphylactoid reaction (0.5% of patients). Can be immediate or delayed up to 1 hour after injection and can last for minutes to several hours or longer. Watch for hypotension and bronchospasm. These may lead to laryngeal edema, arrhythmias, cardiac arrest, coma, and death. Other signs of allergic response include erythema, pilomotor erection, rash, pruritic urticaria, con-

*Liquid form contains alcohol. **May contain tartrazine.

junctivitis, vasomotor rhinitis, angioedema, or various GI disturbances.
- Keep an I.V. line open to permit rapid management of anaphylaxis. Keep epinephrine and steroids readily available.
- Instruct patient to anticipate the possibility of delayed allergic reactions, such as rash, urticaria, or itching, which may occur as late as 15 days after injection. Patient should report these to doctor immediately.
- Patients may experience back pain or involuntary muscle spasm in the lower back for several days after injection. Reassure patient that this is common and will not be chronic.
- Use within 60 minutes after reconstitution. Discard unused drug.

fibrinolysin and desoxyribonuclease

Elase

Pregnancy Risk Category: C

HOW SUPPLIED

Dry powder: 25 units fibrinolysin and 15,000 units deoxyribonuclease in 30-ml vial

Ointment: 30 units fibrinolysin and 20,000 units deoxyribonuclease in 30-g tube

MECHANISM OF ACTION

Desoxyribonuclease attacks DNA and fibrinolysin attacks fibrin of blood clots and fibrinous exudates. Enzymatic action produces clean surfaces and promotes healing.

INDICATIONS & DOSAGE

Debridement of inflammatory and infected lesions (surgical wounds, ulcerative lesions, second- and third-degree burns, circumcision, episiotomy, cervicitis, vaginitis, abscesses, fistulas, and sinus tracts) –

Intravaginally –

Adults and children: 5 ml ointment may be inserted using applicator supplied, once daily h.s. for vaginitis or cervicitis for 5 days or until tube is empty.

Topical use –

Adults and children: apply ointment at intervals as long as enzyme action is desired.

Irrigating agent for infected wounds, empyema cavities, abscesses, otorhinolaryngologic wounds, subcutaneous hematomas –

Adults and children: dilution for irrigation depends on extent and severity of wound.

ADVERSE REACTIONS

Common reactions are in italics; life-threatening reactions are in bold italics.

Local: hyperemia with high doses, allergic reactions.

INTERACTIONS

None significant.

NURSING CONSIDERATIONS

- *Contraindicated* for parenteral use.
- Dense, dry eschar must be removed surgically before enzymatic debridement. Enzyme must be in constant contact with substrate. Accumulated necrotic debris must be removed periodically and the enzyme replenished at least once daily.
- Ensure that wound-dressing techniques are performed carefully under aseptic conditions and that antibiotic therapy is instituted as ordered.
- Cleanse wound with water, normal salines, or peroxide and dry gently; cover with thin layer of Elase. Cover with nonadhering dressing.
- Change dressing at least once and preferably two to three times daily. Flush away necrotic debris and reapply ointment. Frequency of application may be more important than the amount of drug used.
- Solution as wet to dry dressing: mix 1 vial of Elase powder with 10 to 50 ml saline solution; saturate strips of fine gauze with solution. Pack ulcer-

ated area with Elase gauze. Allow gauze to dry in contact with ulcerated lesion for about 6 to 8 hours. Remove dried gauze and repeat 3 to 4 times daily.
• Solution as irrigating agent: Drain cavity and replace Elase every 6 to 10 hours to reduce amount of by-product accumulation and to minimize loss of enzyme activity. Although parenteral use is contraindicated, Elase is used as an irrigating agent in certain specific conditions.
• Prepare solution just before use. Discard after 24 hours.

hyaluronidase

Wydase

Pregnancy Risk Category: C

HOW SUPPLIED

Injection: 150 units/vial, 1,500 units/vial; 150 units/ml in 1-ml, 10-ml vials

MECHANISM OF ACTION

Hydrolyzes hyaluronic acid, thereby promoting diffusion of fluids in the tissues.

INDICATIONS & DOSAGE

Adjunct to increase absorption and dispersion of other injected drugs –
Adults and children: 150 units to injection medium containing other medication.
Hypodermoclysis –
Adults and children over 3 years: 150 units injected S.C. before clysis or injected into clysis tubing near needle for each 1,000 ml clysis solution.
Excretory urography when contrast medium is given S.C. –
Adults and children: with patient in a prone position, give 75 units S.C. over each scapula, followed by injection of contrast medium at same sites.

ADVERSE REACTIONS

Common reactions are in italics; life-threatening reactions are in bold italics.
Skin: rash, urticaria.
Local: irritation.

INTERACTIONS

Local anesthetics: increased potential for toxic local reaction. Use together cautiously.

NURSING CONSIDERATIONS

• *Use cautiously* in patients with blood-clotting abnormalities, severe hepatic or renal disease.
• Not recommended for I.V. use.
• Do not inject into acutely inflamed or cancerous areas.
• In hypodermoclysis, adjust dosage, rate of injection, and type of solution according to patient's response.
• Administration precautions: Perform a skin test for sensitivity. Avoid injecting into diseased areas (may spread infection). Observe injection site for local reactions.
• Avoid getting solution in eyes. If solution does get in eyes, flush with water at once.
• Protect from heat. Do not use cloudy or discolored solution.
• For children, 15 units are added to each 100 ml of solution. The drip rate should not exceed 2 ml/minute.
• Hyaluronidase is incompatible with epinephrine and heparin. Don't add to any solutions containing these drugs.

96

Oxytocics

carboprost tromethamine
dinoprostone
ergonovine maleate
methylergonovine maleate
oxytocin, synthetic injection
oxytocin, synthetic nasal solution

COMBINATION PRODUCTS
None.

carboprost tromethamine
Hemabate

HOW SUPPLIED
Injection: 250 mcg/ml

MECHANISM OF ACTION
Produces strong, prompt contractions of uterine smooth muscle, possibly mediated by calcium and cyclic 3′,5′-adenosine monophosphate. A prostaglandin.

INDICATIONS & DOSAGE
Abort pregnancy between 13th and 20th weeks of gestation –
Adults: initially, 250 mcg is administered deep I.M. Subsequent doses of 250 mcg should be administered at intervals of 1½ to 3½ hours, depending on uterine response. Increments in dosage may be increased to 500 mcg if contractility is inadequate after several 250-mcg doses. Total dosage should not exceed 12 mg.
Postpartum hemorrhage caused by uterine atony that has not responded to conventional management –
Adults: 250 mcg by deep I.M. injection. May administer repeat doses at 15- to 90-minute intervals. Maximum total dosage is 2 mg.

ADVERSE REACTIONS
Common reactions are in italics; life-threatening reactions are in bold italics.
GI: *vomiting, diarrhea,* nausea.
Other: *fever,* chills.

INTERACTIONS
None significant.

NURSING CONSIDERATIONS
- *Contraindicated* in pelvic inflammatory disease or active cardiac, pulmonary, renal, or hepatic disease.
- *Use cautiously* in history of asthma; hypertension; cardiovascular, renal, or hepatic disease; anemia; jaundice; diabetes; seizure disorder; and previous uterine surgery.
- Unlike other prostaglandin abortifacients, carboprost tromethamine is administered by I.M. injection. Injectable form avoids risk of expelling vaginal suppositories, which may occur in the presence of profuse vaginal bleeding.
- Should be used only in a hospital setting by trained personnel.

dinoprostone
Prostin E_2

HOW SUPPLIED
Vaginal suppositories: 20 mg

MECHANISM OF ACTION
Produces strong, prompt contractions of uterine smooth muscle, possibly mediated by calcium and cyclic 3′,5′-adenosine monophosphate. A prostaglandin.

INDICATIONS & DOSAGE
Abort second trimester pregnancy, evacuate uterus in cases of missed abortion, intrauterine fetal deaths up

to 28 weeks of gestation, or benign hydatidiform mole –
Adults: insert 20-mg suppository high into posterior vaginal fornix. Repeat q 3 to 5 hours until abortion is complete.

ADVERSE REACTIONS
Common reactions are in italics; life-threatening reactions are in bold italics.
CNS: headache, *dizziness.*
CV: hypotension (in large doses).
GI: *nausea, vomiting, diarrhea.*
GU: vaginal pain, vaginitis.
Other: *fever, shivering, chills, joint inflammation, nocturnal leg cramps, bronchospasm.*

INTERACTIONS
Alcohol (I.V. infusions of 500 ml of 10% over 1 hour): inhibited uterine activity.

NURSING CONSIDERATIONS
- *Contraindicated* in pelvic inflammatory disease or history of pelvic surgery, incisions, uterine fibroids, or cervical stenosis.
- *Use cautiously* in asthma, seizure disorder, anemia, diabetes, hypertension or hypotension, jaundice, and cardiovascular, renal, or hepatic disease.
- Administer only when critical care facilities are readily available.
- Patient may be pretreated with an antiemetic and an antidiarrheal agent.
- Just before use, warm dinoprostone suppositories in their wrapping to room temperature.
- After administration, patient should remain supine for 10 minutes.
- Store suppositories in freezer at temperature of − 20° C. (− 4° F.).
- Dinoprostone-induced fever is self-limiting and transient and occurs in approximately 50% of all patients. Treat with water or alcohol sponging and increased fluid intake rather than with aspirin.
- Check vaginal discharge daily.
- Abortion should be complete within 30 hours.
- Dinoprostone is being investigated as an agent that promotes cervical inducibility (cervical "ripening") before induction of labor with oxytocin.

ergonovine maleate (ergometrine maleate)
Ergotrate Maleate

HOW SUPPLIED
Tablets: 0.2 mg
Injection: 0.2 mg/ml

MECHANISM OF ACTION
Increases motor activity of the uterus by direct stimulation. Prolonged uterine contraction helps control hemorrhage.

INDICATIONS & DOSAGE
Prevent or treat postpartum and postabortion hemorrhage from uterine atony or subinvolution –
Adults: 0.2 mg I.M. q 2 to 4 hours, maximum of 5 doses; or 0.2 mg I.V. (only for severe uterine bleeding or other life-threatening emergency) over 1 minute while blood pressure and uterine contractions are monitored. I.V. dose may be diluted to 5 ml with normal saline injection. After initial I.M. or I.V. dose, may give 0.2 to 0.4 mg P.O. q 6 to 12 hours for 2 to 7 days. Decrease dosage if severe uterine cramping occurs.

ADVERSE REACTIONS
Common reactions are in italics; life-threatening reactions are in bold italics.
CNS: dizziness, headache.
CV: ***hypertension,*** chest pain.
EENT: tinnitus.
GI: nausea, vomiting.
GU: uterine cramping.
Other: sweating, dyspnea, ***hypersensitivity.***

*Liquid form contains alcohol. **May contain tartrazine.

INTERACTIONS

Regional anesthetics, dopamine, I.V. oxytocin: excessive vasoconstriction. Use together cautiously.

NURSING CONSIDERATIONS

• *Contraindicated* for induction or augmentation of labor, before delivery of placenta, in threatened spontaneous abortion, and in patients with allergy or sensitivity to ergot preparations.
• *Use cautiously* in hypertension, cardiac disease, venoatrial shunts, mitral valve stenosis, obliterative vascular disease, sepsis, and hepatic or renal impairment.
• Administer only under conditions of meticulous observation. Uterine hyperstimulation during labor may lead to uterine tetany, which may impair placental blood flow and cause amniotic fluid embolism.
• Monitor blood pressure, pulse rate, and uterine response. Report sudden changes in vital signs, frequent periods of uterine relaxation, and character and amount of vaginal bleeding.
• Hypocalcemia may decrease patient response. If patient is not also taking digitalis, cautious administration of calcium gluconate I.V. may produce desired oxytocic action.
• Contractions begin 5 to 15 minutes after P.O. administration. May continue 3 hours or more after P.O. or I.M. administration.
• Keep patient warm.
• Store drug in tightly closed, light-resistant container. Discard if discolored.
• **I.V. use:** Contractions begin immediately after I.V. injection and may continue for up to 45 minutes.
• Store I.V. solutions below 8° C (46.4° F). Daily stock may be kept at cool room temperature for 60 days.
• I.V. ergonovine is also used to diagnose coronary artery spasm (Prinzmetal's angina).

methylergonovine maleate

Methergine

HOW SUPPLIED

Tablets: 0.2 mg
Injection: 0.2 mg/ml

MECHANISM OF ACTION

Increases motor activity of the uterus by direct stimulation.

INDICATIONS & DOSAGE

Prevent and treat postpartum hemorrhage caused by uterine atony or subinvolution –
Adults: 0.2 mg I.M. q 2 to 5 hours for maximum of five doses; or I.V. (excessive uterine bleeding or other emergencies) over 1 minute while blood pressure and uterine contractions are monitored. I.V. dose may be diluted to 5 ml with 0.9% sodium chloride solution. Following initial I.M. or I.V. dose, may give 0.2 to 0.4 mg P.O. q 6 to 12 hours for 2 to 7 days. Decrease dosage if severe cramping occurs.

ADVERSE REACTIONS

Common reactions are in italics; life-threatening reactions are in bold italics.
CNS: dizziness, headache, ***seizures.***
CV: ***hypertension, MI,*** transient chest pain, dyspnea, palpitations, peripheral vasoconstriction, gangrene.
EENT: tinnitus.
GI: *nausea, vomiting.*
Other: sweating, ***hypersensitivity, uterine tetany.***

INTERACTIONS

Regional anesthetics, vasoconstrictors, dopamine, I.V. oxytocin: excessive vasoconstriction.

NURSING CONSIDERATIONS

• *Contraindicated* for induction of labor; before delivery of placenta; in patients with hypertension, toxemia, or sensitivity to ergot preparations;

and in threatened spontaneous abortion.
• *Use cautiously* in sepsis; obliterative vascular disease; and hepatic, renal, or cardiac disease.
• Monitor and record blood pressure, pulse rate, and uterine response; report any sudden change in vital signs, frequent periods of uterine relaxation, and character and amount of vaginal bleeding.
• Contractions begin 5 to 15 minutes after P.O. administration; 2 to 5 minutes after I.M. injection. May continue 3 hours or more after P.O. or I.M. administration.
• Store in tightly closed, light-resistant containers. Discard if discolored.
• **I.V. use:** Drug should not be routinely administered I.V. because of the risk of severe hypertension and CVA. If it must be given by this route, administer slowly over 1 minute with careful blood pressure monitoring. Contractions begin immediately after I.V. use and continue for up to 45 minutes.
• Store I.V. solutions below 8° C (46.4° F). Daily stock may be kept at room temperature for 60 to 90 days.

oxytocin, synthetic injection
Oxytocin, Pitocin, Syntocinon

HOW SUPPLIED
Injection: 10 units/ml

MECHANISM OF ACTION
Causes potent and selective stimulation of uterine and mammary gland smooth muscle.

INDICATIONS & DOSAGE
Induction or stimulation of labor –
Adults: initially, 1 ml (10 units) ampule in 1,000 ml of dextrose 5% injection or 0.9% sodium chloride solution I.V. infused at 1 to 2 milliunits/minute. Increase rate at 15- to 30-minute intervals until normal contraction pattern is established. Maximum is 1 to 2 ml (20 milliunits)/minute. Decrease rate when labor is firmly established.
Reduction of postpartum bleeding after expulsion of placenta –
Adults: 10 to 40 units added to 1,000 ml of dextrose 5% in water or 0.9% sodium chloride solution infused at rate necessary to control bleeding, usually 10 to 20 milliunits/minute. Also, 1 ml (10 units) can be given I.M. after delivery of the placenta.
Incomplete or inevitable abortion –
Adults: I.V. infusion with 10 units of oxytocin in 500 ml of 0.9% sodium chloride solution or dextrose 5% in 0.9% sodium chloride solution. Infuse at rate of 10 to 20 milliunits/minute.

ADVERSE REACTIONS
Common reactions are in italics; life-threatening reactions are in bold italics.
Maternal –
Blood: afibrinogenemia; may be related to postpartum bleeding.
CNS: ***subarachnoid hemorrhage*** resulting from hypertension; ***seizures or coma*** resulting from water intoxication.
CV: ***hypertension;*** increased heart rate, systemic venous return, and cardiac output; ***arrhythmias.***
GI: nausea, vomiting.
Other: ***hypersensitivity,*** tetanic contractions, ***abruptio placentae, impaired uterine blood flow,*** pelvic hematoma, ***increased uterine motility, anaphylaxis.***
Fetal –
Blood: hyperbilirubinemia.
CV: bradycardia, tachycardia, ***premature ventricular contractions.***
Other: ***anoxia, asphyxia.***

INTERACTIONS
Cyclopropane anesthetics: less pronounced bradycardia; hypotension.

*Liquid form contains alcohol. **May contain tartrazine.

Thiopental anesthetics: delayed induction reported.
Vasoconstrictors: severe hypertension if oxytocin is given within 3 to 4 hours of vasoconstrictor in patient receiving caudal block anesthetic.

NURSING CONSIDERATIONS
- *Contraindicated* in cephalopelvic disproportion or when delivery requires conversion, as in transverse lie; fetal distress, when delivery isn't imminent; severe toxemia; partial placenta previa; prematurity; and other obstetric emergencies.
- *Use with extreme caution* during first and second stages of labor because cervical laceration, uterine rupture, and maternal and fetal death have been reported.
- *Use cautiously* in history of cervical or uterine surgery (including cesarean section), grand multiparity, uterine sepsis, traumatic delivery, or overdistended uterus and in primiparas over 35 years.
- **I.V. use:** Don't give by I.V. bolus injection. Must administer by infusion; give by piggyback infusion so the drug may be discontinued without interrupting the I.V. line. Use an infusion pump.
- Used to induce or reinforce labor only when pelvis is known to be adequate, when vaginal delivery is indicated, when fetal maturity is assured, and when fetal position is favorable. Should be used only in hospital where critical care facilities and doctor are immediately available.
- Oxytocin should never be given simultaneously by more than one route.
- Do the following every 15 minutes: monitor and record uterine contractions, heart rate, blood pressure, intrauterine pressure, fetal heart rate, and character of blood loss.
- Antidiuretic effect may lead to fluid overload, seizures, and coma. Monitor fluid intake and output.
- If contractions occur less than 2 minutes apart and if contractions above 50 mm Hg are recorded, or if contractions last 90 seconds or longer, stop infusion, turn patient on her side, and notify doctor.
- Not recommended for routine I.M. use. However, 10 units may be given I.M. after delivery of placenta to control postpartum uterine bleeding.
- Should have magnesium sulfate (20% solution) available for relaxation of the myometrium.

oxytocin, synthetic nasal solution
Syntocinon

HOW SUPPLIED
Nasal solution: 40 units/ml

MECHANISM OF ACTION
Stimulates impaired milk ejection.

INDICATIONS & DOSAGE
To promote initial milk ejection; may relieve postpartum breast engorgement –
Adults: 1 spray into one or both nostrils 2 or 3 minutes before breastfeeding or pumping breasts.

ADVERSE REACTIONS
None reported.

INTERACTIONS
None significant.

NURSING CONSIDERATIONS
- *Contraindicated* in patients with hypersensitivity to the drug.
- Instruct patient to clear nasal passages first. With patient's head in vertical position, hold squeeze bottle upright and eject solution into nostril.

97
Spasmolytics

flavoxate hydrochloride
oxybutynin chloride

COMBINATION PRODUCTS
None.

flavoxate hydrochloride
Urispas
Pregnancy Risk Category: C

HOW SUPPLIED
Tablets: 100 mg

MECHANISM OF ACTION
Has a direct spasmolytic effect on smooth muscles of the urinary tract. It also provides some local anesthesia and analgesia.

INDICATIONS & DOSAGE
Symptomatic relief of dysuria, frequency, urgency, nocturia, incontinence, and suprapubic pain associated with urologic disorders –
Adults and children over 12 years: 100 to 200 mg P.O. t.i.d. to q.i.d.

ADVERSE REACTIONS
Common reactions are in italics; life-threatening reactions are in bold italics.
CNS: *mental confusion* (especially in elderly), nervousness, dizziness, headache, drowsiness, difficulty with concentration.
CV: tachycardia, palpitations.
EENT: *dry mouth and throat, blurred vision,* disturbed eye accommodation.
GI: abdominal pain, constipation (with high doses), nausea, vomiting.
Skin: urticaria, dermatoses.
Other: fever.

INTERACTIONS
None significant.

NURSING CONSIDERATIONS
- *Contraindicated* in pyloric or duodenal obstruction, obstructive intestinal lesions or ileus, achalasia, GI hemorrhage, or obstructive uropathies of lower urinary tract.
- *Use cautiously* in patients suspected of having glaucoma.
- Check history for other drug use before giving drugs with anticholinergic adverse reactions.
- Patient should avoid driving and other hazardous activities that require alertness because of possible drowsiness, mental confusion, and blurred vision.
- Tell the patient to report adverse reactions or lack of response to drug.

oxybutynin chloride
Ditropan
Pregnancy Risk Category: C

HOW SUPPLIED
Tablets: 5 mg
Syrup: 5 mg/5 ml

MECHANISM OF ACTION
Has both a direct spasmolytic effect and an atropine-like effect on urinary tract smooth muscles. It increases urinary bladder capacity and provides some local anesthesia and mild analgesia.

INDICATIONS & DOSAGE
Antispasmodic for neurogenic bladder –
Adults: 5 mg P.O. b.i.d. to t.i.d., to maximum of 5 mg q.i.d.
Children over 5 years: 5 mg P.O. b.i.d., to maximum of 5 mg t.i.d.

ADVERSE REACTIONS

Common reactions are in italics; life-threatening reactions are in bold italics.
CNS: *drowsiness,* dizziness, insomnia, *dry mouth,* restlessness, flushing.
CV: *palpitations, tachycardia.*
EENT: *transient blurred vision,* mydriasis, cycloplegia.
GI: nausea, vomiting, *constipation,* bloated feeling.
GU: impotence, *urinary hesitance or urine retention.*
Skin: rash, urticaria, allergic reactions in patients with sensitivity to anticholinergics.
Other: decreased sweating, fever, suppression of lactation.

INTERACTIONS

None significant.

NURSING CONSIDERATIONS

- *Contraindicated* in myasthenia gravis, GI obstruction, glaucoma, adynamic ileus, megacolon, severe or ulcerative colitis, obstructive uropathy, or in elderly or debilitated patients with intestinal atony.
- *Use cautiously* in elderly patients and in autonomic neuropathy, reflux esophagitis, and hepatic or renal disease.
- May aggravate symptoms of hyperthyroidism, coronary artery disease, CHF, cardiac arrhythmias, tachycardia, hypertension, or prostatic hypertrophy.
- Therapy should be stopped periodically to determine whether patient can get along without it. Minimizes tendency toward tolerance.
- Rapid onset of action, peaks at 3 to 4 hours, and lasts 6 to 10 hours.
- Neurogenic bladder should be confirmed by cystometry before oxybutynin is given. Evaluate patient response to therapy periodically by cystometry.
- Rule out partial intestinal obstruction in patients with diarrhea, especially those with colostomy or ileostomy, before giving oxybutynin.
- If urinary tract infection is present, patient should receive antibiotics concomitantly.
- Warn patient that drug may impair alertness or vision. He should avoid driving and other hazardous activities until the adverse CNS effects of the drug are known.
- Since oxybutynin suppresses sweating, its use during very hot weather may precipitate fever or heatstroke.
- Store in tightly closed containers at 59° to 86° F (15° to 30° C).

Gold salts

auranofin
aurothioglucose
gold sodium thiomalate

COMBINATION PRODUCTS
None.

auranofin
Ridaura

Pregnancy Risk Category: C

HOW SUPPLIED
Capsules: 3 mg

MECHANISM OF ACTION
Unknown. Anti-inflammatory effects in rheumatoid arthritis are probably caused by inhibition of sulfhydryl systems, which alters cellular metabolism. Auranofin may also alter enzyme function and immune response and suppress phagocytic activity.

INDICATIONS & DOSAGE
Rheumatoid arthritis –
Adults: 6 mg P.O. daily, administered either as 3 mg b.i.d. or 6 mg once daily. After 6 months, may be increased to 9 mg daily.

ADVERSE REACTIONS
Common reactions are in italics; life-threatening reactions are in bold italics.
Blood: ***thrombocytopenia*** (with or without purpura), ***aplastic anemia, agranulocytosis,*** leukopenia, eosinophilia.
GI: *diarrhea, abdominal pain, nausea, vomiting,* stomatitis, enterocolitis, anorexia, metallic taste, dyspepsia, flatulence.
GU: proteinuria, hematuria, nephrotic syndrome, glomerulonephritis.
Hepatic: jaundice, elevated liver enzymes.
Respiratory: interstitial pneumonitis.
Skin: *rash, pruritus, dermatitis,* ***exfoliative dermatitis.***

INTERACTIONS
Phenytoin: auranofin may increase phenytoin blood levels. Monitor for toxicity.

NURSING CONSIDERATIONS
- *Contraindicated* in patients with history of necrotizing enterocolitis, pulmonary fibrosis, exfoliative dermatitis, bone marrow aplasia, or severe hematologic disorders.
- *Use cautiously* with other drugs that cause blood dyscrasias. Also use cautiously in patients who have preexisting renal disease, liver disease, inflammatory bowel disease, and skin rash.
- Remind patients to see their doctors on schedule for monthly platelet counts. Auranofin should be discontinued if platelet count falls below 100,000/mm³, if hemoglobin drops suddenly, if granulocytes are below 1,500/mm³, and if leukopenia (WBC count below 4,000/mm³) or eosinophilia (eosinophils greater than 75%) is present.
- Reassure patient that beneficial drug effect may be delayed as long as 3 months. However, if response is inadequate after 3 months and after maximum dose is reached, doctor will probably discontinue auranofin.
- Encourage patient to take the drug as prescribed and not to alter the dosage schedule.
- Diarrhea is the most common adverse reaction. Tell patient to continue taking this drug if he experiences mild diarrhea; however, if he notes blood

in his stool he should contact the doctor immediately.
- Tell patient to continue taking concomitant drug therapy, such as NSAIDs, if prescribed.
- Regular urinalysis is advisable. If proteinuria or hematuria is detected, discontinue drug because it can produce a nephrotic syndrome or glomerulonephritis.
- Dermatitis is a common adverse reaction. Advise patient to report any rashes or other skin problems immediately. Pruritus often precedes dermatitis and should be considered a warning of impending skin reactions. Any pruritic skin eruption while a patient is receiving auranofin should be considered a reaction to this drug until proven otherwise. Therapy is stopped until reaction subsides.
- Stomatitis is another common adverse reaction. Tell patient that stomatitis is often preceded by a metallic taste. Advise him to report this symptom to his doctor immediately. Careful oral hygiene is recommended during therapy.
- Auranofin, like injectable gold preparations, should be prescribed only for selected rheumatoid arthritis patients. Warn your patient *not* to give the drug to others.
- Patient should receive a copy of the patient information supplied by the manufacturer.

aurothioglucose
Gold-50‡, Solganal

gold sodium thiomalate
Myochrysine

Pregnancy Risk Category: C

HOW SUPPLIED
aurothioglucose
Injection (suspension): 50 mg/ml in sesame oil with aluminum monostearate 2% and propylparaben 0.1% in a 10 ml container

gold sodium thiomalate
Injection: 10 mg/ml, 50 mg/ml with benzyl alcohol

MECHANISM OF ACTION
Unknown. Anti-inflammatory effects in rheumatoid arthritis are probably caused by inhibition of sulfhydryl systems, which alters cellular metabolism. Gold salts may also alter enzyme function and immune response and suppress phagocytic activity.

INDICATIONS & DOSAGE
Rheumatoid arthritis–
Adults: initially, 10 mg (aurothioglucose) I.M., followed by 25 mg for second and third doses at weekly intervals. Then, 50 mg weekly until 1 g has been given. If improvement occurs without toxicity, continue 25 to 50 mg at 3- to 4-week intervals indefinitely as maintenance therapy.
Children 6 to 12 years: ¼ usual adult dosage. Alternatively, 1 mg/kg I.M. once weekly for 20 weeks.
Rheumatoid arthritis–
Adults: initially, 10 mg (gold sodium thiomalate) I.M., followed by 25 mg in 1 week. Then, 50 mg weekly until 14 to 20 doses have been given. If improvement occurs without toxicity, continue 50 mg q 2 weeks for 4 doses; then, 50 mg q 3 weeks for 4 doses; then, 50 mg q month indefinitely as maintenance therapy. If relapse occurs during maintenance therapy, resume injections at weekly intervals.
Children: 1 mg/kg I.M. weekly for 20 weeks. If response is good, may be given q 3 to 4 weeks indefinitely.

ADVERSE REACTIONS
Common reactions are in italics; life-threatening reactions are in bold italics. Adverse reactions to gold are considered severe and potentially life-threatening. Report any reactions to the doctor immediately.
Blood: ***thrombocytopenia*** (with or without purpura), ***aplastic anemia,***

agranulocytosis, leukopenia, eosinophilia.
CNS: *dizziness,* syncope, sweating.
CV: bradycardia, hypotension.
EENT: corneal gold deposition, corneal ulcers.
GI: *metallic taste, stomatitis,* difficulty swallowing, nausea, vomiting.
GU: albuminuria, proteinuria, ***nephrotic syndrome,*** nephritis, acute tubular necrosis.
Hepatic: hepatitis, jaundice.
Skin: *rash and dermatitis in 20% of patients. (If drug is not stopped, may lead to fatal* ***exfoliative dermatitis.****)*
Other: ***anaphylaxis, angioneurotic edema.***

INTERACTIONS

None significant.

NURSING CONSIDERATIONS

- *Contraindicated* in severe uncontrollable diabetes, renal disease, hepatic dysfunction, hypertension, heart failure, systemic lupus erythematosus, Sjögren's syndrome, skin rash, and drug allergies or hypersensitivities.
- *Use cautiously* with other drugs that cause blood dyscrasias.
- Indicated only in active rheumatoid arthritis that has not responded adequately to salicylates, rest, and physical therapy.
- Should be administered only under constant supervision of a doctor who is thoroughly familiar with the drug's toxicities and benefits.
- Most adverse reactions are readily reversible if drug is stopped immediately.
- Administer all gold salts I.M., preferably intragluteally. Color of drug is pale yellow; don't use if it darkens.
- Observe patient for 30 minutes after administration because of possible anaphylactoid reaction.
- Inform patient that benefits of therapy may not appear for 3 to 4 months or longer.
- Increased joint pain may occur for 1 to 2 days after injection. This usually subsides after a few injections.
- Gold therapy may alter liver function studies.
- Aurothioglucose is a suspension. Immerse vial in warm water and shake vigorously before injecting.
- When giving gold sodium thiomalate, advise patient to lie down and to remain recumbent for 10 to 20 minutes after injection to minimize adverse reactions of hypotension.
- CBC, including platelet count, should be performed before every second injection during therapy.
- Dermatitis is the most common adverse reaction of gold salts. Advise patient to report any skin rashes or problems immediately. Pruritus often precedes dermatitis and should be considered a warning of impending skin reactions. Any pruritic skin eruption while a patient is receiving gold therapy should be considered a reaction until proven otherwise. Therapy is stopped until reaction subsides.
- Exposure to sunlight or artificial ultraviolet light should be minimized.
- Stomatitis is the second most common adverse reaction to gold therapy. Advise patient that stomatitis is often preceded by a metallic taste, which should be reported to the doctor immediately. Careful oral hygiene is recommended during therapy.
- Advise patient of the importance of close medical follow-ups and the need for frequent blood and urine tests during therapy.
- Urine should be analyzed for protein and sediment changes before each injection.
- Platelet counts should be performed if patient develops purpura or ecchymoses.
- If adverse reactions are mild, some rheumatologists resume gold therapy after 2 to 3 weeks' rest.
- Dimercaprol should be kept on hand to treat acute toxicity.

99

Diagnostic skin tests

coccidioidin
histoplasmin
mumps skin test antigen
tuberculin purified protein derivative
tuberculosis multiple-puncture tests

COMBINATION PRODUCTS
None.

coccidioidin

Spherulin

Pregnancy Risk Category: C

HOW SUPPLIED
Injection: 1:100 dilution (1 ml), 1:10 dilution (0.5 ml)

MECHANISM OF ACTION
Causes a cell-mediated immune response.

INDICATIONS & DOSAGE
Suspected coccidioidomycosis; to assess cell-mediated immunity –
Adults and children: 0.1 ml of 1:100 dilution intradermally into the flexor surface of the forearm. Use tuberculin syringe with 26G or 27G ½″ needle. In persons nonreactive to this form, repeat test using 1:10 dilution.

ADVERSE REACTIONS
Common reactions are in italics; life-threatening reactions are in bold italics.
Local: hypersensitivity (vesiculation, ulceration, necrosis).
Other: ***anaphylaxis,*** Arthus reaction.

INTERACTIONS
None significant.

NURSING CONSIDERATIONS
- *Contraindicated* in patients allergic to thimerosal.
- Test is read at 24 and 48 hours. Induration of 5 mm or more indicates a positive reaction (cell-mediated immune response). Erythema is not considered indicative of a delayed hypersensitivity reaction or positive response.
- Obtain history of allergies and reactions to skin tests.
- Tell the patient not to wash off the circle marked on the the skin for serial skin tests, since this aids in the reading of the test results.
- Obtain history of any recent residence or travel to endemic areas – southern California, Arizona, New Mexico, and western Texas.
- Keep epinephrine 1:1,000 available.
- If a patient is suspected of having coccidioidomycosis because of clinical manifestations or X-ray findings and the 1:100 dilution is negative, the 1:10 dilution may be used.
- Reactivity to this test may be depressed or suppressed for as long as 4 to 6 weeks in individuals who have received concurrent or recent immunization with certain virus vaccines (for example, measles or influenza), in those who are receiving corticosteroid or immunosuppressive agents, in malnourished patients, and in those who have had viral infections (rubeola, influenza, mumps, and probably others).

histoplasmin

Histolyn-CYL

Pregnancy Risk Category: C

HOW SUPPLIED
Injection: vials containing 10 doses of 0.1 ml

MECHANISM OF ACTION
Causes a cell-mediated immune response.

INDICATIONS & DOSAGE
Suspected histoplasmosis; to assess cell-mediated immunity –
Adults and children: 0.1 ml intradermally into the flexor surface of the forearm. Use tuberculin syringe with 26G or 27G ½″ needle.

ADVERSE REACTIONS
Common reactions are in italics; life-threatening reactions are in bold italics.
Local: urticaria, ulceration or necrosis in highly sensitive patients.
Other: ***anaphylaxis.***

INTERACTIONS
None significant.

NURSING CONSIDERATIONS
- *Contraindicated* in patients known to be positive reactors.
- Read test within 24 to 48 hours. Induration of 5 mm or more is positive response. In some instances, maximum reactions may not be present until the fourth day.
- A positive reaction may indicate a past infection or a mild subacute or chronic infection with histoplasmosis or such immunologically related organisms as coccidioidomycosis or blastomycosis.
- Obtain history of allergies and reactions to skin tests.
- Cold packs or topical corticosteroids may relieve pain and itching if severe local reaction occurs.
- Serologic titers are often boosted by previous skin test. Draw serologic sample between 48 to 96 hours after skin test administration.
- Tuberculin skin test is advisable concurrently with histoplasmin test.
- Obtain history of any residence or recent travel to endemic areas – central (Ohio Valley) and eastern United States and Africa.
- Reactivity to this test may be depressed or suppressed for as long as 4 to 6 weeks in individuals who have received concurrent or recent immunization with certain virus vaccines (for example, measles or influenza), in those who are receiving corticosteroid or immunosuppressive agents, in malnourished patients, and in those who have had viral infections (rubeola, influenza, mumps, and probably others).

mumps skin test antigen
MSTA

Pregnancy Risk Category: C

HOW SUPPLIED
Injection (suspension): 20 complement-fixing units/ml

MECHANISM OF ACTION
Causes a cell-mediated immune response.

INDICATIONS & DOSAGE
To assess cell-mediated immunity –
Adults and children: 0.1 ml intradermally into the flexor surface of the forearm. Use tuberculin syringe with 26G or 27G ½″ needle.

ADVERSE REACTIONS
Common reactions are in italics; life-threatening reactions are in bold italics.
Local: hypersensitivity (vesiculation, ulceration).
Other: ***anaphylaxis,*** Arthus reaction.

INTERACTIONS
None significant.

NURSING CONSIDERATIONS
- *Contraindicated* in patients allergic to thimerosal.
- *Use cautiously* in patients with hy-

*Liquid form contains alcohol. **May contain tartrazine.

persensitivity to eggs, feathers, or chicken.

- Test is read at 48- and 72-hour intervals. A positive reaction (cell-mediated immune response) is 5 mm or more of induration. Erythema is not considered indicative of a delayed hypersensitivity reaction.
- Obtain history of allergies and reactions to skin tests.
- Keep epinephrine 1:1,000 available.
- Store vials in refrigerator.
- Mumps skin test antigen is *not* used to assess exposure to mumps. This antigen is used in assessing T cell function for immunocompetence.
- Reactivity to this test may be depressed or suppressed for as long as 4 to 6 weeks in individuals who have received concurrent or recent immunization with certain virus vaccines (for example, measles or influenza), in those who are receiving corticosteroid or immunosuppressive agents, in malnourished patients, and in those who have had viral infections (rubeola, influenza, mumps, and probably others).

tuberculin purified protein derivative (PPD)

Aplisol, PPD-stabilized Solution (Mantoux test), Tubersol

Pregnancy Risk Category: C

HOW SUPPLIED

Injection (intradermal): 1 tuberculin unit (TU)/0.1 ml, 5 TU/0.1 ml, 250 TU/0.1 ml

MECHANISM OF ACTION

Causes a cell-mediated immune response.

INDICATIONS & DOSAGE

Diagnosis of tuberculosis, evaluation of immunocompetence in patients with cancer, malnutrition –

Adults and children: initially, 1 TU (0.1 ml of appropriate solution) intradermally into flexor surface of the forearm. Use tuberculin syringe with 26G or 27G ½" needle. Retest with 5 TU and, if negative, 250 TU. If still no response, the individual is nonreactive.

ADVERSE REACTIONS

Common reactions are in italics; life-threatening reactions are in bold italics.

Local: pain, pruritus, vesiculation, ulceration, necrosis.

Other: ***anaphylaxis,*** Arthus reaction.

INTERACTIONS

None significant.

NURSING CONSIDERATIONS

- *Contraindicated* in known tuberculin-positive reactors; severe reactions may occur.
- Read test within 48 to 72 hours. An induration of 10 mm or greater indicates a significant reaction (formerly called positive reaction). Significance of a reaction is determined not only by the size of the reaction but by circumstances. For example, a reaction of 5 mm or more may be considered significant in a close relative of a person with known tuberculosis. A reaction of 2 mm or more may also be considered significant in infants and children. The amount of induration at the site – not erythema – determines the significance of the reaction.
- If reaction is positive, further testing is needed to confirm diagnosis. Report all known cases of tuberculosis to the appropriate public health agency.
- Obtain history of allergies and reactions to skin tests.
- Reactivity to this test may be depressed or suppressed for as long as 4 to 6 weeks in individuals who have received concurrent or recent immunization with certain virus vaccines (for example, measles or influenza), in those who are receiving corticoste-

roid or immunosuppressive agents, in malnourished patients, and in those who have had viral infections (rubeola, influenza, mumps, and probably others).
• Keep epinephrine 1:1,000 available.
• S.C. injection invalidates test results. Bleb (6 to 10 mm in diameter) must form on skin upon intradermal injection.
• Cold packs or topical corticosteroids may relieve pain and itching of severe local reaction.
• Strongly positive tests can result in scarring at test site.
• Never give initial test with second test strength (250 tuberculin units). Use only when a patient has negative response to a 5-tuberculin unit PPD but has the clinical signs and symptoms of tuberculosis.

tuberculosis multiple-puncture tests

Aplitest (dried purified protein derivative [PPD]),
Mono-Vacc Test (liquid Old Tuberculin [OT]), Sclavo Test (dried PPD), Tine Test (dried OT, dried PPD)

Pregnancy Risk Category: C

HOW SUPPLIED
Test: 25 devices/pack, 5 tuberculin units/device

MECHANISM OF ACTION
Causes a cell-mediated immune response.

INDICATIONS & DOSAGE
Screening for tuberculosis –
Adults and children: cleanse skin thoroughly with alcohol; make skin taut on flexor surface of forearm and press points firmly into selected site. Hold device at injection site for about 3 seconds to ensure stabilizing the dried tuberculin B in tissue lymph.

ADVERSE REACTIONS
Common reactions are in italics; life-threatening reactions are in bold italics.
Local: hypersensitivity (vesiculation, ulceration, necrosis).
Other: ***anaphylaxis.***

INTERACTIONS
Virus vaccine: tuberculosis skin-test reaction may be suppressed if test is given within 4 to 6 weeks after immunization with live or attenuated virus.

NURSING CONSIDERATIONS
• *Contraindicated* in known tuberculin-positive reactors.
• Obtain history of allergies, especially to acacia (a stabilizer in the Tine Test), and reactions to skin tests.
• False-positive reaction can occur in sensitive patients.
• Reactivity to this test may be depressed or suppressed for as long as 4 to 6 weeks in persons with concurrent or recent immunization with certain virus vaccines (for example, measles or influenza), in viral infections (rubeola, influenza, mumps, and probably others) or miliary tuberculosis, in those who are receiving corticosteroid or immunosuppressive agents, and in malnourished patients.
• Rarely, minimal bleeding can occur at the puncture site. It does not interfere with interpretation of the test results.
• Read test within 48 to 72 hours. Questionable or positive reactions must be verified by the Mantoux test. Induration – not erythema – at the site determines significance of the reaction. Induration of 1 to 2 mm is significant.
• If vesiculation is present, the test may be interpreted as positive.
• Keep epinephrine 1:1,000 available.
• Report all cases of tuberculosis to appropriate public health agency.
• Cold packs or topical corticosteroids may relieve pain and itching if severe local reaction occurs after test.

100

Miscellaneous antagonists and antidotes

activated charcoal
aminocaproic acid
ammonia, aromatic spirits
apomorphine hydrochloride
deferoxamine mesylate
digoxin immune FAB (ovine)
dimercaprol
doxapram hydrochloride
D-penicillamine
edetate calcium disodium
edetate disodium
flumazenil
ipecac syrup
naloxone hydrochloride
naltrexone hydrochloride
pralidoxime chloride
protamine sulfate
sodium cellulose phosphate
sodium polystyrene sulfonate
succimer
trientine hydrochloride

(See also Chapter 37, ANTICHOLINERGICS.)
(See also Chapter 39, ADRENERGIC BLOCKERS [SYMPATHOLYTICS].)

COMBINATION PRODUCTS
None.

activated charcoal

Actidose-Aqua◇, Charcoaide◇, Charcocaps◇, Liqui-Char◇, Superchar◇

Pregnancy Risk Category: C

HOW SUPPLIED
Tablets: 200 mg‡◇, 300 mg‡◇, 325 mg◇, 650 mg◇
Capsules: 260 mg◇
Powder: 30 g◇, 50 g◇
Oral suspension: 0.625 g/5 ml◇, 0.83 g/5 ml◇, 1 g/5 ml◇, 1.25 g/5 ml◇

MECHANISM OF ACTION
Adheres to many drugs and chemicals, inhibiting their absorption from the GI tract. An adsorbent.

INDICATIONS & DOSAGE
Flatulence or dyspepsia –
Adults: 600 mg to 5 g P.O. t.i.d. or q.i.d.
Poisoning –
Adults: initially, 1g/kg (30 to 100 g) P.O. or 5 to 10 times the amount of poison ingested as a suspension in 180 to 240 ml of water.
Children: 5 to 10 times estimated weight of drug or chemical ingested. Minimum dose is 30 g P.O. in 250 ml water to make a slurry. Give orally, preferably within 30 minutes of poisoning. Larger dose is necessary if food is in the stomach. For treating poisoning or overdosage with acetaminophen, amphetamines, aspirin, antimony, atropine, arsenic, barbiturates, camphor, cocaine, digitalis glycosides, glutethimide, ipecac, malathion, morphine, poisonous mushrooms, opium, oxalic acid, parathion, phenol, phenothiazines, potassium permanganate, propoxyphene, quinine, strychnine, sulfonamides, or tricyclic antidepressants.

ADVERSE REACTIONS
Common reactions are in italics; life-threatening reactions are in bold italics.
GI: black stools, nausea.

INTERACTIONS
Acetylcysteine, ipecac: rendered ineffective. Don't administer together or lavage stomach until all charcoal is removed.

NURSING CONSIDERATIONS

- *Contraindicated* in semiconscious or unconscious patients unless airway is protected and then use cautiously. Can be given by nasogastric tube after lavage.
- Because activated charcoal absorbs and inactivates syrup of ipecac, give after emesis is complete.
- Don't give in ice cream, milk, or sherbert. Reduces absorptive capacity.
- Powder form is most effective. Mix with tap water to form consistency of thick syrup. May add small amount of fruit juice or flavoring to make more palatable.
- May need to repeat dose if patient vomits shortly after administration.
- Space doses at least 1 hour apart from other drugs if activated charcoal is being used for any indication other than poisoning.
- Warn patient that feces will be black.

aminocaproic acid

Amicar

Pregnancy Risk Category: C

HOW SUPPLIED

Tablets: 500 mg
Syrup: 250 mg/ml
Injection: 5 g/20 ml for dilution, 24 g/96 ml for infusion

MECHANISM OF ACTION

Inhibits plasminogen activator substances. To a lesser degree, it blocks antiplasmin activity by inhibiting fibrinolysis.

INDICATIONS & DOSAGE

Excessive bleeding resulting from hyperfibrinolysis –
Adults: initially, 5 g P.O. or slow I.V. infusion, followed by 1 to 1.25 g hourly until bleeding is controlled. Maximum dosage is 30 g daily.

Prevention of hemorrhage after dental surgery in hemophiliacs –
Adults: initially, 6 g P.O. immediately after surgery, then 6 g P.O. q 6 hours for 9 to 10 days.

ADVERSE REACTIONS

Common reactions are in italics; life-threatening reactions are in bold italics.
Blood: generalized thrombosis.
CNS: dizziness, malaise, headache.
CV: hypotension, bradycardia, ***arrhythmias*** (with rapid I.V. infusion).
EENT: tinnitus, nasal stuffiness, conjunctival suffusion.
GI: nausea, cramps, diarrhea.
Skin: rash.
Other: malaise, myopathy.

INTERACTIONS

Oral contraceptives, estrogens: increased probability of hypercoagulability. Use together cautiously.

NURSING CONSIDERATIONS

- *Contraindicated* in active intravascular clotting.
- *Use cautiously* in thrombophlebitis and cardiac, hepatic, or renal disease.
- Monitor coagulation studies, heart rhythm, and blood pressure. Notify doctor of any change immediately.
- **I.V. use:** Dilute solution with sterile water for injection, normal saline injection, dextrose 5% in water, or Ringer's injection. Infuse slowly. Don't give by direct or intermittent injection.
- Drug is sometimes helpful as an adjunct in treating hemophilia.
- Also used as antidote for alteplase, anistreplase, streptokinase or urokinase; not beneficial in treating thrombocytopenia.

ammonia, aromatic spirits◊

Pregnancy Risk Category: C

HOW SUPPLIED

Solution: 30 ml◇, 60 ml◇, 120 ml◇; pints◇; gallons◇
Inhalant: 0.33 ml◇, 0.4 ml◇

MECHANISM OF ACTION

Irritates the sensory receptors in the nasal membranes, producing reflex stimulation of the respiratory centers.

INDICATIONS & DOSAGE

Fainting –
Adults and children: inhale as needed.

ADVERSE REACTIONS

Common reactions are in italics; life-threatening reactions are in bold italics.
EENT: irritation.

INTERACTIONS

None significant.

NURSING CONSIDERATIONS

• Avoid inhaling vapors when administering drug.

apomorphine hydrochloride

Controlled Substance Schedule II
Pregnancy Risk Category: C

HOW SUPPLIED

Soluble tablets for injection: 6 mg

MECHANISM OF ACTION

Acts directly on the chemoreceptor trigger zone in the medulla oblongata to induce vomiting.

INDICATIONS & DOSAGE

To induce vomiting in poisoning –
Adults: 5 to 6 mg S.C. preceded by 200 to 300 ml water or, preferably, evaporated milk. Don't repeat.
Children: 0.07 to 0.1 mg/kg S.C. preceded by up to 2 glasses of water or, preferably, evaporated milk.

ADVERSE REACTIONS

Common reactions are in italics; life-threatening reactions are in bold italics.
CNS: *depression, euphoria,* restlessness, tremor.
CV: ***acute circulatory failure in elderly or debilitated patients,*** tachycardia.
Other: ***depressed respiratory center in large or repeated doses.***

INTERACTIONS

Antiemetics (such as antihistamines, phenothiazines): decreased emetic response, possibly with increased CNS depression.

NURSING CONSIDERATIONS

• *Contraindicated* in patients with hypersensitivity to narcotics; impending shock; corrosive poisoning; narcosis resulting from opiates, barbiturates, alcohol, or other CNS depressants; and in patients too inebriated to stand unaided.
• *Use cautiously* in children and in patients who are debilitated, have cardiac decompensation, or are predisposed to nausea and vomiting.
• Don't give after ingestion of petroleum distillates (for example, kerosene, gasoline) or volatile oils; retching and vomiting may cause aspiration and lead to bronchospasm, pulmonary edema, or aspiration pneumonitis. Vegetable oil will delay absorption of these substances.
• Emetic action is increased if dosage is followed immediately by water or evaporated milk. Evaporated milk is preferred because studies show that water may increase absorption of toxic substances.
• Don't give after ingestion of caustic substances, such as lye; additional injury to the esophagus and mediastinum can occur.
• Keep narcotic antagonists, such as naloxone, available to help stop vomiting and to alleviate drowsiness.
• If delay in giving emetic is ex-

pected, give activated charcoal P.O. immediately. When absorbable poison is ingested, give activated charcoal P.O. immediately after apomorphine hydrochloride.
- Vomiting occurs in 5 to 10 minutes in adults. If vomiting doesn't occur within 15 minutes, gastric lavage should begin. Apomorphine is emetic of choice when rapid removal of poisons is necessary, and when identification of enteric-coated tablets or other ingested toxic material in vomitus is important. Stomach contents are usually expelled completely; vomitus may also contain material from upper portion of intestinal tract.
- Don't administer if solution for injection is discolored green or precipitate is present.

deferoxamine mesylate
Desferal

Pregnancy Risk Category: C

HOW SUPPLIED
Powder for injection: 500 mg

MECHANISM OF ACTION
Chelates iron by binding ferric ions.

INDICATIONS & DOSAGE
Adjunctive treatment of acute iron intoxication –
Adults and children: 1 g I.M. or I.V. followed by 500 mg I.M. or I.V. for two doses, q 4 hours; then 500 mg I.M. or I.V. q 4 to 12 hours. Infusion rate shouldn't exceed 15 mg/kg hourly. Don't exceed 6 g in 24 hours.
Chronic iron overload resulting from multiple transfusions –
Adults and children: 500 mg to 1 g I.M. daily and 2 g slow I.V. infusion in separate solution along with each unit of blood transfused. Maximum dosage is 6 g daily. I.V. infusion rate shouldn't exceed 15 mg/kg hourly.
S.C.: 1 to 2 g via a subcutaneous infusion pump over 8 to 24 hours.

ADVERSE REACTIONS
Common reactions are in italics; life-threatening reactions are in bold italics.
EENT: blurred vision, cataracts, hearing loss.
Local: pain and induration at injection site.
Other: *after rapid I.V. administration: erythema, urticaria, hypotension,* ***shock.***
With long-term use: sensitivity reaction (cutaneous wheal formation, pruritus, rash, ***anaphylaxis***), leg cramps, fever, tachycardia, dysuria, diarrhea, abdominal discomfort.

INTERACTIONS
Ascorbic acid: may enhance the effects of deferoxamine and increase tissue toxicity of iron. Use together with extreme caution and close monitoring.

NURSING CONSIDERATIONS
- *Contraindicated* in severe renal disease or anuria.
- *Use cautiously* in impaired renal function.
- Monitor intake and output carefully.
- I.M. route preferred.
- **I.V. use:** Use I.V. only when patient has cardiovascular collapse or shock.
- Add to 0.9% sodium chloride solution, dextrose 5% in water, or lactated Ringer's solution.
- Reconstituted solution is good for 1 week at room temperature. Protect from light.
- For reconstitution, add 2 ml of sterile water for injection to each ampule. Make sure drug is completely dissolved.
- If giving I.V., change to I.M. as soon as possible.
- Warn patient that urine may be red.
- Have epinephrine 1:1,000 readily available in case of allergic reaction.
- Recommend regular eye examinations during long-term therapy.
- Has been used investigationally to treat aluminum toxicity.

digoxin immune FAB (ovine)

Digibind

Pregnancy Risk Category: C

HOW SUPPLIED

Injection: 40-mg vial

MECHANISM OF ACTION

Binds molecules of digoxin and digitoxin, making them unavailable for binding at site of action on cells in the body.

INDICATIONS & DOSAGE

Treatment of potentially life-threatening digoxin or digitoxin intoxication – **Adults and children:** The I.V. dosage varies according to the amount of digoxin or digitoxin to be neutralized. Each vial binds about 0.6 mg digoxin or digitoxin. Average dosage is 10 vials (400 mg). However, if the toxicity resulted from acute digoxin ingestion, and neither a serum digoxin level nor an estimated ingestion amount is known, 20 vials (800 mg) should be administered. See package insert for complete, specific dosage instructions.

ADVERSE REACTIONS

Common reactions are in italics; life-threatening reactions are in bold italics.

CV: ***CHF,*** rapid ventricular rate (both caused by reversal of the cardiac glycoside's therapeutic effects).

Metabolic: hypokalemia.

Other: ***hypersensitivity.***

INTERACTIONS

None reported.

NURSING CONSIDERATIONS

- *Use cautiously* in patients known to be allergic to ovine proteins. In these high-risk patients, skin testing is recommended because digoxin immune FAB is derived from digoxin-specific antibody fragments obtained from immunized sheep.
- This antidote should be used only for life-threatening overdose in patients in shock or cardiac arrest; with ventricular arrhythmias, such as ventricular tachycardia or fibrillation; with progressive bradycardia, such as severe sinus bradycardia; or with second- or third-degree AV block not responsive to atropine.
- Monitor potassium closely.
- In most patients, signs of digitalis toxicity disappear within a few hours.
- Best to infuse this drug through a 0.22-micron membrane filter. However, give by bolus injection if cardiac arrest is considered imminent.
- **I.V. use:** Administer I.V. over 30 minutes or as bolus if cardiac arrest imminent.
- Refrigerate powder for reconstitution. Reconstituted product should be used immediately, but it may be stored for up to 4 hours in the refrigerator.
- Digoxin immune FAB will interfere with digitalis immunoassay measurements, so standard serum digoxin levels will be misleading until the drug is cleared from the body (about 2 days).
- Total serum digoxin levels may rise after administration of this drug, but this reflects FAB-bound (inactive) digoxin.

dimercaprol

BAL in Oil

Pregnancy Risk Category: D

HOW SUPPLIED

Injection: 100 mg/ml

MECHANISM OF ACTION

Forms complexes with heavy metals.

INDICATIONS & DOSAGE

Severe arsenic or gold poisoning – **Adults and children:** 3 mg/kg deep

I.M. q 4 hours for 2 days, then q.i.d. on third day, then b.i.d. for 10 days.
Mild arsenic or gold poisoning –
Adults and children: 2.5 mg/kg deep I.M. q.i.d. for 2 days, then b.i.d. on third day, then once daily for 10 days.
Mercury poisoning –
Adults and children: 5 mg/kg deep I.M. initially, then 2.5 mg/kg daily or b.i.d. for 10 days.
Acute lead encephalopathy or lead level more than 100 mcg/ml –
Adults and children: 4 mg/kg deep I.M. injection, then q 4 hours with edetate calcium disodium (12.5 mg/kg I.M.). Use separate sites. Maximum dosage is 5 mg/kg per dose.

ADVERSE REACTIONS
Common reactions are in italics; life-threatening reactions are in bold italics.
CNS: pain or tightness in throat, chest, or hands; headache; paresthesias; muscle pain or weakness.
CV: *transient increase in blood pressure, returns to normal in 2 hours; tachycardia.*
EENT: blepharospasm, conjunctivitis, lacrimation, rhinorrhea, excessive salivation.
GI: *halitosis; nausea; vomiting; burning sensation in lips, mouth, and throat; abdominal pain.*
GU: *dysuria;* renal damage if alkaline urine not maintained.
Metabolic: decreased iodine uptake.
Local: sterile abscess, pain at injection site.
Other: *fever (especially in children),* sweating, pain in teeth.

INTERACTIONS
Iron: forms toxic metal complex; concurrent therapy contraindicated. Wait 24 hours after last dimercaprol dose.
^{131}I uptake thyroid tests: decreased; don't schedule patient for this test during course of dimercaprol therapy.

NURSING CONSIDERATIONS
- *Contraindicated* in hepatic dysfunction (except postarsenical jaundice), or in acute renal insufficiency.
- *Use cautiously* in hypertension.
- Should not be used in pregnancy except to treat life-threatening poisoning.
- Don't use for iron, cadmium, or selenium toxicity. Complex formed is highly toxic, even fatal.
- Ephedrine or antihistamine may prevent or relieve mild adverse reactions.
- Ineffective in arsine gas poisoning.
- Solution with slight sediment usable.
- Keep urine alkaline to prevent renal damage. Oral sodium bicarbonate may be ordered.
- Don't give I.V.; give by deep I.M. route only. The injection site can be massaged after drug is given.
- Drug has an unpleasant, garlic-like odor.
- Be careful when preparing and administering drug not to let drug come in contact with skin, as it may cause a skin reaction.

doxapram hydrochloride
Dopram

Pregnancy Risk Category: C

HOW SUPPLIED
Injection: 20 mg/ml (benzyl alcohol 0.9%)

MECHANISM OF ACTION
Acts either directly on the central respiratory centers in the medulla or indirectly on the chemoreceptors.

INDICATIONS & DOSAGE
Postanesthesia respiratory stimulation, drug-induced CNS depression, and chronic pulmonary disease associated with acute hypercapnia –
Adults: 0.5 to 1 mg/kg of body weight (up to 2 mg/kg in CNS depres-

sion), I.V. injection or infusion. Maximum dosage is 4 mg/kg, up to 3 g/day. Infusion rate is 1 to 3 mg/minute (initial: 5 mg/minute for postanesthesia).
Chronic obstructive pulmonary disease –
Adults: infusion, 1 to 2 mg/minute. Maximum is 3 mg/minute for a maximum duration of 2 hours.

ADVERSE REACTIONS
Common reactions are in italics; life-threatening reactions are in bold italics.
CNS: ***seizures,*** *headache,* dizziness, apprehension, disorientation, pupillary dilation, bilateral Babinski's signs, flushing, sweating, paresthesias.
CV: *chest pain and tightness, variations in heart rate, hypertension,* lowered T waves.
GI: nausea, vomiting, diarrhea.
GU: urine retention, or stimulation of the bladder with incontinence.
Other: sneezing, coughing, ***laryngospasm, bronchospasm,*** hiccups, rebound hypoventilation, pruritus, pyrexia, muscle spasms.

INTERACTIONS
MAO inhibitors, sympathomimetics: potentiate adverse cardiovascular effects. Use together cautiously.

NURSING CONSIDERATIONS
- *Contraindicated* in seizure disorders; head injury; cardiovascular disorders; frank uncompensated heart failure; severe hypertension; CVA; respiratory failure or incompetence secondary to neuromuscular disorders, muscle paresis, flail chest, obstructed airway, pulmonary embolism, pneumothorax, restrictive respiratory disease, acute bronchial asthma, or extreme dyspnea; or hypoxia not associated with hypercapnia.
- *Use cautiously* in bronchial asthma, severe tachycardia or cardiac arrhythmias, cerebral edema or increased cerebrospinal fluid pressure, hyperthyroidism, pheochromocytoma, and metabolic disorders.
- Doxapram's use as an analeptic is strongly discouraged by most doctors.
- Establish adequate airway before administering drug. Prevent patient from aspirating vomitus by placing him on his side.
- Monitor blood pressure, heart rate, deep tendon reflexes, and arterial blood gases before giving drug and every 30 minutes afterward.
- Be alert for signs of overdosage: hypertension, tachycardia, arrhythmias, skeletal muscle hyperactivity, and dyspnea. Discontinue if patient shows signs of increased arterial carbon dioxide or oxygen tension, or if mechanical ventilation is started. May give I.V. injection of anticonvulsant.
- Use only in surgical or emergency room situations.
- **I.V. use:** Administer slowly; rapid infusion may cause hemolysis. Do not combine with alkaline solutions such as thiopental sodium; doxapram is acidic.
- Extravasation may lead to thrombophlebitis and local skin irritation.

D-penicillamine
Cuprimine, Depen, D-Penamine‡
Pregnancy Risk Category: D

HOW SUPPLIED
Tablets: 125 mg‡, 250 mg
Capsules: 125 mg, 250 mg

MECHANISM OF ACTION
Mechanism of action in rheumatoid arthritis is unknown but is probably from inhibition of collagen formation. Also chelates heavy metals.

INDICATIONS & DOSAGE
Wilson's disease –
Adults: 250 mg P.O. q.i.d. 30 to 60 minutes before meals. Adjust dosage

to achieve urinary copper excretion of 0.5 to 1 mg daily.
Children: 20 mg/kg P.O. daily divided q.i.d. before meals. Adjust dosage to achieve urinary copper excretion of 0.5 to 1 mg daily.
Cystinuria –
Adults: 250 mg to 1 g P.O. q.i.d. before meals. Adjust dosage to achieve urinary cystine excretion of less than 100 mg daily when renal calculi present, or 100 to 200 mg daily when no calculi present. Maximum dosage is 5 g daily.
Children: 30 mg/kg P.O. daily divided q.i.d. before meals. Adjust dosage to achieve urinary cystine excretion of less than 100 mg daily when renal calculi present, or 100 to 200 mg daily when no calculi present.
Rheumatoid arthritis –
Adults: 125 to 250 mg P.O. daily initially, with increases of 250 mg q 2 to 3 months if necessary. Maximum dosage is 1.5 g daily.

ADVERSE REACTIONS

Common reactions are in italics; life-threatening reactions are in bold italics.
Blood: *leukopenia, eosinophilia, thrombocytopenia, monocytosis, granulocytopenia,* elevated sedimentation rate, lupus-like syndrome.
EENT: tinnitus.
GU: ***nephrotic syndrome, glomerulonephritis,*** proteinuria.
Hepatic: hepatotoxicity.
Metabolic: *decreased pyridoxine (may cause optic neuritis),* decreased zinc and mercury.
Skin: friability, especially at pressure spots; wrinkling; erythema; urticaria; ecchymoses.
Other: reversible taste impairment, especially of salts and sweets; hair loss. *About ⅓ of patients develop allergic reactions (rash, pruritus, fever), arthralgia, lymphadenopathy, or pneumonitis.* With long-term use, myasthenia gravis syndrome.

INTERACTIONS

Antacids, oral iron: decreased effectiveness of D-penicillamine. If used together, give at least 2 hours apart.

NURSING CONSIDERATIONS

- *Contraindicated* in pregnant women with cystinuria.
- *Use cautiously* in penicillin allergy; cross-sensitivity may occur. However, most penicillin-allergic patients can receive penicillamine.
- Rash and fever are important signs of toxicity and should be reported immediately.
- Patient should receive supplemental pyridoxine daily.
- Handle patient carefully to avoid skin damage if patient has a skin reaction.
- Antihistamines may be tried to manage skin reactions.
- Dose should be given on empty stomach to facilitate absorption, preferably 1 hour before or 3 hours after meals.
- Patient should drink large amounts of fluid, especially at night.
- Tell patient that therapeutic effect may be delayed up to 3 months in treatment of rheumatoid arthritis.
- Monitor CBC and renal and hepatic function regularly throughout therapy (every 2 weeks for the first 6 months, then monthly).
- Monitor urinalysis regularly for protein loss.
- Withhold drug and notify doctor if WBC count falls below 3,500/mm³ or platelet count falls below 100,000/mm³ (these are indications to stop drug). A progressive decline in platelet or WBC count in three successive blood tests may necessitate temporary cessation of therapy, even if these counts are within normal limits.
- Advise patient to report fever, sore throat, chills, bruising, and increased bleeding time; may be early signs of granulocytopenia.
- Provide appropriate health teaching

*Liquid form contains alcohol. **May contain tartrazine.

for patients with Wilson's disease and cystinuria.
- Taste impairment usually resolves in 6 weeks without changes in dosage.

edetate calcium disodium

Calcium Disodium Versenate, Calcium EDTA

Pregnancy Risk Category: C

HOW SUPPLIED

Injection: 200 mg/ml

MECHANISM OF ACTION

Forms stable, soluble complexes with metals, particularly lead.

INDICATIONS & DOSAGE

Lead poisoning (blood levels greater than 50 mcg/dl) –

Adults and children: 1 g/m² in dextrose 5% in water or normal saline solution I.V. over 1 to 2 hours daily for 3 to 5 days.

Acute lead encephalopathy or lead levels above 100 mcg/dl –

Adults and children: 1.5 g/m² I.V. daily for 3 to 5 days, usually in conjunction with dimercaprol. A second course may be administered at least 4 days later, but preferably 2 to 3 weeks should elapse between courses.

ADVERSE REACTIONS

Common reactions are in italics; life-threatening reactions are in bold italics.

CNS: headache, paresthesias, numbness.

CV: ***arrhythmias,*** hypotension.

GI: anorexia, nausea, vomiting.

GU: proteinuria, hematuria; ***nephrotoxicity with renal tubular necrosis leading to fatal nephrosis.***

Other: arthralgia, myalgia, hypercalcemia.

4 to 8 hours after infusion: sudden fever and chills, fatigue, excessive thirst, sneezing, nasal congestion.

INTERACTIONS

None significant.

NURSING CONSIDERATIONS

- *Contraindicated* in severe renal disease or anuria. I.V. use contraindicated in lead encephalopathy; may increase intracranial pressure. Use I.M. route instead.
- Force fluids to facilitate lead excretion in all patients except those with lead encephalopathy.
- Monitor intake and output, urinalysis, BUN, and ECGs daily.
- To avoid toxicity, use with dimercaprol.
- Procaine hydrochloride may be added to I.M. solutions to minimize pain. Watch for local reactions.
- **I.V. use:** Infuse slowly, diluted into an established I.V. line.
- I.M. route preferred, especially for children.
- Do not confuse this drug with edetate disodium, which is used for treating hypercalcemia.

edetate disodium

Disodium EDTA, Disotate, Endrate

Pregnancy Risk Category: C

HOW SUPPLIED

Injection: 150 mg/ml

MECHANISM OF ACTION

Chelates with metals, such as calcium, to form a stable, soluble complex.

INDICATIONS & DOSAGE

Hypercalcemic crisis –

Adults: 50 mg/kg by slow I.V. infusion added to 500 ml of dextrose 5% in water or normal saline solution. Maximum dosage is 3 g/day.

Children: 40 to 70 mg/kg by slow I.V. infusion, diluted to a maximum concentration of 30 mg/ml in dextrose 5% in water or normal saline solution. Maximum dosage is 70 mg/kg/day.

ADVERSE REACTIONS
Common reactions are in italics; life-threatening reactions are in bold italics.
CNS: circumoral paresthesias, numbness, headache, malaise, fatigue, muscle pain or weakness.
CV: hypertension, thrombophlebitis, orthostatic hypotension.
GI: nausea, vomiting, diarrhea, anorexia, abdominal cramps.
GU: in excessive doses – nephrotoxicity with urgency, nocturia, dysuria, polyuria, proteinuria, ***renal insufficiency and failure, tubular necrosis.***
Metabolic: ***severe hypocalcemia,*** decreased magnesium.
Local: pain at site of infusion, erythema, dermatitis.

INTERACTIONS
None significant.

NURSING CONSIDERATIONS
- *Contraindicated* in anuria, known or suspected hypocalcemia, significant renal disease, active or healed tubercular lesions, history of seizures or intracranial lesions, and generalized arteriosclerosis associated with aging.
- *Use cautiously* in limited cardiac reserve, CHF, hypokalemia, and diabetes.
- **I.V. use:** Drug must be diluted before use. Avoid rapid I.V. infusion; profound hypocalcemia may occur, leading to tetany, seizures, cardiac arrhythmias, and respiratory arrest. Not recommended for direct or intermittent injection. Avoid extravasation.
- Record I.V. site used, and try to avoid repeated use of the same site, as this increases likelihood of thrombophlebitis.
- Monitor ECG, and test renal function frequently.
- Obtain serum calcium after each dose.
- Keep I.V. calcium available.
- Monitor blood pressure closely.
- Keep patient in bed for 15 minutes after infusion to avoid orthostatic hypotension.
- Don't use to treat lead toxicity; use edetate calcium disodium instead.
- Generalized systemic reactions may occur 4 to 8 hours after drug administration; these include fever, chills, back pain, emesis, muscle cramps, and urinary urgency. Report such reactions to doctor. Treatment is usually supportive. Symptoms generally subside within 12 hours.
- Edetate disodium not currently drug of choice for treatment of hypercalcemia; other treatments are safer and more effective.
- EDTA chelation therapy has been inappropriately recommended for treatment of atherosclerosis and related disorders. There's no scientific evidence that the drug is either safe or effective for these indications.

flumazenil
Romazicon

Pregnancy Risk Category: C

HOW SUPPLIED
Injection: 0.1 mg/ml in 5- and 10-ml multiple-dose vials

MECHANISM OF ACTION
Benzodiazepine antagonist that competitively inhibits the actions of benzodiazepines on the gamma-aminobutyric acid-benzodiazepine receptor complex.

INDICATIONS & DOSAGE
Complete or partial reversal of the sedative effects of benzodiazepines after anesthesia or short diagnostic procedures (conscious sedation) –
Adults: initially, 0.2 mg I.V. over 15 seconds. If patient does not reach the desired level of consciousness after 45 seconds, repeat dose. Repeat at 1-minute intervals until a cumulative dose of 1 mg has been given (initial dose plus four additional doses). Most

patients respond after 0.6 to 1 mg of drug. In case of resedation, dosage may be repeated after 20 minutes; however, no more than 1 mg should be given at any one time, and no more than 3 mg/hour.

Management of suspected benzodiazepine overdose –

Adults: initially, 0.2 mg I.V. over 15 seconds. If patient does not reach the desired level of consciousness after 30 seconds, administer 0.3 mg over 30 seconds. If patient still does not respond adequately, give 0.5 mg over 30 seconds; repeat 0.5-mg doses at 1-minute intervals until a cumulative dose of 3 mg has been given. Most patients suffering from benzodiazepine overdose respond to cumulative doses between 1 and 3 mg; rarely, patients who respond partially after 3 mg may require additional doses. Do not give more than 5 mg over 5 minutes initially. Sedation that persists after this dosage is unlikely to be caused by benzodiazepines. In case of resedation, dosage may be repeated after 20 minutes; however, no more than 1 mg should be given at any one time, and no more than 3 mg/hour.

ADVERSE REACTIONS

Common reactions are in italics; life-threatening reactions are in bold italics.

CNS: *dizziness, abnormal or blurred vision, headache,* ***seizures,*** fatigue, agitation, emotional lability.

CV: ***arrhythmias,*** cutaneous vasodilation.

GI: nausea, vomiting.

Local: *pain at injection site.*

Other: *increased sweating.*

INTERACTIONS

Antidepressants; any drug that can cause seizures or arrhythmias: seizures or arrhythmias can develop after the effects of the benzodiazepine overdose is removed. Use flumazenil with caution in cases of mixed overdose.

NURSING CONSIDERATIONS

- *Contraindicated* in patients with hypersensitivity to flumazenil or benzodiazepines; patients who show evidence of serious tricyclic or tetracyclic antidepressant overdose; those who received the benzodiazepine to treat a potentially life-threatening condition (such as status epilepticus); and in benzodiazepine-dependent patients because the drug may precipitate seizures.
- *Use cautiously* in patients at high risk for developing seizures (including patients undergoing concurrent sedative-hypnotic drug withdrawal; patients who have recently received multiple doses of a parenteral benzodiazepine; patients displaying some signs of seizure activity (such as myoclonus); patients who may be at risk for unrecognized benzodiazepine dependence (such as intensive-care-unit patients); patients with head injury (because of the risk of precipitating seizures); those who have received neuromuscular blockers; and psychiatric patients because the drug has precipitated panic attacks in those with panic disorder.
- Dosage adjustments don't appear necessary in elderly patients. Drug should not be used in children because no studies are available to support safety and effectiveness.
- Drug can be administered by direct injection or diluted with a compatible solution. Unused drug that has been drawn into a syringe or diluted should be discarded within 24 hours.
- **I.V. use:** Administer drug into an I.V. line in a large vein with a free-flowing I.V. solution to minimize pain at the injection site. Compatible solutions include dextrose 5% in water, lactated Ringer's injection, or 0.9% sodium chloride.
- Monitor patients closely for resedation that may occur after reversal of benzodiazepine effects. This reaction may occur because the duration of ac-

tion of flumazenil is shorter than that of all benzodiazepines. The duration of the monitoring period depends on the specific drug being reversed. Monitor closely after long-acting benzodiazepines (such as diazepam) or after high doses of short-acting benzodiazepines (such as 10 mg of midazolam). In most cases, severe resedation is unlikely in patients who fail to show signs of resedation 2 hours after a 1-mg dose of flumazenil.

• Warn patient not to perform hazardous activities, such as operating heavy equipment or driving a car, within 24 hours of the procedure because of the resedation risk.

• Know that patients should not be expected to recall information told to them in the postprocedure period because drug does not reverse the amnesic effects of benzodiazepines. Tell family members important instructions or give instructions to patient in writing.

• Tell patient to avoid alcohol, CNS depressants, and OTC drugs for 24 hours.

ipecac syrup*

Pregnancy Risk Category:C

HOW SUPPLIED

Syrup: 70 mg powdered ipecac/ml* ◊

MECHANISM OF ACTION

Induces vomiting by acting locally on the gastric mucosa and centrally on the chemoreceptor trigger zone.

INDICATIONS & DOSAGE

To induce vomiting in poisoning–

Adults and children over 12 years: 30 ml P.O., followed by 200 to 300 ml of water.

Children 1 year or older: 15 ml P.O., followed by about 200 ml of water or milk.

Children under 1 year: 5 to 10 ml P.O., followed by 100 to 200 ml of water or milk. May repeat dose once after 20 minutes, if necessary.

ADVERSE REACTIONS

Common reactions are in italics; life-threatening reactions are in bold italics.

CNS: depression.

CV: ***arrhythmias, bradycardia, hypotension, atrial fibrillation, or fatal myocarditis after ingestion of excessive dose.***

GI: diarrhea.

INTERACTIONS

Activated charcoal: neutralized emetic effect. Don't give together but may give activated charcoal after vomiting has occurred.

NURSING CONSIDERATIONS

• *Contraindicated* in semicomatose or unconscious patients, or those with severe inebriation, seizures, shock, or loss of gag reflex. Don't give after ingestion of petroleum distillates (for example, kerosene, gasoline) or volatile oils; retching and vomiting may cause aspiration and lead to bronchospasm, pulmonary edema, or aspiration pneumonitis. Vegetable oil will delay absorption of these substances. Don't give after ingestion of caustic substances, such as lye; additional injury to the esophagus and mediastinum can occur.

• Clearly indicate ipecac *syrup,* not single word "ipecac," to avoid confusion with fluidextract. Fluidextract is 14 times more concentrated and, if inadvertently used instead of syrup, may cause death. This is unlikely in the United States, because the fluidextract is no longer commerically available.

• Induces vomiting within 30 minutes in more than 90% of patients; average time usually less than 20 minutes.

• Stomach is usually emptied completely; vomitus may contain some intestinal material as well.

• In antiemetic toxicity, ipecac syrup is usually effective if less than 1 hour

*Liquid form contains alcohol. **May contain tartrazine.

has passed since ingestion of antiemetic.
• Recommend that 1 oz (30 ml) of syrup be readily available in the home when child becomes 1 year old for immediate use in case of emergency.
• No systemic toxicity with doses of 30 ml or less.
• If two doses do not induce vomiting, gastric lavage is necessary.
• Now commonly abused by bulimics who practice "binge-purge."

naloxone hydrochloride

Narcan

Pregnancy Risk Category: B

HOW SUPPLIED

Injection: 0.4 mg/ml, 1 mg/ml

MECHANISM OF ACTION

Displaces previously administered narcotic analgesics from their receptors (competitive antagonism). Has no pharmacologic activity of its own.

INDICATIONS & DOSAGE

Known or suspected narcotic-induced respiratory depression, including that caused by pentazocine and propoxyphene –

Adults: 0.4 to 2 mg I.V., S.C., or I.M. May repeat q 2 to 3 minutes, p.r.n. If no response is observed after 10 mg has been administered, the diagnosis of narcotic-induced toxicity should be questioned.

Postoperative narcotic depression –

Adults: 0.1 to 0.2 mg I.V. q 2 to 3 minutes, p.r.n. Adult concentration is 0.4 mg/ml.

Children: 0.01 mg/kg dose I.M., I.V., or S.C. May repeat q 2 to 3 minutes.

Note: If initial dose of 0.01 mg/kg does not result in clinical improvement, up to 10 times this dose (0.1 mg/kg) may be needed to be effective.

Neonates (asphyxia neonatorum): 0.01 mg/kg I.V. into umbilical vein. May repeat q 2 to 3 minutes for 3 doses.

ADVERSE REACTIONS

Common reactions are in italics; life-threatening reactions are in bold italics.

With higher-than-recommended doses:

CV: tachycardia, hypertension.

GI: nausea, vomiting.

Other: tremors, withdrawal symptoms (in narcotic-dependent patients).

INTERACTIONS

None significant.

NURSING CONSIDERATIONS

• *Contraindicated* in patients with hypersensitivity to the drug.
• *Use cautiously* in cardiac irritability and opiate addiction. Abrupt reversal of opiate-induced CNS depression may result in nausea, vomiting, sweating, tachycardia, CNS excitement, and increased blood pressure.
• Naloxone is only effective in reversing respiratory depression caused by opiates. It's not effective against other drug-induced respiratory depression (such as from barbiturates and sedatives). Flumazenil should be used to treat respiratory depression caused by diazepam or other benzodiazepines.
• Duration of action of a narcotic may exceed that of naloxone. Patient may relapse into respiratory depression.
• Monitor respiratory depth and rate. Be prepared to provide oxygen, ventilation, and other resuscitative measures.
• Respiratory rate increases within 1 to 2 minutes. Effect lasts 1 to 4 hours, but dosage may have to be repeated q 20 minutes.
• **I.V. use:** May be administered by continuous I.V. infusion, which is often necessary to control the adverse effects of epidurally administered morphine. May dilute adult concentration (0.4 mg) by mixing 0.5 ml with 9.5 ml sterile water or saline solution for injection to make neonatal concentration (0.02 mg/ml).

- Can see "overshoot" effect – respiratory rate exceeds the rate before respiratory depression.
- Although generally believed to be ineffective in respiratory depression caused by nonnarcotics, recent reports indicate that it may reverse coma induced by alcohol intoxication.
- Naloxone has been used investigationally to treat the senile dementia of Alzheimer's disease.
- Also has been shown to improve circulation in refractory shock.
- Used by some researchers to relieve certain kinds of chronic constipation.

naltrexone hydrochloride
Trexan

Pregnancy Risk Category: C

HOW SUPPLIED

Tablets: 50 mg

MECHANISM OF ACTION

Reversibly blocks the subjective effects of intravenously administered opioids by occupying opiate receptors in the brain.

INDICATIONS & DOSAGE

As an adjunct for maintenance of an opioid-free state in detoxified individuals –

Adults: initially, 25 mg P.O. If no withdrawal signs occur within 1 hour, give an additional 25 mg. Once patient has been started on 50 mg q 24 hours, flexible maintenance schedule may be used. From 50 to 150 mg may be given daily, depending on the schedule prescribed.

ADVERSE REACTIONS

Common reactions are in italics; life-threatening reactions are in bold italics.

CNS: *insomnia, anxiety, nervousness, headache,* depression.

GI: *nausea, vomiting,* anorexia, *abdominal pain.*

Hepatic: hepatotoxicity.

Other: *muscle and joint pain.*

INTERACTIONS

None significant.

NURSING CONSIDERATIONS

- *Contraindicated* in patients receiving opioid analgesics, opioid-dependent patients, patients in acute opioid withdrawal, and in those with positive urine screen for opioids or acute hepatitis or liver failure.
- *Use cautiously* in mild liver disease or history of recent liver disease.
- Treatment shouldn't begin until patient receives naloxone challenge, a provocative test of opioid dependency. If signs of opioid withdrawal persist after naloxone challenge, don't administer naltrexone.
- Patients must be completely free of opioids before taking naltrexone, or they may experience severe withdrawal symptoms. Those who have been addicted to short-acting opioids (such as heroin and meperidine) must wait at least 7 days after the last opioid dose before starting naltrexone. Those who have been addicted to longer-acting opioids (such as methadone) should wait at least 10 days.
- In an emergency that requires opioid analgesia, a patient receiving naltrexone can be given an opioid analgesic. However, the dose must be higher than usual to surmount naltrexone's effect. Monitor for respiratory depression from the opioid, which may be longer and deeper.
- Naltrexone should be used only as part of a comprehensive rehabilitation program.
- A suggested flexible maintenance dosage regimen: 100 mg on Monday and Wednesday; 150 mg on Friday. This schedule would be preferred for those expected to be poor compliers.
- Advise the patient to carry a medical identification card. Warn him to tell medical personnel that he is tak-

ing naltrexone, if he needs medical treatment.

• Give patient the names of nonopioid drugs that he can continue to take for pain, diarrhea, or cough.

pralidoxime chloride (pyridine-2-aldoxime methochloride; 2-PAM)

Protopam Chloride

Pregnancy Risk Category: C

HOW SUPPLIED

Injection: 1-g/20-ml vial without diluent or syringe; 1-g/20-ml vial with diluent, syringe, needle, alcohol swab (emergency kit); 600-mg/2-ml auto-injector, parenteral

MECHANISM OF ACTION

Reactives cholinesterase that has been inactivated by organophosphorus pesticides and related compounds. It permits degradation of accumulated acetylcholine and facilitates normal functioning of neuromuscular junctions.

INDICATIONS & DOSAGE

Antidote for organophosphate poisoning–

Adults: I.V. infusion of 1 to 2 g in 100 ml of saline solution over 15 to 30 minutes. If pulmonary edema is present, give drug by slow I.V. push over 5 minutes. Repeat in 1 hour if muscle weakness persists. Additional doses may be given cautiously. I.M. or S.C. injection can be used if I.V. is not feasible.

Children: 20 to 40 mg/kg I.V.

To treat cholinergic crisis in myasthenia gravis–

Adults: 1 to 2 g I.V., followed by increments of 250 mg I.V. q 5 minutes.

ADVERSE REACTIONS

Common reactions are in italics; life-threatening reactions are in bold italics.

CNS: dizziness, headache, drowsiness, excitement, and manic behavior following recovery of consciousness.

CV: tachycardia.

EENT: blurred vision, diplopia, impaired accommodation, ***laryngospasm.***

GI: nausea.

Other: muscular weakness, muscle rigidity, hyperventilation.

INTERACTIONS

None significant.

NURSING CONSIDERATIONS

• *Contraindicated* in poisoning with Sevin, a carbamate insecticide, since it increases drug's toxicity.

• *Use with extreme caution* in renal insufficiency or myasthenia gravis (overdosage may precipitate myasthenic crisis); also in asthma or peptic ulcer.

• Use in hospitalized patients only; have respiratory and other supportive measures available. Obtain accurate medical history and chronology of poisoning if possible. Give as soon as possible after poisoning.

• **I.V. use:** I.V. preparation should be given slowly, as diluted solution.

• Dilute with sterile water without preservatives.

• Atropine along with pralidoxime should be given I.V., 2 to 4 mg, if cyanosis is not present. If cyanosis is present, atropine should be given I.M. Give atropine every 5 to 6 minutes until signs and symptoms of atropine toxicity appear (flushing, tachycardia, dry mouth, blurred vision, excitement, delirium, and hallucinations); maintain atropinization for at least 48 hours.

• Initial measures should include removal of secretions, maintenance of patent airway, and artificial ventilation if needed. After dermal exposure to organophosphate, patient's clothing should be removed and his skin and hair should be washed with sodium bicarbonate, soap, water, and alcohol

as soon as possible. A second washing may be necessary. When washing the patient, wear protective gloves and clothes to avoid exposure.
- Drug relieves paralysis of respiratory muscles but is less effective in relieving depression of respiratory center.
- Not effective against poisoning due to phosphorus, inorganic phosphates, or organophosphates with no anticholinesterase activity.
- Difficult to distinguish between toxic effects produced by atropine or by organophosphate compounds and those resulting from pralidoxime. Observe patient for 48 to 72 hours if poison was ingested. Delayed absorption may occur from lower bowel.
- Caution patients treated for organophosphate poisoning to avoid contact with insecticides for several weeks.
- Patients with myasthenia gravis treated for overdose of cholinergic drugs should be observed closely for signs of rapid weakening. These patients can pass quickly from a cholinergic crisis to a myasthenic crisis, and require more cholinergic drugs to treat the myasthenia. Keep edrophonium (Tensilon) available in such situations for establishing differential diagnosis.
- Although not approved, subconjunctival injection of pralidoxime has been used to reverse adverse ocular reactions resulting from splashing into the eye or systemic overdose of organophosphates.
- Treatment is most effective if initiated within 24 hours after exposure.
- Draw blood for cholinesterase levels before giving pralidoxime.

protamine sulfate

Pregnancy Risk Category: C

HOW SUPPLIED
Injection: 10 mg/ml

MECHANISM OF ACTION
A heparin antagonist that forms a physiologically inert complex with heparin sodium.

INDICATIONS & DOSAGE
Heparin overdose –
Adults: dosage based on venous blood coagulation studies, usually 1 mg for each 90 to 115 units of heparin. Give diluted to 1% (10 mg/ml) by slow I.V. injection over 1 to 3 minutes. Maximum dose is 50 mg/10 minutes.

ADVERSE REACTIONS
Common reactions are in italics; life-threatening reactions are in bold italics.
CV: fall in blood pressure, bradycardia.
Other: transitory flushing, feeling of warmth, dyspnea, ***anaphylaxis, anaphylactoid reactions.***

INTERACTIONS
None significant.

NURSING CONSIDERATIONS
- *Use cautiously* after cardiac surgery.
- **I.V. use:** Administer slowly by direct I.V. injection. Have equipment available to treat shock.
- Calculate dosage carefully. 1 mg of protamine neutralizes 90 to 115 units of heparin depending on the salt (heparin calcium or heparin sodium) and the source of heparin (beef or pork).
- Monitor patient continually. Check vital signs frequently.
- Watch for spontaneous bleeding (heparin "rebound"), especially in patients undergoing dialysis and those who have had cardiac surgery.
- Protamine sulfate may act as anticoagulant in very high doses.

*Liquid form contains alcohol. **May contain tartrazine.

sodium cellulose phosphate

Calcibind

Pregnancy Risk Category: C

HOW SUPPLIED

Powder: 2.5-g packets or 300-g bulk. Inorganic phosphate content approximately 34%; sodium content approximately 11%.

MECHANISM OF ACTION

Binds calcium in the GI tract and decreases the amount absorbed.

INDICATIONS & DOSAGE

Treatment of absorptive hypercalciuria type I with recurrent calcium oxalate or calcium phosphate renal stones –
Adults: 15 g/day P.O. (5 g with each meal) in patients with urine calcium greater than 300 mg/day. When urine calcium declines to less than 150 mg/day, reduce dosage to 10 g/day (5 g with dinner, 2.5 g with two remaining meals).

ADVERSE REACTIONS

Common reactions are in italics; life-threatening reactions are in bold italics.
CNS: drowsiness, mood or mental changes, ***seizures,*** trembling.
GI: anorexia, nausea, vomiting, discomfort, diarrhea, dyspepsia.
GU: hyperoxaluria, hypomagnesuria.
Other: acute arthralgias.

INTERACTIONS

Magnesium-containing products: may bind drug. Separate doses by at least 1 hour.

NURSING CONSIDERATIONS

• *Contraindicated* in primary or secondary hyperparathyroidism, including renal hypercalciuria; hypomagnesemic states; bone disease; hypocalcemic states; normal or low intestinal absorption; renal excretion of calcium; or enteric hyperoxaluria.
• *Use cautiously* in CHF or ascites.
• Recommended only for the type of absorptive hypercalciuria in which both intestinal calcium absorption and urine calcium remain abnormally high even with a calcium-restricted diet. When administered inappropriately, it can cause hypocalciuria. This could stimulate parathyroid function and lead to parathyroid bone disease.
• Patient should maintain a calcium-restricted diet and avoid all dairy products.
• Patient taking sodium cellulose phosphate may develop hyperoxaluria and hypomagnesuria, which predispose him to stone formation. Therefore, advise patient to restrict dietary intake of oxalate (found in spinach, rhubarb, chocolate, and tea).
• Avoid vitamin C because it can increase urine oxalate.
• Encourage fluid intake. Urine output should be at least 2 liters/day.
• Patient can mix the powder with 8 oz of fruit juice, water, or a soft drink and take it with meals. Patient should rinse glass and drink all of the fluid to get the full dose.
• Encourage a low-sodium diet. Tell patient to avoid salty foods and to avoid adding salt at the table.
• Because of the difficulty involved in managing sodium cellulose phosphate therapy, many doctors prefer to treat hypercalciuria with a low-calcium diet, high fluid intake, and thiazides, when necessary.

sodium polystyrene sulfonate

Kayexalate, Resonium A, SPS

Pregnancy Risk Category: C

HOW SUPPLIED

Oral powder: 1.25 g/5 ml suspension
Rectal: 1.25 g/5 ml suspension

MECHANISM OF ACTION

The potassium-removing resin exchanges sodium ions for potassium ions in the intestine: 1 g of sodium polystyrene sulfonate is exchanged for 0.5 to 1 mEq of potassium. The resin is then eliminated. Much of the exchange capacity is used for cations other than potassium (calcium and magnesium) and possibly for fats and proteins.

INDICATIONS & DOSAGE

Hyperkalemia–
Adults: 15 g P.O. daily to q.i.d. in water or sorbitol (3 to 4 ml/g of resin).

For rectal administration, 30 to 50 g/100 ml of sorbitol q 6 hours as warm emulsion deep into sigmoid colon (20 cm). In persistent vomiting or paralytic ileus, high retention enema of sodium polystyrene sulfonate (30 g) suspended in 200 ml of 10% methylcellulose, 10% dextrose, or 25% sorbitol solution.

Children: 1 g of resin P.O. for each mEq of potassium to be removed.

Oral administration preferred since drug should remain in intestine for at least 6 hours; otherwise, consider nasogastric administration.

For nasogastric administration, mix dose with appropriate medium—aqueous suspension or diet appropriate for renal failure; instill in plastic tube.

ADVERSE REACTIONS

Common reactions are in italics; life-threatening reactions are in bold italics.

GI: *constipation,* fecal impaction (in elderly patients), anorexia, gastric irritation, nausea, vomiting, *diarrhea (with sorbitol emulsions).*

Other: ***hypokalemia,*** hypocalcemia, hypomagnesemia, sodium retention.

INTERACTIONS

Antacids and laxatives (nonabsorbable cation-donating type, including magnesium hydroxide): systemic alkalosis, reduced potassium exchange capability. Don't use together.

NURSING CONSIDERATIONS

- *Use cautiously* in elderly patients and those on digitalis therapy and with severe CHF, severe hypertension, and marked edema.
- Treatment may result in potassium deficiency. Monitor serum potassium at least once daily. Usually stopped when potassium is reduced to 4 or 5 mEq/liter. Watch for other signs of hypokalemia: irritability, confusion, cardiac arrhythmias, ECG changes, severe muscle weakness and sometimes paralysis, and digitalis toxicity in digitalized patients.
- Monitor for symptoms of other electrolyte deficiencies (magnesium, calcium) since drug is nonselective. Monitor serum calcium in patients receiving sodium polystyrene therapy for more than 3 days. Supplementary calcium may be needed.
- Drug contains about 100 mg sodium/g. Watch for sodium overload. About ⅓ of resin's sodium is retained.
- Premixed forms are available (SPS and others).
- Do not heat resin. This will impair effectiveness of drug. Mix resin only with water or sorbitol for P.O. administration. Above all, *never* mix with orange juice (high potassium content) to disguise taste.
- Chill oral suspension for greater palatability.
- If sorbitol is given, it may be mixed with resin suspension.
- Consider solid form. Resin cookie and candy recipes are available; perhaps pharmacist or dietitian can supply.
- Watch for constipation in oral or nasogastric administration. Use sorbitol (10 to 20 ml of 70% syrup every 2 hours as needed) to produce one or two watery stools daily.
- If preparing manually, mix polysty-

*Liquid form contains alcohol. **May contain tartrazine.

rene resin only with water and sorbitol for rectal use. Do not use other vehicles (that is, mineral oil) for rectal administration to prevent impactions. Ion exchange requires aqueous medium. Sorbitol content prevents impaction.

- Prevent fecal impaction in elderly by administering resin rectally. Give cleansing enema before rectal administration. Explain necessity of retaining enema to patient. Retention for 6 to 10 hours is ideal, but 30 to 60 minutes is acceptable.
- Prepare rectal dose at room temperature. Stir emulsion gently during administration.
- Use #28 French rubber tube for rectal dose; insert 20 cm into sigmoid colon. Tape tube in place. Alternatively, consider a Foley catheter with a 30-ml balloon inflated distal to anal sphincter to aid in retention. This is especially helpful for patients with poor sphincter control (for example, after cerebrovascular accident). Use gravity flow. Drain returns constantly through Y-tube connection. When giving rectally, place patient in knee-chest position or with hips on pillow for a while if back-leakage occurs.
- After rectal administration, flush tubing with 50 to 100 ml of nonsodium fluid to ensure delivery of all medication.
- Flush rectum to remove the resin.
- If hyperkalemia is severe, more drastic modalities should be added; for example, dextrose 50% with regular insulin I.V. push. Do not depend solely on polystyrene resin to lower serum potassium in severe hyperkalemia.

---

succimer

Chemet

Pregnancy Risk Category: C

HOW SUPPLIED

Capsules: 100 mg

MECHANISM OF ACTION

A chelating agent that forms water-soluble complexes with lead and increases its excretion in urine.

INDICATIONS & DOSAGE

Lead poisoning in children with blood lead levels above 45 mcg/dl –

Children: initially, 10 mg/kg or 350 mg/m^2 q 8 hours for 5 days. Round dosage as appropriate to the nearest 100 mg (see chart). Then, decrease frequency of administration to q 12 hours for an additional 2 weeks of therapy.

Weight (kg)	Dose (mg)
8 to 15	100
16 to 23	200
24 to 34	300
35 to 44	400
> 45	500

ADVERSE REACTIONS

Common reactions are in italics; life-threatening reactions are in bold italics.

CNS: *drowsiness, dizziness, sensory motor neuropathy, sleepiness, paresthesia, headache.*

CV: arrhythmias, increased platelet count, intermittent eosinophilia.

EENT: ears plugged, cloudy film in eye, otitis media, watery eyes, sore throat, rhinorrhea, nasal congestion.

GI: *nausea, vomiting, diarrhea, loss of appetite,* abdominal cramps, hemorrhoidal symptoms, *metallic taste in mouth, loose stools.*

GU: decreased urination, difficult urination, proteinuria.

Respiratory: cough, head cold.

Skin: papular rash, herpetic rash, mucocutaneous eruptions, pruritus.

Other: *leg, kneecap, back, stomach, rib, or flank pain; flulike symptoms;* moniliasis; *elevated serum AST (SGOT), ALT (SGPT), alkaline phosphatase, or cholesterol levels.*

INTERACTIONS

None reported.

NURSING CONSIDERATIONS

- *Contraindicated* in patients with hypersensitivity to the drug.
- *Use cautiously* in patients with compromised renal function.
- Concurrent administration of succimer with other chelating agents is not recommended. Patients who have received edetate calcium disodium with or without dimercaprol may use succimer as subsequent therapy after a 4-week interval.
- Young children may not be able to swallow capsules. Capsule can be opened and sprinkled on a small amount of soft food. Alternatively, the medicated beads from the capsules may be poured on a spoon; follow with a flavored beverage, such as a fruit drink.
- Elevated blood lead levels and associated symptoms may return rapidly after drug is discontinued because of redistribution of lead from bone to soft tissues and blood. Monitor patient at least once weekly for rebound blood lead levels.
- Identification and removal of sources of lead in child's environment is critical to successful therapy. Chelation therapy is not a substitute for preventing further exposure and should not be used to permit continued exposure. Succimer is not indicated for prophylaxis of lead poisoning.
- The severity of lead intoxication should be used as a guide for more frequent blood lead monitoring. Severity is measured by the initial blood lead level and the rate and degree of rebound of blood lead level.
- A course of treatment lasts 19 days. Repeated courses may be necessary if indicated by weekly monitoring of blood lead levels.
- A minimum of 2 weeks between courses is recommended unless high blood lead levels indicate need for immediate therapy.
- Transient mild elevations of serum transaminases have also been observed. Monitor serum transaminase before and at least weekly during therapy. Patients with a history of liver disease should be monitored more closely.
- False-positive results for ketones in urine using nitroprusside reagents (Ketostix) and falsely decreased levels of serum uric acid and CPK have been reported.
- Tell patient to consult doctor if rash occurs. The possibility of allergic or other mucocutaneous reactions must be considered each time drug is used, including the initial course.

trientine hydrochloride

Cuprid

Pregnancy Risk Category: C

HOW SUPPLIED

Capsules: 250 mg

MECHANISM OF ACTION

Chelates copper and increases its urinary excretion.

INDICATIONS & DOSAGE

Treatment of Wilson's disease in patients who cannot tolerate penicillamine –
Adults: 750 to 2,000 mg P.O. daily in two, three, or four divided doses.
Children: 500 to 1,500 mg P.O. daily in two, three, or four divided doses.

The optimal long-term maintenance dosage should be determined q 6 to 12 months, according to serum copper analysis.

ADVERSE REACTIONS

Common reactions are in italics; life-threatening reactions are in bold italics.
Blood: iron deficiency anemia.
Other: hypersensitivity (rash), fever.

INTERACTIONS

Mineral supplements (including iron): may block trientine absorption. Administer at least 2 hours apart.

NURSING CONSIDERATIONS

- *Contraindicated* in patients with known or suspected hypersensitivity to the drug. Not recommended for use in patients with rheumatoid arthritis, biliary cirrhosis, or cystinuria.
- *Use cautiously* in patients with or at risk for iron-deficiency anemia. Patients (especially women) should be closely monitored for evidence of iron-deficiency anemia throughout therapy.
- Also use cautiously in patients with idiopathic or penicillamine-induced systemic lupus erythematosus because drug may reactivate the disease.
- Observe patient for signs of hypersensitivity, such as skin rash.
- Tell patient to take trientine on an empty stomach at least 1 hour before meals or 2 hours after meals, and at least 1 hour apart from any other drug, food, or milk.
- Capsules should be swallowed whole with water and should not be opened or chewed.
- Exposure to capsule contents may cause contact dermatitis. If capsule is accidentally opened and contents spilled on the skin, tell patient to wash the site thoroughly.
- Trientine should be prescribed for only patients who cannot tolerate penicillamine, the standard treatment for Wilson's disease.
- Urge patient to faithfully follow his trientine regimen and low-copper diet as prescribed.
- Patient should take his temperature every night and report any fevers or skin eruptions, especially during the first month of therapy.

101

Uncategorized drugs

acetohydroxamic acid
alglucerase
alpha-1 proteinase inhibitor (human)
alprostadil
benzoyl peroxide cleansers
benzoyl peroxide creams
benzoyl peroxide gels
benzoyl peroxide lotions
beractant
capsaicin
clomiphene citrate
colfosceril palmitate
cromolyn sodium
diazoxide, oral
disulfiram
etretinate
finasteride
gallium nitrate
isotretinoin
levocarnitine
masoprocol
mesalamine
mesna
methoxsalen
minoxidil (topical)
nedocromil sodium
nicotine polacrilex
nicotine transdermal system
olsalazine sodium
pamidronate disodium
pentoxifylline
ritodrine hydrochloride
sodium benzoate and sodium phenylacetate
sumatriptan succinate
ticlopidine hydrochloride
tiopronin
tretinoin

COMBINATION PRODUCTS
None.

acetohydroxamic acid
Lithostat
Pregnancy Risk Category: X

HOW SUPPLIED
Tablets (scored): 250 mg

MECHANISM OF ACTION
Prevents formation of renal stones by inhibiting bacterial urease activity.

INDICATIONS & DOSAGE
Treatment of infection-related kidney stones –
Adults: 250 mg P.O. t.i.d. or q.i.d. Administer at 6- to 8-hour intervals at a time when the stomach is empty. Maximum daily dosage is 1.5 g.
Children: 10 mg/kg/day P.O. in two or three divided doses.

ADVERSE REACTIONS
Common reactions are in italics; life-threatening reactions are in bold italics.
Blood: ***hemolytic anemia.***
CNS: *mild headache, depression, anxiety, nervousness.*
CV: phlebitis, palpitations.
GI: *nausea, vomiting, diarrhea, constipation, anorexia.*
Skin: *nonpruritic, macular rash on arms and face.*
Other: alopecia, deep vein thrombosis, malaise.

INTERACTIONS
Methenamine: may produce synergistic effects.
Oral iron supplements: reduce absorption of acetohydroxamic acid. Check with doctor; he may request that iron be administered I.M.

*Liquid form contains alcohol. **May contain tartrazine.

NURSING CONSIDERATIONS

• *Contraindicated* in patients whose physical state and disease are amenable to surgery and appropriate antibiotics, in patients whose urine is infected by nonurease-producing organisms in pregnancy, and in poor renal function.
• *Use cautiously* in patients predisposed to deep vein thrombosis.
• Coombs'-negative hemolytic anemia has occurred in patients receiving acetohydroxamic acid.
• Monitor CBC, including reticulocyte count, after 2 weeks of therapy. Thereafter, monitor at 3-month intervals for the duration of treatment. If laboratory findings indicate hemolytic anemia, discontinue drug.
• Skin rash more common during prolonged use and with concomitant use of alcoholic beverages. The rash appears 30 to 45 minutes after ingestion of alcoholic beverages; disappears spontaneously in 30 to 60 minutes. Although skin rash doesn't usually require treatment, advise patient to avoid alcohol.
• Reduced dosage may be necessary in renal impairment.

alglucerase (glucocerebrosidase, glucosylceramidase, glucocerebrosidase-beta-glucosidase)

Ceredase

Pregnancy Risk Category: C

HOW SUPPLIED

Injection: 80 IU/ml in 5-ml bottles

MECHANISM OF ACTION

Appears to reduce glycolipid accumulation by acting as a catalyst for the hydrolysis of glucocerebroside to glucose and ceramide – part of the normal degradation pathway for lipids.

INDICATIONS & DOSAGE

Long-term endogenous enzyme (glucosylceramidase) replacement therapy in confirmed Type I Gaucher's disease –
Adults and children: dosage should be individualized; initial dose of up to 60 units/kg I.V. may be used. Infusion should run over 1 to 2 hours and be given once q 2 weeks. Frequency of infusion may be adjusted based on severity of disease or patient convenience. Once response is established, reduce dosage for maintenance at 3- to 6-month intervals.

ADVERSE REACTIONS

Common reactions are in italics; life-threatening reactions are in bold italics.
GI: abdominal discomfort, nausea, vomiting.
Other: chills, slight fever, discomfort, burning, swelling at injection site.

INTERACTIONS

None reported.

NURSING CONSIDERATIONS

• *Contraindicated* in patients with hypersensitivity to the drug. Alglucerase is purified from a large pool of human placental tissue collected from selected donors. The risk of viral contamination has been reduced but cannot be totally eliminated. Although the risk of viral contamination from slow-acting or latent viruses is believed to be remote, the risks and benefits of therapy must be carefully assessed before administration.
• Monitor response parameters to use lowest effective dose.
• There is no age restriction for receiving alglucerase.
• Hemoglobin levels may normalize after 6 months of therapy. Improved mineralization may also occur after prolonged treatment.
• **I.V. use:** Prepare fresh solution by diluting the appropriate amount of alglucerase with 0.9% sodium chloride

solution to a final volume not to exceed 100 ml. Use an in-line particulate filter during administration. Because alglucerase is preservative-free, do not store for subsequent use after opening.
• Do not shake bottle. Shaking may denature the glycoprotein and render it biologically inactive.
• Store at 39° F (4° C). Do not use solution that is discolored or that contains particles.

alpha-1 proteinase inhibitor (human)

Prolastin

Pregnancy Risk Category: C

HOW SUPPLIED

Injection: 500 mg, 1,000 mg

MECHANISM OF ACTION

Replaces $alpha_1$-proteinase in patients with $alpha_1$-antitrypsin deficiency.

INDICATIONS & DOSAGE

Chronic replacement therapy in patients with congenital $alpha_1$-antitrypsin deficiency and demonstrable panacinar emphysema –
Adults: 60 mg/kg I.V. once weekly. May be given at the rate of 0.08 ml/kg/minute or greater.

ADVERSE REACTIONS

Common reactions are in italics; life-threatening reactions are in bold italics.
Blood: possible viral transmission.

INTERACTIONS

Cigarette smoke: inactivates drug. Patients should not smoke.

NURSING CONSIDERATIONS

• Explain to the patient that the product has been treated to minimize the risk of transmission of hepatitis and AIDS.
• **I.V. use:** Store powder for injection in the refrigerator (36° to 46° F [2° to 8° C]). Reconstitute using the diluent supplied by the manufacturer (sterile water for injection). After reconstitution, administer within 3 hours. Inject directly into vein at a rate of at least 0.08 ml/minute. Intermittent or continuous infusion is not recommended.
• Many commercial assays for $alpha_1$-proteinase inhibitor measure immunoreactivity of the protein and not inhibitor activity. Monitoring serum level may not accurately reflect clinical response.

alprostadil

Prostin VR Pediatric

HOW SUPPLIED

Injection: 500 mcg/ml

MECHANISM OF ACTION

A prostaglandin derivative which relaxes the smooth muscle of the ductus arteriosus.

INDICATIONS & DOSAGE

Palliative therapy for temporary maintenance of patency of ductus arteriosus until surgery can be performed –
Infants: 0.05 to 0.1 mcg/kg/minute by I.V., intraarterial, or intraaortic infusion. When therapeutic response is achieved, reduce infusion rate to give lowest dosage that will maintain response. Maximum dosage is 0.4 mcg/kg/minute. Alternatively, administer through umbilical artery catheter placed at ductal opening.

ADVERSE REACTIONS

Common reactions are in italics; life-threatening reactions are in bold italics.
Blood: ***disseminated intravascular coagulation.***
CNS: ***seizures.***
CV: *flushing,* bradycardia, hypotension, tachycardia.
GI: diarrhea.
Other: ***apnea, fever, sepsis.***

INTERACTIONS
None reported.

NURSING CONSIDERATIONS
- *Contraindicated* in neonatal respiratory distress syndrome.
- *Use cautiously* in neonates with bleeding tendencies because drug inhibits platelet aggregation.
- Monitor arterial pressure by umbilical artery catheter, auscultation, or Doppler transducer. Slow rate of infusion if arterial pressure falls significantly.
- In infants with restricted pulmonary blood flow, measure drug's effectiveness by monitoring blood oxygenation. In infants with restricted systemic blood flow, measure drug's effectiveness by monitoring systemic blood pressure and blood pH.
- **I.V. use:** This drug is not recommended for direct injection or intermittent infusion. Administer by continuous infusion using a constant-rate pump. Infuse through a large peripheral or central vein or through an umbilical artery catheter placed at the level of the ductus arteriosus.
- Reduce infusion rate if fever or significant hypotension occurs.
- Drug must be diluted before being administered. Fresh solution must be prepared daily. Discard any solution more than 24 hours old.
- Do not use diluents that contain benzyl alcohol. Fatal toxic syndrome may occur.
- Apnea and bradycardia may reflect drug overdose. If the signs occur, stop infusion immediately.
- CV and CNS adverse reactions are more frequent in infants weighing less than 2 kg and in those receiving infusions for longer than 48 hours.
- Keep respiratory support available.
- If flushing occurs from peripheral vasodilation, reposition catheter.

benzoyl peroxide cleansers
Benzac W Wash 5, Benzac W Wash 10, Desquam-X 5 Wash, Desquam-X 10 Wash, Fostex 10% BPO Cleansing◇, Fostex 10% BPO Wash◇, Oxy-10 Wash◇, PanOxyl 5◇, PanOxyl 10◇, Propa P.H. Liquid Acne Soap◇

benzoyl peroxide creams
Acne-Aid◇, Clearasil Maximum Strength◇, Cuticura Acne◇, Dry and Clear Double Strength, Fostex 10% BPO Tinted◇, Oxy 10 Cover◇, phisoAc BP◇

benzoyl peroxide gels
5 Benzagel, 10 Benzagel, Benzac 5, Benzac W 5, Benzac W 10, Benzac W 2 1/2, Ben-Aqua 5, Ben-Aqua 10, Buf-Oxal 10◇, Clear By Design◇, Del Aqua 5◇, Del Aqua 10◇, Desquam-E, Desquam-X 5, Desquam-X 10, Desquam-X 2.5, Fostex 5% BPO◇, Fostex 10% BPO◇, PanOxyl 5, PanOxyl 10, PanOxyl AQ 5, PanOxyl AQ 10, PanOxyl AQ 2 1/2, Persa-Gel, Persa-Gel W 5%, Persa-Gel W 10%, Xerac BP5◇, Xerac BP10◇, Zeroxin-5, Zeroxin-10

benzoyl peroxide lotions
Acne-10◇, Ben-Aqua 5◇, Benoxyl 5◇, Benoxyl 10◇, Clearasil 10◇, Dry and Clear◇, Loroxide ◇, Oxy 5◇, Oxy 10◇, Vanoxide◇

Pregnancy Risk Category: C

HOW SUPPLIED
Cream: 5%◇, 10%◇
Gel: 2.5%◇, 5%◇, 10%◇
Liquid cleanser: 5%, 10%◇
Lotion: 5%◇, 5.5%◇, 10%◇
Soap (bar): 5%◇, 10%◇

MECHANISM OF ACTION
Antimicrobial and comedolytic.

INDICATIONS & DOSAGE

Acne –
Adults and children: apply once daily to q.i.d., depending on tolerance and effect.

ADVERSE REACTIONS

Common reactions are in italics; life-threatening reactions are in bold italics.
Skin: stinging on application, warmth, painful irritation, pruritus, vesicles, allergic contact dermatitis.

INTERACTIONS

Abrasives, medical soaps and cleansers, acne preparations and preparations containing peeling agents, topical alcohol preparations (including cosmetics, after-shave, cologne): cumulative irritation of skin or excessive drying of skin. Use together cautiously.

NURSING CONSIDERATIONS

- *Contraindicated* in sensitivity to any of the drug's ingredients.
- Don't use near the eyes, on mucous membranes, or on denuded or highly inflamed skin.
- Initiate therapy with 2.5% or 5% preparation; change to 10% strength after 3 to 4 weeks or as tolerance develops.
- Patients with fair skin or patients living in very dry climates should begin with one application daily.
- Patient should wash face thoroughly 20 to 30 minutes before applying.
- Dryness, redness, and peeling should occur 3 to 4 days after starting treatment. If these common reactions cause considerable discomfort, discontinue temporarily.
- If painful irritation or vesicles develop, discontinue use.
- May bleach hair or clothing.

beractant (natural lung surfactant)

Survanta

HOW SUPPLIED

Suspension for intratracheal instillation: 25 mg/ml

MECHANISM OF ACTION

Lowers the surface tension on alveolar surfaces during respiration and stabilizes the alveoli against collapse. It mimics the naturally occurring surfactant. An extract of bovine lung containing neutral lipids, fatty acids, surfactant-associated proteins, and phospholipids; palmitic acid, palmitin, and dipalmitoylphosphatidylcholine are added to standardize the composition of the solution.

INDICATIONS & DOSAGE

Prevention of respiratory distress syndrome (RDS or hyaline membrane disease) in premature neonates weighing 1,250 g or less at birth or having symptoms consistent with surfactant deficiency –
Neonates: 4 ml/kg intratracheally; each dose is administered in four quarter-doses, with manual hand-bag ventilation between quarter-doses at a rate of 60 breaths/minute and sufficient oxygen to prevent cyanosis. Give the drug as soon as possible, preferably within 15 minutes of birth. Repeat in 6 hours if there is evidence of continued respiratory distress. Give no more than four doses in 48 hours.
Rescue treatment of RDS in premature infants –
Neonates: 4 ml/kg intratracheally; before administering, increase ventilator rate to 60 breaths/minute with an inspiratory time of 0.5 second and a fraction of inspired oxygen (FIO_2) of 1. Each dose is administered in four quarter-doses, with manual hand-bag ventilation between quarter-doses at a rate of 60 breaths/minute and suffi-

cient oxygen to prevent cyanosis. Give dose as soon as RDS is confirmed by X-ray, preferably within 8 hours of birth. Repeat in 6 hours if there is evidence of continued respiratory distress. Give no more than four doses in 48 hours.

ADVERSE REACTIONS

Common reactions are in italics; life-threatening reactions are in bold italics.

Blood: decreased oxygen saturation, hypocarbia, hypercarbia.

CV: transient bradycardia, vasoconstriction, hypotension.

Other: endotracheal tube reflux, pallor, endotracheal tube blockage, ***apnea.***

INTERACTIONS

None reported.

NURSING CONSIDERATIONS

• The drug should be administered only by persons familiar with the care of clinically unstable premature neonates. Such personnel should have knowledge of neonatal intubation and airway management.

• Accurate determination of weight is essential to proper measurement of dosage.

• Continuous monitoring of ECG and transcutaneous oxygen saturation are essential; frequent arterial blood pressure monitoring and frequent arterial blood gas sampling are highly desirable.

• Continuously monitor the neonate before, during, and after administration of the drug. The endotracheal tube may be suctioned before giving the drug; allow the neonate to stabilize before proceeding with administration of the drug.

• Transient bradycardia and oxygen desaturation are common after dosing.

• Know that the drug can rapidly affect oxygenation and lung compliance. Peak ventilator inspiratory pressures may need to be adjusted if chest expansion improves substantially after administration of the drug. This should be done *immediately* because lung overdistention and fatal pulmonary air leak may result.

• The drug is stored in the refrigerator (36° to 46° F [2° to 8° C]). Warm to room temperature before administration by allowing the drug to stand at room temperature for at least 20 minutes or by holding in hand for at least 8 minutes. Do not use artificial warming methods. Unopened vials that have been warmed to room temperature may be returned to the refrigerator within 8 hours of warming; however, the drug should be warmed and returned to the refrigerator only once. Vials are for single use only – unused drug should be discarded.

• Beractant does not require sonication or reconstitution before use. Inspect the contents before giving; the color should be off white to light brown and the contents uniform. If settling occurs, swirl the vial gently; do not shake. Some foaming is normal.

• Draw up the drug using a large bore needle (20G or larger); do not use a filter. Give the drug using a 5-French end-hole catheter. Premeasure and shorten the catheter before use. Fill the catheter with beractant and discard any excess drug so that only the total dose to be given remains in the syringe. Insert catheter into the neonate's endotracheal tube; the tip of the catheter should protrude just beyond the end of the tube above the neonate's carina. The drug should not be instilled into a mainstem bronchus.

• Homogeneous distribution of the drug is important. In clinical trials, each dose of the drug was given in four quarter-doses, with the patient positioned differently after each administration. Each quarter-dose is given over 2 to 3 seconds; the catheter is removed and the patient is venti-

lated between quarter-doses. With the head and body inclined slightly downward, the first quarter-dose is given with the head turned to the right. The second quarter-dose is given with the head turned to the left. Then the head and body are inclined slightly upward, and the third quarter-dose is given with the head turned to the right. The fourth quarter-dose is given with the head turned to the left.
- Immediately after administration, moist breath sounds and crackles can occur. *Do not* suction the infant for 1 hour unless other signs of airway obstruction are evident.
- The manufacturer has audiovisual materials available describing dosage and administration procedures.

capsaicin

Axsain◇, Zostrix◇

Pregnancy Risk Category: C

HOW SUPPLIED

Cream: 0.025%◇ (Zostrix◇), 0.075%◇ (Axsain◇)

MECHANISM OF ACTION

Exact mechanism unknown, but the drug may deplete substance P (the principle neurotransmitter for pain) in peripheral type C sensory fibers.

INDICATIONS & DOSAGE

Temporary relief of pain after herpes zoster infections –

Adults and children 2 years and over: 0.025% cream applied to affected areas not more than q.i.d.

Relief of neuralgias, such as postsurgical pain and painful diabetic neuropathy; treatment of pain associated with osteoarthritis or rheumatoid arthritis –

Adults and children over 2 years: 0.075% cream applied to affected areas not more than q.i.d.

ADVERSE REACTIONS

Common reactions are in italics; life-threatening reactions are in bold italics.

Local: redness, *stinging or burning upon application.*

INTERACTIONS

None reported.

NURSING CONSIDERATIONS

- Avoid getting drug in the eyes or on broken skin.
- Note that the drug may cause transient burning or stinging with application. This is usually evident at initial therapy and will persist in patients who use the drug less than t.i.d.
- Do not bandage area tightly after applying drug.
- Tell patient who is self-medicating with capsaicin to contact the doctor if symptoms persist beyond 2 to 4 weeks or if they resolve and shortly reappear.
- Tell patient to wash hands frequently after applying drug.

clomiphene citrate

Clomid

Pregnancy Risk Category: X

HOW SUPPLIED

Tablets: 50 mg

MECHANISM OF ACTION

Appears to stimulate release of pituitary gonadotropins, follicle-stimulating hormone, and luteinizing hormone. This results in maturation of the ovarian follicle, ovulation, and development of the corpus luteum.

INDICATIONS & DOSAGE

To induce ovulation –

Women: 50 to 100 mg P.O. daily for 5 days, starting any time; or 50 to 100 mg P.O. daily starting on day 5 of menstrual cycle (first day of menstrual flow is day 1). Repeat until

*Liquid form contains alcohol. **May contain tartrazine.

conception occurs or until three courses of therapy are completed.

ADVERSE REACTIONS
Common reactions are in italics; life-threatening reactions are in bold italics.
CNS: headache, restlessness, insomnia, dizziness, light-headedness, depression, fatigue, tension.
CV: hypertension.
EENT: blurred vision, diplopia, scotoma, photophobia (signs of impending visual toxicity).
GI: nausea, vomiting, bloating, distention, increased appetite, weight gain.
GU: urinary frequency and polyuria; ovarian enlargement and cyst formation, which regress spontaneously when drug is stopped.
Metabolic: hyperglycemia.
Skin: urticaria, rash, dermatitis.
Other: *hot flashes,* reversible alopecia, *breast discomfort.*

INTERACTIONS
None significant.

NURSING CONSIDERATIONS
- *Contraindicated* in undiagnosed abnormal genital bleeding, ovarian cyst, or hepatic disease or dysfunction, or in patients with a history of thrombophlebitis or thromboembolism.
- *Use cautiously* in hypertension, mental depression, migraines, seizures, diabetes mellitus, and gonadotropin sensitivity. Report the development or worsening of these conditions to doctor. May require stopping drug.
- Patient with visual disturbances should report symptoms to doctor immediately.
- Tell patient possibility of multiple births exists with this drug. Risk increases with higher doses.
- Teach patient to take basal body temperature and chart on graph to ascertain whether ovulation has occurred.
- Advise patient to stop drug and contact doctor immediately if abdominal symptoms or pain occurs because these indicate ovarian enlargement or ovarian cyst.
- Reassure patient that response (ovulation) generally occurs after the first course of therapy. If pregnancy does not occur, course of therapy may be repeated twice.
- Since drug may cause dizziness or visual disturbances, caution patient not to perform hazardous tasks until CNS effects of the drug are known.
- Advise patient to stop drug and contact doctor immediately if she suspects she is pregnant (drug may have teratogenic effect).

colfosceril palmitate
Exosurf Neonatal

HOW SUPPLIED
Suspension for intratracheal instillation: 10 ml

MECHANISM OF ACTION
Replaces a major component of naturally occurring lung surfactant (dipalmitoylphosphatidylcholine), which is deficient in premature infants. The mixture also contains cetyl alcohol (which acts as a spreading agent between the air-fluid interface) and tyloxapol, a long chain alcohol polymer (which acts as a dispersant).

INDICATIONS & DOSAGE
Prophylatic treatment of respiratory distress syndrome (RDS) of neonates weighing less than 1,350 g at risk of developing RDS; prophylactic treatment of neonates weighing 1,350 g or more with evidence of pulmonary insufficiency–
Neonates: administer 5 ml/kg intratracheally as soon as possible after delivery. If neonate is maintained on a mechanical ventilator, repeat dosage 12 and 24 hours later.

Rescue treatment of neonates with RDS –
Neonates: administer 5 ml/kg intratracheally as soon as possible after diagnosis of RDS. A second dose of 5 ml/kg should be administered 12 hours later if the neonate is still mechanically ventilated.

ADVERSE REACTIONS
Common reactions are in italics; life-threatening reactions are in bold italics.
Respiratory: ***pulmonary hemorrhage.***

INTERACTIONS
None reported.

NURSING CONSIDERATIONS
- There are no known contraindications to the use of the drug.
- The drug should be administered only by persons familiar with the care of clinically unstable premature neonates. Such personnel should have knowledge of neonatal intubation and airway management.
- Accurate determination of weight is essential to proper measurement of dosage.
- Know that the drug can rapidly affect oxygenation and lung compliance. Peak ventilator inspiratory pressures may need to be adjusted if chest expansion improves substantially after administration of the drug. This should be done *immediately* because lung overdistention and fatal pulmonary air leak may result.
- If the neonate becomes pink and the transcutaneous oxygen saturation exceeds 95%, reduce fraction of inspired oxygen (FIO_2) in a stepwise fashion until the saturation is 90% to 95%. This should be done *immediately* because hyperoxia (an excess of systemic oxygen) may result.
- Reduce ventilator rate immediately if the transcutaneous or arterial carbon dioxide measurements are less than 30 torr. Failure to reduce the rate may result in hypocarbia, which can reduce brain blood flow.
- Monitor neonates for pulmonary hemorrhage.
- Continuous monitoring of ECG and transcutaneous oxygen saturation are essential; frequent arterial blood pressure monitoring and frequent arterial blood gas sampling are highly desirable. Continuously monitor the neonate before, during, and after administration of the drug.
- Use the supplied preservative-free sterile water for injection to reconstitute the drug. Do not use solutions that contain antibacterial preservatives. Because the drug does not contain preservatives, reconstitute drug immediately before use. Once reconstituted, the drug is stable for up to 12 hours at 36° to 86° F (2° to 30° C). Fill a 10-ml syringe with the supplied 8 ml of diluent using an 18G or 19G needle. Then, pierce the top of the vial and allow the vacuum to draw in the sterile water. Do not use vials that do not have a vacuum. Aspirate as much of the 8 ml as possible out of the vial while maintaining the vacuum. Suddenly release the syringe plunger. Repeat this final step at least three or four times to ensure adequate mixing of the contents of the vial.
- When drawing up the dose, use liquid below the froth. Each 8-ml vial contains sufficient material to administer a 5 ml/kg dose to a neonate weighing up to 1,600 g.
- Note that the suspension should have a homogeneous, milky white appearance. Do not use vials that appear to contain large flakes. If the suspension appears to separate, the vial may be shaken or swirled gently to resuspend the material.
- The neonate should be suctioned before the drug is administered. Suctioning should not be performed for 2 hours after dosing unless it is necessary.
- Special endotracheal tube adapters

*Liquid form contains alcohol. **May contain tartrazine.

are available with each kit of surfactant. The adapter used should correspond to the inside diameter of the neonate's endotracheal tube. Insert the adapter into the tube with a twisting motion and connect to the ventilator circuit. To administer the drug (in half-doses), remove the cap from the side port of the adapter and attach syringe. The drug is administered without interrupting mechanical ventilation. After dosing, remember to reattach the cap.

- Instill each half-dose slowly over 1 to 2 minutes (30 to 50 mechanical breaths) in small bursts timed with inspiration. The first half-dose is administered with the neonate in the midline position; then the neonate's head and torso are turned 45 degrees to the right for 30 seconds to assist distribution of the drug. Return the neonate to the midline position for the second half-dose over 1 to 2 minutes as before. After the second half-dose, turn the neonate's head and torso 45 degrees to the left for 30 seconds.
- When administering the drug, monitor the newborn's facial expressions, skin color, chest expansion, heart rate, and endotracheal tube patency and position. If the neonate becomes dusky or agitated, heart rate slows, the drug backs up in the endotracheal tube, or oxygen saturation decreases by more than 15%, discontinue the drug and modify peak inspiratory pressure, ventilator rate, or FIO_2 as ordered. Note that rapid improvements in lung function may require rapid reductions in peak inspiratory pressure, ventilator rate, or FIO_2.

cromolyn sodium (sodium cromoglycate)

Gastrocrom, Intal, Intal Inhaler, Intal Spincaps†, Nalcrom, Nasalcrom, Opticrom, Rynacrom†

Pregnancy Risk Category: B

HOW SUPPLIED

Capsules (for oral solution): 100 mg
Aerosol: 800 mcg/metered spray
Capsules (for inhalation): 20 mg
Nasal solution: 5.2 mg/metered spray (40 mg/ml)
Solution: 20 mg/2 ml for nebulization
Ophthalmic solution: 4% (with benzalkonium chloride 0.01%, EDTA 0.01%, and phenylethyl alcohol 0.4%)

MECHANISM OF ACTION

Inhibits the degranulation of sensitized mast cells that occurs after a patient's exposure to specific antigens. It also inhibits release of histamine and slow-reacting substance of anaphylaxis (SRS-A).

INDICATIONS & DOSAGE

Adjunct in treatment of severe perennial bronchial asthma –
Adults and children over 5 years: contents of 20-mg capsule inhaled q.i.d. at regular intervals. Or administer 2 metered sprays using inhaler q.i.d. at regular intervals. Also available as an aqueous solution administered through a nebulizer.

Prevention and treatment of allergic rhinitis –
Adults and children over 5 years: 1 spray in each nostril t.i.d or q.i.d. May give up to 6 times daily.

Prevention of exercise-induced bronchospasm –
Adults and children over 5 years: contents of 20-mg capsule or 2 metered sprays inhaled no more than 1 hour before anticipated exercise.

Allergic ocular disorders –
Adults and children 4 years and older: 1 to 2 drops in each eye 4 to 6 times daily at regular intervals.

Systemic mastocytosis –
Adults: 100 to 200 mg P.O. q.i.d.

Food allergy –
Adults: 200 mg P.O. q.i.d. 15 to 20 minutes before meals. Dosage may be

doubled in 2 to 3 weeks if results are not satisfactory.
Children 2 to 13 years: 100 mg P.O. q.i.d. 15 to 20 minutes before meals. Dosage may be doubled in 2 to 3 weeks if results are not satisfactory. Do not exceed 40 mg/kg daily.
Children under 2 years: up to 20 mg/kg P.O. daily.
Inflammatory bowel disease –
Adults: 200 mg P.O. q.i.d. 15 to 20 minutes before meals.
Children 2 to 14 years: 100 mg P.O. q.i.d. 15 to 20 minutes before meals.

ADVERSE REACTIONS
Common reactions are in italics; life-threatening reactions are in bold italics.
CNS: dizziness, headache.
EENT: *irritation of the throat and trachea, cough,* ***bronchospasm after inhalation of dry powder;*** esophagitis; nasal congestion; pharyngeal irritation; wheezing.
GI: nausea.
GU: dysuria, urinary frequency.
Skin: rash, urticaria.
Other: joint swelling and pain, lacrimation, swollen parotid gland, ***angioedema,*** *eosinophilic pneumonia.*

INTERACTIONS
None significant.

NURSING CONSIDERATIONS
- *Contraindicated* in acute asthma attacks and status asthmaticus because the drug is useful only in preventing attacks.
- *Use cautiously* in coronary artery disease or history of cardiac arrhythmias.
- Should be discontinued if patient develops eosinophilic pneumonia.
- Capsule for inhalation not to be swallowed; insert capsule into inhaler provided; follow manufacturer's directions.
- Watch for recurrence of asthmatic symptoms when dosage is decreased, especially when corticosteroids are also used.
- Use only when acute episode has been controlled; airway is cleared; and patient is able to inhale.
- Teach correct use of Spinhaler: insert capsule in device properly, exhale completely before placing mouthpiece between lips, then inhale deeply and rapidly with a steady, even breath; remove inhaler from mouth, hold breath a few seconds, and then exhale. Repeat until all powder has been inhaled.
- Store capsules for inhalation at room temperature in a tightly closed container; protect from moisture and temperatures higher than 104° F(40° C).
- Instruct patient to avoid excessive handling of capsule for inhalation.
- Esophagitis may be relieved by antacids or a glass of milk.
- Don't confuse capsules for oral solution with capsules for inhalation.
- Powder in capsules for oral dose must be dissolved in hot water. May be further diluted with cold water before ingestion. Do not mix with fruit juice, milk, or food.
- Use of oral forms is still investigational.

diazoxide, oral
Proglycem
Pregnancy Risk Category: C

HOW SUPPLIED
Capsules: 50 mg
Oral suspension: 50 mg/ml in 30-ml bottle

MECHANISM OF ACTION
Inhibits the release of insulin from the pancreas and decreases peripheral utilization of glucose.

*Liquid form contains alcohol. **May contain tartrazine.

INDICATIONS & DOSAGE
Management of hypoglycemia from a variety of conditions resulting in hyperinsulinism –
Adults and children: 3 to 8 mg/kg P.O. daily, in three equally divided doses q 8 hours.
Infants and newborns: 8 to 15 mg/kg P.O. daily, in two or three equally divided doses q 8 to 12 hours.

ADVERSE REACTIONS
Common reactions are in italics; life-threatening reactions are in bold italics.
Blood: leukopenia, thrombocytopenia.
CV: arrhythmias.
EENT: diplopia.
GI: nausea, vomiting, anorexia, taste alteration.
Metabolic: sodium and fluid retention, ketoacidosis and hyperosmolar nonketotic syndrome, hyperuricemia.
Other: *severe hypertrichosis (hair growth) in 25% of adults and higher percentage of children.*

INTERACTIONS
Alpha-adrenergic blocking agents: antagonize inhibition of insulin release by diazoxide.
Anticoagulants: increased anticoagulant effect. Adjust dosage of anticoagulant.
Antigout agents: increased serum uric acid. Adjust dosage of antigout agent.
Antihypertensive agents, peripheral vasodilators: additive hypotensive effects.
Beta-adrenergic blocking agents: increased hypotensive effect.
Hydantoin anticonvulsants: decreased anticonvulsant effects and decreased hyperglycemic effect of diazoxide. Don't use together.
Thiazide diuretics: may potentiate hyperglycemic, hyperuricemic, and hypotensive effects. Monitor appropriate laboratory values.

NURSING CONSIDERATIONS
- *Contraindicated* in thiazide hypersensitivity and functional hypoglycemia.
- Oral diazoxide does not significantly lower blood pressure in dosages used to treat hypoglycemia.
- Most important use is in management of hypoglycemia from hyperinsulinism in infants and children.
- Monitor urine regularly for glucose and ketones; report any abnormalities to doctor.
- If not effective after 2 or 3 weeks, drug should be stopped.
- Reassure patient that hair growth on arms and forehead is a common adverse reaction that subsides when drug treatment is completed.
- Explain importance of following dietary restrictions for successful therapy.
- Advise patient to report any adverse reactions, including excessive thirst, fruity breath odor, or urinary frequency.

disulfiram
Antabuse, Cronetal, Ro-Sulfiram-500

Pregnancy Risk Category: X

HOW SUPPLIED
Tablets: 250 mg, 500 mg

MECHANISM OF ACTION
Blocks oxidation of alcohol at the acetaldehyde stage. Excess acetaldehyde produces a highly unpleasant reaction in the presence of even small amounts of alcohol.

INDICATIONS & DOSAGE
Adjunct in management of chronic alcoholism –
Adults: maximum of 500 mg P.O. q morning for 1 to 2 weeks. Can be taken in evening if drowsiness occurs. Maintenance: 125 to 500 mg P.O. daily (average dose 250 mg) until per-

manent self-control is established. Treatment may continue for months or years.

ADVERSE REACTIONS

Common reactions are in italics; life-threatening reactions are in bold italics.
CNS: drowsiness, headache, fatigue, delirium, depression, neuritis.
EENT: optic neuritis.
GI: metallic or garlic-like aftertaste.
GU: impotence.
Skin: acneiform or allergic dermatitis.
Other: peripheral neuritis; polyneuritis; disulfiram reaction, which may include flushing, throbbing headache, dyspnea, nausea, copious vomiting, sweating, thirst, chest pain, palpitations, hyperventilation, hypotension, syncope, anxiety, weakness, blurred vision, confusion. ***In severe reactions, respiratory depression, cardiovascular collapse, arrhythmias, myocardial infarction, acute CHF, seizures, unconsciousness, and even death can occur.***

INTERACTIONS

Alfentanil: prolonged duration of effect.
Anticoagulants: increased anticoagulant effect. Adjust dosage of anticoagulant.
Ascorbic acid: may interfere with disulfiram-alcohol interaction.
Bacampicillin: use with caution, because its metabolism produces low concentrations of alcohol and acetaldehyde.
CNS depressants: increased CNS depression.
Isoniazid (INH): ataxia or marked change in behavior. Don't use together.
Metronidazole: psychotic reaction. Do not use together.
Midazolam: increased plasma levels of midazolam.
Paraldehyde: toxic levels of the acetaldehyde. Don't use together.
Tricyclic antidepressants, especially amitriptyline: transient delirium.

NURSING CONSIDERATIONS

- *Contraindicated* in alcohol intoxication and within 12 hours of alcohol ingestion; in psychoses, myocardial disease, or coronary occlusion; in patients receiving metronidazole, paraldehyde, alcohol, or alcohol-containing preparations; and in pregnancy.
- *Use cautiously* in diabetes mellitus, hypothyroidism, seizure disorder, cerebral damage, nephritis, hepatic cirrhosis or insufficiency, abnormal EEG, and multiple drug dependence.
- Used only under close medical and nursing supervision. Never administer until patient has abstained from alcohol for at least 12 hours. Patient should clearly understand consequences of disulfiram therapy and give permission. Drug should be used only in patients who are cooperative, well motivated, and are receiving supportive psychiatric therapy.
- Complete physical examination and laboratory studies, including CBC, SMA-12, and transaminase, should precede therapy and be repeated regularly.
- Warn patient to avoid all sources of alcohol (for example, sauces and cough syrups). Even external application of liniments, shaving lotion, and back-rub preparations may precipitate disulfiram reaction. Tell him that alcohol reaction may occur as long as 2 weeks after single dosage of disulfiram; the longer the patient remains on drug, the more sensitive he will become to alcohol.
- Patient should wear a bracelet or carry a card supplied by drug manufacturer identifying him as disulfiram user.

Note: Mild reactions may occur in sensitive patients with blood alcohol level of 5 to 10 mg/100 ml; symptoms are fully developed at 50 mg/100 ml; unconsciousness usually occurs at 125

to 150 mg/100 ml level. Reaction may last half an hour to several hours, or as long as alcohol remains in blood.
- Caution patient's family that disulfiram should never be given to the patient without his knowledge; severe reaction or death could result if such a patient then ingested alcohol.
- Reassure patient that disulfiram-induced adverse reactions, such as drowsiness, fatigue, impotence, headache, peripheral neuritis, and metallic or garlic taste, subside after about 2 weeks of therapy.

etretinate

Tegison

Pregnancy Risk Category: X

HOW SUPPLIED

Capsules: 10 mg, 25 mg

MECHANISM OF ACTION

Unknown.

INDICATIONS & DOSAGE

Treatment of severe recalcitrant psoriasis, including the erythrodermic and generalized pustular types in patients unresponsive to standard therapy (topical tar plus UVB light, psoralens plus UVA light, systemic corticosteroids, and methotrexate) –

Adults: initially, 0.75 to 1 mg/kg P.O. daily in divided doses. Don't exceed maximum initial dose of 1.5 mg/kg daily. After initial response, begin maintenance dosage of 0.5 to 0.75 mg/kg daily (usually after 8 to 16 weeks).

ADVERSE REACTIONS

Common reactions are in italics; life-threatening reactions are in bold italics.

Blood: ***blood dyscrasias,*** anemia, altered prothrombin time.

CNS: *benign intracranial hypertension (pseudotumor cerebri), fatigue, headache,* dizziness, lethargy.

CV: thrombosis, edema.

EENT: *eye pain, sore tongue, chapped lips.*

GI: *appetite change, nausea, dry mouth.*

Hepatic: ***hepatitis,*** elevated liver enzymes.

GU: *white blood cells in urine,* proteinuria, hematuria.

Metabolic: *hypokalemia or hyperkalemia, hyperlipidemia.*

Skin: *peeling, itching.*

Other: *bone pain,* dyspnea, photosensitivity.

INTERACTIONS

Alcohol: increased risk of hypertriglyceridemia.

Hepatotoxic medications (including methotrexate): increased risk of hepatotoxicity.

Milk, high-fat diet: increases etretinate's absorption.

Tetracyclines: increased risk of pseudotumor cerebri.

Vitamin A: additive toxic effects. Avoid concomitant use.

NURSING CONSIDERATIONS

- *Contraindicated* in patients who are pregnant, who intend to become pregnant, or who may not use reliable contraception during and after treatment because drug causes severe birth defects.
- Women of childbearing age must not receive etretinate unless pregnancy is excluded by a pregnancy test within 2 weeks before initiating therapy. Therapy may begin on the 2nd or 3rd day of the next normal menstrual period.
- Patient should use effective contraception for 1 month before therapy begins, during treatment, and for an indefinite time after treatment is discontinued.
- Significant residual blood levels of etretinate have been reported as long as 2.9 years after discontinuation of treatment. Consequently, the period of time after treatment during which

pregnancy must be avoided to prevent teratogenicity is unknown.
• Sugarless gum or hard candy or ice may help relieve dry mouth. Check with dentist if this continues beyond 2 weeks.
• Monitor liver function tests at 1- to 2-week intervals for the first 1 to 2 months of therapy, and thereafter at intervals of 1 to 3 months. Suspected hepatotoxicity requires discontinuation of etretinate.
• Monitor blood lipids every 1 to 2 weeks during treatment.
• Tell patient to promptly report headache, nausea and vomiting, and visual disturbances (possible early signs of pseudotumor cerebri). These reactions require immediate check for papilledema. If present, discontinue drug immediately.
• Advise patient not to take vitamin A supplements to avoid possible additive adverse reactions.
• Reassure patient that transient exacerbation of psoriasis is common during the beginning of therapy.
• Advise patient to expect dry skin and possible difficulty tolerating contact lenses during treatment.
• Advise patient to take this drug with milk or fatty food to enhance absorption. Otherwise, patient should follow a low-fat diet.
• Patient should take a missed dose as soon as possible, with milk or fatty food. If it's nearly time for the next dose, he should skip the missed dose and resume schedule. Never double dose.
• May cause photosensitivity. Patient should avoid excess bright sun and use a sunscreen.
• If a decrease in night vision occurs, patient should contact doctor.
• Diabetic patients should monitor blood glucose closely. Adjustments of hypoglycemic medications may be necessary.

finasteride

Proscar

Pregnancy Risk Category: X

HOW SUPPLIED

Tablets: 5 mg

MECHANISM OF ACTION

Competitively inhibits steroid 5α-reductase, an enzyme responsible for formation of the potent androgen 5α-dihydrotestosterone (DHT) from testosterone. Because DHT influences development of the prostate gland, decreasing levels of this hormone in adult males should relieve the symptoms associated with benign prostatic hyperplasia (BPH).

INDICATIONS & DOSAGE

Symptomatic BPH –
Adults: 5 mg P.O. daily.

ADVERSE REACTIONS

Common reactions are in italics; life-threatening reactions are in bold italics.
GU: impotence, decreased volume of ejaculate.
Other: decreased libido.

INTERACTIONS

Theophylline: small, clinically insignificant increases in theophylline clearance and decreases in theophylline half-life (10%) have been observed.

NURSING CONSIDERATIONS

• *Contraindicated* in patients with hypersensitivity to the drug, in pregnant and breast-feeding women, and in children.
• *Use cautiously* in patients with hepatic dysfunction because drug is metabolized extensively in the liver. No dosage adjustments are necessary in renal impairment; decreased urinary excretion of metabolites is associated with increased excretion of metabolites in the feces.

*Liquid form contains alcohol. **May contain tartrazine.

• Crushed tablets shouldn't be handled by women who are or may become pregnant because of the risk of adverse effects on a male fetus.
• Although drug's elimination rate is decreased in elderly patients, dosage adjustments aren't necessary.
• Baseline and periodic digital rectal examinations are recommended. This drug will decrease serum prostate-specific antigen (PSA) levels, even in prostate cancer. However, in clinical trials, this drug didn't appear to decrease the rate of prostate cancer detection.
• Before therapy, closely evaluate patient for conditions that might mimic BPH, including hypotonic bladder, prostate cancer, infection, stricture, or relevant neurologic conditions.
• Because it's impossible to identify prospectively which patients will respond to finasteride, a minimum of 6 months of therapy may be necessary.
• Carefully monitor patients who have a large residual urine volume or severely diminished urine flow. Because not all patients respond to this drug, such patients may not be candidates for finasteride therapy.
• Long-term effects of this drug on the complications of BPH, including acute urinary obstruction, and the incidence of surgery are unknown.
• Sustained increases in serum PSA levels should be carefully evaluated in patients receiving finasteride therapy. This could indicate noncompliance with therapy.
• A patient whose sexual partner is or may become pregnant should take precautions to avoid exposing her to his semen or should discontinue the drug.
• Patients should understand that finasteride may decrease the volume of ejaculate but doesn't appear to impair normal sexual function. However, impotence and decreased libido have occurred in less than 4% of patients treated with this drug.
• Investigators are currently determining the drug's effectiveness as adjuvant therapy after radical prostatectomy; as adjuvant treatment of prostate cancer; and as treatment of male pattern baldness, acne, and hirsutism.

gallium nitrate
Ganite

Pregnancy Risk Category: C

HOW SUPPLIED
Injection: 25 mg/ml

MECHANISM OF ACTION
Precise mechanism unknown; the drug has no cytotoxic effects in animals. It appears to reduce hypercalcemia by inhibiting the resorption of bone and reducing bone turnover in patients with increased bone turnover.

INDICATIONS & DOSAGE
Treatment of symptomatic, unresponsive hypercalcemia caused by cancer–
Adults: 200 mg/m² I.V. daily for 5 consecutive days or until serum calcium is normal. Administer as a constant infusion over 24 hours. Lower doses (100 mg/m²) may be given to patients with mild hypercalcemia.

ADVERSE REACTIONS
Common reactions are in italics; life-threatening reactions are in bold italics.
Blood: anemia, leukopenia.
CNS: lethargy, confusion.
CV: tachycardia, lower extremity edema, decreased mean systolic and diastolic blood pressures.
GI: nausea and vomiting, diarrhea, constipation.
GU: ***acute renal failure,*** *increased BUN and creatinine levels.*
Respiratory: dyspnea, crackles and rhonchi, pulmonary infiltrates, pleural effusion.
Metabolic: *hypophosphatemia, hypo-*

calcemia, decreased serum bicarbonate.
Other: visual or hearing impairment, acute optic neuritis.

INTERACTIONS
Nephrotoxic drugs, such as aminoglycosides or amphotericin B: increased risk of nephrotoxicity. Avoid concomitant use.

NURSING CONSIDERATIONS
- *Contraindicated* in patients with severe renal impairment. Keep in mind the association of hypercalcemia with decreased renal function in cancer patients. This drug should *not* be used in patients with asymptomatic hypercalcemia (generally, serum calcium levels of < 12 mg/dl).
- Be sure the patient is adequately hydrated, either with oral fluids or I.V. saline, before using the drug and during the infusion. It is important to establish an adequate urine flow (2 liters per day) before treatment. Diuretic therapy is not recommended before the correction of hypovolemia. Avoid overhydration, especially in patients with decreased CV function.
- **I.V. use:** Dilute the daily dose in 1 liter of 0.9% sodium chloride injection or dextrose 5% in water. Because the drug contains no preservatives, discard the unused portion.
- Rapid I.V. infusion or dosage over 200 mg/m² may increase the risk of nephrotoxicity or cause nausea and vomiting.
- If patient requires treatment with a potentially nephrotoxic drug, such as an aminoglycoside, discontinue gallium nitrate therapy and continue hydration for several days after administration of the nephrotoxic drug. Monitor renal function closely.
- Monitor renal function, including intake and output and BUN and serum creatinine levels, during therapy. Discontinue the drug if serum creatinine rises above 2.5 mg/dl.
- Monitor serum calcium levels, and assess patient for signs of hypocalcemia (including a positive Chvostek's sign). If hypocalcemia occurs, discontinue the drug. Treatment of hypocalcemia may be required.
- Overdosage is usually treated with vigorous hydration, sometimes with diuretics, for 2 to 3 days. Carefully monitor the patient's intake and output and renal function. Short-term therapy with I.V. calcium may be needed.
- Transient hypophosphatemia is common. Patients may require oral phosphorus supplements.
- Advise patient to report hearing or vision problems.

isotretinoin
Accutane, Roaccutane‡

Pregnancy Risk Category: X

HOW SUPPLIED
Capsules: 10 mg, 20 mg, 40 mg

MECHANISM OF ACTION
Normalizes keratinization, reversibly decreases the size of sebaceous glands, and alters the composition of sebum to a less viscous form that's less likely to cause follicular plugging.

INDICATIONS & DOSAGE
Severe cystic acne unresponsive to conventional therapy –
Adults and adolescents: 0.5 to 2 mg/kg P.O. daily given in two divided doses and continued for 15 to 20 weeks.

ADVERSE REACTIONS
Common reactions are in italics; life-threatening reactions are in bold italics.
Blood: anemia, elevated platelet count.
CNS: headache, fatigue, *pseudotumor cerebri* (benign intracranial hypertension).

EENT: *conjunctivitis,* corneal deposits, dry eyes.
Endocrine: hyperglycemia.
GI: nonspecific GI symptoms, gum bleeding and inflammation.
Hepatic: elevated AST (SGOT), ALT (SPGT), and alkaline phosphatase.
Skin: *cheilosis, rash, dry skin,* peeling of palms and toes, skin infection, photosensitivity.
Other: *hypertriglyceridemia, musculoskeletal pain (skeletal hyperostosis),* thinning of hair.

INTERACTIONS
Abrasives, medicated soaps and cleansers, acne preparations containing peeling agents, topical alcohol preparations (including cosmetics, after-shave, cologne): cumulative irritation of skin or excessive drying of skin. Use together cautiously.
Alcohol: increased risk of hypertriglyceridemia.
Tetracyclines: increased risk of pseudotumor cerebri.
Vitamin A and vitamin supplements containing vitamin A: increase in isotretinoin's toxic effects. Don't use together without doctor's permission.

NURSING CONSIDERATIONS
- *Contraindicated* in women of childbearing age unless the patient has had a negative serum pregnancy test within 2 weeks before beginning therapy; will begin drug therapy on the 2nd or 3rd day of the next menstrual period; and will comply with stringent contraceptive measures for 1 month before therapy, during therapy, and for at least 1 month after therapy. *Severe fetal abnormalities may occur if used during pregnancy.*
- Also *contraindicated* in patients hypersensitive to parabens, which are used as preservatives.
- If used with other photosensitivity agents, may have additive effect. Tell patient to avoid prolonged exposure to the sun; use sunscreen.
- Tell patient to immediately report any visual disturbances and bone or skeletal pain.
- Patients who experience headache, nausea and vomiting, or visual disturbances should be screened for papilledema. Signs and symptoms of pseudotumor cerebri require immediate discontinuation of therapy and prompt neurologic intervention.
- Perform serum lipid studies and liver function tests before therapy begins and then at regular intervals until response to drug is established, usually about 4 weeks.
- Monitor blood glucose regularly.
- Monitor creatine phosphokinase levels in patients who undergo vigorous physical activity.
- Warn patient that contact lenses may feel uncomfortable during isotretinoin therapy.
- If a second course of therapy is needed, it shouldn't be started until at least 8 weeks after the completion of the first course because improvement may continue after withdrawal of the drug.
- Most adverse reactions appear to be dose-related, occurring at dosages greater than 1 mg/kg daily. They are generally reversible when therapy is discontinued or dosage is reduced.
- Advise patient to take drug with or shortly after meals to ensure adequate absorption.

levocarnitine (L-carnitine)
Carnitor, Vitacarn
Pregnancy Risk Category: B

HOW SUPPLIED
Tablets: 330 mg
Capsules: 250 mg
Oral liquid: 100 mg/ml

MECHANISM OF ACTION
Facilitates the transport of fatty acids into cellular mitochondria. The fatty acids are then used to produce energy.

INDICATIONS & DOSAGE
Primary systemic carnitine deficiency –
Adults: 990 mg (three tablets) P.O. b.i.d. or t.i.d. Alternatively, may give enteral liquid 10 to 30 ml (1 to 3 g) daily.
Children: 50 to 100 mg/kg/day P.O. in divided doses of either the tablet or enteral liquid form.

All dosages depend upon the clinical response. Higher dosages may be given. However, for children, the maximum dosage is 3 g/day.

ADVERSE REACTIONS
Common reactions are in italics; life-threatening reactions are in bold italics.
GI: *nausea, vomiting, cramps, diarrhea.*
Other: body odor.

INTERACTIONS
D,L-*carnitine (sold as vitamin B_T in vitamin stores):* inhibits levocarnitine and can cause deficiency.
Valproic acid: increased requirement for carnitine.

NURSING CONSIDERATIONS
- Monitor patient's tolerance during the first week of therapy and after increasing dosage.
- Monitor blood chemistries and plasma carnitine concentrations periodically, as well as vital signs and patient's overall clinical condition.
- May give enteral liquid alone or dissolved in drinks or liquid food.
- Space doses evenly every 3 to 4 hours if possible. Best to give with or after meals.
- Tell patient to consume enteral liquid slowly to minimize GI distress. If GI intolerance persists, dosage may have to be reduced.
- Warn patient to avoid so-called "vitamin B_T" in health food stores. This will interact with the drug and render it ineffective.
- Caution patient not to share drug with others. Some people have used it to improve athletic performance.
- The entire or partial contents of the containers of liquid should be used immediately after opening. Discard any unused contents of opened containers.
- Do not refrigerate solution.

masoprocol
Actinex
Pregnancy Risk Category: B

HOW SUPPLIED
Cream: 10%

MECHANISM OF ACTION
Unknown. The drug has antiproliferative activity against keratinocytes in vitro.

INDICATIONS & DOSAGE
Topical treatment of actinic (solar) keratoses –
Adults: apply a sufficient amount of cream to cover the area b.i.d. (in the morning and evening) for 28 days.

ADVERSE REACTIONS
Common reactions are in italics; life-threatening reactions are in bold italics.
EENT: eye irritation.
Skin: *erythema, flaking, dryness, itching, burning, soreness,* bleeding, crusting, oozing, rash, irritation, stinging, tightness, tingling.

INTERACTIONS
None reported.

NURSING CONSIDERATIONS
- *Contraindicated* in patients with hypersensitivity to the drug or any component of the formulation. The drug contains sulfites, which may precipitate allergic reactions in certain sensitive individuals.
- *Use cautiously* in areas near the eyes because drug may cause pain and burning if it comes into contact with

*Liquid form contains alcohol. **May contain tartrazine.

the eyes. If such contact occurs, rinse with plenty of water.

- Teach patient how to apply drug: wash and dry the area, then gently massage in the cream (avoiding the eyes and mucous membranes of the nose and mouth) until it's evenly distributed. Tell patient not to use occlusive dressings or to apply makeup or any other skin product without the doctor's approval.
- Local skin reactions are common but don't interfere with drug's effectiveness. Explain to patient that these reactions will clear within 2 weeks of discontinuing drug. However, if severe reactions occur, such as oozing or blistering, patient should discontinue using drug and contact doctor immediately.
- Instruct patient to wash his hands after applying drug with his fingers.
- Explain the importance of avoiding unnecessary exposure to the sun during treatment. Advise patient to wear protective clothing and use a sunscreen.

mesalamine

Rowasa

Pregnancy Risk Category: B

HOW SUPPLIED

Rectal suspension: 4 g/60 ml
Suppositories: 500 mg

MECHANISM OF ACTION

Exact mechanism unknown; mesalamine is one of the active metabolites of sulfasalazine. Probably acts topically by inhibiting prostaglandin production in the colon.

INDICATIONS & DOSAGE

Treatment of active mild to moderate distal ulcerative colitis, proctitis, or proctosigmoiditis –

Adults: 500 mg P.R. (suppository) b.i.d., or 1 rectal unit as a retention enema once daily (preferably h.s.). Drug should be retained overnight (for about 8 hours). Usual course of therapy is 3 to 6 weeks.

ADVERSE REACTIONS

Common reactions are in italics; life-threatening reactions are in bold italics.

CNS: headache, dizziness, fatigue, malaise.

GI: abdominal pain, cramps, discomfort, flatulence, diarrhea, rectal pain, bloating, nausea, *pancolitis.*

Skin: itching, rash, urticaria, hair loss.

Other: wheezing, ***anaphylaxis*** (rare), fever.

INTERACTIONS

None significant.

NURSING CONSIDERATIONS

- *Contraindicated* in patients sensitive to the drug or its components.
- *Use cautiously* in renal impairment. Problems have not been documented, but the nephrotoxic potential from absorbed mesalamine exists. Patients on long-term mesalamine therapy should have periodic renal function studies.
- Mesalamine may rarely cause allergic reactions in patients sensitive to sulfites, because it contains potassium metabisulfite.
- Instruct patient to carefully follow instructions supplied with medication.
- Patients intolerant of sulfasalazine may also be hypersensitive to mesalamine. Instruct these patients to discontinue drug if they have a fever or rash.

mesna

Mesnex

Pregnancy Risk Category: B

HOW SUPPLIED

Injection: 100 mg/ml

MECHANISM OF ACTION
Prevents ifosfamide-induced hemorrhagic cystitis by reacting with urotoxic ifosfamide metabolites.

INDICATIONS & DOSAGE
Prophylaxis of hemorrhagic cystitis in patients receiving ifosfamide –
Adults: dosage varies with amount of ifosfamide administered. Usual dosage is 240 mg/m² administered as an I.V. bolus with administration of ifosfamide. Repeat dosage at 4 hours and 8 hours after administration of ifosfamide.

ADVERSE REACTIONS
Common reactions are in italics; life-threatening reactions are in bold italics.

Note: Because it is used concomitantly with ifosfamide and other chemotherapeutic agents, it is difficult to determine adverse reactions attributable solely to mesna.
EENT: dysgeusia.
GI: soft stools, nausea, vomiting, diarrhea.

INTERACTIONS
None reported.

NURSING CONSIDERATIONS
- *Contraindicated* in patients with hypersensitivity to mesna or thiol-containing compounds. Not effective in preventing hematuria from other causes (such as thrombocytopenia). Although formulated to prevent hemorrhagic cystitis from ifosfamide, it will not protect against other toxicities associated with ifosfamide therapy.
- Monitor urine samples in patients receiving mesna for hematuria daily.
- Up to 6% of patients may not respond to the drug's protective effects.
- May interfere with diagnostic tests for urine ketones.
- **I.V. use:** Prepare I.V. solutions by diluting commercially available ampules with dextrose 5% in water solution, dextrose 5% and normal saline injection, normal saline injection, or lactated Ringer's solution.
- Diluted solutions are stable for 24 hours at room temperature, but they should be refrigerated after preparation and used within 6 hours. After the ampule is opened, any unused drug should be discarded because it decomposes quickly into an inactive compound.
- Mesna I.V. is incompatible with cisplatin.

methoxsalen
Oxsoralen**, Oxsoralen-Ultra
Pregnancy Risk Category: C

HOW SUPPLIED
Capsules: 10 mg**
Lotion: 1%

MECHANISM OF ACTION
May enhance melanogenesis, either directly or secondarily, to an inflammatory process.

INDICATIONS & DOSAGE
To induce repigmentation in vitiligo; psoriasis –
Adults and children over 12 years: 0.6 mg/kg P.O. 1.5 to 2 hours before measured periods of high-intensity long-wave ultraviolet exposure, 2 to 3 times weekly at least 48 hours apart.
Topical solution:
Apply to small, well-defined vitiliginous lesions and allow to dry (1 to 2 minutes) and reapply: 2 to 2.5 hours before measured periods of long-wave ultraviolet exposure. After exposure, wash lesions with soap and water. Protect area with opaque sunscreen. Although manufacturer recommends treatment weekly, some clinicians may treat q 3 to 5 days.

ADVERSE REACTIONS
Common reactions are in italics; life-threatening reactions are in bold italics.

*Liquid form contains alcohol. **May contain tartrazine.

CNS: nervousness, insomnia, depression, vertigo, headache.
GI: *discomfort, nausea, diarrhea.*
Skin: edema, erythema, painful blistering, burning, peeling, pruritus.

INTERACTIONS
Photosensitizing agents: do not use together. May increase toxicity.

NURSING CONSIDERATIONS
- *Contraindicated* in hepatic insufficiency, porphyria, acute lupus erythematosus, or hydromorphic and polymorphic light eruptions.
- *Use cautiously* in patients with familial history of sunlight allergy, GI diseases, and chronic infection.
- Regulate therapy carefully. Overdosage or overexposure to light can cause serious burning or blistering. Patients should avoid excessive sunlight during therapy.
- Drug should be taken with meals or milk. Patient should avoid the following foods: limes, figs, parsley, parsnips, mustard, carrots, and celery.
- During light exposure treatments, protect eyes and lips.
- Monthly liver function tests should be done on patients with vitiligo (especially at beginning of therapy).

minoxidil (topical)
Rogaine

Pregnancy Risk Category: C

HOW SUPPLIED
Topical solution: 2%

MECHANISM OF ACTION
Stimulation of hair growth may be related to dilation of arterial microcapillaries around hair follicles.

INDICATIONS & DOSAGE
Treatment of male or female pattern baldness (alopecia androgenetica) of the vertex and scalp –
Adults: apply 1 ml of 2% solution to affected area twice daily. Total daily dosage should not exceed 2 ml.

ADVERSE REACTIONS
Common reactions are in italics; life-threatening reactions are in bold italics.
CNS: headache, dizziness, faintness, light-headedness.
CV: edema, chest pain, increased or decreased blood pressure, palpitations, increased or decreased pulse rate.
EENT: sinusitis.
GU: urinary tract infections, renal calculi, urethritis.
Metabolic: edema, weight gain.
Respiratory: bronchitis, upper respiratory infection.
Skin: irritant dermatitis, allergic contact dermatitis, eczema, hypertrichosis, local erythema, pruritus, dry skin or scalp, flaking, alopecia, exacerbation of hair loss.
Other: back pain, tendinitis.

INTERACTIONS
Topical corticosteroids, petrolatum, topical retinoids, or other drugs that may enhance skin absorption: increased risk of systemic effects of minoxidil. Do not apply minoxidil with other drugs.

NURSING CONSIDERATIONS
- *Contraindicated* in patients with hypersensitivity to any component of the topical solution. Adverse effects are uncommon.
- Tell patient to avoid inhalation of any spray or mist from the drug. Avoid spraying around the eyes, because the solution contains alcohol and may be irritating.
- Patient needs to have a normal, healthy scalp before beginning therapy, because absorption of the drug through irritated skin may cause adverse systemic effects.
- Treatment with topical minoxidil is most likely to be successful in patients

with balding area smaller than 4″ (10 cm) within the last 10 years.

- Patients with a history of heart disease should be aware that this drug may exacerbate their illness.
- Teach patient to monitor pulse rate and body weight.
- Patients need medical follow-ups 1 month after initiation of therapy and every 6 months thereafter.
- Teach patient how to correctly apply topical minoxidil. Hair and scalp should be thoroughly dry before application, and the drug should not be applied to any other areas of the body. Patient should not use the drug on irritated or sunburned scalp, or with any other medication on the scalp. Tell patient to thoroughly wash his hands after application.
- Advise patient that therapy will be prolonged and will continue for at least 4 months before clinical effects appear. About 40% of patients will see moderate to dense hair growth.
- Discontinuing the drug may result in the loss of new hair growth. New hair growth is usually fine and may be colorless, but will resemble existing hair after continued treatment.

nedocromil sodium

Tilade

Pregnancy Risk Category: C

HOW SUPPLIED

Inhalation aerosol: 1.75 mg/activation

MECHANISM OF ACTION

Reduces inflammatory changes in the airway by blocking the release of mediators of inflammation, such as leukotrienes, histamine, and prostaglandins from mast cells, eosinophils, monocytes, neutrophils, macrophages, and other immune cells.

INDICATIONS & DOSAGE

Maintenance therapy in mild-to-moderate reversible obstructive airway disease –

Adults: 2 inhalations q.i.d., preferably at regular intervals.

ADVERSE REACTIONS

Common reactions are in italics; life-threatening reactions are in bold italics.

CNS: headache.

GI: nausea, vomiting.

Other: *unpleasant taste.*

INTERACTIONS

None reported.

NURSING CONSIDERATIONS

- *Contraindicated* in patients with hypersensitivity to the formulation or in patients with an acute asthmatic attack or acute bronchospasm.
- Be sure patient understands that nedocromil has no direct bronchodilating action. It shouldn't replace bronchodilators during an acute asthmatic attack.
- Nedocromil should be added to patient's regular bronchodilator regimen. This drug may reduce patient's need for corticosteroids or bronchodilators.
- Be sure patient understands how to use the inhaler. Emphasize that regular use of the drug will help him feel better. Most patients report benefits after 1 week of use; some require longer treatment before any improvement.
- In some patients, bronchospasm may be prevented by a single dose of the drug before activities that precipitate asthma, such as exercise or exposure to cold air, pollutants, or allergens.

nicotine polacrilex (nicotine resin complex)

Nicorette

Pregnancy Risk Category: X

HOW SUPPLIED

Chewing gum: 2 mg/square

MECHANISM OF ACTION

Stimulates receptors in the CNS and causes the release of catecholamines from the adrenal medulla.

INDICATIONS & DOSAGE

Temporary aid to the cigarette smoker seeking to give up smoking while participating in a behavior modification program under medical supervision – **Adults:** chew one piece of gum slowly and intermittently for 30 minutes whenever the urge to smoke occurs. Most patients require approximately 10 pieces of gum daily during the first month. Don't exceed 30 pieces of gum daily.

ADVERSE REACTIONS

Common reactions are in italics; life-threatening reactions are in bold italics.

CNS: dizziness, light-headedness.
CV: atrial fibrillation.
EENT: throat soreness, jaw muscle ache (from chewing).
GI: nausea, vomiting, indigestion.
Other: hiccups.

INTERACTIONS

None significant.

NURSING CONSIDERATIONS

- *Contraindicated* in nonsmokers, during the immediate postmyocardial infarction period; in life-threatening arrhythmias, severe or worsening angina pectoris, and active temporomandibular joint disease; or in pregnancy.
- *Use cautiously* in hyperthyroidism, pheochromocytoma, or insulin-dependent diabetes.
- Nicotine resin complex is the only smoking cessation aid that has been proven safe and effective.
- Smokers most likely to benefit from nicotine gum are those with a high "physical" nicotine dependence. Such smokers show the following characteristics: smoke more than 15 cigarettes daily; prefer brands of cigarettes with high nicotine levels; usually inhale the smoke; smoke the first cigarette within 30 minutes of arising; find the first morning cigarette the hardest to give up; smoke most frequently during the morning; find it difficult to refrain from smoking in places where it's forbidden; or smoke even when they are so ill that they are confined to bed during the day.
- Instruct patient to chew gum slowly and intermittently (chew several times, then place between cheek and gums) for about 30 minutes to promote slow and even buccal absorption of nicotine. Fast chewing tends to produce more adverse reactions.
- Successful abstainers will begin gradually withdrawing gum usage after 3 months. Use of the gum for longer than 6 months is not recommended. For gradual withdrawal, cut gum in halves or quarters and mix with other sugar-free gum.
- Emphasize the importance of withdrawing the gum gradually.
- The gum is sugar-free and usually doesn't stick to dentures.
- Patient who stops smoking may require dosage adjustments of propoxyphene, propranolol, beta-blocking agents, and xanthine bronchodilators because decreased metabolism of these agents may increase their therapeutic effects.
- A patient instruction sheet is included in the package dispensed to the patient.

nicotine transdermal system

Habitrol, Nicoderm, Prostep

Pregnancy Risk Category: D

HOW SUPPLIED

Transdermal system: designed to release nicotine at a fixed rate.
Habitrol – 21 mg/day, 14 mg/day, 11 mg/day
Nicoderm – 21 mg/day, 14 mg/day, 11 mg/day
Prostep – 22 mg/day, 11 mg/day

MECHANISM OF ACTION

Provides nicotine, the chief alkaloid found in tobacco products, which stimulates nicotinic acetylcholine receptors in the CNS, neuromuscular junction, autonomic ganglia, and adrenal medulla.

INDICATIONS & DOSAGE

Relief of nicotine withdrawal symptoms in patients undergoing smoking cessation –
Adults: 1 transdermal patch applied to a nonhairy part of the upper trunk or upper outer arm. After 24 hours, the patch should be removed and a new one applied to a different site. Dosage varies slightly with product selected.
Nicoderm, Habitrol – initially, apply 1 21-mg/day patch daily for 6 weeks. Then, taper dosage to 14 mg/day for 2 to 4 weeks. Finally, taper dosage to 7 mg/day if necessary. Nicotine substitution and gradual withdrawal should take 8 to 12 weeks. Patients who weigh under 100 lb (45.5 kg), patients who have cardiovascular disease, and those who smoke less than half a pack of cigarettes per day should start therapy with the 14-mg/day system.
Prostep – initially, apply 1 22-mg/day patch daily for 4 to 8 weeks. Patients who weigh under 100 lb should start therapy with the 11-mg/day system. Those who have successfully stopped smoking during this period may discontinue the drug. If therapy was initiated with the 22-mg/day system, patient may be treated for an additional 2 to 4 weeks at the lower dosage (11 mg/day). Nicotine substitution and gradual withdrawal should take 6 to 12 weeks.

ADVERSE REACTIONS

Common reactions are in italics; life-threatening reactions are in bold italics.
CNS: somnolence, dizziness, *headache, insomnia.*
EENT: pharyngitis, sinusitis.
GI: abdominal pain, constipation, dyspepsia, nausea.
GU: dysmenorrhea.
Skin: *erythema, pruritus, burning at application site, local erythema,* cutaneous hypersensitivity, rash, sweating.
Other: back pain, myalgia.

INTERACTIONS

Acetaminophen, caffeine, imipramine, oxazepam, pentazocine, propranolol, theophylline: cessation of smoking may decrease induction of hepatic enzymes responsible for metabolizing certain drugs. Dosage reduction may be necessary.
Adrenergic agonists (such as isoproterenol or phenylephrine): cessation of smoking may decrease circulating catecholamines. Dosage increase may be necessary.
Adrenergic antagonists (such as prazosin or labetalol): cessation of smoking may decrease circulating catecholamines. Dosage reduction may be necessary.
Insulin: cessation of smoking may increase amount of subcutaneous insulin absorbed. Dosage reduction may be necessary.

NURSING CONSIDERATIONS

- *Contraindicated* in patients with hypersensitivity to nicotine or any component of the transdermal system.
- *Use with extreme caution* and only after educational and behavioral interventions have failed in patients with recent MI, serious arrhythmias, or worsening angina pectoris or during pregnancy.
- *Use cautiously* in elderly patients and those with renal or hepatic insufficiency, endocrine disease, peptic ulcer disease, or hypertension.
- Because nicotine can be addictive and toxic, use cautiously in all patients. The risks of nicotine administration must be weighed against the hazards associated with patient's likelihood of continued smoking while using the transdermal system. Patients should be warned not to smoke. If they continue to smoke while using the system, they may experience adverse effects because peak serum nicotine levels will be substantially higher than those achieved by smoking alone.
- Health care workers' exposure to the nicotine within the transdermal systems is probably minimal; however, avoid unnecessary contact with the system. Wash hands with water alone because soap can enhance absorption.
- Tell patient to immediately discontinue use of the patch and contact the doctor is he experiences persistent or severe local skin reactions (pruritus, edema, or erythema) or a generalized rash.
- Use of the transdermal system for more than 3 months should be discouraged. Chronic nicotine consumption by any route can be dangerous and habit-forming.
- Patients who cannot stop cigarette smoking during the initial 4 weeks of therapy will probably not benefit from the continued use of the drug. Patients who were unsuccessful may benefit from counseling to identify factors that led to treatment failure. Encourage patient to minimize or eliminate the factors that contributed to treatment failure and to try again, possibly after some interval before the next attempt.
- Patients should understand that the nicotine can evaporate from the transdermal system once it is removed from its protective packaging. The patch should not be altered in any way (folded or cut) before it is applied. Apply promptly after removing the system from its protective packaging. Do not store in temperatures above 86° F (30° C).
- Teach patient proper disposal of the transdermal system. After removal, fold the patch in half, bringing the adhesive sides together. If the system comes in a protective pouch, place the used patch in the pouch that contained the new system. Careful disposal is necessary to prevent accidental poisoning of children or pets.
- Drug therapy alone is usually not sufficient to wean patients from use of tobacco. Better results may be obtained when patient receives behavior modification therapy.
- Patient information is dispensed with the drug at the time the prescription is filled. Be sure that patient reads and understands this material.

olsalazine sodium

Dipentum

Pregnancy Risk Category: C

HOW SUPPLIED

Capsules: 250 mg

MECHANISM OF ACTION

After oral administration, converted to 5-aminosalicylic acid (5-ASA or mesalamine) in the colon. Acts as a local anti-inflammatory agent in the colon.

INDICATIONS & DOSAGE
Maintenance of remission of ulcerative colitis in patients intolerant of sulfasalazine –
Adults: 500 mg P.O. b.i.d. with meals.

ADVERSE REACTIONS
Common reactions are in italics; life-threatening reactions are in bold italics.
CNS: headache, depression, vertigo, dizziness.
GI: *diarrhea,* nausea, abdominal pain, heartburn.
Skin: rash, itching.
Other: arthralgia.

INTERACTIONS
None reported.

NURSING CONSIDERATIONS
- *Contraindicated* in patients hypersensitive to salicylates.
- *Use cautiously* in patients with preexisting renal disease. Regularly monitor BUN and creatinine levels and urinalysis in these patients. Although problems have not been reported for this drug, the possibility of renal tubular damage from absorbed mesalamine or its metabolites must be considered.
- Clinical trials showed that 17% of all patients reported diarrhea sometime during therapy. Although diarrhea appears dose-related, it is difficult to distinguish from a worsening of the symptoms of the disease. Exacerbation of the disease has been noted with similar drugs.
- Teach the patient to take the drug in evenly divided doses, with food.

pamidronate disodium
Aredia
Pregnancy Risk Category: C

HOW SUPPLIED
Injection: 30 mg/vial

MECHANISM OF ACTION
An antihypercalcemic agent that inhibits the resorption of bone. Adsorbs to hydroxyapatite crystals in bone and may directly block dissolution of calcium phosphate. Drug apparently doesn't inhibit bone formation or mineralization.

INDICATIONS & DOSAGE
Moderate to severe hypercalcemia associated with cancer (with or without metastases) –
Adults: dosage depends on severity of hypercalcemia. Serum calcium levels should be corrected (CCa) for serum albumin:

$$\text{Corrected serum calcium (CCa) (in mg/dl)} = \text{serum calcium (in mg/dl)} + 0.8\,(4 - \text{serum albumin (in g/dl)})$$

Patients with moderate hypercalcemia (CCa levels of 12 to 13.5 mg/dl) may receive 60 to 90 mg by I.V. infusion over 24 hours. Patients with severe hypercalcemia (CCa levels over 13.5 mg/dl) may receive 90 mg as the initial dose.

ADVERSE REACTIONS
Common reactions are in italics; life-threatening reactions are in bold italics.
Blood: *anemia.*
CNS: ***seizures.***
CV: *fluid overload, hypertension.*
GI: *abdominal pain, anorexia, constipation, nausea, vomiting.*
GU: *urinary tract infection.*
Local: *redness, swelling, redness, pain.*
Other: *hypophosphatemia, hypokalemia, hypomagnesemia, hypocalcemia, bone pain, fever.*

INTERACTIONS
Calcium-containing solutions: precipitate formation. Don't mix together.

NURSING CONSIDERATIONS
- *Contraindicated* in patients with hypersensitivity to the drug or other bi-

phosphonates, such as etidronate. *Use with extreme caution* and consider the risks and benefits in patients with renal impairment.

• Drug should be used only after patient has been vigorously hydrated with sodium chloride solution. In patients with mild to moderate hypercalcemia, hydration alone may be sufficient.

• Because drug can cause electrolyte disturbances, careful monitoring of serum electrolytes (especially calcium, phosphate,and magnesium) is essential. Short-term administration of calcium may be necessary in patients with severe hypocalcemia. Also monitor creatinine, CBC, differential, hematocrit, and hemoglobin levels.

• Patients with preexisting anemia, leukopenia, or thrombocytopenia should be carefully monitored during the first 2 weeks after therapy.

• Monitor patient's temperature. In clinical trials, 27% of patients experienced an elevation of 1° C for 24 to 48 hours after therapy.

• **I.V. use:** Reconstitute vial with 10 ml sterile water for injection. Once drug is completely dissolved, add to 1,000 ml 0.45% or 0.9% sodium chloride injection or dextrose 5% in water. Do not mix with infusion solutions that contain calcium, such as Ringer's injection or lactated Ringer's injection. Visually inspect for precipitate before administering.

• Solution is stable for 24 hours at room temperature. Give only by I.V. infusion. Animal studies have shown evidence of nephropathy when drug is given as a bolus.

pentoxifylline

Trental

Pregnancy Risk Category: C

HOW SUPPLIED

Tablets (extended-release): 400 mg

MECHANISM OF ACTION

Improves capillary blood flow by increasing erythrocyte flexibility and lowering blood viscosity.

INDICATIONS & DOSAGE

Treatment of intermittent claudication caused by chronic occlusive vascular disease –

Adults: 400 mg P.O. t.i.d. with meals.

ADVERSE REACTIONS

Common reactions are in italics; life-threatening reactions are in bold italics.

CNS: headache, dizziness.

GI: dyspepsia, nausea, vomiting.

INTERACTIONS

Anticoagulants: increased anticoagulant effect.

Antihypertensives: increased hypotensive effect. Dosage adjustments may be necessary.

NURSING CONSIDERATIONS

• *Contraindicated* in patients who are intolerant to methylxanthines such as caffeine, theophylline, and theobromine.

• Pentoxifylline should be taken for a minimum of 8 weeks to achieve clinical effects. Tell patient not to discontinue the drug during this period unless directed by doctor.

• Advise patient to take with meals to minimize GI upset.

• Patient should report any GI or CNS adverse reactions. Doctor may reduce dosage.

• Pentoxifylline therapy is useful in patients who are not good surgical candidates.

• Patient should avoid smoking because nicotine causes vasoconstriction that can worsen the condition.

• Patient should swallow medication whole, without breaking, crushing, or chewing.

• Elderly patients may be more sensitive to this drug's effects.

ritodrine hydrochloride

Yutopar

Pregnancy Risk Category: B

HOW SUPPLIED

Tablets: 10 mg
Injection: 10-mg/ml, 15-mg/ml ampules

MECHANISM OF ACTION

A beta-receptor agonist that stimulates the $beta_2$-adrenergic receptors in uterine smooth muscle, inhibiting contractility.

INDICATIONS & DOSAGE

Management of preterm labor –
Women: dilute 150 mg (3 ampules) in 500 ml of fluid, yielding a final concentration of 0.3 mg/ml. Usual initial dose is 0.1 mg/minute I.V., to be gradually increased according to the results by 0.05 mg/minute q 10 minutes until desired result obtained. Effective dosage usually ranges from 0.15 to 0.35 mg/minute.

Note: I.V. infusion should be continued for 12 to 24 hours after contractions have stopped. Oral maintenance: 1 tablet (10 mg) may be given approximately 30 minutes before termination of I.V. therapy. Usual dosage for first 24 hours of maintenance is 10 mg P.O. q 2 hours. Thereafter, usual dosage is 10 to 20 mg P.O. q 4 to 6 hours. Total daily dosage should not exceed 120 mg.

ADVERSE REACTIONS

Common reactions are in italics; life-threatening reactions are in bold italics.
I.V.:
CNS: nervousness, anxiety, headache.
CV: *dose-related alterations in blood pressure, palpitations,* ***pulmonary edema,*** *tachycardia,* ECG changes.
GI: nausea, vomiting.
Metabolic: *hyperglycemia,* hypokalemia.
Other: erythema.
Oral:
CNS: tremors, nervousness.
CV: palpitations.
GI: nausea, vomiting.
Skin: rash.

INTERACTIONS

Beta-adrenergic blockers: may inhibit ritodrine's action. Avoid concurrent administration.
Corticosteroids: may produce pulmonary edema in mother. When these drugs are used concomitantly, monitor closely.
Inhalational anesthetics: potentiated adverse cardiac effects, arrhythmias, hypotension.
Sympathomimetics: additive effects. Use together cautiously.

NURSING CONSIDERATIONS

- *Contraindicated* before 20th week of pregnancy and in the following conditions: antepartum hemorrhage, eclampsia, intrauterine fetal death, chorioamnionitis, maternal cardiac disease, pulmonary hypertension, maternal hyperthyroidism, or uncontrolled maternal diabetes mellitus.
- **I.V. use:** Because cardiovascular responses are common and more pronounced during I.V. administration, cardiovascular effects – including maternal pulse rate and blood pressure, and fetal heart rate – should be closely monitored. A maternal tachycardia of over 140 beats/minute or persistent respiratory rate of over 20 breaths/minute may be a sign of impending pulmonary edema.
- Monitor amount of fluids administered I.V., to prevent circulatory overload.
- Don't use ritodrine I.V. if solution is discolored or contains a precipitate.
- Monitor blood glucose concentrations during ritodrine infusions, especially in diabetic mothers.
- Discontinue drug if pulmonary edema develops.

*Liquid form contains alcohol. **May contain tartrazine.

• Drug's effectiveness in preterm labor is currently being reviewed by the FDA.

sodium benzoate and sodium phenylacetate

Ucephan

Pregnancy Risk Category: C

HOW SUPPLIED

Oral solution: 10 g sodium benzoate and 10 g sodium phenylacetate per 100 ml

MECHANISM OF ACTION

Activates metabolic pathways that are ineffective in patients with urea cycle enzymopathies, resulting in decreased ammonia formation.

INDICATIONS & DOSAGE

Prevention or treatment of hyperammonemia in patients with urea cycle enzymopathy –

Children: 2.5 ml/kg P.O. daily in three to six equally divided doses. Total daily dosage should not exceed 100 ml.

ADVERSE REACTIONS

Common reactions are in italics; life-threatening reactions are in bold italics.

GI: nausea and vomiting.

INTERACTIONS

Penicillin, probenecid: may impair renal excretion of conjugated metabolites.

NURSING CONSIDERATIONS

• *Contraindicated* in patients with hypersensitivity to sodium benzoate or sodium phenylacetate.

• *Use cautiously* in neonates with hyperbilirubinemia.

• Benzoic acid may compete with bilirubin for binding sites on serum albumin.

• Not intended as sole therapy for patients with urea cycle enzymopathies. Most effective when combined with dietary modification (low-protein diet) and amino acid supplementation.

• Dilute each dose in 4 to 8 oz of infant formula or milk and administer with meals. Inspect the mixture for compatibility if other liquids are used. The drug may precipitate in some solutions (especially acidic solutions like fruit juice), depending upon concentration and pH.

• Carefully measure the required dosage because the stock solution is very concentrated (10 g of sodium benzoate and 10 g of sodium phenylacetate per 100 ml).

• Avoid getting the solution on skin or clothing. The lingering odor of the drug may be offensive.

• Benzoic acid is structurally similar to salicylates.

• Watch for adverse reactions associated with salicylates, including mild respiratory alkalosis and exacerbation of peptic ulcers.

sumatriptan succinate

Imitrex

Pregnancy Risk Category: C

HOW SUPPLIED

Injection: 6 mg/0.5 ml (12 mg/ml) in 0.5-ml prefilled syringes and vials

MECHANISM OF ACTION

Selectively activates vascular serotonin (5-hydroxytryptamine, 5-HT) receptors. The specific receptor subtype, 5-HT_1, is present on cranial arteries and the dura mater. Receptor stimulation causes vasoconstriction of these cerebral vessels but has minimal effects on systemic vessels, tissue perfusion, and blood pressure.

INDICATIONS & DOSAGE

Acute migraine attacks (with or without aura) –

Adults: 6 mg S.C. May be repeated after a minimum of 1 hour. Maximum recommended dosage is two 6-mg injections daily.

ADVERSE REACTIONS

Common reactions are in italics; life-threatening reactions are in bold italics.

CNS: *dizziness, vertigo,* drowsiness, headache, anxiety, malaise, fatigue, weakness.

CV: ***atrial fibrillation, ventricular fibrillation, ventricular tachycardia, MI, ECG changes such as ischemic ST-segment elevation*** (rare).

EENT: discomfort of the throat, nasal cavity or sinus, mouth, jaw, or tongue; visual alterations.

GI: abdominal discomfort, dysphagia.

Skin: local reactions, flushing.

Other: *tingling; warm or hot sensation; burning sensation; heaviness, pressure or tightness;* feeling strange; tight feeling in head; cold sensation; pressure or tightness in chest; neck pain; myalgia; muscle cramps; sweating.

INTERACTIONS

Ergot and ergot derivatives: prolonged vasospastic effects. Don't use these drugs and sumatriptan within 24 hours of each other.

NURSING CONSIDERATIONS

- *Contraindicated* in patients with hypersensitivity to the drug; in patients with ischemic heart disease, such as angina pectoris, Prinzmetal's angina, history of MI, or documented silent ischemia; in those with hypertension; in those taking ergotamine; and in patients with hemiplegic or basilar migraine.
- *Use cautiously* in patients who may have unrecognized coronary artery disease (CAD), such as postmenopausal women; male patients over age 40; or those with risk factors such as hypertension, hypercholesterolemia, obesity, diabetes, smoking, or a family history of CAD.
- Serious adverse cardiac effects can follow a dose of this drug, but such events are extremely rare. When giving the drug to patients at risk for unrecognized CAD, consider administering the first dose in the doctor's office.
- Onset of pain relief is often rapid (within 10 minutes). In clinical trials, up to 70% of patients experienced relief within 1 hour and 82% within 2 hours.
- Although patients may receive a second dose after a minimum of 1 hour, studies haven't confirmed benefit from this second dose.
- An information leaflet about therapy with this drug is available for the patient.
- Drug is available in a spring-loaded injector system that facilitates self-administration by the patient. Detailed patient information is available with the system; however, it's advisable to review this information with patient. Be sure patient understands how to load the injector, administer the injection, and dispose of the used syringes.
- Be sure patient understands that drug is intended only as a treatment for a migraine attack, not to prevent or reduce the number of attacks.
- Tell female patients not to use this drug when they are pregnant or intending to become pregnant. Advise them to discuss with the doctor the risks and benefits of using the drug during pregnancy.
- Patients should understand that drug may be given at any time during a migraine attack, preferably as soon as symptoms appear.
- Tell patient to call doctor immediately if he feels persistent or severe chest pain. If he feels pain or tightness in the throat or has wheezing; heart throbbing; swelling of the eyelids, face, or lips; or a rash, lumps, or hives, he should stop using the drug and call the doctor.

• Redness or pain at the injection site should subside within 1 hour after the injection.
• Drug has been used investigationally to treat cluster headaches.

ticlopidine hydrochloride

Ticlid

Pregnancy Risk Category: B

HOW SUPPLIED
Tablets: 250 mg

MECHANISM OF ACTION
An antiplatelet agent that blocks adenosine diphosphate (ADP)-induced platelet-fibrinogen and platelet-platelet binding.

INDICATIONS & DOSAGE
To reduce the risk of thrombotic stroke in patients with a history of stroke or who have experienced stroke precursors –
Adults: 250 mg P.O. b.i.d. with meals.

ADVERSE REACTIONS
Common reactions are in italics; life-threatening reactions are in bold italics.
Blood: neutropenia, ***pancytopenia, hemolytic anemia, immune thrombocytopenia,*** *increased serum cholesterol levels.*
CNS: dizziness, anorexia.
CV: ***vasculitis.***
EENT: epistaxis, conjunctival hemorrhage.
GI: diarrhea, *nausea, dyspepsia,* vomiting, flatulence, *pain,* bleeding.
GU: hematuria, ***nephrotic syndrome.***
Respiratory: ***allergic pneumonitis.***
Skin: *rash,* purpura, pruritus, ecchymosis, maculopapular rash, urticaria, thrombocytopenic thrombotic purpura.
Other: allergic reactions, postoperative bleeding, systemic lupus erythematosus, ***serum sickness,*** arthropathy, hepatitis, cholestatic jaundice, myositis, ***hyponatremia,*** peripheral neuropathy.

INTERACTIONS
Antacids: decreased plasma levels of ticlopidine. Separate administration times by at least 2 hours.
Aspirin: ticlopidine potentiates aspirin's effects on platelets. Avoid concomitant use.
Cimetidine: decreased clearance of ticlopidine and increased risk of toxicity. Avoid concomitant use.
Digoxin: slight decrease in serum digoxin levels. Monitor serum digoxin levels.
Theophylline: decreased theophylline clearance and risk of toxicity. Monitor closely and adjust theophylline dosage as ordered.

NURSING CONSIDERATIONS
• *Contraindicated* in patients with hypersensitivity to the drug; in patients with hematopoietic disorders, such as neutropenia, thrombocytopenia, or disorders of hemostasis; in patients with active pathologic bleeding, such as peptic ulcer or active intracranial bleeding; and in those with severe liver impairment.
• *Use cautiously* and with close monitoring of CBC and WBC differentials. Moderate to severe neutropenia and agranulocytosis have occurred in patients taking ticlopidine, usually within the first 3 weeks to 3 months of therapy. CBC and WBC differential determinations must be made beginning the second week of therapy and repeated every 2 weeks until the end of the third month of therapy. Increase the frequency of tests in any patient showing signs of declining neutrophil count or if the count is 30% less than baseline. After the first 3 months of therapy, CBC and WBC differential determinations need to be performed only in patients showing signs of infection.
• Thrombocytopenia has occurred

rarely. Drug should be discontinued in patients with platelet counts of 80,000 cells/mm³ or less. If necessary, methylprednisolone 20 mg I.V. can be given to normalize the bleeding time within 2 hours. Platelet transfusions may also be used.

- If ticlopidine is being substituted for a fibrinolytic or anticoagulant drug, discontinue those drugs before starting ticlopidine therapy.
- Patients should discontinue drug 10 to 14 days before undergoing elective surgery.
- Perform baseline liver function tests and repeat whenever liver dysfunction is suspected. Monitor closely, especially during the first 4 months of treatment.
- Stress the importance of regular blood tests. Neutropenia can result in an increased risk of infection. Tell patient to immediately report any signs of infection, such as fever, chills, or sore throat.
- Several other types of adverse reactions should also be reported immediately: yellow skin or sclera, severe or persistent diarrhea, skin rashes, subcutaneous bleeding, light-colored stools, or dark urine.
- Explain to patient that drug will increase bleeding time. Any unusual or prolonged bleeding should be reported. Advise patient to tell dentists and other doctors that he is taking ticlopidine.
- Tell patient to avoid aspirin and aspirin-containing products. Because many OTC medications contain aspirin, patient should not take these drugs without first checking with the doctor or pharmacist.
- Tell patient to take drug with meals. Taking drug with food substantially increases bioavailability and improves GI tolerance.
- Ticlopidine has been investigated for use in many conditions, including intermittent claudication, chronic arterial occlusion, subarachnoid hemorrhage, primary glomerulonephritis, and sickle cell disease. When used preoperatively, it may decrease the incidence of graft occlusion in patients receiving coronary artery bypass grafts and reduce the severity of the dropin platelet count in patients receiving extracorporeal hemoperfusion during open heart surgery.

tiopronin

Thiola

Pregnancy Risk Category: C

HOW SUPPLIED

Tablets: 100 mg

MECHANISM OF ACTION

Forms a water-soluble chemical complex with cysteine in the urine, increasing cysteine solubility and preventing the formation of urinary cysteine stones.

INDICATIONS & DOSAGE

Prevention of urinary cysteine stone formation in patients with severe homozygous cysteinuria (urinary cysteine excretion exceeding 500 mg/day) unresponsive to other therapies –

Adults: 800 mg P.O. daily, divided t.i.d.

Children: 15 mg/kg P.O. daily, divided t.i.d.

ADVERSE REACTIONS

Common reactions are in italics; life-threatening reactions are in bold italics.

EENT: hypogeusia.

Skin: rash, pruritus, wrinkling and friability.

Other: drug fever, lupus erythematous-like reaction.

INTERACTIONS

None reported.

NURSING CONSIDERATIONS

- *Contraindicated* in patients with a history of agranulocytosis, aplastic

anemia, or thrombocytopenia with tiopronin therapy.
- Dosage is usually adjusted to keep urine cysteine levels below 250 mg/liter.
- Conservative measures to treat cysteinuria should be attempted before tiopronin is administered. Patients should drink at least 3 liters of fluid daily, including at least two 8-oz glasses of water at each meal and at bedtime. Patient's urine output should be at least 3 liters daily, and urine pH should be 6.5 to 7. Excessive alkalization of urine may precipitate calcium stones. Urine pH should not exceed 7.
- Whenever possible, tiopronin should be administered at least 1 hour before or 2 hours after meals.
- Routine monitoring tests are recommended at 3- to 6-month intervals during treatment, including CBC, platelet counts, hemoglobin, serum albumin, liver functions tests, 24-hour urine protein, and routine urinalysis.
- Urine cysteine should be frequently monitored during the first 6 months of treatment (to identify optimal dosage level) and then at least every 6 months.
- An abdominal X-ray is advised annually to assess for the presence of stones.
- Tell patient to report any signs or symptoms of hematologic abnormalities, including fever, sore throat, bleeding or bruising, and chills. Blood dyscrasias have been reported in patients receiving other drugs for cysteinuria.
- Rare complications seen with other drugs used to treat cysteinuria include Goodpasture's syndrome (evidenced by abnormal urine findings, pulmonary infiltrates, and hemoptysis), myasthenia (evidenced by severe muscle weakness), and pemphigus-like reactions (bullous skin eruptions).
- Drug fever may develop, especially during the first month of therapy. Discontinue drug until fever subsides, then therapy will probably be reinstituted at lower dosages.
- Skin rashes have been noted with tiopronin therapy. A generalized rash with mild pruritus that develops in the first few months of therapy may be controlled with antihistamines, and disappears after discontinuing the drug. A less common rash that appears after at least 6 months of therapy appears on the trunk and is accompanied by intense pruritus. This form of rash disappears slowly after discontinuing the drug.
- Some clinicians prefer to use penicillamine for cysteinuria therapy, but patients may not tolerate it well. Studies indicate about two-thirds of patients who cannot tolerate penicillamine will tolerate tiopronin.

tretinoin (vitamin A acid, retinoic acid)

Retin-A, StieVAA†

Pregnancy Risk Category: B

HOW SUPPLIED

Cream: 0.025%, 0.05%, 0.1%
Gel: 0.025%, 0.01%
Solution: 0.05%

MECHANISM OF ACTION

Inhibits comedones by increasing epidermal cell mitosis and turnover.

INDICATIONS & DOSAGE

Acne vulgaris (especially grades I, II, and III), treatment of fine wrinkles from photodamaged skin –
Adults and children: cleanse affected area and lightly apply solution once daily h.s.

ADVERSE REACTIONS

Common reactions are in italics; life-threatening reactions are in bold italics.
Skin: *feeling of warmth, slight stinging, local erythema, peeling,* chap-

ping, swelling, blistering, crusting, temporary hyperpigmentation or hypopigmentation.

INTERACTIONS

Topical preparations containing sulfur, resorcinol, or salicylic acid: increased risk of skin irritation. Don't use together.

NURSING CONSIDERATIONS

- *Contraindicated* in hypersensitivity to any tretinoin component. *Use cautiously* in eczema.
- Avoid contact with eyes, mouth, and mucous membranes.
- Cleanse area thoroughly before application.
- May cause transient exacerbation of inflammatory lesions; it's not necessary to discontinue the drug. If severe local irritation develops, discontinue temporarily and readjust dosage when application is resumed.
- Some redness and scaling are normal reactions.
- Beneficial effects should be seen within 6 weeks of treatment.
- Relapses generally occur within 3 to 6 weeks after treatment.
- Patient should wash face with a mild soap no more than two or three times a day. Warn against using strong or medicated cosmetics, soaps, or other skin cleansers. Patient should also avoid topical products containing alcohol, astringents, spices, and lime since these may interfere with drug.
- Exposure to sunlight or ultraviolet rays should be minimal during treatment. If patient is sunburned, delay therapy until sunburn subsides.
- Patient who can't avoid exposure to sunlight should use a SPF 15 sunscreen and wear protective clothing.
- Patient may experience increased sensitivity to wind or cold temperatures.
- No medicated cosmetics may be used.

102
Investigational drugs

amsacrine
azacytidine
domperidone
enoxaparin sodium
felbamate
flunarizine hydrochloride
halofantrine
hexoprenaline sulfate
ketotifen fumarate
metformin
mifepristone
semustine
tacrine hydrochloride
tolrestat
trimebutine maleate
trimetrexate gluconate
vindesine sulfate

COMBINATION PRODUCTS
None.

amsacrine (m-AMSA)
Amsidyl†

HOW SUPPLIED
Available only through investigational protocols
Injection: 50 mg/ml†

MECHANISM OF ACTION
Intercalates DNA and inhibits DNA synthesis, producing a cytotoxic effect.

INDICATIONS & DOSAGE
Ovarian carcinoma, lymphomas –
Adults: 30 to 50 mg/m²/day I.V. for 3 days, or 90 to 180 mg/m² as a single dose.
Acute myelogenous leukemia –
Adults: 75 to 120 mg/m²/day for 5 days given by I.V. or intra-arterial infusion.

ADVERSE REACTIONS
Common reactions are in italics; life-threatening reactions are in bold italics.
Blood: *leukopenia (usually dose-limiting),* mild thrombocytopenia.
CNS: ***seizures*** *at dosages as low as 40 mg/m²/day.*
CV: ***ventricular arrhythmias*** (rare) *and* ***cardiac arrest,*** possibly caused by the diluent.
GI: infrequent and mild nausea and vomiting, stomatitis at higher doses.
Other: *local irritation and mild phlebitis,* abnormal liver function tests.

INTERACTIONS
Heparin: don't mix. May form a precipitate.

NURSING CONSIDERATIONS
- *Use cautiously* in impaired hepatic function.
- To prepare solution for administration, two sterile liquids are combined. Add 1.5 ml from the amsacrine ampule (50 mg/ml) to the vial containing 13.5 ml of lactic acid. The combined solution will contain 5 mg/ml of amsacrine and is stable for at least 48 hours at room temperature.
- Use glass syringes for combining the amsacrine and lactic acid. The diluent in the amsacrine may dissolve plastic syringes.
- The solution may be further diluted for infusion with dextrose 5% in water (D_5W) to minimize vein irritation. Administer doses of less than 100 mg in at least 100 ml of D_5W, doses from 100 to 199 mg in 250 ml D_5W, and doses 200 mg or greater in a minimum of 500 ml D_5W. Solutions for infusion are stable at least 48 hours at room temperature.
- Solutions should be infused slowly

over several hours to minimize vein irritation.
• Do not add amsacrine to 0.9% sodium chloride or other chloride-containing solution. Precipitation may occur.
• Do not administer amsacrine through membrane-type in-line filters. The diluent may dissolve the filter.
• Inform the patient that the drug may turn the urine orange.
• Monitor CBC and liver function tests.
• Monitor patient closely for CNS and cardiac toxicity during administration.
• Avoid direct contact of amsacrine with skin to prevent possible sensitization.
• Preparation of parenteral form is associated with carcinogenic, mutagenic, and teratogenic risks for personnel. Follow institutional policy to reduce risks.

azacytidine (5-azacytidine)

HOW SUPPLIED
Available only through investigational protocols
Injection: 100-mg vials

MECHANISM OF ACTION
An antimetabolite that disrupts the translation of nucleic acid sequences into protein.

INDICATIONS & DOSAGE
Acute lymphocytic and acute myelogenous leukemia –
Adults and children: 200 to 300 mg/m^2 I.V. daily for 5 to 10 days. Repeated at 2- to 3-week intervals.

ADVERSE REACTIONS
Common reactions are in italics; life-threatening reactions are in bold italics.
Blood: *leukopenia (usually dose-limiting), thrombocytopenia.*
CNS: infrequent neurologic toxicities, including generalized muscle pain and weakness.
CV: *hypotension from rapid infusion.*
GI: *severe nausea and vomiting, diarrhea.*
Other: rare hepatotoxicity and drug fever.

NURSING CONSIDERATIONS
• *Contraindicated* in liver disease.
• Information based on current literature. Dosage, indications, and adverse effect profile may change with additional clinical experience.
• For stability reasons, azacytidine should be infused only in lactated Ringer's solution.
• After the drug is diluted for infusion, it is stable for 8 hours.
• **I.V. use:** Give by slow I.V. infusion to prevent severe hypotension. Monitor blood pressure before infusion and at 30-minute intervals during infusion. If systolic blood pressure falls below 90 mm Hg, stop infusion and notify doctor.
• Nausea and vomiting may be reduced with continuous infusions. Tolerance to nausea and vomiting develops during prolonged treatment.
• Instruct patient to report any signs of neurotoxicity, for example, muscle pain and weakness.
• If necessary, drug may be given S.C. Drug should be mixed in a smaller quantity of diluent (3 to 5 ml for a 100-mg vial) for S.C. administration.
• Monitor temperature, CBC, and liver function tests.

domperidone
Motilium†‡

HOW SUPPLIED
Tablets: 10 mg†‡

MECHANISM OF ACTION
Blocks peripheral dopamine receptors, including those in the medullary chemoreceptor trigger zone (located outside the blood-brain barrier). In the GI tract, it enhances motility in the stomach and small intestine.

INDICATIONS & DOSAGE
Symptomatic treatment of upper GI motility disorders associated with gastritis and diabetic gastroparesis; prevention of nausea and vomiting caused by antiparkinsonian medications –
Adults: 10 mg P.O. t.i.d. to q.i.d. 30 minutes before meals and h.s. Maximum dose is 20 mg P.O. q.i.d.

ADVERSE REACTIONS
Common reactions are in italics; life-threatening reactions are in bold italics.
CNS: headache.
GI: dry mouth.
Metabolic: galactorrhea, gynecomastia, menstrual irregularities, hot flashes.
Skin: rash.

INTERACTIONS
Antacids, H_2 antagonists: may impair absorption of domperidone.
Anticholinergic agents: decreased domperidone effectiveness.

NURSING CONSIDERATIONS
- *Contraindicated* in patients with hypersensitivity to the drug, mechanical obstruction of the GI tract, or GI hemorrhage.
- Information based on current literature. Dosage, indications, and adverse effect profile may change with additional clinical experience.
- Parenteral domperidone has also been tested as an antiemetic for patients receiving chemotherapy. Dosage up to 1 mg/kg appears to be effective and well tolerated.
- Because domperidone enhances gastric emptying and small intestine motility, it may alter the absorption of other orally administered drugs and may require dosage adjustments.

enoxaparin sodium
Lovenox
Pregnancy Risk Category: B

HOW SUPPLIED
Injection: 30 mg/0.3 ml

MECHANISM OF ACTION
A low molecular weight heparin derivative with antithrombotic properties. It has a higher ratio of anti-Factor Xa to anti-Factor IIa than heparin and doesn't significantly alter bleeding time, platelet function, prothrombin time, or activated partial thromboplastin time (APTT).

INDICATIONS & DOSAGE
Prevention of deep vein thrombosis after hip replacement –
Adults: 30 mg S.C. b.i.d. Initiate therapy as soon as possible, but no later than 24 hours, after surgery. Most patients receive the drug for 7 to 10 days.

ADVERSE REACTIONS
Common reactions are in italics; life-threatening reactions are in bold italics.
Blood: thrombocytopenia, hemorrhage, hypochromic anemia.
Local: mild irritation, pain, hematoma, erythema.
Other: fever, ecchymosis, peripheral edema.

INTERACTIONS
Oral anticoagulants: increased risk of bleeding. Use cautiously.

NURSING CONSIDERATIONS
- *Contraindicated* in patients with hypersensitivity to the drug, heparin, or pork products; patients with active major bleeding episodes; or those with thrombocytopenia associated with antiplatelet antibody.

• *Use cautiously* in patients with uncontrolled hypertension, bleeding diathesis, or conditions that increase the risk of hemorrhage, such as bacterial endocarditis; in those with a history of GI ulceration or hemorrhagic stroke; or shortly after brain, eye, or spinal surgery.
• Perform baseline hematologic studies, including CBC and platelet count, and repeat periodically during therapy. Usually there's no need to check hematologic parameters daily in patients with normal baseline studies.
• Alternate injection sites between the left and right anterolateral and posterolateral abdominal wall. Administer with patient lying down.
• To administer by deep S.C. injection, grasp a fold of abdominal skin between the thumb and forefinger. Introduce the full length of the needle into the skin fold. Hold the skin fold throughout the injection.
• If overdose occurs, enoxaparin may be neutralized by protamine sulfate. Give 1 mg of protamine sulfate for each mg of enoxaparin administered. Although hemorrhagic complications may be corrected by such treatment, the APTT may remain prolonged.
• Have resuscitation equipment readily available when administering protamine sulfate because hypotensive and anaphylactoid reactions have occurred.

felbamate
Felbamyl

MECHANISM OF ACTION
A dicarbamate anticonvulsant; mechanism of action is unclear. Drug may act by elevating the seizure threshold or preventing the spread of seizure activity.

INDICATIONS & DOSAGE
Refractory partial seizures; Lennox-Gastaut syndrome –
Adults: initially, 1,200 mg P.O. daily in two divided doses. Increase in increments of 1,200 mg daily to a maximum of 3,600 mg daily.

ADVERSE REACTIONS
Common reactions are in italics; life-threatening reactions are in bold italics.
CNS: dizziness, *somnolence*.
EENT: blurred or double vision.
GI: *nausea, vomiting*.
Skin: rash.
Other: anorexia.

NURSING CONSIDERATIONS
• Information is based on current literature and may change with further clinical experience.
• Felbamate is generally well tolerated by most patients, and early trials indicate that it has a broad spectrum of antiseizure activity.

flunarizine hydrochloride
Sibelium†

HOW SUPPLIED
Capsules: 5 mg†

MECHANISM OF ACTION
A calcium channel blocker that blocks the entry of calcium ions into specialized channels within the membrane of smooth muscle cells. Unlike many other calcium channel blockers, flunarizine doesn't affect the SA or AV node of the heart and doesn't cause peripheral vasodilation. Drug also has weak antihistamine activity.

INDICATIONS & DOSAGE
Prophylaxis of vascular headache –
Adults: 10 mg P.O. daily, in the evening.

ADVERSE REACTIONS
Common reactions are in italics; life-threatening reactions are in bold italics.
CNS: *drowsiness, sedation, fatigue,* depression, extrapyramidal symp-

*Liquid form contains alcohol. **May contain tartrazine.

toms, sleep disturbances, insomnia, anxiety, dizziness, vertigo.
GI: nausea, vomiting, heartburn, discomfort, dry mouth.
Skin: rash.
Other: *weight gain, increased appetite,* asthenia, muscle aches.

INTERACTIONS
Mephenytoin, other anticonvulsants: flunarizine lowers steady-state levels of mephenytoin and other anticonvulsants. Monitor anticonvulsant blood levels.
Oral contraceptives: some patients have exhibited galactorrhea. Monitor closely.

NURSING CONSIDERATIONS
- Information is based on current literature and may change with further clinical experience.
- *Contraindicated* in patients with hypersensitivity to the drug and in patients with Parkinson's disease, other preexisting extrapyramidal disorders, or a history of mental depression.
- *Use cautiously* in patients with hepatic failure. Elderly patients may require lower dosage.
- Drug is used to reduce the frequency of migraine attacks. To a lesser extent, it reduces the severity of the attack; it doesn't appear to change duration. Patients should understand that drug isn't useful in the treatment of acute attacks and that daily use is necessary for best drug effect.
- Sedation or drowsiness may occur, especially at start of therapy. Tell patient to avoid hazardous activities that require mental alertness, such as driving, until adverse CNS effects of drug are known.
- Extrapyramidal symptoms may develop during therapy. Elderly patients are particularly at risk. Advise patients to report movement or coordination disturbances.

halofantrine
Halfan

MECHANISM OF ACTION
A phenanthrenemethanol derivative structurally similar to mefloquine. Halofantrine is an antimalarial agent active against multidrug-resistant *Plasmodium falciparum.*

INDICATIONS & DOSAGE
P. falciparum *malaria* –
Adults and children over 40 kg: 500 mg P.O. q 6 hours for three doses. A second course of therapy may be recommended after 7 days.

ADVERSE REACTIONS
Common reactions are in italics; life-threatening reactions are in bold italics.
GI: *abdominal pain, vomiting, diarrhea.*
Skin: pruritus, rash.

NURSING CONSIDERATIONS
- Information is based on current literature and may change with further clinical experience.
- Drug's effectiveness in the treatment of *P. ovale, P. vivax,* or *P. malariae* infections hasn't been determined.
- Absorption after oral administration is erratic and variable. Diet, genetic factors, and racial factors may also influence bioavailability.

hexoprenaline sulfate
Delaprem

MECHANISM OF ACTION
A $beta_2$-selective adrenergic agonist that stimulates uterine $beta_2$ receptors, resulting in a decrease in the frequency or intensity of uterine muscle contractions.

INDICATIONS & DOSAGE

Tocolysis in preterm labor –

Women: Dosage is individualized. Some studies employed I.V. bolus injections of 7.5 mcg, resulting in decreased uterine activity within 13 minutes, lasting about 33 minutes. Other studies used continuous I.V. infusion of 0.38 mcg/minute for 20 minutes.

ADVERSE REACTIONS

Common reactions are in italics; life-threatening reactions are in bold italics.

CV: tachycardia (maternal and fetal), supraventricular or ventricular arrhythmias, myocardial ischemia, hypotension.

Metabolic: hyperglycemia, hypokalemia.

Respiratory: pulmonary edema.

Other: tremor.

NURSING CONSIDERATIONS

- Information is based on current literature and may change with further clinical experience.
- Hexoprenaline appears to cause fewer adverse effects than currently used tocolytic agents, such as ritodrine or terbutaline.
- Closely monitor maternal and fetal heart rates during therapy.
- Drug has also been used to treat fetal heart rate disturbances, a measure of fetal distress, during labor. Increases in fetal heart rate probably aren't caused by a direct action of the drug because animal studies have shown that less than 1% of a dose crosses the placenta.

ketotifen fumarate

Zaditen*

HOW SUPPLIED

Tablets: 1 mg
Capsules: 1 mg
Elixir: 1 mg/5 ml*

MECHANISM OF ACTION

Like cromolyn, ketotifen stabilizes mast cells. However, it has a number of other pharmacologic effects that may contribute to its action, including antihistamine, phosphodiesterase-inhibiting, and calcium channel blocking effects. It may also have some activity on $beta_2$-adrenergic receptors.

INDICATIONS & DOSAGE

Asthma prophylaxis; treatment of allergic rhinitis and conjunctivitis –

Adults: 1 mg P.O. b.i.d. with food. May be increased to 2 mg b.i.d.

ADVERSE REACTIONS

Common reactions are in italics; life-threatening reactions are in bold italics.

CNS: sedation, tiredness, dizziness, headache.

GI: dry mouth, nausea.

Other: increased appetite and weight gain, exacerbation of asthma, ***bronchospasm, status asthmaticus.***

INTERACTIONS

Alcohol: may potentiate adverse reactions. Avoid concomitant use.

Oral antidiabetic agents: reversible fall in platelet count has been reported. Avoid concomitant use.

NURSING CONSIDERATIONS

- Information is based upon current literature and may change with further clinical experience. Ketotifen is currently available in Europe.
- Long-term therapy is necessary for asthma prophylaxis. Studies lasting less than 4 weeks have not shown consistent benefits, but patients taking the drug for 3 months or more consider the drug effective.
- Ketotifen may produce drowsiness. Warn patients not to perform hazardous activities requiring alertness (such as operating heavy machinery or driving) until the adverse CNS effects of the drug are known.

*Liquid form contains alcohol. **May contain tartrazine.

metformin

Glucophage†

HOW SUPPLIED

Tablets: 500 mg†

MECHANISM OF ACTION

A substituted biguanide that produces its antidiabetic effects only in the presence of insulin. It facilitates insulin's action on peripheral receptor sites and may increase the number of insulin receptors. It has no effect on pancreatic beta cells.

INDICATIONS & DOSAGE

To control diabetes in stable, mild, nonketosis-prone type II diabetics –
Adults: initially, 500 mg P.O. t.i.d., preferably with food. Adjust dosage upward as necessary, not to exceed 2.5 g daily.

ADVERSE REACTIONS

Common reactions are in italics; life-threatening reactions are in bold italics.
EENT: metallic taste.
GI: epigastric discomfort, nausea, vomiting, diarrhea, anorexia.
Other: *lactic acidosis.*

INTERACTIONS

Anticoagulants: metformin may increase the elimination of oral anticoagulants. Monitor prothrombin times carefully during changes in metformin dosage.
Diuretics, corticosteroids, oral contraceptives, nicotinic acid: may produce hyperglycemia and reduce effectiveness of metformin therapy.

NURSING CONSIDERATIONS

- *Contraindicated* in patients allergic to the drug and in insulin-dependent diabetes; in patients with a history of ketoacidosis; in those with liver disease, lactic acidosis or a history of lactic acidosis, or renal dysfunction; during acute stress (surgery, severe infections, or trauma); in pregnant patients; and in patients undergoing pyelography or angiography, which may precipitate temporary oliguria.
- Information is based on current literature and may change with further clinical experience.
- Lactic acidosis is a potentially fatal complication of biguanide therapy. Phenformin (DBI), a similar compound, was withdrawn from the U.S. market in the mid-1970s after it was associated with this adverse reaction. If vomiting occurs, drug should be discontinued immediately and patient assessed for lactic acidosis.
- Drug should be discontinued 2 days before elective surgery or angiographic exams. Renal function should be assessed before drug is restarted.
- Metformin will not prevent the development of complications from diabetes mellitus.
- Patients should be advised of the importance of good dietary management to control their diabetes. Metformin therapy should not be used in place of good diet.
- Advise taking metformin with food to minimize gastric irritation.
- Advise patients to avoid excessive alcohol consumption while taking metformin to prevent excessive elevation of blood lactate.
- Impaired absorption of vitamin B_{12} and folic acid have been reported in some patients on long-term therapy. Serum levels of these cofactors should be measured every 1 or 2 years.
- The drug should be temporarily discontinued once or twice a year to assess the need for continued therapy.

mifepristone (RU 486)

Mifegyne

MECHANISM OF ACTION

Blocks progesterone and glucocorticoid receptors, but doesn't block estrogen or mineralocorticoid receptors.

Has weak antagonist activity at androgen receptors.

INDICATIONS & DOSAGE
Early termination of pregnancy –
Women: 600 mg P.O.
Postcoital contraception –
Women: 600 mg P.O. within 3 days of unprotected intercourse.
Cushing's syndrome –
Adults: 20 mg/kg P.O. daily.

ADVERSE REACTIONS
Common reactions are in italics; life-threatening reactions are in bold italics.
CNS: headache.
GI: *abdominal pain, nausea, vomiting, diarrhea.*
GU: *excessive bleeding.*

NURSING CONSIDERATIONS
- Information is based on current literature and may change with further clinical experience.
- When used as an abortifacient, drug should be used within 60 days of first missed period. Usually administered with a prostaglandin analog, which will increase uterine activity.
- Drug has been investigated for several uses, including tamoxifen-resistant breast cancer with evidence of progesterone receptors, open-angle glaucoma, and induction of labor.

semustine (methyl CCNU)

MECHANISM OF ACTION
A nitrosourea compound that probably acts as an alkylating agent. The drug cross-links DNA and also inhibits several key enzymatic processes.

INDICATIONS & DOSAGE
Advanced GI tumors, brain tumors, Hodgkin's and non-Hodgkin's lymphomas –
Adults: 150 to 200 mg/m² P.O. q 6 to 8 weeks.

ADVERSE REACTIONS
Common reactions are in italics; life-threatening reactions are in bold italics.
Blood: *delayed thrombocytopenia (about 4 weeks) and leukopenia (about 6 weeks). Myelosuppression may be cumulative.*
GI: *acute nausea and vomiting 2 to 6 hours after administration, anorexia.*
GU: renal toxicity.
Hepatic: elevated liver enzymes.
Other: pulmonary fibrosis with prolonged use.

NURSING CONSIDERATIONS
- *Use cautiously* with other nephrotoxic drugs.
- Monitor renal and liver function.
- Capsules are usually stored in the refrigerator but are stable for 1 year at room temperature. Avoid high temperatures and excessive moisture.
- Drug should be taken on an empty stomach to ensure absorption.
- Monitor CBC for delayed myelosuppression, up to 4 weeks for the onset of thrombocytopenia and 6 weeks for leukopenia.

tacrine hydrochloride (tetrahydroaminoacridine, THA)
Cognex

HOW SUPPLIED
Available only through investigational protocols
Capsules: 10 mg, 20 mg, 30 mg, 40 mg

MECHANISM OF ACTION
A centrally acting anticholinesterase agent. Probably acts by preventing the breakdown of acetylcholine in the CNS, prolonging its actions and enhancing central cholinergic function. Drug also blocks central potassium channels, alters phosphorylation, and blocks presynaptic and postsynaptic cholinergic receptors.

INDICATIONS & DOSAGE
Adjunctive treatment of Alzheimer's disease –
Adults: initially, 40 to 80 mg P.O. daily in divided doses. If no evidence of hepatotoxicity exists, dosage is increased to 120 mg daily.

ADVERSE REACTIONS
Common reactions are in italics; life-threatening reactions are in bold italics.
GI: *diarrhea, increased salivation.*
GU: *increased urination.*
Other: ***hepatotoxicity,*** *sweating.*

INTERACTIONS
Anticholinergics: decreased effectiveness. Adjust dosage as ordered.
Cholinergic agonists: enhanced effects. Monitor closely.
Cimetidine: may interfere with metabolism of tacrine, resulting in increased plasma levels of tacrine. Adjust dosage as ordered.
Theophylline: decreased hepatic clearance of theophylline. Adjust theophylline dosage as ordered.

NURSING CONSIDERATIONS
- Information is based on current literature and may change with further clinical experience.
- *Contraindicated* in patients with hypersensitivity to the drug.
- Cholinergic adverse effects are common. Addition of anticholinergic medications, such as glycopyrrolate, may block these adverse effects.

tolrestat
Alderase

MECHANISM OF ACTION
Blocks the enzyme aldose reductase, and prevents the intracellular formation of sorbitol from glucose and galactitol from galactose. This metabolic pathway is active in patients with diabetes and may be responsible for late diabetic complications.

INDICATIONS & DOSAGE
Prevention of late complications of diabetes, including diabetic retinopathy and neuropathy –
Adults: dosage not clearly established. Early studies have used 50 to 200 mg P.O. once or twice daily.

ADVERSE REACTIONS
Common reactions are in italics; life-threatening reactions are in bold italics.
CNS: dizziness.
Skin: rash.
Other: elevations of liver enzymes.

INTERACTIONS
Salicylates, tolbutamide: increased plasma levels of active tolrestat by displacing the drug from protein-binding sites.

NURSING CONSIDERATIONS
- Information is based on current literature and may change with further clinical experience.
- Aldose reductase inhibitors have no effect on blood glucose, and patients must continue antidiabetic agents as instructed. The purpose of therapy is to prevent late complications of diabetes that may be secondary to chronic elevation of blood sugar.
- The benefits of tolrestat therapy have been difficult to establish because of the slow onset of complications of diabetes. The drug appears to be well tolerated in clinical trials.

trimebutine maleate
Modulon†

HOW SUPPLIED
Tablets: 100 mg†
Injection: 50 mg/5 ml†

MECHANISM OF ACTION
Acts on intestinal opiate and serotonin receptors to regulate normal intestinal motility.

INDICATIONS & DOSAGE
Symptomatic relief of irritable bowel syndrome –
Adults: 100 to 200 mg P.O. t.i.d. before meals.
Postoperative paralytic ileus –
Adults: 50 to 100 mg I.M. t.i.d. May also be given by slow I.V. push, or infused I.V. over 1 hour.

ADVERSE REACTIONS
Common reactions are in italics; life-threatening reactions are in bold italics.
CNS: dizziness, syncope, drowsiness, tiredness, headache.
CV: hypotension.
GI: constipation, diarrhea, nausea, vomiting, abdominal pain.

INTERACTIONS
Antihypertensives: possibly excessive hypotension, especially after rapid I.V. injection of trimebutine maleate. Use together cautiously.
Tubocurarine: Animal studies have shown that trimebutine maleate may prolong neuromuscular blockade.

NURSING CONSIDERATIONS
- Information is based upon current literature and may change with further clinical experience.
- **I.V. use:** Rapid I.V. injection may cause hypotension. Inject drug over 1 minute. I.V. infusions may be mixed with normal saline solution or dextrose 5% in water.

trimetrexate gluconate
Pregnancy Risk Category: C

HOW SUPPLIED
Information about use of trimetrexate under the treatment IND available from the National Information Center for Orphan Drugs and Rare Diseases (NICODARD) at (800) 336-4797, or (202) 565-4167 in the Washington, D.C., metropolitan area.
Injection: 25-mg vials

MECHANISM OF ACTION
Prevents reduction of folic acid to tetrahydrofolate by binding to dihydrofolate reductase.

INDICATIONS & DOSAGE
Neoplastic disorders –
Adults: dosage and indication will vary with protocol.
Treatment of Pneumocystis carinii *pneumonia in patients with AIDS (approved as a treatment IND) –*
Adults: dosage may vary with protocol. 30 mg/m² I.V. bolus daily for 21 days, administered with leucovorin (20 mg/m² I.V. or P.O. daily).

ADVERSE REACTIONS
Common reactions are in italics; life-threatening reactions are in bold italics.
Blood: ***neutropenia, thrombocytopenia.***
Skin: rash.
Other: ***hepatotoxicity,*** *peripheral neuropathy.*

INTERACTIONS
Leucovorin: precipitate will form if mixed with trimetrexate. Administer separately.

NURSING CONSIDERATIONS
- *Contraindicated* in patients with hypersensitivity to the drug.
- Avoid I.M. injections in patients with thrombocytopenia.
- Warn patient to watch for signs of infection (fever, sore throat, fatigue) and bleeding (easy bruising, nosebleeds, bleeding gums, melena). Take temperature daily.
- Store intact vials in refrigerator.
- **I.V. use:** Reconstitute 25-mg vial with 2 ml sterile water for injection to yield a solution of 12.5 mg/ml. Incompatible with chloride-containing solutions (including 0.9% sodium chloride solution). Only dextrose 5% in water is recommended for I.V. infusion.
- Preparation of parenteral form is as-

*Liquid form contains alcohol. **May contain tartrazine.

sociated with carcinogenic, mutagenic, and teratogenic risks for personnel. Follow institutional policy to reduce risks.

vindesine sulfate

Eldisine†

HOW SUPPLIED

Available only through investigational protocols

Injection: 5-mg vials†

MECHANISM OF ACTION

Arrests mitosis in metaphase, blocking cell division.

INDICATIONS & DOSAGE

Acute lymphoblastic leukemia, breast cancer, malignant melanoma, lymphosarcoma, non-small-cell lung carcinoma –

Adults: 3 to 4 mg/m² I.V. q 7 to 14 days, or continuous I.V. infusion of 1.2 to 1.5 mg/m² daily for 5 days q 3 weeks.

ADVERSE REACTIONS

Common reactions are in italics; life-threatening reactions are in bold italics.

Blood: *leukopenia, thrombocytopenia.*

CNS: *paresthesias, decreased deep tendon reflex, muscle weakness.*

GI: *constipation, abdominal cramping,* nausea, vomiting.

Local: *phlebitis,* necrosis on extravasation.

Other: ***acute bronchospasm,*** *reversible alopecia,* jaw pain, fever with continuous infusions.

NURSING CONSIDERATIONS

- **I.V. use:** Do not give as a continuous infusion unless patient has a central I.V. line.
- Avoid extravasation. Drug is a painful vesicant. Give 10-ml 0.9% sodium chloride solution flush before drug to test vein patency and after drug is given to flush tubing.
- When reconstituted with the 10-ml diluent provided or 0.9% sodium chloride solution, the drug is stable for 30 days under refrigeration.
- Do not mix vindesine with other drugs; compatibility with other drugs has not yet been determined.
- After administering, monitor for life-threatening acute bronchospasm. If this occurs, notify doctor immediately. Reaction most likely in patient who is also receiving mitomycin.
- To prevent paralytic ileus, encourage patient to drink fluids, increase ambulation, and use stool softeners.
- Instruct patient to report any symptoms of neurotoxicity: numbness and tingling of extremities, jaw pain, constipation (may be an early symptom).
- Assess for depression of Achilles tendon reflex, footdrop or wristdrop, and slapping gait (late signs of neurotoxicity).
- To detect neuropathy, record patient signatures before each course of therapy and observe for deterioration of handwriting.
- Monitor CBC.

Appendices and Index

Topical agents

DRUG	INDICATIONS & DOSAGE
Antibacterials and antifungals	
alcohol, ethyl and isopropyl	*To disinfect skin, instruments, and ampules:* disinfect as needed. Isopropyl alcohol is superior to ethyl alcohol as an anti-infective (70%). *Antipyresis:* apply 25% solution. *Anhidrosis:* apply 50% solution p.r.n.
hydrogen peroxide	*Cleansing wounds:* use 1.5% to 3% solution, p.r.n. *Mouthwash for necrotizing ulcerative gingivitis:* gargle with 3% solution, p.r.n. *Cleansing douche:* use 2% solution q.i.d., p.r.n.
Antiseptics and germicidals	
benzalkonium chloride (Benza, Germicin, Spensomide, Zephiran)	*Preoperative disinfection of unbroken skin:* apply 1:750 tincture or spray. *Disinfection of mucous membranes and denuded skin:* apply 1:10,000 to 1:5,000 aqueous solution. *Irrigation of vagina:* instill 1:5,000 to 1:2,000 aqueous solution. *Irrigation of deep infected wounds:* instill 1:20,000 to 1:3,000 aqueous solution. *Preservation of metallic instruments, ampules, thermometers, and rubber articles:* wipe with or soak objects in 1:5,000 to 1:750 solution. *Disinfection of operating room equipment:* wipe with 1:5,000 solution.
chlorhexidine gluconate (Hibiclens, Hibistat, Peridex)	*Surgical hand scrub, hand wash, hand rinse, skin wound cleanser:* use p.r.n. *Gingivitis:* use 0.12% strength (Peridex oral rinse), p.r.n.
hexachlorophene (pHisoHex, pHisoScrub, Septisol, Septsoft)	*Surgical scrub, bacteriostatic skin cleanser:* use p.r.n. in 0.25% to 3% concentrations.
iodine (Sepp)	*Preoperative disinfection of skin (small wounds and abraded areas):* apply p.r.n.

*Available in Canada only

ACTION	SPECIAL CONSIDERATIONS
Antibacterial effect through reduction of surface tension of bacterial cell walls, inhibiting bacterial growth. Also antipyretic and astringent effects.	• Avoid contact with eyes and mucous membranes. • Contraindicated in patients taking disulfiram if used over large surface area. • Do not apply to open wounds.
Antibacterial effect through oxidation.	• Do not instill into closed body cavities or abscesses because released gas cannot escape. • Store in tightly capped, dark container in cool, dry place. • Do not confuse with peroxide (6% to 20%) used for bleaching hair.
Cationic surface action producing bacteriostatic or bacteriocidal effect depending on the concentration used.	• Do not use with occlusive dressings or packs. • Use only in proper diluted strength for each use. • Inactivated by anionic compounds such as soap. • Rinse area thoroughly after each application. • Skin inflammation and irritation may require lower concentration or discontinuation.
Persistent antimicrobial effect against gram-negative and gram-positive bacteria.	• Avoid contact with eyes, ears, and mucous membranes. Rinse well if drug enters eyes or ears. • May cause deafness if drug enters middle ear.
Bacteriostatic effect against staphylococci and other gram-positive bacteria, probably due to inhibition of bacterial membrane-bound enzymes.	• Do not use on broken skin, skin lesions, burns, wounds, or under occlusive dressings to prevent increased absorption and neurotoxicity. • Do not use around eyes or mucous membranes. • Use for at least 3 days preoperatively for optimum effect. • Rinse thoroughly after use. • Do not use in infants; use cautiously in children. • May be toxic if ingested.
Germicidal effect against bacteria, fungi, and viruses, probably due to disruption of micro-organism proteins.	• Cleanse area before applying. • Do not cover after application to avoid irritation. • Iodine stains skin and clothing. • Do not use near eyes or on mucous membranes. • Toxic if ingested; sodium thiosulfate is antidote.

(continued)

Topical agents *(continued)*

DRUG	INDICATIONS & DOSAGE
Antiseptics and germicidals *(continued)*	
povidone-iodine (Acu-dyne, Betadine, Biodine, Efodine, Frepp, Iodex, Iso-dine, Operand, Pharmadine, Polydine, Proviodine*, Sepp)	*Preoperative skin preparation and scrub; germicide for surface wounds; postoperative application to incisions; prophylactic application to urinary meatus of catheterized patients; miscellaneous disinfection:* apply p.r.n., or use as scrub p.r.n.
Astringents	
calamine	*Astringent and protectant; itching, poison ivy and poison oak, nonpoisonous insect bites, mild sunburn, minor skin irritations:* apply p.r.n. three or four times a day.
hamamelis water, witch hazel (Mediconet, Tucks)	*Anal discomfort, itching, burning, minor external hemorrhoidal or outer vaginal discomfort, diaper rash:* apply t.i.d. or q.i.d.
Emollients	
petrolatum (Vaseline)	*Dry rough skin; temporary relief of discomfort due to sunburn, windburn, or any drying of epithelial tissue:* topical protection and emollience: use alone or with other drugs, apply p.r.n.
Keratolytics	
podophyllum resin (Pod-Ben 25, Podoben, Pudofin)	*Venereal warts:* apply podophyllum resin preparation to the lesion, cover with waxed paper, and bandage. Leave covered for 4 to 6 hours, then wash lesion to remove medication. Repeat at weekly intervals, if indicated. *Multiple superficial epitheliomatosis and keratosis:* apply daily with applicator and allow to dry. Remove necrotic tissue before each application.
salicylic acid (Calicylic, Compound W, Derma-Soft Creme, Freezone, Gordofilm, Hydrisalic, Keralyt, Occlusal, Off-Ezy, Salacid, Salonil, Wart-Off)	*Scaling dermatoses, hyperkeratosis, callouses, warts:* apply to affected area and place under an occlusive dressing at night.
Protectants	
collodion, flexible collodion	*Protectant; vehicle for other medicinal agents; sealant for small wounds:* apply to dry skin, p.r.n., or use flexible collodion when a flexible film is desired.

*Available in Canada only

ACTION	SPECIAL CONSIDERATIONS
Germicidal effect against bacteria, fungi, and viruses; has same action as iodine without its irritating effects.	• Contraindicated in known sensitivity to iodine. • Do not use around eyes; do not use full strength solution on mucous membranes. • May stain skin and mucous membranes.
Antipruritic and astringent activity through drying effect.	• Avoid use on eyes and mucous membranes. • Do not apply to raw, oozing areas. • Cleanse and dry area before each application.
Soothing, cooling effect of superficial irritation through astringent action.	• Avoid use around eyes. • Cleanse area before use.
Protective and emollient effect through formation of moisture barrier, increasing the natural retention of moisture.	• Avoid use in eyes. • May stain clothing. • May cause body surfaces to become slippery. • Apply sparingly; is not absorbed, so coating is all that is necessary.
Caustic and erosive action due to disruption of cell division of the epithelium.	• Avoid eye contact. • May be toxic if applied to large surface area or applied too frequently. • Should not be used in pregnant women. • Wash hands thoroughly after applying. • Protect surrounding area with petrolatum. • Wash off thoroughly with soap and water after prescribed time period. • May cause abnormal pigmentation.
Causes desquamation of cornified epithelium by increasing hydration.	• Avoid use on eyes and mucous membranes. • Do not use in aspirin-sensitive patients. • Apply emollient to surrounding skin for protection. • Do not use on birthmarks, moles, or areas with hair follicle involvement. • Wash off thoroughly, after overnight use.
Protects wounds from the environment by forming an occlusive seal and excluding air.	• Do not use on deep or puncture wounds; may promote growth of anaerobic bacteria. • Avoid use on eyes and mucous membranes. • May be painful on application or cause dry skin. • Use alcohol or acetone as solvent for removal.

(continued)

Topical agents *(continued)*

DRUG	INDICATIONS & DOSAGE
Protectants *(continued)*	
compound benzoin tincture	*Demulcent and protectant (cutaneous ulcers, bedsores, cracked nipples, fissures of lips and anus):* apply locally once daily or b.i.d.
zinc gelatin (Dome-Paste, Unna's Boot, Unna's Powder)	*Protectant (lesions or injuries of lower legs or arms):* Wrap the wet bandage in place and retain for about 1 week. Dome-Paste, in 3″ to 4″ (8 to 10 cm) bandages, can be applied directly to arm or leg.
Wet dressings, soaks	
aluminum acetate, aluminum sulfate (Bluboro Powder, Burow's solution, Domeboro powder, Pedi-Boro Soak Paks)	*Mild skin irritation from exposure to soaps, chemicals, diaper rash, acne, eczema:* apply p.r.n. *Skin inflammation, contact dermatoses:* mix powder or tablet with 1 pint of lukewarm water. Apply to loose dressing q 15 to 30 minutes for 4 to 8 hours.
Miscellaneous agents	
hydroquinone (Eldoquin, Esoterica, Porcelana, Solaquin Forte)	*Treatment of hyperpigmentation in conditions such as freckling, inactive chloasma, lentigo, photosensitization:* apply uniformly to desired area b.i.d., until desired depigmentation occurs, then as needed to maintain depigmentation.
methyl salicylate (Ben-Gay, Icy Hot Balm/Cream, Deep Heating Rub)	*Counterirritant (minor pains of osteoarthritis, rheumatism, sprains, muscle and tendon soreness and tightness, lumbago, sciatica):* apply with gentle massage several times daily for adults.
para-aminobenzoic acid (PABA) (Pabanol)	*Topical protectant; sunburn protection, sun-sensitive skin, slow tanning:* apply evenly to dry skin indoors before exposure to sun. Reapply after swimming.
selenium sulfide (Exsel, Selsun, Selsun Blue)	*Treatment of tinea versicolor:* massage into affected area; rinse after 10 minutes. Apply daily for 7 days. *Dandruff, seborrheic scalp dermatitis:* massage 1 to 2 teaspoonfuls into wet scalp. After 2 to 3 minutes, rinse thoroughly, and repeat application.

ACTION	SPECIAL CONSIDERATIONS
Protects skin from external environment by coating action.	• Avoid contact with eyes and mucous membranes. • Cleanse and dry area before application. • Useful in protection of skin from adhesive.
Protects skin by forming occlusive barrier.	• Avoid contact with eyes and mucous membranes. • Watch for signs of infection. • Warn patient not to shower or bathe with gel on. • Remove by soaking in warm water. Remove all of previous application before reapplication. • Apply with nap of hair to avoid folliculitis. • Do not use with constrictive bandage.
Reduces friction and provides soothing relief through astringent action.	• Avoid use around eyes and mucous membranes. • Do not apply under occlusive dressings. • Discontinue if irritation occurs.
Depigmenting action.	• Avoid use near eyes and on broken skin. • Sunscreen and protective clothing should be used during and after use to prevent repigmentation. • Should not be used in children or pregnant women. • May be toxic if ingested.
Acts as counterirritant, replacing pain perception with another sensation that blocks pain temporarily.	• Avoid use in patients allergic to salicylates around eyes, on mucous membranes, or on broken skin, or in children. • May be toxic if ingested. • Do not use with heating pad or hot water.
Provides sun screening action by absorbing ultraviolet rays.	• Avoid use in eyes and on mucous membranes. • May discolor clothing. • Not recommended for infants.
Antiseborrheic effect through cytostatic action on epithelial cells, which inhibits corneocyte production.	• Avoid use in eyes and on mucous membranes or inflamed areas. • May damage jewelry. • Should not be used in pregnant women. • May discolor hair or cause increased hair loss.

Orphan drugs and biologicals

As defined by the Orphan Drug Act, an orphan drug is one that is useful for the diagnosis, treatment, or prevention of a rare disease or disorder. This act defines a rare disease as one that affects fewer than 200,000 persons in the United States, or one for which the expected sales will not recover the cost of developing and making the drug available. The following list includes the drugs and biologicals that have received orphan drug designation.*

GENERIC NAME	TRADE NAME	DESIGNATED USE
Drugs		
aconiazide	Not established	Treatment of tuberculosis.
adenosine	Not established	Treatment of brain tumors.
AI-RSA	Not established	Treatment of autoimmune uveitis.
allopurinol	Zyloprim	For use in the ex vivo preservation of cadaveric kidneys for transplantation.
allopurinol riboside	Not established	Treatment of cutaneous and visceral leishmaniasis and Chagas' disease.
anagrelide	Not established	Treatment of polycythemia vera and thrombocytosis in chronic myelogenous leukemia.
antiepilepsirine	Not established	Treatment of refractory generalized tonic-clonic seizures.
antipyrine	Not established	Antipyrine test as an index of hepatic drug-metabolizing capacity.
AS-101	Not established	Treatment of AIDS.
3′ azido-2, 3′dideoxyuridine	Not established	Treatment of AIDS.
bacitracin zinc	Altracin	Treatment of antibiotic-associated pseudomembranous enterocolitis caused by toxins A and B from *Clostridium difficile*.
bethanidine sulfate	Not established	Prevention or treatment of primary ventricular fibrillation.
BMY-45622	Not established	Treatment of ovarian cancer.
bromhexine	Not established	Treatment of keratoconjunctivitis sicca in patients with Sjögren's syndrome.
BW B759U	Not established	Treatment of severe human CMV infections in specific immunosuppressed patient populations (for example, bone marrow transplant, AIDS).

**USP DI* 13(1): 2817-2941, 1993.

Orphan drugs and biologicals *(continued)*

GENERIC NAME	TRADE NAME	DESIGNATED USE
Drugs *(continued)*		
BW 12C	Not established	Treatment of sickle cell disease crisis.
C1-esterase-inhibitor, human	Not established	Prevention and treatment of acute attacks of hereditary angioedema.
566C80	Not established	Treatment of *Pneumocystis carinii* pneumonia in patients with AIDS.
calcium gluconate gel 2.5%	H-F Gel	Emergency topical treatment of hydrogen fluoride (hydrofluoric acid) burns.
carbovir	Not established	Treatment of AIDS and symptomatic HIV infection.
ceramide trihexosidase/alpha galactosidase A	Not established	Treatment of Fabry's disease.
cetiedil citrate	Not established	Treatment of sickle cell disease crisis.
2-chlorodeoxyadenosine	Not established	Treatment of chronic lymphocytic leukemia and hairy-cell leukemia.
2-chloro-2′-deoxyadenosine	Not established	Treatment of acute myeloid leukemia.
citric acid, glucono-delta-lactone, and magnesium carbonate	Renacidin	Treatment of apatite or struvite renal or bladder calculi.
copolymer 1 (COP 1)	Not established	Treatment of multiple sclerosis.
cyproterone acetate	Androcur, Cyproteron	Treatment of severe hirsutism.
cysteamine hydrochloride (2-aminoethanethiol)	Not established	Treatment of nephropathic cystinosis.
cystic fibrosis transmembrane conductance regulator gene	Not established	Treatment of cystic fibrosis.
decitabine (5-AZA-2′-deoxycytidine; DAC)	Not established	Treatment of acute leukemias.
defibrotide	Not established	Treatment of thrombotic thrombocytopenic purpura.
deslorelin	Somagard	Treatment of central precocious puberty.
dextran and deferoxamine	Bio-Rescue	Treatment of acute iron poisoning.

(continued)

Orphan drugs and biologicals *(continued)*

GENERIC NAME	TRADE NAME	DESIGNATED USE
Drugs *(continued)*		
dextran sulfate aerosol inhalation	Uendex	Adjunctive treatment of cystic fibrosis.
dextran sulfate sodium (UA001)	Not established	Treatment of AIDS.
3,4-diaminopyridine	Not established	Treatment of Eaton-Lambert (myasthenic) syndrome.
diaziquone	Not established	Treatment of primary brain malignancies (grades III to IV astrocytomas).
2′-3′-dideoxy-adenosine	Not established	Treatment of AIDS.
2′-3′-dideoxycytidine	Not established	Treatment of AIDS.
2′-3′-dideoxyinosine	Not established	Treatment of AIDS.
diethyldithiocarbamate (DTC)	Imuthiol	Treatment of AIDS.
dihematoporphyrin ethers	Photofrin II	Photodynamic treatment of primary or recurrent obstructive esophageal carcinoma; treatment of transitional cell carcinoma of the bladder.
2,3-dimercaptosuccinic acid (DMSA)	Not established	Treatment of lead poisoning in children.
dimethyl sulfoxide (DMSO)	Sclerosol	Treatment of cutaneous manifestations of scleroderma.
disodium clodronate tetrahydrate	Bonefos	Treatment of bone resorption caused by malignant tumors.
disodium silibinin dihemisuccinate	Legalon Sil	Treatment of hepatic intoxication by *Amanita phalloides* (mushroom poisoning).
dynamine	Not established	Treatment of Eaton-Lambert (myasthenic) syndrome.
enisoprost	Not established	Adjunctive treatment (with cyclosporine) to reduce rejection and decrease cyclosporine nephrotoxicity in transplant recipients.
epidermal growth factor (human)	Not established	Acceleration of corneal epithelial regeneration and healing of stromal tissue in patients with nonhealing corneal defects or following corneal transplant surgery, and promotion of cutaneous wound healing in extreme burn treatment protocols.

Orphan drugs and biologicals *(continued)*

GENERIC NAME	TRADE NAME	DESIGNATED USE
Drugs *(continued)*		
epoprostenol	Cyclo-Prostin	Replacement of heparin in patients requiring hemodialysis and who are at increased risk for hemorrhage.
ethiofos	Ethyol	Adjunctive therapy (chemoprotective agent) with cisplatin or cyclophosphamide in the treatment of cancer.
fatty acid solution, short chain	Not established	Treatment of ulcerative colitis (active phase) with involvement restricted to the left side of the colon.
fibronectin (plasma derived)	Not established	Treatment of corneal ulcers or epithelial defects refractory to conventional therapy.
flumecinol	Zixoryn	Hyberbilirubinemia in neonates unresponsive to phototherapy.
fosphenytoin	Not established	Acute treatment of status epilepticus.
gangliosides (sodium salts)	Cronassial	Treatment of retinitis pigmentosa.
gentamicin-impregnated PMMA beads on surgical wire	Septopal	Treatment of chronic osteomyelitis.
gossypol	Not established	Treatment of adrenal cortex cancer.
herpes simplex virus gene	Not established	Treatment of primary and metastatic brain tumors.
HPA-23	Not established	Treatment of AIDS.
human growth hormone-releasing factor	Not established	Treatment of children with growth failure caused by lack of endogenous growth hormone secretion.
humanized anti-TAC	Not established	Prevention of acute renal allograft rejection and acute graft-versus-host disease after bone marrow transplantation.
hydroxycobalamin/ sodium thiosulfate	Not established	Treatment of severe acute cyanide poisoning.
iloprost	Not established	Treatment of heparin-induced thrombocytopenia and Raynaud's phenomenon secondary to systemic sclerosis.
inosine pranobex	Isoprinosine	Treatment of subacute sclerosing panencephalitis.

(continued)

Orphan drugs and biologicals *(continued)*

GENERIC NAME	TRADE NAME	DESIGNATED USE
Drugs *(continued)*		
interferon beta, recombinant human	Not established	Treatment of primary brain tumors and AIDS.
interleukin-1 receptor antagonist, human recombinant	Antril	Prevention and treatment of graft-versus-host disease in transplant recipients.
iodine ^{131}I 6B-iodomethyl-19-norcholesterol	Not established	Adrenocortical imaging.
iodine ^{131}I iodobenzylguanidine	Not established	Diagnostic adjunct in patients with pheochromocytoma.
isobutyramide	Not established	Treatment of beta-hemoglobinopathies and beta-thalassemia syndromes.
leupeptin	Not established	Adjunctive treatment of microsurgical nerve repair.
levocabastine hydrochloride	Not established	Treatment of vernal keratoconjunctivitis.
LHRH [(des-gly^{10})-d-tri^{8}-Pro^{9}-n-ethylamide]	Not established	Treatment of central precocious puberty.
L-5 hydroxytryptophan (L-5-HTP)	Not established	Treatment of postanoxic intention myoclonus.
L-leucine, L-isoleucine, and L-valine	Not established	Treatment of amyotrophic lateral sclerosis.
L-leucovorin	Isovorin	Palliative treatment (with fluorouracil) of metastatic adenocarcinoma of the colon and rectum.
L-threonine	Threostat	Treatment of amyotropic lateral sclerosis.
lysine acetylsalicylate	Aspegic	Treatment of pain and fever associated with sickle cell disease crisis.
methotrexate with laurocapram	Not established	Treatment of mycosis fungoides.
4-methylpyrazole (4-MP)	Not established	Treatment of poisoning from methanol, ethylene glycol, 2-methoxyethanol, or 2-butoxyethanol.
mitodrine hydrochloride	Midamine	Treatment of idiopathic orthostatic hypotension.
mitolactol (dibromodulcitol, DBD)	Not established	Treatment of invasive cervical carcinoma.
modafinil	Not established	Treatment of narcolepsy.

Orphan drugs and biologicals *(continued)*

GENERIC NAME	TRADE NAME	DESIGNATED USE
Drugs *(continued)*		
n-acetylprocainamide (NAPA)	Not established	Adjunctive treatment of ventricular fibrillation in patients with automatic implantable cardioverter defibrillators.
NG-29	Somatrel	Assessment of pituitary function in children with suspected growth hormone deficiency.
ovine corticotropin-releasing hormone (oCRH)	Not established	To differentiate pituitary and ectopic production of corticotropin in patients with corticotropin-dependent Cushing's syndrome.
oxaliplatin	Not established	Treatment of ovarian cancer.
PEG-adenosine deaminase (PEG-ADA)	Imudon	Enzyme replacement therapy for ADA deficiency in patients with severe combined immunodeficiency.
phosphocysteamine	Not established	Treatment of cystinosis.
piracetam	Nootropil	Treatment of myoclonus.
piritrexim isethionate	Not established	Treatment of infections caused by *Pneumocystis carinii, Toxoplasma gondii,* and *Mycobacterium avium-intracellulare.*
poloxamer 188	Rheoth Rx Copolymer	Treatment of sickle cell disease crisis and severe burns.
poloxamer 331	Protox	Initial treatment of toxoplasmosis in patients with AIDS.
polymer implant containing carmustine	Biodel	Localized treatment of recurrent malignant melanoma in the brain.
potassium citrate and citric acid	Polycitra-K	Dissolution and control of uric acid and cystine calculi in the urinary tract.
PR-122 (redox-phenytoin)	Not established	Emergency treatment of status epilepticus.
PR-225 (redox acyclovir)	Not established	Treatment of herpes simplex encephalitis in patients with AIDS.
PR-239 (redox penicillin G)	Not established	Treatment of neurosyphilis associated with AIDS.
PR-320 (molecusol-carbamazepine)	Not established	Emergency treatment of status epilepticus.
prednimustine	Sterecyt	Treatment of non-Hodgkin's lymphomas.

(continued)

Orphan drugs and biologicals *(continued)*

GENERIC NAME	TRADE NAME	DESIGNATED USE
Drugs *(continued)*		
propamidine isethionate 0.1%	Brolene Eye Drops	Treatment of *Acanthamoeba* keratitis.
protirelin (TRH)	Thymone	Treatment of amyotrophic lateral sclerosis.
rifampin, isoniazid, pyrazinamide	Rifater	Short-course treatment of tuberculosis.
riluzole	Not established	Treatment of amyotrophic lateral sclerosis.
secalciferol (24, 25 dihydroxycholecalciferol)	Not established	Treatment of uremic osteodystrophy.
sermorelin acetate	Geref	Treatment of idiopathic growth hormone deficiency in children and ovulatory failure in women who fail to respond to clomiphene or gonadotropin.
sodium dichloroacetate	Not established	Treatment of homozygous familial hypercholesterolemia and congenital lactic acidosis.
sodium monomercap-toundecahydro-closo-dodeca-borate	Borolife	Treatment of gliobastoma multiforme as an alternative to conventional photon therapy.
sodium oxybate (sodium gamma hydroxy-butyrate)	Not established	Treatment of narcolepsy and the auxiliary symptoms of cataplexy, sleep paralysis, hypnagogic hallucinations, and automatic behavior.
sodium tetradecyl sulfate	Sotradecol	Treatment of bleeding esophageal varices.
spiramycin	Rovamycine	Symptomatic relief and parasitic cure of chronic cryptosporidosis in patients with immunodeficiency.
superoxide dismutase (recombinant, human)	Not established	Protection of donor organ tissue from damage or injury mediated by oxygen-derived free radicals that are generated during the necessary periods of ischemia (hypoxia) and especially reperfusion and anoxia associated with the operative procedure; prevention of bronchopulmonary dysplasia in premature neonates (under 1,500 g).
T4 endonuclease V, liposome encapsulated	T4N5 Liposomes	Prevention of skin abnormalities such as cutaneous neoplasms in patients with xeroderma pigmentosum.

Orphan drugs and biologicals *(continued)*

GENERIC NAME	TRADE NAME	DESIGNATED USE
Drugs *(continued)*		
teriparatide	Parathar	To aid diagnosis in patients with clinical and laboratory evidence of hypocalcemia due to either hypoparathyroidism or pseudohypoparathyroidism.
terlipressin	Glypressin	Treatment of bleeding esophageal varices.
thalidomide	Not established	Prevention and treatment of graft-versus-host disease in patients receiving bone marrow transplant; treatment and maintenance of reactional lepromatous leprosy; treatment of clinical manifestations of mycobacterial infection.
thymoxamine hydrochloride	Not established	Reversal of phenylephrine-induced mydriasis in patients who have narrow anterior angles and are at risk for developing an acute attack of angle-closure glaucoma after mydriasis.
tocophersolan oral solution (vitamin E, d-alpha tocopheryl polylene glycol-1000 succinate, TPGS)	Not established	Treatment of vitamin E deficiency in patients with malabsorption caused by prolonged cholestatic hepatobiliary disease.
topiramate	Topimax	Treatment of Lennox-Gastaut syndrome.
tranexamic acid	Cyklokapron	Treatment of hereditary angioneurotic edema, patients undergoing prostatectomy where there is hemorrhage or risk of hemorrhage from increased fibrinolysis or fibrinogenolysis, and patients with congenital coagulopathies who are undergoing surgical procedures, such as dental extractions.
transforming growth factor beta-2	Not established	Treatment of full-thickness macular hole disease.
tretinoin	Not established	Treatment of squamous metaplasia of the ocular surface epithelia (conjunctiva or cornea) with mucous deficiency and keratinization.
triptorelin pamoate	Decapeptyl Injection	Palliative treatment of advanced ovarian carcinoma of epithelial origin.
troleandomycin	Not established	Adjunctive treatment of severe steroid-dependent asthma.

(continued)

Orphan drugs and biologicals *(continued)*

GENERIC NAME	TRADE NAME	DESIGNATED USE
Drugs *(continued)*		
tumor necrosis factor-binding protein I	Not established	Treatment of AIDS.
tumor necrosis factor-binding protein II	Not established	Treatment of AIDS.
urofollitropin	Metrodin	Induction of ovulation in patients with polycystic ovarian disease who have an elevated luteinizing hormone to follicle-stimulating hormone ratio and who have failed to respond to adequate clomiphene therapy.
viloxazine hydrochloride	Catatrol	Treatment of narcolepsy and cataplexy.
zinc acetate	Not established	Treatment of Wilson's disease.

Biologicals

GENERIC NAME	TRADE NAME	DESIGNATED USE
alpha-1-antitrypsin (recombinant DNA origin)	Not established	Supplementation therapy for alpha-1-antitrypsin deficiency in the ZZ phenotype population.
ancrod	Arvin	Treatment of heparin-induced thrombosis or thrombocytopenia.
anticytomegalovirus monoclonal antibodies	Not established	Prevention or treatment of CMV infection in patients with AIDS, and in organ transplant or bone marrow transplant recipients.
antihemophilic factor (recombinant DNA origin)	Not established	Prophylaxis and treatment of bleeding in patients with hemophilia A.
antimelanoma antibody XMMME-001-RTA	Not established	Treatment of Stage III melanoma not amenable to surgical resection.
anti-TAP-72 immunotoxin	Xomazyme-791	Treatment of metastatic colorectal cancer adenocarcinoma.
benzylpenicillin, benzylpenicilloic acid, and benzylpenilloic acid	Pre-Pen/MDM	For assessing the risk of administering penicillin when it's the drug of choice in adults who have a history of clinical hypersensitivity.
botulism immune globulin	Not established.	Treatment of infant botulism.
bovine colostrum	Not established	Treatment of AIDS-related diarrhea.
CD4, human recombinant soluble	Receptin	Treatment of AIDS.

Orphan drugs and biologicals *(continued)*

GENERIC NAME	TRADE NAME	DESIGNATED USE
Biologicals *(continued)*		
CD4, human truncated-369 AA polypeptide (recombinant CHO cells)	Soluble T4	Treatment of AIDS.
CD4 immunoglobulin G (recombinant human)	Not established	Treatment of AIDS.
CD-45 monoclonal antibodies	Not established	Prevention of rejection of human organ transplants.
CD5-T lymphocyte Immunotoxin	Xomazyme-H65	Ex vivo treatment to eliminate mature T cells from potential bone marrow grafts, in vivo treatment of bone marrow recipients to prevent graft rejection and graft-versus-host disease (GVHD), and treatment of GVHD or rejection in patients who have received bone marrow transplants.
chimeric M-T412 (human-murine) IgG monoclonal anti-CD4	Not established	Treatment of multiple sclerosis.
C1-inhibitor	C1-inhibitor (human) vapor treated, Immuno	Prevention or treatment of acute attacks of angioedema.
deoxyribonuclease, recombinant human	rhDNase	To reduce the viscosity of mucus secretions and enhance airway clearance in patients with cystic fibrosis.
disaccharide tripeptide glycerol dipalmitoyl	Immther	Treatment of hepatic and pulmonary metastases in patients with colorectal adenocarcinoma.
epoetin beta (recombinant-human)	Marogen	Treatment of anemia associated with end-stage renal disease.
factor VIIa (recombinant, DNA origin)	Not established	Treatment of von Willebrand's disease and of patients with hemophilia A and B with and without antibodies against factor VIII and IX.
factor XIII	Fibrogammin	Congenital factor XIII deficiency.
fibronectin (human plasma derived)	Not established	Treatment of epithelial defects or nonhealing corneal ulcers unresponsive to conventional therapy.
group B streptococcus immune globulin	Not established	Treatment of disseminated group B streptococcus infection in neonates.
heme arginate	Normosang	Treatment of acute, symptomatic porphyria.

(continued)

Orphan drugs and biologicals *(continued)*

GENERIC NAME	TRADE NAME	DESIGNATED USE
Biologicals *(continued)*		
hemin	Panhematin	Amelioration of recurrent attacks of acute intermittent porphyria temporally related to the menstrual cycle in susceptible women and similar symptoms that occur in other patients with acute intermittent porphyria, porphyria variegata, and hereditary coproporphyria.
human IgM monoclonal antibody (C-58) to cytomegalovirus (CMV)	Centovir	Prophylaxis and treatment of CMV infections in bone marrow transplant recipients.
human immunodeficiency virus (HIV-1) immune globulin (human) I.V.	Not established	Treatment of AIDS.
human monoclonal antibody against hepatitis B virus	Not established	Prophylaxis against reinfection with hepatitis B in patients undergoing liver transplant secondary to end-stage chronic hepatitis B infection.
human T-lymphotropic virus type III gp160 antigens, recombinant vaccine, alum absorbed	VaxSyn HIV-1	Treatment of AIDS.
interferon beta (recombinant, human)	Betaseron	Treatment of AIDS and multiple sclerosis.
interleukin-1 alpha (recombinant, human)	Not established	Promotion of graft acceptance in patients undergoing bone marrow transplant.
interleukin-3 (recombinant, human)	Not established	Promotion of erythropoiesis in patients with congenital pure cell aplasia (Diamond-Blackfan anemia).
iodine ^{131}I Lym-1 monoclonal antibody	Not established	Treatment of B-cell lymphoma.
iodine ^{131}I murine monoclonal antibody to human alpha-fetoprotein	AFP-I 131	Treatment of hepatocellular carcinoma, hepatoblastoma, and alpha-fetoprotein-producing germ cell tumors.
iodine ^{131}I murine monoclonal antibody to human chorionic gonadotropin	hCG-I 131	Treatment of human chorionic gonadotropin-producing tumors, including germ cell and trophoblastic cell tumors.

Orphan drugs and biologicals *(continued)*

GENERIC NAME	TRADE NAME	DESIGNATED USE
Biologicals *(continued)*		
iodine ^{131}I murine monoclonal antibody IgG^{2a} to B cell	LL-2-I 131	Treatment of B-cell leukemia and lymphoma.
lactobin	Lactobin	Treatment of refractory diarrhea associated with AIDS.
melanoma vaccine	Melaccine	Treatment of melanoma (stage III or IV).
monoclonal antibodies (murine or human) recognizing B-cell lymphoma idiotypes	Not established	Treatment of B-cell lymphoma.
monoclonal antibodies PM-81 and AML-2-23	Not established	Treatment of patients with acute myelogenous leukemia undergoing bone marrow transplant.
monoclonal antibody 17-1A	Panorex	Treatment of pancreatic cancer.
monoclonal antibody PM-81	Not established	Adjunctive treatment of acute myelogenous leukemia.
monoclonal antibody for immunization against lupus nephritis	Not established	Treatment of lupus nephritis.
monoclonal factor IX	Not established	Treatment of hemophilia B.
mucoid exopolysaccharide *Pseudomonas* hyperimmune globulin	MEPIG	Prevention or treatment of *Pseudomonas aeruginosa* pulmonary infections in patients with cystic fibrosis.
myelin	Not established	Treatment of multiple sclerosis.
PEG-interleukin 2	Not established	Treatment of immunodeficiencies associated with T-cell defects.
PEG-L-asparaginase	Not established	Treatment of acute lymphocytic leukemia.
pentastarch	Pentaspan	Adjunctive use in leukapheresis, to improve the harvesting and increase the yield of leukocytes by centrifugal means.
poly I:poly C12U	Ampligen	Treatment of renal cell carcinoma.
polyribonucleotide	Ampligen	Treatment of AIDS.
respiratory syncytial virus immune globulin (human)	Hyperimmune RSV	Prophylaxis and treatment of respiratory syncytial virus infections in hospitalized infants and children.

(continued)

Orphan drugs and biologicals *(continued)*

GENERIC NAME	TRADE NAME	DESIGNATED USE
Biologicals *(continued)*		
ricin (blocked) conjugated murine monoclonal antibody (anti-B4) to B cell (CD19)	Not established	Treatment of B-cell leukemia and B-cell lymphoma.
ricin (blocked) conjugated murine monoclonal antibody (anti-My9) to myeloid cells (CD-33)	Anti-My9-bR	Treatment of myeloid leukemias.
ricin (blocked) conjugated murine monoclonal antibody (N901)	Not established	Treatment of small-cell lung cancer.
secretory leukocyte protease inhibitor, recombinant	Not established	Treatment of congenital deficiency of alpha-1-antitrypsin; treatment of cystic fibrosis.
Serratia marcescens extract (ribosomes and lipid vesicles)	ImuVert	Treatment of primary malignant brain tumors.
ST1-RTA immunotoxin (SR 44163)	Not established	Prevention of acute graft-versus-host disease in allogenic bone marrow transplantation and treatment of patients with B-chronic lymphocytic leukemia.
teceleukin	Not established	Treatment of metastatic malignant melanoma (with interferon alfa-2a).
thymosin alpha-1	Not established	Adjunctive treatment of active chronic hepatitis B.
trisaccharides A and B	Not established	Treatment of moderate to severe clinical forms of hemolytic disease of the newborn arising from placental transfer of antibodies against blood group substances A and B; use in ABO-incompatible solid organ transplantation, including kidney, heart, liver, and pancreas; and treatment of moderate-to-severe clinical forms of transfusion reactions arising from ABO-incompatible transfusion of blood, blood products, and blood derivatives.

Cancer chemotherapy: Acronyms and protocols

Combination chemotherapy is well established for treatment of cancer. The chart below lists commonly used acronyms and protocols, including standard dosages for specific cancers.

ACRONYM & INDICATION	DRUG: Generic name	DRUG: Trade name	DOSAGE
AA (Leukemia – AML, induction)	cytarabine (ara-C)	Cytosar-U	100 mg/m² daily by continuous I.V. infusion for 7 to 10 days
	doxorubicin	Adriamycin	30 mg/m² I.V., days 1 to 3
ABVD (Hodgkin's lymphoma)	doxorubicin	Adriamycin	25 mg/m² I.V., days 1 and 15
	bleomycin	Blenoxane	10 units/m² I.V., days 1 and 15
	vinblastine	Velban	6 mg/m² I.V., days 1 and 15
	dacarbazine	DTIC-Dome	375 mg/m² I.V., days 1 and 15 *Repeat cycle q 28 days.*
AC (Multiple myeloma)	doxorubicin	Adriamycin	30 mg/m² I.V., day 1
	carmustine	BiCNU	30 mg/m² I.V., day 1 *Repeat cycle q 21 to 28 days.*
AC (Bony sarcoma)	doxorubicin	Adriamycin	75 to 90 mg/m² by 96-hour continuous I.V. infusion
	cisplatin	Platinol	90 to 120 mg/m² IA or I.V., day 6 *Repeat cycle q 28 days.*
AFM (Breast cancer)	doxorubicin	Adriamycin	25 mg/m² by continuous I.V. infusion, days 1 to 3
	fluorouracil (5-FU)	Adrucil	400 mg/m² I.V., days 1 to 5
	methotrexate	Folex	250 mg/m² I.V., day 18
	leucovorin calcium	Wellcovorin	15 mg/m² P.O. q 6 hours, days 19 to 20 *Repeat cycle q 21 days for four cycles.*
AP (Ovarian cancer, epithelial)	doxorubicin	Adriamycin	50 to 60 mg/m² I.V., day 1
	cisplatin	Platinol	50 to 60 mg/m² I.V., day 1 *Repeat cycle q 21 days.*
APE (EAP) (Gastric cancer)	doxorubicin	Adriamycin	20 mg/m² I.V. daily, days 1 and 7
	cisplatin	Platinol	40 mg/m² I.V. daily, days 2 and 8
	etoposide (VP-16)	VePesid	120 mg/m² I.V. daily, days 4, 5, and 6 *Repeat cycle q 8 weeks.*
ASHAP (Non-Hodgkin's lymphoma)	doxorubicin	Adriamycin	10 mg/m² daily by continuous I.V. infusion, days 1 to 4
	cisplatin	Platinol	25 mg/m² daily by continuous I.V. infusion days 1 to 4
	cytarabine (ara-C)	Cytosar-U	1,500 mg/m² I.V. immediately after completion of doxorubicin and cisplatin therapy
	methylprednisolone	Solu-Medrol	500 mg I.V. daily, days 1 to 5 *Repeat cycle q 21 to 25 days.*

(continued)

Cancer chemotherapy: Acronyms and protocols *(continued)*

ACRONYM & INDICATION	DRUG Generic name	Trade name	DOSAGE
BACON (Non-small-cell lung cancer)	bleomycin	Blenoxane	30 units I.V. q 6 weeks, day 2
	doxorubicin	Adriamycin	40 mg/m² I.V. q 4 weeks, day 1
	lomustine (CCNU)	CeeNU	65 mg/m² P.O. q 8 weeks, day 1
	vincristine	Oncovin	0.75 to 1 mg/m² I.V. q 6 weeks, day 2
	mechlorethamine (nitrogen mustard)	Mustargen	8 mg/m² I.V. q 4 weeks, day 1
BACOP (Non-Hodgkin's lymphoma)	bleomycin	Blenoxane	5 units/m² I.V. daily, days 15 and 22
	doxorubicin	Adriamycin	25 mg/m² I.V., days 1 and 8
	cyclophosphamide	Cytoxan	650 mg/m² I.V., days 1 and 8
	vincristine	Oncovin	1.4 mg/m² (2 mg maximum) I.V., days 1 and 8
	prednisone	Deltasone	60 mg/m² P.O., days 15 to 28 *Repeat cycle q 28 days.*
BCP (Multiple myeloma)	carmustine	BiCNU	75 mg/m² I.V., day 1
	cyclophosphamide	Cytoxan	400 mg/m² I.V., day 1
	prednisone	Deltasone	75 mg P.O., days 1 to 7 *Repeat cycle q 28 days.*
BEP (Genitourinary cancer)	bleomycin	Blenoxane	30 units I.V., days 2, 9, and 16
	etoposide (VP-16)	VePesid	100 mg/m², days 1 to 5
	cisplatin	Platinol	20 mg/m² I.V., days 1 to 5
BHD (Malignant melanoma)	carmustine	BiCNU	100 to 150 mg/m² I.V. q 6 weeks
	hydroxyurea	Hydrea	1,480 mg/m² P.O. q 3 weeks, days 1 to 5
	dacarbazine	DTIC-Dome	100 to 150 mg/m² I.V. q 3 weeks, days 1 to 5
CA (Breast cancer)	cyclophosphamide	Cytoxan	200 mg/m² P.O., days 3 to 6
	doxorubicin	Adriamycin	40 mg/m² I.V., day 1 *Repeat cycle q 21 to 28 days.*
CAE (ACE) (Small-cell lung cancer)	cyclophosphamide	Cytoxan	1 g/m² I.V., day 1
	doxorubicin	Adriamycin	50 mg/m² I.V., day 1
	etoposide (VP-16)	VePesid	80 to 120 mg/m² I.V., day 1 *Repeat cycle q 21 days.*
CAF (FAC) (Breast cancer)	cyclophosphamide	Cytoxan	100 mg/m² P.O., days 1 to 14
	doxorubicin	Adriamycin	30 mg/m² I.V., days 1 and 8
	fluorouracil (5-FU)	Adrucil	400 to 500 mg/m² I.V., days 1 and 8 *Repeat cycle q 28 days.*
or	cyclophosphamide	Cytoxan	500 mg/m² I.V., day 1
	doxorubicin	Adriamycin	50 mg/m² I.V., day 1
	fluorouracil (5-FU)	Adrucil	500 mg/m² I.V., day 1 *Repeat cycle q 21 days.*

Cancer chemotherapy: Acronyms and protocols *(continued)*

ACRONYM & INDICATION	DRUG Generic name	DRUG Trade name	DOSAGE
CAMP (Non-small-cell lung cancer)	cyclophosphamide	Cytoxan	300 mg/m² I.V., days 1 and 8
	doxorubicin	Adriamycin	20 mg/m² I.V., days 1 and 8
	methotrexate sodium	Folex	15 mg/m² I.V., days 1 and 8
	procarbazine	Matulane	100 mg/m² P.O., days 1 to 10 *Repeat cycle q 28 days.*
CAP (Genitourinary cancer)	cisplatin	Platinol	60 mg/m² I.V., day 1
	doxorubicin	Adriamycin	40 mg/m² I.V., day 1
	cyclophosphamide	Cytoxan	400 mg/m² I.V., day 1 *Repeat cycle q 21 days.*
CAP (Non-small-cell lung cancer)	cyclophosphamide	Cytoxan	400 mg/m² I.V., day 1
	doxorubicin	Adriamycin	40 mg/m² I.V., day 1
	cisplatin	Platinol	60 mg/m² I.V., day 1 *Repeat cycle q 28 days.*
CAP (PAC) (Ovarian cancer, epithelial)	cisplatin	Platinol	50 mg/m² I.V., day 1
	doxorubicin	Adriamycin	50 mg/m² I.V., day 1
	cyclophosphamide	Cytoxan	500 mg/m² I.V., day 1 *Repeat cycle q 21 days for eight cycles.*
CAV (Small-cell lung cancer)	cyclophosphamide	Cytoxan	750 mg/m² I.V., day 1
	doxorubicin	Adriamycin	50 mg/m² I.V., day 1
	vincristine	Oncovin	2 mg/m² I.V., day 1 *Repeat cycle q 3 weeks.*
CAVe (Hodgkin's lymphoma)	lomustine (CCNU)	CeeNU	100 mg/m² I.V., day 1
	doxorubicin	Adriamycin	60 mg/m² I.V., day 1
	vinblastine	Velban	5 mg/m² I.V., day 1 *Repeat cycle q 6 weeks.*
CC (Ovarian cancer, epithelial)	carboplatin	Paraplatin	300 mg/m² I.V., day 1
	cyclophosphamide	Cytoxan	600 mg/m² I.V., day 1 *Repeat cycle q 20 days.*
CD (DC) (Leukemia – ANLL, consolidation)	cytarabine (ara-C)	Cytosar-U	3,000 mg/m² I.V. q 12 hours for 6 days
	daunorubicin	Cerubidine	30 mg/m² I.V. daily for 3 days, after cytarabine therapy

(continued)

Cancer chemotherapy: Acronyms and protocols *(continued)*

ACRONYM & INDICATION	DRUG		DOSAGE
	Generic name	Trade name	
CDC (Ovarian cancer, epithelial)	carboplatin	Paraplatin	300 mg/m² I.V., day 1
	doxorubicin	Adriamycin	40 mg/m² I.V., day 1
	cyclophosphamide	Cytoxan	500 mg/m² I.V., day 1 *Repeat cycle q 28 days.*
CF (Head and neck cancer)	cisplatin	Platinol	100 mg/m² I.V., day 1
	fluorouracil (5-FU)	Adrucil	1,000 mg/m² daily by continuous I.V. infusion, days 1 to 5 *Repeat cycle q 21 to 28 days.*
or	carboplatin	Paraplatin	400 mg/m² I.V., day 1
	fluorouracil (5-FU)	Adrucil	1,000 mg/m² daily by continuous I.V. infusion, days 1 to 5 *Repeat cycle q 21 to 28 days.*
CFL (Head and neck cancer)	cisplatin	Platinol	100 mg/m² I.V., day 1
	fluorouracil (5-FU)	Adrucil	600 to 800 mg/m² daily by continuous I.V. infusion, days 1 to 5
	leucovorin calcium	Wellcovorin	200 to 300 mg/m² I.V. daily, days 1 to 5 *Repeat cycle q 21 days.*
CFM (Breast cancer)	cyclophosphamide	Cytoxan	500 mg/m² I.V., day 1
	fluorouracil (5-FU)	Adrucil	500 mg/m² I.V., day 1
	mitoxantrone	Novantrone	10 mg/m² I.V., day 1 *Repeat cycle q 21 days.*
CFPT (Breast cancer)	cyclophosphamide	Cytoxan	150 mg/m² I.V., days 1 to 5
	fluorouracil (5-FU)	Adrucil	300 mg/m² I.V., days 1 to 5
	prednisone	Deltasone	10 mg P.O. t.i.d. for first 7 days of each course
	tamoxifen	Nolvadex	10 mg P.O. b.i.d. (daily through each course) *Repeat cycle q 6 weeks.*
CHAP (Ovarian cancer, epithelial)	cyclophosphamide	Cytoxan	300 to 500 mg/m² I.V., day 1
	altretamine	Hexalen	150 mg/m² P.O., days 1 to 7
	doxorubicin	Adriamycin	30 to 50 mg/m² I.V., day 1
	cisplatin	Platinol	50 mg/m² I.V., day 1 *Repeat cycle q 28 days.*
ChlVPP (Hodgkin's lymphoma)	chlorambucil	Leukeran	6 mg/m² P.O., days 1 to 14 (10 mg/day maximum)
	vinblastine	Velban	6 mg/m² I.V., days 1 to 8 (10 mg/day maximum)
	procarbazine	Matulane	50 mg P.O., days 1 to 14 (150 mg/day maximum)
	prednisone	Deltasone	40 mg/m² P.O., days 1 to 14 (25 mg/m² for child)

Cancer chemotherapy: Acronyms and protocols *(continued)*

ACRONYM & INDICATION	DRUG: Generic name	DRUG: Trade name	DOSAGE
CHOP (Non-Hodgkin's lymphoma)	cyclophosphamide	Cytoxan	750 mg/m² I.V., day 1
	doxorubicin	Adriamycin	50 mg/m² I.V., day 1
	vincristine	Oncovin	1.4 mg/m² (2 mg maximum) I.V., day 1
	prednisone	Deltasone	100 mg/m² P.O., days 1 to 5 *Repeat cycle q 21 days.*
CHOP-Bleo (Non-Hodgkin's lymphoma)	cyclophosphamide	Cytoxan	750 mg/m² I.V., day 1
	doxorubicin	Adriamycin	50 mg/m² I.V., day 1
	vincristine	Oncovin	2 mg I.V., days 1 and 5
	prednisone	Deltasone	100 mg P.O., days 1 to 5
	bleomycin	Blenoxane	15 units I.V., days 1 and 5 *Repeat cycle q 21 days.*
CISCA (Genitourinary cancer)	cyclophosphamide	Cytoxan	650 mg/m² I.V., day 1
	doxorubicin	Adriamycin	50 mg/m² I.V., day 1
	cisplatin	Platinol	70 to 100 mg/m² I.V., day 2 *Repeat cycle q 21 to 28 days.*
CMF (Breast cancer)	cyclophosphamide	Cytoxan	100 mg/m² P.O., days 1 to 14, or 400 to 600 mg/m² I.V., day 1
	methotrexate	Folex	40 to 60 mg/m² I.V., days 1 and 8
	fluorouracil (5-FU)	Adrucil	400 to 600 mg/m² I.V., days 1 and 8 *Repeat cycle q 28 days.*
CMFVP (Cooper's) (Breast cancer)	cyclophosphamide	Cytoxan	2 to 2.5 mg/kg P.O. daily for 9 months
	methotrexate	Folex	0.7 mg/kg/week I.V. for 8 weeks, then every other week for 7 months
	fluorouracil (5-FU)	Adrucil	12 mg/kg/week I.V. for 8 weeks, then weekly for 7 months
	vincristine	Oncovin	0.035 mg/kg (2 mg/week maximum) I.V. for 5 weeks, then once monthly
	prednisone	Deltasone	0.75 mg/kg P.O. daily, days 1 to 10, then taper over next 40 days and discontinue
CMFVP (SWOG) (Breast cancer)	cyclophosphamide	Cytoxan	60 mg/m² P.O. daily for 1 year
	methotrexate	Folex	15 mg/m² I.V. weekly for 1 year
	fluorouracil (5-FU)	Adrucil	300 mg/m² I.V. weekly for 1 year
	vincristine	Oncovin	0.625 mg/m² I.V. weekly for 1 year
	prednisone	Deltasone	30 mg/m² P.O., days 1 to 14; 20 mg/m², days 15 to 28; 10 mg/m², days 29 to 42 *Repeat cycle q 42 days.*

(continued)

Cancer chemotherapy: Acronyms and protocols *(continued)*

ACRONYM & INDICATION	DRUG		DOSAGE
	Generic name	Trade name	
COAP (Leukemia – AML, induction)	cyclophosphamide	Cytoxan	100 mg/m² I.V. or P.O., days 1 to 5
	vincristine	Oncovin	2 mg/m² I.V., day 1
	cytarabine (ara-C)	Cytosar-U	100 mg/m² I.V., days 1 to 5
	prednisone	Deltasone	100 mg P.O., days 1 to 5
COB (Head and neck cancer)	cisplatin	Platinol	100 mg/m² I.V., day 1
	vincristine	Oncovin	1 mg I.V., days 2 and 5
	bleomycin	Blenoxane	30 units by continuous I.V. infusion, days 2 to 5 *Repeat cycle q 21 days.*
COMLA (Non-Hodgkin's lymphoma)	cyclophosphamide	Cytoxan	1,500 mg/m² I.V., day 1
	vincristine	Oncovin	1.4 mg/m² (2.5 mg maximum) I.V., days 1, 8, and 15
	methotrexate	Folex	120 mg/m² I.V., days 22, 29, 36, 43, 50, 57, 64, and 71
	leucovorin calcium	Wellcovorin	25 mg/m² P.O. q 6 hours for four doses, beginning 24 hours after methotrexate dose
	cytarabine (ara-C)	Cytosar-U	300 mg/m² I.V., days 22, 29, 36, 43, 50, 57, 64, and 71 *Repeat cycle q 21 days.*
COP (Non-Hodgkin's lymphoma)	cyclophosphamide	Cytoxan	800 to 1,000 mg/m² I.V., day 1
	vincristine	Oncovin	1.4 mg/m² (2 mg maximum) I.V., day 1
	prednisone	Deltasone	60 mg/m² P.O., days 1 to 5 *Repeat cycle q 21 days.*
COP-BLAM (Non-Hodgkin's lymphoma)	cyclophosphamide	Cytoxan	400 mg/m² I.V., day 1
	vincristine	Oncovin	1 mg/m² I.V., day 1
	prednisone	Deltasone	40 mg/m² P.O., days 1 to 10
	bleomycin	Blenoxane	15 mg I.V., day 14
	doxorubicin	Adriamycin	40 mg/m², day 1
	procarbazine	Matulane	100 mg/m², days 1 to 10
COPE (Small-cell lung cancer)	cyclophosphamide	Cytoxan	750 mg/m² I.V., day 1
	cisplatin	Platinol	20 mg/m² I.V., days 1 to 3
	etoposide (VP-16)	VePesid	100 mg/m² I.V., days 1 to 3
	vincristine	Oncovin	2 mg/m² I.V., day 3 *Repeat cycle q 21 days.*
COPP (Non-Hodgkin's lymphoma)	cyclophosphamide	Cytoxan	400 to 650 mg/m² I.V., days 1 and 8
	vincristine	Oncovin	1.4 to 1.5 mg/m² (2 mg maximum) I.V., days 1 and 8
	procarbazine	Matulane	100 mg/m² P.O., days 1 to 10 or 1 to 14
	prednisone	Deltasone	40 mg/m² P.O., days 1 to 14 *Repeat cycle q 28 days.*

Cancer chemotherapy: Acronyms and protocols *(continued)*

ACRONYM & INDICATION	DRUG: Generic name	DRUG: Trade name	DOSAGE
CP (Ovarian cancer, epithelial)	cyclophosphamide	Cytoxan	1,000 mg/m² I.V., day 1
	cisplatin	Platinol	50 to 60 mg/m² I.V., day 1 *Repeat cycle q 21 days.*
CV (Small-cell lung cancer)	cisplatin	Platinol	50 mg/m² I.V., day 1
	etoposide (VP-16)	VePesid	60 mg/m² I.V., days 1 to 5 *Repeat cycle q 21 to 28 days.*
CV (Non-small-cell lung cancer)	cisplatin	Platinol	60 to 80 mg/m² I.V., day 1
	etoposide (VP-16)	VePesid	120 mg/m² I.V., days 4, 6, and 8 *Repeat cycle q 21 to 28 days.*
CVEB (Genitourinary cancer)	cisplatin	Platinol	40 mg/m² I.V., days 1 to 5
	vinblastine	Velban	7.5 mg/m² I.V., day 1
	etoposide (VP-16)	VePesid	100 mg/m² I.V., days 1 to 5
	bleomycin	Blenoxane	30 units I.V. weekly *Repeat cycle q 21 days.*
CVI (VIC) (Non-small-cell lung cancer)	carboplatin	Paraplatin	300 mg/m² I.V., day 1
	etoposide (VP-16)	VePesid	60 to 100 mg/m² I.V., day 1
	ifosfamide	Ifex	1.5 g/m² I.V., days 1, 3, and 5
	mesna	Mesnex	Dosage is 20% of ifosfamide dose, given immediately before and at 4 and 8 hours after ifosfamide infusion *Repeat cycle q 28 days.*
CVP (Leukemia – CLL, blast crisis)	cyclophosphamide	Cytoxan	300 mg/m² P.O., days 1 to 5
	vincristine	Oncovin	1.4 mg/m² (2 mg maximum) I.V., day 1
	prednisone	Deltasone	100 mg/m² P.O., days 1 to 5 *Repeat cycle q 21 days.*
CVP (Non-Hodgkin's lymphoma)	cyclophosphamide	Cytoxan	400 mg/m² P.O., days 1 to 5
	vincristine	Oncovin	1.4 mg/m² (2 mg maximum) I.V., day 1
	prednisone	Deltasone	100 mg/m² P.O., days 1 to 5 *Repeat cycle q 21 days.*
CVPP (Hodgkin's lymphoma)	lomustine (CCNU)	CeeNU	75 mg/m² P.O., day 1
	vinblastine	Velban	4 mg/m² I.V., days 1 and 8
	procarbazine	Matulane	100 mg/m² P.O., days 1 to 14
	prednisone	Deltasone	30 mg/m² P.O., days 1 to 14 (cycles 1 and 4 only) *Repeat cycle q 28 days.*
CYADIC (Soft-tissue sarcoma)	cyclophosphamide	Cytoxan	600 mg/m² I.V., day 1
	doxorubicin	Adriamycin	15 mg/m² by continuous I.V. infusion, days 1 to 4
	dacarbazine	DTIC-Dome	250 mg/m² by continuous I.V. infusion, days 1 to 4

(continued)

Cancer chemotherapy: Acronyms and protocols *(continued)*

ACRONYM & INDICATION	DRUG: Generic name	DRUG: Trade name	DOSAGE
CYVADIC (Bony sarcoma)	cyclophosphamide	Cytoxan	600 mg/m² I.V., day 1
	vincristine	Oncovin	1.4 mg/m² (2 mg maximum) I.V. weekly for 6 weeks, then on day 1 of future cycles
	doxorubicin	Adriamycin	15 mg/m² by continuous I.V. infusion, days 1 to 4
	dacarbazine	DTIC-Dome	250 mg/m² by continuous I.V. infusion, days 1 to 4 *Repeat cycle q 21 to 28 days.*
CYVADIC (Soft-tissue sarcoma)	cyclophosphamide	Cytoxan	500 mg/m² I.V., day 1
	vincristine	Oncovin	1.4 mg/m² (2 mg maximum) I.V., days 1 and 5
	doxorubicin	Adriamycin	50 mg/m² I.V., day 1
	dacarbazine	DTIC-Dome	250 mg/m² I.V., days 1 to 5 *Repeat cycle q 21 days.*
DC (Leukemia – pediatric AML, induction)	daunorubicin	Cerubidine	45 to 60 mg/m² I.V., days 1 to 3
	cytarabine (ara-C)	Cytosar-U	100 mg/m² I.V. or S.C. q 12 hours for 5 to 7 days
DCPM (Leukemia – pediatric AML, induction)	daunorubicin	Cerubidine	25 mg/m² I.V., day 1
	cytarabine (ara-C)	Cytosar-U	80 mg/m² I.V., days 1 to 3
	prednisone	Deltasone	40 mg/m² P.O. daily
	mercaptopurine (6-MP)	Purinethol	100 mg/m² P.O. daily
DCT (Leukemia – ANLL, induction)	daunorubicin	Cerubidine	60 mg/m² I.V., days 1 to 3
	cytarabine (ara-C)	Cytosar-U	200 mg/m² daily by continuous I.V. infusion, days 1 to 5
	thioguanine (6-TG)		100 mg/m² P.O. q 12 hours, days 1 to 5
DHAP (Hodgkin's lymphoma)	dexamethasone	Decadron	40 mg P.O. or I.V., days 1 to 4
	cisplatin	Platinol	100 mg/m² by continuous I.V. infusion, day 1
	cytarabine (ara-C)	Cytosar-U	2 g/m² I.V. q 12 hours for two doses, day 2 *Repeat cycle q 3 to 4 weeks.*
DTIC-ACTD (Malignant melanoma)	dacarbazine	DTIC-Dome	750 mg/m² I.V., day 1
	dactinomycin (actinomycin D)	Cosmegen	1 mg/m² I.V., day 1 *Repeat cycle q 28 days.*
DVP (Leukemia – ALL, induction)	daunorubicin	Cerubidine	45 mg/m² I.V., days 1 to 4
	vincristine	Oncovin	2 mg/m² (2 mg maximum) I.V. weekly for 4 weeks
	prednisone	Deltasone	45 mg/m² P.O., for 28 to 35 days

Cancer chemotherapy: Acronyms and protocols *(continued)*

ACRONYM & INDICATION	DRUG Generic name	DRUG Trade name	DOSAGE
EP (Small-cell or non-small-cell lung cancer)	cisplatin	Platinol	75 to 100 mg/m² I.V., day 1
	etoposide (VP-16)	VePesid	75 to 100 mg/m² I.V., days 1 to 3 *Repeat cycle q 21 to 28 days.*
ESHAP (Non-Hodgkin's lymphoma)	etoposide (VP-16)	VePesid	40 mg/m² by continuous I.V. infusion, days 1 to 4
	cisplatin	Platinol	25 mg/m² daily by continuous I.V. infusion, days 1 to 4
	cytarabine (ara-C)	Cytosar-U	2 g/m² I.V. immediately after completion of etoposide and cisplatin therapy
	methylprednisolone	Solu-Medrol	500 mg I.V. daily, days 1 to 4 *Repeat cycle q 21 to 28 days.*
EVA (Hodgkin's lymphoma)	etoposide (VP-16)	VePesid	100 mg/m² I.V., days 1 to 3
	vinblastine	Velban	6 mg/m² I.V., day 1
	doxorubicin	Adriamycin	50 mg/m² I.V., day 1 *Repeat cycle q 28 days.*
FAC (CAF) (Breast cancer)	fluorouracil (5-FU)	Adrucil	500 mg/m² I.V., days 1 and 8
	doxorubicin	Adriamycin	50 mg/m² I.V., day 1
	cyclophosphamide	Cytoxan	500 mg/m² I.V., day 1 *Repeat cycle q 21 days.*
FAM (Colon cancer; gastric cancer)	fluorouracil (5-FU)	Adrucil	600 mg/m² I.V., days 1, 8, 29, and 36
	doxorubicin	Adriamycin	30 mg/m² I.V., days 1 and 29
	mitomycin	Mutamycin	10 mg/m² I.V., day 1 *Repeat cycle q 8 weeks.*
FAM (Non-small-cell lung cancer)	fluorouracil (5-FU)	Adrucil	600 mg/m² I.V., days 1, 8, 28, and 36
	doxorubicin	Adriamycin	30 mg/m² I.V., days 1 and 28
	mitomycin	Mutamycin	10 mg/m² I.V., day 1 *Repeat cycle q 8 weeks.*
FAM (Pancreatic cancer)	fluorouracil (5-FU)	Adrucil	600 mg/m² I.V., days 1, 8, 29, and 36
	doxorubicin	Adriamycin	30 mg/m² I.V., days 1 and 29
	mitomycin	Mutamycin	10 mg/m² I.V., day 1 *Repeat cycle q 8 weeks.*
FAME (Gastric cancer)	fluorouracil (5-FU)	Adrucil	350 mg/m² I.V., days 1 to 5 and 36 to 40
	doxorubicin	Adriamycin	40 mg/m² I.V., days 1 and 36
	semustine (methyl CCNU)		150 mg/m² P.O., day 1 *Repeat cycle q 10 weeks.*
FCE (Gastric cancer)	fluorouracil (5-FU)	Adrucil	900 mg/m² by continuous I.V. infusion, days 1 to 5
	cisplatin	Platinol	20 mg/m² I.V., days 1 to 5
	etoposide (VP-16)	VePesid	90 mg/m² I.V., days 1, 3, and 5 *Repeat cycle q 21 days.*

(continued)

Cancer chemotherapy: Acronyms and protocols *(continued)*

ACRONYM & INDICATION	DRUG: Generic name	DRUG: Trade name	DOSAGE
F-CL (Colon cancer)	fluorouracil (5-FU)	Adrucil	370 to 400 mg/m² I.V., days 1 to 5
	leucovorin calcium	Wellcovorin	200 mg/m² daily I.V., days 1 to 5, begun 15 minutes before fluorouracil infusion *Repeat cycle q 21 days.*
5 + 2 (Leukemia – ANLL, consolidation)	cytarabine (ara-C)	Cytosar-U	100 mg/m² I.V. q 12 hours for 6 days
	daunorubicin	Cerubidine	45 mg/m² I.V., days 1 and 2
FL (Genitourinary cancer)	flutamide	Eulexin	250 mg P.O. t.i.d.
	leuprolide acetate	Lupron	1 mg S.C. daily
or	flutamide	Eulexin	250 mg P.O. t.i.d.
	leuprolide acetate	Lupron Depot	7.5 mg I.M. q 28 days
FLe (Colon cancer)	levamisole	Ergamisol	50 mg P.O. t.i.d. for 3 days, repeated q 2 weeks for 1 year
	fluorouracil (5-FU)	Adrucil	450 mg/m² I.V. for 5 days, then, after a pause of 4 weeks, 450 mg/m² I.V. weekly for 48 weeks
FMS (Pancreatic cancer)	fluorouracil (5-FU)	Adrucil	600 mg/m² I.V., days 1, 8, 29, and 36
	mitomycin	Mutamycin	10 mg/m² I.V., day 1
	streptozocin	Zanosar	1 g/m² I.V., days 1, 8, 29, and 36 *Repeat cycle q 8 weeks.*
FMV (Colon cancer)	fluorouracil (5-FU)	Adrucil	10 mg/kg I.V., days 1 to 5
	semustine (methyl CCNU)		175 mg/m² P.O., day 1
	vincristine	Oncovin	1 mg/m² (2 mg maximum) I.V., day 1 *Repeat cycle q 35 days.*
FZ (Genitourinary cancer)	flutamide	Eulexin	250 P.O. t.i.d.
	goserelin acetate	Zoladex	3.6 mg implant S.C. q 28 days
HDMTX (high-dose methotrexate) (Bony sarcoma)	methotrexate	Folex	12 g/m² I.V. (20 g maximum)
	leucovorin calcium	Wellcovorin	15 mg I.V. or P.O. q 6 hours for 10 doses, beginning 24 hours after methotrexate dose (serum methotrexate levels must be monitored) *Repeat cycle q 4 to 16 weeks.*
Hexa-CAF (Ovarian cancer, epithelial)	altretamine	Hexalen	150 mg/m² P.O., days 1 to 14
	cyclophosphamide	Cytoxan	150 mg/m² P.O., days 1 to 14
	methotrexate	Folex	40 mg/m², days 1 and 8
	fluorouracil (5-FU)	Adrucil	600 mg/m² I.V., days 1 and 8 *Repeat cycle q 28 days.*
HiDAC (Leukemia – ANLL, consolidation)	cytarabine (ara-C)	Cytosar-U	3,000 mg/m² I.V. q 12 hours, days 1 to 6

Cancer chemotherapy: Acronyms and protocols *(continued)*

ACRONYM & INDICATION	DRUG: Generic name	DRUG: Trade name	DOSAGE
IMF (Breast cancer)	ifosfamide	Ifex	1.5 g/m² I.V., days 1 and 8
	mesna	Mesnex	Dosage is 20% of ifosfamide dose, given immediately before and at 4 and 8 hours after ifosfamide infusion
	methotrexate	Folex	40 mg/m² I.V., days 1 and 8
	fluorouracil (5-FU)	Adrucil	600 mg/m² I.V., days 1 and 8 *Repeat cycle q 28 days.*
L-VAM (Genitourinary cancer)	leuprolide acetate	Lupron	1 mg S.C. daily
	vinblastine	Velban	1.5 mg/m² by continuous I.V. infusion, days 2 to 7
	doxorubicin	Adriamycin	50 mg/m² by 24-hour continuous I.V. infusion, day 1
	mitomycin	Mutamycin	10 mg/m² I.V., day 2 *Repeat VAM cycle q 28 days.*
MACC (Non-small-cell lung cancer)	methotrexate	Folex	30 to 40 mg/m² I.V., day 1
	doxorubicin	Adriamycin	30 to 40 mg/m² I.V., day 1
	cyclophospamide	Cytoxan	400 to 600 mg/m² I.V., day 1
	lomustine (CCNU)	CeeNU	30 to 40 mg/m² P.O., day 1 *Repeat cycle q 21 to 28 days.*
MACOP-B (Non-Hodgkin's lymphoma)	methotrexate	Folex	100 mg/m² I.V., weeks 2, 6, and 10; then 300 mg/m² I.V. for 4 hours, weeks 2, 6, and 10
	leucovorin calcium	Wellcovorin	15 mg P.O.q 6 hours for 6 doses, beginning 24 hours after methotrexate
	doxorubicin	Adriamycin	50 mg/m² I.V., weeks 1, 3, 5, 7, 9, and 11
	cyclophospamide	Cytoxan	350 mg/m² I.V., weeks 1, 3, 5, 7, 9, and 11
	vincristine	Oncovin	1.4 mg/m² I.V. (2 mg maximum), weeks 2, 4, 8, 10, and 12
	bleomycin	Blenoxane	10 mg/m² I.V., weeks 4, 8, and 12
	prednisone	Deltasone	75 mg P.O. daily
MAID (Bony sarcoma)	mesna	Mesnex	Uroprotection 1.5 g/m² by continuous I.V. infusion, days 1 to 4
	doxorubicin	Adriamycin	15 mg/m² by continuous I.V. infusion, days 1 to 3
	ifosfamide	Ifex	1.5 g/m² by continuous I.V. infusion, days 1 to 3
	dacarbazine	DTIC-Dome	250 mg/m² by continuous I.V. infusion, days 1 to 3 *Repeat cycle q 21 to 28 days.*
MAID (Soft-tissue sarcoma)	mesna	Mesnex	1.5 g/m² by continuous I.V. infusion, days 1 to 4
	doxorubicin	Adriamycin	15 mg/m² by continuous I.V. infusion, days 1 to 3
	ifosfamide	Ifex	1.5 g/m² by continuous I.V. infusion, days 1 to 3
	dacarbazine	DTIC-Dome	250 mg/m² by continuous I.V. infusion, days 1 to 3 *Repeat cycle q 21 to 28 days.*

(continued)

Cancer chemotherapy: Acronyms and protocols *(continued)*

ACRONYM & INDICATION	DRUG: Generic name	DRUG: Trade name	DOSAGE
MAP (Head and neck cancer)	mitomycin	Mutamycin	8 mg/m² I.V., day 1
	doxorubicin	Adriamycin	40 mg/m² I.V., day 1
	cisplatin	Platinol	60 mg/m² I.V., day 1 *Repeat cycle q 28 days.*
m-BACOD (Non-Hodgkin's lymphoma)	bleomycin	Blenoxane	4 units/m² I.V., day 1
	doxorubicin	Adriamycin	45 mg/m² I.V., day 1
	cyclophosphamide	Cytoxan	600 mg/m² I.V., day 1
	vincristine	Oncovin	1 mg/m² I.V., day 1
	dexamethasone	Decadron	6 mg/m² I.V., days 1 to 5
	methotrexate	Folex	200 mg/m² I.V., days 8 and 15
	leucovorin calcium	Wellcovorin	10 mg/m² P.O. q 6 hours for 8 doses, beginning 24 hours after methotrexate dose *Repeat cycle q 21 days.*
m-BACOS (Non-Hodgkin's lymphoma)	doxorubicin	Adriamycin	50 mg/m² by 24-hour continuous I.V. infusion, day 1
	vincristine	Oncovin	1.4 mg/m² (2 mg maximum) I.V., day 1
	bleomycin	Blenoxane	10 units/m² I.V., day 1
	cyclophosphamide	Cytoxan	750 mg/m² I.V., day 1
	methotrexate	Folex	1 g/m² I.V., day 2
	leucovorin calcium	Wellcovorin	15 mg P.O. q 6 hours for 8 doses starting 24 hours after methotrexate dose *Repeat cycle q 21 to 25 days.*
MBC (Head and neck cancer)	methotrexate	Folex	40 mg/m² I.M. or I.V., days 1 and 15
	bleomycin	Blenoxane	10 units I.M. or I.V. weekly
	cisplatin	Platinol	50 mg/m² I.V., day 1 *Repeat cycle q 21 days.*
MC (Leukemia – ANLL, consolidation)	mitoxantrone	Novantrone	12 mg/m² I.V. daily, days 1 and 2
	cytarabine (ara-C)	Cytosar-U	100 mg/m² daily by continuous I.V. infusion, days 1 to 5 *Repeat cycle.*
MC (Leukemia – ANLL, induction)	mitoxantrone	Novantrone	12 mg/m² I.V., days 1 to 3 and 17 to 18
	cytarabine (ara-C)	Cytosar-U	100 mg/m² daily by continuous I.V. infusion, days 1 to 7 and 17 to 21
MF (Head and neck cancer)	methotrexate	Folex	125 to 150 mg/m² I.V., day 1
	fluorouracil (5-FU)	Adrucil	600 mg/m² I.V., beginning 1 hour after methotrexate dose
	leucovorin calcium	Wellcovorin	10 mg/m² I.V. or P.O. q 6 hours for 5 doses, beginning 24 hours after methotrexate dose *Repeat cycle weekly.*

Cancer chemotherapy: Acronyms and protocols *(continued)*

ACRONYM & INDICATION	DRUG: Generic name	DRUG: Trade name	DOSAGE
MICE (ICE) (Small-cell and non-small-cell lung cancer)	mesna	Mesnex	Dosage is 20% of ifosfamide doses given I.V. immediately before and at 4 and 8 hours after ifosfamide infusion
	ifosfamide	Ifex	2,000 mg/m² I.V., days 1 to 3
	carboplatin	Paraplatin	300 to 350 mg/m² I.V., day 1
	etoposide (VP-16)	VePesid	60 to 100 mg/m² I.V., days 1 to 3
MINE (Non-Hodgkin's lymphoma)	mesna	Mesnex	1.3 to 1.5 g/m² I.V., days 1 to 3
	ifosfamide	Ifex	1.3 to 1.5 g/m² I.V., days 1 to 3
	mitoxantrone	Novantrone	8 to 10 mg/m² I.V., day 1
	etoposide (VP-16)	VePesid	65 to 80 mg/m² I.V., days 1 to 3
MM (Leukemia – ALL, maintenance)	mercaptopurine (6-MP)	Purinethol	50 mg/m² P.O. daily
	methotrexate	Folex	20 mg/m² P.O. or I.V. weekly
MOF (Colon cancer)	fluorouracil (5-FU)	Adrucil	10 mg/kg/day I.V., days 1 to 5
	semustine (methyl CCNU)		175 mg/m² P.O., day 1
	vincristine	Oncovin	1 mg/m² (2 mg maximum) I.V., day 1 *Repeat cycle q 35 days.*
MOP (Pediatric brain tumors)	mechlorethamine (nitrogen mustard)	Mustargen	6 mg/m² I.V., days 1 and 8
	vincristine	Oncovin	1.4 mg/m² (2 mg maximum) I.V., days 1 and 8
	procarbazine	Matulane	100 mg/m² P.O., days 1 to 14 *Repeat cycle q 28 days.*
MOPP (Hodgkin's lymphoma)	mechlorethamine (nitrogen mustard)	Mustargen	6 mg/m² I.V., days 1 and 8
	vincristine	Oncovin	1.4 mg/m² (2 mg maximum) I.V., days 1 and 8
	procarbazine	Matulane	100 mg/m² P.O., days 1 to 14
	prednisone	Deltasone	40 mg/m² P.O., days 1 to 14 *Repeat cycle q 28 days.*
MP (Multiple myeloma)	melphalan (L-phenylalanine mustard)	Alkeran	8 mg/m² P.O., days 1 to 4
	prednisone	Deltasone	40 mg/m² P.O., days 1 to 7 *Repeat cycle q 28 days.*
m-PFL (Genitourinary cancer)	methotrexate	Folex	60 mg/m², day 1
	cisplatin	Platinol	25 mg/m² by continuous I.V. infusion, days 2 to 6
	fluorouracil (5-FU)	Adrucil	800 mg/m² by continuous I.V. infusion, days 2 to 6
	leucovorin calcium	Wellcovorin	500 mg/m² by continuous I.V. infusion, days 2 to 6 *Repeat cycle q 28 days for four cycles.*

(continued)

Cancer chemotherapy: Acronyms and protocols *(continued)*

ACRONYM & INDICATION	DRUG Generic name	DRUG Trade name	DOSAGE
M-2 (Multiple myeloma)	vincristine	Oncovin	0.03 mg/kg (2 mg maximum) I.V., day 1
	carmustine	BiCNU	0.5 mg/kg I.V., day 1
	cyclophosphamide	Cytoxan	10 mg/kg I.V, day 1
	melphalan (L-phenylalanine mustard)	Alkeran	0.25 mg/kg P.O., days 1 to 14
	prednisone	Deltasone	1 mg/kg, days 1 to 7, then taper over next 14 days *Repeat cycle q 35 days.*
MV (Leukemia – AML, induction)	mitoxantrone	Novantrone	10 mg/m² I.V., days 1 to 5
	etoposide (VP-16)	VePesid	100 mg/m² I.V., days 1 to 3
MVAC (Genitourinary cancer)	methotrexate	Folex	30 mg/m² I.V., days 1, 15, and 22
	vinblastine	Velban	3 mg/m² I.V., days 2, 15, and 22
	doxorubicin	Adriamycin	30 mg/m² I.V., day 2
	cisplatin	Platinol	70 mg/m² I.V., day 2 *Repeat cycle q 28 days.*
MVP (Non-small-cell lung cancer)	mitomycin	Mutamycin	8 mg/m² I.V., days 1, 29, and 71
	vinblastine	Velban	4.5 mg/m² I.V., days 15, 22, and 29, then q 2 weeks
	cisplatin	Platinol	120 mg/m² I.V., days 1 and 29, then q 6 weeks
MVPP (Hodgkin's lymphoma)	mechlorethamine (nitrogen mustard)	Mustargen	6 mg/m² I.V., days 1 and 8
	vinblastine	Velban	6 mg/m² I.V., days 1 and 8
	procarbazine	Matulane	100 mg/m² P.O., days 1 to 14
	prednisone	Deltasone	40 mg/m² P.O., days 1 to 14 *Repeat cycle q 42 days for six cycles.*
OPEN (Non-Hodgkin's lymphoma)	vincristine	Oncovin	2 mg I.V., day 1
	prednisone	Deltasone	100 mg P.O. daily for 5 days
	etoposide (VP-16)	VePesid	100 mg/m² I.V. daily for 3 days
	mitoxantrone	Novantrone	10 mg/m² I.V., day 1
PCV (Pediatric brain tumors)	procarbazine	Matulane	60 mg/m² P.O., days 18 to 21
	lomustine (CCNU)	CeeNU	110 mg/m² P.O., day 1
	vincristine	Oncovin	1.4 mg/m² (2 mg maximum), days 8 and 29 *Repeat cycle q 6 to 8 weeks.*
PFL (Head and neck cancer)	cisplatin	Platinol	25 mg/m² by continuous I.V. infusion, days 1 to 5
	5-fluorouracil (5-FU)	Adrucil	800 mg/m² by continuous I.V. infusion, days 2 to 6
	leucovorin calcium	Wellcovorin	500 mg/m² by continuous I.V. infusion, days 1 to 6 *Repeat cycle q 28 days.*

Cancer chemotherapy: Acronyms and protocols *(continued)*

ACRONYM & INDICATION	DRUG: Generic name	DRUG: Trade name	DOSAGE
PFL (Non-small-cell lung cancer)	cisplatin	Platinol	25 mg/m² I.V., days 1 and 15
	fluorouracil (5-FU)	Adrucil	800 mg/m² by continuous I.V. infusion, days 1 to 5
	leucovorin calcium	Wellcovorin	500 mg/m² by continuous I.V. infusion, days 1 to 5 *Repeat cycle q 28 days.*
ProMACE (Non-Hodgkin's lymphoma)	prednisone	Deltasone	60 mg/m² P.O., days 1 to 14
	methotrexate	Folex	1.5 g/m² I.V., day 14
	leucovorin calcium	Wellcovorin	50 mg/m² I.V. q 6 hours for 5 doses, beginning 24 hours after methotrexate dose
	doxorubicin	Adriamycin	25 mg/m² I.V., days 1 and 8
	cyclophosphamide	Cytoxan	650 mg/m² I.V., days 1 and 8
	etoposide (VP-16)	VePesid	120 mg/m² I.V., days 1 and 8 *Repeat cycle q 28 days; MOPP therapy to begin after the required number of ProMACE cycles are completed.*
ProMACE/ cytaBOM (Non-Hodgkin's lymphoma)	cyclophosphamide	Cytoxan	650 mg/m² I.V., day 1
	doxorubicin	Adriamycin	25 mg/m² I.V., day 1
	etoposide (VP-16)	VePesid	120 mg/m² I.V., day 1
	prednisone	Deltasone	60 mg/m² P.O., days 1 to 14
	cytarabine (ara-C)	Cytosar-U	300 mg/m² I.V., day 8
	bleomycin	Blenoxane	5 mg/m² I.V., day 8
	vincristine	Oncovin	1.4 mg/m² I.V., day 8
	methotrexate	Folex	120 mg/m² I.V., day 8
	leucovorin calcium	Wellcovorin	25 mg/m² P.O. q 6 hours for 4 doses *Repeat cycle q 28 days.*
(pulse) VAC (Soft-tissue sarcoma)	vincristine	Oncovin	1.5 g/m² (2 mg maximum) I.V., day 1 or weekly, starting on day 1
	dactinomycin (actinomycin D)	Cosmegen	0.4 mg/m² I.V., day 1
	cyclophosphamide	Cytoxan	1,000 mg/m² I.V., day 1 *Repeat cycle q 3 to 4 weeks.*
7 + 3 (A + D) (Leukemia – AML, induction)	cytarabine (ara-C)	Cytosar-U	100 or 200 mg/m² by continuous I.V. infusion, days 1 to 7
	daunorubicin	Cerubidine	45 mg/m² I.V., days 1 to 3
TC (Leukemia – ANLL, maintenance)	thioguanine (6-TG)		40 mg/m² P.O. q 12 hours for 8 doses, days 1 to 4
	cytarabine (ara-C)	Cytosar-U	60 mg/m² S.C. day 5 *Repeat cycle weekly.*

(continued)

Cancer chemotherapy: Acronyms and protocols *(continued)*

ACRONYM & INDICATION	DRUG: Generic name	DRUG: Trade name	DOSAGE
T-10 (Pediatric bony sarcoma)	methotrexate	Folex	12 g/m² I.V. for 12 or 16 doses
	leucovorin calcium	Wellcovorin	15 mg I.V. or P.O. q 6 hours for 10 doses, each starting 20 hours after methotrexate dose
	doxorubicin	Adriamycin	30 mg/m² I.V. for 2 to 3 days
	cisplatin	Platinol	120 mg/m² I.V. for 1 day
	bleomycin	Blenoxane	15 units/m² I.V. for 2 days
	cyclophosphamide	Cytoxan	600 mg/m² I.V. for 2 days
	dactinomycin (actinomycin D)	Cosmegen	0.6 mg/m² I.V. for 2 days
VA (Wilms' tumor)	vincristine	Oncovin	1.5 mg/m² (2 mg maximum) weekly
	dactinomycin (actinomycin D)	Cosmegen	0.4 mg/m² q 2 weeks
VAB (Genitourinary cancer)	vinblastine	Velban	4 mg/m² I.V., day 1
	dactinomycin (actinomycin D)	Cosmegen	1 mg/m² I.V., day 1
	bleomycin	Blenoxane	30 units I.V. push, then 20 units/m² by continuous I.V. infusion, days 1 to 3
	cisplatin	Platinol	120 mg/m² I.V., day 4
	cyclophosphamide	Cytoxan	600 mg/m² I.V., day 1 *Repeat cycle q 21 days.*
VAC (Small-cell lung cancer)	vincristine	Oncovin	2 mg I.V., day 1
	doxorubicin	Adriamycin	50 mg/m² I.V., day 1
	cyclophosphamide	Cytoxan	750 mg/m² I.V., day 1 *Repeat cycle q 21 days for four cycles.*
VAC (Ovarian cancer, germ-cell)	vincristine	Oncovin	1.2 to 1.5 mg/m² (2 mg maximum) I.V. weekly for 10 to 12 weeks, or q 2 weeks for 12 doses
	dactinomycin (actinomycin D)	Cosmegen	0.3 to 0.4 mg/m² I.V., days 1 to 5
	cyclophosphamide	Cytoxan	150 mg/m² I.V., days 1 to 5 *Repeat cycle q 28 days.*
VAC (Wilms' tumor)	vincristine	Oncovin	1.5 mg/m² (2 mg maximum) weekly
	dactinomycin (actinomycin D)	Cosmegen	1.25 g/m² q 3 weeks
	cyclophosphamide	Cytoxan	1,000 mg/m² q 3 weeks
VAD (Multiple myeloma)	vincristine	Oncovin	0.4 mg by continuous I.V. infusion, days 1 to 4
	doxorubicin	Adriamycin	9 to 10 mg/m² by continuous I.V. infusion, days 1 to 4
	dexamethasone	Decadron	40 mg P.O. on days 1 to 4, 9 to 12, and 17 to 20 *Repeat cycle q 25 to 35 days.*

Cancer chemotherapy: Acronyms and protocols *(continued)*

ACRONYM & INDICATION	DRUG: Generic name	DRUG: Trade name	DOSAGE
VAP (VP + A) (Leukemia – pediatric ALL, induction)	vincristine	Oncovin	1.5 to 2 mg/m² (2 mg maximum) I.V. weekly for 4 weeks
	asparaginase	Elspar	10,000 units I.M., days 1 and 8 (other doses include 6,000 units/m² I.M. for 3 days/week or 25,000 units/m²)
	prednisone	Deltasone	40 mg/m² P.O., days 1 to 28, then taper over 7 days
VATH (Breast cancer)	vinblastine	Velban	4.5 mg/m² I.V., day 1
	doxorubicin	Adriamycin	45 mg/m² I.V., day 1
	thiotepa	Thiotepa	12 mg/m² I.V., day 1
	fluoxymesterone	Halotestin	30 mg P.O. (daily through each course) *Repeat cycle q 21 days.*
VB (Genitourinary cancer)	vinblastine	Velban	3 to 4 mg/m² I.V., day 1
	methotrexate	Folex	30 to 40 mg/m² I.V., day 1 *Repeat cycle weekly.*
VBAP (Multiple myeloma)	vincristine	Oncovin	1 mg I.V., day 1
	carmustine	BiCNU	30 mg/m² I.V., day 1
	doxorubicin	Adriamycin	30 mg/m² I.V., day 1
	prednisone	Deltasone	100 mg P.O., days 1 to 4 *Repeat cycle q 21 days.*
VBC (Malignant melanoma)	vinblastine	Velban	6 mg/m² I.V., days 1 and 2
	bleomycin	Blenoxane	15 units/m² by continuous I.V. infusion, days 1 to 5
	cisplatin	Platinol	50 mg/m² I.V., day 5 *Repeat cycle q 28 days.*
VBP (Genitourinary cancer)	vinblastine	Velban	6 mg/m² I.V., days 1 and 2
	bleomycin	Blenoxane	30 units I.V. weekly
	cisplatin	Platinol	20 mg/m² I.V., days 1 to 5 *Repeat cycle q 21 to 28 days.*
VC (Small-cell lung cancer)	etoposide (VP-16)	VePesid	100 to 200 mg/m² I.V., days 1 to 3
	carboplatin	Paraplatin	50 to 125 mg/m² I.V., days 1 to 3 *Repeat cycle q 28 days.*
VCAP (Multiple myeloma)	vincristine	Oncovin	1 mg I.V., day 1
	cyclophosphamide	Cytoxan	100 mg/m² P.O., days 1 to 4
	doxorubicin	Adriamycin	25 mg/m² I.V., day 2
	prednisone	Deltasone	60 mg/m² P.O., days 1 to 4 *Repeat cycle q 28 days.*

(continued)

Cancer chemotherapy: Acronyms and protocols *(continued)*

ACRONYM & INDICATION	DRUG: Generic name	DRUG: Trade name	DOSAGE
VDP (Malignant melanoma)	vinblastine	Velban	5 mg/m² I.V., days 1 and 2
	dacarbazine	DTIC-Dome	150 mg/m² I.V., days 1 to 5
	cisplatin	Platinol	75 mg/m² I.V., day 5 *Repeat cycle q 21 to 28 days.*
VIP (Genitourinary cancer)	vinblastine	Velban	0.11 mg/kg I.V., days 1 and 2
	ifosfamide	Ifex	1.2 g/m² I.V., days 1 to 5
	cisplatin	Platinol	20 mg/m², days 1 to 5
	mesna	Mesnex	400 mg I.V., 15 minutes before ifosfamide, then 1.2 g by continuous I.V. infusion, days 1 to 5 *Repeat cycle q 3 weeks for four cycles.*
or	etoposide (VP-12)	VePesid	75 mg/m² I.V., days 1 to 5
	ifosfamide	Ifex	1.2 g/m² I.V., days 1 to 5
	cisplatin	Platinol	20 mg/m², days 1 to 5
	mesna	Mesnex	400 mg I.V., 15 minutes before ifosfamide, then 1.2 g by continuous I.V. infusion, days 1 to 5 *Repeat cycle q 3 weeks for four cycles.*

Index

A

t refers to a table.

t refers to a table.

t refers to a table.

t refers to a table.

t refers to a table.

B

t refers to a table.

t refers to a table.

C

t refers to a table.

t refers to a table.

t refers to a table.

t refers to a table.

t refers to a table.

D

t refers to a table.

t refers to a table.

t refers to a table.

t refers to a table.

E

t refers to a table.

t refers to a table.

F

t refers to a table.

t refers to a table.

G

t refers to a table.

H

t refers to a table.

t refers to a table.

I

t refers to a table.

t refers to a table.

J

K

t refers to a table.

t refers to a table.

t refers to a table.

t refers to a table.

t refers to a table.

t refers to a table.

t refers to a table.

t refers to a table.

t refers to a table.

t refers to a table.

t refers to a table.

t refers to a table.

t refers to a table.

t refers to a table.

t refers to a table.

t refers to a table.

Q

R

t refers to a table.

t refers to a table.

t refers to a table.

t refers to a table.

t refers to a table.

t refers to a table.

t refers to a table.

t refers to a table.

U

t refers to a table.

V

t refers to a table.

W

t refers to a table.

t refers to a table.

TABLE OF EQUIVALENTS

Frequently used equivalents in the metric system

Metric Weight		Metric Volume	
1 kilogram	= 1,000 grams (g or gm)	1 liter (l or L)	=1,000 milliliters (ml)*
1 gram	= 1,000 milligrams (mg)	1 milliliter	=1,000 microliters (μl)
1 milligram	= 1,000 micrograms (μg or mcg)		

Frequently used equivalents in the apothecaries' system

Apothecaries' Weight			Apothecaries' Volume	
20 grains (gr)	=	1 scruple (℈)	60 minims (♏)†	=1 fluidram (f℥)
3 scruples	=	1 dram (ʒ)	8 fluidrams	=1 fluidounce (f℥)
8 drams	=	1 ounce (℥)	16 fluidounces	=1 pint (pt)
12 ounces	=	1 pound (lb)	2 pints	=1 quart (qt)
			4 quarts	=1 gallon (gal)

Approximate metric and apothecaries' weight equivalents

Metric		Apothecaries'	Metric		Apothecaries'
1 gram (g) (1,000 mg)	=	15 grains	0.05 g (50 mg)	=	¾ grain
0.6 g (600 mg)	=	10 grains	0.03 g (30 mg)	=	½ grain
0.5 g (500 mg)	=	7½ grains	0.015 g (15 mg)	=	¼ grain
0.3 g (300 mg)	=	5 grains	0.001 g (1 mg)	=	1/60 grain
0.2 g (200 mg)	=	3 grains	0.6 mg	=	1/100 grain
0.1 g (100 mg)	=	1½ grains	0.5 mg	=	1/120 grain
0.06 g (60 mg)	=	1 grain	0.4 mg	=	1/150 grain

Approximate household, apothecaries', and metric volume equivalents

Household		Apothecaries'		Metric
1 teaspoon (tsp)	=	1 fluidram (fʒ)	=	4 or 5 ml‡
1 tablespoon (T or tbs)	=	½ fluidounce (f℥)	=	15 ml
2 tablespoons	=	1 fluidounce	=	30 ml
1 measuring cupful	=	8 fluidounces	=	240 ml
1 pint (pt)	=	16 fluidounces	=	473 ml
1 quart (qt)	=	32 fluidounces	=	946 ml
1 gallon (gal)	=	128 fluidounces	=	3,785 ml

Conversions

Temperature

Centigrade → Fahrenheit: $(°C \times 9/5) + 32 = °F$

Fahrenheit → Centigrade: $(°F - 32) \times 5/9 = °C$

Weight 1 oz = 30 g 1 lb = 453.6 g 2.2 lb = 1 kg

*1 ml = 1 cubic centimeter (cc); however, ml is the preferred measurement term today.

†A minim is *almost equal* to a drop. When a drug is prescribed in minims, it is best to measure it in minims. The minim is measured with a minim glass; a drop, with a medicine dropper.

‡Although the fluidram is approximately 4 ml, in prescriptions it is considered equivalent to the teaspoon (which is 5 ml).